Treatment of Skin Disease

Commissioning Editor: Claire Bonnett
Development Editor: Joanne Scott
Editorial Assistant: Rachael Harrison
Project Manager: Alan Nicholson
Design: Charles Gray
Illustration Manager: Gillian Richards
Marketing Manager: Courtney Ingram

Treatment of Skin Disease

COMPREHENSIVE THERAPEUTIC STRATEGIES

THIRD EDITION

MARK G LEBWOHL MD

Professor and Chairman

Department of Dermatology
The Mount Sinai School of Medicine
New York, NY, USA

WARREN R HEYMANN MD

Professor of Medicine and Pediatrics
and Head, Division of Dermatology

University of Medicine and Dentistry of New Jersey–Robert
Wood Johnson Medical School at Camden
Clinical Professor of Dermatology, University of Pennsylvania
School of Medicine
Camden, NJ, USA

JOHN BERTH-JONES FRCP

Consultant Dermatologist

Department of Dermatology
University Hospital
Coventry, UK

IAN COULSON BSc MB FRCP

Consultant Dermatologist

Dermatology Unit
Burnley General Hospital
Casterton Avenue
Burnley, UK

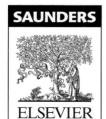

SAUNDERS

ELSEVIER

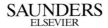

SAUNDERS
ELSEVIER

First edition published 2002
Reprinted 2002 (twice), 2003 (twice), 2004
Second edition 2006
Third edition 2010
© 2010 Elsevier Limited. All rights reserved.

The chapter entitled 'Xeroderma Pigmentosum' was written by Federal employees and is therefore in the public domain.

The rights of Mark G Lebwohl, Warren R Heymann, John Berth-Jones, and Ian Coulson to be identified as authors of this work has been asserted by them in accordance with the Copyright, Designs and Patents Act 1988.

British Library Cataloguing in Publication Data

Treatment of skin disease. - 3rd ed.
  1. Dermatology 2. Skin - Diseases - Treatment
  I. Lebwohl, Mark
  616.5'06

ISBN: 978-0-7020-3121-2

Library of Congress Cataloging in Publication Data
A catalog record for this book is available from the Library of Congress

---

Notice

Medical knowledge is constantly changing. Standard safety precautions must be followed, but as new research and clinical experience broaden our knowledge, changes in treatment and drug therapy may become necessary or appropriate. Readers are advised to check the most current product information provided by the manufacturer of each drug to be administered to verify the recommended dose, the method and duration of administration, and contraindications. It is the responsibility of the practitioner, relying on experience and knowledge of the patient, to determine dosages and the best treatment for each individual patient. Neither the Publisher nor the author assume any liability for any injury and/or damage to persons or property arising from this publication.

The Publisher

ELSEVIER | your source for books, journals and multimedia in the health sciences

www.elsevierhealth.com

Working together to grow
libraries in developing countries

www.elsevier.com | www.bookaid.org | www.sabre.org

ELSEVIER   BOOK AID International   Sabre Foundation

The publisher's policy is to use **paper manufactured from sustainable forests**

Printed in China
Last digit is the print number: 9 8 7 6 5 4 3 2 1

Contents

Contents

Contents

Contents

Preface

"Now What Do I Do?"

With this question we introduced our first and second editions of *Treatment of Skin Disease*. No matter what advances are made and regardless of how many editions of this textbook are written, dermatologists will always focus on that question. Since the last edition, there have been major innovations in our specialty. Biologic therapies, in their infancy when our second edition was published, have now been used to treat tens of thousands of psoriasis patients and have been tried off-label in numerous skin diseases. New devices and new drugs are introduced on a regular basis.

The third edition of *Treatment of Skin Disease* contains updates and new references in all chapters, and new figures in nearly all chapters. Based on feedback from dermatologists, we have added chapters on atypical nevi, autoimmune progesterone dermatitis, Jessner's lymphocytic infiltrate, mucoceles, notalgia paresthetica, papular urticaria, pyogenic granulomas, and Well's syndrome. We encourage our colleagues to continue to suggest improvements, changes, or additional chapters for future editions. We have also added a chapter on a newly described disease entity, nephrogenic systemic fibrosis. And with the emergence of methicillin-resistant *Staphylococcus aureus* as a leading cause of skin and soft tissue infections, we have added a separate chapter on this important infectious disease. Finally, in response to comments about our previous editions, we have separated the previous chapter on herpes simplex virus into two separate chapters on herpes genitalis and herpes labialis.

We have retained successful features of our previous editions, namely our evidence-based rating scales and our separation of treatments into first-line, second-line, and third-line therapies. New technology has allowed us to change our electronic version of *Treatment of Skin Disease* from a PDA to a completely web-accessible textbook.

In our third edition, we continue to emphasize the importance of double-blind, placebo-controlled trials, but also continue to stress the value of case reports and series, particularly in rare disorders for which large trials are not practical.

As we go to press with our third edition, it is our hope that medical progress will continue at such a fast pace that we will soon need a fourth edition. Even as this edition goes to print, reports of progressive multifocal leukoencephalopathy are emerging in patients treated with efalizumab leading to the withdrawal of this biologic agent, and new biologics such as ustekinumab are poised for approval. Our goal, as in previous editions, is to help our colleagues manage their patients in the safest and most effective ways possible.

Mark G Lebwohl MD
Warren R Heymann MD
John Berth-Jones FRCP
Ian Coulson, BSc MB FRCP
2009

Contributors

Anthony Abdullah BSc (Hons) MBChB (Hons) FRCP DTM&H
Consultant Dermatologist
The Birmingham Skin Centre
Birmingham, UK

Robert E Accordino MSc
Research Assistant
Department of Dermatology
Mount Sinai School of Medicine
New York NY, USA

Imtiaz Ahmed BSc MBBS FRCP
Consultant Dermatologist
Department of Dermatology
University Hospitals Coventry and
Warwickshire
Coventry, UK

Hanadi Abdallah Al Quran MD
Consultant Dermatologist
Mount Sinai Medical Center
New York NY, USA

Anwar Al Hammadi MD FRCPC FAAD
Consultant Dermatologist
Clinical Assistant Professor
College of Medicine
University of Sharjah
United Arab Emirates

Sandra Albert MBBS MD DNB
Visiting Fellow
St John's Institute of Dermatology
St Thomas' Hospital
London, UK

Lauren Alberta-Wszolek MD
Dermatologist
Division of Dermatology
UMass Memorial Medical Center
Worcester MA, USA

Robert A Allen MD
Clinical Assistant Professor of Dermatology
Drexel University College of Medicine
Philadelphia PA, USA

Mahreen Ameen MD DTM&H
St John's Institute of Dermatology
Guy's and St Thomas' Hospital
London, UK

Sadegh Amini MD
Clinical Research Fellow
Department of Dermatology and
Cutaneous Surgery
University of Miami Miller School of Medicine
Miami FL, USA

Caroline Angit MBBS MRCP(UK)
Dermatologist
Burnley General Hospital
Burnley, UK

Grant J Anhalt MD
Professor of Dermatology and Pathology
Department of Dermatology
Johns Hopkins University Hospital
Baltimore MD, USA

Sarah Asch MD
Dermatologist
Temple University School of Medicine
Philadelphia PA, USA

Eanas Bader MRCP
Dermatologist
Department of Dermatology
University Hospital Coventry
Coventry, UK

Donald J Baker MD
Clinical Assistant Professor of Medicine
Division of Dermatology
UMDNJ-Robert Wood Johnson Medical
School
Gibbsboro NJ, USA

Periasamy Balasubramaniam
MD MRCP(UK)
Consultant Dermatologist
Department of Dermatology
Maelor Hospital
North Wales NHS Trust
Wrexham, UK

Ali Banki DO
Dermatologist
St Barnabas Hospital
Bronx NY, USA

Robert L Baran MD
Consultant Dermatologist
Gustave Roussy Cancer Institute
Cannes, France

Melissa C Barkham MBChB MRCP
Consultant Dermatologist
Department of Dermatology
St Peter's Hospital
Surrey, UK

Brenda L Bartlett MD
Clinical Research Fellow
Center for Clinical Studies
University of Texas Health Science Center
Houston TX, USA

Leah Belazarian MD
Clinical Instructor in Medicine and
Pediatric Dermatology Fellow
University of Massachusetts Medical School
Worcester MA, USA

Ysabel Bello MD
Dermatologist
Department of Dermatology and
Cutaneous Surgery
University of Miami School of Medicine
Miami FL, USA

Emma C Benton MBChB MRCP
Dermatologist
St John's Institute of Dermatology
St Thomas' Hospital
London, UK

E Claire Benton BSc MBChB FRCPE
Consultant Dermatologist
Honorary Clinical Senior Lecturer
Department of Dermatology
The Royal Infirmary
Edinburgh, UK

Wilma F Bergfeld MD FAAD
Senior Dermatologist and Co-Director
Dermatopathology
Departments of Dermatology and
Pathology
Cleveland Clinic Foundation
Cleveland OH, USA

Eric Berkowitz MD
Assistant Clinical Professor
Department of Medicine (Dematology)
Albert Einstein College of Medicine
Bronx NY, USA

Brian Berman MD PhD
Professor of Dermatology and Internal
Medicine
Departments of Dermatology and
Cutaneous Surgery and Internal
Medicine
University of Miami
Miller School of Medicine
Miami FL, USA

Jeffrey D Bernhard MD
Professor Emeritus
University of Massachusetts Medical
School
Worcester MA, USA

John Berth-Jones FRCP
Consultant Dermatologist
Department of Dermatology
University Hospital
Coventry, UK

Yuval Bibi MD PhD
Dermatologist
Department of Dermatology
Boston University Medical Center
Boston MA, USA

Jonathan E Blume MD
Instructor
Department of Dermatology
Columbia University–College of
Physicians and Surgeons
New York NY, USA

Paul H Bowman MD
Fellow
Department of Dermatology
St Louis University
St Louis MO, USA

Gary J Brauner MD
Associate Clinical Professor
Mount Sinai School of Medicine
New York NY, USA

Robert T Brodell MD
Professor of Internal Medicine
Dermatology Section
Clinical Professor of Dermatopathology in
Pathology
Permanent Master Teacher
Northeastern Ohio Universities College of
Medicine
Associate Clinical Professor of Dermatology
Case Western Reserve University School of
Medicine
Instructor in Dermatology
University of Rochester School of Medicine
and Dentistry
Rochester NY, USA

Rebecca CC Brooke MBChB MRCP
Consultant Dermatologist
Dermatology Centre
University of Manchester
Salford Royal Hospital
Manchester, UK

Marc David Brown MD
Professor of Dermatology
Department of Dermatology
University of Rochester School of Medicine
Rochester NY, USA

Alison J Bruce MD MBChB
Assistant Professor of Dermatology
Department of Dermatology
The Mayo Clinic
Rochester MN, USA

Robert Burd MBChB MRCP
Consultant Dermatologist
Department of Dermatology
Leicester Royal Infirmary NHS Trust
Leicester, UK

Anne E Burdick MD MPH
Professor of Dermatology and Director
Telemedicine Program
Department of Dermatology and Cutaneous
Surgery
University of Miami School of Medicine
Miami FL, USA

Susan Mary Burge BSc BM BCh FRCP DM
Consultant Dermatologist
Department of Dermatology
Churchill Hospital
Headington
Oxford, UK

Jeffrey P Callen MD FACP FAAD
Professor of Medicine (Dermatology)
Chief, Division of Dermatology
University of Louisville School of Medicine
Louisville KY, USA

Ivan D Camacho MD
Fellow
Department of Dermatology and Cutaneous
Surgery
University of Miami
Miller School of Medicine
Miami FL, USA

Mitchell S Cappell MD PhD
Chief
Division of Gastroenterology
William Beaumont Hospital
Royal Oak MI, USA

John A Carucci MD PhD
Assistant Professor and Chief
Mohs Micrographic and
Dermatologic Surgery
Weill Medical College of Cornell University
New York NY, USA

Leslie Castelo-Soccio MD PhD
Dermatologist
Department of Dermatology
University of Pennsylvania
Philadelphia PA, USA

Bridgette Cave BM MRCS(London)
Dermatologist
The Birmingham Skin Centre
City Hospital NHS Trust
Birmingham, UK

Samuel L Chachkin MD
Physician
Department of Dermatology
University of Pennsylvania School of
Medicine
Philadelphia PA, USA

Robert J G Chalmers MB FRCP
Consultant Dermatologist
The Dermatology Centre
University of Manchester
Salford Royal Hospital
Manchester, UK

Loi-yuen Chan MBBS MRCPI Dip Derm
(London) FHKAM
Consultant Dermatologist
Quality HealthCare Medical Service
Hong Kong, China

Lawrence S Chan MD
Professor and Head
Department of Dermatology
University of Illinois College of
Medicine
Chicago IL, USA

Pamela Chayavichitsilp MD
Research Fellow
Pediatric and Adolescent
Dermatology
University of California
San Diego
Rady Children's Hospital
San Diego
San Diego CA, USA

Fiona J Child BSc MD FRCP
Consultant Dermatologist
Department of Dermatology
Royal Free Hospital
London, UK

Anthony C Chu FRCP
Consultant Dermatologist/Honorary
Senior Lecturer
Head of Dermatology
Unit of Dermatology
Imperial College School of Medicine
London, UK

Timothy Howel Clayton FRCP(Edin) MBChB
MRCPCH
Consultant Paediatric Dermatologist
Royal Liverpool Children's Trust
Alder Hey Children's Hospital
Liverpool, UK

Carrie Wood Cobb MD
Dermatologist
Division of Dermatology
UMDNJ Robert Wood Johnson Medical
School at Camden
Camden NJ, USA

Steven Cohen MD MPH
Professor and Chief
Division of Dermatology
Albert Einstein College of Medicine
Bronx NY, USA

Clara-Dina Cokonis MD RPh
Dermatologist
Harvard Vanguard Medical Associates
Newton MA, USA

Elizabeth A Cooper BESc HBSc
Senior Clinical Research Scientist
Mediprobe Research
London ON, Canada

Susan M Cooper MD MBChB MRCGP MRCP
Consultant Dermatologist
Department of Dermatology
Churchill Hospital
Oxford, UK

Ian Coulson BSc MB FRCP
Consultant Dermatologist
Dermatology Unit
Burnley General Hospital
Burnley, UK

Shawn E Cowper MD
Assistant Professor of Dermatology and
Pathology
Department of Dermatology and Pathology
Yale University School of Medicine
New Haven CT, USA

Neil H Cox BSc(Hons) MBChB FRCP(Lond)
FRCP(Edin)
Consultant Dermatologist
Dermatology Department
Cumberland Infirmary
Carlisle, UK

Nicholas M Craven BM BCh MA FRCP
Consultant Dermatologist
East Cheshire NHS Trust
Department of Dermatology
Macclesfield District General Hospital
Macclesfield
Cheshire, UK

Daniel Creamer BSc MD FRCP
Consultant Dermatologist
Department of Dermatology
King's College Hospital
London, UK

Ponciano D Cruz Jr MD
Professor and Vice Chair
Department of Dermatology
The University of Texas Southwestern
Medical Center
Dallas TX, USA

Bahar Dasgeb MD
Fellow in Dermatology
Department of Dematology
Boston University School of Medicine
Boston MA, USA

Rosemary Davis MRCP
Dermatologist
Department of Dermatology
Leicester Royal Infirmary
Leicester, UK

Mark D P Davis MD
Professor of Dermatology
Department of Dermatology
College of Medicine
Rochester MN, USA

Robert S Dawe MD FRCP
Consultant Dermatologist
Photobiology Unit
Department of Dermatology
Ninewells Hospital and Medical School
Dundee, UK

David de Berker BA MBBS MRCP
Associate Clinical Director Dermatology
Consultant Dermatologist and Honorary
Senior Lecturer
Bristol Dermatology Centre
Bristol Royal Infirmary Hospital
Bristol, UK

Danielle M DeHoratius MD
Clinical Associate
Department of Dermatology
Hospital of the University of Pennsylvania
Philadelphia PA, USA

Sasha J K Dhoat MBBS BSc(Hons) MRCP
Locum Consultant Dermatologist
South House Royal Free Hospital
London, UK

John J DiGiovanna MD PhD
Director
Division of Dermatopharmacology
Professor at Brown Medical School
Providence, RI
and Investigator
DNA Repair Section
Center for Cancer Research
Bethesda MD, USA

Alexander Doctoroff DO MS
Dermatologist
Clinical Assistant Professor of Medicine
University of Medicine and Dentistry of
New Jersey
School of Osteopathic Medicine
Springfield NJ, USA

Lisa A Drage MD
Assistant Professor of Dermatology
The Mayo Medical School
Department of Dermatology
The Mayo School
Rochester MN, USA

Lawrence F Eichenfield MD
Chief
Pediatric and Adolescent Dermatology
Professor of Pediatrics and Medicine
(Dermatology)
Rady Children's Hospital San Diego
University of California
San Diego School of Medicine
San Diego CA, USA

Drore Eisen MD DDS
Dermatology Associates of Cincinnati
Cincinnati OH, USA

Dirk M Elston MD
Director
Department of Dermatology
Geisinger Medical Center
Danville PA
USA

Patrick OM Emanuel MD
Assistant Professor Pathology and
Dermatology
Mount Sinai Medical Center
New York NY, USA

Anna F Falabella MD CWS
Voluntary Associate Professor
Department of Dermatology and Cutaneous
Surgery
Miami School of Medicine
Miami FL, USA

Anat Feingold MD MPH
Assistant Professor
Department of Pediatrics
UMDNJ–Robert Wood Johnson Medical
School at Camden
Camden NJ, USA

James Ferguson MD FRCP
Consultant Dermatologist
Photobiology Unit
Department of Dermatology
Ninewells Hospital
Dundee, UK

Geover Fernández MD
Dermatologist
Department of Dermatology
New Jersey Medical School
Newark NJ, USA

Pascal G Ferzli MD MSc
Dermatologist
Division of Dermatology
UMDNJ–Robert Wood Johnson Medical
School at Camden
Camden NJ, USA

Andrew Y Finlay MBBS FRCP
Professor of Dermatology
Department of Dermatology
Cardiff University
School of Medicine
Cardiff, UK

Bahar F Firoz MD MPH
Dermatologist
Dermatology Surgery Fellow
DermSurgery Associates
Houston TX, USA

Elnaz F Firoz BA
Dermatologist
Columbia University College of Physicians
and Surgeons
Short Hills NJ, USA

James E Fitzpatrick MD
Professor of Dermatology
Department of Dermatology
University of Colorado, Denver
Aurora CO, USA

Richard G Fried MD PhD
Clinical Director
Yardley Dermatology and Yardley Skin
Enhancement and Wellness Center
Yardley PA, USA

Adam Friedman MD
Dermatologist
Division of Dermatology
Albert Einstein College of Medicine
New York NY, USA

Brian S Fuchs MD
Research Assistant
Department of Dermatology
The Mount Sinai School of Medicine
New York NY, USA

L Claire Fuller MA FRCP
Consultant Dermatologist
Kent and Canterbury Hospital
Kent, UK

Joanna E Gach MD FRCP
Consultant Dermatologist
Department of Dermatology
University Hospital Coventry and
Warwickshire NHS Trust
Coventry, UK

Loma S Gardner MBChB BSc(Med Sci) MRCP
Dermatologist
Department of Dermatology
Burnley General Hospital
Burnley
Lancashire, UK

Amit Garg MD FAAD
Director, Dermatology Training Program
Boston University School of Medicine
Assistant Professor of Dermatology
Boston Medical Center
Boston MA, USA

Joel M Gelfand MD MSCE
Medical Director, Clinical Studies Unit
Assistant Professor of Dermatology
Associate Scholar, Center for Clinical
Epidemiology and Biostatistics
University of Pennsylvania
Philadelphia PA, USA

Carlo Gelmetti MD
Professor and Head
Department of Anesthesiology, Intensive
Care and Dermatological Sciences of the
University of Milan
Foundation I.R.C.C.S. Ospedale Maggiore
Policlinico, Mangiagalli e Regina Elena di
Milano
Milan, Italy

Aron J Gewirtzman MD
Clinical Research Fellow
Center for Clinical Studies
Houston TX, USA

Leonard H Goldberg MD FRCP
Clinical Professor, Dept of Dermatology,
Weill Medical College of Cornell University,
Clinical Professor in Dermatology
MD Anderson Cancer Center
University of Texas Medical School at Houston
Houston TX, USA

Mark J D Goodfield MD FRCP
Consultant Dermatologist
Department of Dermatology
Leeds General Infirmary
Leeds, UK

Marsha L Gordon MD
Professor of Dermatology
Mount Sinai School of Medicine
New York, USA

Patricia Mary Gordon MBChB MRCP(UK)
Consultant Dermatologist
Honorary Senior Lecturer
Department of Dermatology
Royal Infirmary
Edinburgh, UK

Robin A C Graham-Brown BSc MBBS FRCP
FRCPCH
Consultant Dermatologist
Spire Leicester Hospital
Leicester, UK

Clive E H Grattan MD FRCP
Consultant Dermatologist
Dermatology Centre
Norfolk and Norwich University Hospital
Norfolk, UK

Malcolm W Greaves MD PhD FRCP
Emeritus Professor of Dermatology
Cutaneous Allergy Clinc
St Johns Institute of Dermatology
St Thomas' Hospital
London, UK

Justin J Green MD
Assistant Professor of Dermatology
Division of Dermatology
University of Medicine and Dentistry of
New Jersey
Robert Wood Johnson School of
Medicine
Marlton NJ, USA

Christopher E M Griffiths BSc MBBS MD
FRCP FRCPath
Professor of Dermatology
Dermatology Centre
University of Manchester
Salford, UK

Charles A Gropper MD
Associate Professor, Department of
Dermatology, Mount Sinai School of
Medicine
Chief, Division of Dermatology
Saint Barnabas Hospital,
New York NY, USA

Arpeta Gupta MBBS
Dermatologist
All India Institute of Medical Sciences
New Delhi, India

Aditya Gupta MD PhD MA CCI CCTI CCRP DABD
FAAD FRCPC
Professor, Division of Dermatology
Department of Medicine
Sunnybrook and Women's Health
Science Center and the University of Toronto
London ON, Canada

Alejandra Gurtman MD
Director, Clinical Research
Wyeth Vaccine Research
Pearl River NY, USA

Suhail M Hadi MBChB MD MPhil
Assistant Professor of Dermatology
Department of Dermatology
The Mount Sinai Medical Center
New York NY, USA

Abdul Hafejee MBChB MRCP(UK)
Dermatologist
Department of Dermatology
Hope Hospital
Salford, UK

Joanne Hague MBB MRCP
Consultant in Dermatology
Worcester Royal Hospital
Worcester, UK

Julia E Haimowitz MD
Dermatologist
Department of Dermatology
Kaiser Permanente Medical Center
San Rafael CA, USA

Bethany R Hairston MD
Dermatologist
Mayo School of Graduate Medical
Education
Mayo Clinic College of Medicine
Rochester MN, USA

Analisa Vincent Halpern MD
Assistant Professor of Medicine
Division of Dermatology
UMDNJ–Robert Wood Johnson Medical
School at Camden
Camden NJ, USA

Susan E Handfield-Jones BM FRCP
Consultant Dermatologist
Department of Dermatology
West Suffolk Hospital
Bury St Edmunds, UK

Shannon Harrison MBBS MMed FACD
Clinical Research Fellow
Department of Dermatology
Cleveland Clinic Foundation
Cleveland OH, USA

John L M Hawk BSc MD FRCP
Emeritus Professor of Dermatological
Photobiology
St John's Institute of Dermatology
St Thomas' Hospital
London, UK

Adrian H M Heagerty BSc MD FRCP
Department of Dermatology
Solihull Hospital
West Midlands, UK

Adelaide A Hebert MD
Professor of Dermatology and Pediatrics
Department of Dermatology
University of Texas Health Science Center,
Houston
Houston TX, USA

Amy E Helms MD
Dermatologist
Department of Dermatology
University Hospitals Case Medical
Center
Cleveland OH, USA

Stephen E Helms MD
Associate Professor of Internal Medicine,
Northeastern Ohio University College of
Medicine
Assistant Clinical Professor of Dermatology
Case Western Reserve University School of
Medicine
Warren OH, USA

Patricia A Henry DO
Dermatologist
Department of Medicine
Cooper University Hospital
Cherry Hill NJ, USA

Warren R Heymann MD
Professor of Medicine and Pediatrics
and Head, Division of Dermatology
University of Medicine and Dentistry of
New Jersey–Robert Wood Johnson Medical
School at Camden
Clinical Professor of Dermatology, University
of Pennsylvania School of Medicine
Camden NJ, USA

Doris Hexsel MD
Formerly Professor of Medicine
School of Medicine
University of Passo Fundo
Porto Alegre, Brazil

Elisabeth M Higgins MBBS MA BA MRCP
Consultant Dermatologist
Department of Dermatology
King's College Hospital
London, UK

Herbert Hönigsmann MD
Professor of Dermatology, Chairman
Department of Dermatology
Medical University of Vienna
Vienna, Austria

Marcelo G Horenstein MD
Director of Dermatopathology
The Dermatology Group
Verona NJ, USA

Laura Houk MD
Dermatologist
Department of Dermatology and Cutaneous
Biology
Thomas Jefferson University
Philadelphia PA, USA

Frances Humphreys MBBS FRCP
Consultant and Honorary Associate Professor
Department of Dermatology
Warwick Hospital
Warwick, UK

Ran Huo MD
Clinical Research Fellow
Department of Dermatology and Cutaneous
Surgery
University of Miami, Miller School of Medicine
Miami FL, USA

Walayat Hussain BSc(Hons) MBChB MRCP
Dermatologist
The Dermatology Unit
Burnley General Hospital
Burnley, UK

Linda Y Hwang MD
Dermatologist
Department of Dermatology
Kaiser Permanente Medical Center
San Rafael CA, USA

Sherrif F Ibrahim MD PhD
Dermatologic Surgeon
Department of Dermatology
University of California–San Francisco
San Francisco CA, USA

Andrew Ilchyshyn MBChB FRCP
Consultant Dermatologist
Walsgrave Hospital NHS Trust
Coventry, UK

Stefania Jablonska MD
Professor of Dermatology
Department of Dermatology and Venereology
Warsaw School of Medicine
Warsaw, Poland

William D James MD FAAD
Vice Chair and Professor, Department of
Dermatology
Director of Residency Program and Clinical
Practices
Hospital of the University of Pennsylvania
Philadelphia PA, USA

Gregor B E Jemec MD DMedSc
Associate Professor and Chairman
Department of Dermatology
Roskilde Hospital
Health Sciences Faculty
University of Copenhagen
Roskilde, Denmark

Graham Johnston MBChB MRCP
Consultant Dermatologist
Department of Dermatology
Leicester Royal Infirmary
Leicester, UK

Stephen K Jones MD FRCP
Consultant Dermatologist
Department of Dermatology
Clatterbridge Hospital
Wirral, UK

Joseph L Jorizzo MD
Professor and Former (Founding) Chair
Department of Dermatology
Wake Forest University School of Medicine
Winston-Salem NC, USA

Jacqueline M Junkins-Hopkins MD
Associate Professor of Dermatology
Department of Dermatology
University of Pennsylvania
Philadelphia PA, USA

Wolfgang Jurecka MD
Professor of Dermatology and Head
Department of Dermatology
Wilhelminenspital der Stadt Wien
Vienna, Austria

Antonios Kanelleas MD
Clinical and Research Fellow
Department of Dermatology
University Hospitals of Coventry and
Warwickshire NHS Trust
George Eliot Hospital NHS Trust
Nuneaton, UK

Ruwani P Katugampola MD
Consultant Dermatologist
Department of Dermatology
University Hospital of Wales
Cardiff, UK

Bruce E Katz MD
Clinical Professor of Dermatology
Mount Sinai School of Medicine
Director
JUVA Skin and Laser Center
JUVA Skin and Laser Center
New York NY, USA

Manjit Kaur BSc(Hons) BMBS MRCP
PGCMedEd
Consultant Dermatologist
Department of Dermatology
Solihull Hospital
Birmingham, UK

Martin Keefe MC ChB DM FRCP
Consultant Dermatologist
Department of Dermatology
Royal South Hants Hospital
Southampton, UK

Kevin F Kia MD
Dermatologist
Department of Dermatology
The University of Texas Southwestern
Medical Center
Dallas TX, USA

George G Kihiczak MD
Dermatologist
New Jersey Medical School
Newark NJ, USA

Brian Kirby MB MRCPI
Consultant/Lecturer in Dermatology
Department of Dermatology
Adelaide and Meath Hospital
Dublin, Ireland

Gudula Kirtschig MD PhD
Consultant Dermatologist
Department of Dermatology
VU Medisch Centrum
Amsterdam, The Netherlands

Rebecca Kleinerman MD
Department of Dermatology
Mount Sinai School of Medicine
New York NY, USA

Eleanor A Knopp MD
Dermatologist
Department of Dermatology
Yale University
New Haven CT, USA

Sandra R Knowles RPh BScPhm
Drug Safety Pharmacist and Lecturer
Faculty of Pharmacy
University of Toronto
Toronto ON, Canada

Dimitra Koch MD MRCP
Dermatologist
Department of Dermatology
Birmingham Children's Hospital
Birmingham, UK

John Koo MD FAAD
Director, University of California San
Francisco
Medical Center Department of Dermatology
UCSF Psoriasis Treatment Center
San Francisco CA, USA

Neil J Korman MD PhD
Professor of Dermatology
Department of Dermatology
University Hospitals Case Medical Center
Case Western Reserve University
Cleveland OH, USA

Kenneth H Kraemer MD
Senior Investigator
Head, DNA Repair Section
National Cancer Institute
Bethesda MD, UK

Bernice R Krafchik MBChB FRCP(C)
Professor Emeritus
University of Toronto
Hospital for Sick Children
Toronto ON, Canada

Andrew C Krakowski MD
Fellow in Pediatric Dermatology
Division of Pediatrics and Adolescent
Dermatology at
Rady Children's Hospital San Diego
San Diego CA, USA

Karthik Krishnamurthy DO
Dermatologist
Division of Dermatology
Saint Barnabas Hospital, Bronx, NY
Kew Gardens Hill NY, USA

Knut Kvernebo MD PhD
Professor of CardioThoracic Surgery
Department of Cardiothoracic Surgery
University of Oslo
Oslo, Norway

James A A Langtry MBBS FRCP
Consultant Dermatologist and
Dermatological Surgeon
Department of Dermatology
Royal Victoria Infirmary
Newcastle Upon Tyne, UK

Amir A Larian MD
Department of Dermatology
Mount Sinai School of Medicine
New York NY, USA

Frances Lawlor MD FRCP DCHObst RCOG
Consultant Dermatologist
Division of Cutaneous Allergy
St John's Hospital for Diseases of the Skin
London, UK

Naomi Lawrence MD
Director, Procedural Dermatology
Department of Medicine
Cooper University Hospital
Marlton NJ, USA

Clifford M Lawrence MD FRCP
Consultant Dermatologist
Royal Victoria Infirmary
Newcastle, UK

Mark G Lebwohl MD
Professor and Chairman
Department of Dermatology
The Mount Sinai School of Medicine
New York NY, USA

Oscar Lebwohl MD
Clinical Professor of Medicine
Department of Medicine
Columbia University College of Physicians
and Surgeons
New York NY, USA

Andrew D Lee MD
Dermatologist
Department of Dermatology
Wake Forest Medical Center
Winston-Salem NC, USA

Julia S Lehman MD
Dermatologist
Department of Dermatology
Mayo Clinic
Rochester MN, USA

Stuart R Lessin MD
Director
Dermatology, Melanoma Family Risk
Assessment Program
Fox Chase Cancer Center
Philadelphia PA, USA

Jacob O Levitt MD FAAD
Assistant Clinical Professor
Department of Dermatology
Mount Sinai Medical Center
New York NY, USA

Thomas A Luger MD
Professor of Dermatology
Department of Dermatology
University of Münster
Münster, Germany

Calum C Lyon MA FRCP
Clinical Lecturer
University of Manchester, Hull and York
Medical Schools
Department of Dermatology
York Hospital Foundation Trust
York, UK

Chrystallas Macedo MBBS BSc MRCP
Dermatologist
Chelsea and Westminster Hospital
Isleworth, Middlesex, UK

Slawomir Majewski MD
Professor of Dermatology
Department of Dermatology and
Venereology
Warsaw School of Medicine
Warsaw, Poland

Vallari Majmudar MBBS
Dermatologist
Basildon and Thurrock University
Hospitals NHS Foundation Trust
Nethermayne, UK

Richard B Mallett MB FRCP
Consultant Dermatologist, Peterborough and
Stamford Hospitals NHS Foundation Trust
Department of Dermatology
Edith Cavell Hospital
Peterborough, UK

Steven M Manders MD
Professor of Medicine and Pediatrics
Cooper University Hospital
UMDNJ–Robert Wood Johnson Medical
School at Camden
Camden NJ, USA

Ranon Mann MD
Instructor of Medicine
Department of Dermatology
Albert Einstein College of Medicine
Bronx NY, USA

David J Margolis MD PhD
Associate Professor
Centre for Epidemiology and
Biostatistics
University of Pennsylvania
Philadelphia PA, USA

Sarah Markoff
Research Assistant
Department of Dermatology
The Mount Sinai School of Medicine
New York NY, USA

Orit Markowitz MD
Assistant Clinical Professor of
Dermatology
Department of Dermatology
Mount Sinai School of Medicine
New York, NY, USA

Ellen S Marmur MD
Associate Professor
The Mount Sinai Medical Center
New York NY, USA

Najat A Y Marraiki BSc MSc PhD
Assistant Professor in Immunology
Virology and Microbiology
King Saud University
Saudi Arabia

Jeremy R Marsden FRCP
Consultant Dermatologist
University Hospital Birmingham
Birmingham, UK

Agustin Martin-Clavijo MRCP
Dermatologist
Department of Dermatology
George Eliot Hospital
Nuneaton, UK

Andrew J G McDonagh FRCP
Consultant Dermatologist
Royal Hallamshire Hospital and Honorary
Clinical Senior Lecturer
Department of Dermatology
Royal Hallamshire Hospital
Sheffield, UK

Brandie J Metz MD
Assistant Clinical Professor of Pediatrics
and Medicine
Department of Dermatology
Children's Hospital San Diego
San Diego CA, USA

Giuseppe Micali MD
Professor and Chairman
Clinica Dermatologica
Universita' di Catania
Catania, Italy

Leslie G Millard MD FRCP
Consultant Dermatologist
Queens Medical Centre
Nottingham, UK

Jason H Miller MD
Dermatologist
Department of Dermatology
University of Texas Health Science Center at
Houston and MD Anderson Cancer Center
Houston TX, USA

Christian R Millett MD
Dermatologist
Division of Dermatology
UMDNJ–Robert Wood Johnson Medical
School at Camden
Camden NJ, USA

Alex Milligan FRCP
Consultant Dermatologist
Department of Dermatology
Leicester Royal Infirmary
Leicester, UK

Daniel Mimouni MD
Faculty
Department of Dermatology
Rabin Medical Center
Israel and the Sackler Faculty of Medicine
Tel Aviv University
Petah-Tikva, Israel

John Minni DO
Private Practice
Stuart FL, USA

Ginat W Mirowski DMD MD
Associate Professor of Dermatology
Department of Oral Pathology, Medicine,
Radiology
Indiana University School of Dentistry
Indianapolis IN, USA

Sonja Christine Molin MD
Department of Dermatology and Allergology
Ludwig-Maximilians University
Munich, Germany

Dwayne Montie DO FAOCD
Dermatologist
Martin Memorial Hospital
Stuart FL, USA

Patrice Morel MD
Professor of Dermatology
Department of Dermatology
Hôpital St Louis
Paris, France

Warwick L Morison MBBS MD FRCP
Professor
Department of Dermatology
Johns Hopkins Hospital
Lutherville MD, USA

Cato Mørk MD PhD
Professor and Consultant Dermatologist
Department of Dermatology
Oslo University Hospital
Oslo, Norway

Richard J Motley MA MD FRCP
Consultant in Dermatology and Cutaneous
Surgery
Welsh Institute of Dermatology University
Hospital of Wales
Cardiff, UK

Christen M Mowad MD
Associate Professor
Department of Dermatology
Geisinger Medical Center
Danville PA, USA

Megan Mowbray MBChB BSc(Hons) MD
Consultant Dermatologist
Department of Dermatology
Queen Margaret Hospital
Dunfermline, UK

Anna E Muncaster MBChB FRCP
Consultant Dermatologist
Department of Dermatology
Rotherham General Hospital
Rotherham, UK

George J Murakawa MD PhD
Professor, Department of Internal Medicine,
Michigan State University
Somerset Skin Center
Dermcenter
Troy MI, USA

Michele E Murdoch BSc FRCP
Consultant Dermatologist
Department of Dermatology
Watford General Hospital
Watford, UK

Stuart C Murray BM BS BSc BEc FACD
Consultant Dermatologist
Department of Dermatology
Flinders Medical Centre
Adelaide SA, Australia

Maria R Nasca MD PhD
Assistant Professor Dermatology Clinic
University of Catania
AOU Policlinico 'G. Rodolico'
Catania, Italy

Sallie Neill MBChB FRCP
Consultant Dermatologist
St John's Institute of Dermatology
St Thomas Hospital
London, UK

Kenneth H Neldner MD
Professor and Chairman Emeritus
Department of Dermatology
Texas Tech University Health Sciences Center
Lubbock, TX, USA

Glenn C Newell MD FACP
Attending Physician, Camden County STD
Clinic
Associate Professor of Medicine
Cooper University Hospital
Camden NJ, USA

Rosemary L Nixon BSc(Hons) MBBS MPH
FACD FAFOM
Director
Occupational Dermatology Research and
Education Centre
Carlton VIC, Australia

Carlos H Nousari MD
Director
Institute for Immunofluorescence
Pompano Beach FL, USA

Nuala O'Donoghue MBChB MRCPI
Locum Consultant Dermatologist
St John's Institute of Dermatology
Guy's Hospital
London, UK

Stephanie Ogden MBChB MRCP
Dermatologist
Dermatology Centre
University of Manchester
Salford, UK

Caroline M Owen MBChB FRCP
Consultant Dermatologist
Department of Dermatology
Burnley General Hospital
Burnley, UK

Roy A Palmer MA MRCP PhD
Consultant Dermatologist
Department of Dermatology
King Edward VII Hospital
Windsor, UK

Katherine Panting MBChB MRCP
Dermatologist
Royal Liverpool Children's NHS Trust
Alder Hey Children's Hospital
Liverpool, UK

Jennifer L Parish MD
Assistant Professor of Dermatology and
Cutaneous Biology
Jefferson Medical College of Thomas
Jefferson University
Philadelphia PA, USA

Lawrence Charles Parish MD (Hon)
Clinical Professor of Dermatology and
Cutaneous Biology
Department of Dermatology
Jefferson Medical College of Thomas
Jefferson University
Philadelphia PA, USA

Rakesh Patalay BSc MBBS MRCP
Dermatologist
Imperial College Healthcare NHS Trust
Hammersmith Hospital
London, UK

Gopi Patel MD
Instructor, Division of Infectious Diseases
Department of Medicine
Mount Sinai School of Medicine
New York NY, USA

Nisha C Patel MD
Dermatologist
Georgetown University Hospital
Pittsburgh PA, USA

Christopher Rowland Payne
Consultant Dermatologist
The London Clinic
London, UK

Gary L Peck MD
Director, Melanoma Center
Melanoma Center
Washington Cancer Institute
Washington DC, USA

William Perkins MBBS FRCP
Consultant Dermatologist
Queens Medical Centre
Nottingham, UK

Clifford S Perlis MD
Teaching Fellow in Mohs Micrographic Surgery
Department of Dermatology
Brown Medical School
Department of Dermatology
Rhode Island Hospital
Providence RI, USA

Robert George Phelps MD
Professor of Dermatology and Pathology
Director of Dermatopathology
Departments of Dermatology and Pathology
Mount Sinai School of Medicine
New York NY, USA

Tania J Phillips MD FRCP FRCPC
Clinical Professor of Dermatology
Dermatology Department
Boston University School of Medicine
Boston MA, USA

Bianca Maria Piraccini MD PhD
Researcher in Dermatology
Department of Dermatology
University of Bologna
Bologna, Italy

Maureen B Poh-Fitzpatrick MD
Professor Emerita of Dermatology
(Columbia University) and Professor of
Medicine in Dermatology
Division of Dermatology
University of Tenessee College of
Medicine
Memphis TN, USA

Lori D Prok MD
Assistant Professor of Pediatric Dermatology
and Dermatopathology
Department of Dermatology and
Pediatrics
University of Colorado, Denver and
The Children's Hospital
Aurora CO, USA

Sajjad F Rajpar MBChB(Hons) MRCP
Dermatologist
Department of Dermatology
Selly Oak Hospital, University Hospital
Birmingham
Birmingham, UK

Ronald P Rapini MD
Professor and Chair
Department of Dermatology
University of Texas Medical School and MD
Anderson Cancer Center
Houston TX, USA

Ravi Ratnavel DM FRCP
Consultant Dermatologist
Buckinghamshire Hospitals Trust
Buckinghamshire, UK

Larisa Ravitskiy MD
Dermatologist
Division of Dermatology
Cooper University Hospital
Camden NJ, USA

Jean Revuz MD
Professor of Dermatology
Chairman, Department of Dermatology
Service de Dermatologie
Hôpital Henri Mondor
Creteil, France

Gabriele Richard MD FACMG
Medical Director
Gene DX Inc
Gaithersburg MD, USA

Darrell S Rigel MD
Clinical Professor of Dermatology
New York University Medical Centre
Rigel Dermatology
New York NY, USA

Wanda Sonia Robles MBBS MD PhD
Consultant Dermatologist
Department of Dermatology
Barnet and Chase Farm Hospitals NHS Trust
Middlesex, UK

Roy S Rogers III MD
Professor of Dermatology
Department of Dermatology
The Mayo Clinic
Rochester MN, USA

Alain H Rook MD
Professor of Dermatology
Department of Dermatology
University of Pennsylvania Hospital
Philadelphia PA, USA

Donald Rudikoff MD
Chief of Dermatology, Bronx Lebanon Hospital
Associate Professor of Clinical Medicine
(Dermatology)
Albert Einstein College of Medicine
Adjunct Associate Professor of Dermatology
Mount Sinai School of Medicine
New York, NY, USA

Malcolm H A Rustin BSc MD FRCP
Consultant
Dermatology
King Edward VII's Hospital
London, UK

Thomas Ruzicka MD
Professor of Dermatology and Allergology
Department of Dermatology
Ludwig-Maximilians-Universität
Munich, Germany

Heather L Salvaggio MD
Dermatologist
Department of Dermatology
Penn State / Milton S Hershey Medical Center
Hershey PA, USA

Miguel R Sanchez MD
Director, Bellevue Hospital Center
Associate Professor of Clinical Dermatology
Department of Dermatology
NYU Medical Center
New York NY, USA

Lawrence A Schachner MD
Harvey Blank Professor and Chairman
Department of Dermatology and Cutaneous
Surgery
University of Miami School of Medicine
Miami FL, USA

Noah Scheinfeld MD JD
Department of Dermatology
St Lukes Roosevelt Hospital Center and
Assistant Clinical Professor of Dermatology
Columbia University
New York NY, USA

Bethanee J Schlosser MD PhD
Assistant Professor of Dermatology
Department of Dermatology
Northwestern University Feinberg School of
Medicine
Chicago IL, USA

Rhonda E Schnur MD FACMG
Associate Professor of Pediatrics
Head, Division of Genetics
Department of Pediatrics
Cooper University Hospital
Robert Wood Johnson Medical School
Camden NJ, USA

Olivia M V Schofield MBBS FRCP
Consultant Dermatologist
Department of Dermatology
Royal Infirmary of Edinburgh
Edinburgh, UK

Robert A Schwartz MD MPH
Professor and Head, Dermatology
Professor of Pathology, Medicine, Pediatrics
and Preventive Medicine
Department of Dermatology
New Jersey Medical School
Newark NJ, USA

Joslyn Sciacca Kirby MD
Assistant Professor of Dermatology
Department of Dermatology
Penn State Milton S Hershey Medical
Center
Philadelphia PA, USA

Bryan A Selkin MD
Dermatologist
Dermatology Center of Plano
Plano TX, USA

Christopher R Shea BA MD
Professor and Chief of Dermatology
Department of Medicine
Section of Dermatology
University of Chicago Medical Center
Chicago IL, USA

Neil H Shear BSc MD FRCP(C) FACP
Professor and Chief of Dermatology
Department of Dermatology
University of Toronto
Toronto ON, Canada

Hiroshi Shimizu MD PhD
Professor and Chairman
Department of Dermatology
Hokkaido University Graduate School of
Medicine
Sapporo, Japan

Robert Silverman MD
Clinical Associate Professor
Department of Pediatrics
Pasquerilla Healthcare Center
Washington DC, USA

Saurabh Singh MD
Dermatologist
Georgetown University
Washington Hospital Center
Washington DC, USA

Michael Sladden
Dermatologist, Launceston
Honorary Senior Lecturer
Department of Medicine
University of Tasmania
Legana, Tasmania, Australia

Najwa Somani MD FRCPC
Dermatologist
Departments of Dermatology and Pathology
Cleveland Clinic
Cleveland OH, USA

Christine Soon MRCP
Dermatologist
Department of Dermatology
Walsgrave Hospital
Coventry, UK

Nicholas A Soter MD
Professor of Dermatology
Ronald O Perelman Department of Dermatology
New York University Medical Center
New York NY, USA

James M Spencer MD MS
Associate Professor of Clinical Dermatology
Department of Dermatology
Mount Sinai School of Medicine
St Petersburg FL, USA

Richard L Spielvogel MD
Clinical Assistant Professor of Dermatology
and Pathology
Drexel University College of Medicine
Institute for Dermatopathology
Haddon Heights NJ, USA

Richard C D Staughton MA MBBChir FRCP
Consultant Dermatologist
Daniel Turner Clinic
Department of Dermatology
Chelsea and Westminster Hospital
London, UK

Jane C Sterling MB BChir MA FRCP PhD
Senior Lecturer and Honorary Consultant
Dermatologist
Department of Dermatology
Addenbrooke's Hospital
Cambridge, UK

Adam S Stibich MD
Fellow in Dermatology
Department of Dermatology
Stough Clinic
Hot Springs AR, USA

Brett T Summey Jr MD
Dermatologist and Dermatopathologist
Department of Dermatology
Drexel University
Boone NC, USA

Cord Sunderkötter MD
University Professor
Clinic for Dermatology and Venerology
University Clinic Münster
Münster, Germany

Saleem M Taibjee MBBCh BMedSci MRCPCH
DipRCPath
Consultant Paediatric Dermatologist
Honorary Senior Lecturer
Department of Dermatology
Birmingham Children's Hospital
Birmingham, UK

Anita Takwale MD MRCP
Consultant Dermatologist
Department of Dermatology
Gloucestershire Royal Hospital
Goucester, UK

Deborah Tamura MS RN APNG
Research Nurse
National Institutes of Health
National Cancer Institute
Bethesda MD, USA

Eunice Tan MRCP
Consultant Dermatologist
Department of Dermatology
Norfolk and Norwich University Hospitals
Norwich, UK

William Y–M Tang MBBS FHKCP FHKAM
(Medicine) FRCP(Edin) FRCP(Glas)
Consultant Dermatologist
Shatin International Medical Centre
Union Hospital
Hong Kong, China

Mordechai M Tarlow MD
Dermatologist
Department of Dermatology
UMNDJ–New Jersey Medical School
Newark NJ, USA

Nicholas R Telfer FRCP
Consultant Dermatological and Mohs
Micrographic Surgeon
Department of Dermatology
Hope Hospital
Salford
Manchester, UK

Maryanna C Ter Poorten MD
General and Pediatric Dermatology
Dermatology Group of the Carolinas
Concord NC, USA

Bruce H Thiers MD
Professor and Chairman
Department of Dermatology and
Dermatologic Surgery
Medical University of South Carolina
Charleston SC, USA

Michelle A Thomson MRCP
Consultant Dermatologist
Birmingham Skin Centre
City Hospital
Birmingham, UK

Anne-Marie Tobin MB BSc MRCPI
Dermatologist
Department of Dermatology
Adelaide and Meath Hospital
Dublin, Ireland

Antonella Tosti MD
Professor of Dermatology
Department of Dermatology
University of Bologna
Bologna, Italy

Anne Marie Tremaine MD
Clinical Research Fellow
Dermatology Research
University of California, Irvine
Irvine CA, USA

Fragkiski Tsatsou MD MSc BSc
Dermatologist
Departments of Dermatology, Venereology,
Allergology and Immunology
Dessau Medical Center
Dessau, Germany

Yukiko Tsuji-Abe MD PhD
Instructor
Department of Dermatology
Hokkaido University Graduate School of
Medicine
Sapporo, Japan

William F G Tucker MB FRCP
Consultant Dermatologist
Department of Dermatology
Alexandra Hospital
Worcestershire Acute NHS Trust
Redditch, UK

Stephen K Tyring MD PhD MBA
Professor of Dermatology, Microbiology/
Molecular Genetics and Internal Medicine
Department of Dermatology
University of Texas Health Science Center
Houston TX, USA

Walter Unger MD
Clinical Professor
Department of Dermatology
Mount Sinai School of Medicine
New York NY, USA

Robin H Unger MD
Assistant Clinical Professor
Department of Dermatology
Mount Sinai Medical School
New York NY, USA

Peter C M van de Kerkhof MD PhD
Professor and Chairman
Department of Dermatology
University Hospital Nijmegen
Nijmegen, Netherlands

Abby S Van Voorhees MD
Assistant Professor, Director of Psoriasis
and Phototherapy
Department of Dermatology
University of Pennsylvania
Philadelphia PA, USA

Claudia Irene Vidal MD PhD
Fellow, Dermatopathology
Division of Dermatology
Mount Sinai School of Medicine
New York NY, USA

Martha Viera MD
Senior Clinical Research Fellow
Department of Dermatology and
Cutaneous Surgery
University of Miami, Miller School of
Medicine
Miami FL, USA

Carmela C Vittorio MD
Assistant Profesor
Department of Dermatology
University of Pennsylvania
Philadelphia PA, USA

Christina Vlachou MRCP
Dermatologist
Department of Dermatology
Watford General Hospital
Watford, UK

Heidi A Waldorf MD
Associate Clinical Professor
Director, Laser and Cosmetic
Dermatology
The Mount Sinai Hospital, New York, NY
Waldorf Dermatology and Laser
Associates, PC
Nanuet NY, USA

Frances Wallach MD
Clinical Associate Professor
The Mount Sinai Hospital
New York NY, USA

Joanna Wallengren MD
Department of Dermatology
Malmö General Hospital
University of Lund, Sweden

Gabriele Weichert MD PhD
Dermatologist
Brickyard Medical Clinic
Nanaimo BC, Canada

Jeffrey M Weinberg MD
Director, Clinical Research Center
Department of Dermatology
St Luke's–Roosevelt Hospital Center
New York NY, USA

Victoria P Werth MD
Professor of Dermatology
Department of Dermatology
University of Pennsylvania
Philadelphia PA, USA

Carlos K Wesley MD
Surgical Associate
Private Practice
New York NY, USA

Contributors

Dennis West PhD FCCP
Professor of Dermatology
Department of Dermatology and Chair for
Administrative Review
Institutional Review Board
North Western University
Chicago IL, USA

Lucile E White MD
Dermatologist
Pearland Dermatology
Pearland TX, USA

Sean J Whittaker MD FRCP
Consultant Dermatologist
Skin Tumor Unit
St John's Institute of Dermatology
London, UK

Adam H Wiener DO
Physician
Somerset Skin Center
Dermcenter
Troy MI, USA

Nathaniel K Wilkin MD
Assistant Professor
UNC Dermatology
Chapel Hill NC, USA

Jonathan K Wilkin MD
Dermatologist
Private Practice
Columbus OH, USA

Jason Williams MBChB MRCP
Consultant Dermatologist
Hope Hospital
Salford, UK

Karen Wiss MD
Director, Pediatric Dermatology and
Professor of Medicine (Dermatology) and
Pediatrics
Dermatology Department
UMass Memorial Medical Center
Worcester MA, USA

Joseph A Witkowski MD FACP
Clinical Professor of Dermatology
University of Pennsylvania School of
Medicine
Philadelphia PA, USA

Fenella Wojnarowska FRCP DM
Professor of Dermatology
Department of Dermatology
Churchill Hospital
Oxford, UK

Andrew L Wright MedSci MRCS MBChB FRCP
Honourary Senior Research Fellow,
University of Bradford and Consultant
Dermatologist
Dermatology Department
St Luke's Hospital
Bradford, UK

Andrea L Zaenglein MD
Associate Professor of Dermatology and
Pediatrics
Department of Dermatology
Penn State/Milton S Hershey Medical Center
Hershey PA, USA

Sameh S Zaghloul MBBCh DDSc MSc MD
Clinical Research Fellow and Lecturer in
Dermatology
Leeds General Infirmary
University of Leeds, School of Medicine
Leeds, UK

Irshad Zaki BMedSci(Hons) BMBS FRCP
Consultant Dermatolgist
Department of Dermatology
Solihull Hospital
West Midlands, UK

Joshua A Zeichner MD
Instructor
Department of Dermatology
The Mount Sinai School of
Medicine
New York NY, USA

John J Zone MD
Professor and Chair
Department of Dermatology
University of Utah
Salt Lake City UT, USA

Christos C Zouboulis MD Prof Dr med
Professor of Dermatology and Venereology
Director, Departments of Dermatology
Venereology, Allergology and Immunology
Dessau Medical Center
Dessau, Germany

Acknowledgements

The editors want to thank their families for continued support and patience through the many months of writing and editing. We are also fortunate to have worked with outstanding staff at Elsevier and are grateful to Joanne Scott, Rachael Harrison, Thu Nguyen, and Claire Bonnett for their constant assistance. This book could not have come to fruition without the help of our staff, Marion Rodriguez and Victoria White.

It is difficult to make an excellent product even better, but that is precisely what authors of the third edition have done. In thanking them we must acknowledge the authors of prior editions whose chapters were the foundation onto which new information was added.

Finally, we never forget to thank our patients who participate in clinical trials that lead to new therapies and volunteer for photographs that appear in this and many other books. Hopefully, they will ultimately benefit from *Treatment of Skin Disease*.

Dedication

Dedicated to our parents:

the late Harold and Elizabeth Berth-Jones

Alan and the late Verna Coulson

Ruth Heymann and the late Horace Heymann

The late Zachary and Jennie Lebwohl

Evidence Levels

Each therapy covered has been assigned a letter from A (most evidence) to E (least evidence) signifying the amount of published evidence available to support its use. The following table shows the criteria used in making this classification.

A DOUBLE-BLIND STUDY

At least one prospective randomized, double-blind, controlled trial without major design flaws (in the author's view)

B CLINICAL TRIAL ≥ 20 SUBJECTS

Prospective clinical trials with 20 or more subjects; trials lacking adequate controls or another key facet of design, which would normally be considered desirable (in the author's opinion)

C CLINICAL TRIAL < 20 SUBJECTS

Small trials with less than 20 subjects with significant design limitations, very large numbers of case reports (at least 20 cases in the literature), retrospective analyses of data

D SERIES ≥ 5 SUBJECTS

Series of patients reported to respond (at least 5 cases in the literature)

E ANECDOTAL CASE REPORTS

Individual case reports amounting to published experience of less than 5 cases

Acanthosis nigricans

Kevin F Kia, Ponciano D Cruz, Jr

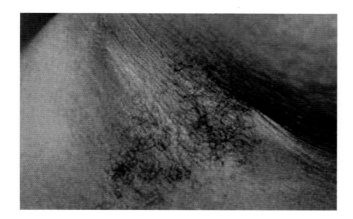

Acanthosis nigricans is characterized by hyperpigmented, verrucous or velvety plaques which usually appear on flexural surfaces and in intertriginous regions. It is most commonly seen in individuals with insulin resistance states, especially obesity, and less frequently in association with other metabolic disorders, drugs, and malignancy. Although hyperinsulinemia, hyperandrogenemia, circulating anti-insulin receptor antibodies, and activating mutations in fibroblast growth factor receptor (especially for syndromes associated with skeletal dysplasia) have been implicated as causal factors, the precise pathogenesis is not yet known.

MANAGEMENT STRATEGY

The management of patients with acanthosis nigricans depends on the underlying cause, the identification of which requires a salient history, a targeted physical examination, and a finite set of laboratory tests.

Relevant historical information includes age at onset, presence or absence of a family history, medications, and presence or absence of symptoms related to hyperinsulinemia (with or without diabetes mellitus), hyperandrogenemia (with or without virilism) and internal malignancy (with or without weight loss).

Drugs reported in association with acanthosis nigricans include nicotinic acid, corticosteroids, estrogens, insulin, fusidic acid, protease inhibitors, triazinate, diethylstilbestrol, palifermin, and recombinant growth hormone.

Physical examination should document obesity, masculinization, lymphadenopathy, and organomegaly. Initial laboratory screening should include fasting blood glucose and insulin tested concurrently to confirm or exclude insulin resistance (insulin value inappropriately high for the glucose level).

Because obesity is the most common cause of both insulin resistance and acanthosis nigricans, it is reasonable to assume that it is the cause of acanthosis nigricans in obese patients with no historical or physical examination evidence of malignancy or of suspect drugs.

Rare causes of insulin resistance and acanthosis nigricans include the type A and B syndromes, the former characterized by defective insulin receptors and manifested typically in young girls with masculinized features, and the latter reported mostly in women with circulating anti-insulin receptor antibodies in association with autoimmune disorders such as lupus erythematosus. Other causes of insulin resistance and acanthosis nigricans are polycystic ovarian disease, HAIR-AN syndrome (hyperandrogenism, insulin resistance and acanthosis nigricans), familial lipodystrophies, and various endocrinopathies. If insulin resistance is present, then the possibility of malignancy becomes unlikely.

The most common malignancy associated with acanthosis nigricans is gastric adenocarcinoma. Less frequently reported are endocrine, genitourinary and lung carcinomas, and melanoma. Malignant acanthosis nigricans may coexist with other cutaneous markers of internal malignancy, such as tripe palms, the sign of Leser–Trelat, florid cutaneous papillomatosis, and hyperkeratosis of the palms and soles (tylosis). If malignancy-associated acanthosis nigricans is suspected, the initial laboratory screen may include a complete blood count, stool test for occult blood, chest and gastrointestinal radiographs, as well as gastrointestinal endoscopy. Pelvic and rectal examinations, including pelvic ultrasonography, may be warranted in women and men depending on their age.

In the absence of objective evidence for a specific cause, the acanthosis nigricans may be labeled as idiopathic, which may or may not be familial. *Treatment of the underlying cause* often leads to resolution of the acanthosis nigricans. Otherwise, most published modes of treatment are *symptomatic* and/or *cosmetic*, and testimony to their efficacy has been anecdotal.

SPECIFIC INVESTIGATIONS

> ▶ Document obesity based on ideal body weight
> ▶ Determine fasting blood glucose and insulin levels in parallel
> ▶ Depending on historical clues, screen for other endocrine disease
> ▶ Consider malignancy; if suspected refer to appropriate specialist for the best diagnostic procedure
> ▶ Consider drugs as a cause

Prevalence and significance of acanthosis nigricans in an adult population. Hud J, Cohen J, Wagner J, Cruz P. Arch Dermatol 1992; 128: 941–4.

Up to 74% of obese adult patients seen at the Parkland Memorial Hospital Adult Obesity Clinic in Dallas, Texas, had acanthosis nigricans. The skin disorder predicted the existence of hyperinsulinemia.

Prevalence of obesity, acanthosis nigricans and hyperinsulinemia in an adolescent clinic. Bolding J, Wratchford T, Perkins K, Ogershok P. WV Med J 2005; 101: 112–15.

The prevalence of obesity (37%) and acanthosis nigricans (17%) was established in this adolescent population of West Virginia.

Juvenile acanthosis nigricans. Sinha S, Schwartz RA. J Am Acad Dermatol 2007; 57: 502–8.

A review of the evaluation of children presenting with acanthosis nigricans.

Acanthosis nigricans associated with insulin resistance: pathophysiology and management. Hermanns-Le T, Scheen A, Pierard G. Am J Clin Dermatol 2004; 5: 199–203.

A review of the pathogenesis and treatment of acanthosis nigricans.

Genes, growth factors and acanthosis nigricans. Torleyu D, Bellus G, Munro C. Br J Dermatol 2002; 147: 1096–101.

Craniosynostosis and skeletal dysplasia syndromes with acanthosis nigricans are associated with activating mutations in fibroblast growth factor receptors, particularly FGFR3.

Characterization of groups of hyperandrogenic women with acanthosis nigricans, impaired glucose tolerance and/or hyperinsulinemia. Dunaif A, Graf M, Mandeli J, Laumas V, Dobrjansky A. J Clin Endocrinol Metab 1987; 65: 499–507.

Among obese women with polycystic ovaries 50% had acanthosis nigricans.

Malignant acanthosis nigricans: a review. Rigel D, Jacobe M. J Dermatol Surg Oncol 1980; 6: 923–7.

Gastric carcinoma was reported in 55% of 227 cases of acanthosis nigricans associated with an internal malignancy. Other intra-abdominal malignancies accounted for 18% of cases, and the remaining 27% had extra-abdominal sites of malignancy.

Acanthosis nigricans: a new manifestation of insulin resistance in patients receiving treatment with protease inhibitors. Mellor-Pita S, Yebra-Bango M, Alfaro-Martinez J, Suarez E. Clin Infect Dis 2002; 34: 716–17.

A man with HIV infection developed insulin resistance, diabetes mellitus, and acanthosis nigricans soon after starting treatment with protease inhibitors.

Acanthosis nigricans-like lesions from nicotinic acid. Tromovitch T, Jacobs P, Kern S. Arch Dermatol 1964; 89: 222–3.

A man treated with nicotinic acid (4 g/day) developed acanthosis nigricans, which cleared after discontinuation of the drug.

Somatotrophin-induced acanthosis nigricans. Downs A, Kennedy C. Br J Dermatol 1999; 141: 390–1.

A boy with achondroplasia treated long-term with recombinant growth hormone (3–4 units of subcutaneous somatotropin weekly for 7 years) developed acanthosis nigricans in the groin and axilla.

FIRST-LINE THERAPY

▶ Treat the underlying cause	D

Acanthosis nigricans: a cutaneous marker of tissue resistant to insulin. Rendon M, Cruz P, Sontheimer R, Bergstresser P. J Am Acad Dermatol 1989; 21: 461–9.

In a woman with systemic lupus erythematosus and the type B syndrome of insulin resistance, the acanthosis nigricans cleared after treatment with oral corticosteroids and subcutaneous injection of insulin. Her circulating anti-insulin antibodies also disappeared with treatment of the autoimmune disease.

Clearance of acanthosis nigricans associated with the HAIR-AN syndrome after partial pancreatectomy: an 11-year follow up. Pfeifer SL, Wilson RM, Gawkrodger DJ. Postgrad Med J 1999; 75: 421–2.

An obese woman with HAIR-AN syndrome was diagnosed a year later with insulinoma. One year after resection of the tumor the patient's virilism resolved, and 9 years after the surgery the acanthosis nigricans was much improved.

Acanthosis nigricans in association with congenital adrenal hyperplasia: resolution after treatment. Kurtoglu S, Atabek ME, Keskin M, Canöz O. Turk J Pediatr 2005; 47: 183–7.

A 3-day-old girl with the salt-wasting type of 21-hydroxylase deficient congenital adrenal hyperplasia presented with acanthosis nigricans of both axillae. Following corticosteroid and mineralocorticoid therapy for disease, the acanthosis nigricans resolved.

SECOND-LINE THERAPY

▶ Topical tretinoin and ammonium lactate	D
▶ Oral metformin E -Topical vitamin A	E
▶ Topical tazarotene	E
▶ Topical calcipotriol	E

Topical therapy with tretinoin and ammonium lactate for acanthosis nigricans associated with obesity. Blobstein SH. Cutis 2003; 71: 33–4.

Five obese patients with acanthosis nigricans were successfully treated with 12% ammonium lactate cream twice daily and tretinoin 0.05% cream nightly to one side of the neck (the other side serving as control).

There was no mention of whether the obese patients lost weight during the treatment period, which could have contributed to the improvement.

Acanthosis nigricans and hypovitaminosis A. Response to topical vitamin A acid. Montes L, Hirschowitz B, Krumdieck C. J Cutan Pathol 1974; 1: 88–94.

A teenage girl had acanthosis nigricans, deafness, steatorrhea, peripheral sensory nerve demyelination, and hypovitaminosis A. The skin condition improved within 2 weeks of applying retinoic acid ointment 0.1% twice daily.

Successful symptomatic tazarotene treatment of juvenile acanthosis nigricans of the familial obesity-associated type in insulin resistance. Weisshaar E, Bonnekoh B, Franke I, Gollnick H. Hautarzt 2001; 52: 499–503 [in German].

A single report of a boy suffering from morbid obesity since infancy. In a right–left comparison the affected skin of one body side was treated with tazarotene 0.05% versus urea 10%, once daily each. A great benefit for the tazarotene-treated side was seen after 3 weeks.

Treatment of mixed-type acanthosis nigricans with topical calcipotriol. Bohm M, Luger T, Metze D. Br J Dermatol 1998; 139: 932–3.

An obese patient with metastatic transitional cell carcinoma of the bladder, insulin resistance, and acanthosis nigricans was treated with topical calcipotriol 0.005% twice daily for 3 months, which led to improvement of her skin condition.

Therapeutic approach in insulin resistance with acanthosis nigricans. Tankova T, Koev D, Dakovska L, Kirilov G. Int J Clin Pract 2002; 56: 578–81.

Five obese patients (two children and three adults with diabetes mellitus) were treated with metformin daily for 6 months, resulting in significant reduction in plasma insulin, body weight, and body fat mass. Both children and one adult showed improvement of acanthosis nigricans.

THIRD-LINE THERAPY

▶ Oral isotretinoin	E
▶ Oral ketoconazole	E
▶ Palliative chemotherapy	E
▶ Cyproheptadine	E
▶ Dietary fish oil	E
▶ Oral contraceptives	E
▶ Dermabrasion	E
▶ Long-pulsed alexandrite laser	E
▶ Continuous wave carbon dioxide laser	E

Treatment of acanthosis nigricans with oral isotretinoin. Katz R. Arch Dermatol 1980; 116: 110–11.

An obese, hirsute, diabetic woman with acanthosis nigricans was treated with oral isotretinoin (2–3 mg/kg/day for 4 months), producing clearance of the skin problem. However, long-term treatment was required to maintain clearance because the acanthosis nigricans recurred when the retinoid was discontinued.

Because of the side effects of isotretinoin, long-term use for a benign condition may not be practical.

Improvement of acanthosis nigricans on isotretinoin and metformin. Walling HW, Messingham M, Myers LM, Mason CL, Strauss JS. J Drugs Dermatol 2003; 2: 677–81.

An obese man developed acanthosis nigricans, tripe palms, and laryngeal papillomatosis, with no evidence of malignancy after 6 years of follow-up. Isotretinoin (80 mg/day) led to improvement after 2 months of therapy. The addition of metformin produced extra improvement.

Effect of ketoconazole in the hyperandrogenism, insulin resistance and acanthosis nigricans (HAIR-AN) syndrome. Tercedor J, Rodenas JM. J Am Acad Dermatol 1992; 27: 786.

Ketoconazole improved acanthosis nigricans in a patient with HAIR-AN syndrome.

Because of its hepatotoxic effects, oral ketoconazole, which has antiandrogenic effects, is largely avoided nowadays.

Malignant acanthosis nigricans: potential role of chemotherapy. Anderson SH, Hudson-Peacock M, Muller AF. Br J Dermatol 1999; 141: 714–16.

A man with metastatic gastric adenocarcinoma and disseminated acanthosis nigricans was treated with palliative chemotherapy, leading to significant improvement.

Treatment of acanthosis nigricans with cyproheptadine. Greenwood R, Tring F. Br J Dermatol 1982; 106: 697–8.

A man with gastric adenocarcinoma and acanthosis nigricans showed clearance of the skin disease following treatment with cyproheptadine (4 mg three times daily for 3 weeks).

Because the patient underwent palliative gastrectomy 4 months earlier, it is not clear whether removal of the adenocarcinoma or the cyproheptadine was responsible for clearing the acanthosis nigricans.

Acanthosis nigricans. Schwartz RA. J Am Acad Dermatol 1994; 31: 1.

A white woman with lipodystrophic diabetes mellitus and acanthosis nigricans was treated with dietary fish oil supplementation, leading to improvement of the skin condition despite continued elevation of triglyceride levels.

Remission of acanthosis nigricans associated with polycystic ovarian disease and stromal luteoma. Andersen RN, Coleman SA, Fish SA. J Clin Endocrinol Metab 1974; 38: 347–55.

A girl with acanthosis nigricans and polycystic ovaries showed complete clearance of acanthosis nigricans and hyperandrogenism after treatment with OrthoNovum 2 mg/day.

Treatment of acanthosis nigricans of the axillae using a long-pulsed (5-msec) alexandrite laser. Rosenback A, Ram R. Dermatol Surg 2004; 30: 1158–60.

A woman with axillary acanthosis nigricans was treated with long-pulsed alexandrite laser (5 ms) on one axilla, with the other as an untreated control. The treated axilla showed significant improvement.

Continuous-wave carbon dioxide laser therapy of pseudoacanthosis nigricans. Bredlich R, Krahn G, Kunzi-Rapp K, Wortmann S, Peter RU. Br J Dermatol 1998; 139: 937–8.

An obese man with acanthosis nigricans who had failed previous treatments with topical retinoids and salicylic acid was then treated with continuous-wave carbon dioxide laser (three sessions at 4–6-week intervals). His acanthosis nigricans improved after 6 months of treatment.

Acne keloidalis nuchae

William Perkins

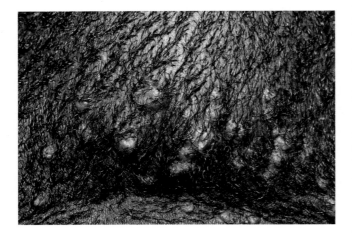

Acne keloidalis nuchae (AKN) is an idiopathic chronic inflammatory process affecting the nape of the neck and the occipital scalp; it occurs predominantly in black males. Initial features consist of papules and pustules on the occiput and posterior neck, which subsequently coalesce into plaques of dense scar tissue with central scarring alopecia. Although the etiology is unknown, the histology of early cases shows evidence of acute and chronic folliculitis, with ruptured follicles, perifolliculitis, and a foreign body granulomatous response. Later cases may show similar features, but additionally there may be hypertrophic scar formation. Close shaving of the hair has been postulated as a cause for AKN, but even during the 1960s and 1970s, with the fashion for longer hair, AKN was still seen. Physical trauma due to collars rubbing and picking by patients have all been suggested as precipitants, but none of these has been investigated in any systematic way. Whether folliculitis leading to ruptured follicles and the subsequent foreign body reaction, or the development of ingrowing hairs is the primary event, the term 'acne keloidalis' is a misnomer. Keloids at other sites or a family history of keloids are not features of AKN, and excision of the area does not result in keloid formation. Pseudofolliculitis barbae was associated with AKN in five of six cases in one series, but clinical or histologic evidence of superficial hair penetration is lacking. Lesions resembling AKN have been reported in those receiving long-term ciclosporin, and sarcoid papules may occasionally mimic the condition.

MANAGEMENT STRATEGY

A clear diagnosis is a prerequisite for the management of AKN. The presence of inflammatory papules, pustules, and hypertrophic scar formation on the occipital scalp and posterior neck in a black male is pathognomonic, but cases have been described in Caucasians, and occasionally in females. Biopsy of the area is not usually required, but concerns about keloidal scarring should not inhibit obtaining histologic confirmation. Folliculitis secondary to bacterial infections, particularly staphylococcal, needs to be excluded. In staphylococcal folliculitis the pustules and papules tend to be more widely distributed across the scalp, especially over the crown. Culture will yield heavy growths of staphylococci, and the condition usually responds well to treatment with *oral antibiotics*, but may recur and require long-term treatment.

In view of the suggested associations with close-cropped hair and picking, it may be worthwhile enquiring about these factors. If present, these practices should be avoided.

Treatment depends on the stage of presentation. Unfortunately, the evidence base for many of the management recommendations is weak. Many patients will prefer no treatment or conservative treatment in the early stages of the disease. This is demonstrated by the fact that only 30% of patients identified in one survey had tried any treatment at all. Early disease with papules and pustules scattered across the posterior neck and occipital scalp may well be best managed by *topical antiseptics*, *antibiotics*, or *potent topical corticosteroids*.

With the development of hypertrophic scar formation, *topical or intralesional corticosteroids* may well be of benefit. Once scarring alopecia, hypertrophic scars, and symptoms related to itch, pain, and discharging sinuses are present, treatment directed at the removal of the follicles from the affected area in their entirety is recommended.

Excisional surgery is the only treatment reported in any significant case series. The factors influencing the use of excision will be the severity of symptoms the patient is experiencing and the confidence the patient and surgeon have in the process of surgery. Scattered papules and pustules across the occipital scalp without confluent areas of hypertrophic scar formation and with only limited symptoms may lead patients to seek a more conservative treatment option.

Prioritization of the following treatments is not meant to be a strict hierarchy; for a well-developed case of AKN, the author's treatment of choice is excision. When this is not acceptable, some of the following non-surgical approaches may be appropriate. Advice to *reduce the picking* (a consistently reported association) *and close cropping* of the hair is the first measure one should employ. This may be aided by the anti-inflammatory effect of potent topical corticosteroids. In mild early cases treatment with a topical antibiotic such as 1% *clindamycin* or *erythromycin* may be helpful. Oral antistaphylococcal antibiotics, such as *flucloxacillin* or *erythromycin*, may be helpful, but this is not a recommendation supported by trial evidence. A very good response to flucloxacillin or erythromycin in the early stages when no scarring is present may suggest staphylococcal folliculitis rather than AKN. Long-term oral *tetracycline* antibiotics may be of help in some cases of early disease. Limited hypertrophic scars may respond to intralesional *triamcinolone*. *Isotretinoin* has been used with success.

SPECIFIC INVESTIGATIONS

▶ Pustule swab
▶ Deep biopsy

Investigations are not particularly helpful in AKN, and even histology tends to be a byproduct of excisional treatment. If the diagnosis is in doubt, a deep biopsy to below the level of the scar tissue and follicular bulbs will confirm the diagnosis. Folliculitis secondary to *Staphylococcus aureus* is worth excluding, largely based on clinical features such as the distribution and the lack of hypertrophic scar formation, but positive cultures from pustules may direct topical and systemic antibiotic therapy. Pustular lesions of AKN may well grow *S. aureus*, but the response to treatment in the context of a simple bacterial folliculitis will be much greater than that seen in AKN.

FIRST-LINE THERAPIES

▶ Dissuade picking, close hair cutting	E
▶ Topical clindamycin	E
▶ Oral antistaphylococcal antibiotics – erythromycin or flucloxacillin	E
▶ Oral tetracycline	E
▶ Topical corticosteroids	B

An open label study of clobetasol propionate 0.05% and betamethasone valerate 0.12% foams in the treatment of mild to moderate acne keloidalis. Callender VD, Young CM, Haverstock CL, Carroll CL, Feldman SR. Cutis 2005; 75: 317–21.

Pseudofolliculitis barbae. Chu T. Practitioner 1989; 233: 307–9.

In a limited open study, 1% topical clindamycin was anecdotally found to be effective for pseudofolliculitis and acne keloidalis.

Acne keloidalis is a form of scarring alopecia. Sperling LC, Homoky C, Pratt L, Sau P. Arch Dermatol 2000; 136: 479–84.

Medical treatment for early papular lesions includes intralesional injections of corticosteroids, topical steroids, and topical or oral antibiotics (usually tetracycline).

SECOND-LINE THERAPIES

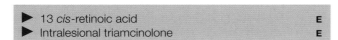

▶ 13 *cis*-retinoic acid	E
▶ Intralesional triamcinolone	E

Folliculitis nuchae scleroticans – successful treatment with 13-cis-retinoic acid (isotretinoin). Stieler W, Senff H, Janner M. Hautarzt 1988; 39: 739–42.

Oral therapy with 13-*cis*-retinoic acid (isotretinoin) in a 23-year-old white man resulted in a remarkable improvement within a few weeks.

If antibiotic treatment fails, oral isotretinoin may be helpful in selected cases. Once hypertrophic scarring has developed, treatment with oral or topical antibiotics is less successful and measures to control the formation of hypertrophic scar need to be employed. Potent topical corticosteroid creams may help, but intralesional injections of corticosteroids such as triamcinolone can reduce the bulk of the scar tissue. Despite these injections the process tends to continue and the treatment will need to be repeated at intervals.

THIRD-LINE THERAPIES

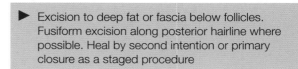

▶ Excision to deep fat or fascia below follicles. Fusiform excision along posterior hairline where possible. Heal by second intention or primary closure as a staged procedure	C

The surgical management of extensive cases of acne keloidalis nuchae. Gloster HM. Arch Dermatol 2000; 136: 1376–9.

Of 25 young African-Caribbean men with extensive AKN who underwent surgical excision of AKN, 20 underwent excision with layered closure in one stage. Four patients underwent two-stage excisions with layered closure. One patient underwent excision with second-intention healing. All rated the cosmetic result of surgery as good to excellent. No patient experienced complete recurrence of acne keloidalis; 15 patients developed tiny pustules and papules within the surgical scar; five developed hypertrophic scars, all of which were successfully treated with high-potency topical and intralesional corticosteroids. Extremely large lesions should be excised in several stages.

Surgical excision of acne keloidalis nuchae with secondary intention healing. Bajaj V, Langtry JA. Clin Exp Dermatol 2008; 33: 53–5.

Anesthesia can be achieved simply with either 0.5% or 1% lidocaine plus epinephrine (adrenaline) 1:200 000 or even 0.1% with epinephrine 1:1 000 000. The advantage of the latter is that it gives excellent longer-term control of bleeding, which can be a problem with large scalp excisions. The use of electrosurgical excision can thus be avoided, as this is associated with increased levels of postoperative pain and an increased risk of wound dehiscence.

Acne vulgaris

Fragkiski Tsatsou, Christos C Zouboulis

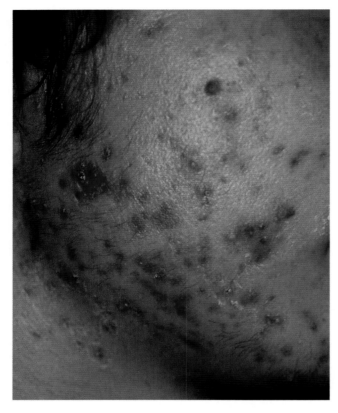

Acne vulgaris is one of the most common dermatologic disorders encountered in everyday clinical practice. It is a disease of the sebaceous follicle, primarily the pilosebaceous units located on the face, chest, and back. Inflammatory and non-inflammatory lesions present with highly variable morphologies.

MANAGEMENT STRATEGY

The treatment of acne vulgaris is tailored to the etiology, type, and severity of the disease.

Several factors contribute to the pathogenesis of acne, the major ones being increased sebaceous gland activity with hyperseborrhea, abnormal follicular differentiation and increased cornification, increased bacterial colonization, inflammation and immunological host reaction. Each of these provides a potential target for treatment; concomitant targeting of these factors is required to treat acne effectively.

Suppression of sebaceous gland hyperactivity can be achieved by systemic administration of anti-androgens or isotretinoin. Increased cornification can be directly influenced through topical retinoids, as well as through topical application of azelaic acid. Agents with anti-inflammatory activity may also reduce comedones. Inflammation can be improved with the use of benzoyl peroxide, and topical and systemic antibiotics. In addition to being comedolytic, retinoids also exhibit anti-inflammatory effects. The tendency for scar formation plays a role in the selection of treatment. Scarring acne usually requires a systemic treatment.

In mild forms of acne, *topical therapy* is most appropriate. According to guidelines developed through an international consensus for the treatment of acne, the Global Alliance to Improve Outcomes in Acne, monotherapy with *topical retinoids* is the treatment of choice for mild comedonal acne. Following successful treatment, topical retinoids are suitable for maintenance therapy. *Topical antimicrobials* with *anti-inflammatory properties* should be used in combination with topical retinoids for mild papulopustular acne only. *Clindamycin phosphate plus benzoyl peroxide* (CDP+BPO) is recommended for the topical treatment of both mild and moderate acne vulgaris and should be considered, with or without topical retinoids, as first-line therapy for the treatment of the majority of cases. *Topical retinoids* are appropriate for the treatment of most types of acne and for maintenance treatment.

Oral antibiotics have been suggested to improve inflammatory acne by inhibiting the growth of *Propionibacterium acnes*. Although there is no correlation between the number of *P. acnes* and the severity of acne, the occurrence of antibiotic-resistant *P. acnes* correlates with poor clinical response. Several antibiotics exhibit anti-inflammatory properties, assisting in the improvement of acne through reduced leukocyte chemotaxis and alteration of cytokine production. *Tetracyclines, erythromycin,* and *nadifloxacin* reduce the formation of reactive oxygen species by neutrophils, and hence acne inflammation. New antibiotics for the treatment of acne include *lymecycline*, a second-generation tetracycline, and *roxithromycin*, a macrolide that exhibits anti-inflammatory and anti-androgenic activities.

Antibiotics with anti-inflammatory properties, such as tetracyclines (*oxytetracycline, tetracycline chloride, doxycycline, minocycline, lymecycline*) and macrolides (*erythromycin, azithromycin*) are the agents of choice for papulopustular acne. Second-generation tetracyclines (*doxycycline, minocycline, lymecycline*) have pharmacokinetic advantages over tetracycline. Dosage is easier owing to their longer half-life, and they can be taken with meals, whereas tetracycline must be taken half an hour before meals.

Doxycycline is used at 100 or 200 mg daily in two equal doses. *Minocycline* is not equally recommendable because of its rare but potentially severe side effects and high cost. An initially higher dose of doxycycline or minocycline (4 weeks 100 mg/po/day, then 50 mg/po/day) is more effective than 50 mg/po/day over 12 weeks. Patients with strong seborrhea may require higher doses (doxycycline and minocycline up to 200 mg daily, lymecycline up to 600 mg daily). At such dosages increased side effects may be expected. Small daily doses with concomitant subinhibitory concentrations may promote resistance. An extended-release minocycline tablet, administered at a dosage of 1 mg/kg daily for 12 weeks, has been approved by the FDA for moderate to severe inflammatory acne vulgaris in patients over 12 years old.

Systemic antibiotic therapy of moderate to severe papulopustular acne should in general be continued for 3 months and should be combined with BPO (either continuously or in intervals) to prevent antibiotic resistance. Combination therapy with topical agents, especially retinoids, BPO or azelaic acid, also increases the efficacy of treatment. It appears that antibiotic therapy for more than 3–6 months brings little additional effect but increases the risk of resistance. Tetracycline resistance encompasses the entire class. There is cross-resistance between erythromycin and clindamycin.

In case of renal failure *doxycycline* is preferred, as it is metabolized in the liver. *Azithromycin*, a methyl derivative of erythromycin, has a favorable safety profile and can be used safely during pregnancy. There have been several reports of failure of oral contraceptives during antibiotic therapy of acne with *rifampicin*; however, that is not the case for other antibiotic drugs.

In severe papulopustular and in nodulocystic or conglobate acne *oral isotretinoin* is the treatment of choice. This is still the only compound that affects all pathogenic factors of acne. It directly suppresses sebaceous gland activity, leading to a significant reduction in sebaceous lipogenesis, normalizes the pattern of keratinization within the pilosebaceous follicle, inhibits inflammation, and – in a secondary manner – reduces the growth of *P. acnes*. Oral isotretinoin is the most effective anti-acne drug available, especially in the treatment of severe recalcitrant nodulocystic acne, and in the prevention of acne scarring. However, despite its undeniable effectiveness, isotretinoin is not curative, and its discontinuation may be followed by relapses.

Identifying the appropriate patient for isotretinoin treatment of acne is important nowadays, as, because it is no longer patent protected, the compound has already drawn the attention of the European Committee on Proprietary Medicinal Products, which released a European directive to ensure harmonization of isotretinoin treatment throughout the European Union. Both European guidelines and the iPLEDGE isotretinoin distribution program of the FDA are aimed at preventing the use of the drug in women during pregnancy.

Isotretinoin is recommended at a dosage of 0.5 mg/kg/day. In most cases of severe acne a 6–12-month course of isotretinoin 0.5–1 mg/kg/day in order to reach 150 mg/kg total cumulative dose is recommended. Higher doses are indicated particularly for severe involvement of the chest and back. Factors contributing to the need for longer treatment schedules include low-dose regimens (0.1–0.5 mg/kg/day), the presence of severe acne, extrafacial involvement, and a prolonged history of the disease.

In addition to our better understanding of its activity, other developments in the application of this potent compound include reduction of the risk of side effects by using low-dose, long-term regimens (0.1–0.3 mg/mL/day, or intermittent use) and a micronized isotretinoin formulation, which exhibits similar efficacy and is associated with a lower risk of adverse events.

Isotretinoin treatment can initially induce inflammatory flares of acne, occasionally leading to acne fulminans. This usually occurs 3–4 weeks after treatment initiation. Mild flares do not require modification of the oral dose and improve spontaneously. Severe episodes should be treated with systemic corticosteroids, and dose reduction or discontinuation of isotretinoin may be required.

The adverse effect profile of oral isotretinoin is closely associated with hypervitaminosis A. It includes characteristic dose-dependent mucocutaneous side effects (cheilitis, xerosis, dry mucosae, conjunctivitis, epistaxis), elevation of serum lipids, hyperostosis, extraskeletal calcification, arthralgia, and myalgia.

The teratogenic potential of isotretinoin, with a high rate of spontaneous abortions and life-threatening congenital malformations, demands the use of secure contraception when it is prescribed for women of childbearing age. Contraception is recommended 1 month before the initiation of treatment, during the entire period of drug administration, and for 3 months after discontinuation of the regimen. Oral isotretinoin is strictly contraindicated in pregnancy, during lactation, and in severe hepatic and renal dysfunction. Relative

contraindications include hyperlipidemia, diabetes mellitus, and severe osteoporosis. Co-administration of vitamin A, tetracycline, and high doses of aspirin is contraindicated. Liver enzymes and blood lipid levels should be monitored.

For acne fulminans a combination of low-dose *oral corticosteroid* (prednisone, prednisolone, or dexamethasone) and *isotretinoin* is indicated.

Infantile and pediatric acne and androgenization signs in female patients with late-onset acne may necessitate an alternative treatment. Women with signs of peripheral hyperandrogenism or with hyperandrogenemia, late-onset or recalcitrant acne who also desire contraception, and women being treated with systemic *isotretinoin* should be treated with *anti-androgens*. For patients with adrenal hyperadrogenism low-dose *oral corticosteroids* combined with *systemic retinoid* are the treatment of choice.

SPECIFIC INVESTIGATIONS

None are required routinely.
▶ Consider microbiology to exclude Gram-positive or -negative folliculitis
▶ Consider endocrine work-up if hyperandrogenemia is suspected

FIRST-LINE THERAPY

Comedonal acne
▶ Topical retinoids   A

Mild papulopustular acne
▶ Benzoyl peroxide (topical) with topical retinoids or with topical antimicrobials (antibiotics or azelaic acid)   A

Moderate papulopustular acne without scarring
▶ Benzoyl peroxide (topical) with topical retinoids and topical antibiotics   A

Moderate papulopustular acne with light scarring
▶ For males use oral antibiotics (tetracyclines, macrolides) with benzoyl peroxide (topical) or topical retinoids   A
▶ For females use an oral anti-androgen contraceptive with benzoyl peroxide (topical) and topical antibiotics   A

Severe papulopustular acne*
▶ Oral isotretinoin   A

Nodulocystic and/or conglobate acne*
▶ Oral isotretinoin   c

Acne fulminans*
▶ Oral isotretinoin with low-dose oral corticosteroids   c

* In women, add an oral anti-androgen contraceptive.

Topical retinoids in acne – an evidence-based overview. Thielitz A, Naser MB, Fluhr JW, Zouboulis CC, Gollnick H. J Dtsch Dermatol Ges 2008 [Epub ahead of print].

A review of the substances approved for topical acne treatment, their differences in efficacy and tolerability, and their adverse effects, according to the currently available evidence (EBM-levels).

A comparison of the efficacy and tolerability of adapalene 0.1% gel versus tretinoin 0.025% gel in patients with acne vulgaris: a meta-analysis of five randomized trials. Cunliffe WJ, Poncet M, Loesche C, Verschoore M. Br J Dermatol 1998; 139: 48–56.

In a meta-analysis of five multicenter studies with a total of 900 patients both adapalene and tretinoin 0.025% gel were equally effective in reducing the total number of acne lesions after 12 weeks of treatment. Adapalene demonstrated more rapid efficacy and was associated with significantly less skin irritation than tretinoin.

Emerging topical antimicrobial options for mild-to-moderate acne: a review of the clinical evidence. Del Rosso J. J Drugs Dermatol 2008; 7: 2–7.

A review of the wide array of topical antimicrobial agents used as first-line treatment for mild to moderate acne vulgaris. Antibacterial agents, topical antibiotics, topical retinoids, azelaic acid, and new formulations with improved efficacy and tolerability are discussed.

Efficacy and safety of stabilized hydrogen peroxide cream (Crystacide) in mild-to-moderate acne vulgaris: a randomized controlled trial versus benzoyl peroxide gel. Milani M, Bigardi A, Zattarelli M. Curr Med Res Opin 2003; 19: 135–8.

A new formulation of hydrogen peroxide stabilized (HPS) in monoglyceride cream (Crystacide 1%) was shown to be as effective as benzoyl peroxide (BP) in reducing both inflammatory and non-inflammatory acne vulgaris lesions in patients with mild to moderate disease. HPS cream showed a better local tolerability profile than BP 4% gel.

A randomized, single-blind comparison of topical clindamycin + benzoyl peroxide and adapalene in the treatment of mild to moderate facial acne vulgaris. Langner A, Chu A, Goulden V, Ambroziak M. Br J Dermatol 2008; 158: 122–9.

Clindamycin phosphate plus benzoyl peroxide 0.5% (CDP+BPO) ready-mixed gel once daily and once-daily gel containing adapalene 0.1% are both effective treatments for acne, but CDP+BPO has a significantly earlier onset of action, is significantly more effective against inflamed and total lesions, and is better tolerated, which should improve patient compliance.

The combination formulation of clindamycin 1% plus benzoyl peroxide 5% versus 3 different formulations of topical clindamycin alone in the reduction of *Propionibacterium acnes*. An in vivo comparative study. Leyden J, Kaidbey K, Levy SF. Am J Clin Dermatol 2001; 2: 263–6.

Comparison of the in vivo effectiveness of the combination of clindamycin 1% plus benzoyl peroxide 5% in a gel formulation to that of each of three clindamycin 1% preparations (gel, lotion, and solution) with respect to reduction in counts of *P. acnes* cultured from the foreheads of healthy volunteers. The combination of clindamycin 1% plus benzoyl peroxide 5% gel produced more rapid and highly significant reductions in *P. acnes* compared with formulations containing clindamycin alone.

A randomized, single-blind comparison of topical clindamycin + benzoyl peroxide (Duac) and erythromycin + zinc acetate (Zineryt) in the treatment of mild to moderate facial acne vulgaris. Langner A, Sheehan-Dare R, Layton A. J Eur Acad Dermatol Venereol 2007; 21: 311–19.

Comparison of the clinical effectiveness of two combination treatments for facial acne: a ready-mixed once-daily gel containing clindamycin phosphate (1%) plus benzoyl peroxide (5%) (CDP+BPO) and a twice-daily solution of erythromycin (4%) plus zinc acetate (1.2%) (ERY+Zn). CDP+BPO and ERY+Zn are effective treatments for acne, but CDP+BPO has an earlier onset of action that should improve patient compliance.

A review of the use of combination therapies for the treatment of acne vulgaris. Leyden JJ. J Am Acad Dermatol 2003; 49: 200–10.

The major classes of topical and systemic therapeutic agents in the treatment of acne are discussed. Combination therapy, initial therapy, and long-term maintenance therapy are revisited.

Update and future of systemic acne treatment. Zouboulis CC, Piquero-Martin J. Dermatology 2003; 206: 37–53.

A review of all compounds used in the systemic treatment of acne, including new developments and future therapeutic trends.

Management of acne: a report from a Global Alliance to Improve Outcomes in Acne. Gollnick H, Cunliffe W, Berson D, Dreno B, Finlay A, Leyden JJ, et al. J Am Acad Dermatol 2003; 49: S1–37.

Guidelines developed through an international consensus for the treatment of acne, the Global Alliance to Improve Outcomes in Acne.

Isotretinoin: state of the art treatment for acne vulgaris. Ganceviciene R, Zouboulis CC. Exp Rev Dermatol 2007; 2: 693–706.

The multiple modes of action of isotretinoin, such as suppression of sebaceous gland activity and of the growth of *Propionibacterium acnes* in a secondary manner, alteration of the pattern of keratinization within the follicle, inhibition of inflammation, and as currently shown, normalization of the expression of matrix tissue metalloproteinases and their inhibitors, make this compound the most effective in the treatment of severe recalcitrant nodulocystic acne, in the prevention of acne scarring, and in seborrhea.

Treatment of acne with antiandrogens – An evidence-based overview. Zouboulis CC. J Dtsch Dermatol Ges 2003; 1: 535–46.

Anti-androgen treatment should be limited to female patients with additional signs of peripheral hyperandrogenism or hyperandrogenemia. Women with late-onset or recalcitrant acne who also desire contraception can be treated with anti-androgens, as well as those being treated with systemic isotretinoin. Anti-androgen treatment is not appropriate primary monotherapy for non-inflammatory and mild inflammatory acne.

Efficacy and safety of 3 mg drospirenone/20 mcg ethinylestradiol oral contraceptive administered in 24/4 regimen in the treatment of acne vulgaris: a randomized, double-blind, placebo-controlled trial. Koltun W, Lucky AW, Thiboutot D, Niknian M, Sampson-Landers C, Korner P, et al. Contraception 2008; 77: 249–56.

The drospirenone 3 mg, ethinylestradiol 20 μg combined oral contraceptive (COC) was significantly more effective than placebo in treating moderate acne vulgaris.

Evidence Levels: **A** Double-blind study **B** Clinical trial ≥ 20 subjects **C** Clinical trial < 20 subjects **D** Series ≥ 5 subjects **E** Anecdotal case reports

This new non-androgenic progestin-containing contraceptive with strong anti-androgenic activity (drospirenone 3 mg) but reduced concentration of ethinyl estradiol (20 µg) has been shown to be effective in acne vulgaris and may replace the classic cyproterone acetate/ethinyl estradiol and chlormadinone acetate/ethinyl estradiol oral contraceptives because of its improved side-effect profile.

Systemic antibiotic therapy of acne vulgaris. Ochsendorf F. J Dtsch Dermatol Ges 2006; 4: 828–41.

A review of the systemic antibiotics used for the treatment of inflammatory, medium to severe acne vulgaris; their efficacy, side effects, resistance rates, and cost are discussed. Systemic antibiotics should not be used as monotherapy. Systemic antibiotic therapy of widespread papulopustular acne not amenable to a topical therapy is effective and well tolerated. Therapy can be carried out for 3 months and should be combined with benzoyl peroxide.

Expert Committee recommendations for acne management. Zaenglein AL, Thiboutot DM. Pediatrics 2006; 118: 1188–99.

Consensus guidelines for the treatment of acne from the Global Alliance to Improve Outcomes in Acne induced significant changes in management routines. Acne treatments should be combined to target as many pathogenic factors as possible. A topical retinoid should be the foundation of treatment for most patients. Oral antibiotics should be used only in moderate to severe acne, should not be used as monotherapy, and should be discontinued as soon as possible, usually within 8–12 weeks. Because of their effect on the microcomedo, topical retinoids are recommended as an important facet of maintenance therapy.

Is antibiotic resistance in cutaneous propionibacteria clinically relevant?: implications of resistance for acne patients and prescribers. Eady AE, Cove JH, Layton AM. Am J Clin Dermatol 2003; 4: 813–31.

A review presenting a decision tree for acne management that provides an alternative to existing treatment algorithms by placing topical retinoids and not antibiotics at the centre of management.

Recurrence rates and relapse risk factors of acne treatment with oral isotretinoin. Zouboulis CC. Dermatology 2006; 212: 99–100.

An overview of the history of oral isotretinoin therapy, the drug's characteristics, efficacy, and adverse events.

A review of the European Directive for prescribing systemic isotretinoin for acne vulgaris. Layton AM, Dreno B, Gollnick HPM, Zouboulis CC. J Eur Acad Dermatol Venereol 2006; 20: 773–6.

A review of the new recommendations of the European Directive concerned with the prescription of oral isotretinoin and the impact of these changes on clinical practice.

Acne flare-up and deterioration with oral isotretinoin. Chivot M. Ann Dermatol Venereol 2001; 128: 224–8.

Isotretinoin treatment for acne can lead to inflammatory flares or an aggravation, occasionally leading to acne fulminans. Factors predictive of aggravation were shown to be young age, male gender, and sebaceous retention. Systemic corticosteroids are generally required, together with a lower daily dose of isotretinoin and local care.

SECOND-LINE THERAPY

Mild to moderate acne	
▶ Azelaic acid	A
▶ Picolinic acid	C
▶ Dapsone gel	C
▶ Oral zinc	C
▶ Photodynamic therapy	C
▶ Blue light	C
▶ Blue/red light combinations	C
▶ 1450-nm diode laser	C
▶ Topical cyproterone acetate	A
▶ Zileuton	D
▶ Prebiotic cosmetics	E
Moderate to severe acne	
▶ Oral antibiotics (tetracyclines, macrolides)	A

Efficacy of topical azelaic acid gel in the treatment of mild-moderate acne vulgaris. Iraji F, Sadeghinia A, Shahmoradi Z, Siadat AH, Jooya A. Indian J Dermatol Venereol Leprol 2007; 73: 94–6.

An evaluation of the efficacy of 20% azelaic acid gel compared to vehicle gel alone in patients with mild to moderate acne vulgaris. Azelaic acid gel was shown to be effective in the treatment of mild to moderate acne vulgaris.

A pilot study of the safety and efficacy of picolinic acid gel in the treatment of acne vulgaris. Heffernan MP, Nelson MM, Anadkat MJ. Br J Dermatol 2007; 156: 548–52.

Picolinic acid gel 10% applied twice daily may be safe and effective in the treatment of mild to moderate acne vulgaris.

Picolinic acid, an intermediate metabolite of tryptophan, is safe and effective in the treatment of mild to moderate acne vulgaris and is available as 10% picolinic acid gel for twice-daily application.

Dapsone gel 5% for the treatment of acne vulgaris: safety and efficacy of long-term (1 year) treatment. Lucky AW, Maloney JM, Roberts J, Taylor S, Jones T, Ling M, et al. J Drugs Dermatol 2007; 6: 981–7.

In a 12-month, open-label, long-term safety study dapsone gel 5% was shown to be safe and effective for long-term treatment of acne vulgaris, with a rapid onset of action.

Dapsone is a sulfone with anti-inflammatory and antimicrobial properties. Dapsone gel 5% delivers clinically effective doses of dapsone with minimal systemic absorption. This topical formulation of dapsone has a rapid onset of action and appeared to be safe and effective for long-term treatment of acne vulgaris.

New and emerging treatments in dermatology: acne. Katsambas A, Dessinioti C. Dermatol Ther 2008; 21: 86–95.

An overview of the therapeutic alternatives in the treatment of all types of acne, including the classic, long-used treatments as well as new therapies and future perspectives.

Zinc sulfate and zinc gluconate have been used for the treatment of inflammatory acne vulgaris with conflicting results. Zinc acts via inhibition of polymorphonuclear cell chemotaxis and inhibition of growth of P. acnes. Its anti-inflammatory activity could also be related to a reduction in tumor necrosis factor-α production, the modulation of the expression of integrins, and the inhibition of TLR2 surface expression by keratinocytes. Zinc salts have been used at a dosage of 30–150 mg of elemental zinc daily for 3 months.

Zinc gluconate does not induce bacterial resistance, has a favorable safety profile, and can be administered to pregnant women.

Photodynamic therapy of acne vulgaris using 5-aminolevulinic acid versus methyl aminolevulinate. Wiegell SR, Wulf HC. J Am Acad Dermatol 2006; 54: 647–51.

A comparison of the treatment effect and tolerability of ALA-PDT versus MAL-PDT in the treatment of acne vulgaris in a controlled randomized investigator-blinded trial. PDT appeared to be an effective treatment for inflammatory acne vulgaris, with no significant differences in the response rate between ALA-PDT and MAL-PDT. ALA-PDT resulted in more prolonged and severe adverse effects after treatment.

Photodynamic therapy in dermatology – an update 2008. Klein A, Babilas P, Karrer S, Landthaler M, Szeimies RM. J Dtsch Dermatol Ges 2008 [Epub ahead of print].

An overview of new indications for photodynamic therapy, as in acne vulgaris, the mechanism of action, and its advantages in comparison to other treatment modalities.

Photodynamic therapy of acne vulgaris using methyl aminolaevulinate: a blinded, randomized, controlled trial. Wiegell SR, Wulf HC. Br J Dermatol 2006; 154: 969–76.

Evaluation of the efficacy and tolerability of methyl aminolevulinate-based photodynamic therapy (MAL-PDT) in patients with moderate to severe facial acne vulgaris in a randomized, controlled and investigator-blinded trial. MAL-PDT proved to be an efficient treatment for inflammatory acne, but was associated with severe pain during treatment and severe adverse effects after treatment.

Long-pulsed dye laser versus long-pulsed dye laser-assisted photodynamic therapy for acne vulgaris: A randomized controlled trial. Haedersdal M, Togsverd-Bo K, Wiegell SR, Wulf HC. J Am Acad Dermatol 2008; 58: 387–94.

Evaluation of the efficacy and safety of LPDL alone versus LPDL in photodynamic therapy with methylaminolevulinic acid (MAL-LPDL) for acne vulgaris in 15 patients receiving a series of three full-face LPDL treatments and half-face prelaser MAL treatments. Limited sample size; the split-face design in this randomized controlled trial does not allow conclusions to be drawn about the efficacy of the LPDL, only about the efficacy of MAL-LPDL compared to LPDL alone.

Photodynamic therapy (PDT) with the porphyrin precursor 5-aminolevulinic acid (ALA) or its methyl ester (MAL) is used in the treatment of inflammatory acne vulgaris for the stimulation of immunomodulatory effects. ALA or MAL are applied topically as photosensitizers. Side effects are transient: usually pain and erythema. There have been no significant differences seen in the response rate between ALA-PDT and methyl aminolevulinate (MAL-PDT), but ALA-PDT resulted in more prolonged and severe adverse effects after treatment. Randomized, placebo-controlled studies are still lacking.

For moderate to severe acne vulgaris, ALA-PDT with photoactivation by intense pulsed light (IPL) appears to provide greater, longer-lasting and more consistent improvement than either radiofrequency-intense pulsed light (RF-IPL) or blue light activation. MAL-LPDL was shown slightly superior to long-pulsed dye laser (LPDL) for the treatment of inflammatory acne.

An assessment of the efficacy of blue light phototherapy in the treatment of acne vulgaris. Ammad S, Gonzales M, Edwards C, Finlay AY, Mills C. J Cosmet Dermatol 2008; 7: 180–8.

Significant improvement was demonstrated in this uncontrolled study with 21 subjects.

Handheld LED array device in the treatment of acne vulgaris. Sadick NS. J Drugs Dermatol 2008; 7: 347–50.

Evaluation of the efficacy of alternate blue light (415 nm) and red light (633 nm) treatments in the reduction of inflammatory lesions on the face of patients with mild to moderate acne vulgaris.

Blue light (405–420 nm wavelength), blue/red light combinations, 1450-nm diode laser and intense pulsed light (IPL, 600–850 nm) are thought to enhance the therapeutic response to routine medical management.

Clinical evaluation of a 1,450-nm diode laser as adjunctive treatment for refractory facial acne vulgaris. Astner S, Tsao SS. Dermatol Surg 2008; 34: 1054–61.

The 1450-nm diode laser provides moderate improvement of refractory acne vulgaris and can be used as an adjunctive treatment for acne management.

Cyproterone acetate loading to lipid nanoparticles for topical acne treatment: particle characterisation and skin uptake. Stecová J, Mehnert W, Blaschke T, Kleuser B, Sivaramakrishnan R, Zouboulis CC, et al. Pharm Res 2007; 24: 991–1000.

The efficacy of topical cyproterone acetate alcohol lotion versus placebo in the treatment of the mild to moderate acne vulgaris: a double blind study. Iraji F, Momeni A, Naji SM, Siadat AH. Dermatol Online J 2006; 12: 26.

Topical cyproterone acetate (CPA) treatment with a particulate system vehicle to increase skin penetration is an additional therapeutic option. The attachment of CPA to solid lipid nanoparticles, or its incorporation into the lipid matrix of nanostructured lipid carriers and microspheres, increases penetration into the follicular canal. Males are not excluded from topical treatment of CPA, and contraceptive measures in females may not be demanded. CPA alcohol lotion was shown to be effective in the treatment of mild to moderate acne vulgaris and could be used as one of the main treatments, or as an adjuvant treatment for moderate to severe acne vulgaris.

A new concept for acne therapy: a pilot study with zileuton, an oral 5-lipoxygenase inhibitor. Zouboulis CC, Nestoris S, Adler YD, Orth M, Orfanos CE, Picardo M, et al. Arch Dermatol 2003; 139: 668–70.

A pilot clinical study of 10 patients with papulopustular acne. Treatment with zileuton 4 × 600 mg/day po reduced the acne severity index, being 41% of the initial score at week 12 (p<0.05) with reduction of the inflammatory lesions of 29% (p<0.01). Total sebum lipids significantly decreased (35%, p<0.05), and the proinflammatory free fatty acids (22%) and lipoperoxides (26%) were markedly diminished in the sebum of patients' under treatment.

Prebiotic cosmetics: an alternative to antibacterial products. Bockmühl D, Jassoy C, Nieveler S, Scholtyssek R, Wadle A, Waldmann-Laue M. Int J Cosmet Sci 2007; 29: 63–4.

Prebiotic substances have the potential to provide a well-tolerated alternative approach to existing topical antibacterial agents. A prebiotic product for treatment of inflamed (or acne-prone) skin reduced levels of *Propionibacterium acnes*.

THIRD-LINE THERAPY

Mild to moderate acne

▶ Chemical peels (α-hydroxy acid or 30% glycolic acid peels), (β-hydroxy acid or 30% salicylic acid peels)   C
▶ Microdermabrasion   C

Acne sinuses and scars

▶ Intralesional steroids   C
▶ Dermabrasion   C

Procedural therapies are adjunctive to medical therapy for the treatment of moderate to severe inflammatory acne vulgaris in particular. They include intralesional steroids, chemical peels (α-hydroxy acid or 30% glycolic acid peels, and β-hydroxy acid or 30% salicylic acid peels) and microdermabrasion.

Acrodermatitis enteropathica

Kenneth H Neldner

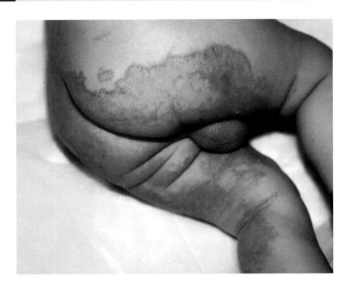

Acrodermatitis enteropathica (AE) is a rare, inherited disorder of zinc deficiency caused by defective intestinal absorption. It occurs worldwide, without apparent predilection for race or gender. AE manifests itself shortly after birth in a bottle-fed infant, and sometime soon after weaning in a breast-fed infant. Characteristic clinical signs are lesions in acral and periorificial sites; the first signs are often large areas of severe dermatitis commonly in the diaper area, where it can resemble the severe diaper dermatitis of infancy. Proper supplementation of zinc in the infant's diet generally results in a rapid and dramatic cure. If left untreated, AE usually causes diarrhea, irritability, alopecia, and secondarily infected lesions in infants, and impaired physical and mental development in older children and adults.

The diagnosis of AE is applied only to *inherited* zinc deficiency; non-inherited zinc deficiency is called acquired zinc deficiency. Long-term therapy and management of zinc deficiency vary depending on the severity of the disorder.

The genetics of AE have been studied extensively in recent years; most current reports indicate autosomal recessive transmission caused by a mutation in the intestinal zinc-specific transporter gene SLC39A4. A mouse model with zinc deficiency has been developed for future studies. It is possible that with further research other genes may be found to account for other cases of acrodermatitis.

MANAGEMENT STRATEGY

Chronic dermatitis in an acral area should suggest the possibility of zinc deficiency, but establishing the diagnosis of AE may be difficult. The first step is laboratory determination of blood plasma or serum zinc levels. Follow-up with other laboratory tests may be necessary but not definitive. If the diagnosis of zinc deficiency has been confirmed, management becomes relatively simple: oral zinc supplementation produces dramatic resolution of the problem. Dermatitis clears rapidly without the need for other medications.

The patient or their family must understand the need for lifelong management of the disorder in terms of zinc supplementation and medical supervision. Discuss foods rich in zinc, such as seafood and meat. Cereal grains should be avoided because of their phytate content. Phytates are known chelators of zinc. With age and a more varied diet, the dose of daily zinc supplementation may be reduced.

SPECIFIC INVESTIGATIONS

> ▶ Blood plasma or serum zinc levels
> ▶ Urine zinc excretion
> ▶ General physical examination and routine laboratory tests, including a complete lipid profile and serum copper levels
> ▶ Genetic studies; family history for evidence of similar problems

The normal plasma zinc level is 70–110 µg/dL and serum is 80–120 µg/dL. When drawing blood for zinc studies, it is important that it be a fasting specimen drawn in a trace-element free collection tube. Laboratory determination of blood plasma or serum zinc levels may be subject to error from zinc contamination.

Urinary zinc can be measured but is not definitive for diagnosis. Serum copper levels can be temporarily depressed by hypozincemia.

Homozygosity mapping places the acrodermatitis enteropathica gene on chromosomal regions 8q24.3. Wang K, Pugh EW, Griffen S, Doheny KF, Mostafa WZ, al-Aboosi MM, et al. Am J Hum Genet 2001; 68: 1055–70.

Identification of SLC39A4, a gene involved in acrodermatitis enteropathica. Küry S, Dréno B, Bézieau S, Giraudet S, Kharfi M, Kamoun R, et al. Nature Genet 202; 31: 239–40.

FIRST-LINE THERAPY

> ▶ Oral zinc supplementation   **A**

In most cases, oral supplementation with two to three times the recommended daily allowance of zinc salts in doses of 30–55 mg of elemental Zn^{2+} will be sufficient to restore normal zinc status within days to a few weeks, depending on the degree of depletion. The dose of elemental zinc must be determined by the patient's blood or plasma zinc levels, and by body weight. Available forms of zinc supplementation include zinc sulfate, zinc acetate, zinc gluconate, and zinc propionate. Dosage must be based on the amount of elemental zinc present in the preparation, which varies between compounds. For example, a standard 220 mg capsule of a commercial zinc preparation contains approximately 55 mg Zn^{2+}, which is an adequate daily dose for most deficient individuals. A commonly used preparation is Zincate, which is $ZnSO_4.7H_2O$.

Zinc deficiency in acrodermatitis enteropathica: multiple dietary intolerance treated with synthetic diet. Barnes PM, Moynahan EJ. Proc Roy Soc Med 1973; 66: 327–9.

Evidence Levels: **A** Double-blind study **B** Clinical trial ≥ 20 subjects **C** Clinical trial < 20 subjects **D** Series ≥ 5 subjects **E** Anecdotal case reports

The history of zinc therapy in AE is interesting. In 1973, Barnes and Moynahan were treating children with chronic, unresponsive AE-type acral dermatoses and having poor results. They then tried different medications, one of which was oral zinc. To their surprise, the patients receiving the zinc supplements cleared rapidly and completely. The authors reported these results in the medical literature.

Zinc therapy of acrodermatitis enteropathica. Neldner KH, Hambidge KM. N Engl J Med 1975; 292: 879–82.

At this time, Neldner and Hambidge were treating a 15-year-old patient with severe AE using a variety of medications currently in use, but with poor results. After reading the London article on zinc therapy, oral zinc was tried on the patient and produced rapid, dramatic total clearing of all acral lesions.

Acrodermatitis enteropathica and other zinc deficiency disorders. Neldner KH. In: Freedberg IM, Eisen AZ, Wolff K, et al., eds. Fitzpatrick's dermatology in general medicine, 6th edn. New York: McGraw-Hill, 2003; 412–18.

The article contains an overview of zinc deficiency, including a list of chronic disorders with nutrient deficiencies that can result in signs of marginal zinc deficiency.

Acrodermatitis enteropathica and an overview of zinc metabolism. Maverakis E, Fung MA, Lynch PJ, Draznin M, Michael DJ, Ruben B, Fazel N. J Am Acad Dermatol 2007; 56: 116–24.

An excellent review of AE and other zinc deficiency disorders.

Actinic keratoses

Sherrif F Ibrahim, Marc D Brown

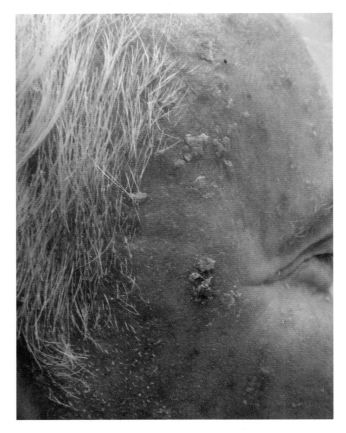

Actinic keratoses (AK) are ill-defined pink to skin-colored, scaly papules found on chronically sun-exposed areas in light-skinned individuals. They are most frequently found on the face, ears, balding scalp, extensor forearms, and dorsal hands. AKs represent a strong predictor for subsequent squamous cell carcinoma and, to a lesser extent, basal cell carcinoma. Australians have the highest reported prevalence: up to 60%. In the United States, AKs are the second most common reason for visits to the dermatologist.

MANAGEMENT STRATEGY

Actinic keratoses are common dysplastic intraepidermal lesions that are considered to be precursors to squamous cell carcinoma (SCC). Reports have varied as to the rates of progression to invasive SCC, from 0.025% to over 25% per year, and AKs are commonly located adjacent to SCC histologically. For these reasons, most practitioners advocate the treatment of AKs, as considerable morbidity and potential mortality can be associated with invasive disease. However, there have been no randomized controlled studies demonstrating a reduction in the frequency of SCC with treatment of AK.

The diagnosis of AK is primarily clinical, and a variety of effective management approaches exist. Biopsy of suspected AKs is typically not warranted; however, in patients with a history of multiple skin cancers, immunosuppressed patients,

and lesions in high-risk areas such as the lip or ear, clinicians should have a low threshold for biopsy to rule out invasive SCC. Indications for biopsy include tenderness, rapid growth or thickening of lesions, bleeding, hyperkeratosis, and failure to respond to treatment.

Prevention of AKs through sun avoidance and diligent use of broad-spectrum sunscreens and blocking agents is an important aspect of management. This has been shown to prevent the development of new AKs and reduce the incidence of non-melanoma skin cancers.

With cumulative sun exposure and advancing age, rates of AK development increase, necessitating either *ablative* or *topical treatment*. *Cryotherapy* with liquid nitrogen is by far the most commonly employed therapeutic modality because it can be performed quickly and effectively in the office setting. However, given the common appearance of AKs in a background of diffuse actinic damage, individual lesions may be poorly defined, requiring field treatment with topical agents such as *5-fluorouracil* (5-FU) or *imiquimod*. The latter has recently been shown to have high rates of treatment success with durable results and has become an accepted first-line therapy. The advantages of topical approaches are that they are non-invasive with little risk of scarring or pigmentary change, and can be used for anatomically difficult or cosmetically sensitive areas. However, the majority of these agents must be used for weeks to months and require adequate patient compliance. *Photodynamic therapy* with aminolevulinic acid (ALA) or methyl aminolevulinate (MAL) has become more widespread, given its proven therapeutic results and excellent cosmetic outcome. Variations in the light dose, light source, sensitizing agent and its application time, and frequency of treatments may improve efficacy. Recently, there has been a growing trend towards *combination therapy*, such as topical agents either before or after cryotherapy, or concurrent use of multiple topical modalities. Other approaches such as *laser resurfacing*, *chemical peels*, and *dermabrasion* may be considered in certain situations when lesions have failed the above treatments, or if extensive photodamage is present. Finally, for recalcitrant or hyperkeratotic lesions, *curettage* or *excision* may be appropriate.

SPECIFIC INVESTIGATIONS

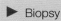 Biopsy

Actinic keratoses and the incidence of occult squamous cell carcinoma: a clinical–histopathologic correlation. Ehrig T, Cockerell C, Piacquadio D, Dromgoole S. Dermatol Surg 2006; 32: 1261–5.

Two hundred and seventy-one clinically diagnosed AKs were biopsied. Clinical diagnosis was in agreement with histology 91% of the time, with about 1 in 25 lesions revealing invasive squamous cell carcinoma.

Clinical recognition of actinic keratoses in a high-risk population: how good are we? Venna SS, Lee D, Stadecker MJ, Rogers GS. Arch Dermatol 2005; 141: 507–9.

Seventeen of 23 lesions (74%) with classic features of AK in patients with a history of previous skin cancer were confirmed histologically. Five lesions (22%) were shown to be squamous cell carcinoma.

Actinic keratoses are typically diagnosed clinically. However, there should be a low threshold to biopsy tender, hyperkeratotic, large, and recalcitrant lesions to exclude malignancy.

FIRST-LINE THERAPIES

▶ Sunscreens	A
▶ Cryosurgery	B
▶ Topical 5-FU	A
▶ Imiquimod	A

A randomized controlled trial to assess sunscreen application and beta carotene supplementation in the prevention of solar keratoses. Darlington S, Williams G, Neale R, Frost C, Green A. Arch Dermatol 2003; 139: 451–5.

In this Australian study, 1621 adults were randomized to either daily use of sunscreen or application at their usual discretionary rate. There was a 24% reduction in AKs in the daily use group.

Reduction of solar keratoses by regular sunscreen use. Thompson SC, Jolley D, Marks R. N Engl J Med 1993; 14: 1147–51.

In a 6-month randomized, placebo-controlled trial of 588 patients in Australia, SPF 17 sunscreen applied daily was found to both reduce the development of new AKs and increase the remission of existing AKs compared to a vehicle cream.

A prospective study of the use of cryosurgery for the treatment of actinic keratoses. Thai K, Fergin P, Freeman M, Vinciullo C, Francis D, Spelman L, et al. Int J Dermatol 2004; 43: 687–92.

In this prospective multicenter study, 90 patients with 421 AKs on the face and scalp were treated with cryotherapy with a single freeze–thaw cycle using different freeze times. The patients were reviewed 3 months later. Overall, the complete response (CR) rate was 67.2%, varying from 39% for freeze times less than 5 s to 83% for times longer than 20 s. The authors also found that hypopigmentation was present in 29% of CR lesions. Patients rated cosmetic outcomes as good to excellent for 94% of CR lesions.

Effect of a 1 week treatment with 0.5% topical fluorouracil on occurrence of actinic keratosis after cryosurgery. Jorizzo J, Weiss J, Furst K, VandePol C, Levy SF. Arch Dermatol 2004; 140: 813–16.

This study demonstrates that there is a role for the combination of therapeutic modalities in the treatment of AKs. In this prospective, double-blind, randomized controlled trial, 144 patients, each with at least five AKs on the face, were randomized to receive 1 week of treatment with 0.5% 5-FU cream daily for 7 days or placebo cream. Patients were then treated with single freeze–thaw cycle cryotherapy using liquid nitrogen, with a thaw time of 10 s. These patients were then followed up at 4 weeks and 6 months. The authors found that at 4 weeks, 16.7% of patients in the 5-FU group were completely clear of lesions, compared to 0% in the vehicle group (p<0.001). At 6 months post treatment 30% of patients in the 5-FU group were clear of lesions, compared to 7.7% of patients in the vehicle group (p<0.001).

Effective treatment of actinic keratosis with 0.5% fluorouracil cream for 1, 2 or 4 weeks. Weiss J, Menter A, Hevia O, Jones T, Ling M, Rist T, et al. Cutis 2002; 70: 22–9.

In this randomized, double-blind, parallel-group vehicle-controlled study, 177 patients with at least five AKs were treated with topical 0.5% 5-FU cream daily for 1, 2, or 4 weeks. In patients who were treated for 4 weeks, complete clearance of lesions was observed in 47.5%, compared to 26% who were treated for 1 week (p<0.001 vs vehicle). Moderate to severe irritation of the skin was noted in 90% of these patients.

Imiquimod 5% cream for the treatment of actinic keratosis: results from two phase III, randomized, double-blind, parallel group, vehicle-controlled trials. Lebwohl M, Dinehart S, Whiting D, LeePK, Tawfik N, Jorizzo J, et al. J Am Acad Dermatol 2004; 50: 714–21.

In this report of two phase III double-blind, vehicle-controlled studies, 436 subjects at 24 centers in the US were randomized to either 5% imiquimod or vehicle applied once daily, two days per week, for 16 weeks. The complete clearance rate for the treated arm was 45%, as opposed to 3.2% for the vehicle group. The median percent reduction in AK lesions was 83% for the treated group and 0% for the vehicle group, indicating that a reduced frequency of imiquimod application is quite effective.

A randomised study of topical 5% imiquimod vs. topical 5-fluorouracil vs. cryosurgery in immunocompetent patients with actinic keratoses: a comparison of clinical and histological outcomes including 1-year follow-up. Krawtchenko N, Roewert-Huber J, Ulrich M, Mann I, Sterry W, Stockfleth E. Br J Dermatol 2007; 157 Suppl 2: 34–40.

This study compared the baseline and 1-year follow-up rates of clinical clearance, histological clearance, and cosmetic outcomes of imiquimod, 5-FU, and cryosurgery for the treatment of AKs. Patients were randomized to one of the three treatment groups. Clinical clearance was achieved in 68% of those treated with cryosurgery, 96% with 5-FU, and 85% with imiquimod. Histological clearance rate was 32% for cryosurgery, 67% for 5-FU, and 73% for imiquimod. The 1-year sustained clearance rate was 28% for cryosurgery, 54% for 5-FU, and 73% for imiquimod. The patients treated with imiquimod were also judged to have superior cosmetic outcomes.

Imiquimod for actinic keratosis: systematic review and meta-analysis. Hadley G, Derry S, Moore RA. J Invest Dermatol 2006; 126: 1251–5.

There have been several well-designed vehicle-controlled, randomized, double-blind studies assessing the efficacy of imiquimod 5% cream in the treatment of AKs. This systematic review was the first comparison of these trials, comprising 1293 patients. Although optimal frequency and duration of treatment remain to be established, it is clear that imiquimod results in comparable outcomes to other more widely used treatment modalities, and has now become a first-line agent. Complete clearance occurred in 50% of patients treated with imiquimod, and the number needed to treat (NNT) for one patient to have AKs completely and partially cleared after 12–16 weeks were 2.2 and 1.8, respectively. This compares with NNTs of 3.7 and 2.0 for topical diclofenac and 5-FU. Adverse events were local, most frequently erythema, scabbing, and flaking.

Open-label study to assess the safety and efficacy of imiquimod 5% cream applied once daily three times per week in cycles for treatment of actinic keratoses on the head. Rivers JK, Rosoph L, Provost N, Bissonnette R. J Cutan Med Surg 2008; 12: 97–101.

In this study, imiquimod was administered three times per week for 4 weeks, followed by 4 weeks of rest. If AKs were present after this cycle, a second cycle was instituted. Fifty percent (30 of 60) of patients experienced complete clearance of

AK lesions, and 75% (30 of 40) experienced partial clearance of lesions after imiquimod treatment at the end of cycle 2. Additionally, 77% of patients who achieved complete clearance had no visible AK lesions 12 weeks post treatment. This article demonstrates the utility of cycle therapy for the treatment of AKs.

Long-term clinical outcomes following treatment of actinic keratosis with imiquimod 5% cream. Lee PK, Harwell WB, Loven KH, Phillips TJ, Whiting DA, Andres KL, et al. Dermatol Surg 2005; 31: 659–64.

This paper looked to obtain long-term safety and efficacy data for imiquimod in the treatment of AKs. One hundred and forty-six patients from 30 study centers were evaluated for clinical evidence of AK after a median follow-up period of 16 months. Only 25% of the patients who received imiquimod three times per week and 43% of patients who received imiquimod twice per week had a recurrence of AK. The median number of lesions present was one for both groups, compared to six at baseline. This study supports the long-term clinical benefit in a large number of patients treated with imiquimod for AK, possibly secondary to immune modification.

SECOND-LINE THERAPIES

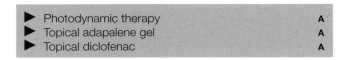

▶ Photodynamic therapy	A
▶ Topical adapalene gel	A
▶ Topical diclofenac	A

Guidelines on the use of photodynamic therapy for nonmelanoma skin cancer: An international consensus. Braathen LR, Szeimies R, Basset-Seguin N, Bissonnette R, Foley P, Pariser D, et al. J Am Acad Dermatol 2007; 56: 125–43.

This is a comprehensive evidence-based review and treatment recommendations for the use of PDT to treat nonmelanoma skin cancers, including AKs. The authors review each of the main clinical trials using PDT to treat AKs, and conclude that PDT with MAL and ALA is highly effective, offering excellent cosmetic results, and should be considered as first-line therapy.

Intraindividual, right-left comparison of topical methyl aminolaevulinate-photodynamic therapy and cryotherapy in subjects with actinic keratoses: a multicentre, randomized controlled study. Morton C, Campbell S, Gupta G, Keohane S, Lear J, Zaki I, et al. Br J Dermatol 2006; 155: 1029–36.

In this 24-week study subjects received one treatment session of PDT to one side of their face and two cycles of freeze–thaw cryosurgery to the other. Of the 1501 lesions treated, PDT resulted in a higher rate of cure (87% vs 76% reduction from baseline). Both subjects and investigators preferred PDT and also felt it had a better cosmetic outcome. Both treatment regimens were deemed safe and well tolerated.

Multicentre intraindividual randomized trial of topical methyl aminolaevulinate–photodynamic therapy vs. cryotherapy for multiple actinic keratoses on the extremities. Kaufmann R, Spelman L, Weightman W, Reifenberger J, Szeimies RM, Verhaeghe E, et al. Br J Dermatol 2008; 158: 994–9.

This was another intraindividual trial that treated one side of the body (non-face/scalp) with a single course of PDT and the other with cryotherapy. For the 1343 lesions treated, both treatment modalities had high efficacy rates at 24 weeks, although cryosurgery performed better (78% for PDT and 88% for cryosurgery). Investigator and patient assessment of cosmetic outcome was much higher for PDT than for cryosurgery (79% vs 56% of lesions having 'excellent cosmetic outcome' based on investigator evaluation, 50% vs 22% based on patient evaluation).

Photodynamic therapy with aminolevulinic acid topical solution and visible blue light in the treatment of multiple actinic keratoses of the face and scalp: investigator-blinded, phase 3, multicenter trials. Piacquadio DJ, Chen DM, Farber HF, Fowler JF Jr, Glazer SD, Goodman JJ, et al. Arch Dermatol 2004; 140: 41–6.

In this randomized, placebo-controlled study 243 patients were randomized to receive vehicle or aminolevulinic acid (ALA) followed by PDT within 14–18 hours. Clinical response rate was based on complete clearing of 75% of lesions measured at weeks 8 and 12. Of the PDT-treated group, 77% had a complete response by week 8 and 89% by week 12. This compared to 18% and 13% for the placebo group. Most patients experienced erythema and edema at the treated sites, which improved within 4 weeks of therapy. Stinging, burning, or pain occurred during the treatments, but resolved within 24 hours.

Assessment of adapalene gel for the treatment of actinic keratoses and lentigines: a randomized trial. Kang S, Goldfarb MT, Weiss JS, Metz RD, Hamilton TA, Voorhees JJ, Griffiths CE. J Am Acad Dermatol 2003; 49: 83–90.

In this prospective randomized, vehicle-controlled study 90 patients received either 0.1% adapalene gel, 0.3% adapalene gel or vehicle gel, initially daily for 4 weeks, then twice daily for up to 9 months. Overall, 62% (p<0.01) of those who received 0.1% adapalene gel and 66% (p<0.01) of those who received 0.3% adapalene gel showed at least a moderate improvement of their AKs, compared to 34% of patients receiving a vehicle cream. Adapalene gel recipients reported a higher level of mild erythema, peeling and dryness compared to control groups.

Three percent diclofenac in 2.5% hyaluronan gel in the treatment of actinic keratoses: a meta-analysis of the recent studies. Pirard D, Vereecken P, Melot C, Heenen M. Arch Dermatol Res 2005; 297: 185–9.

This meta-analysis pooled 364 patients from three studies that compared diclofenac to hyaluronan vehicle gel. Overall, patients treated with diclofenac had a significantly higher rate of complete clearance of lesions. They concluded that complete response rates were 39% with a mean treatment duration of 75 ± 21 days. Mild-to-moderate skin irritation was the major side effect of the treatment group.

Diclofenac sodium 3% gel in the treatment of actinic keratoses postcryosurgery. Berlin JM, Rigel DS. J Drugs Dermatol 2008; 7: 669–73.

This prospective, double-arm, multicenter, open-label, phase 4 study aimed to determine the efficacy of sequential therapy of AKs with cryosurgery followed by diclofenac for 90 days. Forty-six percent of subjects who underwent combination treatment achieved 100% lesion clearance, compared to 21% in the cryosurgery-alone arm. This is a good example of newly emerging strategies involving combinations of established treatment modalities.

Phase IV open-label assessment of the treatment of actinic keratosis with 3.0% diclofenac sodium topical gel (Solaraze). Nelson C, Rigel D, Smith S, Swanson N, Wolf J. J Drugs Dermatol 2004; 3: 401–7.

This study evaluated the treatment and efficacy of diclofenac applied twice daily for 90 days with a 30-day follow-up. Of the 67 patients who completed the study, 78% had ≥75% clearance of AKs, which improved to 85% by the 30-day follow-up. Dry skin and rash at the application site were the most common side effects of treatment.

THIRD-LINE THERAPIES

▶ Curettage	E
▶ Excision	E
▶ Ablative lasers	B
▶ Chemical peels	D
▶ Dermabrasion	D

Guidelines for the management of actinic keratoses. de Berker D, McGregor JM, Hughes BR. Br J Dermatol 2007; 156: 222–30.

Recalcitrant treatment-resistant AKs may be treated with curettage or surgical excision. Both techniques enable tissue to be obtained for the purposes of histological analysis. Curettage can be used alone or in conjunction with electrosurgery, cryotherapy, or chemical applications. Surgical excision is particularly useful in lesions suspected of being SCC because this technique enables the clinician to treat the lesion and establish the diagnosis.

Widespread, extensive AKs may benefit from field treatments of a physical nature. These include ablative laser resurfacing, dermabrasion and chemical peels. Photodynamic therapy with an intense pulsed light source has also been used in this manner.

Full face laser resurfacing: Therapy and prophylaxis for actinic keratoses and non-melanoma skin cancer. Iyer S, Friedli A, Bowes L, Kricorian G, Fitzpatrick RE. Lasers Surg Med 2004; 34: 114–19.

In this retrospective study of 24 patients with over 30 AKs on the face treated with full-face ultrapulse CO_2 laser or erbium Er:YAG laser resurfacing, the authors found that 21 patients remained lesion free for at least 1 year.

Long-term efficacy of carbon dioxide laser resurfacing for facial actinic keratosis. Sherry SD, Miles BA, Finn RA. J Oral Maxillofac Surg 2007; 65: 1135–9.

A retrospective chart analysis of 31 patients who underwent full-face CO_2 laser resurfacing for AK showed that 58% were free of lesions for an average of 27 months.

Recurrence rates and long-term follow-up after laser resurfacing as a treatment for widespread actinic keratoses on the face and scalp. Ostertag JU, Quaedvlieg PJ, Neumann MH, Krekels GA. Dermatol Surg 2006; 32: 261–7.

A retrospective case–control study of 25 patients who underwent laser resurfacing for widespread AKs on the scalp and/or face. Forty-four percent had no recurrences in an average follow-up period of 39 months (range 7–70 months).

A clinical comparison and long-term follow-up of topical 5-fluorouracil versus laser resurfacing in the treatment of widespread actinic keratoses. Ostertag JU, Quaedvlieg PJ, van der Geer S, Nelemans P, Christianen ME, Neumann MH, Krekels GA. Lasers Surg Med 2006; 38: 731–9.

A prospective randomized trial of 55 patients comparing 5-FU with Er:YAG laser resurfacing. At 3, 6, and 12 months there were significantly fewer recurrences in the laser group than in the 5-FU group. Side effects were more common in the group treated with laser resurfacing, and included erythema and hypopigmentation.

Long-term efficacy and safety of Jessner's solution and 35% trichloroacetic acid vs 5% fluorouracil in the treatment of widespread facial actinic keratoses. Witheiler DD, Lawrence N, Cox SE, Cruz C, Cockerell CJ, Freemen RG. Dermatol Surg 1997; 23: 191–6.

In this prospective study, 15 patients with severe facial AKs were treated on one side of the face with a single application of Jessner's solution – a medium-depth chemical peel – and the other side with twice-daily applications of topical 5-FU 5% for 3 weeks. The authors found that both treatments resulted in a similar reduction of AKs at 12 months, with an increase in the number of AKs in both groups from 12 to 32 months. The authors concluded that both treatments were similarly efficacious in the treatment of AK, and that retreatment for recurrences might be necessary after 12 months.

Dermabrasion for prophylaxis and treatment of actinic keratoses. Coleman WP, Yardborough JM, Mandy SH. Dermatol Surg 1996; 22: 17–21.

In this retrospective study, 23 patients who had undergone dermabrasion for facial AKs were followed for 2–5 years. The authors found that the benefits of dermabrasion diminished with time: 1 year post dermabrasion, 22 patients remained clear of AKs. Of 13 patients who were followed up for 5 years, seven remained clear. The authors concluded that dermabrasion provided long-term clearance of AKs in some patients.

Actinic prurigo

James Ferguson, Robert S Dawe

(Synonyms: hereditary polymorphic light eruption of American Indians, Hutchinson's summer prurigo, photodermatitis in North American Indians)

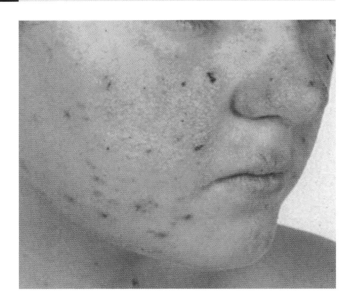

Actinic prurigo is a distinct photodermatosis, diagnosed on the basis of characteristic clinical features including perennial (albeit worse in summer) nature, vesiculopapular eruption during acute flares, persistent eroded nodules and/or dermatitic patches (sometimes affecting covered sites), scarring, dorsal nose involvement, cheilitis and conjunctivitis. Abnormal photosensitivity (UVA, UVB) is frequently severe, but generally gradually improves, especially when (as is usual) it presents before the age of 10 years.

MANAGEMENT STRATEGY

Diagnosis is normally straightforward, but the differential diagnosis can include severe polymorphic light eruption or photoaggravated atopic dermatitis. Although differences between European and Amerindian forms of actinic prurigo have been noted, these appear to be closely related conditions. Phototesting and HLA typing may be helpful in cases of diagnostic uncertainty. Possible coexisting conditions such as sunscreen allergic contact dermatitis or photocontact reactions should be considered, as their presence will affect the recommended treatments.

Once the diagnosis is established, initial treatment consists of advice on *sunlight avoidance* measures (behavioral, clothing, and topical sunscreen), and the use of potent or very potent *topical corticosteroids*. This approach alone is often insufficient, and many patients require the addition of a springtime course of TL-01 UVB or PUVA. When *phototherapy* is administered for this indication, only normally sunlight-exposed sites should be treated. It is helpful to apply a potent topical steroid to the treated areas immediately after each exposure, to reduce the risk of actinic prurigo flares.

In Scotland systemic treatment is rarely required, but is more often necessary where the availability of phototherapy is limited and in countries with more intense year-round sunlight exposure. *Antimalarials* and *β-carotene* are sometimes tried, but it remains uncertain whether they are truly of value. *Thalidomide* may be more useful, but its value is restricted by teratogenicity and the risk of irreversible peripheral neuropathy. *Pentoxifylline* has anti-TNF-α effects and, although listed as a third-line therapy here, may be worth considering before thalidomide because of its more attractive safety profile.

SPECIFIC INVESTIGATIONS

> ▶ Phototesting
> ▶ HLA-typing
> ▶ Histopathology of cheilitis

Actinic prurigo – a specific photodermatosis? Addo HA, Frain-Bell W. Photodermatology 1984; 1: 119–28.

This study showed that almost 60% of actinic prurigo patients have abnormal delayed erythemal responses on monochromator phototesting.

Phototest abnormalities tend to be more severe in actinic prurigo than in polymorphic light eruption.

Actinic prurigo among the Chimila Indians in Colombia: HLA studies. Bernal JE, Duran de Rueda MM, Ordonez CP, Duran C, de Brigard D. J Am Acad Dermatol 1990; 22: 1049–51.

In this population, the HLA class 1 antigen Cw4 was more frequent in actinic prurigo patients than in controls.

Actinic prurigo: an update. Hojyo-Tomoka T, Vega-Memije E, Granados J, Flores O, Cortes-Franco R, Teixeira F, Dominguez-Soto L. Int J Dermatol 1995; 34: 380–4.

HLA-DR4 may determine expression of actinic prurigo in British patients. Menage H du P, Vaughan RW, Baker CS, Page G, Proby CM, Breathnach SM, Hawk JL. J Invest Dermatol 1996; 106: 362–7.

Actinic prurigo and HLA-DR4. Dawe RS, Collins P, O'Sullivan A, Ferguson J. J Invest Dermatol 1997; 108: 233–4.

An even stronger association with the HLA class 2 antigen HLA-DR4 was shown and, more specifically, with HLA-DRB1*0407.

Association of HLA subtype DRB10407 in Colombian patients with actinic prurigo. Suárex A, Valbuena MC, Rey M, de Porras Quintana L. Photodermatol Photoimmunol Photomed 2006; 22: 55–8.

*These associations are not a feature of polymorphic light eruption. The absence of HLA-DR4 can help to rule out the diagnosis of AP, whereas the presence of HLA-DRB1*0407 helps to rule in the diagnosis.*

Actinic prurigo: clinical features and HLA associations in a Canadian Inuit population. Wiseman MC, Orr PH, MacDonald SM, Schroeder ML, Toole JW. J Am Acad Dermatol 2001; 44: 952–6.

No statistically significant association of AP with HLA-DR4 (frequent in the studied population) or HLA-DRB1*0407 was detected, and another HLA type (DRB1*14) was found more commonly than expected, although it was only present in 19 of 37 AP subjects. The authors acknowledge the possibility that they were studying a different condition from AP in other populations. Nevertheless, these findings suggest we should be cautious in attempting to use HLA typing as a diagnostic test, especially in populations in which strong HLA associations have not been confirmed. The diagnosis should still be based on the characteristic constellation of clinical features.

Actinic prurigo of the lower lip – review of the literature and report of five cases. Mounsdon T, Kratochvil F, Auclair P, Neale J, Lee L. Oral Surg Oral Med Oral Pathol 1988; 65: 327–32.

Follicular cheilitis – a distinctive histopathologic finding in actinic prurigo. Herrera-Geopfert R, Magana M. Am J Dermatopathol 1995; 17: 357–61.

Actinic prurigo cheilitis: clinicopathologic analysis and therapeutic results in 116 cases. Vega-Memije ME, Mosqueda-Taylor A, Irigoyen-Camacho ME, Hojyo-Tomoka MT, Dominguez-Soto L. Oral Surg Oral Med Oral Pathol Oral Radiol Endod 2002; 94: 83–91.

A 'follicular cheilitis' has been reported to be characteristic of actinic prurigo. Thirty-two of 116 patients attending a dermatology clinic in Mexico City had cheilitis as their sole manifestation of disease.

Lip histopathology may be helpful diagnostically, especially in patients presenting with cheilitis without cutaneous features at presentation. Where other typical features (skin, eyes) are present it is arguable how much lip histopathology will contribute to diagnosis.

Augmentation of ultraviolet erythema by indomethacin in actinic prurigo: evidence of mechanism of photosensitivity. Farr PM, Diffey BL. Photochem Photobiol 1988; 47: 413–17.

Topical indomethacin was found to augment the erythemal response on phototesting.

This study has not been replicated in the literature, and has not developed into a routine diagnostic test.

FIRST-LINE THERAPIES

▶ Sunlight avoidance – environmental, behavioral, clothing, topical sunscreen	C
▶ Potent/very potent topical corticosteroids	C
▶ Narrowband (TL-01 lamp) UVB phototherapy	C

Topical photoprotection for hereditary polymorphic light eruption of American Indians. Fusaro RM, Johnson JA. J Am Acad Dermatol 1991; 24: 744–6.

The authors of this open study found 18 of 30 patients with hereditary polymorphic light eruption of American Indians (with described features indistinguishable from actinic prurigo) to show 'good to excellent results' with use of a broad-spectrum sunscreen.

Although broad-spectrum sunscreens are useful, advice on other sunlight avoidance measures, including appropriate clothing and behavioral avoidance, is equally important.

Actinic prurigo deterioration due to degradation of DermaGard window film. Kerr AC, Ferguson J. Br J Dermatol 2007; 157: 619–20.

Window films that reduce the transmission of ultraviolet rays can be used as a method of environmental photoprotection. This case report describes an exacerbation of actinic prurigo explained by increased transmission through such a window film as it aged.

Treatment of actinic prurigo with intermittent short-course topical 0.05% clobetasol 17-propionate – a preliminary report. Lane PR, Moreland AA, Hogan DJ. Arch Dermatol 1990; 126: 1211–13.

Seven out of eight patients treated with intermittent 3–14-day courses of topical 0.05% clobetasol 17-proprionate cream or ointment cleared or markedly improved. All had previously found less potent topical steroids ineffective.

Narrow-band UVB (TL-01) phototherapy: an effective preventative treatment for the photodermatoses. Collins P, Ferguson J. Br J Dermatol 1995; 132: 956–63.

Six patients with actinic prurigo were included in this open study. All reported at least a sixfold increase in tolerable duration of sunlight exposure, which was sustained 4 months after treatment. In one patient, whose phototesting (severely abnormal before treatment) was repeated after treatment, the test results normalized.

SECOND-LINE THERAPIES

▶ Psoralen–UVA photochemotherapy	C
▶ Thalidomide	C

Controlled trial of methoxsalen in solar dermatitis of Chippewa Indians. Schenck RR. JAMA 1960; 172: 1134–7.

This small (13 patients recruited, eight completed) placebo-controlled, crossover study showed no benefit. However, the psoralen dose was low (10 mg), the irradiation source was uncontrollable (the sun), and the study was conducted during summer.

Treatment of actinic prurigo with PUVA: mechanism of action. Farr PM, Diffey BL. Br J Dermatol 1989; 120: 411–18.

Five patients were treated in this open study. Clinical improvement was accompanied by an increase of UVA minimal erythemal doses to within the normal range on phototesting. Corroboration that PUVA worked through a local effect was provided by before and after phototesting of areas kept covered during treatment. The UVA minimal erythema dose did not increase in these areas.

In the absence of any controlled study comparisons of PUVA and TL-01 phototherapy for this condition, PUVA should generally be reserved for those who fail to benefit from TL-01.

Thalidomide in the treatment of actinic prurigo. Londoño F. Int J Dermatol 1973; 12: 326–8.

Thirty-four patients were treated, with a starting dose of 300 mg thalidomide daily, gradually reducing to a minimum of 15 mg; 32 had good results while on the drug, but relapsed on stopping.

Thalidomide in actinic prurigo. Lovell CR, Hawk JL, Calnan CD, Magnus IA. Br J Dermatol 1983; 108: 467–71.

Of 14 patients treated with thalidomide (adult starting dose 100–200 mg daily), 13 (one could not tolerate the drug owing to dizziness) reported improvement. This benefit was sustained in 11, of whom eight required maintenance doses of between 50 mg weekly and 100 mg daily.

Includes a review of earlier open studies reporting the use of thalidomide in actinic prurigo.

THIRD-LINE THERAPIES

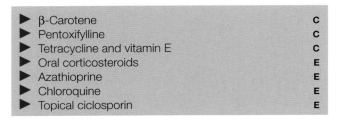

▶ β-Carotene	C
▶ Pentoxifylline	C
▶ Tetracycline and vitamin E	C
▶ Oral corticosteroids	E
▶ Azathioprine	E
▶ Chloroquine	E
▶ Topical ciclosporin	E

Hereditary polymorphic light eruption in American Indians – photoprotection and prevention of streptococcal pyoderma and glomerulonephritis. Fusaro RM, Johnson JA. JAMA 1980; 244: 1456–9.

Seventeen of 54 patients who participated in this open study were reported to have achieved complete photoprotection, and 16 'marked improvement.' The plasma carotene level tended to be higher in those who benefited. The authors also comment on their use of dihydroxyacetone and lawsone cream, with apparent benefit.

The clinical features of the study patients were not reported, but the authors' introductory description of hereditary polymorphic light eruption suggests that they probably included actinic prurigo.

Pentoxifylline in the treatment of actinic prurigo: a preliminary report of 10 patients. Torres-Alvarez B, Castanedo-Cazares JP, Moncada B. Dermatology 2004; 208: 198–201.

Clinical improvement was reported in all 10 participants in this 6-month open-label uncontrolled study.

Treatment of actinic prurigo in Chimila Indians. Duran MM, Ordonez CP, Prieto JC, Bernal J. Int J Dermatol 1996; 35: 413–16.

One group of eight patients was treated with tetracycline (1.5 g daily), and another eight with vitamin E (100 IU daily). On follow-up analysis comparing signs and itch, no difference was found between the groups. Both treatments were considered promising, and the possibility of using a tetracycline–vitamin E combination therapy raised.

These treatments need further investigation, but may be worth considering if first-line therapies are inadequate and thalidomide is contraindicated or not tolerated.

The clinical features and management of actinic prurigo: a retrospective study. Lestarini D, Khoo LS, Goh CL. Photodermatol, Photoimmunol Photomed 1999; 15: 183–7.

This was a review of the features and clinical course of 11 patients. Of three treated with systemic corticosteroids, one improved slightly. Intralesional steroids helped one. Three patients were treated with azathioprine: two appeared to benefit.

Actinic prurigo: clinico-pathological correlation. Hojyo-Tomoka MT, Dominguez-Soto L, Vargasocamp F. Int J Dermatol 1978; 17: 706–10.

In this review, the authors comment that chloroquine 'seems to give temporary relief,' and also suggest that antihistamines and tranquilizers may be of some benefit.

Use of topical ciclosporin for conjunctival manifestations of actinic prurigo. McCoombes JA, Hirst LW, Green WR. Am J Ophthalmol 2000; 130: 830–1.

Topical ciclosporin in the treatment of ocular actinic prurigo. Ortiz-Castillo JV, Boto-De-Los-Bueis A, De-Lucas-Laguna R, Pastor-Nieto B, Peláez-Restrepo N, Fonseca-Sandomingo A. Arch Soc Esp Oftalmol 2006; 81: 661–4.

In these two case reports topical 2% ciclosporin eye drops were associated with improvement in chronic AP conjunctivitis.

Actinomycosis

Jonathan E Blume

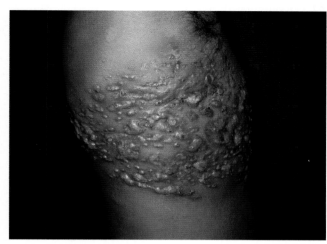

Courtesy of Dr Hema Jerajani

Actinomycosis is an infection caused by *Actinomyces* spp., anaerobic or microaerophilic Gram-positive, filamentous bacteria that reside in the human oropharynx and gastrointestinal tract. The infection typically affects immunocompetent patients and has multiple forms (e.g., cervicofacial, thoracic, abdominopelvic, primary cutaneous). 'Lumpy jaw', the cervicofacial variant, often presents as 'wooden' induration with draining sinuses at the angle of the jaw or submandibular region. This is the most common form of the disease, and is likely to be the most common type seen by dermatologists.

MANAGEMENT STRATEGY

Mild disease can usually be fully cured with antibiotics, whereas more extensive disease often requires a combination of antibiotics and surgery. Except for minor cases, most patients are initially treated with parenteral antibiotics, followed by a course of oral therapy. Although recently many antibiotics have shown both in-vitro and in-vivo activity against *Actinomyces* spp., *penicillin* has remained the drug of choice since the 1940s.

Historically, actinomycosis was treated with long courses of antibiotics. However, there is mounting evidence that, if diagnosed in an early stage, actinomycosis can be successfully treated with brief courses (<6 months) of therapy. Ultimately, the patient's condition and response to therapy will dictate the duration of treatment.

Treatment failures with penicillin are extremely rare, but when they occur they are likely to be due to β-lactamase-producing bacteria that accompany *Actinomyces* spp. and help initiate infection. When faced with such a case, modifying the antibiotic regimen to cover these accomplices is warranted (e.g., switching to *imipenem* or *clindamycin*).

Short-term treatment of actinomycosis: two cases and a review. Sudhakar SS, Ross JJ. Clin Infect Dis 2004; 38: 444–7.

Susceptibility of pathogenic actinomycetes to antimicrobial compounds. Lerner PI. Antimicrob Agents Chemother 1974; 5: 302–9.

SPECIFIC INVESTIGATIONS

▶ Gram stain
▶ Biopsy with special stains
▶ Culture and measurement of physiological and biochemical characteristics
▶ Immunofluorescent staining
▶ Direct immunoperoxidase technique
▶ Ribosomal RNA gene sequencing
▶ Computed tomography (CT) and magnetic resonance imaging (MRI)

Diagnostic methods for human actinomycosis. Holmberg K. Microbiol Sci 1987; 4: 72–8.

An excellent review of the diagnosis of actinomycosis.

The most accurate way to diagnose actinomycosis is via culture – usually a difficult task, which requires thioglycolate or brain–heart-enriched agar at 37°C under anaerobic or microaerophilic conditions. 'Molar-tooth' and 'breadcrumb' colonies may take up to 3 weeks to grow. Unfortunately, definitive identification cannot be based on colony morphology and requires the measurement of physiological and biochemical characteristics (e.g., sensitivity to oxygen, presence of preformed enzymes).

Because cultures of Actinomyces spp. are often unsuccessful, observation of 'sulfur granules' on a peripheral smear or histology often helps make the diagnosis. The granules are bacterial colonies which on hematoxylin and eosin staining have a basophilic central area surrounded by a zone of eosinophilic 'clubs'. Other typical histologic findings include extensive fibrosis, chronic granulation tissue, sinus tracts, and scattered microabscesses.

Immunofluorescent staining of Actinomyces spp. is available and can be used on clinical material, granules, and formalin-fixed tissues. The direct immunoperoxidase technique can specifically show Actinomyces spp. in formalin-fixed sections via light microscopy. These techniques, as well as gene sequencing (see below), are promising diagnostic modalities given the difficulty of culture and histologic identification.

Cervicofacial actinomycosis: diagnosis and management. Oostman O, Smego RA. Curr Infect Dis Resp 2005; 7: 170–4.

Culture isolation of *Actinomyces* species and microscopic visualization of Gram-positive, non-acid-fast, thin, branching filaments remain the best methods of diagnosing cervicofacial actinomycosis.

Diagnosis of pelvic actinomycosis by 16s ribosomal RNA gene sequencing and its clinical significance. Woo PCY, Fung AMY, Lau SKP, Hon E, Yuen KY. Diagn Microbiol Infect Dis 2002; 43: 113–18.

Actinomyces odontolyticus was identified by rRNA gene sequencing. Because the 16S ribosomal RNA gene is conserved within a species, it can be used to identify a specific species of bacteria.

Cervicofacial actinomycosis: CT and MR imaging findings in seven patients. Park JK, Lee HK, Ha HK, Choi HY, Choi CG. AJNR Am J Neuroradiol 2003; 24: 331–5.

Findings on CT and MRI may be helpful in distinguishing cervicofacial actinomycosis from malignant neoplasms, tuberculosis, and fungal infections.

FIRST-LINE THERAPIES

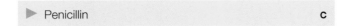

▶ Penicillin	C

Antimicrobial susceptibility testing of *Actinomyces* species with 12 antimicrobial agents. Smith AJ, Hall V, Thakker B, Gemmell CG. J Antimicrob Chemother 2005; 56: 407–9.

The authors tested the susceptibility of 87 strains of *Actinomyces* to 12 different antimicrobial agents. All isolates were susceptible to penicillin and amoxicillin.

Actinomycosis. Smego RA, Foglia G. Clin Infect Dis 1998; 26: 1255–63.

The authors recommend 2 months of oral penicillin V or a tetracycline (e.g., oral doxycycline 100 mg twice daily) for mild cervicofacial disease. For more complicated infections, parenteral penicillin G (10–20 million U/day divided every 6 h) for 4–6 weeks, followed by 6–12 months of oral penicillin V (2–4 g/day divided every 6 h) is suggested. A tetracycline, erythromycin, clindamycin, or cephalosporins are advocated for patients allergic to penicillin.

Actinomycosis and nocardiosis. A review of basic differences in therapy. Peabody JW, Seabury JH. Am J Med 1960; 28: 99–115.

The authors review the treatment of actinomycosis and state that penicillin is the drug of choice.

SECOND-LINE THERAPIES

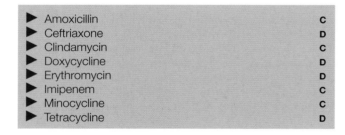

▶ Amoxicillin	C
▶ Ceftriaxone	D
▶ Clindamycin	C
▶ Doxycycline	D
▶ Erythromycin	D
▶ Imipenem	C
▶ Minocycline	C
▶ Tetracycline	D

The use of oral amoxycillin for the treatment of actinomycosis: a clinical and in vitro study. Martin MV. Br Dent J 1984; 156: 252–4.

Ten patients with cervicofacial actinomycosis were cured in less than 6 weeks with a combination of amoxicillin (500 mg four times daily) and surgery.

Actinomycosis abscess of the thyroid gland. Cevera JJ, Butehorn HF, Shapiro J, Setzen G. Laryngoscope 2003; 113: 2108–11.

A 39-year-old woman who developed actinomycosis of the thyroid gland after tooth extraction was cured with thyroidectomy and 6 months of ceftriaxone.

Successful treatment of thoracic actinomycosis with ceftriaxone. Skoutelis A, Petrochilos J, Bassaris H. Clin Infect Dis 1994; 19: 161–2.

A 38-year-old patient with pulmonary actinomycosis was successfully treated with a 3-week course of daily ceftriaxone followed by 3 months of daily oral ampicillin.

Mandibular actinomycosis treated with oral clindamycin. Badgett JT, Adams G. Pediatr Infect Dis J 1987; 6: 221–2.

Clindamycin in the treatment of cervicofacial actinomycosis. de Vries J, Bentley KC. Int J Clin Pharmacol 1974; 9: 46–8.

A 60-year-old man with cervicofacial actinomycosis that was resistant to penicillin and tetracycline responded fully to a 1-month course of clindamycin (150 mg four times a day).

Clindamycin in the treatment of serious anaerobic infections. Fass RJ, Scholand JF, Hodges GR, Saslaw S. Ann Intern Med 1973; 78: 853–9.

Four patients with cervicofacial actinomycosis and one with thoracic actinomycosis were successfully treated with a combination of intravenous and oral clindamycin.

Primary actinomycosis of the hand: a case report and literature review. Mert A, Bilir M, Bahar H, Torun M, Tabak F, Ozturk R, et al. Int J Infect Dis 2001; 5: 112–14.

A 35-year-old man with primary actinomycosis of the hand was cured with 1 month of intravenous ampicillin (12 g/day) followed by 11 months of oral doxycycline (200 mg/day).

Actinomycosis of the prostate. de Souza E, Katz DA, Dworzack DL, Longo G. J Urol 1985; 133: 290–1.

A case of acute prostatitis due to *Actinomyces* spp. was cured with long-term erythromycin, chosen because of its excellent penetration into prostatic secretions.

Actinomycosis of the temporomandibular joint. Bradley P. Br J Oral Surg 1971; 9: 54–6.

A 58-year-old man with actinomycosis of the temporomandibular joint was cured with a 12-week course of erythromycin (500 mg six times a day).

Use of imipenem in the treatment of thoracic actinomycosis. Yew WW, Wong PC, Wong CF, Chau CH. Clin Infect Dis 1994; 19: 983–4.

Report of eight cases of pulmonary actinomycosis and their treatment with imipenem–cilastatin. Yew WW, Wong PC, Lee J, Fung SL, Wong CF, Chan CY. Monaldi Arch Chest Dis 1994; 54: 126–9.

Seven of eight patients with pulmonary actinomycosis were successfully treated with a 4-week course of parenteral imipenem–cilastatin.

Cutaneous disseminated actinomycosis in a patient with acute lymphocytic leukemia. Takeda H, Mitsuhashi Y, Kondo S. J Dermatol 1998; 25: 37–40.

A patient with primary cutaneous disseminated actinomycosis was cured with a 3-month course of intravenous minocycline (2 mg/kg/day).

Antibiotic treatment of cervicofacial actinomycosis for patients allergic to penicillin: a clinical and in vitro study. Martin MV. Br J Oral Maxillofac Surg 1985; 23: 428–34.

Six patients with cervicofacial actinomycosis were cured with 8–16 weeks of oral minocycline (250 mg four times a day). There were no recurrences after 1 year.

Primary actinomycosis of the quadriceps. Langloh JT, Lauerman WC. J Pediatr Orthop 1987; 7: 222–3.

Surgical drainage followed by a 6-week course of oral tetracycline cured a case of actinomycosis of the quadriceps.

THIRD-LINE THERAPIES

► Ciprofloxacin	E
► Levofloxacin	E
► Rifampin	E
► Hyperbaric oxygen	E

Treatment of recalcitrant actinomycosis with ciprofloxacin. Macfarlane DJ, Tucker LG, Kemp RJ. J Infection 1993; 27: 177–80.

Treatment of pulmonary actinomycosis with levofloxacin. Ferreira D de F, Amado J, Neves S, Taveira N, Carvalho A, Nogueira R. J Bras Pneumol 2008; 34: 245–8.

Treatment of pulmonary actinomycosis with rifampin. Morrone N, De Castro Pereira CA, Saito M, Dourado AM, Pereira Da Silva Mendes ES. G Ital Chemioter 1982; 29: 121–4.

Pulmonary actinomycosis. Rapid improvement with isoniazid and rifampin. King JW, White MC. Arch Intern Med 1981; 141: 1234–5.

Adjunctive hyperbaric oxygen therapy for actinomycotic lacrimal canaliculitis. Shauly Y, Nachum Z, Gdal-On M, Melamed S, Miller B. Graefes Arch Clin Exp Ophthalmol 1993; 231: 429–31.

A 52-year-old patient with treatment-resistant lacrimal canaliculitis due to *A. israelii* was cured with hyperbaric oxygen.

Hyperbaric oxygen in the treatment of actinomycosis. Manheim SD, Voleti C, Ludwig A, Jacobson JH. J Am Med Assoc 1969; 210: 552–3.

After failing to respond to surgery and intravenous penicillin, a 63-year-old patient with perirectal actinomycosis was cured with hyperbaric oxygen.

Acute generalized exanthematous pustulosis

Walayat Hussain, Ian Coulson

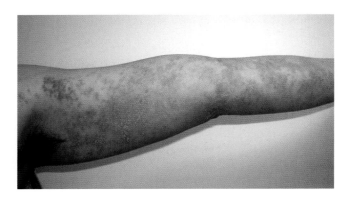

Acute generalized exanthematous pustulosis (AGEP) is characterized by the acute onset of numerous small, non-follicular, sterile pustules arising on a diffuse erythematous base in a febrile patient with an accompanying blood neutrophilia. The majority of cases occur in the context of drug ingestion (commonly within 24 hours). Rapid resolution following drug withdrawal is the usual outcome.

MANAGEMENT STRATEGY

Treatment of AGEP involves establishing the correct diagnosis (Table 1) coupled with the *withdrawal of any implicated medication* (Table 2). Pustular psoriasis is its main differential diagnosis. A comprehensive drug history and a personal or family history of psoriasis is therefore required.

Intraepidermal or subcorneal pustules in conjunction with a leukocytoclastic vasculitis, focal necrosis of keratinocytes, marked edema of the papillary dermis, and an infiltrate of eosinophils are histological features that help distinguish AGEP from pustular psoriasis; biopsy is thus an integral facet of management.

Differentiation of AGEP from other inflammatory, toxic, or infectious conditions, such as Sneddon–Wilkinson disease (subcorneal pustular dermatosis) or, in severe cases, toxic epidermal necrolysis, is often readily apparent both clinically and histologically. The clinician should, however, be aware that erythema multiforme-like targetoid lesions, mucus membrane involvement, facial edema, purpura, and vesicobullous lesions have all been documented in the context of AGEP.

Antibiotics (primarily penicillin or macrolide based) are the most frequently implicated medications. Numerous case reports have cited various other causative agents, including calcium channel blockers, non-steroidal anti-inflammatory drugs (NSAIDs), angiotensin-converting enzyme (ACE) inhibitors and anticonvulsants (Table 2). Acute enterovirus infection, cytomegalovirus, parvovirus B19, spider bites, Chinese herbal compounds (ginkgo biloba), contrast media, and mercury exposure have also been reported as possible causes.

There is no specific therapy for AGEP. A skin swab establishes the sterile nature of the pustules and drug withdrawal, if feasible, results in rapid spontaneous resolution. *Supportive therapy* is all that is required. A superficial desquamation often occurs during this time and may be treated with *simple emollients*. Several case reports cite the use of patch testing to confirm the causative medication. Only a single case report supports the use of *systemic corticosteroids* for this self-limiting condition.

SPECIFIC INVESTIGATIONS

- ▶ Detailed history
- ▶ Hematology
- ▶ Skin swab of pustule
- ▶ Microscopy, culture, Gram stain
- ▶ Skin biopsy

FIRST-LINE THERAPIES

▶ Drug withdrawal	E

Risk factors for acute generalized exanthematous pustulosis (AGEP)-results of a multinational case-control study (EuroSCAR). Sidoroff A, Dunant A, Viboud C. Br J Dermatol 2007; 157: 6.

A multinational case–control study (97 cases of AGEP and 1009 controls) which assessed the risk for different drugs of causing severe cutaneous adverse reactions.

The most frequently implicated drugs were pristinamycin (a macrolide marketed in France), ampicillin/amoxicillin, quinolones, (hydroxy)chloroquine, anti-infective sulfonamides, terbinafine, and dilitiazem. Infections and a personal or family history of psoriasis were not deemed to be significant risk factors for developing AGEP. Of note, the median treatment duration was 1 day for antibiotics and 11 days for all other associated drugs.

Acute generalized exanthematous pustulosis. Analysis of 63 cases. Roujeau JC, Bioulac-Sage P, Bourseau C, Guillaume JC, Bernard P, Lok C, et al. Arch Dermatol 1991; 127: 1333–8.

Table 1 Diagnostic criteria for AGEP (from Roujeau et al. Arch Dermatol 1991; 127: 1333–8)

Numerous, small (<5 mm), non-follicular pustules arising on a widespread oedematous erythema
Pathology reveals intraepidermal/subcorneal pustules associated with one or more of the following:
    Dermal edema
    Vasculitis
    Perivascular eosinophils
    Focal necrosis of keratinocytes
Fever >38°
Blood neutrophil count >7 × 10^9/L
Acute progression with spontaneous recovery within 15 days

Although an alternative diagnostic algorithm has been proposed by Sidoroff et al. (J Cutan Pathol 2001; 28: 113–19), we feel the above criteria remain the most succinct and practical clinical guide for diagnosing AGEP.

Evidence Levels: **A** Double-blind study **B** Clinical trial ≥ 20 subjects **C** Clinical trial < 20 subjects **D** Series ≥ 5 subjects **E** Anecdotal case reports

Table 2 Drugs reported to cause AGEP

Acetaminophen	Clemastine	Iohexol	Pneumococcal vaccine
Acetazolamide	Clindamycin	Iopamidol	Prednisolone
Acetylsalicyclic acid	Clobazam	Isepamicin sulfate	Progestins
Allopurinol	Clozapine	Isoniazid	Proguanil
Amoxapine	Co-trimoxazole	Itraconazole	Propafenone
Amoxicillin	Codeine	Lamivudine	Propicillin
Ampicillin	Corticosteroids	Lansoprazole	Prostaglandin E1
Amphotericin	Cytaribine	Lopinavir	Protease inhibitors
Aspirin	Dalteparin	Lincomycin	Pseudoephidrine
Azathioprine	Dexamethasone	Mercury	Psoralen plus UV-A
Azithromycin	Dextropropoxyphene	Metamizole	Pyrimethamine
Bacampicillin	Diaphenylsulphone	Methylprednisolone	Quinidine
Bamifylline	Diltiazem	Metronidazole	Ranitidine
Bleomycin	Disulfiram	Minocycline	Rifampicin
Bufenin	Doxycycline	Morphine	Ritonavir
Bufexamac	Enalapril	Nadoxolol	Salbutiamine
Cadralazine	Eperisone hydrochloride	Naproxen	Sennoside
Calcium channel blockers	Eprazinone	Nifedipine	Sertraline
Captopril	Erythromycin	Nifuroxazide	Simvastatin
Carbamazepine	Etoricoxib	Nimesulide	Streptomycin
Carbimazole	Famotidine	Nimodipine	Sulfamethoxazole
Carbutamide	Fenoterol	Nitrazepam	Sulfasalazine
Cefaclor	Fluconazole	Norfloxacin	Tazobactam
Cefazolin	Fluindione	Nystatin	Teicoplanin
Cefuroxime	Furosemide	Ofloxacin	Terazosin
Celecoxib	Gefitinib	Omeprazole	Terbinafine
Cephalexin	Gentamicin	Paracetamol	Tetracycline
Cephradine	Hydrochlorothiazide	Penicillins	Tetrazepam
Chloramphenicol	Hydroxychloroquine	Pentoxifylline	Thalidomide
Chloroquine	Hydroxyzine	Phenobarbital	Ticlopidine
Chlorpromazine	Ibuprofen	Phenylbutazone	Valdecoxib
Chromium picolinate	Icodextrin	Phenytoin	Vancomycin
Cimetidine	Imatinib	Pipemidic acid	Zidovudine
Ciprofloxacin	Imipenem/cilastatin	Piperacillin	
	Interferon	Piperazine	

A thorough retrospective review of cases of AGEP. Almost 90% of cases were attributable to drugs, with 50% of reactions occurring within 24 hours of ingestion.

AGEP is distinct from pustular psoriasis based on histological differences, drug induction in most cases, a more acute course of fever and pustulosis, blood neutrophilia, and rapid spontaneous healing (within 15 days).

Acute generalized exanthematous pustulosis (AGEP) – a clinical reaction pattern. Sidoroff A, Halevy S, Bavinck JN, Vaillant L, Roujeau JC. J Cutan Pathol 2001; 28: 113–19.

A very useful clinicopathologic review of AGEP which proposes a diagnostic algorithm for validating cases.

Acute generalized exanthematous pustulosis. Manders SM, Heymann WR. Cutis 1994; 54: 194–6.

Two of the three cases reported in this series were attributable to penicillin. This succinct overview of AGEP also provides the reader with useful clinicopathologic features that may help distinguish AGEP from pustular psoriasis.

Pustular eruption after drug exposure: is it pustular psoriasis or a pustular drug eruption? Spencer JM, Silvers DN, Grossman ME. Br J Dermatol 1994; 130: 514–19.

Another series highlighting the diagnostic challenge when confronted with a patient with pustulosis and fever. One of the four cases of AGEP occurred in a patient with known psoriasis who was given trimethoprim for a urinary tract infection. An awareness of the condition, eosinophils in the biopsy, and rapid resolution following drug withdrawal prevented unnecessary treatment for pustular psoriasis.

Generalized pustular psoriasis or drug-induced toxic pustuloderma? The use of patch testing. Whittam LR, Wakelin SH, Barker JNWN. Clin Exp Dermatol 2000; 25: 122–4.

Patch testing to a 1% and 5% amoxicillin preparation confirmed a type 4 hypersensitivity reaction in a patient with long-standing plaque psoriasis who developed a generalized pustular eruption when treated with amoxicillin for an episode of epididymo-orchitis.

A systemic reaction to patch testing for the evaluation of acute generalized exanthematous pustulosis. Mashiah J, Brenner S. Arch Dermatol. 2003; 139: 1181–3.

The authors report a generalized AGEP-like reaction caused by patch tests carried out to determine the drug eliciting AGEP. Interestingly, negative results were obtained with the drug in question.

SECOND-LINE THERAPIES

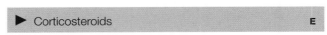

▶ Corticosteroids   E

Acute generalised exanthematous pustulosis. Criton S, Sofia B. Indian J Dermatol Venereol Leprol 2001; 67: 93–5.

A case report in which the authors claim that parenteral corticosteroids hastened the resolution of AGEP presumptively caused by benzylpenicillin.

Allergic contact dermatitis and photoallergy

Rosemary L Nixon

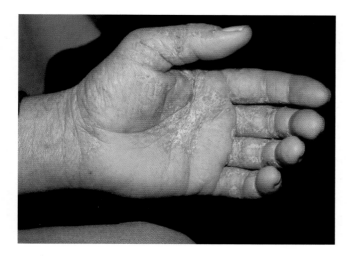

Allergic contact dermatitis (ACD) is a delayed hypersensitivity reaction, usually to the topical application of an allergen to which the sufferer is sensitized. At first, the rash is localized to the site of contact with the causative allergen, but it may spread to other areas, either from transfer of the allergen to other sites or because of an 'id' or hypersensitivity eruption. Spread of the rash to other areas is very characteristic of ACD and clinically may help to differentiate it from an irritant contact dermatitis.

In photoallergy, a substance does not become allergenic until exposed to UV light. The most important photoallergens are currently sunscreens, and perhaps some pesticides, but in the past fragrances (especially musk ambrette), halogenated salicylanilides, and topical non-steroidal agents (such as ketoprofen) were common photoallergens.

Some patients with an airborne contact dermatitis to sesquiterpene lactones, found in the Compositae group of plants, will develop photosensitivity, as evidenced by abnormal results on monochromator testing. This condition is generally termed chronic actinic dermatitis (CAD).

Localization may give clues to the causative allergen, for example involvement of the hands in cases of ACD caused by rubber accelerators in gloves; the ears and neck caused by nickel in costume jewelry; eyelid and neck dermatitis from preservatives or perfumes in moisturizing creams.

Determinants of whether sensitization will occur include the nature of the allergen involved, the duration and concentration of skin contact with the allergen, and individual susceptibility.

MANAGEMENT STRATEGY

The primary responsibility is to *identify and avoid further contact* with the offending allergen, as well as any potentially cross-reacting agents. *Patch testing* is required to elucidate this.

From a public health perspective it is important to reduce exposure to known allergens. In parts of Europe, legislation has been enacted to reduce the nickel content of jewelry that comes in contact with the skin. The addition of ferrous sulfate to cement, initially in Denmark, effectively reduces the available chromate through chemical reduction. Higher molecular weight epoxy resins are preferred to lower weight resins because of their decreased allergenicity.

In the workplace other measures should be undertaken to reduce exposure to known allergens, such as substitution of known allergens, changing the design of an engineering process to limit skin contact with chemicals, installation of appropriate ventilation to reduce airborne exposure to substances, and the use of personal protective equipment.

It is most important to wear gloves that are appropriate for handling a particular chemical. In addition, it is often suggested that cotton gloves be worn underneath rubber or leather gloves to prevent sensitization to rubber accelerators and chromate, respectively. This is especially important in the context of work in hot environments, where sweating and leaching of allergens is likely.

The initial treatments use the general principles of eczema therapy, including *avoidance of skin irritants*, such as water, soap, solvents, oils, heat, sweating, dust, and friction. Use of *soap substitutes* and *moisturizing creams*, together with *topical corticosteroids*, is recommended.

The use of *barrier creams* to prevent dermatitis has had limited success; however, the development of *topical skin protectants* in the US has had encouraging results when used experimentally to prevent allergic reactions caused by poison ivy. The use of chelating agents in skin creams may be helpful. Short courses of *oral corticosteroids*, such as prednisolone 25–50 mg daily for 1 week, are sometimes required in severe cases. Occasionally the dermatitis may become secondarily infected, so a course of *antibiotics*, such as *cephalosporin, erythromycin*, or *flucloxacillin* may be required. *Topical antibiotics* such as *mupirocin* or *fusidic acid* are often helpful, particularly for the treatment of persistently cracked or fissured skin that becomes infected.

Once the cause of ACD has been identified, long-term treatments other than avoidance of the allergen(s) are usually not required. Desensitization, commonly used in the treatment of allergies caused by immediate hypersensitivity reactions, has been of extremely limited value when employed in delayed hypersensitivity.

Occasionally, severe episodes of dermatitis may precipitate a recurring eczematous condition, termed persisting post-occupational dermatitis.

In persistent cases *ultraviolet light therapy* may be considered, such as with hand UVB or PUVA (psoralen plus UVA).

Systemic immunosuppression using *azathioprine or ciclosporin* may be considered. Other agents, such as *methotrexate or acitretin* (particularly if the hands are hyperkeratotic), are less often used. Newer topical treatments include *tacrolimus* and *pimecrolimus*. *Disulfiram* has been used in the treatment of nickel dermatitis with equivocal success. Chelation of nickel topically with *clioquinol* may be a more useful approach, but has been little studied. *Superficial X-ray* and *Grenz ray* treatments have been successfully used in some cases.

In photoallergy, identification and avoidance of the photoallergen is of major importance. In the case of allergy to chemical sunscreening agents, this may involve substitution with physical sunscreening agents such as titanium dioxide.

In CAD, treatments have centered on reduction of UV exposure, including hospitalization and use of *plastic films* for windows to reduce UV transmission. The use of *topical tacrolimus* has recently been reported. Systemic therapies include *azathioprine, prednisolone, hydroxychloroquine, ciclosporin, PUVA or UVB, and combinations of UV with prednisolone.*

SPECIFIC INVESTIGATIONS

> ▶ Patch testing to appropriately diluted allergens
> ▶ Photopatch testing if photoallergic dermatitis is suspected – duplicate sets of allergens are applied, and after 48 hours one set is exposed to 5 J/cm UVA; results are read after a further 48 hours

Contact dermatitis: Allergic. Beck MH, Wilkinson SM. In: Burns DA, Breathnach SM, Cox N, Griffiths C, eds. Rook's Textbook of Dermatology, 7th edn. Oxford: Blackwell Science, 2004; Chapter 20.

This comprehensive chapter from a major dermatology text is a great source of information.

FIRST-LINE THERAPIES

Contact allergic dermatitis	
▶ Prevent contact with allergen	C
▶ Topical corticosteroids	B
▶ Emollients and soap substitutes	C
▶ Barrier creams	B
▶ Tacrolimus	B
▶ Pimecrolimus	B
▶ Topical clioquinol (nickel dermatitis)	D
▶ Prednisolone	D
▶ Antibiotics – topical and systemic	D
Photoallergy/CAD	
▶ Reduction of ultraviolet light	C
▶ Sunscreens – physical agents	E
▶ Tacrolimus	D

A double-blind randomized placebo-controlled pilot study comparing topical immunomodulating agents and corticosteroids for treatment of experimentally induced nickel contact dermatitis. Bhardwaj SS, Jaimes JP, Liu A, Warshaw EM. Dermatitis 2007; 18: 26–31.

Twenty-one nickel-allergic volunteers had patch test reaction sites treated with pimecrolimus, tacrolimus, clobetasol, triamcinolone, and control moisturizing cream and ointment, in order to assess the relative efficacies of these agents. In fact, it was demonstrated that these studies are difficult to perform, as most pairwise comparisons were not statistically significant. Nevertheless, clobetasol was more effective than petrolatum, pimecrolimus, and tacrolimus.

Efficacy of topical corticosteroids in nickel-induced contact allergy. Hachem JP, De Paepe K, Vanpe'e E, Bogaerts M, Kaufman L, Rogiers V, et al. Clin Exp Dermatol 2002; 27: 47–50.

Twenty nickel-allergic female volunteers had patch tests applied with nickel on one forearm and control saline on the other. Topical corticosteroid was applied twice daily after day 4. Transepidermal water loss values were significantly reduced on the topical corticosteroid-treated sites in the early phase of ACD.

The effect of two moisturisers on skin barrier damage in allergic contact dermatitis. Hachem J-P, De Paepe K, Vanpee E, Kaufman L, Rogiers V, Roseeuw D, et al. Eur J Dermatol 2002; 12: 136–8.

Fifteen female volunteers with known nickel allergy had two different moisturizers, with both highly and poorly hydrating formulations, applied to nickel-induced ACD on their forearms. Transepidermal water loss measurements were significantly increased on the sites pretreated with the poorly hydrating moisturizer.

A cream containing the chelator DTPA (diethylenetriamine-penta-acetic acid) can prevent contact allergic reactions to metals. Wohrl S, Kriechbaumer N, Hemmer W, Focke M, Brannath W, Götz M, et al. Contact Dermatol 2001; 44: 224–8.

Patients with known allergies to nickel, cobalt, and copper had abrogation of their patch test reactions with pretreatment with DTPA cream.

Assessment of the ability of the topical skin protectant (TSP) to protect against contact dermatitis to urushiol (Rhus) antigen. Vidmar DA, Iwane MK. Am J Contact Dermatol 1999; 10: 190–7.

Fifty Rhus-sensitive subjects underwent paired open patch tests to urushiol, with and without prior skin application of TSP. TSP-protected sites were associated with significantly less dermatitis. TSP is composed of polytetrafluoroethylene resins mixed in a perfluorinated polyether oil (similar to Teflon).

Prevention of poison ivy and poison oak allergic contact dermatitis by quaternium-18 bentonite. Marks JG, Fowler JF, Sheretz EF. J Am Acad Dermatol 1995; 33: 212–16.

Quaternium-18 bentonite 5% lotion was applied to the skin 1 hour before patch testing to urushiol in a large group of poison ivy-allergic individuals. Non-pretreated sites were used as controls. Pretreated sites had absent or significantly reduced reactions to the urushiol compared to controls.

Tacrolimus ointment in the treatment of nickel-induced allergic contact dermatitis. Saripelli YV, Gadzia JE, Belsito DV. J Am Acad Dermatol 2003; 49: 477–82.

Of 19 volunteers with known nickel sensitivity, 18 had improvement in signs and symptoms of ACD with topical tacrolimus compared to 10 using vehicle.

Topical tacrolimus 0.1% ointment (Protopic®) reverses nickel contact dermatitis elicited by allergen challenge to a similar degree to mometasone furoate 0.1% with greater suppression of late erythema. Alomar A, Puig L, Gallardo CM, Valenzuela N. Contact Dermatol 2003; 49: 185–8.

Twenty-eight female volunteers who were allergic to nickel had patch tests removed at day 2 and then applied either tacrolimus or mometasone furoate under occlusion for 48 hours. The reactions were assessed with visual scores and measurement of erythema.

SDZ ASM 981 is the first non-steroid that suppresses established nickel contact dermatitis elicited by allergen challenge. Queille-Roussel C, Graeber M, Thurston M, Lachapelle JM, Decroix J, de Cuyper C, et al. Contact Dermatol 2000; 42: 349–50.

Sixty-six nickel-sensitive subjects were exposed to nickel, and the ensuing dermatitis was treated twice daily with SDZ ASM 981 (pimecrolimus) at 0.2% and 0.6%. This was significantly more effective than treatment with the corresponding vehicle, and similar in effectiveness of treatment to use of 0.1% betamethasone-17 valerate cream.

Treatment of chronic actinic dermatitis with tacrolimus ointment. Uetsu N, Okamoto H, Fujii K, Doi R, Horio T. J Am Acad Dermatol 2002; 47: 881–4.

Six patients with CAD unresponsive to other topical agents, including topical corticosteroids and sunscreens, and also oral antihistamines, improved with application of 0.1% tacrolimus ointment applied twice daily. Improvement was moderate after 2 weeks, and greater after 4 weeks.

The inhibitory effects of topical chelating agents and antioxidants on nickel-induced hypersensitivity reactions. Memon AA, Molokhia MM, Friedmann PS. J Am Acad Dermatol 1994; 30: 560–5.

Clioquinol ointment 3% applied to a coin completely abolished the allergic reaction to it in all 29 nickel-sensitive subjects. In clinical use, sites treated with a cream containing 3% clioquinol and 1% hydrocortisone showed marked clinical improvement in all 10 subjects. Clioquinol is a potent inhibitor of nickel-induced hypersensitivity reactions, and it is feasible to use it as a barrier ointment to block the allergenic effects of nickel in sensitive patients.

SECOND-LINE THERAPIES

Contact dermatitis	
▶ Ultraviolet light	B
▶ Azathioprine	C
▶ Ciclosporin	D
▶ Methotrexate	D
▶ Acitretin	E
▶ Superficial X-ray and Grenz ray therapy	C
▶ Low-nickel diet	C
Photoallergy/chronic actinic dermatitis	
▶ Azathioprine	C
▶ Prednisolone	D
▶ Hydroxychloroquine	D
▶ Ciclosporin	B
▶ PUVA/UVB	D
▶ PUVA/UVB and prednisolone	D

Chronic eczematous dermatitis of the hands: a comparison of PUVA and UVB treatment. Rosen K, Mobacken H, Swanbeck G. Acta Dermatol Venereol 1987; 67: 48–54.

Thirty-five patients were randomly allocated to PUVA or UVB, with one hand acting as an untreated control. Although there was statistically significant improvement in both groups, PUVA was superior to UVB.

Azathioprine in the treatment of *Parthenium* dermatitis. Sharma VK, Chakrabarti A, Mahajan V. Int J Dermatol 1998; 37: 299–302.

Avoidance of this allergen is almost impossible. Twenty patients with chronic *Parthenium* dermatitis, with relative contraindications to systemic corticosteroids or their side effects, were treated with oral azathioprine 100–150 mg daily for 6 months. Ten showed near-total clearance, and three showed more than 50% eczema reduction.

Oral cyclosporin inhibits the expression of contact hypersensitivity in man. Higgins EM, McLelland J, Friedmann PS, Matthews JN, Shuster S. J Dermatol Sci 1991; 2: 79–83.

The expression of delayed contact hypersensitivity was studied in six patients with chronic contact dermatitis treated with

ciclosporin 5 mg/kg/day. Quantitative patch test reactions were diminished in all six; responses were reduced over the whole range of allergen concentrations. In addition, the clinical manifestations of ACD underwent complete resolution within 2–3 weeks of ciclosporin therapy.

Low-dose oral methotrexate treatment for recalcitrant palmoplantar pompholyx. Egan CA, Rallis TM, Meadows KP, Krueger GG. J Am Acad Dermatol 1999; 40: 612–14.

Five patients with severe pompholyx who did not respond to conventional therapy or who had debilitating side effects from corticosteroids responded to low-dose methotrexate with clearing of their dermatitis and a reduction in their need for oral corticosteroid therapy.

A double-blind study of Grenz ray therapy in chronic eczema of the hands. Lidelof B, Wrangso K, Liden S. Br J Dermatol 1987; 117: 77–80.

Grenz rays at 3 Gy were applied to hand eczema on six occasions at intervals of 1 week, with significant improvement in the treated compared to the sham treated control hand.

Low nickel diet: an open prospective trial. Veien NK, Hattel T, Laurberg G. J Am Acad Dermatol 1993; 29: 1002–7.

Ninety nickel-sensitive patients who had previously flared with oral nickel challenge were treated with a nickel-free diet. Fifty-eight improved, and 40 had had long-term benefit when followed 1–2 years later. Those with moderately positive patch test reactions rather than strongly positive appeared to benefit more from the diet.

Chronic actinic dermatitis: An analysis of 51 patients evaluated in the United States and Japan. Lim HW, Morison WL, Kamide R, Buchness MR, Harris R, Soter NA. Arch Dermatol 1994; 130: 1284–9.

The clinical features of 51 patients were detailed. Topical corticosteroids were helpful for minor eruptions. Nine patients were treated with hydroxychloroquine sulfate (200 mg once to twice daily), with a partial to good response in some patients.

Azathioprine treatment in chronic actinic dermatitis: a double-blind controlled trial with monitoring of exposure to ultraviolet radiation. Murphy GM, Maurice PD, Norris PG, Morris RW, Hawk JL. Br J Dermatol 1989; 121: 639–46.

Azathioprine 150 mg/day was compared with placebo in 18 severely affected patients. Five of eight patients treated with azathioprine, but none of 10 patients on placebo, achieved remission within 6 months.

Successful treatment of musk ketone-induced chronic actinic dermatitis with cyclosporine and PUVA. Gardeazabal J, Arregui MA, Gil N, Landa N, Ratón JA, Diáz-Pérez JL. J Am Acad Dermatol 1992; 27: 838–42.

A single case of musk ambrette persistent light reaction responding to ciclosporin and PUVA.

Actinic reticuloid: response to cyclosporin. Norris P, Camp RDR, Hawk JLM. J Am Acad Dermatol 1989; 21: 307–9.

Two patients responded to treatment with ciclosporin after failure of azathioprine.

Psoralen plus UVA protocol for Compositae photosensitivity. Burke DA, Corey G, Storrs FJ. Am J Contact Dermatol 1996; 7: 171–6.

Two elderly men received prednisolone-assisted PUVA for their chronic photodistributed dermatitis associated with Compositae sensitivity, which resolved with this treatment and in one instance remained clear for 18 months without needing further PUVA therapy.

THIRD-LINE THERAPIES

▶ Pentoxifylline

Prevention of nickel-induced contact reactions with pentoxifylline. Saricaoglu H, Tunali S, Bulbul E, White IR, Palali Z. Contact Dermatol 1998; 39: 244–7.

A guinea-pig study showing that oral pentoxifylline inhibits nickel contact dermatitis elicitation. Others have questioned the effects in humans.

Alopecia areata

Joanne Hague, John Berth-Jones

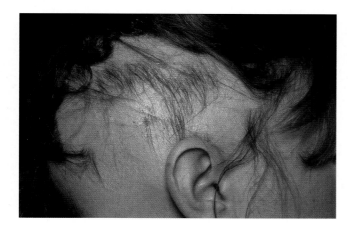

Alopecia areata (AA) is a T lymphocyte-mediated autoimmune disease of the hair follicle. It is characterized by patchy hair loss developing in otherwise normal skin, with 'exclamation mark' hairs around margins of expanding areas. Most cases are limited to one or more coin-sized patches, but in severe cases there may be complete baldness of the scalp (alopecia totalis, AT) or of the entire body (alopecia universalis, AU). The alopecia is non-cicatrizing, and in most cases resolves spontaneously after a few months.

MANAGEMENT STRATEGY

Leaving alopecia areata untreated is a reasonable option for many patients. Spontaneous remission often occurs, and no treatment has been shown to alter the long-term prognosis. Treatment can be time-consuming, uncomfortable, and potentially toxic, and relapse after treatment may be difficult to cope with. On the other hand, some patients are affected to such an extent that they require psychological support and counselling. Contact with other sufferers and support groups may also help. Patients should receive a thorough explanation of the natural history of the disease, and a realistic expectation of treatment outcome.

The treatments listed as first line are the most consistently effective and safe; however, the response to any treatment is variable and depends largely on the extent and duration of the alopecia. This is one reason why the results of trials are often conflicting. Trials involving recent-onset patchy alopecia may have a high rate of spontaneous remission, whereas trials limited to severe longstanding disease that is resistant to treatment do not exclude efficacy in mild alopecia. The term 'percentage regrowth' used in this chapter refers to hair regrowth in the lesional area compared to baseline.

Intralesional corticosteroid injections are considered first-line treatment for adult patients when only one or two small patches of alopecia are present, but can be used on up to 50% of the scalp if patients can tolerate the discomfort. The authors most frequently use triamcinolone acetonide aqueous suspension (2.5–10 mg/mL) injected intradermally in 0.05–0.1 mL doses, and repeated on a monthly basis. At a concentration

of 5 mg/mL a maximum of 3 mL can be used on the scalp in one visit. A concentration of 2.5 mg/mL should be used on the beard and eyebrow area. The main side effect is minimal, often transient, pitting atrophy.

Topical immunotherapy is the induction of contact allergy on the scalp. Contact sensitizers include dinitrochlorobenzene (DNCB, now considered potentially carcinogenic and therefore no longer used), squaric acid dibutyl ester (SADBE; this has limited stability), and diphencyprone (DPCP, diphenylcyclopropenone). The latter compound combines efficacy and safety with a practical shelf-life and has become the most widely used. *Diphencyprone* can initially be applied as 2% lotion to a small area (2–4 cm²) of scalp until the site of application becomes pruritic and erythematous. Treatment is then continued over a larger area with weekly applications of lower concentrations, typically ranging from 0.001% to 0.1%. The lowest concentration that maintains mild erythema or pruritus should be used. Our patients usually have half of their scalp treated initially, until a favorable result means treatment can then be extended to the contralateral scalp. This is one of the best-documented therapies for AA, and is the one most likely to be effective in extensive longstanding disease. The timing of the response is quite unpredictable, however, so the authors treat patients for as long as they wish to continue. Relapse rates may be high. Side effects include regional lymphadenopathy and rarely autosensitization, resulting in generalized eczema or even an eruption resembling erythema multiforme. Vitiligo may develop, although this is usually confined to the treated areas. For this reason, sensitization therapy is best avoided in patients with pigmented skin types.

Topical corticosteroids have demonstrated efficacy in some studies of patchy alopecia areata, particularly those using potent steroids with occlusion. They are fairly inexpensive and practical to use, and the main side effect is transient folliculitis. Results are variable, however, and they do not appear effective in AT or AU.

Psoralen plus ultraviolet A treatment (PUVA) has been studied in several trials with variable results. The relapse rate following treatment is high, and continued treatment appears to be necessary for maintenance of hair growth.

Irritants, including *anthralin (dithranol)* and *retinoic acid*, are safe and practical to use, although the evidence for their efficacy is weak. For patients with dark hair, anthralin has the advantage of camouflaging a pale area of scalp by staining it brown. Application needs to be frequent and at a fairly high concentration, as it needs to induce significant irritation to be effective. Retinoic acid is more practical for use in patients with fair hair.

Topical minoxidil is a safe treatment, but most studies have failed to demonstrate a response of cosmetic value in most patients.

Systemic corticosteroids are effective in some cases if high enough doses are used, and the use of pulsed regimens has had some limited success. AT, AU, and ophiasiform AA do not respond well, however, and high relapse rates make this potentially toxic treatment hard to justify.

Systemic ciclosporin also appears effective if given in high dosage, but the response is not maintained on cessation of therapy, so again it is difficult to justify its use.

Topical tacrolimus trials have shown encouraging results in rats and mice, but so far there is no evidence to suggest it is effective in humans.

By way of *camouflage*, many patients feel much happier wearing a wig. Both acrylic and real hair wigs are available in the UK on the NHS. Tattooing (dermatography) of the eyebrows may lead to a more socially acceptable image for some patients.

SPECIFIC INVESTIGATIONS

> ► Consider complete blood count, thyroid function tests, serum B$_{12}$ and autoantibodies as a screen for associated autoimmune conditions.

No routine investigation is normally necessary and the diagnosis is essentially clinical. However, in patients with symptoms or a family history of autoimmune diseases, such as thyroiditis, pernicious anemia, or Addison's disease, autoantibody screening and further investigation may be indicated.

FIRST-LINE THERAPIES

> ► Intralesional steroids   **A**
> ► Topical immunotherapy   **B**

Intralesional treatment of alopecia areata with triamcinolone acetonide by jet injector. Abell E, Munro DD. Br J Dermatol 1973; 88: 55–9.

A report of 84 patients treated with 0.1 mL needleless injections of triamcinolone acetonide 5 mg/mL and normal saline controls. After 6 weeks regrowth was observed in 86% of patients treated with triamcinolone and 7% of controls. Mild transient atrophy was frequently observed.

A comparison of intralesional triamcinolone hexacetonide and triamcinolone acetonide in alopecia areata. Porter D, Burton J. Br J Dermatol 1971; 85: 272–3.

Tufts of hair grew in 33 of 34 sites injected with hexacetonide in 11 patients with alopecia areata. In another group of 17 patients 16 of 25 sites injected with triamcinolone acetonide regrew. Growth continued for 18 months, even in two patients in whom the alopecia had progressed over the rest of the scalp to AT.

Prognostic factors in the treatment of alopecia areata with diphenylcyclopropenone. Van der Steen PHM, Van Baar HMJ, Happle R, Boezeman JBM, Perret CM. J Am Acad Dermatol 1991; 24: 227–30.

An open study of DPCP in 139 patients: 40% of 85 patients with alopecia of >90% of the scalp achieved subtotal or total regrowth; 75% of 54 patients with scalp involvement of 40–90% responded. The duration of AA and nail changes were independent risk factors for a poorer prognosis, but atopy, age of onset, and gender did not affect the outcome of treatment.

The use of topical diphenylcyclopropenone for the treatment of extensive alopecia areata. Cotellessa C, Peris K, Caracciolo E, Mordenti C, Chimenti S., et al. J Am Acad Dermatol 2001; 44: 73–6.

In this open study 56 patients with alopecia of more than 12 months' duration (mean 6 years) were treated on half of their scalp with DPCP. Forty-two had >90% hair loss, 14 had 30–90% patchy alopecia. Four atopic patients withdrew because of the development of widespread eczema. Of the 52 completing the study 25 (48%) achieved total regrowth at 6 months. After 6–18 months' follow-up 15 (29%) maintained full regrowth. Five of the 10 patients who relapsed achieved complete regrowth with a second course.

Predictive model for immunotherapy of alopecia areata with diphencyprone. Wiseman M, Shapiro J, MacDonald N, Lui H. Arch Dermatol 2001; 137: 1063–8.

A retrospective review of 148 patients with alopecia for a mean duration of 9.6 years (range 0.5 months to 55 years). Patients were treated on half of their scalp, and a response was defined as >75% regrowth or a cosmetically acceptable result. Response rates were 22.5% at 6 months, 52.0% at 12 months, and 77.9% after 32 months. Response rates were 100% in those with AA affecting 25–49% of their scalp, but only 17.8% in AT/AU. A relapse (loss of >25% of the regrowth) occurred in 63% of responders after 37 months' follow-up, irrespective of ongoing maintenance treatment.

SECOND-LINE THERAPIES

> ► Topical corticosteroids   **B**
> ► Topical minoxidil   **B**
> ► Phototherapy   **B**
> ► Anthralin/dithranol   **B**
> ► Retinoic acid   **E**

Randomised double-blind placebo-controlled trial in the treatment of alopecia areata with 0.25% desoximetasone cream. Charuwichitratana S, Wattanakrai P, Tanrattanakorn S. Arch Dermatol 2000; 136: 1276–7.

Seventy patients with patchy alopecia, mean duration 8.8 weeks, had twice-daily application of either active cream or placebo for 12 weeks; 54 completed the study. Fifteen out of 26 in the active group and 11 out of 28 in the placebo group achieved complete regrowth, which was not statistically significant. Nineteen non-responders were then treated with intralesional triamcinolone, and 13 achieved complete regrowth.

Clobetasol propionate 0.05% under occlusion in the treatment of alopecia totalis/universalis. Tosti A, Piraccini B, Pazzaglia M, Vincenzi C. J Am Acad Dermatol 2003; 49: 96–8.

Twenty-eight patients with AT/AU of 3–12 years' duration who had not responded to immunotherapy were treated on half of their scalp with 2.5 g of clobetasol propionate ointment under plastic film on 6 nights per week for 6 months. Regrowth started at 6–14 weeks, and eight patients (28.5%) achieved >75% regrowth, which was then extended to the other side of the scalp. Eleven patients developed painful folliculitis, including five of the six who withdrew from the study. After a further 6 months' follow-up 17.8% of the 28 patients retained complete regrowth.

Efficacy of betamethasone valerate foam formulation in comparison with betamethasone diproprionate lotion in the treatment of mild-moderate alopecia areata; a multicentre, prospective, randomised, controlled, investigator-blinded trial. Mancuso G, Balducci A, Casadio C, Farina P, Staffa M, Valenti L, et al. Int J Dermatol 2003; 42: 572–5.

In this investigator-blinded study 61 patients with mild to moderate hair loss (<26%) were treated with twice-daily applications of foam or lotion for 12 weeks. At week 20 more than 75% regrowth was achieved in 19 of the 31 patients treated with betamethasone valerate foam (61%), compared to eight out of 30 treated with betamethasone diproprionate lotion (27%), which was statistically significant.

Efficacy and safety of a new clobetasol proprionate 0.05% foam in alopecia areata: a randomised, double-blind, placebo-controlled trial. Tosti A, Iorizzo M, Botta G, Milani M. J Eur Acad Dermatol Venerol 2006; 20: 1243–7.

Thirty-four patients with moderate to severe AA (mean 50–75% scalp hair loss) were enrolled in this double-blind trial. Clobetasol foam or placebo foam was applied twice daily for 12 weeks using an inpatient design (right vs left) for 12 weeks, followed by extension of the most effective treatment to both sides of the scalp for a further 12 weeks. At 12 weeks 20% of clobetasol-treated sites achieved >50% regrowth, compared to 3% of placebo-treated sites. More than 75% regrowth occurred in only 9% of clobetasol-treated sites at week 24.

Alopecia areata: Current therapy. Fiedler VC. J Invest Dermatol 1991; 96(suppl): 69S.

A double-blind study of 5% minoxidil, 0.05% betamethasone dipropionate, both treatments and placebo. After 16 weeks response was fair to good in 13% of patients on placebo, 22% on betamethasone dipropionate, 27% on minoxidil, and 56% on the combined treatment (subject numbers and statistical analysis were not reported).

Alopecia areata treated with topical minoxidil. Fenton DA, Wilkinson JD. Br Med J 1983; 287: 1015–17.

A double-blind, crossover trial in which 30 subjects applied 1% minoxidil (lotion or ointment) and placebo twice daily, each for 3 months. By the end of the study 16 patients had grown cosmetically acceptable terminal hair, only one of them while on placebo.

A trial of 1% minoxidil used topically for severe alopecia areata. Vesty JP, Savin JA. Acta Dermatol Venereol 1986; 66: 179–80.

In this double-blind, placebo-controlled trial, 48 patients with severe AA, AT, and AU were treated for 32 weeks. There was no significant difference in response between the minoxidil and the placebo groups.

Topical minoxidil solution (1% and 5%) in the treatment of alopecia areata. Fiedler-Weiss VC. J Am Acad Dermatol 1987; 16: 745–8.

Sixty-six patients with >75% scalp hair loss applied treatments twice daily. Even in the high-dose group only 6% showed a cosmetically acceptable response. Occlusion of the treated area with white petrolatum at night was necessary to achieve maximum results.

PUVA treatment of alopecia totalis. Larko O, Swanbeck G. Acta Dermatol Venereol 1983; 63: 546–9.

Forty patients with AT were treated twice weekly with oral 8-methoxypsoralen and whole body or local irradiation. Fourteen patients responded, eight of whom experienced complete remission. This latter group required a mean of 44.5 sessions and 431 joules to achieve complete remission that lasted for a median of 10 weeks before relapse. Whole body treatment was not considered superior to local irradiation.

Treatment of alopecia areata with three different PUVA modalities. Lassus A, Eskelinen A, Johansson E. Photodermatology 1984; 1: 141–4.

Seventy-six patients with severe alopecia areata were treated with local or oral 8-methoxypsoralen and local or whole body UVA irradiation. In 43 cases (57%) a good-to-excellent result was obtained, with 20–40 treatments being sufficient in most cases. No particular treatment method was significantly superior. Patients with circumscribed or ophiasic alopecia responded better than patients with AT or AU. Disease duration, onset before the age of 20 years, and atopy were poor prognostic factors. During a follow-up period of 6–68 months, 22 patients had a relapse.

Effects of psoralen-UVA-turban in alopecia areata. Broniarczyk-Dyla G, Wawrzycka-Kaflik A, Dubla-Berner M, Prusinska-Bratos M. Skinmed 2006; 5: 64–8.

Twenty patients with treatment-resistant AA of 1–35 years' duration had 8-methoxypsoralen solution applied for 20 minutes with a cotton towel turban, followed by UVA. Treatment was performed two to three times weekly for a mean of 54 treatments, cumulative dose 48–253 J/cm². More than 80% regrowth occurred in 30% of patients; four of nine patients with AA, and two of 11 patients with AU/AT.

Treatment of alopecia areata by anthralin-induced dermatitis. Schmoeckel C, Weissmann I, Plewig G, Braun-Falco O. Arch Dermatol 1979; 115: 1254–5.

Anthralin 0.2–0.8% was applied daily to maintain dermatitis over involved areas of the scalp. A cosmetically good result was seen in 18 of 24 cases of AA and two of eight patients with AT. Untreated 'control' sites did not regrow. Regrowth was first visible after 5–8 weeks.

Evaluation of anthralin in the treatment of alopecia areata. Fiedler-Weiss VC, Buys CM. Arch Dermatol 1987; 123: 1491–3.

In this study using 0.5% and 1.0% concentrations of anthralin, the mean time to response was 11 weeks and the mean time to cosmetic response was 23 weeks (range 8–60 weeks). Cosmetic response was achieved in 29% (11/38) of patients with <75% scalp hair loss and in 20% (6/30) of patients with >75% scalp hair loss. Approximately 75% of responders maintained adequate hair growth with continued treatment.

Topical tretinoin as an adjunctive therapy with intralesional triamcinolone acetonide for alopecia areata. Clinical experience in northern Saudi Arabia. Kubeyinje EP, C'Mathur M. Int J Dermatol 1997; 36: 320.

In this open study 58 patients with mainly patchy alopecia were treated with monthly triamcinolone injections; 28 patients also had daily application of 0.05% tretinoin cream. More than 90% regrowth was achieved in 66.7% of patients with triamcinolone alone, and in 85.7% of patients with both treatments, which was statistically significant.

Allergic and irritant contact dermatitis compared in the treatment of alopecia totalis and universalis. A comparison of the value of topical diphencyprone and tretinoin gel. Ashworth J, Tuyp E, Mackie RM. Br J Dermatol 1989; 120: 397–401.

Seventeen patients (eight AT, nine AU) were treated by maintaining on one side of the scalp an allergic contact dermatitis induced by DPCP, and on the other side an irritant contact dermatitis using tretinoin gel. After 20 weeks, treatment with tretinoin was stopped and DPCP was applied bilaterally for a further 10 weeks. Some patients improved on DPCP, but there was no response to the tretinoin.

THIRD-LINE THERAPIES

▶ Systemic corticosteroids	B
▶ Systemic ciclosporin	C
▶ Topical ciclosporin	E
▶ Oral minoxidil	B
▶ Inosiplex (inosine pranobex)	B
▶ Nitrogen mustard	C
▶ Dermatography	B
▶ Cryotherapy	B
▶ Sulphasalazine	D
▶ Pulsed infrared diode laser	C
▶ Excimer laser	C
▶ Aromatherapy	B
▶ Onion juice	B

Placebo-controlled oral pulse prednisolone therapy in alopecia areata. Kar BR, Handa S, Dogra S, Kumar B. J Am Acad Dermatol 2005; 53: 1100–1.

Forty-three patients were randomized to receive oral prednisolone 200 mg weekly (23) or placebo (20) for 3 months. All patients had more than 40% scalp hair loss or more than 10 patches of AA, for more than 9 months. Eight of 23 in the treatment group showed more than 30% regrowth, compared to none in the placebo group. More than 60% regrowth occurred in only two patients (both in the treatment group). Side effects occurred in 55% of the treatment group, compared to 11% in the placebo group, although all were temporary.

Pulse corticosteroid therapy for alopecia areata: study of 139 patients. Nakajima T, Inui S, Itami S. Dermatology 2007; 215: 320–4.

In this uncontrolled study 139 patients, 73% of whom had more than 50% scalp hair loss, were treated with intravenous methylprednisolone 500 mg on 3 consecutive days. At 6 months' follow-up >75% regrowth was observed in 60% of patients with alopecia of <6 months' duration, but only 16% with alopecia for longer than 6 months. Of patients with AT for less than 6 months, 21% responded.

High-dose pulse corticosteroid therapy in the treatment of severe alopecia areata. Seiter S, Ugurel S, Tilgen W, Reinhold U. Dermatology 2001; 202: 230–4.

In this prospective open study 30 patients with >30% hair loss were treated with IV methylprednisolone (8 mg/kg) on 3 consecutive days at 4-week intervals for three courses. Twelve of 18 AA patients achieved >50% regrowth. None of four patients with AT, five with AU, or three with ophiasic AA responded. Ten patients retained the growth at 10 months' follow-up.

Oral cyclosporine for the treatment of alopecia areata. Gupta AK, Ellis CN, Cooper KD, Nickoloff BJ, Ho VC, Chan LS, et al. J Am Acad Dermatol 1990; 22: 242–50.

Six patients with alopecia were treated with oral ciclosporin, 6 mg/kg/day, for 12 weeks. Two had AA, one had AT, and three AU. Hair regrowth in the scalp of all patients occurred within the second and fourth weeks of therapy, but cosmetically acceptable regrowth occurred in only three. In no case did this persist 3 months after stopping the drug.

Systemic cyclosporine and low dose prednisolone in the treatment of chronic severe alopecia areata: a clinical and immunopathologic evaluation. Shapiro J, Lui H, Tron V, Ho V. J Am Acad Dermatol 1997; 36: 114–17.

Eight patients with alopecia involving at least 95% of the scalp were treated with a combination of ciclosporin 5 mg/kg/day and prednisolone 5 mg/day. Only two demonstrated a cosmetically satisfactory response. The addition of low-dose prednisolone did not produce any obvious benefit.

Placebo-controlled trial of topical cyclosporine in alopecia areata. deProst Y, Teillac D, Paquez F, Carrugi L, Bachelez H, Touraine R. Lancet 1986; 2: 803–4.

Forty-three patients with severe alopecia applied ciclosporin solution 100 mg/mL or placebo to their scalp once daily for 6 months. Small tufts of terminal hairs developed in seven subjects using ciclosporin, but in none of the controls. Regrowth was 'mild' and never complete.

Is topical tacrolimus effective in alopecia areata universalis? Feldmann KA, Kunte C, Wollenberg A, Wolff H. Br J Dermatol 2002; 147: 1031–2.

None of five patients with treatment-resistant and extensive AA treated with 0.1% topical tacrolimus showed evidence of hair regrowth.

Evaluation of oral minoxidil in the treatment of alopecia areata. Fiedler-Weiss VC, Rumsfield J, Buys CM, West DP, Wendrow A. Arch Dermatol 1987; 123: 1488–90.

Sixty-five patients with severe AA were treated with oral minoxidil 5 mg twice daily. Cosmetic response was reported in 18%. The drug was well tolerated at this dose, provided the recommended restriction on sodium intake (2 g daily) was observed. Higher sodium intake increased the risk of fluid retention.

Inosiplex for treatment of alopecia areata: a randomized placebo-controlled study. Georgala S, Katoulis AC, Befon A, Georgala K, Stavropoulos PG. Acta Dermatol Venereol 2006; 86: 422–4.

In this double-blind trial 32 subjects were randomized to receive oral inosiplex 50 mg/kg/day in five divided doses for 12 weeks, or placebo. Patients had treatment-resistant disease for 11–34 months, 22 with AA, nine with ophiasis, two with AT. In the 15 treatment patients who completed the trial 33% achieved full regrowth and 53% achieved more than 50% regrowth. None of the 14 placebo patients responded completely, and 28.5% achieved more than 50% regrowth. After a further 6 months tapering to half dose, no recurrences occurred.

A parallel study of inosine pranobex, diphencyprone and both treatments combined in the treatment of alopecia totalis. Berth-Jones J, Hutchinson PE. Clin Exp Dermatol 1991; 16: 172–5.

Thirty-three subjects with AT were randomized into three groups and treated with inosine pranobex 50 mg/kg/day, topical DPCP, or both. There was no response to inosine pranobex in the 22 subjects who received this treatment. Only two of 22 patients responded to DPCP.

Treatment of alopecia areata with topical nitrogen mustard. Arrazola JM, Sendagorta E, Harto A, Ledo A. Int J Dermatol 1985; 9: 608–10.

Cosmetically acceptable hair regrowth was seen in seven of 11 patients (including two of six with AT) after 4–8 weeks' self-treatment with mechlorethamine hydrochloride 0.2 mg/mL once daily. Two patients became sensitized and treatment was discontinued.

Topical nitrogen mustard in the treatment of alopecia areata: a bilateral comparison study. Bernardo O, Tang L, Lui H, Shapiro J. J Am Acad Dermatol 2003; 49: 291–4.

In this half-head controlled study 10 patients with AA for at least 1 year and >50% head involvement applied nitrogen mustard three times weekly for 16 weeks. A significant change was seen in only one patient, and another four did not complete the trial.

Dermatography as a new treatment for alopecia areata of the eyebrows. Van der Velden EM, Drost RHIM, Ijsselmuiden OE, Baruchin AM, Hulsebosch HJ. Int J Dermatol 1998; 37: 617–21.

Thirty-three patients with AA of the eyebrows were treated with dermatography. The eyebrow areas were covered with a halftone pattern of tiny dots of color pigments, using a Van der Velden Derma-injector, without anesthesia. On average, two or three dermatography sessions of 1 hour each were required. The follow-up was 4 years. The results were excellent in 30 patients and good in three.

Effect of superficial hypothermic cryotherapy with liquid nitrogen on alopecia areata. Lei Y, Nie Y, Zhang JM, Liao DY, Li HY, Man MQ. Arch Dermatol 1991; 127: 1851–2.

Seventy-two patients with AA involving >25% of their scalp (disease duration 3 days to 15 years) were treated with liquid nitrogen on a cotton swab for 2–3 seconds on a double freeze–thaw cycle. This was repeated weekly for 4 weeks. Forty comparable controls were treated with glacial acetic acid in a bland emollient vehicle three times a day for 4 weeks. More than 60% regrowth occurred in 70 (97.2%) of the active group, compared to 14 (35%) of the controls.

Sulfasalazine for alopecia areata. Ellis CN, Brown MF, Voorhees JJ. J Am Acad Dermatol 2002; 46: 541–4.

In this series of 39 patients treated with sulfasalazine, 11 withdrew treatment because of side effects and nine were lost to follow-up. Seven patients had cosmetically acceptable results. Based on the authors' experience, starting doses of 500 mg/day were suggested, increasing the dose steadily to achieve a dose of 3 g/day for at least 4 months. For an adequate trial of sulfasalazine, non-responding patients should receive 4 g/day for at least 3 additional months.

Topical photodynamic therapy with 5-aminolaevulinic acid does not induce hair regrowth in patients with extensive alopecia areata. Bissonnette R, Shapiro J, Zeng H, McLean DI, Lui H. Br J Dermatol 2000; 143: 1032–5.

This was a double-blind study with six patients having extensive AA. Topical ALA lotion at 5%, 10% and 20% as well as the vehicle lotion alone were applied separately to different scalp areas, followed 3 hours later by exposure to red light. No significant hair growth was observed after 20 twice-weekly treatment sessions. A significant increase in erythema and pigmentation was observed for the three concentrations of ALA lotion versus the vehicle, implying that a phototoxic PDT effect was achieved in the skin.

Use of the pulsed infrared diode laser (904 nm) in the treatment of alopecia areata. Waiz M, Saleh AZ, Hayani R, Jubory SO. J Cosmet Laser Ther 2006; 8: 27–30.

This was an open study of 16 patients with 34 patches of treatment-resistant alopecia, duration 12 months to 6 years. Patients were treated once weekly for four sessions with the 904 nm pulsed diode laser. Seven patients had control patches. Regrowth occurred in 32 patches (94%) but not in the seven control patches, and was maintained for the 2 months of follow-up.

308-nm excimer laser for the treatment of alopecia areata. Al-Mutairi N. Dermatol Surg 2007; 33: 1483–7.

Eighteen patients with 42 patches in of alopecia present for more than 6 months were treated twice weekly with the 308 nm excimer laser for 24 sessions. One patch in each patient was not treated; 41.5% of treated patches and 76.5% of scalp patches had cosmetically acceptable regrowth. No untreated patches regrew. Two patients relapsed at 6 months (number of patches not stated).

Randomized trial of aromatherapy. Successful treatment for alopecia areata. Hay IC, Jamieson M, Ormerod AD. Arch Dermatol 1998; 134: 1349–52.

In this double-blind controlled trial 86 patients were randomized into two groups. The active group massaged essential oils (thyme, rosemary, lavender and cedarwood) in a mixture of carrier oils (jojoba and grapeseed) into their scalp daily. The control group used only carrier oils for their massage. Nineteen (44%) of 43 patients in the active group showed improvement, compared to six (15%) of 41 patients in the control group.

Perhaps the nicest-smelling treatment!

Onion juice (*Allium cepa* L.), a new topical treatment for alopecia areata. Sharquie KE, Al-Obaidi HK. J Dermatol 2002; 29: 343–6.

Sixty-two patients with patchy alopecia were randomized to either topical onion juice or tap water twice daily for 2 months. Mean duration of disease was 3 weeks and 2.7 weeks, respectively. Twenty-three of the 45 onion juice group completed the trial, with full regrowth occurring in 20. In the tap water-treated group hair regrowth occurred in two of 17 patients. Mild erythema occurred in 14 of the onion juice group.

Probably the worst-smelling treatment!

Androgenetic alopecia

Walter P Unger, Robin H Unger, Carlos K Wesley

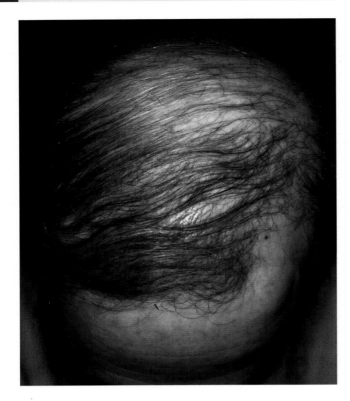

Since the 1940s male pattern baldness (MPB) has been recognized as an androgen-dependent condition. Eventually, dihydrotestosterone (DHT) was established as the key androgen involved in (a) the shortening of the anagen growth phase, and (b) the progressive follicular miniaturization that accompanies each hair growth, loss, and regrowth cycle – the two hallmarks of MPB. The role of androgens in female pattern hair loss (FPHL), however, remains uncertain and prevents us from defining pattern hair loss in both genders as androgenetic alopecia (AGA). Both MPB and FPHL are often familial and have a polygenetic inheritance pattern.

MANAGEMENT STRATEGY

Accurate diagnosis is a prerequisite for the effective treatment of MPB and FPHL. Alternative causes of alopecia that may mimic pattern hair loss must be ruled out and include diffuse alopecia areata, hair loss secondary to metabolic derangements, telogen effluvium, as well as other forms of temporary alopecia. Once this is accomplished through a review of patient history, clinical findings, and laboratory analyses, the objectives of stopping hair loss and promoting regrowth may be addressed.

Men may begin experiencing MPB any time after puberty. The frequency and severity increase with age, resulting in nearly 80% of Caucasian men having MPB by age 70. MPB may involve bitemporal, frontal, mid-scalp, or vertex scalp areas, and is most often described according to Hamilton–Norwood patterns of severity. FPHL tends to occur in either a 'Ludwig type' of diffuse central thinning or in a 'Christmas tree' pattern, with the wide base of the 'tree' located just posterior to the frontal hairline. Dawber found that 87% of a clinic sampling of premenopausal women *without hair loss as a complaint* had Ludwig type I–III loss. A male pattern of hair loss may also occur in women, with 79% of postpubertal women developing Hamilton–Norwood type II MPB that progresses to Hamilton–Norwood type IV MPB in 25% by age 50, and in 50% of them by age 60.

Medical therapy is appropriate first-line management for both MPB and FPHL. The goal is to slow the rate of hair loss and/or to reverse the miniaturization process. Currently, two medications have been approved by the US FDA for these purposes: topical *minoxidil* (a biological response modifier) and oral *finasteride* (a hormone modifier). Topical 2–5% minoxidil increases the duration of the anagen hair growth phase, enlarges miniaturized follicles, and has a vasodilatory effect. Application of 1 mL to the scalp twice daily results in peak hair growth after 26–52 weeks, with the crown showing the best response and the frontal area the least. Although 5% minoxidil is superior to 2% in increasing hair count and hair weight for MPB, adverse dermatologic effects, most commonly scalp irritation, are more common with the 5% solution (a side effect seen less frequently when the 5% is in a 'foam' base). Currently, only the 2% strength is FDA approved for use on women. Cessation of treatment results in reversal of the positive effect within 4–6 months. Anecdotally, combining topical minoxidil with finasteride (see below) sometimes produces superior results to those seen with either of these medications alone.

Finasteride is a competitive inhibitor of type 2 5α-reductase, the enzyme involved in converting testosterone to its metabolite, DHT. An almost 70% reduction in serum and scalp DHT levels can be achieved with finasteride therapy in men. In clinical trials of crown MPB, after 5 years hair counts were increased in 65% of the subjects (versus 0% of those on placebo), and further loss was slowed in 90% (versus 25% of the corresponding placebo group). In other studies, the best response was again seen in the crown and the least in the frontal area. Finasteride is a teratogen, and has been shown to be ineffective in postmenopausal women. Side effects in men are infrequent, affecting less than 2% of patients. They are completely reversed after discontinuation of the drug and often resolve during continued treatment. A 7-year clinical trial demonstrated a 24.8% reduction in the overall incidence of prostate cancer in patients on finasteride versus the placebo. Subsequent analyses revealed finasteride-related risk reductions of 30% for prostate cancer in general and 27% for high-grade prostate cancer, as well as suggesting increased prostate biopsy sensitivity with finasteride use.

Although there is a dearth of well-controlled clinical trials involving other anti-androgens, such as *spironolactone* and *cyproterone acetate*, in women, it appears that the value of these medications is most pronounced in women with hyperandrogenism.

Fortunately, for many patients with MBP and FPHL that is refractory to medical therapy, advances in surgical techniques make *hair transplantation* a reliably effective option. The perfecting and worldwide adoption of 'follicular unit transplanting' (FUT) has yielded natural-appearing results combined with cosmetically good hair density per session, that was not possible until approximately 5–10 years ago. Improvements in the surgical approach now allow many female patients, as well as men in the early stages of MPB, to benefit from this procedure. Furthermore, previously 'pluggy' transplants can now often be 'retrofitted' to make them appear natural in patients who chose to address their hair loss surgically prior to the evolution of FUT.

Cosmetic aids can also provide relief to patients with hair loss if medical treatments are either ineffective, not indicated, or if they are simply preferred as an adjuvant by the patient. Thinning hair can be camouflaged by coloring the scalp with tinted powders or sprays, as well as by the wearing of wigs and hair pieces. On the other hand, hair 'extension,' in which bunches of hairs are attached to individual scalp hairs, is generally discouraged owing to the potential for the development of permanent scarring traction alopecia.

SPECIFIC INVESTIGATIONS FOR FEMALES

> ▶ Work-up for polycystic ovarian syndrome
> ▶ Free testosterone, DHT serum levels
> ▶ Serum ferritin
> ▶ Thyroid function tests
> ▶ 4 mm diameter scalp biopsy

Evaluation and treatment of male and female pattern hair loss. Olsen EA, Messenger AG, Shapiro J, Bergfeld WF, Hordinsky MK, Roberts JL, et al. J Am Acad Dermatol 2005; 52: 301–11.

A thorough review providing current information on the potential pathophysiology, clinical presentation, and histology of MPB and FPHL. Also includes a consensus opinion of an approach to the evaluation and treatment of these conditions.

Hair loss in women. Shapiro J. N Engl J Med 2007; 357: 1620–30.

Using a case vignette, this review emphasizes effective evaluation of FPHL through history taking and clinical findings. Characteristics of non-scarring alopecia and investigative strategies are highlighted.

Androgens and alopecia. Kaufman KD. Mol Cell Endocrinol 2002; 198: 89–95.

An analysis of advances in our understanding of the role of androgens in the development of MPB and FPHL that suggests a pathophysiologic distinction between the two conditions.

MEDICAL THERAPIES

> ▶ Topical minoxidil (2% and 5%) once or twice daily   **A**
> ▶ Finasteride 1 mg once a day   **A**
> ▶ Spironolactone 100 to 200 mg/day   **B**
> ▶ Cyproterone acetate 50–100 mg/day for days 5 to 10 of menstrual cycle, combined with oral estinyl 20 mg twice daily, days 5–24 of cycle   **B**

The finasteride male pattern hair loss study group: Long-term (5 year) multinational experience with finasteride 1 mg in the treatment of men with androgenetic alopecia. Kaufman KD. Eur J Dermatol 2002; 12: 38–49.

Finasteride reduces tissue and circulating levels of DHT by two-thirds. A 5-year double-blind, placebo-controlled study of 588 men with AGA revealed that finasteride 1 mg daily was well tolerated, led to durable improvements in scalp hair growth, and slowed further progression of hair loss that occurred without treatment (p<0.001).

Although the mean hair count was higher in treated patients versus those on placebo, the improvement from baseline tapered off near the conclusion of the study.

A randomized, placebo-controlled trial of 5% and 2% topical minoxidil solutions in the treatment of female pattern hair loss. Lucky AW, Piacquadio DJ, Ditre CM, Dunlap F, Kantor I, Pandya AB, et al. J Am Acad Dermatol 2004; 50: 541–53.

Treatment with both 5% and 2% minoxidil resulted in significantly enhanced hair counts and investigator assessment versus treatment with placebo after 48 weeks. Although patient perception of hair growth was statistically superior in the 5% versus the 2% treatment, no unequivocal dose-dependent improvement was demonstrated in either non-vellus hair count or investigator-rated hair density. Interestingly, the peak efficacy in both treatment groups was noted at the 16-week evaluation, with counts beginning to decline progressively at weeks 32 and 48.

Minoxidil versus finasteride in the treatment of men with androgenetic alopecia. Saraswat A, Kumar B. Arch Dermatol 2003; 139: 1219–21.

In the first efficacy comparison of the only two FDA-approved agents that promote hair regrowth (topical 2% minoxidil and oral finasteride) both treatments were similarly effective in halting progression of moderate AGA in 99 men. Over this 12-month trial, minoxidil produced a faster initial improvement, whereas finasteride's marginal augmentation of both total hair and thick hair counts increased with duration of treatment.

Treatment of female pattern hair loss with oral anti-androgens. Sinclair R, Wewerinke M, Jolley D. Br J Dermatol 2005; 152: 466–73.

The results of this study of 80 women treated with either spironolactone or cyproterone acetate indicated a positive effect with treatment. In the treatment group 44% of women showed regrowth, 44% demonstrated no progression of hair loss, and 12% continued with progressive hair loss. Women with more severe baseline FPHL were more likely to be responders. This study does not compare results with a placebo group, nor were the investigators blinded.

The influence of finasteride on the development of prostate cancer. Thompson IM, Goodman PJ, Tangen CM, Lucia SM, Miller GJ, Ford LG, et al. N Engl J Med 2003; 349: 215–24.

A long-term (7-year) prostate cancer prevention trial (PCPT) of 18882 men comparing 5 mg finasteride with placebo revealed a 24.8% reduction in prostate cancer for those on finasteride. However, finasteride-treated men developed histologically high-grade cancer more frequently (6.4% vs 5.1%). Sexual side effects were more common among men taking finasteride, whereas urinary symptoms were more frequent in the placebo group.

A follow-up study by the same group of investigators revealed finasteride biases to increase prostate cancer detection and more accurate grading of prostate cancer at biopsy.

Finasteride does not increase the risk of high-grade prostate cancer: A bias-adjusted modeling approach. Redman MW, Tangen CM, Goodman PJ, Lucia MS, Coltman CA, Thompson IM. Cancer Prev Res 2008; Online First 2008.

Extending PCPT data analysis to eliminate the effect of aforementioned biases on prostate cancer detection, this group found a 30% risk reduction in prostate cancer in finasteride (5 mg)-treated patients, a 27% risk reduction of high-grade cancer when integrating prostatectomy data, and a likely increased biopsy sensitivity with finasteride.

SURGICAL THERAPIES

▶ Follicular unit transplantation	A
▶ Alopecia reduction	C
▶ Follicular unit extraction	C
▶ Camouflage	D

Hair transplanting: An important but often forgotten treatment for female pattern hair loss. Unger WP, Unger RH. J Am Acad Dermatol 2003; 853–60.

Women can consistently expect natural-appearing and significantly thicker hair with the improved current surgical techniques of hair transplantation. The vast majority of women are candidates for surgery, and this option should be considered in women presenting with female pattern hair loss who do not respond to medical treatment or find such treatments unsatisfactory.

The interview: patient selection. Unger WP. In: Unger WP, Shapiro R, eds. Hair transplantation, 4th edn. New York: Marcel Dekker, 2004; 165–88.

In addition to educating the patient, the initial meeting establishes patient–doctor compatibility and can foster a mutual understanding of realistic short- and long-term goals.

Evolution of techniques in hair transplantation: a 12-year perspective. Epstein JS. Facial Plast Surg 2007; 23: 51–9.

A retrospective analysis of the evolution of hair restoration surgery, including the technical refinements, increased breadth of application, and maturation of the surgical field itself.

Follicular unit extraction: minimally invasive surgery for hair transplantation. Rassman WR, Bernstein RM, McClellan R, Jones R, Worton E, Uyttendaele H. Dermatol Surg 2002; 28: 720–8.

An exploration of the nuances, limitations, and practical aspects of this surgical technique, which circumvents the need for linear donor strip excision.

Correction of cosmetic problems in hair transplanting. Unger WP. In: Unger WP, Shapiro R, eds. Hair transplantation, 4th edn. New York: Marcel Dekker, 2004; 663–87.

The adoption of micro-minigrafting and follicular unit transplanting allows for effective correction of 'pluggy' transplants performed over a decade ago.

Angiolymphoid hyperplasia with eosinophilia

William Y-M Tang, Loi-yuen Chan

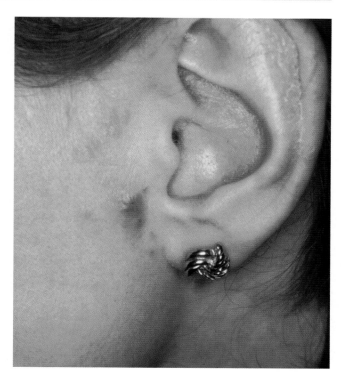

Angiolymphoid hyperplasia with eosinophilia (ALHE) was first described by Wells and Whimster in 1969. Synonyms include epithelioid hemangioma, pseudo- or atypical pyogenic granuloma, inflammatory angiomatous nodule, and histiocytoid hemangioma. It is a benign vascular proliferation of unknown etiology with a characteristic component of epithelioid endothelial cells. It is an uncommon disease, so data on its natural course and treatment response are based on a small number of patients.

ALHE usually affects women in their third decade and presents as cutaneous papules or subcutaneous nodules, sometimes with inflammatory features, on the head, neck, and periauricular region. Involvement elsewhere is rare. Approximately 20% of patients have blood eosinophilia. Malignant transformation has not been observed. Although benign in nature, there may be disfigurement, bleeding, and pain. The etiology of ALHE is unknown, but neoplastic proliferation of vascular tissue, or reactive hyperplasia of vascular tissue secondary to trauma, infection, renin, or hyperestrogenic states have been proposed as causal factors.

The previous alleged overlap with Kimura's disease is incorrect: ALHE and Kimura's disease are separate clinico-pathological entities. Kimura's disease is a chronic inflammatory condition of unknown etiology often affecting young male Orientals, and typically presents as cervical lymphadenopathy and subcutaneous nodules in the head and neck region. It is often associated with blood and tissue eosinophilia, and raised serum immunoglobulin E (IgE).

MANAGEMENT STRATEGY

Treatment is usually required for ALHE, as spontaneous remission is rare. Complete *surgical excision* is preferred for persistent lesions. Recurrence may occur if excision is incomplete. *Laser ablation, electrosurgery,* and *cryotherapy* are alternative surgical options. Other agents that have positive therapeutic effects include *topical and intralesional corticosteroids, topical imiquimod, topical tacrolimus, isotretinoin, intralesional interferon-α_{2b}* and *intravenous anti-IL-5 antibody. Systemic corticosteroid* and *radiotherapy* would seem appropriate only for severely disabling disease unresponsive to less toxic therapies.

SPECIFIC INVESTIGATIONS

> ▶ Histopathology
> ▶ Imaging

Microscopically, ALHE is characterized by a proliferation of capillaries and small vessels with plump, round, oval, or cuboidal endothelial cells that protrude into the lumen, creating a cobblestone appearance. There is also an accompanied perivascular lymphocytic and eosinophilic infiltrate.

The location and extent of underlying vascular anomalies may be assessed by angiography, angiomagnetic resonance imaging, and angio-computed tomography.

Owing to its predominant occurrence in females, hyperestrogenic states may have a causative role in ALHE. However, successful treatment of ALHE using hormonal therapy has not yet been reported.

Angiolymphoid hyperplasia with eosinophilia associated with pregnancy: a case report and review of the literature. Zarrin-Khameh N, Spoden JE, Tran RM. Arch Pathol Lab Med 2005; 129: 1168–71.

The authors report a 33-year-old woman who developed ALHE in her right ear during the second trimester of pregnancy. The lesion was completely excised. The authors also reviewed a total of five other ALHE cases associated with pregnancy, some of which improved with discontinuation of oral contraceptive pills.

FIRST-LINE THERAPIES

> ▶ Surgery   **D**
> ▶ Laser therapy   **D**
> ▶ Corticosteroid, topical or intralesional   **E**
> ▶ Cryotherapy   **E**
> ▶ Electrosurgery   **E**

Angiolymphoid hyperplasia with eosinophilia and vascular tumors of the head and neck. Don DM, Ishiyama A, Johnstone AK, Fu YS, Abemayor E. Am J Otolaryngol 1996; 17: 240–5.

A review of eight patients with confirmed ALHE showed that low-dose irradiation, intralesional corticosteroids, and cryotherapy were not successful. The authors suggested that the preferred treatment is complete surgical extirpation. Recurrence is common when the lesions are inadequately excised.

Eradication of angiolymphoid hyperplasia with eosinophilia by copper vapor laser. Fosko SW, Glaser DA, Rogers CJ. Arch Dermatol 2001; 137: 863–5.

Two patients with ALHE were successfully treated with copper vapor laser (578 nm). In the first case, five treatments were given to each lesion. A spot size of 267 μm, dwell time 100 ms on and 100 ms off, and power 660 mW were used. Three treatments were given to another patient using a spot size of 150 μm or 267 μm, dwell time of 75 ms on and 100 ms off, and power from 750 to 960 mW. The first patient showed gross clearing of lesions. In the second patient there was no recurrence after 6 years.

Treatment of angiolymphoid hyperplasia with eosinophilia with the carbon dioxide laser. Kaur T, Sandhu K, Gupta S, Kanwar AJ, Kumar B. J Dermatol Treat 2004; 15: 328–30.

A 35-year-old woman presented with a 1×1.5 cm ALHE lesion on her left external ear canal for 1 year was treated with CO_2 laser, energy 6 J and pulse duration 0.01 s, repeated at 0.1 s intervals for a total of 140 pulses. There was no recurrence during the 3-month follow-up period after this single treatment session.

Angiolymphoid hyperplasia with eosinophilia responsive to pulsed dye laser. Abrahamson TG, Davis DA. J Am Acad Dermatol 2003; 49: S195–6.

A 41-year-old woman with ALHE over her right ear received four treatments with a 585 nm pulsed dye laser with a 5 mm spot size at energy densities 6.5–7.25 J/cm^2 at 6-week intervals, and showed clearing of lesions. There was no clinical recurrence at 7 months after the fourth treatment.

Rapid remission of severe pruritus from angiolymphoid hyperplasia with eosinophilia by pulsed dye laser therapy. Nomura T, Sato-Matsumura KC, Kikuchi T, Abe M, Shimizu H. Clin Exp Dermatol 2003; 28: 595–6.

A 48-year-old Japanese woman presented with multiple pruritic, tender, slowly growing ALHE lesions over her right ear and postauricular region. She was treated with a 585 nm flashlamp pulsed dye laser with a spot size of 7 mm at energy densities 7 J/cm^2. The severe pruritus improved immediately after the first treatment. A total of five treatments were given over approximately 4 months. No clinical recurrence was noted 1 year after completion of treatment.

Angiolymphoid hyperplasia successfully treated with an ultralong pulsed dye laser. Angel CA, Lewis AT, Griffin T, Levy EJ, Benedetto AV. Dermatol Surg 2005; 31: 713–16.

A 72-year-old man with ALHE for 1 year not responding to intralesional steroid was successfully treated with two sessions of ultralong pulsed dye laser (595 nm). There was no recurrence 3 years after treatment. The longer wavelength produces deeper penetration into dermal tissue and more uniform coagulation necrosis across the entire diameter of the targeted blood vessel.

Treatment using pulsed dye laser is based on the principle of selective photothermolysis, causing destruction of blood vessels in the lesions. It appears that long-pulsed tunable dye laser, which can deliver a longer target wavelength with wider pulse duration, enables destruction of deeper and larger vessels and provides a higher chance of cure. Carbon dioxide and argon laser have also been used with success in treating ALHE, but their use is limited because of the greater chance of post-treatment scarring.

SECOND-LINE THERAPIES

► Imiquimod	E
► Tacrolimus	E
► Isotretinoin	E

Angiolymphoid hyperplasia with eosinophilia successfully treated with imiquimod. Redondo P, Del Olmo J, Idoate M. Br J Dermatol 2004; 151: 1110–11.

A 37-year-old white woman presented with ALHE lesions on her left ear and preauricular area for 8 years. She was treated with 5% imiquimod cream five times a week. After 16 weeks of treatment there was almost complete clinical resolution. There was erythema, pain, and tenderness during the second week, and treatment was withdrawn for 7 days.

Angiolymphoid hyperplasia with eosinophilia successfully treated with imiquimod. A case report. Gencoglan G, Karaca S, Ertekin B. Dermatology 2007; 215: 233–5.

A 48-year-old man with several ALHE lesions behind his right ear, measuring 0.5–1 cm in diameter, was treated with 5% imiquimod cream twice daily, 5 days per week for 2 weeks. He had complete clinical resolution, and no recurrence was observed during 2 years of follow-up. The underlying mechanism may be related to the immunomodulating and anti-angiogenic effect of imiquimod.

A case of angiolymphoid hyperplasia with eosinophilia successfully treated with tacrolimus ointment. Mashiko M, Yokota K, Yamanaka Y, Furuya K. Br J Dermatol 2006; 154: 803–4.

A 33-year-old Japanese woman with ALHE over her left ear for a year was treated with 0.1% tacrolimus ointment twice daily. The lesions disappeared within 4 months. Continuous application resulted in no recurrence in 9 months. The underlying mechanism may be due to tacrolimus ointment reducing eosinophil counts in tissue and suppressing eosinophil function.

As the number of patients treated with imiquimod and tacrolimus is still small, further studies are required to clarify their therapeutic role in ALHE.

Angiolymphoid hyperplasia with eosinophilia: efficacy of isotretinoin? El Sayed F, Dhaybi R, Ammoury A, Chababi M. Head Face Med 2006; 2: 32.

The authors report a 32-year-old man with multiple ALHE lesions treated with isotretinoin 0.5 mg/kg/day for 1 year with complete resolution of scalp nodules. Other lesions on the cheeks and preauricular region remained stable and were surgically removed. The success of isotretinoin was due to its anti-angiogenic properties via a reduction of vascular endothelial growth factor production by keratinocytes.

THIRD-LINE THERAPIES

► Interferon-α$_{2b}$	E
► Anti-IL-5 antibody	E
► Suplatast tosilate	E
► Radiotherapy	E
► Systemic corticosteroid	E

Evidence Levels: **A** Double-blind study **B** Clinical trial ≥ 20 subjects **C** Clinical trial < 20 subjects **D** Series ≥ 5 subjects **E** Anecdotal case reports

Angiolymphoid hyperplasia with eosinophilia responding to interferon-alpha 2B. Oguz O, Antonov M, Demirkesen C. J Eur Acad Dermatol Venereol 2007; 21: 1277–8.

Interferon-α is the first-line treatment in benign angioproliferative disorders. Local intralesional injection of interferon-α$_{2b}$ is an effective treatment for ALHE, but recurrence of lesions 9 years later shows a poor response to repeated treatment.

Including this one, two cases of ALHE treated by interferon-α$_{2b}$ have been reported so far. In both cases the efficacy was reduced when treating recurrent lesions.

Angiolymphoid hyperplasia with eosinophilia treated with anti-interleukin-5 antibody (mepolizumab). Braun-Falco M, Fischer S, Plötz SG, Ring J. Br J Dermatol 2004; 151: 1103–4.

Interleukin-5 is the major cytokine involved in the production, mobilization, and activation of eosinophils. A single intravenous dose of anti-IL-5 antibody therapy was given to a 76-year-old Caucasian man with a painful, pulsatile 7 × 6 × 3 cm ALHE nodule behind his left ear. The patient became asymptomatic the next day, and there was a slight softening of the lesion. The benefit lasted for approximately 3 weeks.

Angiolymphoid hyperplasia with eosinophilia: successful treatment with the antiallergic agent suplatast tosilate. Harada K, Kambe Y, Takeda H, Nakano H, Hanada K. Dermatology 2004; 208: 176–7.

Suplatast tosilate is an anti-allergic agent on the market in Japan. It was reported to exert an inhibitory effect of IL-4 and -5 production in helper T cells, resulting in reduced eosinophil infiltration and suppression of IgE production in B cells. A 32-year-old man with ALHE not responding to topical steroid, cryotherapy, indomethacin farnesil, and oral betamethasone received suplatast tosilate 300 mg/day. A reduction of pruritus was noted after 1 week and a reduction of nodule size after 1 month of treatment. The skin lesions almost disappeared after 5 months of treatment and the dose was reduced to 200 mg/day.

The role of suplatast tosilate in ALHE is at present unclear.

Angiolymphoid hyperplasia with eosinophilia of the nail bed and bone: successful treatment with radiation therapy. Conill C, Toscas I, Mascaro J Jr, Vilalta A, Mascaro J. J Eur Acad Dermatol Venereol 2004; 18: 584–5.

The authors reported a 32-year-old Caucasian woman with multiple ALHE nodules involving the skin, subcutaneous tissue, and bone of the distal phalanx of the fingers treated successfully with orthovoltage radiation therapy (40 Gy in 20 fractions) and without any side effects after 9 years of follow-up.

Considering the benign nature of ALHE and the potential carcinogenicity of radiotherapy, the latter should only be given when other treatment modalities have failed. Systemic steroids can be tried, but abrupt withdrawal may precipitate recurrence.

Angular cheilitis

Alison J Bruce, Roy S Rogers, III

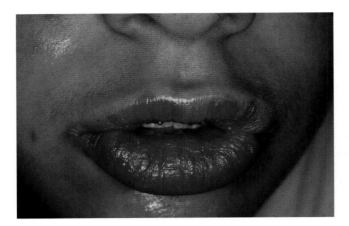

Angular cheilitis is a chronic inflammatory condition of the commissures of the lips characterized by atrophy, fissures, crusting, erythema, and scaling. Angular cheilitis is a reaction pattern with one or more causes, including mechanical (intertrigo), infectious, nutritional, or inflammatory disease. Angular cheilitis may be the sign of a systemic disease such as diabetes mellitus or HIV infection.

MANAGEMENT STRATEGY

Successful therapy is based on identifying and correcting each and all factors of this multifactorial condition. Examination for dentures and palatal erythema and edema suggests candidiasis and denture stomatitis. A pale, depapillated, atrophic tongue suggests iron deficiency. A tender, glossy, depapillated tongue suggests folate or vitamin B_{12} deficiency. An eczematous dermatitis of the lower face suggests a staphylococcal infection.

Unilateral lesions are usually short-lived and induced by trauma. Bilateral lesions tend to be chronic and caused by infection or nutritional deficiency, and are more likely to be associated with an underlying disease process.

Maceration of the commissural epithelium and adjacent skin is a common, non-infectious cause of mechanical angular cheilitis. Trauma from dental flossing, habitual lip licking, and excessive salivation all contribute. Periods of oral hydration and then dryness disrupt epithelial integrity, with fissuring of the commissures. This provides an ideal environment for low-grade candidiasis and infectious eczematoid dermatitis.

Other traumatic factors are denture wearing, loss of vertical dimension of the jaws, sagging skin folds, xerostomia, orofacial granulomatosis, and perioral dermatitis.

Infectious causes must be sought. Angular cheilitis is frequently present in patients with HIV disease, where 10% may have localized candidiasis. Both *Candida albicans* and *Staphylococcus aureus* can colonize the fissures. Anemia, nutritional deficiencies, diabetes mellitus, Crohn's disease, and acrodermatitis enteropathica may be present.

Recurrence of angular cheilitis may be prevented by eliminating offending organisms from their reservoirs. Denture stomatitis, candidiasis, and nasal colonization of staphylococci should be sought. The organisms are treated with *topical miconazole cream* after meals and at bedtime. *Topical mupirocin* is valuable in treating staphylococcal colonization. Dentures should be removed from the mouth at night and cleansed well before being reinserted in the morning. *New dentures* may restore facial contours, increasing the vertical dimension of the jaws and face. *Injection of collagen* into the commissures may alleviate causative mechanical factors.

SPECIFIC INVESTIGATIONS

> ▶ Culture for candidiasis
> ▶ Culture for bacteria
> ▶ Medical evaluation as per burning mouth syndrome
> ▶ HIV testing
> ▶ Patch testing

Diseases of the lips. Rogers RS III, Bekic M. Semin Cutan Med Surg 1997; 16: 325–36.

A discussion of the multifactorial nature and evaluation of angular cheilitis.

Angular cheilosis: An analysis of 156 cases. Konstantinidis AB, Hatziotis JH. J Oral Med 1984; 39: 199–205.

A careful analysis of the cause(s) of angular cheilitis in 156 patients.

Emphasizes that more than a single cause was often present.

Angular cheilitis. In: Scully C, Bagan J-V, Eisen D, Porter S, Rogers RS III, eds. Dermatology of the lips. Oxford: Isis Medical, 2000; 68–73.

Excellent clinical photographs and summary.

Nickel-induced angular cheilitis due to orthodontic braces. Yesudian PD, Memon A. Contact Dermatitis 2003; 48: 287–8.

Down syndrome: lip lesions (angular stomatitis and fissures) and *Candida albicans*. Scully C, can Bruggen W, Diz Dios P, Casal B, Porter S, Davison MF. Br J Dermatol 2002; 147: 37–40.

Angular cheilitis was seen in 25% of patients with trisomy 21.

FIRST-LINE THERAPIES

> ▶ Topical miconazole cream   **D**
> ▶ Topical fusidic acid, polymyxin B or mupirocin ointments   **D**
> ▶ Remove dentures at night and cleanse before reinserting   **D**

Clinical management of oral and perioral candidiasis. Fotos PG, Lilly JP. Dermatol Clin 1996; 14: 273–80.

An excellent description of topical and systemic therapy of candidiasis.

Diseases of the lips. Rogers RS III, Bekic M. Semin Cutan Med Surg 1997; 16: 325–36.

Discussion of the multifactorial nature, evaluation, and treatment of angular cheilitis.

Angular cheilitis. Schoenfeld RJ, Schoenfeld FI. Cutis 1977; 19: 213–16.

Discussion of the differential diagnosis, causes, and management of angular cheilitis.

Treatment of angular cheilitis. The significance of microbial analysis, antimicrobial treatment and interfering factors. Ohman SC, Jentell M. Acta Odontol Scand 1988; 46: 267–72.

SECOND-LINE THERAPIES

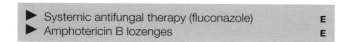

► Systemic antifungal therapy (fluconazole)	E
► Amphotericin B lozenges	E

Treatment of oral *Candida* mucositis infections. Garber GE. Drugs 1994; 47: 734–40.

Reviews the treatment of infections due to *Candida*, high-lighting challenges in the immunocompromised patient.

THIRD-LINE THERAPIES

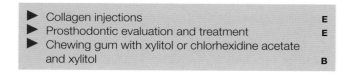

► Collagen injections	E
► Prosthodontic evaluation and treatment	E
► Chewing gum with xylitol or chlorhexidine acetate and xylitol	B

Microlipoinjection and autologous collagen. Pinski KS, Coleman III WP. Dermatol Clin 1995; 13: 339–51.

Although these procedures may need to be repeated, mechanical correction of the deep furrows at the oral commissures can be very rewarding for the patient.

Prosthodontic management of angular cheilitis and persistent drooling: a case report. Lu DP. Compend Coutin Educ Deut 2007; 28: 572–7.

This paper describes a case of persistent drooling and angular cheilitis, which is not uncommon in the elderly. Drug therapy and the temporomandibular joint aspect of the vertical dimension of occlusion during prosthodontic evaluation and construction are discussed. The author describes a method to incorporate a cannula into the denture prosthesis to channel the saliva toward the oropharyngeal area, suitable for geriatric handicapped patients who suffer from chronic drooling and angular cheilitis.

The effects of medicated chewing gums on oral health in frail older people: a 1 year clinical trial. Simons D, Brailsford SR, Kidd EA, Beighton D. J Am Geriatr Soc 2002; 50: 1348–53.

A controlled, double-blind trial of 111 dentate patients in residential homes assessed the effect of a medicated chewing gum on oral health. The reductions in denture stomatitis and angular cheilitis in the group using chlorhexidine acetate/xylitol gums were significant.

Anogenital warts

Brian Berman, Sadegh Amini, Ran Huo

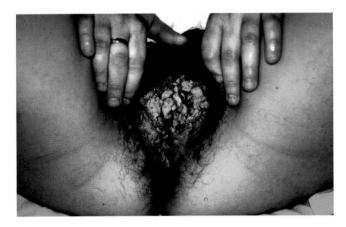

External anogenital warts develop on the skin and mucosal surfaces of the genitalia and perianal areas. They are caused by the human papillomavirus (HPV), with at least 40 of the more than 100 types identified capable of infecting the genital tract. Condyloma acuminata (CA), the classic form of anogenital wart, and the more difficult to detect flat condylomata, are frequently associated with 'benign' HPV types 6 and 11 (up to 95%), but may also be caused by oncogenic HPV types such as 16, 18, 31, 33, and 35.

MANAGEMENT STRATEGY

Most cases of genital warts are asymptomatic; however, they can be disfiguring, lead to physical discomfort, induce psychological suffering, guilt, anger and doubt, and severely affect the patient's quality of life. Untreated genital warts may increase in size or number, remain unchanged, or resolve spontaneously.

The treatment of external genital warts depends on several factors, including the patient's preference, resource availability, and healthcare provider experience.

Current trends in treatment focus on stimulation of the host's immune system response to enhance virus recognition. Available treatments can be categorized as either patient-applied or provider-administered. The former includes *podofilox 0.5% solution or gel* and *imiquimod 5% cream*. Podofilox (podophyllotoxin) is applied twice daily for 3 days, then no treatment for 4 days, for four to six cycles, if necessary.

Imiquimod 5% cream stimulates the host's immune response via cytokine induction and Langerhans' cell activation. It is applied overnight and washed off 6–10 h after application, three times a week, until clearance of the warts or a maximum of 16 weeks.

The provider-administered therapies are either topically applied or surgical. Topical modalities include *podophyllin resin 10–25%, podofilox (podophyllotoxin), bichloroacetic acid (BCA)* and *trichloroacetic acid (TCA)*. Surgical treatments include *cryotherapy, surgical removal* either by tangential shave using a cold knife or tangential scissor excisions, *curettage* with or without electrosurgery and *lasers* (CO_2 and pulsed dye laser – PDL). Intralesional interferon-α has also been reported to be effective. Podophyllin-applied resin is applied for 1–6 h and is less effective on dry areas such as the penile shaft, scrotum, and labia majora.

The safety of podofilox (category C) and imiquimod 5% (category C) during pregnancy has not been established. Both TCA and BCA 80–90% solutions are applied weekly as needed.

Cryotherapy causes thermolysis and necrosis of keratinocytes hosting HPV. Liquid nitrogen, either with cryospray or cryoprobe, usually requires one to two free–thaw cycles per session for two to three sessions. However, HPV DNA is detectable up to 1 cm from the wart's periphery, limiting the practicality of destructive modalities.

Surgery and CO_2 lasers are useful for treating extensive, intraurethral, and recalcitrant warts.

Recombinant HPV quadrivalent (6–11–16–18) vaccine is safe and efficacious in reducing the incidence of persistent anogenital warts and cervical cancer by 90%, and is approved by the Food and Drug Administration for females 9 to 26 years of age. Currently, it is not recommended in males.

Sinecatechin extract of green tea from *Camellia sinensis* was recently approved by the FDA for the treatment of external genital and perianal warts. It contains epigallocatechin gallate, which protects cells from oxidative damage, induces apoptosis, and inhibits telomerase activity.

Estimates of clearance and recurrence rates with various therapies are difficult owing to differences in method of analysis, patient population, and duration of follow-up. Over the years many treatment modalities have emerged, but no single treatment has proved superior to the others. No available therapy can be guaranteed to clear genital warts without any recurrence. Combination therapy using an immunomodulator after a physical ablative therapy has shown to reduce recurrence rates, but the possibility of additive adverse events should be taken in consideration.

SPECIFIC INVESTIGATIONS

▶ Papanicolaou (Pap) smear
▶ HPV typing (not standard of care)

Evaluation of human papillomavirus testing in primary screening for cervical abnormalities: comparison of sensitivity, specificity, and frequency of referral. Kulasingam SL, Hughes JP, Kiviat NB, Mao C, Weiss NS, Kuypers JM, Koutsky LA. JAMA 2002; 288: 1749–57.

Testing for HPV has higher sensitivity but lower specificity than thin-layer Pap screening. In some settings, particularly where screening intervals are long or haphazard, screening for HPV DNA may be a reasonable alternative to cytology-based screening in women of reproductive age.

FIRST-LINE THERAPIES

▶ Imiquimod 5% cream	A
▶ Podofilox (podophyllotoxin)	A
▶ Sinecatechin extract of green tea	A
▶ Podophyllin	B
▶ Cryotherapy	B

Imiquimod, a patient-applied immune response modifier for treatment of external genital warts. Beutner KR, Tyring SK, Trofatter KF, Douglas JM Jr, Spruance S, Owens ML, et al. Antimicrob Agents Chemother 1998; 42: 789–94.

A multicenter, double-blind, randomized, vehicle-controlled trial involving 279 patients evaluating the efficacy and safety of daily patient-applied imiquimod. At week 16, 52% of patients treated with 5% imiquimod, 14% with 1% imiquimod, and 4% of vehicle-treated patients cleared the warts (p<0.0001). Recurrence rate after a complete response was 19% with 5% imiquimod.

Patient-applied 5% imiquimod cream has a favorable safety profile and is effective for the treatment of external genital warts.

Human papillomavirus (HPV) viral load and HPV type in the clinical outcome of HIV-positive patients treated with imiquimod for anogenital warts and anal intraepithelial neoplasia. Sanclemente G, Herrera S, Tyring SK, Rady PL, Zuleta JJ, Correa LA, et al. J Eur Acad Dermatol Venereol 2007; 21: 1054–60.

Imiquimod 5% was evaluated in 37 HIV-positive males with anogenital warts or anal intraepithelial neoplasia (AIN). After 20 weeks, 46% of patients cleared 100%, whereas 14 patients had >50% clearance. Recurrences occurred in 29% of patients who cleared 100%. Clearance was independent of patients' CD4 counts, wart location, HIV viral load, or HPV viral load. Imiquimod appeared to be effective in treating AIN in HIV-positive patients.

Safety and efficacy of 0.5% podofilox gel in the treatment of anogenital warts. Tyring S, Edwards L, Cherry LK, Ramsdell WM, Kotner S, Greenberg MD, et al. Arch Dermatol 1998; 134: 33–8.

In a double-blind, randomized, multicenter, vehicle-controlled trial, 326 patients with anogenital warts received 0.5% podofilox gel. After 8 weeks, 88.4% of the warts in the vehicle-treated group and only 35.9% of warts treated with 0.5% podofilox gel remained after treatment (p=0.001). Podofilox 0.5% gel was safe and significantly more effective than vehicle gel in the treatment of anogenital warts.

Randomised controlled trial and economic evaluation of podophyllotoxin solution, podophyllotoxin cream, and podophyllin in the treatment of genital warts. Lacey CJ, Goodall RL, Tennvall GR, Maw R, Kinghorn GR, Fisk PG, et al. Sex Transm Infect 2003; 79: 270–5.

To evaluate the efficacy of self-applied podophyllotoxin 0.5% solution and podophyllotoxin 0.15% cream, compared to clinic-applied 25% podophyllin in the treatment of their genital warts, 358 immunocompetent patients with genital warts of =3 months were included. Self-treatment podophyllotoxin was more clinically and cost-effective than office-based podophyllin treatment.

Veregen: a botanical for treatment of genital warts. Med Lett Drugs Ther 2008; 50: 15–16.

In controlled clinical trials, 604 patients with genital warts were randomized to apply sinecatechin extract 15% ointment or placebo. At week 16, 53.6% vs 35.3% of patients respectively had complete clearance of all warts. Recurrence rates 12 weeks after complete clearance were 6.8% and 5.8%, respectively. Adverse events included erythema, pruritus, burning, pain, erosion or ulceration, edema, induration and vesicular rash.

Treatment of external genital warts: a randomized clinical trial comparing podophyllin, cryotherapy, and electrodesic-cation. Stone KM, Becker TM, Hadgu A, Kraus SJ. Genitourin Med 1990; 66: 16–19.

After evaluating 450 patients, complete clearance was observed in 41% treated with podophyllin, 79% treated with cryotherapy, and 94% treated with electrodesiccation. The 3-month clearance rates were 17%, 55%, and 71%, respectively. Cryotherapy with cryoprobe is only used for patients who do not have extensive disease.

Cryotherapy is safe to use during pregnancy. Podophyllin, however, has been demonstrated to have severe systemic toxicity and should not be used in pregnant women.

Comparison of the effectiveness of commonly used clinic-based treatments for external genital warts. Sherrard J, Riddell L. Int J STD AIDS 2007; 18: 365–8.

Patients (n=409) presenting with new or recurrent genital warts randomly received one of five treatments on a weekly basis: podophyllin 25%, TCA cryotherapy, TCA plus podophyllin, or cryotherapy plus podophyllin. Clearance rates were 82.1%, 84.5%, 92.4%, 94.0%, and 100%, respectively. Seventy-five percent of patients in the podophyllin 25% plus cryotherapy group required only two treatments to clear their warts. All had clearance in fewer than eight treatments. Single therapy with either TCA or podophyllin 25% resulted in longer time to clearance and more persistent warts.

SECOND-LINE THERAPIES

▶ Surgical excision (with cold knife or scissors)	B
▶ Lasers (CO_2 and PDL)	B
▶ Loop electrosurgical excisional procedure	B
▶ Electrodesiccation (see also above)	B
▶ TCA (see also above)	B

Comparison of podophyllin application with simple surgical excision in clearance and recurrence of perianal condyloma acuminata. Jensen SL. Lancet 1985; 2: 1146–8.

In 60 patients randomized to receive podophyllin or surgery, complete clearance was seen in 76.6% and 93.3%, respectively. At 3 months the cumulative recurrence rates were 43% for podophyllin and 18% for surgical excision.

Study of persistence and recurrence rates in 106 patients with condyloma and intraepithelial neoplasia after CO_2 laser treatment. Aynaud O, Buffet M, Roman P, Plantier F, Dupin N. Eur J Dermatol 2008; 18: 153–8.

Patients (n=106) were treated with CO_2 laser for condylomatous or neoplastic anogenital lesions. At 6 months 83% of patients were in remission after an average of 1.4 laser treatments. The excision of HPV-induced anogenital lesions using CO_2 laser remains an efficient treatment for longstanding lesions, even if it needs to be repeated when lesions recur or persist.

Treatment of genital warts in males by pulsed dye laser. Badawi A, Shokeir HA, Salem AM, Soliman M, Fawzy S, Samy N, et al. J Cosmet Laser Ther 2006; 8: 92–5.

A total of 174 adult males with 550 uncomplicated anogenital warts underwent treatment with the flashlamp-pumped pulsed dye laser. Complete resolution was achieved in 96% of lesions, with a recurrence rate of 5%, and minimal, transient, and infrequent side effects.

Treating vaginal and external anogenital condylomas with electrosurgery vs. CO$_2$ laser ablation. Ferenczy A, Behelak Y, Haber G, Wright TC Jr, Richart RM. J Gynecol Surg 1995; 148: 9–12.

In 208 patients the efficacy and adverse effects of loop electrosurgical excision procedure (LEEP) were similar to those associated with laser ablation. LEEP adverse events included bleeding and scarring.

Scarring of the penis can result in dysfunction; therefore most physicians prefer CO$_2$ laser ablation or cryotherapy for penile warts.

Treatment of external genital warts comparing cryotherapy and trichloroacetic acid. Abdullah AN, Walzman M, Wade A. Sex Transm Dis 1993; 20: 344–5.

In this randomized trial of 86 patients, after up to six treatments complete clearance was noted in 86% of the cryotherapy-treated patients compared to 70% of the TCA-treated patients. Ulcerations at the site of application developed in 30% of the TCA-treated patients.

THIRD-LINE THERAPIES

▶ Intralesional interferon-α	A
▶ Interferon-β gel	A
▶ Oral isotretinoin	B
▶ Intralesional fluorouracil/epinephrine gel	A
▶ Cidofovir	C

Natural interferon-alfa for treatment of condyloma acuminata. Friedman-Kien AE, Eron LJ, Conant M, Growdon W, Badiak H, Bradstreet PW, et al. JAMA 1988; 259: 533–8.

In this double-blind, placebo-controlled trial, complete clearance was experienced by 62% of patients in the treatment group and only 21% of those in the placebo group after intralesional interferon-α injections twice weekly for up to 8 weeks. The results of combining interferon treatment with cryosurgery, podophyllin, or laser ablation have been promising.

Recombinant interferon beta gel as an adjuvant in the treatment of recurrent genital warts: results of a placebo-controlled double-blind study in 120 patients. Gross G, Rogozinski T, Schöfer H, Jabłońska S, Roussaki A, Wöhr C, et al. J Dermatol 1998; 196: 330–4.

This double-blind, placebo-controlled study reported that topical application of recombinant interferon-β gel is safe and slightly reduces the recurrence of condyloma acuminata after surgical treatment.

Treatment of condyloma acuminata with oral isotretinoin. Tsambaos D, Georgiou S, Monastirli A, Sakkis T, Sagriotis A, Goerz G. J Urol 1997; 158: 1810–12.

Oral isotretinoin acheived complete response in 39.6% of 56 male patients with history of refractory condyloma acuminata. Oral isotretinoin may be considered an effective and fairly well tolerated alternative treatment for immature and small condyloma acuminata.

Comparative study of systemic interferon alfa-2a plus isotretinoin versus isotretinoin in the treatment of recurrent condyloma acuminatum in men. Cardamakis E, Kotoulas IG, Relakis K, Metalinos K, Michopoulos J, et al. Urology 1995; 45: 857–60.

Eighty-six men were randomized to receive isotretinoin 1 mg/kg orally (n=2), or isotretinoin plus interferon-$α_{2a}$ subcutaneously (n=44). The combination of isotretinoin plus interferon-$α_{2a}$ achieved lower recurrence rates (4 of 44 versus 16 of 42) and a shorter duration of treatment than isotretinoin alone.

Intralesional fluorouracil/epinephrine injectable gel for the treatment of condyloma acuminata. A phase 3 clinical study. Swinehart JM, Sperling M, Phillips S, Kraus S, Gordon S, McCarty JM, et al. Arch Dermatol 1997; 133: 67–73.

In this randomized, double-blind, placebo-controlled study, 401 patients were treated with fluorouracil/epinephrine (adrenaline) gel, fluorouracil gel alone, or placebo. Complete response rates were 61%, 43%, and 5%, respectively. Recurrence rates were between 50% and 60% for both treatment groups.

Intralesional or topical cidofovir (HPMPC, VISTIDE) for the treatment of recurrent genital warts in HIV-1-infected patients. Orlando G, Fasolo MM, Beretta R, Signori R, Adriani B, Zanchetta N, et al. AIDS 1999; 13: 1978–80.

Twelve HIV-positive patients with extensive or relapsing warts were treated with either topical cidofovir gel alone or a combination of topical gel and intralesional cidofovir. Although the addition of intralesional cidofovir did not seem to affect the extent of the lesions, topical gel cidofovir appeared to flatten lesions in the 10 evaluable patients. Four of the 10 patients had complete remission. The effectiveness of the therapy seemed to be independent of the stage of HIV disease.

Antiphospholipid syndrome

Julia S Lehman, Mark DP Davis

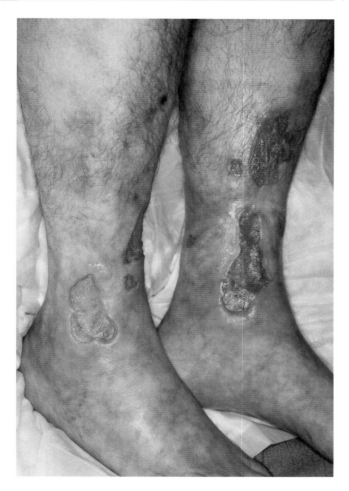

Antiphospholipid syndrome (APS) is characterized by the propensity for recurrent venous and arterial thrombosis in the presence of circulating antibodies against phospholipid-binding proteins. Cutaneous manifestations of APS, such as livedo reticularis, superficial thrombophlebitis, and ulceration, are nonspecific and result from thrombo-occlusion of the cutaneous vasculature. Histopathologic examination of involved skin reveals pauci-inflammatory thrombosis of the dermal vasculature.

MANAGEMENT STRATEGY

Revised Sapporo diagnostic criteria for APS require that patients experience vascular thrombosis (venous or arterial) or pregnancy morbidity (i.e., one or more unexplained deaths or premature births due to eclampsia, severe pre-eclampsia, or placental insufficiency in a morphologically normal fetus, or three or more unexplained consecutive spontaneous abortions before the 10th week of gestation with exclusion of other causes), and harbor at least one serum antiphospholipid (aPL) antibody (i.e., lupus anticoagulant, anticardiolipin, anti-β_2 glycoprotein-1) on two or more occasions over a 12-week period. Other clinical features of APS not included in diagnostic criteria include: heart valve disease, livedo reticularis, thrombocytopenia, nephropathy, and neurologic abnormalities. The term 'catastrophic antiphospholipid syndrome' (CAPS) refers to the development of widespread thromboses with associated end-organ damage in APS, and is associated with a 50% mortality rate.

In some cases APS may represent a primary condition. However, a search for underlying causes, such as infection, prothrombotic medications, primary hematologic coagulopathies (e.g., Factor V Leiden, prothrombin G20210A gene mutation), and connective tissue diseases (e.g., systemic lupus erythematosus (SLE)), is warranted. Because patients with APS are at increased risk for recurrent thromboembolism, the goal of therapy is secondary thromboprophylaxis.

The approach to treatment is guided by the patient's age and comorbidities, the presence of correctable prothrombotic factors, and coagulation history. In patients with persistently elevated aPL antibodies but no history of thrombosis (thereby not meeting strict criteria for APS), *aspirin* has not been shown to be effective in preventing future thromboembolic events. In patients with definitive APS and a history of venous thromboembolism the mainstay of treatment is long-term *warfarin* therapy. The optimal duration of warfarin therapy has not been established. Based on limited available data, indefinite treatment with warfarin appears to be associated with reduced rates of recurrent thromboembolism without an elevated risk for hemorrhagic complications, compared to treatment discontinuation after 6 months. Decisions regarding termination of warfarin therapy should be individualized. Long-term *heparin* use is discouraged because of the risk of heparin-induced osteopenia. *Inferior vena cava filters* may be required in patients with recurrent venous thromboembolism to prevent pulmonary embolism.

In patients with APS who have experienced arterial thromboembolism or have developed recurrent thrombosis despite achieving target international normalized ratio (INR) on warfarin, other treatment options must be pursued. These modalities, such as *rituximab, intravenous immunoglobulin,* and *plasmapheresis,* address circulating pathogenic antibodies directly rather than the resultant coagulopathy.

In patients with SLE and APS, *hydroxychloroquine* has been shown to reduce aPL antibody levels and to have intrinsic anticoagulative properties. Future APS therapies may include *low-dose warfarin, antiplatelet agents,* and *statins,* although these remain to be tested in APS. Correction of reversible prothrombotic factors, such as oral contraceptive use and smoking, is advisable.

Warfarin is contraindicated in pregnancy, a particularly high-risk state for patients with APS. Women with APS should be treated with aspirin prior to conception, with the introduction of low molecular weight heparin thereafter.

In acute thrombosis, monitored intravenous *unfractionated heparin* or subcutaneous *low molecular weight heparin* with or without subsequent initiation of *warfarin* is standard therapy. Thrombolytic medications (e.g., *streptokinase, tissue plasminogen activator,* tPA) or *percutaneous or surgical interventions* may be necessary in life- or limb-threatening thrombotic events. Patients with CAPS require intensive multidisciplinary interventions to halt disease progression and to reverse end-organ damage. *Plasma exchange* may have a role in the treatment of CAPS.

SPECIFIC INVESTIGATIONS

> ► Inquiry into history of thromboembolism, pregnancy morbidity and medication use
> ► aPL antibodies (i.e., lupus anticoagulant, anticardiolipin IgG and IgM antibodies, anti-β_2-glycoprotein 1 antibodies)
> ► Coagulopathy screen (i.e., INR, PTT, protein C, protein S, antithrombin III, prothrombin G20210A gene mutation, anti-prothrombin antibodies, Factor V Leiden, homocysteine level)
> ► Screening for underlying disease state (hematology, fasting blood glucose, fasting lipids, connective tissue serology, HIV testing, hepatitis serology)

International consensus statement on an update of the classification criteria for definite antiphospholipid syndrome (APS). Miyakis S, Lockshin MD, Atsumi T, Branch DW, Brey RL, Cervera R, et al. J Thromb Haemost 2006; 4: 295–306.

Consensus guidelines require a history of thromboembolism and documentation of elevated aPL antibodies on at least two occasions separated by at least 12 weeks for definitive diagnosis of APS.

Controversies and unresolved issues in antiphospholipid syndrome pathogenesis and management. Baker WF Jr, Bick RL, Fareed J. Hematol Oncol Clin North Am 2008; 22: 155–74.

Thorough investigation into underlying (and potentially correctable) conditions is recommended.

FIRST-LINE THERAPIES

> ► Observation (persistent aPL elevation but no thromboembolic events)   **A**
> ► Long-term warfarin, target INR 2.0–3.0   **A**
> ► Correction of reversible prothrombotic factors   **B**
> ► Long-term warfarin, target INR >3.0 (recurrent or arterial thrombosis)   **B**
> ► Low molecular weight heparin and low-dose aspirin (pregnancy)   **B**
> ► Heparin followed by warfarin (acute thrombosis)   **C**
> ► Thrombolytic therapy or percutaneous/surgical intervention (critical thrombosis)   **E**

Aspirin for primary thrombosis prevention in the antiphospholipid syndrome. Erkan D, Harrison MJ, Levy R, Peterson M, Petri M, Sammaritano L. Arthritis Rheum 2007; 56: 2382–91.

A randomized, double-blind, placebo-controlled trial of aspirin versus placebo in asymptomatic patients with persistently positive aPL antibodies found no benefit of aspirin in primary thromboprophylaxis.

A comparison of two intensities of warfarin for the prevention of recurrent thrombosis in patients with the antiphospholipid syndrome. Crowther MA, Ginsberg JS, Julian J, Denburg J, Hirsch J, Douketis J, et al. N Engl J Med 2003; 349: 113–18.

A randomized clinical trial of high-intensity warfarin vs. conventional antithrombotic therapy for the prevention of recurrent thrombosis in patients with the antiphospholipid syndrome. Finazzi G, Marchioli R, Brancaccio V, Schinco P, Wisloff F, Musial J, et al. Thromb Haemost 2005; 3: 848–53.

These two randomized, double-blind trials comparing high-intensity warfarin (target INR 3.0–4.0) and moderate-intensity warfarin (target INR 2.0–3.0) in patients with APS found no significant difference in preventing secondary thrombosis between the two treatment regimens.

A systematic review of secondary thromboprophylaxis in patients with antiphospholipid antibodies. Ruiz-Irastorza G, Hunt BJ, Khamashta MA. Arthritis Rheum 2007; 57: 1487–95.

In several cohort studies of patients with APS, INR at the time of recurrent thromboembolism on warfarin was <3.0 in 86%. The authors propose that the target INR should be >3.0 in patients with recurrent or arterial thrombosis.

Treatment of antiphospholipid antibody syndrome (APS) in pregnancy: a randomized pilot trial comparing low-molecular-weight heparin to unfractionated heparin. Stephenson MD, Ballem PJ, Tsang P, Purkiss S, Ensworth S, Houlihan E, et al. J Obstet Gynaecol Can 2004; 26: 729–34.

In a randomized trial, 28 women with APS received low-dose aspirin and either low molecular weight heparin or unfractionated heparin prior to conception or early in pregnancy. Pregnancy was successful in nine of 13 (69%) women treated with low molecular weight heparin and low-dose aspirin and in four of 13 (31%) women treated with unfractionated heparin and low-dose aspirin.

In addition, the obstetrics literature tends to favor low molecular weight over unfractionated heparin because of its superior safety profile.

Randomized study of subcutaneous low-molecular-weight heparin plus aspirin versus intravenous immunoglobulin in the treatment of recurrent fetal loss associated with antiphospholipid antibodies. Triolo G, Ferrante A, Ciccia F, Accardo-Palumbo A, Perino A, Castelli A, et al. Arthritis Rheum 2003; 48: 728–31.

In this study, 40 pregnant women with APS were randomized to receive low molecular weight heparin plus low-dose aspirin or IVIG. The rate of live births was significantly higher in the former group (84%) than in the latter (57%).

SECOND-LINE THERAPIES

> ► Long-term low molecular weight heparin (recurrent thrombosis)   **D**
> ► Hydroxychloroquine (SLE)   **E**
> ► Rituximab   **E**
> ► IVIG (in pregnancy)   **E**

Evidence-based management of thrombosis in the antiphospholipid antibody syndrome. Petri M. Curr Rheum Rep 2003; 5: 370–3.

Hydroxychloroquine appears to reduce aPL antibody titers and the risk for recurrent thrombosis in patients with SLE.

An excellent evidence-based review of APS treatments.

Effect of rituximab on clinical and laboratory features of antiphospholipid syndrome: a case report and review of literature. Erre GL, Pardini S, Faedda R, Passiu G. Lupus 2008; 17: 50–5.

The authors reviewed 12 case reports documenting the use of rituximab in patients with APS. Each patient had a favorable response to rituximab, as manifested by reduced antiphospholipid antibody titers, lowered lupus anticoagulant titers, absence of further thrombotic events, or recovery of APS-associated thrombocytopenia or autoimmune hemolytic anemia. In most patients rituximab was administered weekly for 4 weeks, with or without subsequent infusions at 3-month intervals.

A multicenter, placebo-controlled pilot study of intravenous immune globulin (IVIG) treatment of antiphospholipid syndrome during pregnancy. Branch DW, Peaceman AM, Druzin M, Silver RK, El-Sayed Y, Silver RM. Gen Obstet Gynecol 2000; 182: 122–7.

In this pilot study of 16 pregnant women with APS, patients were randomized to receive IVIG or placebo. All patients also received heparin and low-dose aspirin. A trend towards decreased fetal growth restriction was observed in the IVIG group compared to the placebo group, but differences were not statistically significant.

THIRD-LINE THERAPIES

▶ Plasma exchange (pregnancy)	**D**
▶ Placement of inferior vena cava filter (refractory, recurrent venous thromboses)	**D**

Plasma exchange in the management of high risk pregnant patients with primary antiphospholipid syndrome. A report of 9 cases and a review of the literature. Ruffatti A, Marson P, Pengo V, Favaro M, Tonello M, Boralati M, et al. Autoimmunity Rev 2007; 6: 196–202.

Nine patients with APS and triple-positive aPL antibodies were treated with plasma exchange for secondary prophylaxis during pregnancy. Authors found that combined plasma exchange and intravenous IG therapy contributed to favorable pregnancy outcomes in high-risk patients.

Insertion of inferior vena cava filters in patients with the antiphospholipid syndrome. Zifman E, Rotman-Pikielny P, Berlin T, Levy Y. Semin Arthritis Rheum 2008 (E-pub).

Ten patients with APS who experienced recurrent thrombosis despite warfarin therapy received IVC filters. One patient had a documented pulmonary embolus (PE) following intervention, and two died suddenly of unknown causes (PE could not be excluded). The authors state that the results were suggestive of a protective effect of IVC filters in refractory APS.

CATASTROPHIC ANTIPHOSPHOLIPID SYNDROME

▶ Anticoagulation, systemic corticosteroids, and plasmapheresis or IVIG	**D**

Catastrophic antiphospholipid syndrome. Clinical and laboratory features of 50 patients. Asherson RA, Cervera R, Piette JC, Font J, Lie JT, Burcoglu A, et al. Medicine (Baltimore) 1998; 77: 195–207.

A review of 50 patients with CAPS revealed a mortality rate of 50%. Of 20 patients who were treated with anticoagulation, systemic corticosteroids, and plasmapheresis or IVIG, 14 (70%) recovered.

Catastrophic antiphospholipid syndrome (CAPS): proposed guidelines for diagnosis and treatment. Asherson RA, Espinosa G, Cervera R, Font J, Carles Reverter J. J Clin Rheumatol 2002; 8: 157–65.

Based on experience from 130 cumulative cases of CAPS, authors recommend heparin, systemic corticosteroids, and plasmapheresis in the treatment of CAPS.

Catastrophic antiphospholipid syndrome presenting with multiorgan failure and gangrenous lesions of the skin. Incalzi RA, Gemma A, Moro L, Antonelli M. Angiology 2008; 59: 517–18.

A 38-year-old woman with CAPS triggered by abrupt withdrawal of systemic corticosteroids recovered completely after treatment with immunosuppressive and antibiotic treatment combined with plasmapheresis.

Aphthous stomatitis

Pascal G Ferzli, Justin J Green

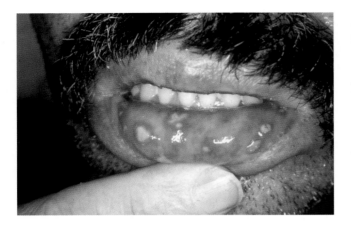

Recurrent aphthous stomatitis (RAS) is the most common cause of oral ulceration. It is characterized by the recurrence of one or more painful, sharply marginated ulcers with a fibrinous coating and an erythematous halo on non-keratinized, mobile oral mucosa. The three main types are minor, major, and herpetiform aphthae.

MANAGEMENT STRATEGY

The therapeutic approach to aphthae is dependent on the frequency of recurrence, duration, and severity of symptoms. In addition, underlying hematologic, viral and systemic diseases may direct appropriate therapy. Because there is no curative treatment, the emphasis is on measures that may afford symptomatic relief.

Topical corticosteroids are the mainstay of therapy. For milder disease, intermediate-strength corticosteroids such as *fluocinonide* are used. Potent corticosteroids such as *clobetasol* or *halobetasol* are appropriate for more severe episodes. Applications can be as frequent as five to 10 times daily. Gel or ointment formulations are preferred. These can be applied in equal parts with an occlusive dressing such as Orabase for better adherence. Drug delivery can be enhanced by cotton-tip applications for 30 seconds and avoidance of eating and drinking for 30 minutes after application. Initial concentrations of 5–10 mg/mL and up to 40 mg/mL of *intralesional triamcinolone acetonide* are helpful for major aphthae. Repeat injections over 2–4-week intervals are advised. *Dexamethasone elixir* 0.5 mg/5 mL three times daily used as a mouthwash or *beclomethasone dipropionate* aerosol spray can target ulcers on the soft palate or oropharynx.

RAS that elicits severe pain may require intermittent *systemic corticosteroid therapy*. Prednisone 40–60 mg daily can be given with a 2-week taper or as 'burst therapy' for shorter periods. Concomitant therapy with topical corticosteroids may be helpful. *Colchicine* 0.6 mg two to three times daily and *thalidomide* 100–200 mg daily are the most effective steroid-sparing agents. *Dapsone* 100 mg daily, *pentoxifylline* 400 mg three times daily, and *levamisole* 50 mg three times daily for 3 days every 2 weeks may also lead to suppression of aphthae. *Anti-tumor necrosis factor (TNF)-α* therapies are effective in recalcitrant cases. Those patients who require suppressive therapy but cannot tolerate the side effects of systemic agents can try medications such as *topical ciclosporin* rinse 500 mg/5 mL three times daily, or *interferon-α_{2a}* 1200 IU daily as a 1-minute rinse and swallow.

Application of amlexanox 5% paste four times daily has been shown to reduce aphthous ulcer healing time, and the application of amlexanox OraDisc four times daily to prodromal areas of the buccal mucosa has shown promise in the prevention of recurrent minor aphthous ulceration.

Topical anesthetics such as *lidocaine, dyclonine,* or *benzocaine* are helpful for pain reduction. Patients must avoid desensitization of the entire oral vault, which may lead to self-induced trauma. A compounded *anesthetic mouthwash* (aluminum hydroxide–magnesium hydroxide, diphenhydramine, and lidocaine) has better mucosal adherence. Systemic *non-steroidal anti-inflammatory drugs (NSAIDs), narcotics, sucralfate suspension,* 0.2% *chlorhexidine gluconate* mouthwash, *tetracycline* suspension 250 mg/5 mL, may provide pain relief and reduce healing time, although these are less effective than potent topical corticosteroids. Bioadhesive *2-octyl cyanoacrylate* forms a protective film and reduces healing time.

Trigger avoidance can be useful. Predisposing factors include food (nuts, chocolate, tomatoes, and spices), trauma, menstruation, and stress. A *food diary* may be of value in identifying an offending agent. Certain medications, such as β-blockers, NSAIDs, and antioxidants, as well as sensitivity to sodium lauryl sulfate found in toothpaste, may contribute to the recurrence of aphthae. *Hormonal therapy* may alleviate RAS associated with menstruation.

SPECIFIC INVESTIGATIONS

> ► Complete blood count
> ► Vitamins B$_1$, B$_2$, B$_6$ and B$_{12}$, folate, zinc, and iron levels
> ► Culture/polymerase chain reaction of aphthae to exclude herpes simplex virus (HSV)

Recurrent aphthous stomatitis. Akintoye SO, Greenberg MS. Dent Clin North Am 2005; 49: 31–47, vii-viii.

Systemic factors associated with recurrent aphthae include Behçet's disease, cyclic neutropenia, mouth and genital ulcers with inflamed cartilage (MAGIC syndrome), inflammatory bowel disease, celiac disease, and HIV infection. Local factors such as trauma and food allergies may also cause aphthae.

HSV infection may simulate recurrent aphthous stomatitis, but frequently involves keratinized attached mucosa. In patients with HIV infection one should consider other viruses, fungi, acid-fast bacilli, and neoplasia in the differential diagnosis.

Recurrent aphthous stomatitis. Ship JA, Chavez EM, Doerr PA, Henson BS, Sarmadi M. Quintessence Int 2000; 31: 95–112.

Causes of RAS are unknown, but local and systemic conditions, genetic, immunologic, and infectious factors have all been identified as potential etiopathogenic agents.

Effects of zinc treatment in patients with recurrent aphthous stomatitis. Orbak R, Cicek Y, Tezel A, Dogru Y. Dent Materials J 2003; 22: 21–9.

Of 40 patients, 42.5% had reduced serum zinc levels. An open trial of 220 mg zinc sulfate daily for 1 month resulted in an 80–100% reduction in the frequency of episodes.

Evidence Levels: **A** Double-blind study **B** Clinical trial ≥ 20 subjects **C** Clinical trial < 20 subjects **D** Series ≥ 5 subjects **E** Anecdotal case reports

Celiac disease in patients having recurrent aphthous stomatitis. Aydemir S, Tekin NS, Aktunc E, Numanoğlu G, Ustündağ Y. Gastroenterology 2004; 15: 192–5.

Of the 41 patients with RAS studied, two (4.8%) were diagnosed with celiac disease. In serum samples of both patients, antibodies to gliadin IgA and antibodies to endomysium were found to be positive. Antibodies to gliadin IgG were positive in only one of these two patients. None of the 49 patients in the control group were diagnosed as having celiac disease.

Serum iron, ferritin, folic acid, and vitamin B12 levels in recurrent aphthous stomatitis. Piskin S, Sayan C, Durukan N, Senol M. J Eur Acad Dermatol Venereol 2002; 16: 66–7.

Serum iron, ferritin, folic acid and vitamin B_{12} levels were investigated in 35 patients with RAS and in 26 healthy controls. Vitamin B_{12} was found to be significantly lower in subjects with RAS than in controls. No significant differences were found in other parameters.

In another study, vitamin B_{12}, iron and folate were deficient in 17.7% of patients with RAS.

Oxidant/antioxidant status in patients with recurrent aphthous stomatitis. Cimen MY, Kaya TI, Eskandari G, Tursen U, Ikizoglu G, Atik U. Clin Exp Dermatol 2003; 28: 647–50.

In 22 patients with RAS and 23 healthy controls, superoxide dismutase, glutathione peroxidase (GSHPx), and catalase (CAT) activities, and malondialdehyde (MDA) and antioxidant potential (AOP) levels were measured in plasma and erythrocytes. Reduced CAT and GSHPx activities and AOP levels in the erythrocytes, and decreased AOP and increased MDA plasma levels were found in patients with RAS compared to controls.

Recurrent aphthous ulceration: vitamin B1, B2, and B6 status and response to replacement therapy. Nolan A, McIntosh WB, Allam BF, Lamey P-J. J Oral Pathol Med 1991; 20: 389–91.

Seventeen of 60 (28.2%) patients with RAS were deficient in one or more of these B vitamins. Significant sustained improvement occurred in those patients with vitamin B deficiencies who received replacement compared to patients without documented deficiencies.

FIRST-LINE THERAPIES

▶ Vitamin and mineral deficiency replacement	B
▶ Topical corticosteroids	A
▶ Intralesional corticosteroids	B
▶ Amlexanox 5% paste in OraDisc	A
▶ Tetracycline	A
▶ Doxycycline	D
▶ Antimicrobial mouth rinses	A
▶ Sucralfate	A
▶ Hydroxypropyl cellulose/carboxymethylcellulose	C

The treatment of oral aphthous ulcerations or erosive lichen planus with topical clobetasol propionate in three preparations: a clinical and pilot study on 54 patients. Lo Muzio LL, della Valle A, Mignogna MD, Pannone G, Bucci P, Bucci E, et al. J Oral Pathol Med 2001; 30: 611–17.

In this double-blind study, topical clobetasol in adhesive denture paste significantly reduced healing time vs clobetasol in Orabase or clobetasol alone.

A controlled clinical trial of the efficacy of topically applied fluocinonide in the treatment of recurrent aphthous ulceration. Pimlott SJ, Walker DM. Br Dent J 1983; 154: 174–7.

In a single-blind clinical trial fluocinonide 0.05% ointment in Orabase applied up to five times daily was more effective than Orabase alone in reducing the duration of ulcers and increasing the number of ulcer-free days.

In some countries, triamcinolone in Orabase is more readily available.

Topical triamcinolone acetonide in recurrent aphthous stomatitis. Browne RM, Fox EC, Anderson RJ. Lancet 1968; 1: 565–7.

Twenty-six patients underwent a double-blind study in which triamcinolone acetonide 0.1% in Orabase was compared to Orabase alone and aqueous triamcinolone alone. Subjective and objective improvement was best in the triamcinolone with Orabase group.

Treatment of aphthous ulcers in AIDS patients. Friedman M, Brenski A, Taylor L. Laryngoscope 1994; 104: 566–70.

Intralesional triamcinolone acetonide 40 mg/mL was used in patients with AIDS having major aphthae that were present for at least 2 weeks and were culture negative for bacteria, viruses, fungi or acid-fast bacilli. Quantities of 0.5–1.0 mL were administered every 2 weeks. Pain relief was achieved within 2 days in 94% of patients. One half of affected patients had complete resolution after one injection.

5% Amlexanox oral paste, a new treatment for recurrent minor aphthous ulcers. Khandwala A, Van Inwegan RG, Alfano MC. Oral Surg Oral Med Oral Pathol 1997; 83: 222–30.

Amlexanox 5% oral paste applied four times daily was studied in four randomized, controlled, double-blind trials involving 1335 patients with minor aphthae. Significant acceleration in healing of ulcers and reduction in pain were achieved with amlexanox therapy.

Amlexanox oral paste: a novel treatment that accelerates the healing of aphthous ulcers. Binnie WH, Curro FA, Khandwala A, Van Inwegan RG. Compend Contin Educ Dent 1997; 18: 1116–18, 1120–2, 1124.

In three controlled clinical studies that evaluated 1124 immunocompetent patients with mild to moderate aphthous ulcers, 5% amlexanox oral paste was shown to accelerate healing of these ulcers.

An evaluation of the efficacy and safety of amlexanox oral adhesive tablets in the treatment of recurrent minor aphthous ulceration in a Chinese cohort: a randomized, double-blind, vehicle-controlled, unparallel multicenter clinical trial. Liu J, Zeng X, Chen Q, Cai Y, Chen F, Wang Y, et al. Oral Surg Oral Med Oral Pathol Oral Radiol Endod 2006; 102: 475–81.

Two hundred and twelve patients with oral aphthae were enrolled in a randomized, double-blind, vehicle-controlled, clinical trial. Amlexanox 5% adhesive tablets or placebo was applied four times daily to the ulcer. Patients were evaluated at day 4 and day 6. The reduction in ulcer pain and lesion size was statistically significant at day 4, and reduction of all parameters, including erythema and exudation, was statistically significant at day 6. No systemic side effects were reported.

The efficacy of amlexanox OraDisc on the prevention of recurrent minor aphthous ulceration. Murray B, Biagioni PA, Lamey PJ. J Oral Pathol Med 2006; 35: 117–22.

Fifty-two patients were randomized to apply OraDisc or vehicle patches four times daily to a prodromal area of the aphthous ulcer. By day 4, 50% of subjects in the OraDisc group developed an ulcer, compared with 69% in the placebo group. Differences in erythema score, ulcer size, and pain score were not statistically significant but showed a trend towards the OraDisc group.

This is the first randomized study designed to determine whether aphthous ulcers can be prevented by intervention. Prodromal areas were identified using patients' self-report and subsequent objective confirmation using infrared thermographic imaging. Only 69% of the vehicle group developed ulcers, as opposed to the expected 100%.

Double-blind trial of tetracycline in recurrent aphthous ulceration. Graykowski EA, Kingman A. J Oral Pathol 1978; 7: 376–82.

A suspension of tetracycline 250 mg/5 mL was used four times daily in patients with RAS. The suspension was held in the mouth for 2 minutes and then swallowed. This study found that tetracycline therapy significantly reduced ulcer duration, size and pain, but did not alter the recurrence rate.

Other studies using tetracycline or its derivatives (topically or orally) have drawn similar conclusions.

Chlorhexidine gluconate mouthwash in the management of minor aphthous ulceration: a double-blind, placebo controlled cross-over trial. Hunter L, Addy M. Br Dent J 1987; 162: 106–10.

This crossover study included 38 patients who used 0.2% chlorhexidine gluconate mouthwash three times daily for 6 weeks. The total number of days with ulcers was significantly reduced, and the interval between successive ulcers was increased.

Gel and mouthwash formulations of 0.1% chlorhexidine have also been efficacious. Chlorhexidine mouthwash is not associated with systemic side effects.

Subantimicrobial dose doxycycline in the treatment of recurrent oral aphthous ulceration: a pilot study. Preshaw PM, Grainger P, Bradshaw MH, Mohammad AR, Powala CV, Nolan A. J Oral Pathol Med 2007; 36: 236–40.

Fifty patients were randomly allocated to receive either doxycycline 20 mg twice daily or placebo for 90 days. Patients receiving doxycycline had more days with no reports of new ulcers.

This pilot study showed a trend towards fewer new ulcers per day over 90 days, and fewer days of pain, but the data were not statistically significant.

Effect of an antimicrobial mouthrinse on recurrent aphthous ulcerations. Meiller TF, Kutcher MJ, Overholser CD, Niehaus C, DePaola LG, Siegel MA. Oral Surg Oral Med Oral Pathol 1991; 72: 425–9.

A 6-month double-blind study compared Listerine antiseptic and a hydroalcoholic control used as a vigorous mouthwash twice daily. The duration of ulcers and pain severity were significantly reduced in the Listerine group. Both the Listerine group and the control group experienced a reduced incidence of ulcers.

Use of proprietary agents to relieve recurrent aphthous stomatitis. Edres MAG, Scully C, Gelbier M. Br Dent J 1997; 182: 144–6.

Retrospective, subjective opinions were taken from 50 patients with aphthae. Of the 10 most frequently used products in this patient population, benzydamine hydrochloride and chlorhexidine gluconate were the most effective.

No significant differences in efficacy have been shown in a trial comparing 0.15% benzydamine hydrochloride, 0.2% aqueous chlorhexidine gluconate, and an alcohol placebo used as mouthwashes.

Sucralfate suspension as a treatment of recurrent aphthous stomatitis. Rattan J, Schneider M, Arber N, Gorsky M, Dayan D. J Intern Med 1994; 236: 341–3.

Sucralfate applied four times daily to ulcers was found to be superior to antacid (aluminum hydroxide and magnesium hydroxide) and placebo with regard to duration of pain, reduction in healing time, response to first treatment, and duration of remission. The 2-year prospective, randomized, double-blind, placebo-controlled, crossover trial included 21 patients unresponsive to conventional therapy.

A randomized, placebo-controlled, double-blind study of sucralfate applied four times daily to oral and genital ulcerations of Behçet's disease resulted in reduced frequency, healing time and pain in oral ulcerations, and reduced healing time and pain in genital ulcerations.

Performance of a hydroxypropyl cellulose film former in normal and ulcerated mucosa. Rodu B, Russell CM. Oral Surg Oral Med Oral Pathol 1988; 65: 699–703.

Zilactin, which contains hydroxypropyl cellulose, led to pain relief after an acidic challenge followed by rechallenge.

Orabase, which contains carboxymethylcellulose, has been beneficial in trials when combined with topical corticosteroids, possibly owing to its adhesive properties.

SECOND-LINE THERAPIES

▶ Oral corticosteroids	C
▶ Colchicine	B
▶ Thalidomide	A

Clinical, historic, and therapeutic features of aphthous stomatitis: literature review and open trial employing steroids. Vincent SD, Lilly GE. Oral Surg Oral Med Oral Pathol 1992; 74: 79–86.

'Burst therapy' with prednisone 40 mg once daily for 5 days, followed by 20 mg every other day for 1 week in addition to topical triamcinolone acetonide 0.1% or 0.2% four times daily, led to complete or partial control of aphthae in 12 of 13 patients.

Prevention of recurrent aphthous stomatitis with colchicine: an open trial. Katz J, Langevitz P, Shemer J, Barak S, Livneh A. J Am Acad Dermatol 1994; 31: 459–61.

Twenty patients with RAS were studied in a 4-month open, prospective trial. During therapy with colchicine 0.5 mg three times daily the mean aphthae count and the mean pain score decreased by 71% and 77%, respectively.

Colchicine has demonstrated efficacy in a double-blinded trial in Behçet's disease, and some clinicians regard recurrent aphthous stomatitis as an incomplete form of Behçet's disease.

Crossover study of thalidomide vs placebo in severe recurrent aphthous stomatitis. Revuz J, Guillaume JC, Janier M, Hans P, Marchand C, Souteyrand P, et al. Arch Dermatol 1990; 126: 923–7.

Evidence Levels: A Double-blind study **B** Clinical trial ≥ 20 subjects **C** Clinical trial < 20 subjects **D** Series ≥ 5 subjects **E** Anecdotal case reports

A multicenter crossover randomized, double-blind trial of thalidomide 100 mg daily versus placebo led to complete remission in 32 of 67 (48%) patients treated with thalidomide and in six of 67 (9%) patients treated with placebo. Side effects, which included drowsiness, constipation, headache, vertigo and neuropathy, resulted in treatment interruptions in 11 patients.

Similar complete remission rates were seen in a double-blind, placebo-controlled study involving patients with HIV infection and oral aphthous ulcers treated with thalidomide 200 mg daily.

Thalidomide for the treatment of oral aphthous ulcers in patients with human immunodeficiency virus infection. Jacobson JM, Greenspan JS, Spritzler J, Ketter N, Fahey JL, Jackson JB, et al. National Institute of Allergy and Infectious Diseases AIDS Clinical Trials Group. N Engl J Med 1997; 336: 1487–93.

Fifty-seven HIV-positive patients were included in this double-blind, randomized, placebo-controlled study of thalidomide 200 mg daily vs placebo as therapy for oral aphthous ulcers in HIV-infected patients. Sixteen of 29 patients in the thalidomide group (55%) had complete healing of their aphthous ulcers after 4 weeks, compared to only two of 28 patients in the placebo group (7%; p<0.001).

Recurrent aphthous stomatitis unresponsive to topical corticosteroids: a study of the comparative therapeutic effects of systemic prednisone and systemic sulodexide. Femiano F, Gombos F, Scully C. Int J Dermatol 2003; 42: 394–7.

Thirty patients with RAS were randomly assigned to one of three study groups: blind therapy with systemic sulodexide, systemic prednisone or control. Systemic prednisone was slightly more effective than sulodexide and both were more effective than placebo.

THIRD-LINE THERAPIES

▶ Dapsone	D
▶ Pentoxifylline	C
▶ Levamisole	A
▶ Topical ciclosporin	C
▶ Oral interferon-α_{2a}	A
▶ Disodium cromoglycate	A
▶ Azathioprine	E
▶ Topical 5-aminosalicylic acid	A
▶ Topical diclofenac in hyaluronan	A
▶ Topical prostaglandin E_2	A
▶ Triclosan	A
▶ Azelastine	B
▶ Longo Vital	A
▶ Phenelzine	E
▶ Aciclovir	C
▶ Etretinate	E
▶ Low-intensity ultrasound	B
▶ CO_2 laser	C
▶ Potassium nitrate/dimethyl isosorbide	C
▶ Penicillin G potassium troches	A
▶ Sulodexide	C
▶ Etanercept	E
▶ Adalimumab	E
▶ Bee propolis	C
▶ Silver nitrate	C

Dapsone use with oral-genital ulcers. Handfield-Jones S, Allen BR, Littlewood SM. Br J Dermatol 1985; 113: 501.

Complete or partial clearing of aphthae was achieved in 11 of 19 patients with previously resistant oral aphthae, oral and genital aphthae, or Behçet's disease using dapsone 100 mg daily. The average duration of treatment was 19 days. Concomitant therapy consisted of zinc sulfate and co-trimoxazole.

A randomized, double-blind, placebo-controlled trial of pentoxifylline for the treatment of recurrent aphthous stomatitis. Thornhill MH, Baccaglini L, Theaker E, Pemberton MN. Arch Dermatol 2007; 143: 463–70.

Twenty-six patients were randomized to pentoxifylline 400 mg three times daily or placebo. Patients taking pentoxifylline had less pain, smaller ulcers, fewer ulcers, and more ulcer-free days, but this was not statistically significant. However, smaller median ulcer size in the treatment group was statistically significant. Adverse events were common and included dizziness, headaches, gastrointestinal symptoms, and fatigue.

According to the study, patients taking the active drug stated that if it was shown to be effective in the treatment of aphthous ulcers, they would not want to use it because of the side effects.

Treatment of recurrent aphthous stomatitis with pentoxifylline. Pizarro A, Navarro A, Fonseca E, Vidaurrazaga C, Herranz P. et al. Br J Dermatol 1995; 133: 659–60.

In patients with minor RAS receiving pentoxifylline 400 mg three times daily over a 6-month period, 50% did not experience a recurrence and 27% experienced a reduced number and duration of ulcers.

In other studies, over 50% of patients noted either complete resolution or a reduction in number and/or duration of ulcers during the treatment period. However, these are open-label trials involving small numbers of patients.

A randomized double-blind trial of levamisole in the therapy of recurrent aphthous stomatitis. De Cree J, Verhaegen H, De Cock W, Verbruggen F. Oral Surg Oral Med Oral Pathol 1978; 45: 378–84.

Eighteen patients with RAS underwent a placebo-controlled, double-blind study in which they were given placebo or levamisole 50 mg three times daily for 3 consecutive days at the start of an aphthous lesion. Statistical evaluation showed reduced frequency of lesions, shorter duration, and diminished pain of lesions in the group receiving levamisole.

Topical cyclosporine for oral mucosal disorders. Eisen D, Ellis CN. J Am Acad Dermatol 1990; 23: 1259–64.

Four of eight patients with severe aphthous stomatitis obtained nearly complete suppression of ulcers during an 8-week course of topical ciclosporin 500 mg/5 mL, swish and rinse three times daily.

Chronic recurrent aphthous stomatitis: oral treatment with low-dose interferon alpha. Hutchinson VA, Angenend JL, Mok WL, Cummins JM, Richards AB. Mol Biother 1990; 2: 160–4.

Oral administration of interferon-α 1200 IU daily resulted in remissions of aphthae within 2 weeks of initiating therapy compared to no improvement in the placebo group.

Di-sodium cromoglycate in the treatment of recurrent aphthous ulceration. Kowolik MJ, Muir KF, MacPhee IT. Br Dent J 1978; 144: 384.

Disodium cromoglycate lozenges, 20 mg four times daily, resulted in an increase in ulcer-free days after a 6-week treatment period in this double-blind crossover trial.

An earlier study found only pain relief was achieved with cromoglycic acid.

Combination immunosuppressant and topical steroid therapy for treatment of recurrent major aphthae. Brown RS, Bottomley WK. Oral Surg Oral Med Oral Pathol 1990; 69: 42–4.

A 32-year-old woman with recurrent major aphthae was successfully treated with azathioprine 50 mg twice daily, ibuprofen 600 mg four times daily, and dexamethasone elixir 0.5 mg/5 mL swish and rinse.

The patient had not used topical corticosteroids prior to azathioprine; hence it is difficult to assess either drug's individual merit.

Topical 5-aminosalicylic acid: a treatment for aphthous ulcers. Collier PM, Neill SM, Copeman PWM. Br J Dermatol 1992; 126: 185–8.

Reduced discomfort and pain, shortened healing time, and reduced difficulty with eating were found with 5-aminosalicylic cream three times daily compared to placebo.

Although this trial was double-blinded and placebo controlled, the duration of treatment was brief – 14 days or until ulcer clearance.

Sustained relief of oral aphthous ulcer pain from topical diclofenac in hyaluronan: a randomized, double-blind clinical trial. Saxen MA, Ambrosius WT, Rehemtula AF, Russell AL, Eckert GJ. Oral Surg Oral Med Oral Pathol Oral Radiol Endod 1997; 84: 356–61.

Gels containing 3% diclofenac in 2.5% hyaluronan, 2.5% hyaluronan, and 2% viscous lidocaine resulted in similar pain relief after application of noxious stimuli. A significant treatment effect was observed with the combination diclofenac and hyaluronan gel 2–6 h after application with respect to pain relief following food/drink consumption.

NSAIDs can be used systemically for analgesia. However, change in ulcer size or suppression of recurrence have not been documented with topical or oral NSAIDs.

A clinical trial of prostaglandin E2 in recurrent aphthous ulceration. Taylor LJ, Walker DM, Bagg J. Br Dent J 1993; 175: 125.

Topical prostaglandin E_2 (PGE_2) gel may exert a prophylactic effect for aphthae.

Treatment time in this randomized, double-blind, placebo-controlled study was only 10 days, and patients experienced fewer new lesions despite applying PGE_2 to active aphthae. No significant differences in speed of healing or pain relief were found. PGE_2 may produce myotonic effects on the uterus, and so pregnancy tests were checked in female patients in this study.

Mouthrinses containing triclosan reduce the incidence of recurrent aphthous ulcers (RAU). Skaare AB, Herlofson BB, Barkvoll P. J Clin Periodontol 1996; 23: 778–81.

In a double-blind crossover study, 0.15% triclosan mouthwash caused a significant reduction in the number of ulcers during the experimental period. Compared to the 7.8% ethanol and triclosan formulation, the efficacy of the mouthwashes was reduced when propylene glycol or a higher concentration of ethanol (15.6%) were used as solubilizing agents.

A clinical trial of azelastine in recurrent aphthous ulceration with an analysis of its actions on leukocytes. Ueta E, Osaki T, Yoneda K, Yamamoto T, Kato I. J Oral Pathol Med 1994; 23: 123–9.

Azelastine hydrochloride was administered orally to 43 patients with RAS. During 6 months after treatment no oral lesions occurred in seven patients, and improvement was exhibited in all but four.

Aphthous ulcers responding to etretinate – a case report. Murphy GM, Griffiths AD. Clin Exp Dermatol 1989; 14: 330–1.

A 34-year-old woman was treated with etretinate 25 mg daily for plantar pustular psoriasis. Two-month remissions of her minor aphthae occurred with two courses of etretinate.

Managing aphthous ulcers: laser treatment applied. Colvard M, Kuo P. J Am Dent Assoc 1991; 122: 51–3.

Pain alleviation was observed in 16 of 18 patients following CO_2 laser therapy of minor aphthae.

The efficacy and safety of 50mg penicillin G potassium troches for recurrent aphthous ulcers. Kerr AR, Drexel CA, Speilman AI. Oral Surg Oral Med Oral Pathol Oral Radiol Endod 2003; 96: 685–94.

Topical application of 50 mg penicillin G troches in 31 patients with minor RAS resulted in a reduction in healing time and earlier pain relief.

The difference between the treatment group and placebo group was borderline in both healing time and pain relief.

Recurrent aphthous stomatitis unresponsive to topical corticosteroids: a study of the comparative therapeutic effects of systemic prednisone and systemic sulodexide. Femiano F, Gombos F, Scully C. Int J Dermatol 2003; 42: 394–7.

A double-blind trial of systemic sulodexide 250 mg twice daily for month 1, then once daily for month 2 vs prednisone taper vs placebo showed reduction in days to re-epithelialization of aphthae that was superior to placebo yet inferior to prednisone.

Recalcitrant, recurrent aphthous stomatitis treated with etanercept. Robinson ND, Guitart J. Arch Dermatol 2003; 139: 1259–62.

A case report of treatment of recalcitrant RAS with subcutaneous etanercept 25 mg twice weekly with a resultant decrease in frequency, severity and duration of flares during the 7 months of therapy.

Treatment of severe, recalcitrant, major aphthous stomatitis with adalimumab. Vujevich J, Zirwas M. Cutis 2005; 76: 129–32.

An 18-year-old man with recalcitrant recurrent severe oral ulcerations responsive only to high-dose prednisone received adalimumab 40 mg subcutaneously every other week. After 2 weeks the patient showed a significant improvement in the ulcerations, which eventually healed. After 4 months there was no recurrence of the ulcerations, and his prednisone was discontinued.

This is the first report demonstrating the effectiveness of adalimumab for the treatment of recurrent aphthous stomatitis.

The effect of bee propolis on recurrent aphthous stomatitis: a pilot study. Samet N, Laurent C, Susarla SM, Samet-Rubinsteen N. Clin Oral Invest 2007; 11: 143–7.

In this randomized, placebo-controlled double-blind study, 19 patients were assigned to receive either propolis 500 mg/day (n=10) or a calcium-based food supplement (n=9). Patients were contacted biweekly and asked to report the frequency of RAS outbreaks. A statistically significant reduction in the number of outbreaks as well as an improvement in quality of life was found.

Silver nitrate cautery in aphthous stomatitis: a randomized controlled trial. Alidaee MR, Taheri A, Mansoori P, Ghodsi SZ. Br J Dermatol 2005; 153: 521–5.

Ninety-seven patients with painful minor aphthae were randomized to receive one stick application of silver nitrate cautery or placebo. After 1 day, a statistically significant reduction in severity of pain was shown. Silver nitrate did not prolong or shorten healing time examined after 7 days. No side effects were noted.

The authors note that the treatment is simple and cost-effective for patients, with few recurrences.

Atopic dermatitis

Andrew C Krakowski, Lawrence F Eichenfield

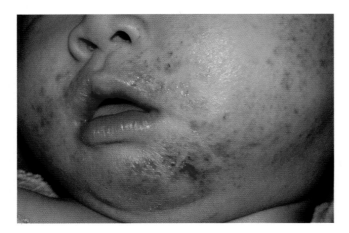

Atopic dermatitis (AD) is a chronic, relapsing, intensely pruritic dermatosis that develops most commonly during early infancy and childhood and is in most cases associated with a personal or family history of atopy (allergic rhinitis, asthma, or eczema). It is frequently associated with abnormalities in skin barrier function and immune dysregulation. Skin involvement ranges from acute, weeping, and crusted areas of eczema to papular lesions or lichenified plaques. Because no single defining clinical feature or laboratory test exists, the diagnosis is based on a constellation of clinical findings.

MANAGEMENT STRATEGY

Successful atopic dermatitis (AD) therapy considers the patient's age and needs, the extent and localization of AD at presentation, and the overall disease course, including previous response to treatment, disease persistence, frequency of flares, and susceptibility to and past history of infection (especially due to *Staphylococcus aureus* and herpes simplex). The goals of management are to educate patients and carers about the disease, promote excellent skin care, reduce the degree and frequency of flares, monitor medication quality/quantity of use and, possibly, modify the overall disease course and the atopic march.

Interventional education

Comprehensive multispecialty 'eczema clinics' are beginning to test the utility of intensive education as a distinct component of long-term AD management. This model, with its longer appointments, focused educational curricula, patient support networks, and the ability to elicit patient/family feedback, parallels strategies shown to be effective for managing asthma, diabetes, and other chronic diseases. Supporters hope to empower patients and carers and improve clinical and quality of life outcomes. Long-term comparative evaluation is required to examine the cost-effectiveness and suitability of these educational programs.

Skin care

Excellent skin care remains a cornerstone of management, and although data to support the notion that moisturizers improve atopic dermatitis directly are limited, these products are widely used because they improve the xerosis associated with AD. With little evidence to recommend the use of one emollient/moisturizer over another, patient and carer preference should drive product selection based on the premise that 'an emollient that is applied works better than one that remains on a shelf.' Very occlusive ointments may not be tolerated during the summer months or very humid climates because of interference with the function of eccrine sweat ducts and the induction of folliculitis; a cream may be a more practical choice. Avoid preparations that contain topical sensitizers (e.g., fragrance, neomycin, benzocaine, etc.). Generally patients should apply emollients/moisturizers after any topical pharmacologic therapies to allow active medications to reach the skin with full effect. The value of *bathing* and the frequency with which it should be undertaken remain controversial. The chief benefits of bathing include cleansing, debridement of infected eczema, improved penetration of topical therapies, and skin hydration (when emollients are used to 'lock in' moisture); potential drawbacks are drying of the skin and disruption of the stratum corneum barrier during water evaporation when emollients are not used. Recent data regarding transepidermal water loss suggest that the frequency of application of emollients/moisturizers may be more important than timing application to coincide strictly with bathing (the traditional 'soak and seal' approach); this finding remains to be confirmed in larger, more controlled studies. Several novel *barrier repair products* have recently been cleared for marketing by the United States Food and Drug Administration as '510(k) medical devices.' These products contain ingredients that may help to replace abnormal epidermal lipids, improve skin hydration, reduce skin barrier dysfunction, and relieve the pruritus, burning, and pain associated with AD. Studies are under way to evaluate the utility of these new products and their potential role in helping to manage AD.

Wet wraps are a useful tool in the intensive treatment of severe AD and/or disease that is refractory to standard topical therapies. They may increase skin hydration, serve as an effective mechanical barrier to scratching, and act as an occlusive layer that promotes penetration of topical corticosteroids into the skin, thereby increasing the amount of medication delivered to the most severely affected areas. Temporary systemic bioactivity of the corticosteroids is a concern. The potential to induce hypothermia should not be forgotten. When wet wraps are overused or used incorrectly, maceration of the skin and secondary infections may occur, and, paradoxically, they may promote skin dryness if sufficient amounts of emollient are not applied concurrently. Because of these concerns wet wraps should only be used under the close supervision of a physician.

Although eliminating specific triggers may not result in clearance of atopic dermatitis, *avoidance of known triggers* is a reasonable approach. Total avoidance of environmental aeroallergens is almost impossible. Where aeroallergens are strongly suspected of having a causative role, mattress covers, low-pile carpet (particularly in sleeping areas), frequent vacuuming, and non-dander-producing pets may be helpful, especially for children who have concomitant asthma and/or allergic rhinitis. Although food allergens may serve as specific triggers in a subpopulation of atopic dermatitis patients,

Evidence Levels: **A** Double-blind study   **B** Clinical trial ≥ 20 subjects   **C** Clinical trial < 20 subjects   **D** Series ≥ 5 subjects   **E** Anecdotal case reports

parents should be cautioned against extreme restriction diets that can lead to serious malnutrition. Likewise, it is important to reintroduce an eliminated trigger food under the supervision of a physician because of the risk of anaphylaxis.

Topical corticosteroids remain first-line therapy for inflammation and pruritus. Variation in corticosteroid-prescribing habits (e.g., quantity, frequency, and duration of therapy) is common even among dermatologists. Some clinicians start treatment with high-potency topical corticosteroid preparations in order to induce remission, followed by a relatively quick tapering-down of potency as the dermatitis improves. Alternatively, some clinicians use short bursts of high-potency corticosteroids followed by moisturizer use only until relapse occurs. Yet another treatment regimen advocates more prolonged continuous treatment with less potent preparations. Drug-specific FDA indications and an expanding body of clinical trial data should help guide clinicians when educating and instructing patients on topical corticosteroid usage.

Topical calcineurin inhibitors (TCIs, tacrolimus and pimecrolimus) have the important advantage that they are not associated with skin atrophy. Current indications for TCI use are as *'second-line therapy* for the short-term and non-continuous chronic treatment' of mild to moderate AD (pimecrolimus) or moderate to severe AD (tacrolimus) in non-immunocompromised adults and children 'who have failed to respond adequately to other topical prescription treatments for atopic dermatitis, or when those treatments are not advisable.' Patients who are especially likely to benefit include those in whom the clinical course of AD is marked by steroid tachyphylaxis (versus simple non-compliance), disease persistence, and/or frequent flares, which would otherwise result in an almost continuous need for topical corticosteroid treatment. TCIs may also be specifically indicated in sensitive thin skin areas, such as around the eye, face, neck, and genital area, where local safety and systemic absorption are of special concern. The safety and efficacy of tacrolimus and pimecrolimus have been studied in several short- (6-week) and long-term (>2 years) clinical trials. Data from these trials demonstrate that pimecrolimus reduces the number and severity of flares, extends the period between major flares, and reduces pruritus and other cutaneous signs associated with AD. Likewise, long-term, intermittent (once daily, two or three times weekly) maintenance use of tacrolimus ointment in patients with stabilized AD has been shown to significantly increase the period between disease exacerbations and the total number of disease-free days compared to vehicle. The incidence of side effects in these studies was generally low and included, most commonly, transient application-site stinging. The currently available data suggest that the use of TCIs is not associated with systemic immunosuppression or an increased risk of skin cancer; nor does it appear to affect the delayed-type hypersensitivity response. In most countries the use of TCIs is not recommended in patients under 2 years of age. Tacrolimus ointment 0.03% is indicated for adults and children aged 2–15 years, whereas tacrolimus ointment 0.1% is indicated only for adults. Long-term prospective studies investigating the clinical use of TCIs in a pediatric population are currently under way and will hopefully help to alleviate safety concerns.

Careful *supervision*, combined with appreciation of the risk–benefit profiles of moisturizers, barrier repair agents, topical corticosteroids, and TCIs, allows for individualized and optimized patient care. Treatment should be readily adjusted on an 'as-needed' basis that takes advantage of available therapeutic modalities. For children with severe flares, this may mean using short-term bursts of mid- to high-potency topical steroids – with or without wet wraps – instead of relying on long-term use of less potent agents. Close re-examination of the patient at regular intervals to evaluate the efficacy and tolerability of local and systemic therapies is warranted. Once control of a flare is achieved, therapy should shift to a less intense regimen with a focus on maintenance and proper skin care at its core. Wet wraps can be stopped and topical corticosteroids can be tapered to a lower-potency agent and/or from daily to intermittent (e.g., thrice- or twice-weekly) application. Transition to TCI therapy for patients with a history of flare recurrence upon discontinuation or tapering of topical corticosteroids may be a good choice at this point. The use of TCI monotherapy to control flare recurrence while limiting patients' extended exposure to corticosteroids is supported by some physicians.

Although they do not appear to have direct effects on the pruritus associated with AD, *sedating systemic antihistamines* such as hydroxyzine and diphenhydramine may be useful in improving sleep in flaring patients. This practice has not been evaluated rigorously in large, randomized, double-blind, placebo-controlled trials, and the drowsiness that may be associated with daytime use is a legitimate concern for schoolchildren. Second-generation antihistamines are less useful in managing atopic dermatitis but may benefit patients with allergic triggers and, with chronic use, are suggested in some studies to reduce the rate of progression to other atopic disease (the atopic march). Importantly, *topical antihistamines* are not recommended because of potential cutaneous sensitization. Oral doxepin hydrochloride, a tricyclic antidepressant with anxiolytic effects, has a high H_1- and H_2-histamine receptor antagonist activity. It is typically used in doses of 10–75 mg orally at night or up to 75 mg twice daily in adult patients; it is not approved for use in children. Because it possesses a side-effect profile that includes daytime sedation, hypotension, tolerance, and an increased risk of depression/suicide, oral doxepin is generally reserved for severe cases. Topical 5% doxepin cream has been reported to reduce pruritus; topical formulations, however, have also been associated with reports of allergic contact dermatitis and sedation.

Patients may have sudden exacerbations of AD due to overgrowth of *S. aureus* that can be independent of clinical signs of bacterial infection, a notion supported by the clinical response of patients with severe AD to anti-staphylococcal *antibiotics*. Honey-colored crusting, folliculitis, and pyoderma are signs of overt infection, and topical and/or oral antibiotic therapy – typically of short duration to avoid the development of bacterial resistance – is indicated. Skin cultures and sensitivity testing should be considered prior to treatment, as methicillin-resistant *S. aureus* (MRSA) may be an important pathogen in some patients. Recurrent, deep-seated *S. aureus* infections should raise the possibility of an immunodeficiency syndrome such as hyper-IgE syndrome.

The addition of *antiseptics* to bath water, e.g., diluted bleach baths ('like swimming in pool water'), may help reduce the number of local skin infections and the need for systemic antibiotics in AD patients with heavily colonized and/or superinfected skin. A bleach bath can be prepared by mixing one-quarter to half a cup of sodium hypochlorite 6% solution (chlorine liquid bleach) in a bathtub full of lukewarm water; the goal is to create a modified Dakin's solution with a final bleach concentration that approximates 0.005%. The patient may soak for 5–10 minutes, rinse their skin thoroughly with fresh water, pat dry, and then apply their topical therapy and/or emollient/moisturizer. Proprietary bath additives containing antiseptics are also available. It is most important that these should be added to the bath water and never applied directly to the skin, to avoid the risk of irritation.

Eczema herpeticum may be easily misdiagnosed as bacterial superinfection and represents a serious risk in patients with widespread AD. Patients can present with multiple vesiculopustular lesions and painful, 'punched-out' erosions that fail to respond to oral antibiotics. Document herpes infection prior to treatment via culture and/or direct fluorescent antibody (DFA), and initiate *antiviral therapy* as soon as possible. Intravenous treatment is certainly indicated in cases of severe disseminated eczema herpeticum. Oral aciclovir (or equivalent dosage of another anti-herpetic medication) may be useful in adults with herpes simplex confined to the skin; 400 mg three times daily for 10 days or 200 mg four times daily for 10 days usually provides a sufficient dosage.

Fungal infections such as those caused by *Trichophyton rubrum* may also be more common in AD patients. *Antifungal therapy* has been shown to reduce the severity of AD lesions exacerbated by *Malassezia furfur*, particularly in the seborrheic areas of the skin and scalp. Patients with documented dermatophyte infection or IgE antibodies to *Malassezia* may benefit from a trial of topical or systemic antifungal therapy.

Owing to a greater understanding of immunologic reaction patterns in the skin, gut, and airways there has been great interest in *probiotics*. Because the findings to date on their utility in preventing or modifying AD are conflicting, however, the long-term significance of probiotics in the treatment of atopic dermatitis warrants further investigation.

Breastfeeding/timing of solid food introduction

In January 2008, the American Academy of Pediatrics' Committee on Nutrition and Section on Allergy and Immunology concluded that there is a lack of evidence to support a major role in AD for maternal dietary restrictions during pregnancy or lactation. For infants at high risk of developing atopic disease, the Committee recommended exclusive breastfeeding for at least 4 months (compared to feeding intact cow's milk protein formula) to help reduce the cumulative incidence of atopic dermatitis in the first 2 years of life; beyond this period exclusive breastfeeding did not seem to lead to additional benefit in the incidence of AD. The Committee also reported that there is no convincing evidence that delaying solid foods beyond 4–6 months of age has a significant protective effect on the development of atopic disease. This includes delaying the introduction of those foods thought to be highly allergic, such as cow's milk, fish, eggs, and peanut-containing foods.

Systemic corticosteroids are commonly prescribed in pediatric outpatient and emergency settings for AD exacerbations, though few clinical trials support their use. The temptation to use systemic corticosteroids can be great, given the dramatic clinical improvement that can occur. The propensity to flare with abrupt discontinuation of treatment and the well-known associated systemic side-effect profile, however, suggest that systemic corticosteroids should be reserved for 'crisis cases' – and even then used with the intent to bridge to another systemic agent or phototherapy.

Although the exact mechanism of action is unknown, *photo-therapy* in AD is thought to suppress proinflammatory cytokines (IL-2, IL-12) and induce T-cell apoptosis.

Broadband UVB, broadband UVA, narrowband UVB (311 nm), UVA-1 (340–400 nm), and combined UV A-B phototherapy have been reported to be useful for widespread or recalcitrant disease. Photochemotherapy with psoralen and UVA light may be indicated in severe cases. Multiple treatments are usually required to be effective, and this can be inconvenient for patients and their families, depending on location and accessibility to a suitable light source. Side effects can include skin pain, erythema, pruritus, and pigment changes. Likewise, UV radiation may increase the long-term risk of premature skin aging and cutaneous malignancies. Shielding and appropriate eye protection may help minimize unnecessary exposure.

Ciclosporin is a calcineurin inhibitor that blocks activation of T lymphocytes and reduces the transcription of cytokines, including IL-2, shown to be involved in the pathogenesis of AD. It may be used as a short-term treatment or as a bridge between other steroid-sparing alternatives. Ciclosporin is typically dosed at 2.5–5 mg/kg/day, and a response may be seen in 2–3 weeks. Alternatively, some experts prefer dosing ciclosporin microemulsion at 3 mg/kg/day in children, or 150 mg (low dose) or 300 mg (high dose) in adults. Flares can occur after discontinuation of therapy, so gradual tapering is recommended. The safety and efficacy of ciclosporin are well documented in both adults and children, and treatment with this agent is associated with reduced skin disease and an improved quality of life. Hypertension and renal toxicity, as well as concerns about malignancy, are limitations to long-term therapy. Continuous therapy is not recommended beyond 1 year, and it is unknown how many short courses may be given safely. Blood pressure, CBC, renal and hepatic function tests, magnesium, and uric acid should be monitored regularly.

Azathioprine (AZA), a 6-mercaptopurine analog that inhibits purine synthesis and demonstrates cytotoxic and immunosuppressive properties, can be effective monotherapy for AD. Marrow suppression and liver toxicity are major concerns, and blood cell counts and liver function tests should be monitored closely. Because one in 300 individuals is homozygous for low metabolic activity alleles (low activity correlates with higher risk of marrow suppression) azathioprine should be dosed according to thiopurine methyltransferase (TPMT) genotype/levels. Drug hypersensitivity and gastrointestinal disturbances have also been reported.

Methotrexate is a folic acid analog that inhibits dihydrofolate reductase and interferes with DNA synthesis and lymphocyte proliferation, leading to anti-inflammatory effects. Controlled trials with methotrexate are lacking, but its greatest advantage may be that, at the relatively low doses used for skin disease, it appears less immunosuppressive than other AD systemic therapies. A recent open, prospective, 24-week trial of adults with AD demonstrated a response plateau at around 12 weeks, with little additional improvement at doses greater than 15 mg weekly; alternatively, some experts dose methotrexate at 2.5 mg daily for 4 days per week. A recent retrospective review of children showed that AD was well controlled with effective dosing of 0.5–0.8 mg/kg/week (either as a single weekly dose or divided 3–4 days/week). There is a long history of use in pediatric and adult inflammatory disease. Nausea and liver function abnormalities/hepatotoxicity may limit dosing. Pulmonary toxicity may be another potential concern. It is unclear what role folic acid supplementation plays in the treatment of AD with methotrexate.

Evidence Levels: **A** Double-blind study **B** Clinical trial ≥ 20 subjects **C** Clinical trial < 20 subjects **D** Series ≥ 5 subjects **E** Anecdotal case reports

Mycophenolate mofetil (MMF) has a good safety profile and represents a possible therapeutic alternative for severe, refractory AD. It is an inhibitor of inosine monophosphate involved in de novo purine synthesis, and has been used as an immunosuppressant in organ transplantation. Several adult studies have demonstrated efficacy at doses up to 2 g daily. A retrospective review of MMF as monotherapy in 14 pediatric AD patients showed MMF to be safe and effective at doses of 40–50 mg/kg/day in younger children (presumably due to increased surface area-to-volume ratios) and 30–40 mg/kg/day in adolescents, with maximal effect after 8–12 weeks of therapy. Patients should be monitored for leukopenia and anemia, and drug levels may be increased in the setting of renal insufficiency. MMF has been loosely linked to herpes retinitis, dose-related bone marrow suppression, and increased infection (*S. aureus*). Further prospective controlled studies are needed for this promising therapy.

Interferon-γ (IFN-γ) is well known to inhibit Th2 cell proliferation/function and to suppress IgE responses. Several adult AD studies have demonstrated efficacy with three-times-weekly high-dose (150 μg/m²) and low-dose (50 μg/m²) therapy. Disadvantages of therapy include flu-like symptoms (especially common early in the treatment course), myelosuppression, neurotoxicity/confusion, hypotension, tachycardia, and cost.

Referral to a pediatric dermatologist or an adult dermatologist/atopic dermatitis specialist may help with comprehensive management of skin care and barrier repair. Likewise, consider referring those patients with a diagnosis of moderate or severe AD; those who are unresponsive to standard treatments (including moderate-potency topical corticosteroids); those with persistent disease and/or frequent flares; those who have been hospitalized as a direct consequence of their AD; and those requiring systemic therapies for flares and/or maintenance. *Allergy testing* is not generally a first-line referral recommendation in the routine evaluation and treatment of uncomplicated AD. Consultation with an allergist can be useful, however, when proper skin care is not working and/or when the clinical picture hints strongly at specific allergic triggers. Immunotherapy with aeroallergens has not been proved effective in the treatment of AD. Referral to immunology or gastroenterology is warranted if underlying systemic infections are frequent or when eosinophilic gastroenteritis/esophagitis becomes a concern in younger children, with concomitant failure to thrive.

Emotional stress can exacerbate AD in some patients who may respond to frustration, anxiety, embarrassment, or other psychologically stressful events with a perceived increase in pruritus and subsequent scratching. This may be particularly important in the adolescent population, where even very mild skin disease may be considered 'disfiguring.' In some cases, patients may use scratching for secondary gain, and in others scratching has simply become habitual. *Relaxation, biofeedback,* and *behavioral modification* techniques may be helpful in such patients. *Psychosocial evaluation* and counseling should be considered in families where emotional triggers appear to function as obstacles to disease management, or where quality of life is clearly affected. Families may also benefit from *support groups* such as the National Eczema Association (US) (*www. nationaleczema.org*) and the National Eczema Society (UK) (*www.eczema.org*).

Hospitalization

Erythrodermic AD patients, those with suspected widespread superinfection, or those with severe recalcitrant disease may benefit from hospitalization. Removal from environmental or emotional stressors, intensive therapy, and carer education should be the goals. Hospitalization may be particularly useful in those patients being transitioned to systemic therapies. It also provides an opportunity for coordinated care between multiple specialty services.

SPECIFIC INVESTIGATIONS

In selected cases only
▶ Skin biopsy
▶ IgE, IgA, IgM, and IgG levels
▶ RAST or intracutaneous allergen testing and oral food challenges
▶ HIV ELISA

Management of atopic dermatitis in the pediatric population. Krakowski AC, Eichenfield LF, Dohil MA. Pediatrics 2008; 122: 812–24.

This paper presents an overview of the strategy for diagnosis and management of AD.

Consensus conference on pediatric atopic dermatitis. Eichenfield LF, Hanifin JM, Luger TA, Stevens SR, Pride HB. J Am Acad Dermatol 2003; 49: 1088–95.

This is a practical set of criteria for the diagnosis of AD, reflecting a consensus meeting by a working group.

Food hypersensitivity and atopic dermatitis: pathophysiology, epidemiology, diagnosis, and management. Sicherer SH, Sampson HA. J Allergy Clin Immunol 1999; 104: S114–22.

Food allergy may play a pathogenic role in a subset of AD patients. Identifying this subset may necessitate appropriate laboratory tests and, in some cases, physician-supervised oral food challenges. Most food allergies resolve in early childhood, and food allergy is rarely of importance in older children and adults.

Seborrheic dermatitis-like and atopic dermatitis-like eruptions in HIV-infected patients. Cockerell CJ. Clin Dermatol 1991; 9: 49–51.

Crusting and lichenification in the flexural areas or in a more widespread distribution, characteristic of an 'AD-like' dermatitis, may represent advanced HIV infection.

FIRST-LINE THERAPIES

▶ Education	B
▶ Emollients	B
▶ Topical corticosteroids	A
▶ Wet wraps	C

Age related, structured educational programmes for the management of atopic dermatitis in children and adolescents: multicentre, randomized controlled trial. Staab D, Diepgen T, Fartasch M, Kupfer J, Lob-Corzilius T, Ring J, et al. Br Med J 2006; 332: 933–8.

This multicenter, randomized controlled trial compared children with AD whose parents had received 6 weeks of intensive AD education to those children whose parents did not. The investigators taught age-appropriate interventions to the parents of AD patients at seven hospitals in Germany. Educational classes were organized according to age, with separate once-weekly sessions for the parents of children aged 3 months to 7 years (n=274), 8–12 years (n=102), and 3–18 years (n=70). Compared to the children of parents who did not receive any extra instruction, patients in all three treatment groups demonstrated significantly improved subjective quality of life scores and objective measures of eczema severity over the 12-month period.

Pediatric atopic eczema: the impact of an educational intervention. Grillo M, Gassner L, Marshman G, Dunn S, Hudson P. Pediatr Dermatol 2006; 23: 428–36.

This longitudinal, controlled study randomized 61 AD patients (0–16 years of age) into an educational treatment group and a control group. Significantly improved objective clinical scores were seen in the treatment group at weeks 4 and 12. Quality of life measures did not significantly improve with reduced severity of eczema, except in the group aged 5–16 years which, despite small numbers, showed a significant improvement in QOL scores.

Psychological and educational interventions for atopic eczema in children. Ersser SJ, Latter S, Sibley A, Satherley PA, Welbourne S. Cochrane Database Syst Rev 2007 Jul 18; CD004054.

This systematic review of five randomized, controlled trials concluded that the lack of rigorously designed trials provides only limited evidence of the effectiveness of educational and psychological interventions in helping to manage AD. The authors state that there is a need for further and comparative evaluation to examine the cost-effectiveness of these programs and their suitability for different health systems.

Emollients improve treatment results with topical corticosteroids in childhood atopic dermatitis: a randomized comparative study. Szczepanowska J, Reich A, Szepietowski JC. Pediatr Allergy Immunol 2008; 19: 614–8.

A randomized study of 52 patients aged 2–12 years found that the use of emollients can significantly improve xerosis and pruritus during corticosteroid treatment of atopic dermatitis and helped maintain clinical improvement after discontinuation of therapy.

A systematic review of the safety of topical therapies for atopic dermatitis. Callen J, Chamlin S, Eichenfield LF, Ellis C, Girardi M, Goldfarb M, et al. Br J Dermatol 2007; 156: 203–21.

This review of topical therapies for atopic dermatitis found that although some systemic exposure to topical steroids does occur, physiologic changes appear to be uncommon and systemic complications are rare when medications are used properly.

Systematic review of treatments of atopic eczema. Hoare C, Li Wan Po A, Williams H. Health Technol Assess 2000; 4: 1–191.

Systematic review of 272 randomized controlled trials covering 47 different classes of AD interventions.

Topical corticosteroids for atopic eczema: clinical and cost effectiveness of once-daily vs. more frequent use. Green C, Colquitt JL, Kirby J, Davidson P. Br J Dermatol 2005; 152: 130–41.

A systematic review found no clear differences in outcomes between once-daily and more frequent application of topical corticosteroids.

Topical fluticasone propionate lotion does not cause HPA axis suppression. Hebert AA, Friedlander SF, Allen DB. J Pediatr 2006; 149: 378–82.

An open-label study of 42 moderate to severe AD patients aged 3 months to 6 years; cortisol stimulation tests were normal in all subjects following 3–4 weeks of twice-daily application (65% mean BSA treated).

Diluted steroid facial wet wraps for childhood atopic eczema. Tang WYM. Dermatology 2000; 200: 338–9.

A short period of diluted steroid wet-wrap dressings – e.g., mometasone 0.1% diluted to 0.01% (one part mometasone cream or ointment to nine parts diluent cream or ointment) – is useful in selected children with dry eczematous facial lesions.

Efficacy and safety of wet-wrap dressings in children with severe atopic dermatitis: influence of corticosteroid dilution. Wolkerstorfer A, Visser RL, De Waard van der Spek FB, Mulder PG, Oranje AP. Br J Dermatol 2000; 143: 999–1004.

In children with severe refractory AD, 5%, 10%, and 25% dilutions of fluticasone propionate 0.05% cream proved highly efficacious, irrespective of dilution, when applied under wet-wrap dressings. Improvement occurred mainly during the first week, and the only significant adverse effect was folliculitis.

Efficacy and safety of wet-wrap dressings as an intervention treatment in children with severe and/or refractory atopic dermatitis: a critical review of the literature. Devillers ACA, Oranje AP. Br J Dermatol 2006; 154: 579–85.

In this review of 24 wet wrap-related publications, 11 were found to be detailed original clinical studies (study design level 2–4); 13 were expert opinions (study design level 5). Evidence levels did not exceed level 4.

SECOND-LINE THERAPIES

▶ Topical immunomodulators	A
▶ Antimicrobials	C
▶ Antihistamines/anxiolytics	C
▶ Barrier repair products	B
▶ Avoidance of triggers	A

Intermittent therapy for flare prevention and long-term disease control in stabilized atopic dermatitis: a randomized comparison of 3-times-weekly applications of tacrolimus ointment versus vehicle. Breneman D, Fleischer AB Jr, Abramovits W, Zeichner J, Gold MH, Kirsner RS, et al. J Am Acad Dermatol 2008; 58: 990–9.

A double-blind study in which 197 clinically clear patients with a history of moderate to severe AD were randomized to three-times weekly topical tacrolimus or vehicle for 40 weeks; tacrolimus ointment was associated with significantly more flare-free days than vehicle, and a significantly longer time until relapse.

Sustained efficacy and safety of pimecrolimus cream 1% when used long-term (up to 26 weeks) to treat children with atopic dermatitis. Langley RG, Eichenfield LF, Lucky AW, Boguniewicz M, Barbier N, Cherill R. Pediatr Dermatol 2008; 25: 301–7.

Two 26-week studies (6 weeks double-blind, followed by 20 weeks' open-label phases) were conducted in 2–17-year-old children with AD. Pimecrolimus was significantly more effective in treating the face and neck than the rest of the body (p<0.0001) and more effective than vehicle (p<0.0001) in the double-blind phase. Disease control was sustained in the pimecrolimus group throughout the whole study.

0.03% Tacrolimus ointment applied once or twice daily is more efficacious than 1% hydrocortisone acetate in children with moderate to severe atopic dermatitis: results of a randomized double-blind controlled trial. Reitamo S, Harper J, Bos JD, Cambazard F, Bruijnzeel-Koomen C, Valk P, et al; European Tacrolimus Ointment Group. Br J Dermatol 2004; 150: 554–62.

Once- or twice-daily tacrolimus ointment 0.03% was significantly more effective than hydrocortisone acetate 1% in treating moderate to severe AD in children. Twice-daily application was particularly effective in patients with severe baseline disease compared to once-daily application.

Efficacy and safety of pimecrolimus cream in the long-term management of atopic dermatitis in children. Wahn U, Bos JD, Goodfield M, Caputo R, Papp K, Manjra A, et al. Pediatrics 2002; 110: e2.

Pimecrolimus prevented progression to flares in more than 50% of patients and reduced or eliminated the need for topical corticosteroids. Benefits were consistently seen at 6 months and were sustained for 12 months.

Safety and efficacy of pimecrolimus (ASM 981) cream 1% in the treatment of mild and moderate atopic dermatitis in children and adolescents. Eichenfield LF, Lucky AW, Boguniewicz M, Langley RG, Cherill R, Marshall K, et al. J Am Acad Dermatol 2002; 46: 495–504.

Skin colonization by Staphylococcus aureus in patients with eczema and atopic dermatitis and relevant combined topical therapy: a double-blind multicentre randomized controlled trial. Gong JQ, Lin L, Lin T, Hao F, Zeng FQ, Bi ZG, et al. Br J Dermatol 2006; 155: 680–7.

Staphylococcus aureus: colonizing features and influence of an antibacterial treatment in adults with atopic dermatitis. Breuer K, Haussler S, Kapp A, Werfel T. Br J Dermatol 2002; 147: 55–61.

Sixty-two of 66 AD adult subjects were found to be carriers of S. aureus; most harbored the bacteria on both skin and anterior nares. Ten of 32 exotoxin-screened patients were colonized with toxigenic strains of bacteria. AD scores decreased in nine of 10 patients who received antimicrobial treatment (p<0.001), and the effect was more pronounced in patients with severe disease at baseline.

Effects of cefuroxime axetil on Staphylococcus aureus colonization and superantigen production in atopic dermatitis. Boguniewicz M, Sampson H, Leung SB, Harbeck R, Leung DY. J Allergy Clin Immunol 2001; 108: 651–2.

An evidence-based review of the efficacy of antihistamines in relieving pruritus in atopic dermatitis. Klein PA, Clark RA. Arch Dermatol 1999; 135: 1522–5.

This review of 16 AD-associated antihistamine trials found that the majority of studies were flawed in terms of sample size or study design.

Addition of fexofenadine to a topical corticosteroid reduces the pruritus associated with atopic dermatitis in a 1-week randomized, multicentre, double-blind, placebo-controlled, parallel-group study. Kawashima M, Tango T, Noguchi T. Br J Dermatol 2003; 148: 1212–21.

In this multicentre, double-blind study, patients aged 16 years with AD were randomized to topical steroid plus fexofenadine HCl 60 mg twice daily (n=201) versus topical steroid plus placebo (n=199) for 1 week. The treatment group demonstrated a significant improvement in pruritus scores versus placebo.

A double-blinded, randomized, placebo-controlled trial of cetirizine in preventing the onset of asthma in children with atopic dermatitis: 18 months' treatment and 18 months' posttreatment follow-up. Warner JO, ETAC Study Group. Early Treatment of the Atopic Child. J Allergy Clin Immunol 2001; 108: 929–37.

Infants between 1 and 2 years of age with AD in this double-blinded trial were randomized to 0.25 mg/kg body weight cetirizine administered twice daily compared with placebo. After 18 months of treatment, follow-up continued for a further 18 months. Although there was no difference in the cumulative prevalence of asthma between active and placebo treatment in the intention-to-treat population (p=0.7), cetirizine did appear to delay (and in some cases to prevent) the development of asthma in those patients sensitized to grass pollen and, to a lesser extent, house dust mites.

Management of sleep disturbance associated with atopic dermatitis. Kelsay K. J Allergy Clin Immunol 2006; 118: 198–201.

The author suggests an algorithm for clinicians treating sleep problems associated with AD.

MAS063DP is effective monotherapy for mild to moderate atopic dermatitis in infants and children: A multicenter, randomized, vehicle-controlled study. Boguniewicz M, Zeichner JA, Eichenfield LF, Hebert AA, Jarratt M, Lucky AW, et al. J Pediatr 2008; 152: 854–9.

This study randomized AD patients (6 months to 12 years of age) into a three-times-daily treatment group (n=72) and a vehicle group (n=70) for 22 days. MAS063DP cream was statistically more effective (p<0.0001) than vehicle for improving objective eczema scores.

Ceramide-dominant barrier repair lipids alleviate childhood atopic dermatitis: changes in barrier function provide a sensitive indicator of disease activity. Chamlin S, Kao J, Frieden I, Sheu MY, Fowler AJ, Fluhr JW, et al. J Am Acad Dermatol 2002; 47: 198–208.

Adjuvant treatment of atopic eczema: assessment of an emollient containing N-palmitoylethanolamine (ATOPA study). Eberlein B, Eicke C, Reinhardt HW, Ring J. J Eur Acad Dermatol Venereol 2008; 22: 73–82.

THIRD-LINE THERAPIES

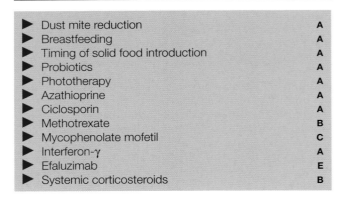

▶ Dust mite reduction	A
▶ Breastfeeding	A
▶ Timing of solid food introduction	A
▶ Probiotics	A
▶ Phototherapy	A
▶ Azathioprine	A
▶ Ciclosporin	A
▶ Methotrexate	B
▶ Mycophenolate mofetil	C
▶ Interferon-γ	A
▶ Efaluzimab	E
▶ Systemic corticosteroids	B

Double-blind controlled trial of effect of housedust-mite allergen avoidance on atopic dermatitis. Tan BB, Weald D, Strickland I, Friedmann PS. Lancet 1996; 347: 15–18.

Measures to reduce house dust mites using a combination of Gore-tex bedcovers, benzyltannate spray, and a high-filtration vacuum cleaner were compared with cotton bedcovers, water spray, and a conventional vacuum cleaner in the households of 48 children and adults with AD. Both active and placebo treatments caused significant reductions in house dust mite antigen concentrations. The severity of eczema decreased in both groups, but the active group showed significantly greater improvement.

A treatment approach for atopic dermatitis. Dohil MA, Eichenfield LF. Pediatr Ann 2005; 34: 201–10.

Rice nightmare: Kwashiorkor in 2 Philadelphia-area infants fed Rice Dream beverage. Katz KA, Mahlberg MJ, Honig PJ, Yan AC. J Am Acad Dermatol 2005; 52: S69–72.

Prolonged exclusive breastfeeding is associated with increased atopic dermatitis: a prospective follow-up study of unselected healthy newborns from birth to age 20 years. Pesonen M, Kallio MJ, Ranki A, Siimes MA. Clin Exp Allergy 2006; 36: 1011–18.

Breastfeeding as prophylaxis against atopic disease: prospective follow-up study until 17 years old. Saarinen UM, Kajosaari M. Lancet 1995; 346: 1065–9.

Timing of solid food introduction in relation to atopic dermatitis and atopic sensitization: results from a prospective birth cohort study. Zutavern A, Brockow I, Schaaf B, Bolte G, von Berg A, Diez U, et al. Pediatrics 2006; 117: 401–11.

Probiotics during pregnancy and breast-feeding might confer immunomodulatory protection against atopic disease in the infant. Rautava S, Kalliomäki M, Isolauri E. J Allergy Clin Immunol 2002; 109: 119–21.

Probiotic supplementation for the first 6 months of life fails to reduce the risk of atopic dermatitis and increases the risk of allergen sensitization in high-risk children: a randomized controlled trial. Taylor AL, Dunstan JA, Prescott SL. J Allergy Clin Immunol 2007; 119: 184–91.

Probiotics in primary prevention of atopic disease: a randomised placebo-controlled trial. Kalliomäki M, Salminen S, Arvilommi H, Kero P, Koskinen P, Isolauri E. Lancet 2001; 357: 1076–9.

Lactobacillus was given orally to mothers predisposed to giving birth to a possible atopic child, and postnatally for 6 months to the child. The frequency of atopic eczema in the treated group was half of that in the placebo group.

Effects of early nutritional interventions on the development of atopic disease in infants and children: The role of maternal dietary restriction, breastfeeding, timing of introduction of complementary foods, and hydrolyzed formulas. Greer FR, Sicherer SH, Burks AW; Committee on Nutrition and Section on Allergy and Immunology. Pediatrics 2008; 121: 183–91.

Phototherapy in the management of atopic dermatitis: a systematic review. [Review] Meduri NB, Vandergriff T, Rasmussen H, Jacobe H. Photodermatol Photoimmunol Photomed 2007; 23: 106–12.

Phototherapy for atopic eczema with narrow-band UVB. Grundmann-Kollmann M, Behrens S, Podda M, Peter RU, Kaufmann R, Kerscher M. J Am Acad Dermatol 1999; 40: 995–7.

Five patients with moderate to severe AD were treated with narrowband UVB for a cumulative dose of 9.2 J/cm^2 over a mean of 19 treatments. Narrowband UVB was effective after 3 weeks in all patients.

The role of psoralen photochemotherapy (PUVA) in the treatment of severe atopic eczema in adolescents. Atherton DJ, Carabott F, Glover MT, Hawk JL. Br J Dermatol 1988; 118: 791–5.

Oral PUVA resulted in initial clearance of eczema in 14 of 15 children, nine of whom achieved complete remission. This was associated with resumption of normal growth in children who were previously growing poorly.

Half-side comparison study on the efficacy of 8-methoxypsoralen bath-PUVA versus narrow-band ultraviolet B phototherapy in patients with severe chronic atopic dermatitis. Der-Petrossian M, Seeber A, Honigsmann H, Tanew A. Br J Dermatol 2000; 142: 39–43.

In this randomized, investigator-blinded, half-side comparison study in 12 patients with severe chronic AD, half-side irradiation with threshold erythemogenic doses of 8-methoxypsoralen bath-PUVA and narrowband UVB was performed three times weekly over a period of 6 weeks. The two modalities were equally effective in equi-erythemogenic doses.

Long-term efficacy of medium-dose UVA1 phototherapy in atopic dermatitis. Abeck D, Schmidt T, Fesq H, Strom K, Mempel M, Brockow K, et al. J Am Acad Dermatol 2000; 42: 254–7.

Thirty-two patients with acute exacerbated AD underwent medium-dose UVA1 therapy consisting of 15 treatments over 3 weeks (cumulative dose 750 J/cm^2). There was a significant improvement in the skin condition at the end of the treatment period; this was still present 1 month later, but by 3 months the condition had returned to pretreatment levels.

Retrospective review of the use of azathioprine in severe atopic dermatitis. Lear JT, English JS, Jones P, Smith AG. J Am Acad Dermatol 1996; 35: 642–3.

A retrospective study of 35 patients who had received azathioprine for severe AD showed a reduction in antibiotic use, fewer outpatient visits and hospital admissions, and reduced use of similar or higher-potency topical steroids in the year after treatment.

Azathioprine in severe adult atopic dermatitis: a double-blind, placebo-controlled, crossover trial. Berth-Jones J, Takwale A, Tan E, Barclay G, Agarwal S, Ahmed I, et al. Br J Dermatol 2002; 147: 324–30.

In this double-blind crossover trial, adult patients with severe AD were treated with azathioprine 2.5 mg/kg daily and placebo for 3 months each. There was a significant difference in favor of azathioprine in the improvement of the Six Area, Six Sign Atopic Dermatitis (SASSAD) sign score, which was the primary endpoint. This decreased by 26% during treatment with azathioprine, versus 3% on placebo. Pruritus, sleep disturbance, and disruption of work/daytime activity all improved significantly on active treatment, but the difference in mean improvement between azathioprine and placebo was statistically significant only for disruption of work/daytime activity. The authors suggested that a longer period of treatment might have further improved the eczema. Gastrointestinal disturbances and deranged liver enzymes were common. Of the 37 patients enrolled, 12 prematurely terminated treatment with azathioprine, and four with placebo.

Parallel-group randomized controlled trial of azathioprine in moderate to severe atopic eczema, using a thiopurine methyltransferase-based dose regimen. Meggitt SJ, Gray JC, Reynolds NJ. Br J Dermatol 2003; 149: 3.

In this study of parallel-group design, 63 patients were randomized. There was again a significant improvement in sign score on azathioprine (39%) relative to placebo (24%). In contrast to the previous study, there was a marked placebo effect. However, pruritus and the physician's global assessment also improved significantly better in the azathioprine group. Six patients withdrew from azathioprine treatment because of nausea or hypersensitivity.

Cyclosporine in the treatment of patients with atopic eczema – a systematic review and meta-analysis. Schmitt J, Schmitt N, Meurer M. J Eur Acad Dermatol Venereol 2007; 21: 606–19.

Double-blind, controlled, crossover study of cyclosporine in adults with severe refractory atopic dermatitis. Sowden JM, Berth-Jones J, Ross J, Motley RJ, Marks R, Finlay AY, et al. Lancet 1991; 338: 137–40.

Cyclosporine greatly improves the quality of life of adults with severe atopic dermatitis. Salek MS, Finlay AY, Luscombe DK, Allen BR, Berth-Jones J, Camp RD, et al. Br J Dermatol 1993; 129: 422–30.

In this study, both sign score and quality of life improved rapidly on 5 mg/kg ciclosporin daily. Whereas the sign score deteriorated rapidly on stopping treatment, the improvement in quality of life was more persistent.

Cyclosporine in atopic dermatitis: time to relapse and effect of intermittent therapy. Granlund H, Erkko P, Sinisalo M, Reitamo S. Br J Dermatol 1994; 132: 106–12.

Forty-three patients with severe AD were treated with a 6-week course of ciclosporin 5 mg/kg daily, and then re-treated after a follow-up of 6–26 weeks (depending on the time to relapse) with an identical course of ciclosporin. A significant reduction in disease activity was observed after 2 weeks of ciclosporin treatment. After both treatment periods, approximately half of the patients relapsed after 2 weeks; after 6 weeks follow-up the relapse rates were 71% and 90%, respectively, for the two treatment periods. Notably, after the first treatment period, five patients did not relapse during the 26-week follow-up, and for the second treatment period two did not relapse. All of these seven patients were still in remission at 1 year.

Long-term efficacy and safety of cyclosporine in severe adult atopic dermatitis. Berth-Jones J, Graham-Brown RAC, Marks R, Camp RD, English JS, Freeman K, et al. Br J Dermatol 1997; 136: 76–81.

An open study of 48 weeks' duration in which 100 patients were enrolled. Improvements in sign score, itch, and sleep disturbance were maintained throughout treatment. Sixty-five subjects completed the trial and only seven were withdrawn due to adverse events considered likely to have been related to treatment.

Cyclosporine in atopic dermatitis: review of the literature and outline of a Belgian consensus. Naeyaert JM, Lachapelle JM, Degreef H, de la Brassinne M, Heenen M, Lambert J. Dermatology 1999; 198: 145–52.

This excellent review summarizes all the major trials of ciclosporin for AD and gives practical recommendations for the clinician.

These authors recommend that ciclosporin be reserved for adults with severe AD and only used in children with recalcitrant disease for short periods. A starting dosage of 2.5 mg/kg daily can be adjusted up after 2 weeks, depending on response, to a maximum dose of 5 mg/kg daily. Screening for gynecologic or prostate malignancy, and skin biopsy to exclude cutaneous T-cell lymphoma, as well as close monitoring of renal function and blood pressure, are recommended.

An open-label, dose-ranging study of methotrexate for moderate-to-severe adult atopic eczema. Weatherhead SC, Wahie S, Reynolds NJ, Meggitt SJ. Br J Dermatol 2007; 156: 346–51.

This 24-week, open-label safety and efficacy study evaluated 12 adults with moderate to severe AD in a dose-ranging, prospective trial of methotrexate.

Treatment of atopic eczema with oral mycophenolate mofetil. Neuber K, Schwartz I, Itschert G, Dieck AT. Br J Dermatol 2000; 143: 385–91.

Ten patients with severe AD were treated with oral mycophenolate mofetil at an initial dose of 1 g/day during the first week and then 2 g daily for a further 11 weeks. Median scores for disease severity improved by 68% (100% in one patient, >75% in three patients, and >50% in the remainder).

Mycophenolate mofetil for severe childhood atopic dermatitis: experience in 14 patients. Heller M, Shin HT, Orlow SJ, Schaffer JV. Br J Dermatol 2007; 157: 127–32.

Recombinant interferon gamma therapy for atopic dermatitis. Hanifin JM, Schneider LC, Leung DY, Ellis CN, Jaffe HS, Izu AE, et al. J Am Acad Dermatol 1993; 28: 189–97.

In this randomized, double-blind study, patients with moderate to severe AD received recombinant human IFN-γ (rIFN-γ; 50 μg/m^2) or placebo by daily subcutaneous injection for 12 weeks. Significant reductions in erythema, pruritus, and excoriation occurred in rIFN-γ-treated patients. Edema, papulation, induration, scaling, dryness, and lichenification showed greater improvement in the rIFN-γ group, but differences were not statistically significant.

Long-term effectiveness and safety of recombinant human interferon gamma therapy for atopic dermatitis despite unchanged serum IgE levels. Stevens SR, Hanifin JM, Hamilton T, Tofte SJ, Cooper KD. Arch Dermatol 1998; 134: 799–804.

Twenty-four of 32 eligible patients who participated in a previously reported 12-week, double-blind, placebo-controlled study, self-administered rIFN-γ, 50 μg/m^2, by daily subcutaneous injection. The initial efficacy and adverse effects reported for rIFN-γ treatment of patients with AD were maintained after 2 years of long-term use.

Do some patients with atopic dermatitis require long term oral steroid therapy? Sonenthal KR, Grammer LC, Patterson R. J Allergy Clin Immunol 1993; 91: 971–3.

Three patients with recalcitrant AD were successfully managed on oral corticosteroids.

Evidence Levels: **A** Double-blind study **B** Clinical trial ≥ 20 subjects **C** Clinical trial < 20 subjects **D** Series ≥ 5 subjects **E** Anecdotal case reports

Atypical nevi

Ronald P Rapini

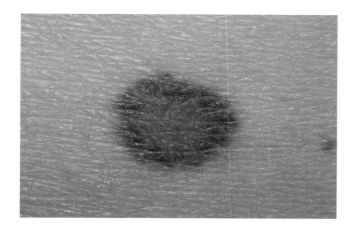

Atypical nevi (atypical moles) are melanocytic neoplasms that deviate from the stereotypical changes expected in benign melanocytic nevi but which do not meet definitive criteria for the diagnosis of malignancy (melanoma). Dermatopathologic terminology is problematic, as there is frequent disagreement about nomenclature and the relative importance of various criteria for distinguishing benign versus malignant lesions. *Dysplastic nevi* (*nevi with architectural disorder, Clark nevi*) might be considered by some to be within this group. Sometimes the term dysplastic nevus is used synonymously with atypical nevus, whereas sometimes it is used instead for those nevi that have more architectural and cytologic atypia at the dermoepidermal junction zone, rather than any dermal atypical cytology. Histologically, dysplastic nevi often have elongated rete ridges, bridging of melanocytes between rete ridges, a predominance of single melanocytes over nested melanocytes, papillary dermal fibroplasia, and a slight inflammatory reaction.

Dysplastic nevi may be considered more of a marker of patients at higher risk of melanoma than as frequent precursors of melanoma within individual lesions. It is not mandatory to remove all nevi that are 'dysplastic' in appearance. It is important to also note that two-thirds of melanomas do not arise from previous nevi, so that removing all atypical nevi does not prevent melanoma. It is helpful to perform total body skin examinations in patients at risk for melanoma, looking for the *'ugling duckling nevus,'* which stands out as different from that patient's typical *'signature nevi.'* The mnemonic ABCDE has been used as a clinical aid (*a*symmetry, *b*order irregularity, *c*olor variegation, *d*iameter >6 mm, and *e*volution or change in a lesion).

Some authorities advocate grading these lesions as mild, moderate, or severe dysplastic nevi (NIH Consensus Conference. Diagnosis and treatment of early melanoma. JAMA 1992; 268: 1314–19). Others have argued that such grading has poor reproducibility, and therefore they do not grade the severity of the atypia. Still others prefer to grade the architectural abnormalities and the cytologic abnormalities separately. *Spitz nevus* (spindle and epithelioid cell nevus, S&E nevus, benign juvenile melanoma) is a benign 'mole' of

children and young adults which can be difficult to distinguish histologically from melanoma.

Because melanoma can metastasize and kill the patient, the treatment of atypical nevi, dysplastic nevi, and Spitz nevi depends on the relative certainty of the diagnosis. *Patients with numerous nevi* (more than 100, for example), a personal melanoma history, and those with a positive *family history of melanoma* are at higher risk. Pathologists have various ways of indicating when they are unsure of the diagnosis: besides using the term atypical nevus they use terms such as *atypical melanocytic proliferation, atypical Spitz tumor, atypical blue nevus,* MELTUMP (*melanocytic tumor of uncertain malignant potential*), SAMPUS (*superficial melanocytic proliferation of uncertain malignant potential*), and others.

MANAGEMENT STRATEGY

The first step in the management of atypical nevi and all of the other indeterminate neoplasms mentioned in the introduction is to determine the relative chances that the lesion is benign rather than malignant.

Handbook of dermoscopy. Malvehy J, Puig S, Braun RP, Marghoob AA, Kopf AW, et al. Andover, UK: Taylor & Francis, 2006.

Atlas of dermoscopy. Marghoob AA, Braun RP, Kopf AW, eds. Boca Raton, FL: Taylor & Francis, 2005.

Color atlas of melanocytic lesions of the skin. Soyer HP, Argenziano G, Hofmann-Wellenhof R, Johr R, eds. Berlin: Springer Verlag, 2007.

Clinical examination of the neoplasm with the dermoscope (dermatoscope) prior to removal can be helpful if the user is experienced in the technique. This can help select lesions that need biopsy and obviate the need for unnecessary procedures. The details of how to perform dermoscopy and the criteria for atypical nevi and melanoma are beyond the scope of this book.

The second step is to consider whether to treat the lesion as the 'worst-case scenario,' that is, as a melanoma rather than less aggressively, yet more so than one would treat a benign nevus. The patient should participate in this decision. Some patients are willing to accept the risks of conservative management, but others want aggressive treatment with no regard for cosmetic and functional implications. For example, some physicians and patients may prefer to excise less tissue in areas around important structures, such as the eyelids, nose, and mouth. If the pathologist and clinician are absolutely certain a lesion is a benign Spitz nevus, for example, they may feel confident enough simply to monitor an incompletely excised lesion. In general, however, it is wise to excise any lesion with an uncertain malignant potential.

The approach to the patient with a difficult melanocytic lesion. Elder DE, Xu X. Pathology 2004; 36: 428–34.

Expert opinion from a dermatopathologist is useful, especially when the histology is equivocal. Sometimes more than one observer is needed, but it is important to recognize that even in expert hands there is frequent disagreement, and even the most seasoned expert can be wrong. Margins of 3–5 mm of normal skin around a lesion are recommended by many clinicians.

Discordance among expert pathologists in diagnosis of melanocytic neoplasms. Ackerman AB. Hum Pathol 1996; 27: 1115–16.

Morphological diagnosis, whether of birds, fish, plants, or pathological processes in humans, is 100% subjective.

Discordance in the histopathologic diagnosis of difficult melanocytic neoplasms in the clinical setting. Lodha S, Saggar S, Celebi JT, Silvers DN. J Cutan Pathol 2008; 35: 349–52.

Discordance in the histopathologic diagnosis of melanoma and melanocytic nevi between expert pathologists. Farmer ER, Gonin R, Hanna MP. Hum Pathol 1996; 27: 528–31.

Thirty-eight percent of the lesions evaluated by experts had two or more discordant interpretations.

SPECIFIC INVESTIGATIONS

▶ Skin biopsy and evaluation of specimen by dermatopathologist	**B**
▶ Dermatoscopic examination	**B**
▶ Photographic documentation	**B**
▶ Genetic testing	**C**

What criteria reliably distinguish melanoma from benign melanocytic lesions? Okun MR, Edelstein LM, Kasznica J. Histopathology 2000; 37: 464–72.

The differential diagnosis of melanocytic lesions is fraught with difficulty and a common source of litigation, either if a lesion misreported as 'benign' recurs locally or re-presents with nodal metastases; if an atypical nevus is called 'malignant,' leading to a cosmetically unsatisfactory wider resection; if there is unwarranted anxiety about the prognosis, or adverse life insurance prospects. The authors regard no one criterion as totally reliable, although pagetoid melanocytosis, uniformity, symmetry, deep maturation, and mitotic activity receive special consideration. Pathological findings must always be integrated with clinical information such as age and site; the presence of a small lesion does not exclude any diagnostic possibility. There is still enormous room to improve classic diagnostic criteria by the audit of known cases of metastatic melanoma. We should admit to the difficulties of melanocytic diagnoses and unashamedly write 'uncertain' in our reports.

Analysis of heterogeneity of atypia within melanocytic nevi. Barr RJ. Arch Dermatol 2003; 139: 289–92.

Although the concept of an atypical nevus is somewhat controversial, there is considerable support for the idea that nevi can be evaluated with respect to the amount of cytologic and architectural atypia present. This grading appears to be a continuous spectrum, ranging from completely benign-appearing nevi to obvious melanoma, both clinically and histopathologically. As with all studies on atypical nevi, it must be recognized that grading the level of atypia is somewhat subjective. The finding that a significant proportion of nevi show heterogeneity of atypia means that a partial biopsy might sample the lesion inadequately and give a false impression as to the overall severity of atypia manifested. Therefore, it appears wise, when possible, to remove suspicious pigmented lesions completely, so that adequate histopathologic analysis may be performed.

Clinical review of 247 case records of Spitz nevus. Dal Pozzo V, Benelli C, Restano L, Gianotti R, Cesana BM. Dermatology 1997; 194: 20–5.

Spitz nevi are pigmented in 72% of cases, and exceptionally may be black like a melanoma. They are usually asymptomatic smooth papules or nodules. Textbooks often emphasize that some Spitz nevi are red and amelanotic, but erythematous lesions account for only a quarter of cases, and these are more common on the head or neck.

Although these authors found the lower extremities to be the most common site, other reviews have found Spitz nevi of the head or neck to be more common. The trunk is also a common site, so that overall they may be found almost anywhere on the body. Most patients are Caucasian.

Spitz nevus or melanoma? Rapini RP. Semin Cutan Med Surg 1999; 18: 56–63.

This review article discusses the clinical and histologic criteria for Spitz nevus, compared to melanoma. The biopsy is best reviewed by an expert dermatopathologist, because the literature is replete with documentation of the difficulty in excluding a melanoma. As Spitz nevus is most common in children and young adults, such a diagnosis should be viewed very suspiciously in middle-aged or older adults. The diagnosis of melanoma should be viewed suspiciously in children. About 73% of Spitz nevi are less than 6 mm in diameter, whereas most melanomas are larger than 6 mm. Ulceration is uncommon in Spitz nevi, unlike melanoma. No single histologic criterion is 100% reliable, so a variety of features must be considered. Compared with melanomas, Spitz nevi are more likely to have: (1) sharp demarcation; (2) symmetry; (3) maturation of smaller, less atypical melanocytes in the deeper portion; (4) epithelial hyperplasia that often clutches melanocytic nests; (5) clefts around the junctional nests; (6) a predominance of spindle or epithelioid melanocytes, with uniform nest size and shape, and less tendency to be confluent in the dermis; (7) Kamino bodies, mitoses, inflammation, and pagetoid cells can be seen in both Spitz nevus and melanoma. A more detailed discussion of histologic minutiae is beyond the scope of this book.

'Atypical' Spitz's nevus, 'malignant' Spitz's nevus, and 'metastasizing' Spitz's nevus: a critique in historical perspective of three concepts flawed fatally. Mones JM, Ackerman AB. Am J Dermatopathol 2004; 26: 310–33.

Some authorities have used the term 'atypical Spitz tumor' to describe cases where the distinction from melanoma was uncertain. 'Malignant Spitz nevus' is a controversial diagnosis that was used by one set of authors to describe cases of 'Spitz nevi' that metastasized to regional lymph nodes but did not spread further, and the patients did well (perhaps these were really childhood melanomas that had a better than average outcome).

'Safe' Spitz and its alternatives. LeBoit PE. Pediatr Dermatol 2002; 19: 163–5.

Lesions with larger diameters, ulceration, abnormal mitoses, necrosis, and other worrisome features ought to be excised with clear surgical margins.

Other sophisticated investigations have been used to help to distinguish Spitz nevi from melanomas, but their use is controversial and sometimes not readily available. Spitz nevi are more likely to have MIB-1 (Ki-67)-positive staining in less than 2% of the cells, whereas in melanoma more than 10% of the cells are positive. HMB-45 staining tends to be diffusely positive. In many melanomas there is more prominent staining of the superficial portion, rather than the deep dermal portion as in Spitz nevi (so-called 'stratification of staining'). Comparative genomic hybridization (CGH) may show a gain or loss of chromosome 9 or 9p in melanoma, but a gain of chromosome 11p in Spitz nevus. BRAF mutations may occur in melanoma, but generally not in Spitz nevi.

The impact of total body photography on biopsy rate in patients from a pigmented lesion clinic. Risser J, Pressley Z, Veledar E, Washington C, Chen SC. J Am Acad Dermatol 2008; 58: 894–5.

Total body photography did not change the biopsy rate in this study. However, it can be useful to monitor changes in nevi, and to help select the best lesions for biopsy, especially in patients with more than 50 atypical nevi. Photography can be useful for monitoring single lesions, but there is some controversy about whether serial photography of an unexcised lesion demonstrating changes may increase the legal risk when the plaintiff claims it should have been removed earlier. Delayed diagnosis of melanoma is a common cause of litigation. Some insurance companies will pay for photography; in the USA, most will not.

FIRST-LINE THERAPIES

▶ Complete excision to adipose with closure by sutures	B
▶ Shave or saucerization removal	C

It is controversial as to whether atypical nevi require clear surgical margins. A general guideline is that those with mild atypia do not need clear margins, those with severe atypia should be completely excised, and those with moderate atypia are in between and should be considered for complete excision. This must always be considered with knowledge of the clinical situation (e.g., if the lesion is continuing to grow), and with knowledge of the terminology and threshold of severe grading on the part of the pathologist. Patients should be followed every 3–12 months, depending on the clinical situation.

My approach to atypical melanocytic lesions. Culpepper KS, Granter, SR, McKee PH. J Clin Pathol 2004; 57: 1121–31.

A 2 mm margin is recommended for dysplastic nevi, or 5 mm for those that are severely atypical. A large number of melanocytic lesions fall into a borderline area that can unnerve the most experienced of pathologists.

Dysplastic naevi: To shave or not to shave? A retrospective study of the use of the shave biopsy technique in the initial management of dysplastic nevi. Armour K, Mann S, Lee S. Australas J Dermatol 2005; 46: 70–5.

Complete excision or punch excision is advocated by some authorities because there is less risk of transecting the base of the lesion and giving an indeterminate Breslow depth in cases where the lesion turns out to be a melanoma. However, in some cases a shallow shave (for macules) or deep shave (saucerization) can avoid incomplete sampling of a lesion by punch excision and may give a superior cosmetic result. In other words, a complete shave of an 11 mm macule might be superior to a 6 mm punch biopsy of only a portion of the lesion.

The surgical management of Spitz nevi. Murphy ME, Boyer JD, Stashower ME, Zitelli JA. Dermatol Surg 2002; 28: 1065–9.

Management of Spitz nevi: a survey of dermatologists in the United States. Gelbard SN, Tripp JM, Marghoob AA, Kopf AW, Koenig KL, Kim JY, et al. J Am Acad Dermatol 2002; 47: 224–30.

Most authorities recommend complete excision with conservative margins (2–5 mm) for the average Spitz nevus. Wider margins may be needed for equivocal cases, but seldom is wide excision with margins of 10–20 mm needed, except in those cases where the possibility of melanoma is a real concern.

SECOND-LINE THERAPIES

▶ Biopsy with no further treatment	C
▶ No treatment with no biopsy	C
▶ Sentinel lymph node biopsy for equivocal cases	D

Spindle and epithelioid cell nevus (Spitz nevus). Natural history following biopsy. Kaye VN, Dehner LP. Arch Dermatol 1990; 126: 1581–3.

Only 39% of 49 Spitz nevi in this study were initially completely excised. Six were re-excised, and no evidence of residual nevus was found in five of these. None of the 49 patients had a recurrence during an average follow-up period of 5 years. Clinical follow-up alone is recommended after a subtotal excision, when the pathologic diagnosis is unequivocal.

The literature does not clearly document the natural history of untreated Spitz nevi. They may have rapid growth for the first 3–12 months, and then often remain static. It is uncertain whether they eventually regress or persist. The rate of spontaneous resolution is not documented. At least some incompletely excised Spitz nevi will recur (average 7–16% in the literature) within an average of 1 year.

Sentinel lymph node biopsy in patients with diagnostically controversial spitzoid melanocytic tumors. Lohmann CM, Coit DG, Brady MS, Berwick M, Busam KJ. Am J Surg Pathol 2002; 26: 47–55.

Sentinel lymph node biopsy for patients with problematic spitzoid melanocytic lesions: a report on 18 patients. Su LD, Fullen DR, Sondak VK, Johnson TM, Lowe L. Cancer 2003; 97: 499–507.

In both of these studies sentinel lymph nodes were used to evaluate problematic spitzoid lesions. Some patients with positive regional nodes had regional lymphadenectomy. All patients in these two studies, even those with positive nodes, remained alive and well.

What do these cells prove? LeBoit PE. Am J Dermatopathol 2003; 25: 355–6.

Even though some reports tell of cases in which diagnostic uncertainty was settled by means of a sentinel node biopsy, the presence of small clusters of melanocytes within nodes does not prove malignancy. Small nests of melanocytes can be found within nodes draining both ordinary benign nevi and apparently benign Spitz nevi.

THIRD-LINE THERAPIES

▶ Cryotherapy	E
▶ Electrodesiccation	E
▶ Laser ablation	E
▶ Imiquimod	D

The use of cryotherapy and electrodessication for various types of melanocytic nevi is casually mentioned in several books, but these methods cannot be relied upon to completely remove atypical nevi, and should be used with caution, if at all.

Treatment of benign and atypical nevi with the normal-mode ruby laser and the Q-switched ruby laser: Clinical improvement but failure to completely eliminate nevomelanocytes. Duke D, Byers HR, Sober AJ, Anderson RR, Grevelink JM. Arch Dermatol 1999; 135: 290–6.

No lesions had complete histologic removal of all nevomelanocytes after one or two treatments; 52% of the lesions had reduced pigment.

Treatment of dysplastic nevi with 5% imiquimod cream, a pilot study. Dusza SW, Delgado R, Busam KJ, Marghoob AA, Halpern AC. J Drugs Dermatol 2006; 5: 56–62.

Imiquimod failed to produce a significant response, and the authors concluded that further study is not warranted.

Evidence Levels: **A** Double-blind study **B** Clinical trial ≥ 20 subjects **C** Clinical trial < 20 subjects **D** Series ≥ 5 subjects **E** Anecdotal case reports

Autoimmune progesterone dermatitis

Laura Houk, Ian Coulson

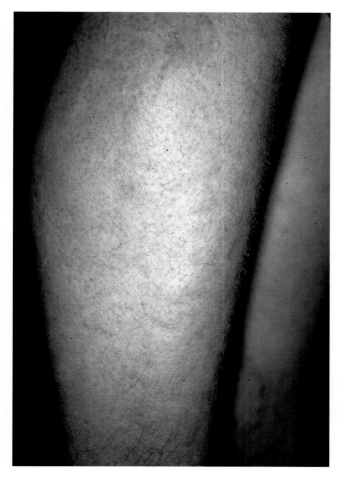

Autoimmune progesterone dermatitis is a rare disorder of cyclical skin eruptions caused by hypersensitivity to progesterone. Multiple skin manifestations have been reported, including urticarial, eczematous, vesicular, papulovesicular, and erythema multiforme-like lesions. Angioedema or anaphylaxis may accompany the skin eruptions. Hypersensitivity following exposure to exogenous progesterone, usually in the form of an oral contraceptive pill, has been implicated in some cases of autoimmune progesterone dermatitis. Endogenous progesterone may also serve as a trigger for autoimmune progesterone dermatitis in cases arising during menarche or pregnancy. The three criteria for diagnosing autoimmune progesterone dermatitis include a cyclical skin eruption during the luteal phase of the menstrual cycle; a positive intradermal progesterone challenge; and prevention of the skin eruption by inhibition of ovulation.

MANAGEMENT STRATEGY

Therapeutic strategies inhibit endogenous progesterone secretion by suppressing ovulation. Classically, *conjugated estrogens* 0.625–1.25 mg daily in a 21-day cycle was a mainstay of therapy, but recently this treatment has been supplanted by *gonadotropin-releasing hormone (GnRH) agonists*. A transient worsening of the skin eruption is expected following initial treatment with GnRH agonists, with improvement thereafter. A major side effect of GnRH agonists is loss of bone density, which generally limits their use to 6 months of therapy. Patients frequently require estrogen replacement while on GnRH agonist therapy.

The antiestrogen *tamoxifen,* 20 mg daily or 10 mg twice a day, exerts its effect by interfering with clinical estrogen sensitivity, possibly by competitive binding of the estrogen receptors.

Oral contraceptive pills have been implicated in triggering some cases of autoimmune progesterone dermatitis. However, in patients naïve to exogenous progesterone, inducing anovulation with oral contraceptive pills may be successful.

Mild cases of autoimmune progesterone dermatitis may be controlled with short courses of systemic *corticosteroids* prior to the luteal phase of the menstrual cycle. Very limited disease may respond to potent *topical corticosteroids* and *oral antihistamines.*

Danazol 200 mg twice daily for 1–2 days prior to menses and continued for 3 days thereafter may prevent the skin eruptions by inhibiting pituitary gonadotropins.

For severe, intractable cases, bilateral oophorectomy is curative.

Autoimmune estrogen dermatitis is a separate entity that can be difficult to distinguish clinically from autoimmune progesterone dermatitis. Intradermal testing that is positive to estrone and negative to progesterone clarifies the diagnosis. Autoimmune estrogen dermatitis responds to tamoxifen, progesterone, and oophorectomy.

SPECIFIC INVESTIGATIONS

> ► Intradermal testing with progesterone
> ► Progesterone challenge
> ► ELISA and ELISpot testing

Different authors have advocated intradermal testing with progesterone in varying amounts and dilutions. One common method of intradermal testing is with 0.1 mL of aqueous progesterone suspension at 100 mg/mL diluted with normal saline to 0.1 mg/mL, 0.01 mg/mL, and 0.001 mg/mL, with normal saline serving as the control. There may be an immediate urticarial reaction within 30 minutes, or a delayed-type hypersensitivity reaction at 24–48 hours.

Progesterone challenge may also be attempted intramuscularly (medroxyprogesterone 10–20 mg) or orally (10 mg) in the first half of the menstrual cycle. Intramuscular skin testing with the depot form of medroxyprogesterone acetate is not advised because of the risk of severe systemic reactions.

ELISA and ELISpot testing can detect elevated levels of IFN-γ-producing peripheral blood mononuclear cells in response to progesterone.

If progesterone testing is negative, consider estrogen sensitivity. Intradermal testing with either estrone (0.1 mL at 1 mg/mL) or conjugated estrogen (0.1 mL of 1, 10, and 100 μg/mL) can be attempted. A positive reaction may be immediate or delayed for several hours, and should persist for more than 24 hours.

The role of intradermal skin testing and patch testing in the diagnosis of autoimmune progesterone dermatitis. Stranahan D, Rausch D, Deng A, Gaspari A. Dermatitis 2006; 17: 39–42.

A case report and a detailed review of the various methods of performing intradermal progesterone testing, highlighting the need for standardization.

Autoimmune progesterone dermatitis and its manifestation as anaphylaxis: A case report and literature review. Snyder JL, Krishnaswamy G. Ann Allergy Asthma Immunol 2003; 90: 469–77.

A case report and review of the current literature, including a summary table and algorithm for the work-up of cyclical anaphylaxis.

Autoimmune progesterone dermatitis. Herzberg AJ, Strohmeyer CR, Cirillio-Hyland VA. J Am Acad Dermatol 1995; 32: 333–8.

A case report accompanied by an excellent review of case reports and current literature.

Progesterone sensitive interferon-γ-producing cells detected by ELISpot assay in autoimmune progesterone dermatitis. Cristaudo A, Bordignon V, Palamara F, De Rocco M, Pietravalle M, Picardo M. Clin Exp Dermatol 2007; 32: 439–41.

Describes the ELISpot technique of diagnosing autoimmune progesterone dermatitis.

Oestrogen dermatitis. Kumar A, Georgouras KE. Australas J Dermatol 1999; 40: 96–8.

A case report comparing progesterone dermatitis and estrogen dermatitis, as well as useful information on the technique and interpretation of intradermal testing for both disorders.

Estrogen dermatitis. Shelley WB, Shelley D, Talanin NY, Santoso-Pham J. J Am Acad Dermatol 1995; 32: 25–31.

An excellent case series and review of estrogen dermatitis, with comparison made to progesterone dermatitis.

FIRST-LINE THERAPIES

▶ Gonadotropin-releasing hormone agonists	A
▶ Tamoxifen	D
▶ Oral contraceptive pill	E
▶ Oral corticosteroids	E
▶ Potent topical corticosteroids	E
▶ Antihistamines	E

Recurrent anaphylaxis in menstruating women: Treatment with a luteinizing hormone-releasing hormone agonist – a preliminary report. Slater JE, Raphael G, Cutler GB, Loriaux DL, Meggs WJ, Kaliner M. Obstet Gynecol 1987; 70: 542–6.

A double-blind, placebo-controlled crossover study of four women with cyclic anaphylaxis associated with progesterone secretion. Two of the subjects experienced dramatic reduction in the severity and number of attacks while receiving an investigational luteinizing hormone-releasing agonist imbzl-D-his6-pro9-NEt-LHRH, 4 μg/kg/day for 4 months. Liaison with a gynecologic endocrinologist may help in the selection of an appropriate GnRH agonist and estrogen combination of therapies.

Autoimmune progesterone dermatitis in a patient with endometriosis: case report and review of the literature. Baptist AP, Baldwin JL. Clin Mol Allergy 2004; 2: 10.

Successful treatment with nafarelin acetate nasal spray, 200 μg twice daily.

Autoimmune progesterone dermatitis. Cocuroccia B, Gisondi P, Gubinelli E, Girolomoni G. Gynecol Endocrinol 2006; 22: 54–6.

Treatment with tamoxifen 20 mg daily produced complete and durable clearing of the eruption after 3 months.

A case of autoimmune progesterone dermatitis in an adolescent female. Kakarla N, Zurawin RK. J Pediatr Adolesc Gynecol 2006; 19: 125–9.

A case report describing a patient with no prior exogenous hormone exposure who cleared on oral contraceptive therapy. For patients naïve to exogenous progesterone, an oral contraceptive pill is considered to be first-line therapy (the preparation used contained 30 μg of ethinyl estradiol and 0.15 mg of levonorgestrel).

Autoimmune progesterone dermatitis. Anderson RH. Cutis 1984; 33: 490–1.

A case successfully treated with prednisolone 20 mg/day for 10 days during menstruation. The dosage of prednisolone was reduced slowly over several cycles and the patient was eventually managed on topical corticosteroids only.

Autoimmune progesterone dermatitis associated with infertility treatment. Jenkins J, Geng A, Robinson-Bostom L. J Am Acad Dermatol 2008; 58: 353–5.

Oral contraceptives and gonadotropin-releasing hormone agonists were contraindicated in this patient undergoing treatment for infertility. The limited disease was well controlled with halobetasol propionate 0.05% cream.

Autoimmune progesterone dermatitis. Case report with histologic overlap of erythema multiforme and urticaria. Walling HW, Scupham RK. Int Soc Dermatol 2008; 47: 380–2.

Durable improvement on cetirizine 10 mg every morning and hydroxyzine 10 mg at bedtime taken on the days of the menstrual cycle previously associated with skin eruptions.

SECOND-LINE THERAPIES

▶ Conjugated estrogens	E
▶ Danazol	E
▶ Azathioprine	E

Autoimmune progesterone anaphylaxis. Bemanian MH, Gharagozlu M, Farashahi MH, Nabavi M, Shirkhoda Z. Iran J Allergy Asthma Immunol 2007; 6: 97–9.

A case report of a patient with perimenstrual urticaria associated with angioedema and respiratory symptoms, all of which improved on conjugated estrogen 0.625 mg once daily.

Autoimmune progesterone dermatitis: effective prophylactic treatment with danazol. Shahar E, Bergman R, Pollack S. Int J Dermatol 1997; 36: 708–11.

Evidence Levels: **A** Double-blind study **B** Clinical trial ≥ 20 subjects **C** Clinical trial < 20 subjects **D** Series ≥ 5 subjects **E** Anecdotal case reports

Successful prophylactic treatment with danazol in two patients at a dose of 200 mg twice daily, starting 1–2 days before menstruation and continuing for 3 days thereafter.

Case 2. Diagnosis: erythema multiforme as a presentation of autoimmune progesterone dermatitis. Warin AP. Clin Exp Dermatol 2001; 26: 107–8.

Successful treatment with azathioprine 100 mg daily.

THIRD-LINE THERAPIES

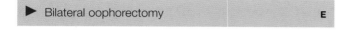

| ▶ Bilateral oophorectomy | E |

Autoimmune progesterone dermatitis: Treatment with oophorectomy. Rodenas JM, Herranz MT, Tercedor J. Br J Dermatol 1998; 139: 508–11.

Oophorectomy was curative in this case of autoimmune progesterone dermatitis that was unresponsive to estrogens, tamoxifen, and a luteinizing-hormone releasing hormone agonist.

Bacillary angiomatosis

Chrystalla Macedo, Richard CD Staughton

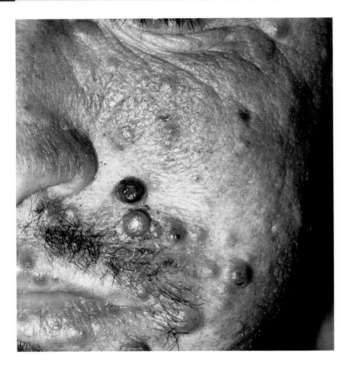

Bacillary angiomatosis was first described in 1983 and typically presents in patients with profound immunocompromise (e.g., advanced HIV infection, post transplant, cytotoxic chemotherapy). Angioproliferative papules, nodules, or plaques can arise in the skin or internally, involving the viscera, bone, central nervous system, and liver, where the condition is termed peliosis hepatis. Lesions are now known to be due to the cat scratch disease infectious agents *Bartonella* (previously *Rochalimaea*, see Cat Scratch Disease), which are also the agents for trench fever, culture-negative endocarditis, neuroretinitis and verruga peruana, a localized cutaneous form of the disease that occurs in South America. The latter continues to plague those in endemic regions and poses a significant threat to travelers in these areas.

MANAGEMENT STRATEGY

Bacillary angiomatosis can present in an indolent manner over several months, and adequate treatment is essential to prevent dissemination, which can be fatal. Clinical suspicion should be aroused in the context of a low CD4 lymphocyte count (<100), especially if there is a history of exposure to cats, the reservoir of infection for *Bartonella henselae* (the cat scratch agent), or the human body louse, the vector for *Bartonella quintana*, the trench fever agent. Lesions can be predominantly cutaneous or subcutaneous and present as multiple brick or cherry-red round papules and nodules, similar to pyogenic granuloma (usually single proud lesions with a hemorrhagic surface and collarette). They can be mistaken for Kaposi sarcoma (dull, dark red cutaneous swellings that are often oval and expanding between tissue planes). In advanced

HIV, differentiation from extensive molluscum contagiosum or deep fungal infection, e.g., cryptococcosis or histoplasmosis, must be made. In-transit metastatic amelanotic melanoma and other malignancies can be hard to differentiate because of the highly vascular and erosive nature of the lesions in skin, bones, and soft tissues. Histology allows easy differentiation and shows a lobular proliferation of small blood vessels, with swollen endothelial cells containing clumps of bacteria.

The response of bacillary angiomatosis to *antibiotic treatment* is usually dramatic, in contrast to the response of cat scratch disease in the immunocompetent. The authors' drugs of first choice are the macrolides (e.g., azithromycin 500 mg daily, clarithromycin 500 mg twice daily, erythromycin 500 mg four times daily), with doxycycline 100 mg twice daily as an alternative. Their use is based on anecdotal experience in the absence of systematic trials. Current recommendations are that treatment should be continued for 2 months where there is skin disease only, and for 4 months where there is bone/visceral involvement or peliosis hepatis. Should relapse occur on the above regimens, then long-term prophylaxis with erythromycin or doxycycline may be indicated. In practice, however, the introduction of highly active antiretroviral therapy (HAART) should reverse immunocompromise and thus alter the response to treatment, making long-term antibiotics less necessary. The patient should be evaluated for parenchymal and osseous disease prior to treatment and warned that a Jarisch–Herxheimer reaction may occur after the first few doses of antibiotic.

A wide variety of therapeutic agents are mentioned in the literature, but there is a lack of correlation between the in-vitro and in-vivo drug susceptibilities of *Bartonella* spp., which reduces the usefulness of laboratory data. The picture is clouded further by the different responses of *Bartonella* to drugs in each of the diseases it causes.

SPECIFIC INVESTIGATIONS

> ▶ Full blood count, liver function tests, and CD4 lymphocyte count
> ▶ Biopsy and Warthin–Starry stains/electron microscopy
> ▶ Prolonged culture of blood and biopsy tissue
> ▶ Polymerase chain reaction (PCR) of biopsy material
> ▶ Serology – indirect fluorescence assay (IFA)

Culture of the fastidious Gram-negative rods of *Bartonella* spp. is extremely difficult, requiring special media and prolonged incubation of up to 45 days; it is invariably negative if antibiotics have been given. Skin biopsy is the essential diagnostic tool and shows characteristic appearances on histology and Warthin–Starry silver stains, which show the organism, as can electron microscopy. Species confirmation can be obtained by PCR. Reliance on serology in the immunosuppressed is hazardous, but the Centers for Disease Control (CDC) definition of a positive test is an indirect fluorescence assay (IFA) titer of over 1:64.

Laboratory diagnosis of *Bartonella* infections. Agan BK, Dolan MJ. Clin Lab Med 2002; 22: 937–62.

Culture methods have improved, but are still prolonged. Serologic testing for *B. henselae* has become the cornerstone for diagnosis in the immunocompetent. Ideal antigens for enzyme immunoassays have yet to be clearly identified. PCR currently offers the ability to establish the diagnosis when other tests fail.

Bacillary angiomatosis and bacillary peliosis in patients infected with human immunodeficiency virus: clinical characteristics in a case–control study. Mohle-Boetani JC, Koehler JE, Berger TG, LeBoit PE, Kemper CA, Reingold AL, et al. Clin Infect Dis 1996; 22: 794–800.

Forty-two cases were compared to 84 matched controls and the distinguishing clinical characteristics were evaluated. Significant differences included the presence of anemia (hematocrit <0.36), raised alkaline phosphatase and aspartate aminotransferase levels, and a low CD4 lymphocyte count (median being 21/mm^3 compared to 186/mm^3 in controls). There was no difference in the white blood cell count, creatinine, bilirubin, and alanine aminotransferase levels. Clinical signs included fever, abdominal pain, and lymphadenopathy.

Bacillary angiomatosis in immunocompromised patients. Gasquet S, Maurin M, Brouqui P, Lepidi H, Raoult D. AIDS 1998; 12: 1793–803.

Diagnosis remains mainly based on histological appearance. On hematoxylin and eosin stains the appearance can be highly variable, and so Warthin–Starry stains are essential to visualize the bacillus and confirm the diagnosis.

Culture of *Bartonella quintana* and *Bartonella henselae* from human samples: a 5-year experience (1993 to 1998). La Scola B, Raoult D. J Clin Microbiol 1999; 37: 1899–905.

From the large number of samples cultured, seven patients were diagnosed with bacillary angiomatosis. PCR was 100% sensitive in diagnosing these cases, in contrast to culture, which isolated *Bartonella* spp. from only three specimens. Serology was of no value, being positive in only one patient.

Rapid identification and differentiation of *Bartonella* species using a single step PCR assay. Jensen WA, Fall MZ, Rooney J, Kordick DL, Breitschwerdt EB. J Clin Microbiol 2000; 38: 1717–22.

The single-step assay described provided a simple and rapid means of identifying *Bartonella* spp.

Use of *Bartonella* adhesin A (BadA) immunoblotting in the serodiagnosis of *Bartonella henselae* infections. Wagner CL, Riess T, Linke D, Eberhardt C, Schäfer A, Reutter S, et al. Int J Microbiol 2008; 298: 579–90.

Two-step serodiagnosis using a combination of an indirect immunofluorescence assay and adhesin A improved identification of *Bartonella henselae* infections.

FIRST-LINE THERAPIES

▶ Azithromycin	C
▶ Clarithromycin	C
▶ Erythromycin	C

Molecular epidemiology of *Bartonella* infections in patients with bacillary angiomatosis-peliosis. Koehler JE, Sanchez MA, Garrido CS, Whitfeld MJ, Chen FM, Berger TG, et al. N Engl J Med 1997; 337: 1876–83.

A case–control study of 49 patients (92% HIV positive) in whom macrolides, doxycycline, tetracycline, and rifampin were found to be effective. This was in contrast to patients treated with trimethoprim-sulfamethoxazole, ciprofloxa-

cin, penicillins, and cephalosporins, in whom *Bartonella* spp. could be isolated on PCR or culture.

MICs of 28 antibiotic compounds for 14 *Bartonella* (formerly *Rochalimaea*) isolates. Maurin M, Gasquet S, Ducco C, Raoult D. Antimicrob Agents Chemother 1995; 39: 2387–91.

The newer macrolides were highly effective in preventing bacterial growth with MIC 90s of 0.03 µg/mL for azithromycin and clarithromycin. Erythromycin, doxycycline, and rifampin all had MIC 90s of 0.25 µg/mL.

AIDS commentary: bacillary angiomatosis and bacillary peliosis in patients infected with human immunodeficiency virus. Koehler JE, Tappero JW. Clin Infect Dis 1993; 17: 612–14.

This review article refers to 50 patients whose lesions and symptoms responded to erythromycin or doxycycline therapy.

Rapid response of AIDS-related bacillary angiomatosis to azithromycin. Guerra LG, Neira CJ, Boman D, Ho H, Casner PR, Zuckerman M, et al. Clin Infect Dis 1993; 17: 264–6.

This documents successful treatment with azithromycin.

Molecular diagnosis of deep nodular bacillary angiomatosis and monitoring of therapeutic success. Schlupen E-M, Schirren CG, Hoegl L, Schaller M, Volkenandt M. Br J Dermatol 1997; 136: 747–51.

An HIV-positive man presented with a 10-month history of bacillary angiomatosis on his ankle and was treated with erythromycin 500 mg four times daily. The swabs became negative on PCR at 12 weeks, at which point treatment was successfully stopped.

Bartonella-associated infections. Spach DH, Koehler JE. Infect Dis Clin North Am 1998; 12: 137–55.

A good review article.

Although azithromycin, clarithromycin, and erythromycin are the authors' first-line treatments for bacillary angiomatosis, their use has been based on anecdotal case reports rather than on controlled clinical trials. Azithromycin has emerged as the first-line treatment for cat scratch disease, for which there are formal trial data.

SECOND-LINE THERAPIES

▶ Doxycycline	C
▶ Tetracycline	D
▶ Rifampin	D

Clarithromycin therapy for bacillary peliosis did not prevent bacillary angiomatosis. Mukunda BN, West BC, Shekar R. Clin Infect Dis 1998; 27: 658.

A patient with AIDS presented with bacillary peliosis and was initially treated for a presumed *Mycobacterium avium intracellulare* complex infection using clarithromycin, ciprofloxacin, and rifabutin. He continued to be febrile and re-presented 15 days later with bacillary angiomatosis. This swiftly responded to doxycycline, which was continued for 6 weeks.

Bacillary angiomatosis: presentation of six patients, some with unusual features. Schwartz RA, Nychay SG, Janniger CK, Lambert WC. Br J Dermatol 1997; 136: 60–5.

This describes a variety of successful treatment regimens, including tetracycline and ciprofloxacin.

Although rifampin has activity in vitro, its efficacy when used alone has not yet been established and so it is recommended as a second-line drug in combination with either erythromycin or doxycycline for severely ill patients, or where there is neurological involvement. It is, however, effective in the treatment of verruga peruana (Bartonella bacilliformis) *and cat scratch disease.*

THIRD-LINE THERAPIES

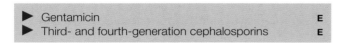

▶ Gentamicin	**E**
▶ Third- and fourth-generation cephalosporins	**E**

Bacillary angiomatosis in a pregnant patient with acquired immunodeficiency syndrome. Riley LE, Tuomala RE. Obstet Gynecol 1992; 79: 818–19.

A pregnant woman was treated with ceftizoxime, a third-generation cephalosporin. However, there are inadequate data to recommend its use at present.

Lack of bactericidal effect of antibiotics except aminoglycosides on *Bartonella (Rochalimaea) henselae*. Musso D, Drancourt M, Raoult D. J Antimicrob Chemother 1995; 36: 101–8.

Aminoglycosides display in-vitro bactericidal activity against *Bartonella* spp., and hence warrant further clinical investigation.

Evidence Levels: **A** Double-blind study **B** Clinical trial ≥ 20 subjects **C** Clinical trial < 20 subjects **D** Series ≥ 5 subjects **E** Anecdotal case reports

Balanitis

Maria Nasca, Giuseppe Micali, Dennis West, Ginat Mirowski

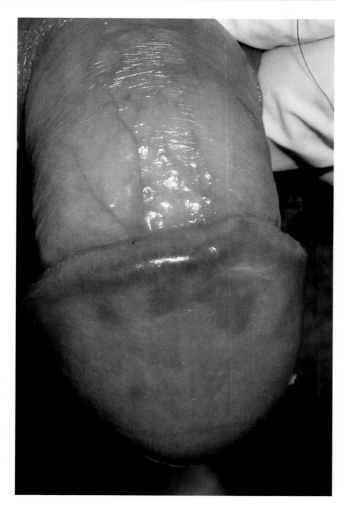

Balanitis is defined as inflammation of the glans penis, and occasionally the prepuce. Most commonly it is of multifactorial etiology. Potential causes include infection, trauma, poor hygiene, contact allergy, dermatoses, cicatricial disorder, malignancy, rheumatologic disease, and fixed drug eruption. This chapter will focus on the treatment of nonspecific balanitis, balanitis xerotica obliterans (BXO), and Zoon's balanitis.

MANAGEMENT STRATEGY

Patients with balanitis commonly complain of itching and irritation of the glans penis. This condition is seen more frequently in uncircumcised men. Clinical manifestations vary from erythematous shiny plaques to white papules or erosions. Complications include phimosis, meatal stenosis, fissures, and involvement of the urethra requiring surgical treatment.

Evaluation of a patient with balanitis should begin with a thorough history. Patients should be asked specifically about sexual practices, use of condoms or spermicidal agents, and symptoms in any partners. The patient's hygiene regimen should be discussed in detail. It is also important to identify potential irritants or allergens, and determine oral and topical medications. A comprehensive physical examination with special attention to mucosal membranes may reveal an underlying dermatosis. Underlying infections should be sought and treated aggressively. Any lesion that is not of an obvious infectious or irritant etiology or not responding to topical therapy should be biopsied.

The initial treatment for balanitis revolves around *hygiene, emollient creams* and *topical corticosteroids*. The patient should be instructed to retract the foreskin and clean the glans penis with a weak saline solution twice a day. Soap, an irritant, should be avoided. All topical agents should be used with caution as they may be irritants or allergens, thereby worsening the condition. Ointments are preferable because they contain fewer preservatives. An emollient applied twice a day after cleansing with clean water will both lubricate and protect the area. A low-potency topical steroid such as 1% hydrocortisone ointment applied twice daily can help to reduce inflammation. If symptoms persist, a higher-potency corticosteroid should be used once or twice daily for 3 weeks. *Carbenoxolone gel, topical testosterone propionate, topical calcineurin inhibitors, topical imiquimod* and *intralesional corticosteroids* may be used judiciously.

Other options for recalcitrant cases are CO_2 or *erbium:YAG laser ablation* and *long-term systemic antibiotics*. The definitive treatment for balanitis of any etiology is *circumcision*. Circumcision is a very effective therapy and is a reasonable option to offer patients early in the treatment of balanitis. It will usually result in complete relief of symptoms, even in refractory cases. In more severe cases leading to BXO, combination with other surgical modalities, including meatotomy, meatoplasty, glans resurfacing, urethroplasty, or definitive perineal urethrostomy, may be required.

SPECIFIC INVESTIGATIONS

> ► Microscopy for fungi and Tzanck smear
> ► Subpreputial swab for *Candida* spp., and viral/bacterial cultures
> ► Fasting blood glucose
> ► Serological tests for syphilis
> ► Biopsy
> ► Patch testing

Mild balanoposthitis. Fornasa CV, Calabro A, Miglietta A, Tarantello M, Biasinutto C, Peserico A. Genitourin Med 1994; 70: 345–6.

Three hundred and twenty-one patients with balanoposthitis were evaluated. An infectious etiology was identified in 185. Organisms isolated included *Candida albicans, Chlamydia trachomatis, Trichomonas vaginalis, Neisseria gonorrhoeae* and β-hemolytic streptococcus. Traumatic/irritant contact dermatitis was the etiology in 17 cases. Allergic contact dermatitis was found in three cases. Neoplasia was found in eight cases. Other etiologies included psoriasis, lichen planus, BXO, Zoon's balanitis, and fixed drug eruption.

Balanitis xerotica obliterans and its differential diagnosis. Neuhaus IM, Skidmore RA. J Am Board Fam Pract 1999; 12: 473–6.

Review of the medical literature showed that BXO was distinguishable from other genital dermatoses through patient history, clinical findings, and laboratory evaluation. Tzanck smear, viral and fungal cultures, a rapid protein reagin test and cutaneous biopsy provided a definitive diagnosis.

FIRST-LINE THERAPIES

► Attention to hygiene	C
► Emollients	C
► Topical pimecrolimus	A
► Topical tacrolimus	E
► Low-potency topical corticosteroids	A

Clinical features and management of recurrent balanitis; association with atopy and genital washing. Birley HD, Walker MM, Luzzi GA, Bell R, Taylor-Robinson D, Byrne M, et al. Genitourin Med 1990; 69: 400–3.

Eighteen patients with a histologic diagnosis of nonspecific balanitis were treated with emollient cream and restriction of soap use. Fifteen had resolution of symptoms. The remaining three responded to 1% hydrocortisone, but two relapsed.

National guidelines for the management of balanitis. Anonymous. Sex Transm Infect 1999; 75: S85–1.

Saline baths and avoidance of soap are recommended for the general management of nonspecific balanitis.

Excellent review.

Plasma cell balanitis and vulvitis (of Zoon). Yoganathan S, Bohl T, Mason G. J Reprod Med 1994; 39: 939–44.

Attention to hygiene combined with topical corticosteroids resulted in improvement of symptoms and signs in six cases of plasma cell balanitis.

Treatment of balanitis xerotica obliterans with topical tacrolimus. Pandher BS, Rustin MHA, Kaisary AV. J Urol 2003; 170: 923.

In a single case, 0.1% tacrolimus ointment applied twice daily to the glans after circumcision reduced the severity and extent of the inflammation and resulted in total resolution of symptoms.

Pimecrolimus 1% cream in non-specific inflammatory recurrent balanitis. Georgala S, Gregoriou S, Georgala C, Papaioannou D, Befon A, Kalogeromitros D, et al. Dermatology 2007; 215: 209–12.

In a randomized controlled study seven of 11 (63.6%) patients with recurrent flares of nonspecific balanitis treated with twice-daily applications of pimecrolimus 1% cream (vs 9% of the placebo group) were symptom free after 7 days. Patients were instructed to resume application at any relapse over the following 3 months.

Two cases of Zoon's balanitis treated with pimecrolimus 1% cream. Bardazzi F, Antonucci A, Savoia F, Balestri R. Int J Dermatol 2008; 47: 198–201.

Two cases of resistant Zoon's balanitis treated with twice-daily applications of topical pimecrolimus 1% for 2 months are reported. Complete clinical regression was achieved in one patient and improvement with persistence of a hyperpigmented patch in the other, with no relapses in both, respectively at a 9- and 10-month follow-up. No local irritation or other side effects were observed.

Topical tacrolimus: an effective therapy for Zoon balanitis. Santos-Juanes J, Sanchez del Rio J, Galache C, Soto J. Arch Dermatol 2004; 140: 1538–9.

Complete remission was reported in three patients with Zoon's balanitis after the application of topical tacrolimus 0.1% twice daily for 3–5 weeks. The only secondary effect reported was mild irritation of the glans penis in one of the patients during the first 4 days of application.

Plasma cell balanitis of Zoon treated successfully with topical tacrolimus. Hernandez-Machin B, Hernando LB, Marrero OB, Hernandez B. Clin Exp Dermatol 2005; 30: 588–9.

One patient responded favorably to twice-daily treatment with topical 0.03% tacrolimus ointment for 2 months. Six months later the lesion recurred, but the condition was again controlled with the same treatment.

SECOND-LINE THERAPIES

► High-potency topical corticosteroids	A
► Moderate-potency topical corticosteroid plus antimicrobials	E
► Intralesional corticosteroids	E
► Carbenoxolone gel	A
► Testosterone propionate	E
► Imiquimod	E

The response of balanitis xerotica obliterans to local steroid application compared with placebo in children. Kiss A, Csontai A, Pirót L, Nyirády P, Merksz M, Király L. J Urol 2001; 165: 219–20.

This double-blind, placebo-controlled, randomized study of 40 boys with clinical BXO showed that the application of a potent topical corticosteroid improves BXO in the histologically early and intermediate stages of disease, and may inhibit progression in the late stage.

The response of clinical balanitis xerotica obliterans to the application of topical steroid-based creams. Vincent MV, Mackinnon E. J Pediatr Surg 2005; 40: 709–12.

This study suggests that the best results may be achieved with topical steroids in mild non-scarring cases of BXO.

Plasma cell balanitis of Zoon; response to Trimovate cream. Tang A, David N, Horton LW. Int J STD AIDS 2001; 12: 216–20.

Ten patients with biopsy-proven plasma balanitis applied a topical mixture comprising oxytetracycline 3%, nystatin 100 000 U/g, and clobetasone butyrate 0.05% (Trimovate) for 3–12 weeks until complete clinical resolution was observed. Three had recurrence within 3 months after cessation of therapy and responded to a second course of treatment. A fourth patient had three recurrences within 12 months, and each time responded to re-treatment within a few days.

Clinical evaluation of carbenoxolone in balanitis. Csonka GW, Murray M. Br J Vener Dis 1971; 47: 179–81.

A controlled double-blind study of 50 patients with non-infectious balanitis showed that carbenoxolone gel was as effective as hydrocortisone cream in treating balanitis. Of patients treated with carbenoxolone gel 73% were fully satisfied, as opposed to 58% treated with hydrocortisone.

Evidence Levels: **A** Double-blind study **B** Clinical trial ≥ 20 subjects **C** Clinical trial < 20 subjects **D** Series ≥ 5 subjects **E** Anecdotal case reports

The treatment of balanitis xerotica obliterans with testosterone propionate ointment. Pasieczny T. Acta Dermatol Venereol 1977; 57: 275–7.

A report of four cases of BXO treated with 2.5% testosterone propionate ointment. Marked improvement was observed after 3–4 months of treatment.

Treatment of Zoon's balanitis with imiquimod 5% cream. Nasca MR, De Pasquale R, Micali G. J Drugs Dermatol 2007; 6: 532–4.

The case is reported of a 43-year-old uncircumcised Caucasian diabetic man with a 4-year history of Zoon's balanitis unresponsive to topical steroids, in whom control of the disease was achieved with imiquimod 5% cream applied three times a week. Clinical but not histological resolution was obtained after 4 months of treatment, with no relapses at an 18-month follow-up. A moderate to marked increased local skin reaction occurred several times throughout the treatment period, necessitating multiple rest periods of several days' duration.

THIRD-LINE THERAPIES

▶ Circumcision	B
▶ CO$_2$ laser	E
▶ Erbium:YAG laser	E
▶ Copper vapor laser	E
▶ Long-term systemic antibiotics	E

Zoon's balanitis treated with erbium:YAG laser ablation. Albertini JG, Holck DE, Farley MF. Lasers Surg Med 2002; 30: 123–6.

A single case of a 67-year-old man who failed prior treatment with 5-fluorouracil, CO$_2$ laser, and 5 months of topical therapy with potent corticosteroids plus mupirocin ointment, but responded to three to six overlapping passes of laser ablation using the lowest power setting (0.5 J/cm^2; 3 mm spot size; 5 Hz). The lesion healed in a week, but recurred and the patient required two more passes of ablation. He remained disease free at 2-year follow-up.

Plasma cell balanitis: clinical and histopathological features – response to circumcision. Kumar B, Sharma R, Rajagopalan M, Radotra BD. Genitourin Med 1995; 71: 32–4.

Twenty-seven patients with plasma cell balanitis were cured with circumcision. There were no recurrences at 3-year follow-up.

Surgical treatment of balanitis xerotica obliterans. Campus GV, Ena P, Scuderi N. Plast Reconstruct Surg 1984; 73: 652–7.

Nineteen patients underwent surgical treatment for BXO. The exact procedure performed was determined by the extent of the disease. All patients experienced relief of symptoms. No relapse was reported in up to 4 years of follow-up.

Balanitis xerotica obliterans in boys. Gargollo PC, Kozakewich HP, Bauer SB, Borer JG, Peters CA, Retik AB, et al. J Urol 2005; 174: 1409–12.

A 10-year experience in 41 pediatric patients with BXO is reported. A combination of circumcision with other surgical procedures, including meatotomy or meatoplasty, tends to be more often required in older patients with a more severe clinical course.

The treatment of Zoon's balanitis with the carbon dioxide laser. Baldwin HE, Geronemus RG. Dermatol Surg Oncol 1989; 15: 491–4.

A case of Zoon's balanitis successfully treated with carbon dioxide laser. The patient was symptom free for 2 years of follow-up.

Plasma cell balanitis treated with a copper vapour laser. Haedersdal M, Wulf HC. Scand J Plast Reconstruct Hand Surg 1995; 29: 357–8.

Report of an uncircumcised male with plasma cell balanitis treated with copper vapor laser. The lesion resolved, but the patient had a minor relapse. No further treatment was required.

Carbon dioxide laser treatment of external genital lesions. Rosemberg SK. Urology 1985; 25: 555–8.

Three cases of BXO were treated with CO$_2$ laser. Complete eradication was achieved after one treatment in two patients. The third patient required a repeat treatment with the laser to achieve cure.

Long-term antibiotic therapy for balanitis xerotica obliterans. Shelley WB, Shelley ED, Grunenwald MA, Anders TJ, Ramnath A. J Am Acad Dermatol 1999; 40: 69–71.

Three patients with BXO were treated with various antibacterial regimens. All showed significant improvement after long-term therapy. The antibiotics used included oral and intramuscular penicillin and dirithromycin.

Basal cell carcinoma

James M Spencer

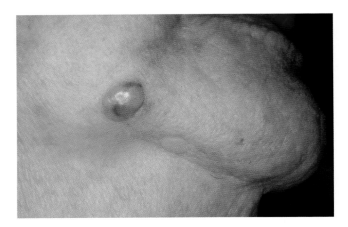

Basal cell carcinoma (BCC) is a slow-growing malignancy originating in the epidermis. It most commonly arises in areas chronically exposed to UV light, especially the head and neck. Although it is very rare for BCC to metastasize, it can produce significant local tissue destruction, including cartilage and bony invasion.

MANAGEMENT STRATEGY

Basal cell carcinoma slowly but relentlessly grows larger and deeper, and therefore therapeutic intervention is geared towards complete eradication of all malignant cells. Local recurrence is the consequence of inadequate therapy. Complete eradication is especially important because recurrent tumors are often larger and more aggressive than the original incompletely treated primary tumor. Although complete eradication is the primary goal, the therapy chosen should achieve this with the maximal preservation of function and the optimal cosmetic result. Most often, therapy uses destructive techniques such as *cryotherapy* or *curettage and electrodesiccation (C&D)*, and more complex tumors may be treated by *excisional surgery, Mohs' surgery*, or *radiation therapy (RT)*. The decision about which therapy to use is best made by considering four factors: tumor size; location; histology; and history (recurrent vs primary). When assessing a tumor, the clinician may wish to consider each of these four factors and decide whether the patient is high risk or low risk for each, to determine whether to use a simple or complex therapeutic strategy.

Most BCCs are discovered as primary tumors when they are still less than 1 cm in diameter. Generally tumors smaller than 1 cm on the face and 2 cm on the body are low risk.

Histologic growth pattern is a separate risk factor. The cytology of BCC does not vary: that is, all BCCs have well-differentiated, relatively monomorphic cell populations, and these tumors are not graded the way other malignancies are. However, the pattern of growth is variable and makes a large difference in choosing therapy. One must consider whether the tumor has a circumscribed or a diffuse growth pattern. Basal cell carcinoma most typically exhibits a circumscribed, cohesive growth pattern known as nodular. Nodular BCCs may show partial differentiation towards other structures, such as cystic or keratotic, but these variants are without therapeutic significance because the growth pattern is still nodular. Morpheaform, micronodular, infiltrating and superficial BCCs are all variants that exhibit a diffuse growth pattern. These lesions are more likely to recur as a result of subclinical extension or more aggressive tumor behavior, or both. Unfortunately, all too often biopsy reports come back to the clinician and simply state 'BCC', with no information about the growth pattern. Inadequately treated nodular BCC often recurs with a more aggressive diffuse growth pattern, such as infiltrating or micronodular.

Location is also an important variable to consider when choosing which therapy to use. Basal cell carcinoma tends to occur in chronically sun-exposed sites, especially the head and neck. Approximately 80% occur on the head and neck, and fully 25% occur on the nose. The central portion of the face, which has the highest incidence of BCC, contains the eyes, nose and mouth, structures of functional and cosmetic importance highly vulnerable to the destructive effects of BCC. These same structures are also highly vulnerable to the destructive effects of therapy directed against BCC. The center of the face extending onto the area around the ears defines a roughly H-shaped area known as the H zone. Tumors in this zone have the highest recurrence rate and thus deserve special therapeutic attention. This zone also contains the most vulnerable structures and has the highest rate of BCC occurrence. Tumors near the ear canal, in the H zone, are of special concern. Extension down the ear canal provides the tumor with access to the brain and other intracranial structures, and when there is evidence of ear canal invasion particularly aggressive therapy is warranted.

Lastly, tumor history is important to consider. Recurrent tumors are more difficult to treat than primary tumors and require more aggressive methods.

When confronted with a BCC, the clinician may wish to consider these four variables in the context of the individual patient. The patient's overall medical status, medical history, and age may influence the therapeutic decision making.

SPECIFIC INVESTIGATIONS

▶ Biopsy with adequate dermal component

An adequate biopsy is critical in assessing the tumor. The tumor growth pattern is important information that is impossible to determine if only a superficial fragment is submitted to the laboratory. Deep shave, punch, incisional or excisional biopsy can all give sufficient dermis for such an evaluation. Because metastasis is so rare, no further evaluation is warranted.

A number of non-invasive imaging technologies are being investigated to delineate tumor depth and extent preoperatively and thus guide treatment. These include confocal microscopy, infrared spectroscopy, and ultrasound, but these all remain experimental and are not part of routine care.

Rarely, a BCC may have been neglected and reached a size such that direct bony invasion has occurred. If this is strongly suspected, a preoperative CT scan should be considered.

The possibility that patients with a BCC have an increased risk of developing subsequent internal malignancies has been suggested over the years, and remains controversial. At present there is no recommendation for extraordinary evaluation for internal malignancies beyond routine medical care in patients with a history of BCC.

Subsequent primary cancers after basal-cell carcinoma: a nationwide study in Finland from 1953 to 1995. Milan T, Pukkala E, Verkasalo PK, Koskenvuo M, Pukkala E. Int J Cancer 2000; 87: 283–8.

A total of 71 924 patients with a diagnosis of BCC were followed during the study period. There was a statistically significant increased risk of developing non-cutaneous malignancies in patients who had a BCC.

Basal cell carcinoma and risk of subsequent malignancies: a cancer registry-based study in southwest England. Bower CP, Lear JT, Bygrave S, Etherington D, Harvey I, Archer CB. J Am Acad Dermatol 2000; 42: 988–91.

A cohort of 13 961 patients diagnosed with BCC between 1981 and 1988 were followed for additional malignancies. There was a significant increased risk of subsequent melanoma, but no increased risk for internal malignancies.

Further complicating the relationship of BCC to other cancers is the argument that vitamin D provides chemoprevention for some visceral cancers. Specifically, it has been theorized that elevated levels of vitamin D lower the incidence of a variety of tumors, including breast, colon, and prostate cancers. As vitamin D is manufactured in the skin following exposure to UVB, it has been suggested that those with high UVB exposure should have a higher incidence of BCC but a lower incidence of breast, colon, and prostate cancers, among others.

Are patients with skin cancer at lower risk of developing colorectal or breast cancer? Soerjomataram I, Louwman WJ, Lemmens VE, Coebergh JW, de Vries E. Am J Epidemiol 2008; 167: 1421–9.

26 916 patients with skin cancer (4089 SCC, 19 319 BCC, and 3508 melanomas) from the Netherlands were identified during the years 1972–2002 and analyzed for their incidence of colorectal and breast cancers. SCC, and BCC of the head and neck only, were associated with a lower incidence of colorectal cancer, but not breast cancer. Patients with melanoma had a higher incidence of breast cancer.

The effect of vitamin D on cancer incidence remains controversial.

FIRST-LINE THERAPIES

▶ Curettage and electrodesiccation	B
▶ Cryosurgery	B
▶ Excisional surgery	B
▶ Mohs' micrographic surgery	B

Recurrence rates of treated basal cell carcinomas. Part 2: Curettage–electrodesiccation. Silverman MK, Kopf AW, Grin CM, Bart RS, Levenstein MJ. J Dermatol Surg Oncol 1991; 17: 720–6.

This retrospective study of 2314 primary BCCs treated by C&D at a university dermatology clinic reports a 13.2% 5-year recurrence rate following C&D. Further analysis showed that size and location were important variables, with 5-year recurrence rates varying from 9.5% in low-risk locations to over 16.3% in high-risk sites. Similarly, 5-year recurrence rates ranged from 8.5% for tumors 0–5 mm in diameter to 19.8% for tumors 20 mm or more.

Long term recurrence rates in previously untreated (primary) basal cell carcinoma: implications for patient follow-up. Rowe DE, Carroll RJ, Day CL. J Dermatol Surg Oncol 1989; 15: 315–28.

Reviewed literature since 1947, and reported a weighted average 5-year recurrence rate of 7.7% of primary BCCs treated with C&D.

Mohs surgery is the treatment of choice for recurrent (previously treated) basal cell carcinoma. Rowe DE, Carroll RJ, Day CL. J Dermatol Surg Oncol 1989; 15: 424–31.

Reports an almost 40% 5-year recurrence rate of recurrent tumors treated by C&D, emphasizing that this modality is not appropriate for recurrent tumors.

Extensive retrospective studies exist supporting the utility of this simple, rapid, and inexpensive method to treat BCC. However, prospective studies directly comparing C&D with other therapeutic modalities are lacking, and drawing conclusions from retrospective studies not controlled for size, histology, location and history makes comparisons impossible.

Cryosurgery of basal cell carcinoma: a study of 358 patients. Bernardeau K, Derancourt C, Cambie M, Salmon-Ehr V, Morel M, Cavenelle F, et al. Ann Dermatol Venereol 2000; 127: 175–9.

A retrospective study of 395 BCCs in 358 patients reports a 5-year recurrence rate of 9%, which is in line with other reports, but that the use of a cryoprobe or other temperature-sensing device made no difference to outcome.

A systematic review of treatment modalities for primary basal cell carcinomas. Thissen MR, Neumann MH, Schouten LJ. Arch Dermatol 1999; 135: 1177–83.

Meta-analysis of published studies evaluating therapeutic methods for treating BCC. Inclusion criteria were prospective studies of at least 50 patients with primary BCC and at least 5 years' follow-up. Four studies of cryosurgery filled these criteria, with recurrence rates ranging from 0 to 20.4%

Several large retrospective reports indicate a greater than 95% cure rate with cryotherapy. However, once again the size, histology, location and history of the tumors are not defined, and hence such reports are difficult to interpret in a clinically useful way. The authors of such series generally recommend two freeze–thaw cycles to maximize cell death and the use of a cryoprobe to assess tissue temperature achieved: −50°C is generally regarded as sufficiently cytotoxic.

Surgical margins for basal cell carcinoma. Wolf DJ, Zitelli JA. Arch Dermatol 1987; 123: 340–4.

Detailed histologic examination following excision with various margins revealed that for BCC <1 cm in diameter in low-risk areas, a surgical margin of 4 mm of normal-appearing skin around the tumor gave a 98% histologic cure rate.

Morpheaform basal-cell epitheliomas: a study of subclinical extensions in a series of 51 cases. Salasche SJ, Amonette RA. J Dermatol Surg Oncol 1981; 7: 387–94.

The average subclinical extension of morpheaform BCC is 7 mm, so a 4 mm margin would be inadequate.

Use the 4 mm margin for primary nodular BCC<1 cm in diameter. Larger tumors, diffuse growth pattern tumors, and recurrent tumors require larger margins or intraoperative histologic control.

Efficacy of curettage before excision in clearing surgical margins of nonmelanoma skin cancer. Chiller K, Passaro D, McCalmont T, Vin-Christian K. Arch Dermatol 2000; 136: 1327–32.

Preoperative curettage to better delineate surgical margins produced a statistically significant reduction in positive margins following surgical excision, suggesting the utility of curettage immediately prior to surgical excision.

Long-term recurrence rates in previously untreated (primary) basal cell carcinoma: implications for patient follow-up. Rowe DE, Carroll RJ, Day CL. J Dermatol Surg Oncol 1989; 15: 315–28.

Retrospective analysis of the literature since 1947 reports a weighted average 5-year recurrence rate of 1% when primary BCCs are treated using the Mohs technique.

Mohs surgery is the treatment of choice for recurrent (previously treated) basal cell carcinoma. Rowe DE, Carroll RJ, Day CL. J Dermatol Surg Oncol 1989; 15: 424–31.

Retrospective analysis of the literature since 1947 reports weighted average 5-year recurrence rate of 5.6% when recurrent BCC are treated using the Mohs technique.

Both this and the previous study are retrospective rather than prospective, and thus direct comparison with other therapeutic modalities is difficult. However, it is most likely that the Mohs technique was used for higher-risk tumors, whereas simple methods such as C&D or cryosurgery are used for low-risk lesions, so the superior results utilizing the Mohs technique may be greater than these numbers would indicate.

Surgical excision vs Mohs' micrographic surgery for basal-cell carcinoma of the face: randomized controlled trial. Smeets NW, Krekels GA, Ostertag JU, Essers BA, Dirksen CD, Nieman FH, et al. Lancet 2004; 364: 1766–72.

A randomized, prospective trial comparing Mohs' surgery with conventional surgical excision has been initiated. In this preliminary report, 408 primary and 204 recurrent facial BCCs were randomized to surgical excision with 3 mm margins or Mohs' surgery. At 18-month follow-up the recurrence rate of primary BCC in the surgical excision group available for analysis was 2.9% (5/171) and 1.9% (3/160) in the Mohs' group. The patients with recurrent tumor were seen at 30 months' follow-up, and the recurrence rate of patients actually seen for follow-up was 3.2% (3/93) for the surgical excision group and 0% (0/95) for the Mohs' group.

This preliminary report gives the suggestion that Mohs' surgery has a lower recurrence rate than conventional surgical excision, but does not reach statistical significance. It is the intention of the authors to continue this study to 5 years of follow-up, at which time any differences may be more obvious.

Mohs micrographic surgery vs. traditional surgical excision: a cost comparison analysis. Bialy TL, Whalen J, Veledar E, Lafreniere D, Spiro J, Chartier T, et al. Arch Dermatol 2004; 140: 736–42.

This analysis suggests the cost of the Mohs technique is comparable to traditional surgical excision when one includes the cost of re-excision for those tumors traditionally excised that have positive margins. If frozen sections are used with traditional excision, then use of the Mohs technique is significantly less costly.

SECOND-LINE THERAPIES

► Radiation therapy	B

Basal cell carcinoma of the face: surgery or radiotherapy? Results of a randomized study. Avril MF, Auperin A, Margulis A, Gerbaulet A, Duvillard P, Benhamou E, et al. Br J Cancer 1997; 76: 100–6.

A randomized trial in which 347 primary BCC <4 cm in size were assigned to surgical excision or radiotherapy (RT). The 4-year recurrence rate was 0.7% for surgical excision and 7.5% for RT. More significantly, cosmesis as judged by the patient and blinded judges was significantly better in the surgery group than in the RT group.

This is a significant result because RT is often recommended as an option for those patients who wish to avoid a scar.

Therapeutic ionizing radiation and the incidence of basal cell carcinoma and squamous cell carcinoma. The New Hampshire Skin Cancer Study Group. Lichter MD, Karagas MR, Mott LA, Spencer SK, Stukel TA, Greenberg ER. Arch Dermatol 2000; 136: 1007–11.

There is a statistically significant increased risk of the development of BCC in the exposure window following therapeutic RT. The development of subsequent tumors is a significant possible side effect.

Radiation therapy is an effective, albeit expensive and time-consuming option for patients unable or unwilling to undergo surgery. Generally, 3000–5000 cGy are given in six to 20 fractionated doses, so therapy may take weeks. Cure rates have repeatedly been reported to be in excess of 90%. BCCs with perineural invasion have a very high local recurrence rate, and postoperative radiation is a wise precaution.

THIRD-LINE THERAPIES

► Intralesional interferon	B
► Retinoids	D
► Topical imiquimod	A
► Photodynamic therapy	A
► Topical 5-fluorouracil (5-FU)	A
► Electrochemotherapy	B
► CO_2 laser	D
► Intralesional interleukin	D
► Systemic chemotherapy	D

Intralesional interferon therapy for basal cell carcinoma. Cornell RC, Greenway HT, Tucker SB, Edwards L, Ashworth S, Vance JC, et al. J Am Acad Dermatol 1990; 23: 694–700.

One hundred and seventy-two patients with nodular or superficial BCC received 1.5 million units of interferon-α three times a week for 3 weeks and had an 80% histologic cure rate 1 year after treatment.

The injection produces transient flu-like symptoms, which are improved with preinjection or oral acetaminophen (paracetamol). An 80% cure rate is not comparable to the >90% cure rate attainable with other modalities, but this may be an option for some patients unable to undergo surgery or RT.

Intralesional recombinant interferon beta-1a in the treatment of basal cell carcinoma: results of an open-label multicentre study. Kowalzick L, Rogozinski T, Wimheuer R, Pilz J, Manske U, Scholz A, et al. Eur J Dermatol 2002; 12: 558–61.

One hundred and thirty-three BCCs were treated with intralesional interferon-β_{1a}, 1 million units three times a week for 3 weeks. At 16 weeks' follow-up, 66.9% were clinically and biopsy clear. At 2-year follow-up, 4.5% of those that had cleared had recurred.

Alternative preparations of interferons have not been as successful as the α_{2a} preparation.

Treatment and prevention of basal cell carcinoma with oral isotretinoin. Peck GL, DiGiovanna JJ, Sarnoff DS, Gross EG, Butkus D, Olsen TG, et al. J Am Acad Dermatol 1988; 19: 176–85.

Evidence Levels: A Double-blind study **B** Clinical trial ≥ 20 subjects **C** Clinical trial < 20 subjects **D** Series ≥ 5 subjects **E** Anecdotal case reports

Twelve patients with multiple BCCs from varying causes were treated with high-dose oral isotretinoin (mean daily dosage 3.1 mg/kg/day) for a mean of 8 months. Of the 270 tumors monitored in these patients, only 8% underwent complete clinical and histologic regression.

Topical tretinoin treatment in basal cell carcinoma. Brenner S, Wolf R, Dascalu DI. J Dermatol Surg Oncol 1993; 19: 264–6.

Case report of patient with multiple superficial BCCs. Four lesions were treated with 0.05% topical tretinoin twice a day for 3 weeks, followed by a 3-week rest. This cycle was repeated twice more. Short-term clinical and histologic evaluation showed clearance in all four lesions, but all four recurred within 9 months.

Topical treatment of basal cell carcinoma with tazarotene: a clinicopathological study on a large series of cases. Bianchi L, Orlandi A, Campione E, Angeloni C, Costanzo A, Spagnoli LG, et al. Br J Dermatol 2004; 151: 148–56.

One hundred and fifty-four small superficial and nodular BCCs were treated daily for 24 weeks with topical tazarotene. At the end of the treatment period, 70.8% of the lesions showed evidence of regression, but only 30.5% actually resolved clinically.

Retinoids, either systemically or topically, have not shown great efficacy in the treatment of BCC. However, retinoids definitely have an effective role in the chemoprevention of future BCCs in high-risk patients.

Imiquimod 5% cream for the treatment of superficial basal cell carcinoma: results from two phase III, randomized, vehicle-controlled studies. Geisse J, Caro I, Lindholm J, Golitz L, Stampone P, Owens M. J Am Acad Dermatol 2004; 50: 722–33.

This paper reports results of multicenter trials of topical imiquimod for superficial BCC with 724 subjects. Patients applied the cream daily five or seven times a week for 6 weeks. Twelve weeks after the treatment period, the area of the tumor was excised and examined histologically. The excised area was tumor free in 82% of the five times a week group and 79% of the seven times a week group.

Open study of the efficacy and mechanism of action of topical imiquimod in basal cell carcinoma. Vidal D, Matias-Guiu X, Alomar A. Clin Exp Dermatol 2004; 29: 518–25.

Fifty-five BCCs measuring more than 8 mm in diameter with superficial, nodular, or infiltrative histologic growth patterns were treated daily, either three times a week for 8 weeks or five times a week for 5 weeks. Punch biopsies were taken 6 weeks after therapy, and patients were followed clinically for 2 years – 4/4 (100%) of superficial BCCs, 7/8 (88%) of nodular BCCs, and 30/43 (70%) of infiltrating BCCs were tumor free following therapy.

This product upregulates interferons α and γ, and interleukin 12, among other cytokines. It seems to be reasonably effective for superficial BCCs, but less so for other histologic growth patterns.

Photodynamic therapy for the treatment of basal cell carcinoma. Wilson BD, Mang TS, Stoll H, Jones C, Cooper M, Dougherty TJ. Arch Dermatol 1992; 128: 1597–1601.

One hundred and fifty-one BCCs in 37 patients were treated with Photofrin, a systemic photosensitizer that preferentially accumulates in tumors, followed by exposure to 630 nm laser light. Overall, complete response rate by clinical observation at 3 months was 88%.

These authors noted that failures tended to be in high-risk areas such as the nose and high-risk histologic variants (morphea-form). Photofrin is a systemic photosensitizer, and some degree of cutaneous and ocular photosensitivity may last up to 4–6 weeks. A variety of other systemic photosensitizers are currently under investigation.

Photodynamic therapy of multiple nonmelanoma skin cancers with verteporfin and red light-emitting diodes: two year results evaluating tumor response and cosmetic outcomes. Lui H, Hobbs L, Tope WD, Lee PK, Elmets C, Provost N, et al. Arch Dermatol 2004; 140: 26–32.

Fifty-four patients with 421 non-melanoma skin cancers, including superficial BCC, nodular BCC, and SCC in situ, were treated with intravenous verteporfin followed by varying doses of red light. Treated areas were biopsied 6 months after treatment, and patients were followed clinically for 2 years. At the highest light dose, 93% of treated tumors were clear on biopsy, and 95% were clinically clear at 2-year follow-up

Like Photofrin, verteporfin is an intravenous medication but has the advantage that patients are photosensitive for only 3–5 days.

Topical photodynamic therapy with δ-aminolevulinic acid (ALA) and its methylated derivative mALA has become more popular, and is commonly used in Europe. Surgical excision remains the gold standard to which other therapies must be compared. Comparison of different therapeutic modalities has been hard because few randomized prospective comparative trials have been performed. One such trial with 5-year follow-up has been completed comparing PDT with mALA to conventional surgical excision.

Five year follow-up of a randomized prospective trial of topical methyl aminolevulinate photodynamic therapy vs. surgery for nodular basal cell carcinoma. Rhodes LE, de Rie MA, Leifsdottir R, Yu RC, Bachmann I, Goulden V, et al. Arch Dermatol 2007; 143: 1131–6.

Fifty-three nodular BCC were treated with two to four sessions of methyl ALA PDT, and 52 nodular BCC were treated by surgical excision. At 5-year follow-up there was a 14% recurrence rate in the PDT group versus 4% in the surgical excision group. However, the cosmetic outcome was rated higher in the PDT group than in the excision group.

Multiple sessions with topical mALA gives a lower cure rate but a better cosmetic outcome than surgical excision.

Treatment of basal cell carcinoma of the skin with 5-fluorouracil ointment. A 10 year follow-up study. Reymann F. Dermatologica 1979; 158: 368–72.

Ninety-five BCCs were treated with 5% 5-FU ointment. At 10-year follow-up there was a 21.4% recurrence rate.

Fluorouracil paste treatment of thin basal cell carcinomas. Epstein E. Arch Dermatol 1985; 121: 207–13.

Forty-four thin BCCs were treated with 25% 5-FU in petrolatum under occlusion for 3 weeks with weekly dressing changes. The 5-year recurrence rate was 21%.

These older papers suggested that topical 5-FU is not a good option for BCC. However, two more recent papers suggest this area may deserve a second look.

5% 5-fluorouracil cream for the treatment of small superficial basal cell carcinoma: efficacy, tolerability, cosmetic outcome, and patient satisfaction. Gross K, Kircik L, Kricorian G. Dermatol Surg 2007; 33: 433–9.

Thirty-one superficial BCC were treated with 5% 5-FU BID for up to 12 weeks. Three weeks after stopping therapy the area of the tumor was excised, which revealed 90% of the treated spots to be tumor free, although 10% had residual tumor.

A pilot study to evaluate the treatment of basal cell carcinoma with 5-fluorouracil using phosphatidylcholine as a transepidermal carrier. Romagosa R, Saap L, Givens M, Salvarrey A, He JL, Hsia SL, et al. Dermatol Surg 2000; 26: 338–40.

Ten moderately thick BCCs were treated with 5% 5-FU in a phosphatidylcholine carrier ointment, and seven similar BCCs were treated with 5% 5-FU in a petrolatum base. The histologic cure rate was 90% in the phosphatidylcholine carrier, but only 57% in the petrolatum vehicle group.

This very small study does not have enough subjects to reach statistical significance, but points out that penetration is the problem with topical 5-FU, and future more penetrant vehicles may solve this problem.

Effective treatment of cutaneous and subcutaneous malignant tumors by electrochemotherapy. Mir LM, Glass LF, Sersa G, Teissié J, Domenge C, Miklavcic D, et al. Br J Cancer 1998; 77: 2336–42.

A variety of cutaneous and subcutaneous tumors, including BCC (32), malignant melanoma (142), adenocarcinoma (30), and squamous cell carcinoma (87), were treated with a novel drug delivery system. Short and intense electrical pulses were applied directly to the tumors shortly after intravenous or intralesional administration of bleomycin. The electrical pulses are thought to increase intracellular drug uptake by altering cell membrane permeability, thereby leading to higher intracellular concentrations of the chemotherapeutic agent bleomycin. Complete clinical resolution was observed in 56.4% of the tumors and a partial response in an additional 28.9%.

Can the carbon dioxide laser completely ablate basal cell carcinomas? A histological study. Horlock N, Grobbelaar AO, Gault DT. Br J Plastic Surg 2000; 53: 286–93.

Use of the continuous-wave CO_2 laser to destroy BCCs was examined by post-laser excision and histologic check. Superficial BCCs of the trunk could be reliably ablated, but nodular and infiltrating (a diffuse growth pattern) could not reliably be treated by this method.

Effect of perilesional injections of PEG-interleukin-2 from one dose a week to four doses a week. Kaplan B, Moy RL. Dermatol Surg 2000; 26: 1037–40.

Intralesional injection of interleukin-2 in varying doses from one dose a week to four doses a week was given to eight patients with 12 BCCs. A complete response was seen in eight of the 12 (66%) tumors.

Preoperative treatment of advanced skin carcinoma with cisplatin and bleomycin. Denic S. Am J Clin Oncol 1999; 22: 32–4.

Five patients with advanced skin cancer of the head and neck were treated with systemic cisplatin and bleomycin before definitive excision to reduce the size of the tumor. Three patients had squamous cell carcinoma, and two had BCC. One patient had clinical but not pathologic resolution, three had a partial response, and one progressed. The surgical resection was reduced from that predicted prior to chemotherapy only in the one patient with a dramatic response.

Systemic chemotherapy has not been extensively investigated for BCC because metastatic disease is so rare. For metastatic disease the response to chemotherapy is generally poor, and there is little reason to believe preoperative systemic chemotherapy for advanced primary BCC would reduce the extent of excisional surgery necessary to achieve a cure.

Evidence Levels: **A** Double-blind study **B** Clinical trial ≥ 20 subjects **C** Clinical trial < 20 subjects **D** Series ≥ 5 subjects **E** Anecdotal case reports

Becker's Nevus

Elnaz F Firoz, Bahar F Firoz, Leonard H Goldberg

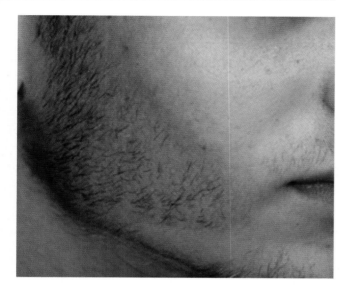

Becker's nevus, also called pigmented hairy epidermal nevus, is a cutaneous hamartoma that can have increased epidermal (melanocyte), dermal (smooth muscle), and appendageal (hair follicle) components. Classically, Becker's nevus is first noticed around puberty on the shoulders and chest in males, but may be congenital, involve any area of the body, and occur in women. The prevalence in postpubertal males is approximated to be 0.5%, or 1 in 200.

MANAGEMENT STRATEGY

Becker's nevus is usually asymptomatic and may come to the attention of a physician for cosmetic or diagnostic reasons. It is important to examine the patient for developmental defects that may accompany Becker's nevus and occur within the spectrum of *Becker's nevus syndrome*, one of several epidermal nevus syndromes. Reported associations include, but are not limited to:

Cutaneous
- acneiform eruptions
- hypohidrosis
- lichen planus
- localized scleroderma
- psoriasiform dermatitis
- unilateral breast hypoplasia

Musculoskeletal
- limb asymmetry
- pectus excavatum or carinatum
- scoliosis, including other vertebral defects.

Associations of Becker's nevus with cutaneous cancers have been reported. Both basal cell carcinoma and intraepithelial squamous cell carcinoma (Bowen's disease) have been described separately in two young women without significant risk factors (i.e., photodamage, papillomavirus infection, arsenic exposure). Although melanoma has been described in patients with Becker's nevus, the risk of malignant transformation appears to be very low. Regular screening for melanoma is unnecessary.

Traditional *surgical* approaches to remove Becker's nevus are either unsuccessful or result in significant scarring. *Laser* technology offers the clinician a means to reduce both the pigmentation and the hypertrichosis often seen in Becker's nevus, and therefore may improve the cosmetic appearance of the lesion. Management of asymptomatic, benign lesions should be based on confirming the diagnosis and fully documenting any associated pathology.

Becker's nevus syndrome revisited. Danarti R, König A, Salhi A, Bittar M, Happle R. J Am Acad Dermatol 2004; 51: 965–9.

A review of ipsilateral breast hypoplasia, other cutaneous anomalies, musculoskeletal abnormalities, and maxillofacial findings that may be observed in Becker's nevus syndrome. The concept of paradominant inheritance is presented to explain occasional familial aggregation in this syndrome.

Becker nevus syndrome. Happle R, Koopman RJ. Am J Med Genet 1997; 68: 357–61.

Proposes the term 'Becker nevus syndrome' to describe the association of Becker's nevus with developmental defects such as unilateral breast hypoplasia and other cutaneous, muscular, or skeletal defects in 23 cases.

Becker's nevus and malignant melanoma. Fehr B, Panizzon RG, Schnyder UW. Dermatologica 1991; 182: 77–80.

Report of nine patients with Becker's nevus and malignant melanoma. Five melanomas were on the same body site as the Becker's nevus, but only one arose within the nevus itself.

SPECIFIC INVESTIGATIONS

The diagnosis of Becker's nevus can be made on clinical examination. Although skin biopsy is diagnostic, it is often unnecessary. Familial Becker's nevus has been regularly reported and it would be prudent to inquire about other family members, especially same-sex siblings.

In some instances, differentiating between large congenital melanocytic nevus and Becker's nevus may be difficult. Dermoscopy may help in equivocal cases. Network, focal hypopigmentation, skin furrow hypopigmentation, hair follicles, perifollicular hypopigmentation, and vessels are the main dermoscopic features of Becker's nevus.

Familial Becker's nevus. Fretzin DF, Whitney D. J Am Acad Dermatol 1985; 12: 589–90.

The first two published cases of familial Becker's nevus.

Dermoscopic features of congenital melanocytic nevus and Becker nevus in an adult male population: an analysis with a 10-fold magnification. Ingordo V, Iannazzone SS, Cusano F, Naldi L. Dermatology 2006; 212: 354–60.

Assesses the use of optical dermoscopy with 10-fold magnification in differentiating between large congenital melanocytic nevus and Becker's nevus.

FIRST-LINE THERAPIES

Treatment requested by patients can be divided into two components:

▶ reduction of hyperpigmentation
▶ removal of excess hair.

Reduction of excess hair

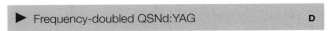

▶ Erbium:YAG laser	C
▶ Erbium-doped fiber laser (Fraxel)	D
▶ Q-switched ruby laser (QSRL)	D

Becker's naevus: a comparative study between erbium:YAG and Q-switched neodynium:YAG: clinical and histopathological findings. Trelles MA, Allones I, Moreno-Arias GA, Vélez M. Br J Dermatol 2005; 152: 308–13.

Twenty-two patients with Becker's nevi were studied, 11 with each laser. Both erbium:YAG and Nd:YAG safely treated the lesions. For pigment removal, one pass with erbium:YAG was superior to three treatment sessions with Nd:YAG.

Fractional resurfacing: a new therapeutic modality for Becker's nevus. Glaich AS, Goldberg LH, Dai T, Kunishige JH, Friedman PM. Arch Dermatol 2007; 143: 1488–90.

Two male patients with Becker's nevi were treated with the 1550-nm wavelength erbium-doped fiber laser between 6 and 10 mJ at 4-week intervals and between five and six treatment sessions. More than 75% of the pigment had faded by 1 month in both patients. There was no improvement in hypertrichosis.

Q-switched ruby laser treatment of tattoos and benign pigmented skin lesions: a critical review. Raulin C, Schönermark MP, Greve B, Werner S. Ann Plast Surg 1998; 41: 555–65.

This review recommends three to 10 treatments at monthly intervals with QSRL at fluences between 7 and 20 J/cm² for hyperpigmentation. Although QSRL for long-term removal of associated hypertrichosis is not recommended, long-pulsed (755 nm) alexandrite laser has produced promising results.

Quality-switched ruby laser treatment of solar lentigines and Becker's nevus: a histopathological and immunohistochemical study. Kopera D, Hohenleutner U, Landthaler M. Dermatology 1997; 194: 338–43.

A single case of Becker's nevus treated with a single 8 J/cm² pulse that resulted in clinical fading within 2 weeks, but reactive patchy hyperpigmentation after 4 weeks.

The removal of cutaneous pigmented lesions with the Q-switched ruby laser and the Q-switched neodymium: yttrium-aluminum-garnet laser. A comparative study. Tse Y, Levine VJ, McClain SA, Ashinoff R. J Dermatol Surg Oncol 1994; 20: 795–800.

An area of Becker's nevus was anesthetized and bisected, and each half treated with either QSRL or QSNd:YAG at 532 nm. Clinical lightening occurred in 63% and 43% of the lesion at fluences of 8.4 and 2.8 J/cm², respectively. QSRL caused intraoperative pain, whereas QSNd:YAG caused postoperative discomfort.

Reduction of hyperpigmentation

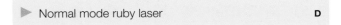

▶ Normal mode ruby laser	D

The ruby laser in the normal or long-pulsed mode has been used for laser epilation. A common side effect is hypopigmentation of adjacent skin, which can be used when treating hypertrichosis of a Becker's nevus.

Treatment of a Becker's nevus using a 694-nm long-pulsed ruby laser. Nanni CA, Alster TS. Dermatol Surg 1998; 24: 1032–4.

A single case report that showed reduction in pigmentation and a 90% reduction in hair growth after three treatments with the long-pulsed ruby laser. Improvement was maintained for 10 months.

SECOND-LINE THERAPIES

Reduction of hyperpigmentation

▶ Frequency-doubled QSNd:YAG	D

The QSNd:YAG laser operating at 532 nm has been shown to reduce pigmentation in Becker's nevus, but does not appear to be as successful as the ruby laser.

Reduction of excess hair

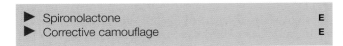

▶ Electrolysis	E

Electrolysis is a well-established method of epilation, but its use in removing hair from Becker's nevus has not been described.

THIRD-LINE THERAPIES

▶ Spironolactone	E
▶ Corrective camouflage	E

Becker's nevus is thought to be an androgen-dependent lesion, as it becomes more prominent after puberty, displays increased hairiness in males, and contains an increased number of androgen receptors and androgen-receptor messenger RNA compared to surrounding skin.

Becker's nevus with ipsilateral breast hypoplasia: improvement with spironolactone. Hoon Jung J, Chan Kim Y, Joon Park H, Woo Cinn Y. J Dermatol 2003; 30: 154–6.

Spironolactone, an anti-androgenic agent, was administered for the treatment of breast hypoplasia associated with Becker's nevus in one case. After 1 month, breast enlargement was observed only in the hypoplastic breast.

Corrective camouflage in pediatric dermatology. Tedeschi A, Dall'Oglio F, Micali G, Schwartz RA, Janniger CK. Cutis 2007; 79: 110–12.

Corrective camouflage using a variety of water-resistant and light to very opaque products was used in two patients with Becker's nevi. Parents were satisfied with the cosmetic cover results. Corrective makeup may be a valid adjunctive therapy for patients undergoing long-term treatment, or in whom conventional therapy is ineffective.

Behçet's disease

Andrew D Lee, Larisa Ravitskiy, Justin J Green, Joseph L Jorizzo

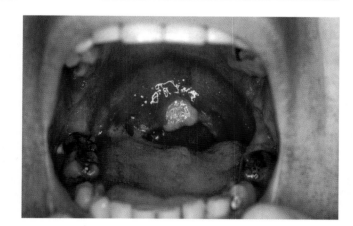

Behçet's disease is a chronic systemic vasculitis characterized by oral and genital aphthae, arthritis, cutaneous lesions (erythema nodosum-like lesions, pyoderma gangrenosum-like lesions, Sweet's syndrome-like lesions, and papulopustular eruptions) and ocular, gastrointestinal, and neurologic manifestations. Many regimens effective for recurrent aphthous stomatitis are used to treat the aphthae of Behçet's disease (see Aphthous stomatitis, page 50).

MANAGEMENT STRATEGY

In the absence of the multisystem disease, the severity and extent of the mucocutaneous manifestations direct the treatment. First-line therapy for oral and genital aphthae is a *high-potency topical corticosteroid* in a gel or ointment formulation. Alternatively, *intralesional corticosteroid* (triamcinolone 5 mg/mL) can be used for major aphthae and severe minor aphthae. Other topical therapies accelerate healing or diminish the pain associated with oral aphthae, and include viscous *lidocaine 2–5%* applied directly to lesions, *chlorhexidine 1–2%*, *amlexanox 5% oral paste*, *sucralfate, tetracycline suspension* and *topical tacrolimus*.

Colchicine 0.6 mg three times daily combined with topical corticosteroid therapy is efficacious in mucocutaneous disease. *Dapsone* 100–200 mg daily is also effective, but requires more rigorous follow-up.

Those patients who fail the more conservative approaches and have severe mucocutaneous disease may require aggressive therapy. *Thalidomide* 100–300 mg daily (pediatric dose varies from 1 mg/kg/week to 1 mg/kg daily) is more effective than low-dose *methotrexate* 7.5–20 mg/week for severe disease. *Prednisone* taper begun at 1 mg/kg daily can be used for severe mucocutaneous flares, but rebound is a possible complication.

Systemic *interferon (IFN)-α_{2a}* and *anti-tumor necrosis factor (TNF)-α* therapies may be best suited for those with severe mucocutaneous lesions and non-ocular systemic manifestations. *Etanercept* 50 mg weekly by subcutaneous injection, or *infliximab* 5 mg/kg in single or multiple intravenous infusions, have been shown to be effective in patients with recalcitrant disease and may be used as monotherapy or as an adjunct to conventional immunosuppressive therapy. Notably, infliximab has demonstrated rapid therapeutic effect, which may be useful in patients with vision-threatening posterior uveitis. These patients should be screened for latent tuberculosis infection prior to initiating anti-TNF therapies. Patients with certain extracutaneous signs (e.g., uveitis, aneurysms) may warrant combination therapy with *prednisone* and an immunosuppressive agent such as *ciclosporin, azathioprine, chlorambucil* or *cyclophosphamide*. Mucocutaneous disease alone rarely warrants this therapy. However, these agents have a beneficial effect on skin and mucous membrane lesions.

SPECIFIC INVESTIGATIONS

> ▶ Pathergy test optimal
> ▶ Culture/polymerase chain reaction of aphthae to exclude herpes simplex virus (HSV)
> ▶ Vitamins B_1, B_2, B_6 and B_{12}, folate, zinc and iron levels
> ▶ anti-DNAse B titer
> ▶ Urinalysis
> ▶ HLA-B27 to exclude that spectrum of disease
> ▶ Exclude inflammatory bowel disease

Behçet's syndrome: immunopathological and histopathological assessment of pathergy lesions is useful in diagnosis and follow-up. Jorizzo JL, Soloman AR, Cavallo T. Arch Pathol Lab Med 1985; 109: 747–51.

This method of pathergy testing may be more sensitive than standard techniques devoid of histologic study.

Behçet's disease and complex aphthosis. Ghate JV, Jorizzo JL. J Am Acad Dermatol 1999; 40: 1–18.

A review of investigations that should be carried out in a patient with complex aphthosis is presented.

HSV, nutritional deficiencies, neutropenia, lymphopenia, reactive arthritis, and inflammatory bowel disease may simulate the oral aphthae of Behçet's disease.

FIRST-LINE THERAPIES

▶ Topical/intralesional corticosteroid	**B**
▶ Topical tacrolimus	**D**
▶ Chlorhexidine gluconate	**D**
▶ Amlexanox 5% paste	**D**
▶ Sucralfate	**A**
▶ Tetracycline suspension	**D**
▶ Colchicine	**A**
▶ Zinc sulfate	**A**

A double-blind trial of colchicine in Behçet's syndrome. Yurdakul S, Mat C, Tuzun Y, Ozyazgan Y, Hamuryudan V, Uysal O, et al. Arthritis Rheum 2001; 44: 2686–92.

A prospective, double-blind, controlled trial of 116 patients treated with colchicine vs placebo. Therapy with colchicine 1–2 mg daily was effective for arthritis and erythema nodosum. Orogenital aphthae were more responsive to treatment in females.

Recurrent aphthous stomatitis: treatment with colchicine. An open trial of 54 cases. Fontes V, Machet L, Huttenberger B, Lorette G, Vaillant L. Ann Dermatol Venereol 2002; 129: 1365–9.

Fifty-four patients were treated with 1–1.5 mg colchicine for at least 3 months. Twelve patients no longer had aphthae and were in complete remission; 22 patients were significantly improved, as the frequency and duration of the lesions had decreased by at least 50%. Treatment failed or tolerance was poor in 20 patients.

Oral zinc sulfate in the treatment of Behcet's disease: a double blind cross-over study. Sharquie KE, Najim RA, Al-Dori WS, Al-Hayani RK. J Dermatol 2006; 33: 541–6.

A prospective, randomized, double-blinded, controlled trial of 27 patients with mucocutaneous and/or joint disease, along with 30 healthy subjects matched for age and gender as a control group, treated with zinc sulfate vs placebo. Zinc sulfate 100 mg three times daily was found to be effective in reducing disease severity, and no adverse effects were reported.

Patients with ocular, neurologic, cardiac, or other systemic manifestations were excluded.

SECOND-LINE THERAPIES

▶ Dapsone	A
▶ Thalidomide	A
▶ Methotrexate	E
▶ Systemic corticosteroid	B

Dapsone in Behçet's disease: a double-blind, placebo-controlled, cross-over study. Sharquie KE, Najim RA, Abu-Raghif AR. J Dermatol 2002; 29: 267–79.

Randomized, double-blind, placebo-controlled, crossover trial of 20 patients treated with either dapsone 100 mg or placebo. There was a significant reduction of orogenital ulcers and other cutaneous manifestations in the dapsone group.

Vitamin E 800 IU daily may reduce the hemolysis induced by dapsone. Other studies have confirmed the utility of dapsone for mucocutaneous Behçet's disease.

Thalidomide in the treatment of the mucocutaneous lesions of Behçet syndrome: a randomized, double-blind, placebo-controlled trial. Hamuryudan V, Mat C, Saip S, Ozyazgan Y, Siva A, Yurdakul S, et al. Ann Intern Med 1998; 128: 443–50.

A randomized, double-blind, controlled trial of 96 males evaluated thalidomide 100 mg daily vs 300 mg daily vs placebo for 24 weeks. Both thalidomide dosages led to a significant suppression of oral ulcers at 4 weeks, and genital ulcers and follicular lesions at 8 weeks. Complete responses were observed in 11% of patients treated with thalidomide.

Thalidomide effects in Behçet's syndrome and pustular vasculitis. Jorizzo JL, Schmalstieg FC, Solomon AR Jr, Schmalstieg FC, Cavallo T. Arch Intern Med 1986; 146: 878–81.

Mechanism-oriented study of four patients with Behçet's syndrome who were given thalidomide in sequential 4-week 'on/off' cycle showed significant clinical benefit.

Treatment of Behçet's disease with thalidomide. Hamza MH. Clin Rheumatol 1986; 5: 365–71.

Thirty male patients were treated with thalidomide. Twenty-six patients with orogenital ulcerations responded (20 completely and six partially), all patients with arthritis responded (13 completely and one partially), and uveitis improved in three patients.

Low-dose weekly methotrexate for unusual neutrophilic vascular reactions: cutaneous polyarteritis nodosa and Behçet's disease. Jorizzo JL, White WL, Wise CM, Zanolli MD, Sherertz EF. J Am Acad Dermatol 1991; 24: 973–8.

Two female patients with oral and genital aphthae, pyoderma gangrenosum-like lesions, and cutaneous pustular vasculitic lesions cleared with methotrexate 15–20 mg/week.

Practical treatment recommendations for pharmacotherapy of Behçet's syndrome. Yazici H, Barnes CG. Drugs 1991; 42: 796–804.

Intravenous pulse methylprednisolone 1 g on 3 alternate days, or 1 mg/kg daily of prednisone for several weeks with subsequent taper, are recommended for severe or life-threatening major ulcerations.

Combined therapy with other immunosuppressants while on maintenance prednisone is found in multiple trials, but prednisone alone vs placebo has not been studied.

THIRD-LINE THERAPIES

▶ IFN-α_{2a}	B
▶ Penicillin	B
▶ Indomethacin	B
▶ Isotretinoin	E
▶ Ciclosporin	A
▶ Azathioprine	A
▶ Cyclophosphamide	E
▶ Chlorambucil	B
▶ Minocycline	C
▶ Plasma exchange	E
▶ Prostaglandin E$_1$	C
▶ IVIG	D
▶ Rebamipide	B
▶ Etanercept	B
▶ Infliximab	C
▶ Adalimumab	D
▶ Peptide 336–351 linked to cholera toxin B	C
▶ Levamisole	C
▶ Adsorption apheresis	E
▶ Azithromycin	C

Differential efficacy of human recombinant interferon-alpha2a on ocular and extraocular manifestations of Behçet disease: results of an open 4-center trial. Kötter I, Vonthein R, Zierhut M, Eckstein AK, Ness T, Günaydin I, et al. Semin Arthritis Rheum 2004; 33: 311–19.

An open, uncontrolled study of 50 patients treated with subcutaneous 6×10^6 U rhIFN-α_{2a} daily resulted in a 92% response rate of ocular manifestations, remission of genital ulcerations and skin lesions, and 36% response of oral aphthae.

There are additional reports substantiating the benefits of IFN-α_{2a} in mucocutaneous Behçet's disease.

Interferon alfa-2a in the treatment of Behçet disease: a randomized placebo-controlled and double-blind study. Alpsoy E, Durusoy C, Yilmaz E, Ozgurel Y, Ermis O, Yazar S, Basaran E. Arch Dermatol 2002; 138: 467–71.

A randomized, double-blinded, placebo-controlled trial of 23 patients receiving interferon-α_{2a} three times a week. After 3 months, 15 of 23 patients demonstrated improvement in oral, genital, and papulopustular lesions.

Evidence Levels: **A** Double-blind study **B** Clinical trial ≥ 20 subjects **C** Clinical trial < 20 subjects **D** Series ≥ 5 subjects **E** Anecdotal case reports

Interferon-alpha treatment of Behçet's disease. O'Duffy JD, Calamia K, Cohen S, Goronzy JJ, Herman D, Jorizzo J, et al. J Rheumatol 1998; 25: 1938–44.

Seven patients underwent daily subcutaneous injections of 3 million units of interferon-α_{2a} This open trial reported a substantial reduction in mucocutaneous lesions and joint disease. Flu-like symptoms, leukopenia, psoriasis, seizure, hyperthyroidism, and psychosis were side effects reported.

Effect of prophylactic benzathine penicillin on mucocutaneous symptoms of Behçet's disease. Calguneri M, Ertenli I, Kiraz S, Erman M, Celik I. Dermatology 1996; 192: 125–8.

A prospective, randomized trial with 60 patients revealed statistically significant decrements in frequency and duration of oral aphthae and erythema nodosum-like lesions and the frequency of genital aphthae with the addition of benzathine penicillin 1.2 million units every 3 weeks to colchicine vs colchicine monotherapy.

This study was apparently non-blinded and not placebo controlled.

Treatment of Behçet disease with indomethacin. Simsek H, Dundar S, Telatar H. Int J Dermatol 1991; 30: 54–7.

An open-label study used indomethacin 25 mg four times daily in 30 patients with articular and skin manifestations. Improvements were seen in reduction of aphthae, erythema nodosum-like lesions, pustular lesions, and joint involvement.

A double-blind, randomized, placebo-controlled study of azapropazone and a few case reports describe unsuccessful treatment of arthritis and leg ulcers with various non-steroidal anti-inflammatory drugs (NSAIDs). When added to colchicine therapy, NSAIDs have been reported to cause an increase in ocular attacks.

Systemic isotretinoin in the treatment of a Behçet's patient with arthritic symptoms and acne lesions. Akyol M, Dogan S, Kaptanoglu E, Ozcelik S. Clin Exp Rheumatol 2002; 20: S-55.

A patient with oral ulcers, acne lesions, and arthritis was treated with 6 months of isotretinoin. He experienced complete resolution of his acne and arthritis, and reduced severity of oral ulcers, controlled with only topical treatment.

Double-masked trial of cyclosporin versus colchicine and long-term open study of cyclosporin in Behçet's disease. Masuda K, Nakajima A, Urayama A, Nakae K, Kogure M, Inaba G. Lancet 1989; 1: 1093–6.

Ciclosporin was more effective than colchicine in reducing the number and frequency of oral aphthae and cutaneous lesions (erythema nodosum-like, subcutaneous thrombophlebitis and folliculitis-like lesions).

Several case reports and open studies corroborate these findings.

Cyclosporine in Behçet's disease: results in 16 patients after 24 months of therapy. Pacor ML, Biasi D, Lunardi C, Cortina P, Caramaschi P, Girelli D, et al. Clin Rheumatol 1994; 13: 224–7.

Sixteen subjects with Behçet's syndrome received 5 mg/kg of ciclosporin daily for 24 months. A marked improvement of the symptoms was observed after 3 months of therapy, and 14 out of 16 patients obtained a complete clinical remission. Two patients dropped out of the study because of anemia and renal dysfunction, which returned to normal when ciclosporin was withdrawn.

Efficacy of cyclosporine on mucocutaneous manifestations of Behçet's disease. Avci O, Gurler N, Gunes AT. J Am Acad Dermatol 1997; 36: 796–7.

Mucocutaneous lesions were markedly suppressed in an open trial involving 24 patients treated for more than 6 months with ciclosporin 5 mg/kg daily. Most responsive to therapy were genital ulcerations, thrombophlebitis, erythema nodosum-like lesions, and acneiform lesions.

A controlled trial of azathioprine in Behçet's syndrome. Yazici H, Pazarli H, Barnes CG, Tüzün Y, Ozyazgan Y, Silman A, et al. N Engl J Med 1990; 322: 281–5.

A randomized, controlled, double-blind trial of azathioprine 2.5 mg/kg daily vs placebo in patients with Behçet's disease resulted in prevention and decreased frequency of ocular disease. The prevalence of oral ulcers and the incidence of genital ulcers were diminished in the azathioprine group.

Cyclophosphamide therapy of Behçet's disease. Buckley CE III, Gillis JP Jr. J Allergy 1969; 64: 105–12.

A single report of oral aphthae and ocular manifestations responding to cyclophosphamide when it was added to prednisone therapy.

Long-lasting remission of Behçet's disease after chlorambucil therapy. Abdalla MI, Bahgat NE. Br J Ophthalmol 1973; 57: 706–11.

Remission of aphthae was achieved in all seven patients treated with oral chlorambucil and corticosteroids, but in a minority of patients treated with corticosteroids alone.

Chlorambucil in the treatment of uveitis and meningoencephalitis of Behçet's disease. O'Duffy JD, Robertson DM, Goldstein NP. Am J Med 1984; 76: 75–84.

In 10 patients treated with either chlorambucil 0.1 mg/kg daily or corticosteroids, uveitis and visual acuities improved in five of seven eyes when the patients were treated with chlorambucil and in only four of 13 eyes when treatment consisted of corticosteroids. Eight of nine patients with meningoencephalitis were treated with chlorambucil and had remission of their disease.

In one controlled study, chlorambucil, when used with corticosteroids, was superior to corticosteroids alone.

Streptococcal infection in the pathogenesis of Behçet's disease and clinical effects of minocycline on the disease symptoms. Kaneko F, Oyama N, Nishibu A. Yonsei Med J 1997; 38: 444–54.

In 11 patients treated with minocycline 100 mg daily the frequency of cutaneous symptoms was reduced by 10% for oral aphthae and by 100% for perifolliculitis.

Behçet's disease with severe cutaneous necrotizing vasculitis: response to plasma exchange – report of a case. Cornelis F, Sigal-Nahum M, Gaulier A, Bleichner G, Sigal S. J Am Acad Dermatol 1989; 21: 576–9.

Oral prostaglandin E1 as a therapeutic modality for leg ulcers in Behçet's disease. Takeuchi A, Hashimoto T. Int J Clin Pharm Res 1987; 7: 283–9.

In five patients, leg ulcers began to regranulate within 2 weeks of using oral prostaglandin E_1 15–30 µg daily.

Intravenous immunoglobulin therapy for resistant ocular Behçet's disease. Seider N, Beiran I, Scharf J, Miller B. Br J Ophthalmol 2001; 85: 1287–8.

Four patients with ocular disease refractory to steroids and ciclosporin were treated with a course of IVIG. Six eyes showed good response to IVIG therapy.

Efficacy of rebamipide as adjunctive therapy in the treatment of recurrent oral aphthous ulcers in patients with Behçet's disease. Matsuda T, Ohno S, Hirohata S, Miyanaga Y, Ujihara H, Inaba G, et al. Drugs R&D 2003; 4: 19–28.

A multicenter, randomized, double-blind, placebo-controlled prospective study of rebamipide 300 mg/kg plus usual therapy (n=19) vs placebo plus usual therapy (n=16) showed moderate to marked improvement of oral aphthae in 65% of the treatment group vs 36% in the placebo group.

Short-term trial of etanercept in Behçet's disease: a double blind, placebo controlled study. Melikoglu M, Fresko I, Mat C, Ozyazgan Y, Gogus F, Yurdakul S, et al. J Rheumatol 2005; 32: 98–105.

A randomized, double-blind, controlled trial of 40 Behçet's patients who received either etanercept 25 mg or placebo subcutaneously twice a week for 4 weeks. Etanercept was found to be effective in suppressing oral ulcers, nodular lesions, and papulopustular lesions.

A patient with neuro-Behçet's disease is successfully treated with etanercept: further evidence for the value of TNF alpha blockade. Alty JE, Monaghan TM, Bamford JM. Clin Neurol Neurosurg 2007; 109: 279–81.

A patient with neuro-Behçet's disease, refractory to conventional immunosuppressive therapy, demonstrated remarkable response when treated with etanercept.

Efficacy, safety, and pharmacokinetics of multiple administrations of infliximab in Behçet's disease with refractory uveoretinitis. Ohno S, Nakamura S, Hori S, Shimakawa M, Kawashima H, Mochizuki M, et al. J Rheumatol 2004; 31–7.

Thirteen patients with refractory uveoretinitis were randomized into 5 mg/kg and 10 mg/kg treatment groups. Five of the patients remained on ciclosporin during the study. After four infusions, the frequency of ocular attacks (ocular attack disappearance rate 71–83%) and improvement of mucocutaneous symptoms were similar in both groups.

Infliximab for the treatment of resistant oral ulcers in Behçet's disease: a case report and review of the literature. Almoznino G, Ben-Chetrit E. Clin Exp Rheumatol 2007; 25: S99–102.

A patient with severe oral lesions refractory to topical and systemic immunosuppressive treatments demonstrated complete recovery and remission after a single administration of infliximab. Five more cases of recalcitrant orogenital ulceration in Behçet's disease responding to infliximab were also summarized.

Infliximab treatment for ocular and extraocular manifestations of Behçet's disease. Accorinti M, Pirraglia MP, Paroli MP, Priori R, Conti F, Pivetti-Pezzi P. Jpn J Ophthalmol 2007; 51: 191–6.

Twelve patients with Behçet's disease and uveitis refractory to conventional immunosuppressive therapy were given infliximab. After a median 15-month follow-up, 11 of the 12 showed a significant reduction in the number of ocular relapses, as well as fewer extraocular manifestations, resulting in less systemic corticosteroid use.

One patient stopped treatment after 2 months because of the development of pulmonary tuberculosis.

Anti-TNF therapy in the management of Behçet's disease-review and basis for recommendations. Sfikakis PP, Markomichelakis N, Alpsoy E, Assaad-Khalil S, Bodaghi B, Gul A, et al. Rheumatology 2007; 46: 736–41.

An evidence-based review of anti-TNF agents in Behçet's disease. This review concluded that etanercept was effective in patients with mucocutaneous and joint involvement, whereas infliximab was more efficacious in patients with ocular, intestinal, and neurologic involvement. Both agents were recommended as adjunctive treatments for patients who are refractory or intolerant to traditional immunosuppressive regimens.

Adalimumab: a new modality for Behçet's disease? van Laar JA, Missotten T, van Daele PL, Jamnitski A, Baarsma GS, van Hagen PM. Ann Rheum Dis 2007; 66: 565–6.

Six patients with severe disease recalcitrant to immunosuppressive therapy were treated with adalimumab. All patients demonstrated improvement, including a complete response in one patient and resolution of severe colitis, unresponsive to infliximab, in another.

Two of the six patients in this series exhibited colitis; we believe, as per the Mayo Clinic O'Duffy criteria, that colitis must be excluded to diagnose Behçet's disease.

Oral tolerization with peptide 336–351 linked to cholera toxin B subunit in preventing relapses of uveitis in Behçet's disease. Stanford M, Whittall T, Bergmeier LA, Lindblad M, Lundin S, Shinnick T, et al. Clin Exp Immunol 2004; 137: 201–8.

Phase I/II clinical trial of oral administration of peptide 336–351 linked to cholera toxin B, three times weekly, followed by gradual withdrawal of all immunosuppressive drugs, can be used to control uveitis and extraocular manifestations of Behçet's disease.

Treatment of Behçet's syndrome with levamisole. De Merieux P, Spitler LE, Paulus HE. Arthritis Rheum 1981; 24: 64–70.

An open study of 11 patients led to complete resolution of orogenital lesions in three and a partial response in six.

Other studies confirm the benefits of levamisole treatment in Behçet's disease.

Remission induction in Behçet's disease following lymphocyte depletion by the anti-CD52 antibody CAMPATH 1-H. Lockwood CM, Hale G, Waldman H, Jayne DR. Rheumatology (Oxford) 2003; 42: 1539–44.

An open prospective study of 18 patients (skin involvement in 67%) treated with lymphocyte-depleting anti-CD52 antibody (total of 134 mg administered by intravenous infusion). Three months after treatment, eight patients were in complete remission, seven in partial remission, and two had worsened. Of 13 patients in remission, seven relapsed after an average of 25 months.

Hypothyroidism and prolonged lymphopenia complicated treatment. There was routine prophylaxis against HSV and fungi.

Treatment of Behçet's disease with granulocyte and monocyte adsorption apheresis. Kanekura T, Gushi A, Fukumaru S, Fukumaru S, Sakamoto R, Kawahara K, et al. J Am Acad Dermatol 2004; 51: S83–7.

A report of successful treatment of orogenital ulceration in two patients who underwent five and eight treatments each.

Clinical and immunological effects of azithromycin in Behçet's disease. Mumcu G, Ergun T, Elbir Y, Eksioglu-Demiralp E, Yavuz S, Atalay T, et al. J Oral Pathol Med 2005; 34: 13–16.

In eight patients treated with azithromycin 500 mg three times per week for 4 weeks, faster healing times of pre-existing oral ulcers, as well as complete resolution of folliculitic lesions, were observed.

Bioterrorism

Donald Rudikoff, Alejandra Gurtman

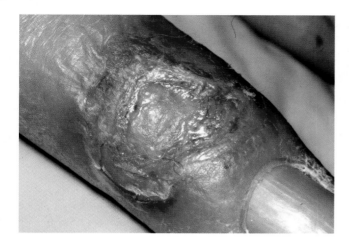

The events of September, 11, 2001 and the subsequent dissemination of anthrax through the US Postal Service heightened concern among public health authorities and physicians regarding the specter of bioterrorist attack on populated areas. The diseases that are of greatest concern are smallpox, anthrax, tularemia, plague, the hemorrhagic fevers, and botulism. Some of these have prominent cutaneous manifestations in their natural setting, but may be less likely to show typical skin lesions when spread by aerosol, which favors pulmonary disease. Dermatologists should familiarize themselves with these disorders, their recognition and treatment, and the measures that can be undertaken to limit the spread of disease. Several of the conditions discussed, including smallpox, pneumonic plague, and viral hemorrhagic fevers, are contagious to caregivers, so appropriate care must be taken to prevent caregivers contracting disease.

SMALLPOX

Naturally occurring smallpox was eradicated in the 1970s and routine vaccination ceased after 1980, so most physicians practicing today have never seen an active case of the disease. Smallpox presents with a febrile prodrome with headache, back pain, and prostration, followed by a normalization of temperature and apparent subjective improvement. The enanthem and characteristic exanthem ensue. Hoarseness may occur, and the eyes can be swollen shut. The deep-seated lesions are firm and umbilicated, and may become multilocular. Around the 10th day of the rash the lesions start to dry, and sticky yellow pus from ruptured blisters forms a crust, imparting a sickening odor. The severe burning in the skin is replaced by itching, which the patient is too weak to scratch.

The diagnosis of smallpox is relatively straightforward. Major criteria for diagnosis are a prodrome of fever for 1–4 days before the onset of rash; classic smallpox lesions – firm, deep-seated papules and pustules, all in the same stage of development. The minor criteria are centrifugal distribution of skin lesions; toxic or moribund appearance; slow evolution of lesions (1–2 days per stage); and palmoplantar lesions.

The conditions most likely to be confused with smallpox are varicella or disseminated herpes zoster, especially if severe, as in immunocompromised individuals. The febrile prodrome is not a usual feature of chickenpox and the patient is not nearly as toxic. Varicella skin lesions are superficial vesicles that appear in crops (in different stages of development), compared to the deep-seated pearly pustules of variola, which are in the same stage of development in any given area of the body. Varicella spares the palms and soles, which are typically involved in variola. Patients with disseminated herpes zoster are often immunosuppressed from chemotherapy, underlying malignancy, or retroviral disease, and typically have concurrent dermatomal lesions. Other conditions that are less likely to be confused with variola are infected molluscum contagiosum in a febrile patient with AIDS, erythema multiforme, pustular drug eruption, purpura fulminans, and hand, foot, and mouth disease. Monkeypox can closely mimic variola.

Smallpox vaccination can cause a wide array of complications in those vaccinated and their close family contacts. Dermatologists are in a unique position to evaluate contraindications to vaccination, such as atopic dermatitis, pemphigus, or Darier's disease in potential vaccinees or their family members. Documented *Vaccinia* transmission to close contacts of vaccinees occurred in recent military vaccination campaigns. Various self-limiting side effects include headache, fatigue, muscle ache, fever, chills, local skin reactions, nonspecific rashes, erythema multiforme, lymphadenopathy, and pain at the inoculation site.

Inoculation vaccinia can occur from inadvertent spread to the eyelids, genitals, or other sites in vaccinees and their close contacts. Eczema vaccinatum, analogous to eczema herpeticum, occurs in vaccinees or contacts with atopic dermatitis or other disturbances of skin integrity. Progressive vaccinia extending from the vaccination site in patients with defective cell-mediated immunity is a relentless, often fatal complication with progressive necrosis and metastatic spread. Other adverse reactions of vaccination include post-vaccinial encephalopathy and encephalomyelitis, fetal vaccinia, and myocarditis.

MANAGEMENT STRATEGY

The management of a smallpox attack would involve recognition of index cases, notification of appropriate government authorities, isolation, treatment, and appropriate public health measures to prevent the spread of disease. Anyone exposed to the patient, if not recently vaccinated, would require immediate vaccination and isolation. So-called 'ring vaccination' – that is, vaccination and isolation of contacts (those with face-to-face exposure to a true case within 2 m) and contacts of contacts, would be instituted. Suspected cases of smallpox should be managed in a negative-pressure isolation room. If there were multiple suspected cases, an 'isolation hospital' or other facility would be designated by public health officials. Strict respiratory and contact isolation and universal precautions are mandatory.

Because *post-exposure vaccination* is part of the currently recommended management, dermatologists must be familiar with the technique now in use, contraindications to vaccination, recognition, and management of vaccine side effects. Treatment of smallpox cases involves *supportive care, management of cutaneous and oral lesions, antibiotic treatment of secondary bacterial infection and sepsis,* and *perhaps use of antiviral medications.*

SPECIFIC INVESTIGATIONS

> ▶ Tzanck smear
> ▶ Direct fluorescent antibody testing for varicella zoster virus (VZV) and herpes simplex virus (HSV)
> ▶ Polymerase chain reaction (PCR) for VZV, *Vaccinia*, variola, other orthopox viruses (monkeypox)
> ▶ Electron microscopy
> ▶ Orthopox virus culture
> ▶ Serology

Laboratory diagnosis to differentiate smallpox, vaccinia, and other vesicular/pustular illnesses. Besser JM, Crouch NA, Sullivan M. J Lab Clin Med 2003; 142: 246–51.

Laboratory testing of low-risk patients can be carried out at standard reference laboratories according to local institutional guidelines. Laboratory testing of moderate- or high-risk patients should be done at a government-designated laboratory. In addition to Tzanck smears for low-risk patients, 'real-time' PCR assays for HSV and VZV can be done locally. Electron microscopy, PCR, orthopox virus culture, and variola serology are carried out at government reference laboratories.

Diagnosis and management of smallpox. Breman JG, Henderson DA. N Engl J Med 2002; 346: 1300–8.

A comprehensive review of the diagnosis and management of smallpox. Postexposure vaccination is crucial, especially if the disease is at an early stage.

Development and experience with an algorithm to evaluate suspected smallpox cases in the United States, 2002–2004. Seward JF, Galil K, Damon I, Norton SA, Rotz L, Schmid S, et al. Clin Infect Dis 2004; 39: 1477–83.

Diagnostic criteria and a Centers for Disease Control and Prevention (CDC) algorithm to evaluate and manage suspected cases of smallpox. Three categories (i.e., those with a low, moderate, or high risk of actually having smallpox) dictate subsequent diagnostic strategies. Specific variola laboratory testing is reserved for high-risk persons. *An interactive version of the algorithm is available online at http://www.bt.cdc.gov/agent/smallpox/diagnosis/riskalgorithm/index.asp.*

FIRST-LINE THERAPIES

> **Suspected cases**
>
> ▶ Isolation – negative-pressure room   E
> ▶ Respiratory and contact isolation   E
> ▶ Vaccination of early-stage patients   E
> ▶ Maintenance of hydration and adequate nutrition E

Large-scale quarantine following biological terrorism in the United States: scientific examination, logistic and legal limits, and possible consequences. Barbera J, Macintyre A, Gostin L, Inglesby T, O'Toole T, DeAtley C, et al. JAMA 2001; 286: 2711–17.

The scientific principles, logistics, and legal issues relevant to quarantine are discussed.

Inactivation of poxviruses by upper-room UVC light in a simulated hospital room environment. McDevitt JJ, Milton DK, Rudnick SN, First MW. PLoS ONE 2008; 3: e3186.

Air disinfection via upper-room 254-nm germicidal UV (UVC) light combined with air mixing with a conventional ceiling fan produced reductions in airborne *Vaccinia* virus concentrations. The greater survival at baseline and greater UVC susceptibility of *Vaccinia* under winter conditions suggest that although the risk from an aerosol attack with smallpox would be greatest in winter, protective measures using UVC may also be most efficient at this time.

> **Vaccination reactions**
>
> ▶ *Vaccinia* immune globulin   D
> ▶ Idoxuridine for corneal lesions   D

Smallpox vaccination and adverse reactions. Guidance for clinicians. Cono J, Casey CG, Bell DM. MMWR Recomm Rep 2003; 52(RR-4): 1–28.

The following people should not be vaccinated unless actually exposed to smallpox: those with a personal history of, or direct household contact with, persons with: a history of atopic dermatitis; active exfoliative skin conditions; pregnant women or women planning to become pregnant in the next month; and persons with systemic immunosuppression.

Outbreak-specific guidance will be disseminated by the CDC regarding populations to be vaccinated and specific contraindications to vaccination

Smallpox vaccination and patients with human immunodeficiency virus infection or acquired immunodeficiency syndrome. Bartlett JG. Clin Infect Dis 2003; 36: 468–71.

The risks associated with both smallpox and *Vaccinia* viruses probably correlate with absolute CD4 cell count. People with HIV infection are advised to decline pre-emptive vaccination, but in the event of an actual smallpox attack such patients exposed to the disease would be advised to be vaccinated.

IMVAMUNE, an attenuated modified *Vaccinia* Ankara virus vaccine for smallpox infection. Jones T. Curr Opin Mol Ther 2008; 10: 407–17.

A new vaccine, IMVAMUNE, based on a live attenuated modified *Vaccinia* Ankara virus, is in phase II trials for potential prevention of smallpox infection, especially in those for whom traditional smallpox vaccines are contraindicated, such as the immunocompromised and those with eczema or dermatitis. Phase III trials are planned for 2009.

Smallpox and live-virus vaccination in transplant recipients. Fishman JA. Am J Transplant 2003; 3: 786–93.

Immunocompromised patients and family members, social contacts, and sexual contacts of immunocompromised persons must not be vaccinated unless actually exposed to smallpox. Should they be vaccinated, they should consider living apart for 3 weeks to avoid transmission to the at-risk individual.

Clinical efficacy of intramuscular *Vaccinia* immune globulin: a literature review. Hopkins RJ, Lane JM. Clin Infect Dis 2004; 39: 819–26.

Vaccinia immunoglobulin (VIG) reduces the morbidity and mortality associated with progressive vaccinia (vaccinia necrosum) and eczema vaccinatum. Indications for treatment include generalized vaccinia, progressive vaccinia, eczema vaccinatum, and some accidental implantations. The use of intramuscular administration of VIG to prevent smallpox in contacts of patients with documented cases of smallpox is also discussed.

Progressive vaccinia. Bray M, Wright ME. Clin Infect Dis 2003; 36: 766–74.

This rare complication (one person per million vaccinees) is characterized by the relentless outward spread of vaccinia from the inoculation site and later spread to other areas on the body. Defective cell-mediated immunity predisposes to this complication, which is lethal in infants with absent cellular immune function. Although one army recruit infected with HIV developed severe vaccinia, it appears that multiple HIV-infected enlistees with asymptomatic HIV infection have been vaccinated without developing the complication.

Ocular complications in the Department of Defense Smallpox Vaccination Program. Fillmore GL, Ward TP, Bower KS, Dudenhoefer EJ, Grabenstein JD, Berry GK, et al. Ophthalmology 2004; 111: 2086–93.

In recent vaccination campaigns, cases of eyelid pustules, blepharitis, periorbital cellulitis, conjunctivitis, conjunctival ulcers, conjunctival membranes, limbal pustules, corneal infiltrates, and iritis occurred 3–24 days after inoculation or contact. Treatment for most cases was topical trifluridine 1%. VIG was used in one case. In all patients, recovery occurred without significant visual sequelae.

Myopericarditis following smallpox vaccination among vaccinia-naive US military personnel. Halsell JS, Riddle JR, Atwood JE, Gardner P, Shope R, Poland GA, et al. JAMA 2003; 289: 3283–9.

Myopericarditis occurred at a rate of slightly less than one in 10 000 military personnel who underwent primary vaccination. Clinicians should consider this diagnosis in patients presenting with chest pain 4–30 days following smallpox vaccination.

Pregnancy discovered after smallpox vaccination: is vaccinia immune globulin appropriate? Napolitano PG, Ryan MA, Grabenstein JD. Am J Obstet Gynecol 2004; 191: 1863–7.

Fetal vaccinia is a rare complication of smallpox vaccination during pregnancy. Although some have suggested that therapeutic treatment with VIG can prevent fetal vaccinia, VIG is currently not approved for such use and a conceivable risk of teratogenicity from mercury in the thimerosal preservative has been cited. VIG should only be given if a pregnant woman develops a condition in which VIG is indicated (e.g., eczema vaccinatum, progressive vaccinia, or serious generalized vaccinia).

SECOND-LINE THERAPIES

> ▶ Penicillinase-resistant antibiotics for secondary skin
>   infection   E
> ▶ Local treatments – manage like a 'burn patient'   E
> ▶ Idoxuridine (topical) treatment of corneal lesions
>   Efficacy is probable in view of use in vaccinia (see
>   above)

THIRD-LINE THERAPIES

> ▶ Cidofovir Experimental evidence only
> ▶ Cidofovir plus VIG Experimental evidence only
> ▶ Cidofovir plus VIG plus ST-246   E

Cidofovir in the treatment of poxvirus infections. De Clercq E. Antiviral Res 2002; 55: 1–13.

Excellent review of the experimental use of cidofovir in poxvirus infections.

Cutaneous infections of mice with vaccinia or cowpox viruses and efficacy of cidofovir. Quenelle DC, Collins DJ, Kern ER. Antiviral Res 2004; 63: 33–40.

In hairless mice, 5% topical cidofovir was more effective than systemic treatment at reducing virus titers in skin, lung, kidney, and spleen.

Severe eczema vaccinatum in a household contact of a smallpox vaccinee. Vora S, Damon I, Fulginiti V, Weber SG, Kahana M, Stein SL, et al. Clin Infect Dis 2008; 46: 1555–61.

A 28-month-old child with refractory atopic dermatitis developed severe eczema vaccinatum after exposure to his father, a member of the US military who had recently received smallpox vaccine. In this first confirmed case of eczema vaccinatum in the United States related to smallpox vaccination since routine vaccination was discontinued in 1972, the child was treated with intravenous *Vaccinia* immunoglobulin, used for the first time in a pediatric patient; cidofovir and ST-246, an investigational drug being studied for orthopoxvirus infection.

This case illustrates the necessity of excluding individuals with a history of remote or active atopic dermatitis from smallpox vaccination or contact with vaccinees. The patient was treated with intravenous VIG and two investigational agents. It is difficult to ascertain the possible contributions of each agent to the patient's recovery because of the close timing of administration.

ANTHRAX

Anthrax typically causes disease in sheep and cattle, but affects humans uncommonly. The 2001 bioterrorist dissemination of anthrax spores in a white powder form through the US Postal Service caused the disease in 22 people and resulted in several fatalities. *Bacillus anthracis* can exist as a stable spore form for years. Human disease usually results from cutaneous inoculation, inhalation of spores, or gastrointestinal ingestion of infected material.

Cutaneous anthrax is generally the most common presentation and follows direct inoculation of material from infected animals into human skin, often in an occupational setting. A painless or itchy papule evolves into a vesicle with surrounding edema, and then into the classic black eschar. Fever and malaise may be present. Numerous cases of inhalational anthrax, the most dangerous form, would most likely follow a bioterrorist attack. Inhaled spores are taken up from alveoli by macrophages and transported via lymphatics to regional lymph nodes, resulting in a hemorrhagic mediastinitis. Initial symptoms are nonspecific or flu-like: fever, malaise, nonproductive cough, and myalgia. Within a few days the bacteria disseminate and, without treatment, hypotension, respiratory failure, obtundation, and death ensue. A gastrointestinal or oropharyngeal form may result from ingestion of inadequately cooked infected meat or meat products.

MANAGEMENT STRATEGY

The diagnosis of anthrax in an urban setting requires a high index of suspicion. The broad differential diagnosis of cutaneous anthrax includes insect bite, brown recluse spider bite, tularemia, the *tache noir* of rickettsial pox, ecthyma gangrenosum, staphylococcal or streptococcal ecthyma, cat scratch disease, orf, and other conditions with eschar or an ulceroglandular presentation. Differentiation of pulmonary anthrax from other community-acquired pneumonias rests mostly on mediastinal widening or pleural effusion on chest radiography.

Universal precautions should be maintained in evaluating a patient with suspected cutaneous anthrax, but a face mask is not necessary. In the absence of spores there is no risk of contracting pulmonary anthrax. Material is obtained for culture using a Dacron or rayon swab, and skin biopsy is performed.

Prophylaxis

The need for prophylaxis is determined by public health officials on the basis of epidemiologic investigation. *Prophylaxis* is indicated for persons exposed to an air space contaminated with aerosolized *B. anthracis*. The optimal duration of prophylaxis is uncertain; however, 60 days has been recommended, primarily on the basis of animal studies of anthrax deaths and spore clearance after exposure.

Vaccine

The currently recommended regimen consists of *three subcutaneous injections at 0, 2, and 4 weeks, followed by three booster doses at 6, 12, and 18 months*. Routine vaccination is indicated for at-risk laboratory workers, workers who handle potentially infected hide or animals, and military personnel. In combination with *antibiotics*, post-exposure vaccination may be effective at preventing disease after exposure to *B. anthracis* spores. Mild local reactions are common (20–30%), but severe adverse events have been rare.

SPECIFIC INVESTIGATIONS

> ▶ Culture and Gram stain of tissue, blood, or other fluids
> ▶ For cutaneous anthrax, use a Dacron or rayon swab (not cotton) to swab the vesicle, ulcer, or eschar edge
> ▶ Punch biopsy fixed in formalin from a papule or vesicular lesion and including adjacent skin
> ▶ Biopsies should be taken from both vesicle and eschar, if present
> ▶ A photograph, digital image, or diagram indicating the site of each biopsy in relation to the lesion
> ▶ Immunohistochemical assays
> ▶ Serology (available through CDC)
> ▶ PCR assay

Recognition and management of anthrax – an update. Swartz MN. N Engl J Med 2001; 345: 1621–6.

A superb overall review of anthrax diagnosis and management.

Cutaneous anthrax management algorithm. Carucci JA, McGovern TW, Norton SA, Daniel CR, Elewski BE, Fallon-Friedlander S, et al. J Am Acad Dermatol 2002; 47: 766–9.

A concise summary of the differential diagnosis and treatment of cutaneous anthrax.

Clinical predictors of bioterrorism-related inhalational anthrax. Kyriacou DN, Stein AC, Yarnold PR, Courtney DM, Nelson RR, Noskin GA, et al. Lancet 2004; 364: 449–52.

In differentiating anthrax from community-acquired pneumonia, the most accurate predictor of anthrax is mediastinal widening or pleural effusion on chest radiography.

The critical role of pathology in the investigation of bioterrorism-related cutaneous anthrax. Shieh WJ, Guarner J, Paddock C, Greer P, Tatti K, Fischer M, et al.; Anthrax Bioterrorism Investigation Team. Am J Pathol 2003; 163: 1901–10.

Two novel immunohistochemical assays have been developed that can detect *B. anthracis* antigens in skin biopsy samples, even after prolonged antibiotic treatment. They are a highly sensitive and specific method for the diagnosis of cutaneous anthrax.

A two-component direct fluorescent-antibody assay for rapid identification of *Bacillus anthracis*. De BK, Bragg SL, Sanden GN, Wilson KE, Diem LA, Marston CK, et al. Emerg Infect Dis 2002; 8: 1060–5.

Direct fluorescent antibody assay, using monoclonal antibodies to *B. anthracis* cell wall and capsule antigens, is sensitive and specific, providing a quick confirmatory test for *B. anthracis* in cultures, and may be useful directly on clinical specimens.

Real-time PCR assay for a unique chromosomal sequence of *Bacillus anthracis*. Bode E, Hurtle W, Norwood D. J Clin Microbiol 2004; 42: 5825–31.

Most real-time PCR assays for *B. anthracis* have been developed to detect virulence genes located on plasmids. This chromosomal assay can verify the presence of *B. anthracis* independently of plasmid occurrence.

FIRST-LINE THERAPIES

> ▶ Ciprofloxacin   E
> ▶ Doxycycline   E

Oral antibiotics are used for cutaneous anthrax below the head and neck if systemic symptoms and malignant edema are absent. If they are present, intravenous antibiotics are used.

Update: investigation of bioterrorism-related anthrax and interim guidelines for exposure management and antimicrobial therapy, October 2001. MMWR Morb Mortal Wkly Rep 2001; 50: 962.

Anthrax as a biological weapon, 2002: updated recommendations for management. Inglesby TV, O'Toole T, Henderson DA, Bartlett JG, Ascher MS, Eitzen E, et al.; Working Group on Civilian Biodefense. JAMA 2002; 287: 2236–52.

These two references provide comprehensive recommendations for managing exposure to anthrax and treating the various forms of the illness.

Anthrax: safe treatment for children. Benavides S, Nahata MC. Ann Pharmacother 2002; 36: 334–7.

A pediatric perspective on the management of anthrax.

Update: interim recommendations for antimicrobial prophylaxis for children and breastfeeding mothers and treatment of children with anthrax. MMWR Morb Mortal Wkly Rep 2001; 50: 1014–16.

Evidence Levels: **A** Double-blind study   **B** Clinical trial ≥ 20 subjects   **C** Clinical trial < 20 subjects   **D** Series ≥ 5 subjects   **E** Anecdotal case reports

Ciprofloxacin or doxycycline are recommended for antimicrobial prophylaxis and treatment of adults and children with *B. anthracis* infection. Amoxicillin is an option for antimicrobial prophylaxis for children and pregnant women, and to complete treatment of cutaneous disease when *B. anthracis* is susceptible to penicillin.

SECOND-LINE THERAPIES

▶ Amoxicillin	E
▶ Penicillin	D
▶ Chloramphenicol	D
▶ Clindamycin	E
▶ Systemic corticosteroids for treatment of edema	E

THIRD-LINE THERAPIES

▶ Macrolides	E
▶ Aminoglycosides	E
▶ Chloroquine – experimental	E

Chloroquine enhances survival in *Bacillus anthracis* intoxication. Artenstein AW, Opal SM, Cristofaro P, Palardy JE, Parejo NA, Green MD, et al. J Infect Dis 2004; 190: 1655–60.

Antibiotics target only replicating organisms, thereby allowing bacterial toxins to cause severe physiological derangements in patients with inhalational anthrax. Chloroquine reduced tissue damage and enhanced survival in mice exposed to anthrax.

PROPHYLAXIS

▶ Antibiotics	E
▶ Vaccination	B

Clinical issues in the prophylaxis, diagnosis, and treatment of anthrax. Bell DM, Kozarsky PE, Stephens DS. Emerg Infect Dis 2002; 8: 222–5.

Management of asymptomatic pregnant or lactating women exposed to anthrax. Committee on Obstetric Practice. Int J Gynaecol Obstet 2002; 77: 293–5.

Asymptomatic pregnant and lactating women who have been exposed to a confirmed environmental contamination or a high-risk source receive prophylactic treatment. Although some of the drugs may pose a risk to the developing fetus, this risk is clearly outweighed by the potential consequences of acquiring anthrax.

Use of anthrax vaccine in the United States. Advisory Committee on Immunization Practices. MMWR Recomm Rep 2000; 49(RR-15): 1–20.

Use of anthrax vaccine in response to terrorism: supplemental recommendations of the Advisory Committee on Immunization Practices. MMWR Morb Mortal Wkly Rep 2002; 51: 1024–6.

Recommendations for pre- and post-exposure prophylaxis are provided and updated in these two references.

Recurrent, localized urticaria and erythema multiforme: a review and management of cutaneous anthrax vaccine-related events. Gilson RT, Schissel DJ. Cutis 2004; 73: 319–25.

This article reviews the latest recommended evaluation and management of anthrax vaccine adverse events.

TULAREMIA

Tularemia is caused by a highly infectious Gram-negative coccobacillus, *Francisella tularensis*. Seven clinical syndromes are described that correspond to the route of inoculation (i.e., respiratory tract, gastrointestinal tract, skin, eye, or other mucous membrane exposure). Because tularemia has no stable spore form, it is a less suitable bioterrorist agent than anthrax. It does not cause person-to-person spread.

Respiratory tularemia, as would occur after a bioterrorist attack, starts as a flu-like illness or atypical pneumonia with fever, chills, myalgia, and cephalalgia. Pulmonary symptoms such as non-productive cough and pleuritic chest pain may not be prominent, but if treatment is not initiated severe pneumonia, hemoptysis, respiratory failure, sepsis, and death can result. There is no specific skin rash with respiratory tularemia, but all of the clinical syndromes can cause bacteremia or tularemia sepsis, with shock, acute respiratory distress syndrome (ARDS), organ failure, disseminated intravascular coagulation, and purpura. Nonspecific eruptions, described below, can occur in a minority of cases, usually on the face and extremities.

Ulceroglandular tularemia, the presentation most familiar to dermatologists, is not likely to occur after a bioterrorist attack. It usually presents with tender localized lymphadenitis. An erythematous, painful papule that then undergoes necrosis develops before, simultaneously with, or shortly after the tender swollen lymph node.

Another form, *oculoglandular tularemia*, could occur after an aerosol attack. It presents with purulent conjunctivitis, periorbital edema, ulceration, and nodules of the conjunctivae, along with tender preauricular or cervical lymphadenopathy.

Water or food contaminated with *F. tularensis* can cause oropharyngeal disease, including stomatitis and exudative pharyngitis. *Typhoidal tularemia* presents as a febrile illness with chills, abdominal pain, nausea, vomiting, and diarrhea, and can be rapidly fatal.

Exanthems have been described in all forms of tularemia. They may be macular, papular, papulovesicular, pustular, or petechial, and are most prominent on the face and extremities. Erythema nodosum occurs most commonly with pulmonary tularemia. Erythema multiforme and Sweet's syndrome have also been described.

MANAGEMENT STRATEGY

A high index of suspicion is necessary for the diagnosis of tularemia outside the natural setting. Ulceroglandular or oculoglandular disease has a rather straightforward presentation, but respiratory tularemia has variable pulmonary symptoms, though subspecies used in a bioterrorist attack would probably cause severe toxicity and cough. *F. tularensis* can be grown in the laboratory, but has stringent growth characteristics. Because laboratory workers are at risk of contracting the disease and routine reference laboratories are not experienced at growing the organism, government health department laboratories should be used. Antibody testing is highly specific, but not useful early on in the disease.

The organism can be detected in clinical specimens (secretions or biopsies) by direct fluorescent antibody or immunohistochemical techniques. PCR is likely to become the diagnostic test of choice in the future.

Although *streptomycin* has been used successfully for many years for tularemia, it is not widely available and has been replaced by *gentamicin*. *Oral ciprofloxacin* has proved effective in tularemia and is the drug of choice for uncomplicated disease. *Doxycycline* is a useful second-line agent for uncomplicated disease. For severe disease, parenteral therapy is indicated. Gentamicin, ciprofloxacin, or doxycycline are the preferred agents in pregnancy.

SPECIFIC INVESTIGATIONS

> ▶ Gram stain
> ▶ Culture
> ▶ Serology – agglutination and enzyme-linked immunosorbent assay (ELISA) testing
> ▶ Direct fluorescent antibody and immunohistochemistry
> ▶ PCR

The development of tools for diagnosis of tularaemia and typing of *Francisella tularensis*. Johansson A, Forsman M, Sjostedt A. APMIS 2004; 112: 898–907.

A detailed description of laboratory diagnostic procedures useful for tularemia.

Methods for enhanced culture recovery of *Francisella tularensis*. Petersen JM, Schriefer ME, Gage KL, Montenieri JA, Carter LG, Stanley M, et al. Appl Environ Microbiol 2004; 70: 3733–5.

Antibiotic supplementation of enriched cysteine heart agar blood culture medium improved recovery of *F. tularensis* from contaminated specimens. Immediate freezing is useful for transport of tissue to achieve enhanced recovery rates.

FIRST-LINE THERAPIES

> ▶ Streptomycin   **D**
> ▶ Gentamicin   **D**
> ▶ Ciprofloxacin for uncomplicated disease   **D**

SECOND-LINE THERAPIES

> ▶ Doxycycline   **D**
> ▶ Chloramphenicol   **D**

Tularaemia: bioterrorism defence renews interest in *Francisella tularensis*. Oyston PC, Sjostedt A, Titball RW. Nature Rev Microbiol 2004; 2: 967–78.

A superb review of the epidemiology, pathophysiology, diagnosis, and treatment of tularemia.

PLAGUE

Plague, caused by *Yersinia pestis*, is a disease of rats that historically has spread to humans by the bite of a flea that has fed on an infected rat. A range of mammals and fleas can serve as vectors. Following exposure to infected humans or to cats with plague pneumonia, respiratory droplet infection occurs. An aerosol attack with plague would cause an abrupt outbreak of fatal pneumonia in an exposed community. Infected fleas could also be used to spread the disease. It is alleged that this was done by the Japanese in China during World War II.

The three main presentations are bubonic plague, a primary pulmonic form, and septicemia. Bubonic plague presents with fever and flu-like symptoms. A painful bubo develops near the site of the infected bite, most often in the cervical, axillary, femoral, or inguinal areas. There is overlying erythema and sometimes vesicles, pustules, eschars, or ulceration. Without antibiotic treatment, secondary pneumonia or septicemia may follow. Bubonic plague would only occur if fleas were used in a bioterrorist attack. Highly contagious pneumonic plague may be primary or may develop from bubonic or septicemic plague. The pneumonic form has no specific skin manifestations, but septicemic plague can cause vasculitis and disseminated intravascular coagulation, with cyanosis, purpura, and gangrene of the nose, fingers, and toes.

MANAGEMENT STRATEGY

A bioterrorist attack with plague would most likely involve aerosol spread. The use of insect vectors would be much less likely. In the event that insect vectors were used, dermatologists would be called upon to evaluate patients with bubonic disease. Buboes, surrounded by edema, typically have adherent overlying erythematous skin. In a bioterrorist scenario, most cases would more likely be of the pneumonic type, many of which would progress to septicemic plague with large areas of ecchymosis and peripheral gangrene. Cervical buboes might occur. High fever, tachycardia, and severe toxicity would be the rule. Pneumonic plague, early on, might be confused with inhalation anthrax; however, chest radiography shows parenchymal disease. Gram-negative rods are evident on sputum Gram staining. Strict respiratory isolation is mandatory for the first 3 days of therapy of pneumonic plague. Prophylactic treatment of at-risk contacts is mandatory.

Skin biopsies of purpuric lesions of plague reveal subepidermal hemorrhage and capillary and venular fibrin thrombi. A diffuse papular eruption sometimes occurs which on biopsy shows a mixed perivascular infiltrate.

Streptomycin has been the mainstay of treatment for plague, but has limited availability in the US. It is ototoxic and nephrotoxic to patients, and if administered to pregnant women can cause fetal hearing loss and kidney damage. *Gentamicin* is also used for plague and is favored in pregnancy. *Tetracyclines*, such as doxycycline, are adequate for uncomplicated plague alone or in combination with other agents. *Chloramphenicol, fluoroquinolones* (e.g., ciprofloxacin) and *sulfonamides* (e.g., sulfadiazine or trimethoprim-sulfamethoxazole) are alternatives.

Yersinia pestis (plague) vaccines. Titball RW, Williamson ED. Expert Opin Biol Ther 2004; 4: 965–73.

Reviews the current status of anti-plague vaccination.

SPECIFIC INVESTIGATIONS

> ▶ Complete blood count and peripheral smear
> ▶ Lactate dehydrogenase
> ▶ Fibrin degradation products, fibrinogen
> ▶ Gram stain and culture of sputum and fluid from buboes
> ▶ Serology – anti-fraction 1 antibody ≥1: 10
> ▶ PCR

Evidence Levels: **A** Double-blind study **B** Clinical trial ≥ 20 subjects **C** Clinical trial < 20 subjects **D** Series ≥ 5 subjects **E** Anecdotal case reports

FIRST-LINE THERAPIES

Aminoglycosides

▶ Intramuscular streptomycin **D**
▶ Intramuscular or intravenous gentamicin **D**

SECOND-LINE THERAPIES

▶ Doxycycline **D**
▶ Ciprofloxacin **E**

THIRD-LINE THERAPIES

▶ Chloramphenicol **D**
▶ Sulfonamides **E**

Bacteria as agents of biowarfare. How to proceed when the worst is suspected. Tjaden JA, Lazarus AA, Martin GJ. Postgrad Med 2002; 112: 57–60,63–4,67–70.

This review covers the bacterial agents of anthrax, plague, and tularemia, and their recognition and treatment.

VIRAL HEMORRHAGIC FEVERS

The viral hemorrhagic fevers are a group of febrile illnesses associated with a bleeding diathesis that are caused by viruses belonging to one of the following families: Filoviridae, Arenaviridae, Bunyaviridae, and Flaviviridae. Ebola, Marburg, Lassa fever, New World arenaviruses, Rift Valley fever, yellow fever, Omsk hemorrhagic fever, and Kyasanur Forest disease have the greatest potential for bioterrorism. The diseases are usually transmitted to humans via contact with infected animal reservoirs or arthropod vectors. The mode of transmission, clinical course, and mortality of these illnesses vary with the specific virus involved, but each is capable of causing a hemorrhagic fever syndrome. Fever, severe toxicity, and hemorrhagic manifestations, with at least two of the following – hemorrhagic or purple rash, epistaxis, hematemesis, hemoptysis, blood in stools – establish the diagnosis.

MANAGEMENT STRATEGY

A high index of suspicion should be maintained for patients presenting with a febrile illness and hemorrhagic manifestations. Cases should be *reported immediately to public health authorities*. Pending definitive diagnosis, patients with suspected hemorrhagic fevers should be classified as low, medium, or high risk. Because of the high risk of contagion to healthcare workers, *stringent universal precautions, appropriate barrier protection, and isolation should be instituted*. Contacts of suspected cases should be closely monitored, and in the case of Lassa fever *ribavirin* should be offered. Diagnostic tests are only available through the CDC or the US Army Medical Research Institute of Infectious Diseases.

SPECIFIC INVESTIGATIONS

▶ Antigen detection by antigen-capture ELISA
▶ IgM antibody detection by antibody-capture ELISA
▶ Reverse transcriptase-PCR
▶ Viral isolation is of limited value because it requires a biosafety level 4 laboratory

Hemorrhagic fever viruses as biological weapons: medical and public health management. Borio L, Inglesby T, Peters CJ, Schmaljohn AL, Hughes JM, Jahrling PB, et al.; Working Group on Civilian Biodefense. JAMA 2002; 287: 2391–405.

Cutaneous manifestations of biological warfare and related threat agents. McGovern TW, Christopher GW, Eitzen EM. Arch Dermatol 1999; 135: 311–22.

A superb overview of the dermatologic manifestations of biowarfare agents.

Management of patients exposed to biologic weapons. Yetman RJ, Parks D, Taft E. J Pediatr Health Care 2002; 16: 256–61.

This review of practice guidelines provides treatment recommendations for children as well as adults, and also includes a comprehensive list of emergency contacts and educational resources.

Diagnosis and management of suspected cases of bioterrorism: a pediatric perspective. Patt HA, Feigin RD. Pediatrics 2002; 109: 685–92.

Review of bioterrorism from a pediatric perspective.

Vaccine to confer to nonhuman primates complete protection against multistrain Ebola and Marburg virus infections. Swenson DL, Wang D, Luo M, Warfield KL, Woraratanadharm J, Holman DH, et al. Clin Vaccine Immunol 2008; 15: 460–7.

There are currently no licensed vaccines available to prevent filovirus outbreaks. This article describes a panfilovirus vaccine that expresses multiple antigens from five different filoviruses which demonstrates 100% protection against infection by two species of Ebola virus and three Marburg virus subtypes in non-human primates.

In the event of a natural hemorrhagic fever outbreak or biological attack, vaccination strategies will probably play a major role.

FIRST-LINE THERAPIES

Supportive care
▶ Intravenous ribavirin pending viral identification **D**

SECOND-LINE THERAPIES

▶ Convalescent plasma **E**

Update: management of patients with suspected viral hemorrhagic fever – United States. MMWR Morb Mortal Wkly Rep 1995; 44: 475–9.

CDC guidelines for the management of suspected cases of viral hemorrhagic fever.

Treatment of Ebola hemorrhagic fever with blood transfusions from convalescent patients. Mupapa K, Massamba M, Kibadi K, Kuvula K, Bwaka A, Kipasa M, et al. J Infect Dis 1999; 179: S18–23.

Eight patients who met the case definition for Ebola hemorrhagic fever were transfused with blood donated by five convalescent patients. Only one transfused patient (12.5%) died, compared to the overall case fatality rate of 80%. It is not entirely clear whether the increased survival resulted from the transfusions or because of the better care received by transfusion recipients.

Bites and stings

Dirk M Elston

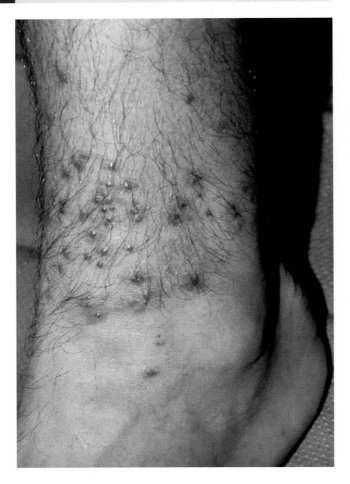

This chapter presents strategies for the prevention and management of bites and stings.

MANAGEMENT STRATEGY

Bite reactions

DEET is effective against a broad range of arthropods. Picaridin is effective against mosquitoes. Permethrin can be used on fabric. A veterinarian should be consulted about flea infestation in pets. Antivenin is available for many arachnid toxins, but most respond to rest, ice, and elevation.

If prevention fails, second-line treatments aim to improve pruritus. *Topical antipruritics*, such as 0.25% camphor and menthol, and *topical anesthetics* such as pramoxine and lidocaine, can be helpful. For persistent bite reactions, topical or intralesional corticosteroids may be helpful.

Anaphylaxis

Individuals who experience anaphylaxis in response to stings should be referred to an allergist for desensitization. They should also carry an epinephrine autoinjector (EpiPen).

Vector-borne disease

Most tick-borne illness responds to doxycycline. For early Lyme disease, evidence suggests that a 10-day course of antibiotic is as effective as longer courses. Babesiosis responds to clindamycin and quinine, but azithromycin and atovaquone may be as effective, with a lower incidence of side effects. Atovaquone-proguanil has been effective in refractory cases in immunocompromised patients.

SPECIFIC INVESTIGATIONS

> ► CBC and fibrin split products after brown recluse spider bite
> ► Rickettsial immunofluorescence and immunoperoxidase
> ► Lyme serologic tests
> ► ELISA, PCR and immunofluorescence for virus such as dengue and Chikungunya

Development and evaluation of one step single tube multiplex RT-PCR for rapid detection and typing of dengue viruses. Saxena P, Dash PK, Santhosh SR, Shrivastava A, Parida M, Lakashmana Roa PV. Virol J 2008; 5: 20.

The authors report a one-step reverse transcription polymerase chain reaction for the detection and typing of dengue virus during the acute phase of illness.

Conventional acute and convalescent antibody titers are of limited value in the acute stage of a febrile illness.

Chikungunya fever in travelers: clinical presentation and course. Taubitz W, Cramer JP, Kapaun A, Pfeffer M, Drosten C, Dobler G, et al. Clin Infect Dis 2007; 45: e1–4.

Chikungunya virus-specific immunoglobulin M or immunoglobulin G antibodies were detected in all patients during a recent outbreak, but testing during the first week of illness yielded negative results in three of five patients.

During the first week of illness, polymerase chain reaction is more reliable than antibody testing.

Complement split products C3a and C4a are early markers of acute Lyme disease in tick bite patients in the United States. Shoemaker RC, Giclas PC, Crowder C, House D, Glovsky MM. Int Arch Allergy Immunol 2008; 146: 255–61.

Acute Lyme disease patients, with or without erythema migrans, had elevated levels of C3a or C4a. The levels were higher in patients with acute Lyme disease than in tick bite patients and controls (p<0.001).

Detection of acute Lyme disease can be problematic. This report suggests that C3a and C4a are useful as markers of acute Lyme disease.

***Loxosceles* venom-induced cytokine activation, hemolysis, and acute kidney injury.** de Souza AL, Malaque CM, Sztajnbok J, Romano CC, Duarte AJ, Seguro AC. Toxicon 2008; 51: 151–6.

Laboratory abnormalities after brown recluse spider bite may include elevated white blood cell count, a decrease in hemoglobin, and abnormalities in international normalized ratio (INR), and D-dimer,

Systemic manifestations of loxoscelism include hemolysis, coagulopathy, acute kidney failure, rhabdomyolysis, and electrolyte disorders. Laboratory testing should be directed by signs and symptoms.

Evidence Levels: **A** Double-blind study **B** Clinical trial ≥ 20 subjects **C** Clinical trial < 20 subjects **D** Series ≥ 5 subjects **E** Anecdotal case reports

A new assay for the detection of *Loxosceles* species (brown recluse) spider venom. Gomez HF, Krywko DM, Stoecker WV. Ann Emerg Med 2002; 39: 469–74.

A sensitive *Loxosceles* venom enzyme-linked immunosorbent assay (ELISA) assay was tested with inoculations of as little as 40 ng of venom.

This assay shows excellent sensitivity and specificity in the range of venom concentration that would actually be found in tissue after a bite.

FIRST-LINE THERAPY

Prevention

▶ DEET	A
▶ Permethrin	A
▶ Picaridin	B

Flea treatments for pets

▶ Lufenuron	A
▶ Fipronil	A
▶ Imidacloprid	A

Anaphylaxis

▶ Epinephrine	A
▶ Immunotherapy	A

Spider bites

▶ Rest, ice, and elevation	B
▶ Tetracycline or triamcinolone for brown recluse spider bites	C
▶ Antivenin for brown recluse spider bites	C
▶ Antivenin for black widow and red-back spider bites	A

Scorpion stings

▶ Antivenin for stings in Arizona	B
▶ Prazosin for Indian red scorpion stings	A

Arthropod-borne infections

▶ Lyme borreliosis	
— Tetracycline	A
— Amoxicillin in children	A
— Intravenous ceftriaxone	A
▶ Rocky Mountain spotted fever	
— Doxycycline	A
▶ Human monocytic ehrlichiosis	
— Doxycycline	A
▶ Human anaplasmosis	
— Doxycycline	A
▶ Babesiosis	
— Azithromycin and atovaquone	A
— Quinine and clindamycin	A

Prevention

Insect repellents: Historical perspectives and new developments. Katz TM, Miller JH, Hebert AA. J Am Acad Dermatol 2008 Feb 11.

EPA (Environmental Protection Agency)-registered repellents approved for application to the skin include DEET (diethyl-3-methyl-benzamide), picaridin, MGK-326, MGK-264, IR3535, and botanical oils including citronella, lemon, and eucalyptus.

DEET retains broad efficacy against ticks, mosquitoes, and chiggers. Picaridin has equal efficacy against mosquitoes. Botanical oils have consumer appeal as natural alternatives, but generally do not perform as well.

Laboratory and field evaluation of the impact of exercise on the performance of regular and polymer-based DEET repellents. Schofield S, Tepper M, Gadawski R. J Med Entomol 2007; 44: 1026–31.

A polymer-based cream and an alcohol-based pump spray formulation were tested against *Ochlerotatus sticticus* (Meigen) and *Aedes vexans* (Meigen). Moderate exercise resulted in a >40% decline in mean protection with both products.

Exercise reduces the efficacy of DEET, including the polymer-based cream.

DEET microencapsulation: a slow-release formulation enhancing the residual efficacy of bed nets against malaria vectors. N'guessan R, Knols BG, Pennetier C, Rowland M. Trans Roy Soc Trop Med Hyg 2008; 102: 259–62.

Microencapsulated DEET on mosquito nets was effective for a period of at least 6 months under laboratory conditions.

Factory-based permethrin impregnation of uniforms: residual activity against *Aedes aegypti* and *Ixodes ricinus* in battledress uniforms worn under field conditions, and cross-contamination during the laundering and storage process. Faulde MK, Uedelhoven WM, Malerius M, Robbins RG. Military Med 2006; 171: 472–7.

Battledress uniforms (BDUs) impregnated by the polymer-coating method were effective for the life of the garment and provided superior protection against *Ixodes* ticks.

Better methods of creating acaricidal clothing are being developed.

Field evaluation of repellent formulations containing deet and picaridin against mosquitoes in Northern Territory, Australia. Frances SP, Waterson DG, Beebe NW, Cooper RD. J Med Entomol 2004; 41: 414–17.

Field testing of picaridin (1-methyl-propyl 2-(2-hydroxyethyl)-1-piperidine carboxylate) (Autan Repel Army 20) and DEET (*N*,*N*,-diethyl-3-methylbenzamide) against *Culex annulirostris*, *Anopheles merankensis*, and *Anopheles bancroftii* showed protection against *Anopheles* spp.

Some species of mosquito remain highly resistant to available repellents. Picaridin has recently been licensed in the US and provides an alternative to DEET.

Efficacy of fipronil-(S)-methoprene on fleas, flea egg collection, and flea egg development following transplantation of gravid fleas onto treated cats. Franc M, Beugnet F, Vermot S. Vet Ther 2007; 8: 285–92.

A combination of fipronil and methoprene produced 93.4% efficacy for up to 6 weeks. The product was 100% ovicidal up to day 56.

Efficacy of selamectin and fipronil-(S)-methoprene spot-on formulations applied to cats against adult cat fleas (*Ctenocephalides felis*), flea eggs, and adult flea emergence. Druden M, Payne P, Smith V. Vet Ther 2007; 8: 255–62.

Selamectin provided greater control of adult fleas and greater reduction in egg production than did fipronil-(S)-methoprene.

Preliminary studies on the effectiveness of the novel pulicide, spinosad, for the treatment and control of fleas on dogs. Snyder DE, Meyer J, Zimmermann AG, Qiao M, Gissendanner SJ, Cruthers LR, et al. Vet Parasitol 2007; 150: 345–51.

Spinosad was compared to topical imidacloprid. Both drugs were highly effective at 30-day intervals.

Efficacy of a novel formulation of metaflumizone for the control of fleas (*Ctenocephalides felis*) on cats. Holzmer S, Hair JA, Dryden MW, Young DR, Carter L. Vet Parasitol 2007; 150: 219–24.

A new topical formulation containing metaflumizone showed efficacy in controlling fleas in cats, providing >90% control for up to 7 weeks.

Dose determination of a novel formulation of metaflumizone plus amitraz for control of cat fleas (*Ctenocephalides felis felis*) and brown dog ticks (*Rhipicephalus sanguineus*) on dogs. Rugg D, Hair JA. Vet Parasitol 2007; 150: 203–8.

The minimum effective dose to provide flea and tick control for at least 30 days was 20 mg/kg.

Ivermectin, fipronil, and imidacloprid have proven efficacy for the prevention of flea infestations in pets. Lufenuron is somewhat less effective. There are several new products under development that appear promising.

Anaphylaxis treatment and prevention

Insect sting anaphylaxis. Golden DB. Immunol Allergy Clin North Am 2007; 27: 261–72, vii.

Studies demonstrate that the efficacy of venom immunotherapy is between 75% and 98%. Most patients can discontinue therapy after about 5 years.

Analysis of the burden of treatment in patients receiving an EpiPen for yellowjacket anaphylaxis. Oude Elberink JN, van der Heide S, Guyatt GH, Dubois AE. J Allergy Clin Immunol 2006; 118: 699–704.

In a study of 94 patients randomized to receive immunotherapy or EpiPen, 91.5% of those receiving immunotherapy were happy with their treatment, compared to 48% of those using the EpiPen.

Venom immunotherapy improves quality of life and is preferred by patients.

Bite treatment

Tetracycline protects against dermonecrosis induced by *Loxosceles* spider venom. Paixão-Cavalcante D, van den Berg CW, Gonçalves-de-Andrade RM, Fernandes-Pedrosa M de F, Okamoto CK, Tambourgi DV. J Invest Dermatol 2007; 127: 1410–18.

In a rabbit model, tetracyclines inhibited dermonecrotic reactions to venom.

Tetracyclines deserve further study for the treatment of cutaneous loxoscelism.

Toxicity of two North American *Loxosceles* (brown recluse spiders) venoms and their neutralization by antivenoms. de Roodt AR, Estevez-Ramírez J, Litwin S, Magaña P, Olvera A, Alagón A. Clin Toxicol (Phila) 2007; 45: 678–87.

A study of anti-*L. boneti* and anti-*L.* recluse antivenins showed efficacy against systemic toxicity and necrosis in mice.

It remains unclear how effective they will be after typical delays in initiating therapy.

Comparison of colchicine, dapsone, triamcinolone, and diphenhydramine therapy for the treatment of brown recluse spider envenomation: a double-blind, controlled study in a rabbit model. Elston DM, Miller SD, Young RJ 3rd, Eggers J, McGlasson D, Schmidt WH, et al. Arch Dermatol 2005; 141: 595–7.

A study in New Zealand White rabbits compared eschar size, depth, inflammation, and thrombosis. The only beneficial outcome was that triamcinolone offered significant protection from thrombosis.

In this animal model, none of the treatment regimens (including dapsone) prevented necrosis. Only intralesional triamcinolone showed any trend towards efficacy.

Scorpion envenomations in young children in central Arizona. LoVecchio F, McBride C. J Toxicol Clin Toxicol 2003; 41: 937–40.

The mean time for abatement of symptoms following antivenin was 31 minutes vs 22.2 hours. There was one acute rash to antivenin and 49 cases (57%) of serum sickness.

Hospital admission was less common among those receiving antivenin.

Utility of scorpion antivenin vs prazosin in the management of severe *Mesobuthus tamulus* (Indian red scorpion) envenoming at rural setting. Bawaskar HS, Bawaskar PH. J Assoc Phys India 2007; 55: 14–21.

Twenty (80%) of those in the antivenin group had acute pulmonary edema vs two (7.5%) in the prazosin group. Four patients in the first group and none in the second group died.

Prazosin remains the standard of care for the management of severe red scorpion stings.

Use of antivenin to treat priapism after a black widow spider bite. Hoover NG, Fortenberry JD. Pediatrics 2004; 114: e128–9.

Priapism is a rare complication of black widow envenomation. In this report, priapism responded to antivenin within hours. Pain abated and opiates were discontinued.

Treatment for black widow envenomation is primarily symptomatic, using opiates and benzodiazepines. Antivenin is effective for refractory symptoms, including priapism.

Arthropod-borne illness

Persistent and relapsing babesiosis in immunocompromised patients. Krause PJ, Gewurz BE, Hill D, Marty FM, Vannier E, Foppa IM, et al. Clin Infect Dis 2008 1; 46: 370–6.

Immunosuppressed patients with babesiosis may not respond to standard therapy with atovaquone and azithromycin or clindamycin and quinine.

In this report, 14 immunosuppressed patients experienced severe morbidity or death despite repeated courses of antibabesial treatment.

Treatment of refractory *Babesia microti* infection with atovaquone-proguanil in an HIV-infected patient: case report. Vyas JM, Telford SR, Robbins GK. Clin Infect Dis 2007; 45: 1588–90.

A patient with AIDS and babesiosis failed treatment with azithromycin and atovaquone as well as with quinine and clindamycin. He responded to atovaquone-proguanil.

Atovaquone-proguanil may be effective against babesiosis in immunosuppressed patients who do not respond to standard therapy.

Doxycycline versus ceftriaxone for the treatment of patients with chronic Lyme borreliosis. Ogrinc K, Logar M, Lotric-Furlan S, Cerar D, Ruzi -Sablji E, Strle F. Wien Klin Wschr 2006; 118: 696–701.

In a study of adult patients who had not been previously treated with antibiotics and lacked pleocytosis in the cerebrospinal fluid, oral doxycycline for 4 weeks was as effective as 2 g of intravenous ceftriaxone daily for 2 weeks followed by 100 mg of doxycycline twice daily for another 2 weeks.

Even in early CNS Lyme disease, oral tetracycline may be as good as intravenous antibiotic therapy.

Duration of antibiotic therapy for early Lyme disease. A randomized, double-blind, placebo-controlled trial. Wormser GP, Ramanathan R, Nowakowski J, McKenna D, Holmgren D, Visintainer P, et al. Ann Intern Med 2003; 138: 697–704.

In patients with erythema migrans, 10-day treatment with oral doxycycline was as effective as 20 days of oral doxycycline and as effective as 10 days of doxycycline plus a single intravenous dose of ceftriaxone.

The response rate based on clinical observations and neurocognitive testing to 30 months was similar in all groups in both on-study and intention-to-treat analyses.

Clinical and laboratory features, hospital course, and outcome of Rocky Mountain spotted fever in children. Buckingham SC, Marshall GS, Schutze GE, Woods CR, Jackson MA, Patterson LE, et al. J Pediatr 2007; 150: 180–4.

A retrospective chart review of 92 patients showed that although 86% sought medical care before admission, only four received effective antibiotic therapy prior to admission. Three patients died, and 13 had neurologic deficits at discharge.

As with adults, any child in an endemic area with fever and a headache should be considered for tetracycline therapy regardless of the presence of rash. Delays in therapy may be fatal. Many of these patients will receive spinal taps to rule out meningitis.

Tick-borne infections in children: epidemiology, clinical manifestations, and optimal management strategies. Buckingham SC. Paediatr Drugs 2005; 7: 163–76.

Doxycycline is the antimicrobial treatment of choice for Rocky Mountain spotted fever, human monocytic ehrlichiosis, and anaplasmosis (human granulocytic ehrlichiosis) in both adults and children.

Analysis of risk factors for fatal Rocky Mountain Spotted Fever: evidence for superiority of tetracyclines for therapy. Holman RC, Paddock CD, Curns AT, Krebs JW, McQuiston JH, Childs JE. J Infect Dis 2001; 184: 1437–44.

Of 6388 patients with RMSF, 213 died. The risk of death was higher for older patients, those treated only with chloramphenicol, and those for whom treatment was delayed for at least 5 days after the onset of symptoms.

Although doxycycline, chloramphenicol, and newer macrolides are all effective for Mediterranean spotted fever, more serious tick-borne illness requires tetracycline therapy. Lyme disease in children can be treated with amoxicillin.

SECOND-LINE THERAPIES

Repellents
▶ Botanicals   B-C

Relief of pruritus
▶ Camphor and menthol   E
▶ Pramoxine   E
▶ Lidocaine   E
▶ Benzocaine   E
▶ Lidocaine/prilocaine   E

Treatment of bite reactions
▶ Superpotent and potent topical corticosteroids   E
▶ For young children: Mild to moderate-strength topical corticosteroids   E

Indian red scorpion stings
▶ Captopril   C
▶ Antivenin   D

Arthropod-borne infections
Babesiosis
▶ Atovaquone-proguanil in immunosuppressed patients   C

THIRD-LINE THERAPIES

Treatment of bites
▶ Intralesional corticosteroids   E

A low-cost repellent for malaria vectors in the Americas: results of two field trials in Guatemala and Peru. Moore SJ, Darling ST, Sihuincha M, Padilla N, Devine GJ. Malar J 2007; 6: 101.

A mixture of para-menthane-diol and lemongrass oil provided >98% protection for at least 5 hours after application

Low-cost repellents may be effective in countries that cannot afford more expensive agents.

Effectiveness of *Zanthoxylum piperitum*-derived essential oil as an alternative repellent under laboratory and field applications. Kamsuk K, Choochote W, Chaithong U, Jitpakdi A, Tippawangkosol P, Riyong D, et al. Parasitol Res 2007; 100: 339–45.

Zanthoxylum piperitum essential oil was inferior to DEET.

Field evaluation of New Mountain Sandalwood Mosquito Sticks and New Mountain Sandalwood Botanical Repellent against mosquitoes in North Queensland, Australia. Ritchie SA, Williams CR, Montgomery BL. J Am Mosq Control Assoc 2006; 22: 158–60.

A botanical repellent containing soybean and geranium oils compared favorably to DEET.

Evaluation of botanicals as repellents against mosquitoes. Das NG, Baruah I, Talukdar PK, Das SC. J Vector Borne Dis 2003; 40: 49–53.

Three plant extracts (*Zanthoxylum limonella* and *Citrus aurantifolia* distillates, and petroleum ether extract of *Z. limonella*) were evaluated against *Aedes albopictus* under laboratory conditions. At 30% concentration, 296–304 minutes' protection time was achieved by the test repellents in mustard oil base.

Captopril in the treatment of cardiovascular manifestations of Indian red scorpion (*Mesobuthus tamulus concanesis* Pocock) envenomation. Krishnan A, Sonawane RV, Karnad DR. J Assoc Phys India 2007; 55: 22–6.

Pulmonary edema resolved in all 15 patients treated with captopril. Of the nine patients with cardiogenic shock, six received captopril and one of these died. The other three patients did not respond to vasopressors and could not be given captopril. All three died.

Although the authors concluded that afterload reduction with oral captopril is safe and effective for the cardiovascular manifestations of scorpion envenomation, there is a selection bias in that patients who did not respond to pressors were not treated with captopril.

Blastomycosis

Wanda Sonia Robles, Mahreen Ameen

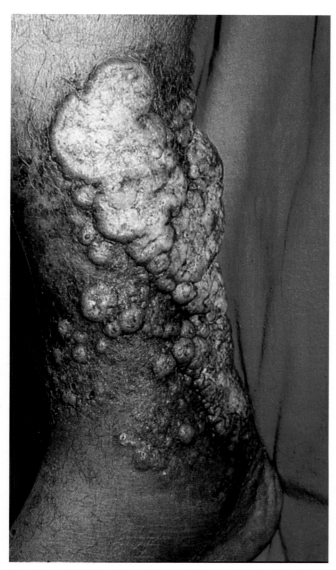

From Lebwohl MG. The Skin and Systemic Disease: A Color Atlas 2nd edn. Churchill Livingstone 2003, with permission of Elsevier.

Blastomycosis is a systemic, suppurative granulomatous infection caused by the thermally dimorphic fungus *Blastomyces dermatitidis*. It is acquired by inhalation of the conidia, which is transformed into the yeast form in the lungs. It is an endemic mycosis that is most prevalent in the North American continent, particularly in the states that border the Mississippi and Ohio rivers, and the Great Lakes region. Cases have also been reported in Latin America, Africa, the Middle East, and India. Consequently, the term 'North American blastomycosis' is now obsolete. Point source epidemics have been reported in endemic regions relating to recreational activities in wooded areas along waterways.

Blastomycosis is associated with a spectrum of disease ranging from subclinical infection to an acute or chronic pneumonia. Most cases are restricted to the respiratory system, and are often asymptomatic; 25–40% develop extrapulmonary

infection, which most commonly affects the skin. Cutaneous lesions range from papules to verrucous and ulcerative lesions. The bones, genitourinary system, and central nervous system (CNS) may also be involved. Dissemination occurs more frequently in the immunocompromised, such as organ transplant recipients and those with HIV infection. The immunocompromised are at high risk of CNS involvement and adult respiratory distress syndrome. Their prognosis is poor, and therefore they require aggressive management. There are also rare reports of primary cutaneous blastomycosis acquired after accidental inoculation, and in some cases infection has been self-limiting.

MANAGEMENT STRATEGY

In the immunocompetent, acute pulmonary blastomycosis may be mild and self-limiting. However, all diagnosed cases are treated in order to prevent extrapulmonary dissemination. *Itraconazole* is the drug of choice for the treatment of non-CNS infection that is not life-threatening. A loading dose of 200 mg three times daily for 3 days, followed by 200 mg once or twice daily for 6–12 months, is recommended. Serum itraconazole levels should be measured 2 weeks after the start of treatment. *Ketoconazole* (400–800 mg daily) and *fluconazole* (400–800 mg daily) are second-line agents as they have lower efficacy against *Blastomyces*. In addition, long-term treatment with ketoconazole is associated with adverse effects. The new generation of azoles, *voriconazole* and *posaconazole*, have demonstrated activity against *B. dermatitidis* both in vitro and in animal studies. There have been reports only of the successful use of voriconazole in the treatment of CNS blastomycosis. *Amphotericin B* (AmB) is the treatment of choice for those who fail on treatment with azoles, those with severe infection, the immunosuppressed, in pregnancy, and with CNS involvement. Experience to date has been largely with the use of AmB deoxycholate. Liposomal AmB is recommended for CNS infection. After an initial response with AmB, step-down therapy to an azole is common practice.

SPECIFIC INVESTIGATIONS

▶ Direct microscopy
▶ Culture
▶ Histopathology
▶ Chest radiography
▶ Bone scanning (radionuclide bone scan/CT/MRI)
▶ Serology for HIV infection (where relevant)

The definitive diagnosis of blastomycosis is based on the identification of characteristic thick-walled, broad-based budding yeasts by direct examination of tissue or the isolation of *Blastomyces* in culture. Specimens for direct microscopy in 10% KOH can be skin scrapings, pus from skin lesions, sputum, and biopsy tissue from any lesion suspicious for infection. Successful culture of sputum, tissue biopsy specimens, cerebrospinal fluid, or urine at 25 °C on Sabouraud's agar produces a white mold, and at 37 °C on blood agar a brown, wrinkled colony. Histopathology of infected tissues reveals a pyogranulomatous response without caseation, and pseudoepitheliomatous hyperplasia. A *Blastomyces* antigen assay is available to test urine, blood, and other fluids, but its role in diagnosis has yet to be established.

FIRST-LINE THERAPIES

| ▶ Itraconazole | **B** |
| ▶ Amphotericin B | **C** |

Itraconazole therapy for blastomycosis and histoplasmosis. Dismukes WE, Badcher RW, Cloud JC, Kauffman CA, Chapman SW, George RB, et al.; NIAID Mycoses Study Group. Am J Med 1992; 93: 489–97.

A prospective, non-randomized, multicenter trial involving 48 patients with pulmonary or disseminated blastomycosis without CNS involvement. Patients were treated with itraconazole 200–400 mg/day for a median of 6.2 months, with a 90% cure rate (43/48). Treatment was very well tolerated, and there was no therapeutic advantage for patients treated with the higher dose.

Endemic blastomycosis in Mississippi: epidemiological and clinical studies. Chapman SW, Lin AC, Hendricks KA, Nolan RL, Currier MM, Morris KR, et al. Semin Respir Infect 1997; 12: 219–28.

This was a review of 326 confirmed cases of blastomycosis from Mississippi. There was involvement of lungs (91.4%), skin (18.1%), bone (4.3%), genitourinary system (1.8%), and CNS (1.2%). Skin or bone disease was associated with multiorgan involvement. A successful outcome without relapse was noted in 86.5% of patients treated with amphotericin B deoxycholate, and in 81.7% of ketoconazole-treated patients. The relapse rate for ketoconazole-treated patients was higher than for amphotericin B-treated patients (14% and 3.9%, respectively).

Recurrent blastomycosis of the central nervous system: case report and review. Chowfin A, Tight R, Mitchell S. Clin Infect Dis 2000; 30: 969–71.

A case of recurrent CNS blastomycosis successfully treated with surgery and liposomal amphotericin B after an inadequate response to amphotericin B alone.

Liposomal amphotericin is the recommended treatment for CNS blastomycosis because it achieves higher CNS penetration and is also better tolerated with prolonged therapy.

Recurrent central nervous system blastomycosis in an immunocompetent child treated successfully with sequential liposomal amphotericin B and voriconazole. Panicker J, Walsh T, Kamani N. Pediatr Infect Dis J 2006; 25: 377–9.

This case report describes the successful treatment of an immunocompetent child who developed CNS infection 18 months after treatment for pulmonary blastomycosis. She was then treated with liposomal amphotericin B, which was stepped downed to oral voriconazole.

There are only reports of a few cases of blastomycosis undergoing treatment with liposomal AmB. It is, however, already successfully used in the management of other invasive fungal infections in the immunocompromised.

Blastomycosis in solid organ transplant recipients. Gauthier GM, Safdar N, Klein BS, Andes DR. Transpl Infect Dis 2007; 9: 310–17.

In this series of 11 cases pneumonia was the most common clinical presentation and seven were complicated by acute respiratory distress syndrome (ARDS). Extrapulmonary disease predominantly involved the skin and spared the CNS. The overall mortality rate was 36%; however, this increased to 67% in those with ARDS. Three of four patients with ARDS treated with liposoomal AmB were cured. The other three patients treated with either AmB deoxycholate (n=2) or voriconazole (n=1) died.

Although the numbers in this study are small, it suggests that liposomal AmB is more effective than AmB deoxycholate for the treatment of severe infection in the immunocompromised.

SECOND-LINE THERAPIES

▶ Ketoconazole	**B**
▶ Fluconazole	**B**
▶ Voriconazole	**E**

Treatment of blastomycosis and histoplasmosis with ketoconazole. Results of a prospective randomized clinical trial. Dismukes WE, Cloud G, Bowles C; National Institute of Allergy and Infectious Diseases Mycoses Study Group. Ann Intern Med 1985; 103: 861–72.

This was a multicenter, prospective, randomized trial. Of 65 patients with blastomycosis treated for 6 months or more, high-dose ketoconazole (800 mg daily) was significantly more effective than low-dose ketoconazole 400 mg daily (100% vs 79% cure rate; p=0.001). Adverse effects occurred in 60% of patients, and were more common in those treated at higher doses. Therefore, the study group recommended that treatment should commence at the lower dose.

Despite its efficacy, ketoconazole is now rarely used because of its associated adverse effects, as well as the availability of better-tolerated azoles.

Treatment of blastomycosis with fluconazole: a pilot study. Pappas PG, Bradsher RW, Chapman SW, Kauffman CA, Dine A, Cloud GA, et al.; The National Institute of Allergy and Infectious Disease Mycoses Study Group. Clin Infect Dis 1995; 20: 267–71.

A multicenter, randomized open-label pilot study compared two doses of fluconazole (200 and 400 mg daily) for the treatment of non-life-threatening blastomycosis. The analysis data included 23 patients who were treated for a minimum of 6 months. There was a successful outcome in 65% of patients (15/23) with no relapse at 7 months' follow-up. Of those who responded, 62% (8/15) had received 200 mg daily and 70% (7/10) received 400 mg daily.

The results of this study were disappointing. However, fluconazole has excellent CNS penetration and may therefore have a better role in the treatment of CNS infection, although there are no studies to support this.

Treatment of blastomycosis with higher doses of fluconazole. Pappas PG, Bradsher RW, Kauffman CA, Cloud GA, Thomas CJ, Campbell GD Jr, et al.; The National Institute of Allergy and Infectious Disease Mycoses Study Group. Clin Infect Dis 1997; 25: 200–5.

This multicentre, randomized, open-label study investigated the efficacy of high-dose fluconazole (400–800 mg daily) for the treatment of non-life-threatening blastomycosis. There was an 87% cure rate (34/39) after a mean treatment period of 8.9 months.

This study demonstrates a much higher efficacy for fluconazole at doses of 400–800 mg daily.

Evidence Levels: A Double-blind study **B** Clinical trial ≥ 20 subjects **C** Clinical trial < 20 subjects **D** Series ≥ 5 subjects **E** Anecdotal case reports

Successful treatment of cerebral blastomycosis with voriconazole. Bakleh M, Aksamit AJ, Tleyjeh IM, Marshall WF. Clin Infect Dis 2005; 40: e69–71.

A case of disseminated infection with CNS involvement in a patient receiving chemotherapy for lymphoma. Treatment with amphotericin B deoxycholate caused nephrotoxicity. A switch to liposomal amphotericin therapy produced chest tightness. However, oral voriconazole (200 mg twice daily for the first month, increasing to 300 mg twice daily) was well tolerated and there was marked clinical and radiographic improvement within 1 month of treatment, which was continued for 12 months.

Animal and human studies indicate that high concentrations of voriconazole can be achieved in the CSF and brain tissue. This case illustrates that it is a useful alternative for CNS infection when amphotericin cannot be tolerated.

Cerebral blastomycosis: a case series incorporating voriconazole in the treatment regimen. Borgia SM, Fuller JD, Sarabia A, El-Helou P. Med Mycol 2006; 44: 659–64.

Three cases from Canada which failed on standard antifungal therapy, two relapsing after treatment with itraconazole. All three cases were subsequently successfully treated with oral voriconazole, which was well tolerated.

Clinical practice guidelines for the management of blastomycosis: 2008 update by the Infectious Diseases Society of America. Chapman SW, Dismukes WE, Proia LA, Bradsher RW, Pappas PG, Threlkeld MG, et al.; Infectious Diseases Society of America. Clin Infect Dis 2008; 46: 1801–12.

This updated evidence-based guideline replaces the previous guidelines published in 2000. Treatment is guided by the extent of infection, CNS involvement, and the immune state of the host. Previously, mild cases of pulmonary blastomycosis were managed conservatively as they are sometimes self-limiting. However, with the advent and high efficacy of oral azoles, primarily itraconazole, most cases are now actively treated in order to prevent extrapulmonary spread and any risk of future reactivation.

- Itraconazole is the drug of choice for the treatment of mild to moderate pulmonary or disseminated infection. The recommended dose is an initial loading dose of 200 mg three times daily for 3 days, followed by 200 mg once or twice daily for 6–12 months. Serum levels should be measure after 2 weeks to ensure adequate drug exposure.
- Amphotericin B is the treatment of choice for those with severe pulmonary or disseminated infection, and in the immunocompromised. Either the lipid formulation (3–5 mg/kg/day) or amphotericin deoxycholate (0.7–1 mg/kg/day) is given for 1–2 weeks or until improvement is noted. Itraconazole is then recommended as step-down therapy (loading dose and then 200 mg twice daily for 6–12 months, except in the immunocompromised, who require at least 12 months of treatment or until immunosuppression has been reversed).
- Liposomal amphotericin B at a dose of 5 mg/kg/day is the recommended treatment for CNS infection. Treatment should be given for 4–6 weeks, followed by an oral azole (fluconazole 800 mg daily/itraconazole 200 mg two to three times daily/voriconazole 200–400 mg twice daily), which should be given for at least 12 months and until there is resolution of CSF abnormalities.
- Amphotericin B is the drug of choice for patients who have failed to respond to azole treatment.
- Amphotericin B is the only drug approved for the treatment of blastomycosis in pregnant women.

Blistering distal dactylitis

Irshad Zaki

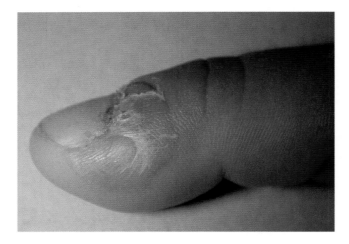

Blistering distal dactylitis (BDD) is a superficial, tender, blistering infection seen in childhood and the early teens. It is usually caused by group A β-hemolytic streptococci, although group B organisms and staphylococci have also been implicated. The distal volar fat pads of the fingers are the most common site of infection, but involvement of the nailfolds and toes can occasionally occur.

MANAGEMENT STRATEGY

Blistering distal dactylitis can cause considerable alarm to parents as large tense blisters rapidly develop. Despite the absence of constitutional symptoms, patients usually seek help soon after the onset of the infection. The condition does not resolve spontaneously, but prompt treatment results in rapid improvement. *Blisters should be incised to release fluid*, which can vary from clear and watery to frank pus. Subsequent application of topical antibiotics can be helpful, but systemic treatment is usually also required. *Penicillin V* is the treatment of choice for streptococcal infection, but *erythromycin* is an effective alternative for patients allergic to penicillin.

The differential diagnosis of the condition includes traumatic blisters, herpetic whitlow, staphylococcal bullous impetigo, and the Weber–Cockayne variant of epidermolysis bullosa.

SPECIFIC INVESTIGATIONS

> ▶ Gram stain of blister fluid
> ▶ Culture of blister fluid
> ▶ Swab of nasopharynx for bacteriology

A clinically recognizable streptococcal infection. Hays GC, Mullard JE. Paediatrics 1975; 56: 129–31.

First large series report describing 13 patients with BDD. Streptococci were found on culture of blister fluid in all cases, and Gram-positive cocci were usually found on Gram staining. This report suggests a link with infection of the nasopharynx, but this has not been confirmed in other case reports.

Staphylococcal blistering dactylitis: a case series in children under nine months of age. Lyon M, Doehring MC. J Emerg Med 2004; 26: 421–3.

Although uncommon under the age of 2, this paper reports three cases under 9 months of age.

These reports highlight the importance of initiating bacteriology prior to commencing treatment. Staphylococcal infection is a relatively rare but recognized cause of BDD.

FIRST-LINE THERAPIES

> ▶ Incision and drainage of blister   C
> ▶ Topical antibiotics   C
> ▶ Systemic penicillin   C

Is blistering distal dactylitis a variant of bullous impetigo? Scheinfeld NS. Clin Exp Dermatol 2007; 32: 314–16.

Good review of literature and treatment. Confirms the importance of incision and drainage, adequate dressings, and the need to consider *Staphylococcus aureus* as a cause if penicillin is ineffective

Group B streptococcal blistering distal dactylitis in an adult diabetic. Benson PM, Solivan G. J Am Acad Dermatol 1987; 17: 310–11.

Report of a diabetic patient who developed BDD as a result of group B β-hemolytic streptococci. Good response to treatment with topical antibiotic and oral dicloxacillin. Infection of skin with group B streptococci is uncommon, although diabetic patients appear to be more susceptible.

SECOND-LINE THERAPIES

> ▶ Systemic erythromycin   D

Blistering distal dactylitis: a manifestation of Group A beta-haemolytic streptococcal infection. Schneider JA, Parlette HL. Arch Dermatol 1982; 118: 879–80.

Short report of the authors' personal experience, suggesting that this is a relatively common problem. Systemic penicillin and erythromycin were both found to be effective. It is likely that many cases of BDD are wrongly diagnosed as bullous impetigo by clinicians not familiar with this disorder.

THIRD-LINE THERAPIES

> ▶ Amoxicillin/clavulanic acid   D
> ▶ Conservative measures for herpetic whitlow   D

A review and report of blistering distal dactylitis due to *Staphylococcus aureus* in two HIV-positive men. Scheinfeld N. Dermatol Online J 2007; 13: 8.

Staphylococcus aureus was found to be the etiologic agent in two HIV-positive patients. The condition improved following treatment with a proprietary mixture of amoxicillin trihydrate and clavulanate potassium. The report highlights that blisters may not always be present and that BDD may present with erosions.

Coexistent infections on a child's distal phalanx: blistering dactylitis and herpetic whitlow. Ney AC, English JC 3rd, Greer KE. Cutis 2002; 69: 46–8.

Consider comorbidity if BDD does not respond to antibiotics.

Evidence Levels: **A** Double-blind study   **B** Clinical trial ≥ 20 subjects   **C** Clinical trial < 20 subjects   **D** Series ≥ 5 subjects   **E** Anecdotal case reports

Bowen's disease and erythroplasia of Queyrat

Carrie Wood Cobb, Naomi Lawrence

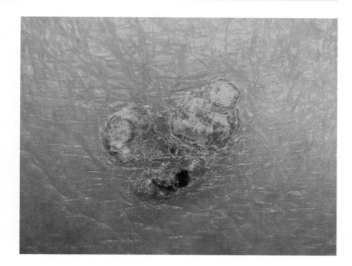

Bowen's disease and erythroplasia of Queyrat (EQ) are defined as intraepidermal squamous cell carcinoma, the latter occurring on the penis. The clinical appearance is that of a sharply demarcated, erythematous patch up to several centimeters in diameter. Risk factors for the development of Bowen's disease and EQ vary according to the site of disease, but generally include sun exposure, HPV infection, arsenic exposure, radiation exposure, and HIV or other forms of immunosuppression.

MANAGEMENT STRATEGY

The goals of treatment in both Bowen's disease and EQ are cure and prevention of progression to invasive squamous cell carcinoma, while maintaining function and cosmesis. Invasive transformation of EQ is more common (10%) and metastasizes earlier than of Bowen's disease (3%). Definitive treatment is *surgical excision* if the lesion is small and well defined. *Mohs' micrographic surgery (MMS)* is recommended over simple excision because the likelihood of recurrence is lower. MMS is also advised in the treatment of larger, ill-defined lesions, especially when preservation of normal tissue is crucial, as with EQ. Surgical ablation may be achieved with *electrodesiccation and curettage, cryotherapy,* or *laser.* Non-surgical options include *imiquimod cream* (a topical immuno-modulator), *topical 5-fluorouracil (5-FU), photodynamic therapy (PDT),* and *radiation therapy.*

Standard of care requires that a follow-up period of no less than 5 years be observed to claim clinical cure of Bowen's disease and EQ. Therefore, the extremely brief duration of follow-up for many studies addressing the treatment for these diseases renders the data difficult to apply in the clinical setting.

SPECIFIC INVESTIGATIONS

▶ Skin biopsy
▶ Dermoscopy
▶ Immunoperoxidase studies for human papillomavirus

Dermoscopy of Bowen's disease. Zalaudek I, Argenziano G, Leinweber B, Citarella L, Hofmann-Wellenhof R, et al. Br J Dermatol 2004; 150: 1112–16.

The small sample size limits the application of this newly described diagnostic tool.

The prevalence of human papillomavirus genotypes in non-melanoma skin cancers of nonimmunosuppressed individuals identifies high-risk genital types as possible risk factors. Iftner A, Klug SJ, Garbe C, Blum A, Blum A, Stancu A, et al. Cancer Res 2003; 63: 7515–19.

The study found an odds ratio of 59 (95% confidence interval 5.4–645) for non-melanoma skin cancer in patients who were DNA positive for the high-risk mucosal HPV types 16, 31, 35, and 51.

FIRST-LINE THERAPIES

▶ Standard excision **B**
▶ Mohs' micrographic surgery **B**

Bowen's disease: a four-year retrospective review of epidemiology and treatment at a university center. Hansen JP, Drake AL, Walling HW. Dermatol Surg 2008; 34: 878–83.

Retrospective analysis of 406 cases of Bowen's disease examining epidemiology, treatment modalities, and histologic recurrence for a 4-year period. Of note, cases of EQ were excluded from the study.

Cutaneous squamous carcinoma in situ (Bowen's disease): treatment with Mohs micrographic surgery. Leibovitch I, Huilgol SC, Selva D, Richards S, Paver R. J Am Acad Dermatol 2005; 52: 997–1002.

A case series evaluating 270 cases of Bowen's disease treated with MMS with 5-year follow-up demonstrating recurrence rates of approximately 6%. The majority of lesions treated were on the head and neck, and many were recurrent at the time of MMS.

Bowen's disease involving the urethra. Yasuda M, Tamura A, Shimizu A, Takahashi A, Ishikawa O. J Dermatol 2005; 32: 210–13.

A case report highlighting the importance of early and definitive treatment of EQ.

Extensive Bowen's disease of the penile shaft treated with fresh tissue Mohs micrographic surgery in two separate operations. Moritz DL, Lynch WS. J Dermatol Surg Oncol 1991; 17: 374–8.

MMS is the only therapy that allows for definitive demonstration of tumor-free margins. Appropriate surgical therapy should be based on lesion size, anatomic location, and history of recurrence.

SECOND-LINE THERAPIES

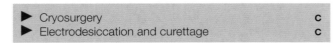

▶ Cryosurgery	**C**
▶ Electrodesiccation and curettage	**C**

Comparison of cryotherapy with curettage in the treatment of Bowen's disease: a prospective study. Ahmed I, Berth-Jones J, Charles-Holmes S, O'Callaghan CJ, Ilchyshyn A. Br J Dermatol 2000; 143: 759–66.

Eighty lesions were randomized to two groups, cryotherapy (n=36) or curettage (n=44) and followed for a median of 2 years. Curettage produced comparable cure rates with more rapid healing, less pain, and fewer complications.

Curettage-cryosurgery for non-melanoma skin cancer of the external ear: excellent 5-year results. Nordin P. Br J Dermatol 1999; 140: 291–3.

Three lesions treated showed no recurrence at 5-year follow-up, with good cosmetic results.

This therapy may be beneficial in areas such as the pinna that are prone to deformity after surgical excision.

THIRD-LINE THERAPIES

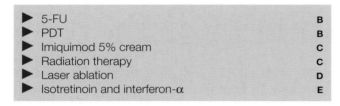

▶ 5-FU	**B**
▶ PDT	**B**
▶ Imiquimod 5% cream	**C**
▶ Radiation therapy	**C**
▶ Laser ablation	**D**
▶ Isotretinoin and interferon-α	**E**

Topical treatment of Bowen's disease with 5-fluorouracil. Bargman H, Hochman J. J Cutan Med Surg 2003; 7: 101–5.

Only two of 26 biopsy-confirmed lesions recurred up to 10 years after treatment.

Guidelines on the use of photodynamic therapy for nonmelanoma skin cancer: an international consensus. International Society for Photodynamic Therapy in Dermatology, 2005. Braathen LR, Szeimies RM, Basset-Seguin N, Bissonnette R, Foley P, Pariser D, et al. J Am Acad Dermatol 2007; 56: 125–43.

A consensus article and review of the literature comparing PDT with other modalities, including 5-FU and cryosurgery. Overall, PDT was found to be equally as effective and as well, if not better, tolerated than other treatments.

Photodynamic therapy with methyl aminolevulinate for atypical carcinoma in situ of the penis. Axcrona K, Brennhovd B, Alfsen GC, Giercksky KE, Warloe T. Scand J Urol Nephrol 2007; 41: 507–10.

A small sample of patients (10) were treated with PDT for EQ with good cosmetic and functional outcome. A high histologic recurrence rate of 3/10 was observed.

Imiquimod 5% cream monotherapy for cutaneous squamous cell carcinoma in situ (Bowen's disease): a randomized, double-blind, placebo-controlled trial. Patel GK, Goodwin R, Chawla M, Laidler P, Price PE, Finlay AY, et al. J Am Acad Dermatol 2006; 54: 1025–32.

Seventy-three percent of patients achieved clinical remission with no recurrence at the 9-month follow-up.

A small sample size (31) limits the validity of this otherwise well-controlled study.

Treatment of Bowen's disease with topical 5% imiquimod cream: retrospective study. Rosen T, Harting M, Gibson M. Dermatol Surg 2007; 33: 427–31.

Forty-two of 49 patients treated with 5% imiquimod cream achieved complete clinical remission at 1.5-year follow-up.

Erythroplasia of Queyrat treated with imiquimod 5% cream Micali G, Nasca MR, De Pasquale R. J Am Acad Dermatol 2006; 55: 901–3.

Case report of an elderly man with EQ treated with 5% imiquimod with clinical and histologically confirmed cure.

Radiation therapy for Bowen's disease of the skin. Lukas VanderSpek LA, Pond GR, Wells W, Tsang RW. Int J Radiat Oncol Biol Phys 2005; 63: 505–10.

Forty-four cases of Bowen's disease treated with radiation therapy were reviewed, demonstrating remission in 42 patients with three recurrences at a mean follow-up period of 2.5 years. A broad range of radiation schedules were used and compared for efficacy and safety. These demonstrated no significant differences between low to medium- and high-dose radiation schedules on disease remission or recurrence.

Concomitant use of a high-energy pulsed CO_2 laser and a long-pulsed (810 nm) diode laser for squamous cell carcinoma in situ. Fader DJ, Lowe L. Dermatol Surg 2002; 28: 97–9.

Three patients showed complete resolution at 4 months, with epidermal and follicular epithelium restored 2 weeks postoperatively.

Use of the diode laser for lesions in non-glabrous skin may enhance the efficacy of the CO_2 laser by targeting lesions that extend down the follicular infundibula.

Treatment of multiple lesions of Bowen's disease with isotretinoin and interferon alpha. Gordon KB, Roenigk HH, Gendleman M. Arch Dermatol 1997; 133: 691–3.

One patient was treated with oral isotretinoin and subcutaneous interferon-α_{2a} with no recurrence at 15 months.

Evidence Levels: **A** Double-blind study **B** Clinical trial ≥ 20 subjects **C** Clinical trial < 20 subjects **D** Series ≥ 5 subjects **E** Anecdotal case reports

Bullous pemphigoid

Brett T Summey Jr, Victoria P Werth

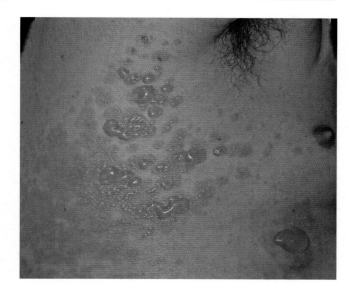

Bullous pemphigoid (BP) is an autoimmune subepidermal blistering disease that mainly affects elderly patients, although childhood cases do occur. Subepidermal blistering is mediated by activation of complement and release of tissue-destructive proteases following IgG autoantibody complex formation with hemidesmosomal antigens BPAg1 (BP230) and BPAg2 (BP180 or collagen XVII). The clinical hallmarks of the eruption are tense bullae with either generalized or localized distribution; however, variants, including urticarial, vesicular, vegetative, erythrodermic, and nodularis, have been described. Pruritus associated with BP can be severe and adversely affect quality of life. Mucosal involvement with small blisters or erosions may exist in a minority of patients. Although there can be relapses and exacerbations, BP is generally self-limiting, with remission in most adults by 5 years, and more rapidly in children. Mortality can be high in patients with poor overall health and advanced age.

MANAGEMENT STRATEGY

The Cochrane Skin Group published its review on the treatment of BP in 2005, a review that focused on only strong evidence from randomized controlled trials (RCT) to help guide physicians with treatment options. Unfortunately, only seven RCTs have been completed on treatment for BP, none of which were blinded, and six of the seven were small in size. The authors showed from the data that doses of prednisolone >0.75 mg/kg/day have no added benefit in efficacy over lower doses, albeit increasing adverse effects. The data also showed that *topical clobetasol propionate 0.05% cream* (40 g/day) was as effective as *oral corticosteroids* in controlling disease, and associated with fewer adverse effects. From an evidence-based medicine perspective, these are the only recommendations with strong evidentiary support.

Patients with localized disease may be successfully treated with clobetasol propionate 0.05% or *intralesional corticosteroids*. Those with generalized disease in which topical therapy is not feasible can be treated with *prednisone*, 0.5–0.75 mg/kg/day, depending on disease severity and considering the overall health of the patient. The risks of both short- and long-term systemic corticosteroid therapy are well known and are heightened in the elderly patient population. Every effort should be made to find the minimum dosage of systemic corticosteroids required to suppress disease. With only a few exceptions, all elderly patients started on systemic corticosteroids should also start calcium, vitamin D, and bisphosphonate therapy at the same time as corticosteroid therapy. All patients on systemic corticosteroids should be screened for tuberculosis and have their blood pressure and serum glucose levels followed closely.

Tetracycline combined with *nicotinamide* can be used for patients unable to tolerate or who have contraindications to corticosteroids. If gastrointestinal side effects manifest, *minocycline* may be substituted. Tetracycline alone has also been used in one case with success. Dapsone is a second-line alternative to systemic corticosteroids and particularly useful when histologic examination reveals a predominance of neutrophils.

Azathioprine may be used alone or as a corticosteroid-sparing agent in more severe disease. Thiopurine methyltransferase (TPMT) is an enzyme that metabolizes this agent. Owing to genetic polymorphisms in the expression of this enzyme, a TPMT level measurement prior to initiation of azathioprine may assist the physician in appropriate dosing. *Azathioprine* has a slow onset of action, and corticosteroids should be started in tandem during the acute stage. Patients usually respond within 3–4 weeks of initiation. *Mycophenolate mofetil*, an immunosuppressive agent, has recently been used as an effective corticosteroid-sparing agent in BP. It is generally well tolerated and does not carry the risk of liver toxicity seen with azathioprine. Methotrexate is another corticosteroid-sparing agent that may be useful in BP. It is given in a weekly, low-dosage protocol in a similar manner to psoriasis therapy.

For severe and refractory BP, a variety of immunosuppressive and immunomodulatory therapies have demonstrated efficacy, including *pulsed intravenous corticosteroids, cyclophosphamide, ciclosporin, chlorambucil, etanercept, intravenous immunoglobulin, rituximab, daclizumab, and plasmapheresis*.

SPECIFIC INVESTIGATIONS

▶ Evaluation of medications to rule out drug-induced cases
▶ Consider patient age and overall medical condition for therapeutic decision making
▶ Biopsy of intact bulla for histologic examination with hematoxylin and eosin
▶ Biopsy of perilesional skin for direct immunofluorescence (send specimen in Michel's transport medium)
▶ Consider BP180 (BPAg2) ELISA or indirect immunofluorescence on blood or blister fluid sample
▶ Consider fasting glucose screening

Drug-induced pemphigoid: bullous and cicatricial. Vassileva S. Clin Dermatol 1998; 16: 379–87.

Many drugs have been recognized to induce BP, including furosemide, bumetanide, spironolactone, phenacetin, penicillins, ibuprofen, D-penicillamine, captopril, fluoxetine, β-adrenergic blockers, terbinafine, gabapentin, risperidone, and PUVA.

Prediction of survival for patients with bullous pemphigoid: a prospective study. Joly P, Benichou J, Lok C, Hellot MF, Saiag P, Tancrede-Bohin E, et al. Arch Dermatol 2005; 141: 691–8.

The only prospective trial evaluating factors that influence survival in 341 BP patients found that increasing age and poor overall health were direct predictors of mortality. They showed that disease activity had no correlation with mortality.

Increased frequency of diabetes mellitus in patients with bullous pemphigoid: a case–control study. Chuang TY, Korkij W, Soltani K, Clayman J, Cook J. J Am Acad Dermatol 1984; 6: 1099–102.

The occurrence rate of diabetes mellitus prior to administration of systemic corticosteroids was significantly higher in patients with BP (20%) than in controls (2.5%).

FIRST-LINE THERAPIES

► Clobetasol propionate 0.05%	B
► Systemic corticosteroids	B
► Tetracycline and nicotinamide	C
► Tetracycline	E
► Minocycline	C

Evaluation of the safety and efficacy of a potent topical corticosteroid in the treatment of bullous pemphigoid. Claudy A. Clin Dermatol 2001; 19: 778–80.

A review of the 111 patients with BP reported in the literature treated with topical clobetasol as monotherapy. Absence of new blisters could be obtained within a few days in more than 80% of patients, with complete re-epithelialization of the affected skin in an average of 13.7 days. This therapy was effective in healing lesions in most of the patients with mild or moderate BP without adverse effects, but is not recommended for patients with severe forms of BP.

A comparison of oral and topical corticosteroids in patients with bullous pemphigoid. Joly P, Roujeau JC, Benichou J, Picard C, Dreno B, Delaporte E, et al. N Engl J Med 2002; 346: 321–7.

A total of 341 patients with BP were enrolled in a non-blinded, randomized, multicenter trial and stratified according to the severity of their disease (moderate or extensive). Patients were randomly assigned to receive either topical clobetasol (40 g/day) or oral prednisolone (0.5 mg/kg for moderate disease and 1 mg/kg for extensive disease). Overall, topical corticosteroid therapy was found to be equal in both survival and efficacy to oral corticosteroids for moderate BP. Topical steroids were superior to oral corticosteroid therapy for extensive disease in terms of survival.

Treatment of bullous pemphigoid with prednisolone only: 0.75 mg/kg/day versus 1.25 mg/kg/day. A multicenter randomized study. Morel P, Guillaume JC. Ann Dermatol Venereol 1984; 11: 925–8.

A randomized, prospective study in 50 patients on two doses of prednisolone found no difference in effectiveness of the higher dosage versus the lower dose.

Nicotinamide and tetracycline therapy of bullous pemphigoid. Fivenson DP, Breneman DL, Rosen GB, Hersh CS, Cardone S, Mutasim D. Arch Dermatol 1994; 130: 753–8.

A randomized open-label trial of 20 patients with BP. The combination of nicotinamide (500 mg three times daily) and tetracycline (500 mg four times daily) was equally efficacious as systemic corticosteroids and resulted in less toxicity.

Minocycline as a therapeutic option in bullous pemphigoid. Loo WJ, Kirtschig G, Wojnarowska F. Clin Exp Dermatol 2001; 26: 376–9.

A retrospective analysis of 22 patients with BP treated with minocycline as an adjuvant therapy. A major response was seen in six patients, a minor response in 11, and no response in five.

Generalized bullous pemphigoid controlled by tetracycline therapy alone. Pereyo NG, Loretta SD. J Am Acad Dermatol 1995; 32: 138–9.

A case report of an 82-year-old woman with generalized BP who responded completely to oral tetracycline (500 mg twice daily) within 2 weeks. The tetracycline was successfully tapered over 6 weeks.

SECOND-LINE THERAPIES

► Dapsone	C
► Azathioprine	B
► Mycophenolate mofetil	B
► Methotrexate	C

Dapsone as first line therapy for bullous pemphigoid. Venning VA, Millard PR, Wojnarowska F. Br J Dermatol 1989; 120: 83–92.

In an open trial of 13 patients placed on dapsone as initial treatment, six were completely controlled with dapsone (50–100 mg daily). Dapsone may be used as initial treatment for BP, particularly when there are contraindications to the use of corticosteroids or immunosuppressants.

A comparison of oral methylprednisolone plus azathioprine or mycophenolate mofetil for the treatment of bullous pemphigoid. Beissert S, Werfel T, Frieling U, Böhm M, Sticherling M, Stadler R, et al. Arch Dermatol 2007; 143: 1536–42.

A randomized controlled, non-blinded trial of 73 BP patients (38 taking azathioprine 2 mg/kg/day and 35 taking mycophenolate mofetil 2 g/day) to assess whether either drug was more effective at reducing the total methylprednisolone dose. They were found to be equal, but azathioprine was associated with more liver toxicity. Both treatment groups had 100% remission of lesions.

Azathioprine in the treatment of bullous pemphigoid. Greaves MW, Burton JL, Marks J. Br Med J 1971; 1: 144–5.

Of 11 patients on long-term maintenance therapy with systemic corticosteroids, nine remained symptom free on azathioprine alone and two were able to have a reduced dosage of prednisone.

Azathioprine plus prednisone in treatment of pemphigoid. Burton J, Harman R, Peachey R, Warin R. Br Med J 1978; 2: 1190–1.

A 3-year controlled trial of 25 patients comparing azathioprine (2.5 mg/kg daily) plus prednisone with prednisone alone showed that azathioprine greatly reduced the need for prednisone and improved outcome.

Evidence Levels: **A** Double-blind study **B** Clinical trial ≥ 20 subjects **C** Clinical trial < 20 subjects **D** Series ≥ 5 subjects **E** Anecdotal case reports

Mycophenolate mofetil; a new therapeutic option in the treatment of blistering autoimmune diseases. Grundmann-Kollmann M, Korting HC, Behrens S, Kaskel P, Leiter U, Krähn G, et al. J Am Acad Dermatol 1999; 40: 957–60.

Mycophenolate mofetil given in combination with prednisone in one patient and as monotherapy in two patients resulted in complete remission of symptoms within 8–11 weeks.

Low-dose methotrexate treatment in elderly patients with bullous pemphigoid. Paul MA, Jorizzo JL, Fleischer AB, White WL. J Am Acad Dermatol 1994; 31: 620–5.

In a retrospective chart review of 34 patients with BP, eight therapy-resistant patients received low-dose weekly methotrexate (average 5–10 mg) combined with oral prednisone. Patients receiving combination therapy required significantly lower doses of prednisone to control their disease at 1 month compared with baseline.

Treatment of bullous pemphigoid by low-dose methotrexate associated with short-term potent topical steroids: an open prospective study of 18 cases. Dereure O. Arch Dermatol 2002; 138: 1255–6.

A prospective review of 18 patients with BP treated with a 2–3-week course of whole-body topical corticosteroid (clobetasol propionate) combined with oral or intramuscular methotrexate. Initial dosages of weekly methotrexate ranged from 7.5 to 10 mg. All 18 patients achieved a complete clinical response during the initial phase of intensive local corticosteroid treatment which was then maintained with methotrexate in monotherapy. Interruption of treatment was tolerated in 13 patients after 6–10 months with an uneventful follow-up for a mean period of 7.8 months.

Low-dose oral pulse methotrexate as monotherapy in elderly patients with bullous pemphigoid. Heilborn JD, Ståhle-Bäckdahl M, Albertioni F, Vassilaki I, Peterson C, Stephansson E. J Am Acad Dermatol 1999; 40: 741–9.

A prospective study of low-dose oral methotrexate (5–12.5 mg/week) in 11 elderly patients with generalized BP. Every patient demonstrated a rapid decrease in disease activity within 4–30 days.

THIRD-LINE THERAPIES

▶ Pulse intravenous corticosteroids	D
▶ Cyclophosphamide	E
▶ Ciclosporin	E
▶ Plasmapheresis	C
▶ Intravenous immunoglobulin (IVIG)	C
▶ Chlorambucil	B
▶ Sulfapyridine	D
▶ Etanercept	E
▶ Rituximab	E
▶ Rituximab + daclizumab	E
▶ Daclizumab	E
▶ Mycophenolate sodium	E
▶ Erythromycin	E

Severe bullous pemphigoid responsive to pulsed intravenous dexamethasone and oral cyclophosphamide. Dawe RS, Naidoo DK, Ferguson J. Br J Dermatol 1997; 137: 826–7.

Refractory BP in a 59-year-old woman with diabetes mellitus cleared with pulsed intravenous dexamethasone therapy (100 mg dexamethasone in 500 mL 5% dextrose infused over 4 hours on 3 consecutive days, monthly) and low-dose oral cyclophosphamide (50 mg/day between pulses).

High-dose methylprednisolone in the treatment of bullous pemphigoid. Siegel J, Eaglstein WH. Arch Dermatol 1984; 120: 1157–65.

Seven of eight hospitalized patients with active BP responded within 24 hours after methylprednisolone pulse therapy (15 mg/kg intravenously over 1 hour daily for 3 days). Moderate doses of oral prednisone (0.4 mg/kg) were required for maintenance.

Successful treatment of bullous pemphigoid with pulsed intravenous cyclophosphamide. Itoh T, Hosokawa H, Shirai Y, Horio T. Br J Dermatol 1996; 134: 931–3.

Case report of a 67-year-old man with refractory BP who responded to monthly pulsed intravenous doses of cyclophosphamide (500–1000 mg) along with low-dose oral cyclophosphamide (50 mg/day).

Effects of cyclosporin on bullous pemphigoid and pemphigus. Thivolet J, Harthelemy H, Rigot-Muller G, Bendelac A. Lancet 1985; 1: 334–5.

Ciclosporin (6 mg/kg daily), adapted to obtain a plasma level of 80–180 μg/L, was successful in treating two patients with BP.

Plasmapheresis as a steroid sparing procedure in bullous pemphigoid. Egan CA, Meadows KP, Zone JJ. Int J Dermatol 2000; 39: 230–5.

A retrospective review of 10 patients, all of whom went into remission with a lower daily dose of oral prednisone at 3 and 6 months after plasmapheresis. The drawbacks of plasmapheresis therapy include cost and procedural complications, such as line infection/sepsis and local thrombus formation.

Intravenous immunoglobulin therapy for patients with bullous pemphigoid unresponsive to conventional immunosuppressive treatment. Ahmed AR. J Am Acad Dermatol 2001; 6: 825–35.

Fifteen patients with recurrent BP who had experienced several significant side effects resulting from conventional therapy were treated with IVIG. In all 15 a rapid initial clinical response was observed, along with a long-term remission. In all subjects oral prednisone and other immunosuppressants could be safely withdrawn without recurrence of disease shortly after initiating IVIG. A gradual withdrawal of IVIG was necessary to prevent relapses.

Consensus statement on the use of intravenous immunoglobulin therapy in the treatment of autoimmune mucocutaneous blistering diseases. Ahmed AR, Dahl MV. Arch Dermatol 2003; 139: 1051–9.

In 27 of 32 cases of BP reported in the literature as unresponsive to conventional therapy, IVIG was of significant benefit and produced lasting clinical benefit with minimal adverse effects.

Chlorambucil as a steroid-sparing agent in bullous pemphigoid. Chave TA, Mortimer NJ, Shah DS, Hutchinson PE. Br J Dermatol 2004; 151: 1107–8.

Of 45 patients, 26 received prednisolone only and 19 received prednisolone and chlorambucil (0.1 mg/kg/day reduced after 2 weeks to 0.05 mg/kg/day, and after 1 month to 2 mg daily). Patients treated with chlorambucil had reduced overall duration of treatment and reduced total steroid requirement.

Bullous pemphigoid responding to sulfapyridine and the sulfones. Person JR, Rogers RS. Arch Dermatol 1977; 113: 610–15.

Of 41 patients with BP, five responded completely to sulfapyridine (500–1000 mg four times daily) and one additional patient showed marked improvement. Histologic examination of skin biopsy specimens from these patients demonstrated a predominance of neutrophils.

Treatment of coexisting bullous pemphigoid and psoriasis with the tumor necrosis factor antagonist etanercept. Yamauchi PS, Lowe NJ, Gindi V. J Am Acad Dermatol 2006; 54: S121–2.

A case report of a 64-year-old man with both psoriasis and bullous pemphigoid. The patient failed mycophenolate mofetil treatment and was started on prednisone 60 mg/day. In an effort to reduce psoriasis rebound, etanercept 50 mg/week was started. Bullae returned as the prednisone was tapered, so the dose of etanercept was increased to 50 mg twice weekly. At this dose, prednisone could be tapered and the psoriasis and BP remained in remission.

A new approach on bullous pemphigoid therapy. Saouli Z, Papadopoulos A, Kaiafa G, Girtovitis F, Kontoninas Z. Ann Oncol 2008; 19: 825–6.

Two cases of BP in women (ages 58 and 78), both in remission for chronic leukemia. Both women received intravenous rituximab 375 mg/m^2 once weekly for 4 weeks. Neither woman had bullae at the end of the cycle. Patients were subsequently treated with one dose every 2 months, with no recurrence in 3 years.

Rituximab in treatment-resistant autoimmune blistering skin disorders. Schmidt E, Bröcker EB, Goebeler M. Clin Rev Allergy Immunol 2008; 34: 56–64.

Four cases of BP treated with rituximab (anti-CD20) are described. A 2-year-old boy had a partial response after four treatments, and complete resolution after re-treatment 9 months later. In the second case the patient died from bacterial pneumonia 6 weeks after the first rituximab infusion, at which time her lesions were resolving. A third BP patient with IPEX syndrome greatly improved with rituximab and oral corticosteroids could be discontinued. The fourth patient had chronic graft-versus-host disease after unrelated cord blood transplantation as a result of B-cell acute precursor lymphocytic leukemia. This patient received anti-CD25 antibody daclizumab in addition to rituximab, and the BP lesions healed completely.

Daclizumab: a novel therapeutic option in severe bullous pemphigoid. Mockenhaupt M, Grosber M, Norganer J. Acta Dermatol Venereol 2005; 85: 65–6.

A case report of a 52-year-old with diffuse BP. The patient failed combination treatment with prednisolone 100 mg/day plus azathioprine 100 mg/day, ciclosporin A 200 mg/day, and mycophenolate mofetil 2 g/day. The steroids were reduced to 5 mg/day secondary to glucose intolerance, so daclizumab was added at 1 mg/kg/day. The patient had six infusions and remained on prednisolone 5 mg/day and azathioprine 50 mg/day, with complete resolution of lesions at 2 weeks.

Treatment of bullous pemphigoid with enteric-coated mycophenolate sodium. Tursen U, Guney A, Kaya T, Ikizoglu G. J Eur Acad Dermatol Venereol 2007; 21: 542–4.

Case report of a 78-year-old woman with BP for 1 year. After failing prednisolone 100 mg plus azathioprine 150 mg and also IVIG, mycophenolate sodium 360 mg twice daily was started with 100 mg prednisolone and the lesions resolved by 8 weeks. Steroid was able to be tapered off, and patient was lesion free at 6 months.

Erythromycin therapy in bullous pemphigoid: possible anti-inflammatory effects. Fox BJ, Odom RB, Findlay RF. J Am Acad Dermatol 1982; 7: 504–10.

Erythromycin was effective in both an 87-year-old woman (at a dosage of 250 mg four times a day) and a 4-year-old girl with BP.

Evidence Levels: **A** Double-blind study **B** Clinical trial ≥ 20 subjects **C** Clinical trial < 20 subjects **D** Series ≥ 5 subjects **E** Anecdotal case reports

Burning mouth syndrome (glossodynia)

Lisa A Drage, Alison J Bruce, Roy S Rogers III

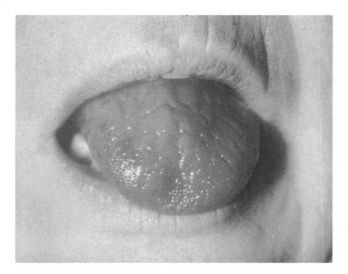

Burning mouth syndrome (BMS) refers to mouth pain in patients who have a normal oral examination. The burning sensation may localize to specific sites such as the tongue, palate, or lip, or it may be a generalized oral pain. BMS has been classified as primary when organic local or systemic causes cannot be identified and a neuropathic cause is probable; and secondary, which results from local or systemic conditions. Secondary BMS is often multifactorial. As many oral mucosal diseases (lichen planus, herpes simplex virus infections, recurrent aphthous stomatitis, aphthous ulcers, etc.) also cause mouth pain, a thorough oral examination to exclude other primary mucosal alterations must be performed prior to considering burning mouth syndrome.

MANAGEMENT STRATEGIES

Identification and treatment of all correctable causes of mouth pain should be emphasized. Conditions most commonly associated with mouth pain include psychiatric illness (depression, anxiety, and cancer phobia), xerostomia (drug related, secondary to connective tissue diseases or ageing), nutritional deficiency (iron, vitamin B_6, B_{12}, folate, zinc, riboflavin, thiamin), and allergic contact stomatitis (particularly to flavorings and food additives). Multiple associated factors are commonly present and demand concurrent treatment.

Geographic tongue is also associated with burning mouth pain. Other less common etiologies include candidiasis, denture-related oral pain, denture sore mouth, menopause, and use of angiotensin-converting enzyme (ACE) inhibitors.

A directed history and physical examination with emphasis on a thorough oral examination must be completed. All medications must be assessed for xerostomic potential. Direct questions should be asked about depression, anxiety, and fear of cancer. Exacerbations with food or other oral preparations (toothpaste, mouthwash, gum, etc.) should be

elicited. A history of pain starting with dental work or dentures, as well as parafunctional behaviors (tongue thrusting, clenching, and bruxism), should be documented.

Treatment should be based on the results of a directed history, a thorough oral examination, and the results of the laboratory investigation, and should be tailored to the individual patient. Initially, treatment should be based on the suspected cause of the mouth pain rather than used in an algorithmic manner. If there were no identifiable causes of the mouth symptoms, then a *trial of a chronic pain protocol*, similar to the medical management of other neuropathic pain conditions, would be appropriate.

SPECIFIC INVESTIGATIONS

▶ A thorough history emphasizing:
  – medications that can cause xerostomia
  – dental work and denture history
  – oral care and habits
  – history or symptoms of depression, anxiety, or fear of cancer
▶ Oral examination specifically checking for any sign of erythema, candidiasis, xerostomia, or abnormal mucosal changes
▶ Laboratory tests
  – complete blood count
  – iron, total iron binding capacity, iron saturation, ferritin
  – vitamin B_6, B_{12}, folate, zinc, riboflavin, thiamin
  – fasting plasma glucose and glycosylated hemoglobin
  – biopsy (only if indicated on the basis of an abnormal oral examination)
▶ Culture for candidiasis
▶ Patch testing (including oral flavors and preservatives)
▶ Psychiatric evaluation if indicated by history and review of systems
▶ Further consultation if indicated by dentistry, neurology, or otorhinolaryngology

Clinical assessment and outcome in 70 patients with complaints of burning or sore mouth. Drage LA, Rogers RS. Mayo Clin Proc 1998; 74: 223–8.

Seventy patients with a burning or sore mouth were retrospectively reviewed. The report lists etiologic agents of burning or sore mouth symptoms. Multiple etiologic factors were present in 37% of patients. The most frequently associated conditions were psychiatric disease (30%), xerostomia (24%), geographic tongue (24%), nutritional deficiency (21%), and allergic contact stomatitis (13%) to food additives. Tables on appropriate management and evaluation are included. Seventy percent of patients improved with tailored therapy.

Management of burning mouth syndrome: systematic review and management recommendations. Patton LL, Siegel MA, Benoliel R, De Laat A. Oral Surg Oral Med Oral Pathol Oral Radiol Endod 2007; 103: e1–13.

The authors review the concept of BMS as an oral dysesthesia or neuropathy and emphasize the need to investigate for treatable secondary causes. Topical clonazepam, cognitive therapy, and α-lipoic acid may be beneficial in some patients.

Interventions for the treatment of burning mouth syndrome. Zakrzewska JM, Forssell, H, Glenny AM. Cochrane Database of Systematic Reviews 2005; 25: CD 002779.

Nine trials on interventions for BMS were included in this review. Only three interventions demonstrated a significant reduction in BMS symptoms: α-lipoic acid, clonazepam, and cognitive behavioral therapy. Lack of efficacy of other interventions may be related to trial design or small sample size.

Psychiatric comorbidity in patients with burning mouth syndrome. Bogetto F, Malina G, Ferro G, Carbone M, Gandolfo S. Psychosom Med 1998; 60: 378–85.

In a case–controlled study 102 patients with burning mouth syndrome (BMS) were evaluated according to the diagnostic criteria of DSM-IV. High rates (71.6%) of comorbid psychiatric diagnoses were found, most commonly depressive disorders and generalized anxiety disorder. BMS also occurred in the absence of psychiatric diagnoses (28.4%).

FIRST-LINE THERAPIES

Tailor treatment to suspected cause of mouth pain:	
▶ Avoidance of irritants, especially alcohol-based mouthwashes and highly flavored dentifrices	E
▶ Avoidance of allergens documented on patch testing, especially flavorings and food additives such as propylene glycol, sorbic acid, cinnamon, mint	E
▶ Discontinuation of ACE inhibitors	D
▶ Sialogogues or artificial saliva for xerostomia	E
▶ Discontinuation of medications that cause xerostomia	E
▶ Assessment for parafunctional habits: clenching, tongue thrusting	E
▶ Reassurance that cancer is not present	E
▶ Denture evaluation and adaptation	C
▶ Replacement of vitamin B_6, B_{12}, iron, zinc, folate, riboflavin, thiamin	C
▶ Anti-yeast agents	C
▶ Appropriate evaluation and treatment of underlying psychiatric disease	C

The burning mouth syndrome. Huang U, Rothe MJ, Grant-Kels JM. J Am Acad Dermatol 1996; 34: 91–8.

Review of burning mouth syndrome with emphasis on contact allergy association. Evaluation and management strategies.

Type III burning mouth syndrome: psychological and allergic aspects. Lamey PJ, Lamb AB, Hughes A, Milligan KA, Forsyth A. J Oral Pathol Med 1994; 23: 216–19.

Of 33 patients with intermittent burning mouth syndrome (type III), 65% had positive patch tests to food additives or flavorings, and 80% of this group improved with avoidance of the documented allergen.

Stomatodynia (burning mouth) as a complication of enalapril therapy. Triantos D, Kanakis P. Oral Dis 2004; 10: 244–5.

A case report of burning mouth syndrome that improved after discontinuing enalapril. Summary of 10 additional cases of ACE inhibitors associated with burning mouth in the literature.

Patients complaining of a burning mouth. Main DMG, Basker RM. Br Dent J 1983; 154: 206–11.

In this study, 50% of cases of burning mouth were attributed to errors in denture design. With replacement of the dentures, the patients improved. Onset of symptoms coincidental with denture implementation or at the site of a denture should prompt referral for a formal dental consultation.

Candidiasis may induce glossodynia without objective manifestation. Osaki T, Yoneda K, Yamamoto T, Ueta E, Kimura T. Am J Med Sci 2000; 319: 100–5.

Of 98 patients, 26 had no objective signs of candidiasis but had hyposalivation and overgrowth of *Candida* on laboratory examination. Glossal pain subsided with treatment (3% amphotericin mouthwash solution).

SECOND-LINE THERAPIES

After evaluation, if no cause of mouth pain is identified, consider one of the following:	
▶ Low doses of tricyclic antidepressant	C
▶ Low-dose benzodiazepines or doxepin	C
▶ Topical capsaicin	E
▶ Topical clonazepam	B
▶ Gabapentin	E
▶ Amisulpride	C

Topical clonazepam in stomatodynia: a randomized placebo-controlled study. Gremeau-Richard C, Woda A, Navez ML, Attal N, Bouhassira D, Gagnieu MC, et al. Pain 2004; 108: 51–7.

Forty-eight BMS patients 'sucked and spit' a 1 mg tablet of clonazepam or placebo three times a day for 14 days. The reduction in pain scores was significantly more pronounced in the clonazepam than in the placebo group. The authors hypothesize that clonazepam acts locally to disrupt the mechanism(s) causing burning.

An open-label dose escalation pilot study of the effect of clonazepam in burning mouth syndrome. Grushka M, Epstein J, Mott A. Oral Surg Oral Med Oral Path Oral Radiol Endod 1998; 86: 557–61.

Clonazepam (a benzodiazepine) was used in increasing doses (starting at 0.25 mg and increasing by 0.25 mg weekly if continued). Seventy percent of patients noted some improvement. The authors propose that the action may be separate from the anxiolytic effect of benzodiazepines.

Oral medicine in practice: burning mouth syndrome. Lamey PJ, Lewis MAO. Br Dent J 1989; 167: 197–200.

These authors recommend doxepin (75–150 mg at night) for patients with depression, anxiety, or parafunctional habits.

Clinical characteristics and management outcome in burning mouth syndrome: an open study of 130 patients. Gorsky M, Silverman S, Chinn H. Oral Surg Oral Med Oral Pathol 1991; 72: 192–5.

Treatment with chlordiazepoxide (a benzodiazepine) was associated with remission in 15% of patients.

Effectiveness of gabapentin for treatment of burning mouth syndrome. White TL, Kent PF Kurtz, DB, Emko P. Arch Otolaryngol Head Neck Surg 2004; 130: 786–8.

Report of a case of burning mouth syndrome responsive to gabapentin.

Evidence Levels: **A** Double-blind study **B** Clinical trial ≥ 20 subjects **C** Clinical trial < 20 subjects **D** Series ≥ 5 subjects **E** Anecdotal case reports

Gabapentin has little or no effect in the treatment of burning mouth syndrome – results of an open-label pilot study. Heckmann SM, Heckmann JG, Ungethüm A, Hujoel P, Hummel T. Eur J Neurol 2006; 13: e6–e7.

Fifteen BMS patients volunteered for this pilot study using gabapentin titrated to a maximum of 2400 mg/day. Results showed little or no effect following treatment for an average of 33 weeks.

Capsaicin in burning mouth syndrome: titration strategies. Spice R, Hagen NA. J Otolaryngol 2004; 33: 53–4.

A commercial hot pepper product is used to combat burning mouth. Clear guidelines on use are included.

Burning mouth syndrome. Grushka M. Am Fam Phys 2002; 65: 615–20.

A practical review on the multiple etiologies and management of BMS.

Comparative efficacy of SSRIs and amisulpride in burning mouth syndrome: a single blind study. Maina G, Vitalucci A, Gandolfo S, Bogetto F. J Clin Psychiatry 2002; 63: 38–43.

Amisulpride was more effective than SSRIs.

THIRD-LINE THERAPIES

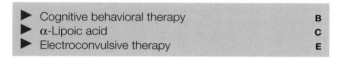

► Cognitive behavioral therapy	B
► α-Lipoic acid	C
► Electroconvulsive therapy	E

Cognitive therapy in the treatment of patients with resistant burning mouth syndrome: a controlled study. Bergdahl J, Anneroth G, Perris H. J Oral Pathol Med 1995; 24: 213–15.

A randomized control study examining the effects of cognitive therapy on resistant BMS in comparison to a 'placebo'

attention program. A statistically significant reduction in pain intensity for those receiving cognitive therapy was found.

Burning mouth syndrome (BMS): double blind controlled study of alpha-lipoic acid (thioctic acid) therapy. Femiano F, Scully C. J Oral Pathol Med 2002; 31: 267–9.

Sixty BMS patients received 200 mg α-lipoic acid (an over-the-counter supplement) or placebo tid for 2 months. Of the treated patients, 74% showed 'decided improvement' compared to 0% of those on placebo. α-Lipoic acid (thioctic acid) is an antioxidant and the authors speculate that BMS is a neuropathy related to free radical production.

Burning mouth syndrome: the efficacy of lipoic acid on subgroups. Femiano F, Gombos F, Scully C. J Eur Acad Dermatol Venereol 2004; 18: 676–8.

This study on two groups of 20 patients with BMS suggests that those not previously treated with tranquilizers respond better to therapy with α-lipoic acid than those who have received prior psychotropic therapy.

Burning mouth syndrome: open trial of psychotherapy alone, medication with alpha-lipoic acid (thioctic) and combination therapy. Fenciano F, Gombos F, Scully C. Medicina Oral 2004; 9: 8–13.

This open study of 192 BMS patients suggested that α-lipoic acid may complement psychotherapy and provide greater benefit than either modality alone.

Alpha-lipoic acid treatment of 31 patients with sore, burning mouth. Steele JC, Bruce AJ, Drage LA, Rogers RS 3rd. Oral Dis 2008; 14: 529–32.

In this retrospective study, 11 of 31 BMS patients benefited from taking α-lipoic acid.

Calcinosis cutis

Caroline Angit, Ian Coulson

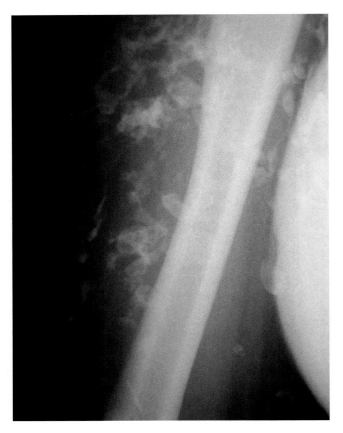

Calcinosis cutis is a rare disease of aberrant calcium deposition in the skin. There are four major types:

1. **Idiopathic** (occurs without tissue injury or metabolic defect)
2. **Dystrophic** (secondary to tissue damage/inflammation/neoplastic or necrotic skin but normal calcium and phosphate, e.g., scleroderma and dermatomyositis)
3. **Metastatic** (secondary to abnormal calcium and phosphate metabolism, e.g., renal failure, hyperparathyroidism)
4. **Iatrogenic** (secondary to treatment or procedure).

Other rare variants of calcinosis cutis that have been described including *calcinosis cutis circumscripta* (occurs earlier, tends to involve extremities), *calcinosis universalis* (occurs later, usually more widespread), *tumoral calcinosis* (often familial, autosomal recessive trait) and *transplant-associated calcinosis cutis* (in transplant recipients, mostly renal transplant, etiology unknown). Most lesions present as asymptomatic firm dermal papules, plaques, nodules, or subcutaneous nodules. Lesions may ulcerate, extrude chalky white material, or become infected. Stiffening of the skin can limit joint mobility and function, and fingertip lesions may be painful. Cutaneous gangrene and a diminished pulse can occur in severe cases.

Classification of calcinosis cutis

Box 1 types and examples

Type	Examples
Idiopathic	Calcinosis of scrotum, vulva
Dystrophic	Scleroderma, dermatomyositis
Metastatic	Renal failure, hyperparathyroidism
Iatrogenic	Calcium-containing paste for EMG electrodes, parenteral calcium administration

MANAGEMENT STRATEGY

The first step in management is to identify any underlying cause. Dystrophic calcification occurs in up to 10% of patients with scleroderma and 10–40% of patients with juvenile dermatomyositis, but is rare in systemic lupus erythematosus. Examination and investigations for connective tissue disease are therefore strongly recommended. Skin biopsy can help to distinguish cutaneous calcification from ossification.

A number of malignancies have been implicated in causing metastatic calcification (e.g., leukemia and multiple myeloma). However, successful treatment of the underlying cause does not always have an impact on calcinosis cutis, which frequently requires other treatment modalities. There are no large studies for the treatment of calcinosis cutis, and most therapies are based on case reports.

Spontaneous extrusion of calcium salts may occur; this may need *surgical* encouragement when calcification results in overlying ulceration (occasionally seen around chronic venous stasis ulcers). *Intralesional corticosteroids, aluminum hydroxide supplements, bisphosphonates, diltiazem, colchicine,* and *probenecid* have shown success, mostly in calcinosis associated with dermatomyositis. Low-dose *minocycline* has been reported to reduce the frequency of ulceration and inflammation associated with cutaneous calcinosis in patients with limited systemic sclerosis. The mechanism of action may be mainly through inhibition of matrix metalloproteinases and anti-inflammatory effects.

Warfarin has been advocated in both dermatomyositis and systemic sclerosis-associated calcinosis. *Carbon-dioxide laser vaporization* and *extracorporeal shock wave lithotripsy* are recent approaches that have been tried in cutaneous calcinosis secondary to CREST syndrome.

SPECIFIC INVESTIGATIONS

- ► Full blood count
- ► Urea and creatinine
- ► Serum calcium and phosphate
- ► Serum electrophoresis
- ► Creatine kinase
- ► Autoantibodies (e.g., antinuclear antibody, Scl 70)
- ► Parathyroid hormone levels
- ► Skin biopsy
- ► Soft tissue radiology

Evidence Levels: **A** Double-blind study **B** Clinical trial ≥ 20 subjects **C** Clinical trial < 20 subjects **D** Series ≥ 5 subjects **E** Anecdotal case reports

FIRST-LINE THERAPIES

▶ No treatment/self-healing	E
▶ Aluminum hydroxide	E E
▶ Intralesional corticosteroid	E

Self-healing dystrophic calcinosis following trauma with transepidermal elimination. Pitt AE, Ethington JE, Troy JL. Cutis 1990; 45: 28–32.

A case of dystrophic calcinosis following trauma that resolved over 8 weeks with spontaneous transepidermal elimination.

Calcinosis cutis and renal failure. Koltan B, Pederson J. Arch Dermatol 1974; 110: 256–7.

A 47-year-old man with metastatic calcinosis cutis secondary to chronic renal failure was successfully treated with oral aluminum hydroxide gel, 30 mL four times a day. After 8 weeks of treatment the patient had complete clearance of calcinosis cutis in all areas except the scrotum.

Calcinosis cutis in juvenile dermatomyositis: remarkable response to aluminum hydroxide therapy. Wang WJ, Lo WL, Wong CK. Arch Dermatol 1988; 124: 1721–2.

A 13-year-old girl with juvenile dermatomyositis complicated by calcinosis cutis was successfully treated with oral aluminum hydroxide and magnesium trisilicate administered four times a day. Clinical improvement of the calcification was observed within 8 months, and near complete clearance by the end of 1 year's therapy.

Calcinosis cutis in juvenile dermatomyositis responsive to aluminum hydroxide treatment. Nakagawa T, Takaiwa T. J Dermatol 1993; 20: 558–60.

A case of calcinosis cutis in juvenile dermatomyositis was successfully treated with oral aluminum hydroxide; near complete clearance was observed after 8 months of therapy. No adverse effects were reported.

Calcinosis cutis circumscripta. Treatment with an intralesional corticosteroid. Lee SS, Felsenstein J, Tanzer FR. Arch Dermatol 1978; 114: 1080–1.

A case report of a teenager with idiopathic calcinosis cutis over the knees, elbows, popliteal fossae, and wrist, successfully treated with intralesional triamcinolone diacetate (25 mg/mL) administered at monthly intervals via Dermojet injector and syringe and needle.

SECOND-LINE THERAPIES

▶ Bisphosphonates	E
▶ Diltiazem	D
▶ Probenecid	E
▶ Colchicine	E
▶ Minocycline	E

Disodium etidronate therapy for dystrophic cutaneous calcification. Rabens SF, Bethune JE. Arch Dermatol 1975; 111: 357–61.

A case report of a patient with extensive disabling dystrophic calcinosis cutis and possible scleroderma treated with oral disodium etidronate 10 mg/kg daily, showing arrest and partial reversal of the calcific process.

Regression of calcinosis associated with adult dermatomyositis following diltiazem therapy. Vinen CS, Patel S, Bruckner FE. Rheumatology 2000; 39: 333–40.

Case report of a patient with disabling calcinosis cutis secondary to dermatomyositis showing marked improvement following diltiazem therapy over 2.5 years. The dose was increased from 60 mg daily to 360 mg daily over 17 months.

An extremely severe case of cutaneous calcinosis with juvenile dermatomyositis, and successful treatment with diltiazem. Ichiki Y, Akiyama T, Shimozawa N, Suzuki Y, Kondo N, Kitajima Y. Br J Dermatol 2001; 144: 894–7.

A 3-year-old girl with a 2-year history of dermatomyositis developed multiple calcified nodules in the subcutaneous tissues and intermuscular fascia despite continual therapy with steroids and aluminium hydroxide. Treatment with diltiazem 30 mg/day completely suppressed the development of calcinosis and resulted in improvement of the calcinosis both clinically and radiologically 1 year after treatment.

Treatment of calcinosis with diltiazem. Palmieri GM, Sebes JI, Aelion JA, Moinuddin M, Ray MW, Wood GC, et al. Arthritis Rheum 1995; 38: 1646–54.

Diltiazem 240–480 mg/day was given to four patients with idiopathic or CREST-related calcinosis for 1–12 years. A fifth patient, who did not tolerate diltiazem, received verapamil 120 mg/day for 18 months. All patients taking diltiazem had a reduction or disappearance of the calcinosis, with striking clinical improvement. One patient developed a large calcific lesion while receiving verapamil for hypertension, but after verapamil was replaced with diltiazem there was a dramatic response. Verapamil was ineffective in the fifth patient.

Clinical significance of subcutaneous calcinosis in patients with systemic sclerosis. Does diltiazem induce its regression? Vayssairat M, Hidouche D, Abdoucheli-Baudot N, Gaitz JP. Ann Rheum Dis 1998; 57: 252–4.

Twelve patients with systemic sclerosis-associated subcutaneous calcinosis were treated with diltiazem 60 mg three times a day and had sequential hand radiographs (differential time between the two radiographs: 7.84 years); there was a slight radiological improvement in three patients only.

Calcinosis in dermatomyositis treated with probenecid. Skuterud E, Sydnes OA, Haavik TK. Scand J Rheumatol 1981; 10: 92–4.

Case report of childhood dermatomyositis with calcinosis responding to treatment with probenecid 250 mg daily. Resorption of soft tissue calcification was observed soon after the start of therapy.

Ulcerated dystrophic calcinosis cutis secondary to localised linear scleroderma. Vereecken P, Stallenberg B, Tas S, de Dobbeleer G, Heenen M. Int J Clin Pract 1998; 52: 593–4.

Case report of a 62-year-old woman with ulcerated dystrophic calcinosis cutis secondary to linear scleroderma. The ulceration healed after 4 months of treatment with colchicine 1 mg/day, without modification of the calcinosis.

Treatment of cutaneous calcinosis in limited systemic sclerosis with minocycline. Robertson LP, Marshall RW, Hickling P. Ann Rheum Dis 2003; 62: 267–9.

In an open-label study, eight out of nine patients with limited cutaneous systemic sclerosis prescribed minocycline 50 or 100 mg daily have shown definite improvement. The frequency of ulceration and inflammation associated with the calcinosis deposits decreased with treatment. The size of the calcinosis deposits also decreased but was less dramatic than expected. Improvement occurred at the earliest after 1 month of treatment with a mean of 4.8 months. The mean length of treatment was 3.5 years. Darkening of the calcinosis deposits to a blue/black colour was noted. One patient had unacceptable nausea and dizziness. None of the patients had changes in renal function, serology or developed a lupus-like illness.

THIRD-LINE THERAPIES

► Warfarin	C
► Surgery	C
► Carbon dioxide laser	E
► Extracorporeal shock wave lithotripsy	E
► Parathyroidectomy	E

Treatment of calcinosis universalis with low-dose warfarin. Berger RG, Featherstone GL, Raasch RH, McCartney WH, Hadler NM. Am J Med 1987; 83: 72–6.

A randomized double-blind study of eight patients with subcutaneous calcification secondary to either dermatomyositis or systemic sclerosis. Patients were treated with either warfarin 1 mg daily or placebo for 18 months. All patients had clinical assessment, plain radiographs, and whole-body bone scintigraphy to detect extraskeletal uptake. Two of the three patients in the warfarin-treated group had a reduction in extraskeletal uptake, as indicated by the bone scan scores, compared to none in the control group. No patient had a change in either clinical examination or plain radiographs.

Low dose warfarin treatment for calcinosis in patients with systemic sclerosis. Cukierman T, Elinav E, Korem M, Chajek-Shaul T. Ann Rheum Dis 2004; 63: 1341–3.

Three patients with disseminated subcutaneous calcinosis were treated with low doses of warfarin (1 mg/day) for 1 year. Two patients (relatively small lesions up to 2 cm in diameter) had complete resolution within 2 months. The other patient (larger and longer-standing lesions reaching up to 5 cm) did not respond to treatment. None of the patients showed a prolongation of prothrombin time, partial thromboplastin time, or an increased tendency for bleeding.

Surgical treatment of calcinosis cutis in the upper extremity. Mendelson BC, Linsheid RL, Dobyns JH, Muller SA. J Hand Surg 1977; 2: 318–24.

A case series of surgical experience on 11 patients with calcinosis cutis in the upper extremity, seven with systemic scleroderma and four with dermatomyositis. Four patients healed without complications and were not followed up. Of the seven follow-up patients, six found the procedure definitely beneficial.

Surgical management of calcinosis cutis universalis in systemic lupus erythematosus. Cousins M, Jones DB, Whyte M, Monafo WW. Arthritis Rheum 1997; 40: 570–2.

A case report of a 43-year-old woman with a 12-year history of SLE who presented with a large ulcerated calcinosis cutis lesion on her left hip which interfered with her waist and hip movement. Prednisone, colchicine, and hydroxychloroquine were ineffective. The lesion ($10 \times 20 \times 20$ cm calcified mass) was excised and the wound closed with split-thickness skin grafts. She began walking on the eight postoperative day, and the area was pain free and devoid of gross calcification at 6 months.

Successful palliation and significant remission of cutaneous calcinosis in CREST syndrome with carbon dioxide laser. Chamberlain AJ, Walker NP. Dermatol Surg 2003; 29: 968–70.

Six affected digits in a patient with CREST syndrome, having failed various medical therapies, received a single treatment with carbon dioxide laser vaporization using the Sharplan 1040 SilkTouch system. Treated digits healed over a 6-week period and led to a significant remission in symptoms, with an average remission time of at least 3 years, allowing the patient to remain in full-time employment.

Treatment of cutaneous calcinosis in CREST syndrome by extracorporeal shock wave lithotripsy. Sparsa A, Lesaux N, Kessler E, Bonnetblanc JM, Blaise S, Lebrun-Ly V, et al. J Am Acad Dermatol 2005; 53: S263–5.

A case report of a 78-year-old woman with extensive and painful leg wound ulcerations and calcifications secondary to CREST syndrome. After failure of various medical and surgical treatments and because of the severity of her symptoms, she was treated by extracorporeal shock-wave lithotripsy. The size of the ulcers and the pain diminished after the first session, and 1 month after treatment she was stone free on radiography. Two other sessions were performed after 2 months, resulting in reduced microcalcification and healing of the ulcer (ulcer size decreased from 20×12 cm to 12×7 cm). Unfortunately, the patient died after a femoral fracture.

Metastatic calcinosis cutis with renal hyperparathyroidism. Posey RE, Ritchie EB. Arch Dermatol 1967; 95: 505–8.

A case report of a 28-year-old woman with metastatic calcinosis cutis secondary to renal failure, which showed rapid resolution following panparathyroidectomy.

Calciphylaxis

Alexander Doctoroff

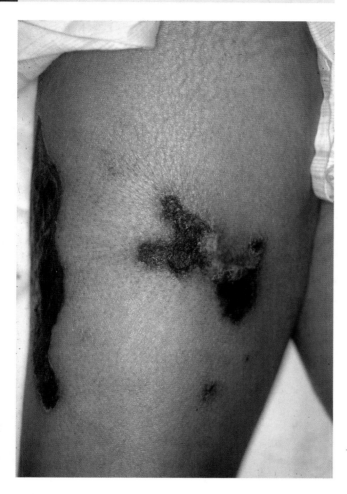

Calciphylaxis (calcific uremic arteriolopathy, uremic small-artery disease with medial calcification and intimal hyperplasia, vascular calcification–cutaneous necrosis syndrome, calcifying panniculitis) is a serious and often lethal condition that mainly affects patients with renal disease. Calciphylaxis may be considered the cutaneous equivalent of myocardial infarction. Medial calcification and subintimal fibrosis of arterioles result in arteriolar stenosis. This is followed by thrombotic occlusion and cutaneous necrosis. Calciphylaxis can present with either tender subcutaneous plaques, or skin ulcers reflecting various stages of the progression of disease.

MANAGEMENT STRATEGY

Because calciphylaxis is a deadly disease with a mortality rate of up to 80%, early diagnosis via skin biopsy and aggressive treatment are essential. Monitoring the patient's metabolic environment is of utmost importance. Hyperphosphatemia must be controlled with non-calcium-containing phosphate binders. A phosphorus-restricted diet should be introduced, and vitamin D supplementation stopped. Aggressive wound debridement needs to be initiated without delay. Monitoring

for infection and appropriate use of antibiotics are a mainstay of treatment, as most patient deaths occur from sepsis.

Intravenous sodium thiosulfate recently emerged as a promising new treatment for calciphylaxis. This medication is currently used as an antidote for the treatment of cyanide poisoning and the prevention of toxicity in cancer therapies. The mechanism of action is believed to be chelation of calcium, resulting in dissolution of calcium deposits. Additionally, sodium thiosulfate appears to act as an antioxidant, reducing damage from intravascular reactive oxygen species. The evidence in favor of sodium thiosulfate is limited to multiple case reports, yet it appears to be safe and nontoxic, and therefore deserves a trial as a first-line therapy for calciphylaxis.

If the patient's calciphylaxis is uncovered at an early stage (indurated plaques without ulcerations), oral prednisone appears to be helpful.

The use of zero- or low-calcium dialysate with induction of hypocalcemia and calcium shift into intravascular space appears to be a reasonable therapy. If hyperbaric oxygen therapy is available, it can be very helpful to some patients.

Parathyroidectomy, which improves calcium, phosphate, and parathyroid hormone levels, is a useful therapy for those patients with high parathyroid hormone levels. Despite being a subject of controversy, for many patients it results in rapid healing of ulcerations. Cinacalcet may also be used for patients with elevated parathyroid hormone. Parathyroid hormone should be monitored throughout the treatment to minimize the risk of adynamic bone disease associated with cinacalcet therapy.

The treatment of calciphylaxis should be a multidisciplinary effort with internists, critical care specialists, nephrologists, dermatologists, infectionists, surgeons, and pain specialists being involved.

SPECIFIC INVESTIGATIONS

▶ Skin biopsy
▶ Serum parathyroid hormone, calcium, phosphate
▶ Bone scan
▶ Measurements of transcutaneous oxygen saturation
▶ X-ray or xeroradiography
▶ Discussion of treatment

FIRST-LINE THERAPIES

▶ Debridement of necrotic tissue and aggressive wound care	C
▶ Discontinuation of calcium and vitamin D supplementation	C
▶ Reduction of serum phosphorus	C
▶ Treatment of low serum albumin	C
▶ Monitoring for infection	C
▶ Intravenous sodium thiosulfate	D
▶ Prednisone (for patients without ulcerations only)	C

Calcium use increases risk of calciphylaxis: a case-control study. Zacharias JM, Fontaine B, Fine A. Perit Dial Int 1999; 19: 248–52.

A retrospective case–control study of eight patients suggests an increased risk of calciphylaxis with calcium ingestion.

Risk factors and mortality associated with calciphylaxis in end-stage renal disease. Mazhar AR, Johnson RJ, Gillen D, Stivelman JC, Ryan MJ, Davis CL, et al. Kidney Int 2001; 60: 324–32.

A retrospective case–control study of 19 cases demonstrated female gender, hyperphosphatemia, high alkaline phosphatase, and low serum albumin to be risk factors for calciphylaxis.

Calciphylaxis: natural history, risk factor analysis, and outcome. Weenig RH, Sewell LD, Davis MD, McCarthy JT, Pittelkow MR. J Am Acad Dermatol 2007; 56: 569–79.

Retrospective case–control study of 64 cases showed that obesity, liver disease, systemic corticosteroid use, elevated calcium-phosphate product and serum aluminum were risk factors for calciphylaxis.

The evolving pattern of calciphylaxis: therapeutic considerations. Llach F. Nephrol Dial Transplant 2001; 16: 448–51.

This and other reviews suggest aggressive lowering of serum phosphorus with non-calcium-containing phosphate binders (such as Renagel), dietary control of calcium and phosphorus intake, as well as aggressive wound debridement and monitoring for infection. Six out of eight patients had a significant improvement with zero-calcium dialysate.

Sodium thiosulfate as first-line treatment for calciphylaxis. Ackermann F, Levy A, Daugas E, Schartz N, Riaux A, Derancourt C, et al. Arch Dermatol 2007; 143: 1336–7.

This is one of several case reports of successful calciphylaxis therapy with IV infusions of sodium thiosulfate (25 g IV infusions three times per week).

Calciphylaxis is usually non-ulcerating: risk factors, outcome and therapy. Fine A, Zacharias J. Kidney Int 2002; 61: 2210–17.

A review of 36 patients who presented without ulcerations but with subcutaneous indurated plaques in the legs demonstrated improvement with steroid therapy (prednisone 30–50 mg po daily for 3–8 weeks) in 80% of cases. Contraindications to steroid therapy include ulceration anywhere (related to PVD or calciphylaxis) or high risk of infection.

SECOND-LINE THERAPIES

► Parathyroidectomy (for patients with elevated parathyroid hormone)	C
► Hyperbaric oxygen therapy	D
► Low-calcium dialysate	D
► Cinacalcet	D
► Vitamin K supplementation in patients who are deficient	E
► Pamidronate	E
► Tissue plasminogen activator	E

Calciphylaxis: a syndrome of skin necrosis and acral gangrene in chronic renal failure. Hafner J, Keusch G, Wahl C, Burg G. Vasa 1998; 27: 137–43.

Meta-analysis of all case reports of calciphylaxis from 1936 to 1996 revealed that 70% of patients who were parathyroidectomized survived, compared to 43% of those who did not receive the operation.

This study did not stratify patients into those with and without hyperparathyroidism.

Hyperbaric oxygen in the treatment of calciphylaxis: A case series. Podymow T, Wherrett C, Burns KD. Nephrol Dial Transplant 2001; 16: 2176.

In this retrospective study, two out of five patients with calciphylaxis had complete resolution of their ulcers with hyperbaric oxygen therapy.

Successful treatment of severe calciphylaxis in a hemodialysis patient using low-calcium dialysate and medical parathyroidectomy: case report and literature review. Wang HY, Yu CC, Huang CC. Renal Failure 2004; 26: 77–82.

This is one of several case reports of successful calciphylaxis treatment with low-calcium dialysis.

Proximal calciphylaxis treated with calcimimetic 'Cinacalcet'. Mohammed IA, Sekar V, Bubtana AJ, Mitra S, Hutchison AJ. Nephrol Dial Transpl 2008; 23: 387–9.

A case report of successful calciphylaxis treatment with 3 mg/day of cinacalcet. Doses from 30 mg to 120 mg/day have been used in other cases.

Skin necrosis and protein C deficiency associated with vitamin K depletion in a patient with renal failure. Soundararajan R, Leehey DJ, Yu AW, Miller JB. Am J Med 1992; 93: 467–70.

Vitamin K replacement resulted in reversal of calciphylaxis in a vitamin K-deficient patient.

Rapid improvement of calciphylaxis after intravenous pamidronate therapy in a patient with chronic renal failure. Monney P, Nguyen QV, Perroud H, Descombes E. Nephrol Dial Transplant 2004; 19: 2130–2.

Five intravenous doses of 30 mg pamidronate resulted in healing of ulcerations in a patient whose clinical condition was worsening despite other medical therapy. When, 6 weeks after discharge, the calciphylaxis returned, an additional 30 mg pamidronate dose aborted the recurrence.

Low-dose tissue plasminogen activator for calciphylaxis. Sewell LD, Weenig RH, Davis MD, McEvoy MT, Pittelkow MR. Arch Dermatol 2004; 140: 1045–8.

Tissue plasminogen activator (tPA; alteplase) in 10-mg intravenous daily dose for 14 days, followed by warfarin anticoagulation, resulted in eventual healing of ulcerations.

THIRD-LINE THERAPIES

► Maggot therapy and pentoxyfillin	E
► Ozonetherapy	E
► Cryofiltration apheresis	E

Painful ulcers in calciphylaxis – combined treatment with maggot therapy and oral pentoxyfillin. Tittelbach J, Graefe T, Wollina U. J Dermatol Treat 2001; 12: 211–14.

Maggot therapy and 800 mg/day of oral pentoxyfillin were successful in healing of ulcers over a 6-month period.

Ozone therapy in a dialyzed patient with calcific uremic arteriolopathy. Biedunkiewicz B, Tylicki L, Lichodziejewska-Niemierko M, Liberek T, Rutkowski B. Kidney Int 2003; 64: 367–8.

Evidence Levels: **A** Double-blind study **B** Clinical trial ≥ 20 subjects **C** Clinical trial < 20 subjects **D** Series ≥ 5 subjects **E** Anecdotal case reports

Fifteen sessions of treatment with ozonated autohemotherapy (O3-AHT) with ozone concentration of 50–70 µg/mL over 3 weeks, accompanied by local wound lavage with ozonated water, led to healing of necrotic areas.

Intensive tandem cryofiltration apheresis and hemodialysis to treat a patient with severe calciphylaxis, cryoglobulinemia, and end-stage renal disease. Siami GA, Siami FS. J Am Soc Artif Intern Org 1999; 45: 229–33.

This is a report on tandem cryofiltration apheresis (CFA) and hemodialysis (HD) in a critically ill patient with type II mixed cryoglobulinemia, hepatitis C virus, calciphylaxis, and end-stage renal disease. The patient received 18 tandem CFA/HD treatments, and four extra HD treatments in 1 month. His plasma cryoglobulin level dropped and his calciphylaxis also improved.

Cutaneous candidiasis and chronic mucocutaneous candidiasis

Ali Banki, Steven R Cohen

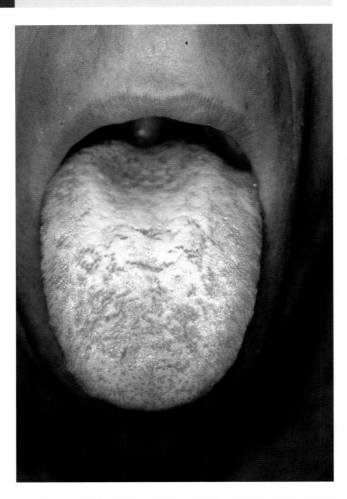

CUTANEOUS CANDIDIASIS

Cutaneous candidiasis is typically caused by *Candida albicans*, which exists as normal flora of human skin as well as in the gastrointestinal and genitourinary systems. Overgrowth of *Candida* species is suppressed by normal bacterial flora. Other *Candida* species occasionally cause mucocutaneous infections, the second most common being *Candida tropicalis*. Under certain conditions these *Candida* species overgrow and become pathogens. Warmth and moisture of the intertriginous skin (axilla, inguinal folds, abdominal creases, inframammary creases), an increased skin pH, and the administration of antibiotics can disrupt the normal bacterial flora, allowing *Candida* to proliferate. Clinically, candidiasis presents as scaly erythematous patches with satellite papules and pustules. The diagnosis is made either microscopically with a potassium hydroxide (KOH) preparation revealing spores and pseudo-hyphae, or by culture.

MANAGEMENT STRATEGY

Topical antifungal agents include but are not limited to polyenes, azoles, allylamines, and ciclopirox olamines.

Topical corticosteroids are a source of controversy. Although the addition of corticosteroids to local antifungal therapy may reduce local inflammation in acute candidiasis, their use should be limited to 1 or 2 days because of their immunosuppressant properties.

Systemic therapy, including amphotericin B, fluconazole, ketoconazole, voriconazole, and caspofungin, is indicated primarily for systemic candidiasis; however, oral administration of the appropriate drug is essential for cutaneous infections in immunosuppressed patients, or in the setting of extensive disease not responding to topical therapy.

SPECIFIC INVESTIGATIONS

> ▶ KOH
> ▶ Culture
> ▶ Urinalysis for sugar

Prospective aetiological study of diaper dermatitis in the elderly. Foureur N, Vanzo B, Meaume S, Senet P. Br J Dermatol 2006; 155: 941–6.

Of 46 patients, all over 85 years of age with dermatitis of the diaper area, 24 (63%) were due to candidiasis, six (16%) were attributed to irritant contact dermatitis, and the remaining cases were due to 'eczema' and 'psoriasis.' Concerning the patients with candidiasis, eight (33%) were cured after 1 month of topical therapy, three (12.5%) improved, and 13 (54%) were cured after the addition of oral fluconazole. This study identifies cutaneous candidiasis as the main cause of diaper dermatitis in the elderly. Although topical antifungal drugs represent the first line of treatment, more than half the patients in this study required an oral antifungal to achieve a complete cure.

***Candida parapsilosis* infection in a rose thorn wound.** Turkal NW, Baumgardner DJ. J Am Board Fam Pract 1995; 8: 484–5.

Candida parapsilosis should be recognized as an important nosocomial pathogen, which is also frequently associated with sporadic skin and appendage infections. Its association with environmentally acquired skin ulcers can mimic fixed cutaneous sporotrichosis. This report of soft tissue infection caused by *Candida parapsilosis* following a rose thorn puncture provides a brief review of *C. parapsilosis* infections, which account for up to 27% of fungemias in a large, hospital-based series. The frequent associations with medical devices and invasive procedures are emphasized.

FIRST-LINE THERAPIES

▶ Topical antifungal	A
▶ Topical antifungal combined with topical corticosteroids	A
▶ Systemic antifungal in immunosuppressed host	A

Evidence Levels: **A** Double-blind study **B** Clinical trial ≥ 20 subjects **C** Clinical trial < 20 subjects **D** Series ≥ 5 subjects **E** Anecdotal case reports

A multicenter, open-label study to assess the safety and efficacy of ciclopirox topical suspension 0.77% in the treatment of diaper dermatitis due to *Candida albicans*. Gallup E, Plott T. J Drugs Dermatol 2005; 4: 29–34.

A multicenter, open-label study which included 44 male and female subjects aged 6–29 months. The study medication was applied topically to the affected diaper area twice daily for 1 week. Subjects were clinically evaluated at baseline and at days 3, 7, and 14. The results showed a statistically significant improvement in both the rate of mycological cure and the reduction of severity score at each time point compared to baseline. Ciclopirox was safe and effective in the treatment of diaper dermatitis due to *C. albicans*.

Topical treatment of dermatophytosis and cutaneous candidiasis with flutrimazole 1% cream: double-blind, randomized comparative trial with ketoconazole 2% cream. Del Palacio A, Cuetara S, Perez A, Garau M, Calvo T, Sánchez-Alor G. Mycoses 1999; 42: 649–55.

A double-blind, randomized study in which the efficacy and tolerance of flutrimazole 1% cream was compared with ketoconazole 2% cream, applied once daily for 4 weeks, in 60 patients with culture-proven dermatophytosis (47 patients) or cutaneous candidiasis (13 patients). The results of this study showed that flutrimazole 1% cream is as safe and effective as ketoconazole 2% cream for *Candida* and dermatophyte skin infections.

Naftifine cream in the treatment of cutaneous candidiasis. Zaias N, Astorga E, Cordero CN, Day RM, de Espinoza ZD, DeGryse R, et al. Cutis 1988; 42: 238–40.

In a double-blind, parallel-group clinical trial, 60 patients with cutaneous candidiasis were randomly assigned to receive naftifine cream 1% or its vehicle twice a day for 3 weeks. Two weeks after the end of therapy, 77% of the naftifine-treated patients were mycologically cured (negative results on potassium hydroxide preparations and culture) and had no clinically apparent disease, compared to only 3% of patients treated with vehicle alone. Side effects reported with naftifine cream were few and minor.

A comparison of nystatin cream with nystatin/triamcinolone acetonide combination cream in the treatment of candidal inflammation of the flexures. Beveridge GW, Fairburn E, Finn OA, Scott OL, Stewart TW, Summerly R. Curr Med Res Opin 1977; 4: 584–7.

In a multicenter double-blind trial, 31 patients with bilateral candidal lesions of the flexures were treated for 14 days with nystatin cream on one side and with a combination of nystatin and triamcinolone acetonide cream on the other side. Both treatments proved equally effective in terms of mycological cure rate and clinical improvement. There was a weak trend by both patients and physicians to favor the combination preparation because symptoms resolved more rapidly.

Fluconazole versus ketoconazole in the treatment of dermatophytoses and cutaneous candidiasis. Stengel F, Robles-Soto M, Galimberti R, Suchil P. Int J Dermatol 1994; 33: 726–9.

In this multicenter, randomized, double-blind comparative trial patients were stratified into two groups: group 1 comprised patients with mycologically proven tinea corporis, tinea cruris, or cutaneous candidiasis treated for 2–4 weeks. Group 2 comprised patients with tinea pedis treated for 2–6

weeks. One hundred and fifty-eight patients were randomly assigned to receive one of the two treatment regimens: fluconazole 150 mg once weekly plus daily placebo (lactose), or ketoconazole 200 mg once daily plus weekly placebo for 2–6 weeks. Both treatments were clinically effective, with sites of infection responding equally to treatment with fluconazole and ketoconazole. Mycologic cure rates were seen in 68 of 73 fluconazole-treated patients and in 70 of 77 ketoconazole-treated patients. However, fluconazole offered the advantage of once-weekly oral administration.

SECOND-LINE THERAPIES

▶ Systemic antifungals	B

Antifungal activity of itraconazole and terbinafine in human stratum corneum. A comparative study. Pierard GE, Arrese JE, De Doncker P. J Am Acad Dermatol 1995; 32: 429–35.

Itraconazole 200 mg daily for 7 days was compared with terbinafine 250 mg daily for 14 days in the treatment of cutaneous candidiasis caused by *C. albicans*. Fifteen patients were included in each group. On follow-up, the treatment cure rate was 87% in the itraconazole group and 27% in the terbinafine group. Data correlated with previous stratum corneum ex vivo studies comparing both agents.

Clinical trials and double-blind studies of oral antifungals for cutaneous candidiasis are sparse.

THIRD-LINE THERAPIES

▶ Lavender oil	E
▶ Topical mupirocin	C

Antifungal activity of *Lavandula angustifolia* essential oil against *Candida albicans* yeast and mycelial form. D'Auria FD, Tecca M, Strippoli V, Salvatore G, Battinelli L, Mazzanti G. Med Mycol 2005; 43: 391–6.

The antifungal activity of the essential oil of *Lavandula angustifolia* Mill (lavender oil) and its main components, linalool and linalyl acetate, was studied for its effectiveness against 50 clinical isolates of *Candida albicans* (28 oropharyngeal strains, 22 vaginal strains). Growth inhibition, killing time, and inhibition of germ tube formation were evaluated. Lavender oil showed both fungistatic and fungicidal activity against *C. albicans* strains. At lower concentrations lavender oil inhibits germ tube formation and hyphal elongation, indicating that it is effective against *C. albicans* dimorphism and may thus reduce fungal progression and the spread of infection in host tissues.

Perianal candidosis – a comparative study with mupirocin and nystatin. De Wet PM, Rode H, Van Dyk A, Millar AJ. Int J Dermatol 1999; 38: 618–22.

A clinical trial to assess the efficacy and clinical outcome of 2% mupirocin in a polyethylene glycol base and nystatin cream as treatment regiments in diaper candidiasis. Eradication of all *Candida* organisms was achieved within 2–6 days (mean 2.6 days) in 10 patients receiving topical mupirocin therapy. Ten patients received topical nystatin cream, and in each case *Candida* was successfully cleared within 5 days (mean, 2.8 days). Both agents eradicated *Candida*, the major difference being in the marked response of the diaper dermatitis to mupirocin. Mupirocin should be applied topically three to four times daily or with each diaper change, and is an excellent antifungal agent.

CHRONIC MUCOCUTANEOUS CANDIDIASIS

Chronic mucocutaneous candidiasis (CMC) is a heterogeneous group of disorders with progressive and recurrent infections of the skin, nails, and mucosal surfaces with *Candida albicans*. Affected individuals have a defect in cell-mediated immunity that appears to be correlated with abnormalities in type 1 cytokines (reduction in IL-12, IL-2, and IFN-γ), as well as natural killer (NK) cells. CMC typically presents in childhood, with half of those affected developing autoimmune polyendocrinopathy candidiasis ectodermal dystrophy (APECED). APECED is characterized by hypoparathyroidism, hypothyroidism, and adrenal or gonadal failure. Malabsorption, gastric cell atrophy, or autoimmune hepatitis occur in about a third of patients. Alopecia, vitiligo, dental enamel dysplasia, and keratopathy are frequent associations.

MANAGEMENT STRATEGY

The work-up for CMC should start with positive identification of *C. albicans* by culture and sensitivities. Further tests include CBC with differential, HIV antibody test, and serum immunoglobulins (IgG, IgA, IgM, and IgE). Endocrine function tests should be assessed, including thyroid-stimulating hormone (TSH), fasting blood glucose, serum iron and ferritin levels, morning plasma cortisol levels, parathyroid hormone levels, and serum calcium levels. In HIV-negative patients with adult-onset CMC, a chest CT scan should be obtained to explore for thymoma.

Treatment options include systemic therapy with azoles (ketoconazole, itraconazole, and fluconazole), and amphotericin B. Newer second-generation azoles (voriconazole) and echinocandins (caspofungin) may be used for treatment-resistant candidiasis. Relapse occurs after withdrawal of these agents as the inherited immune defect remains. Therefore, therapeutic strategies that augment the immune response can be very beneficial, including transfer factor (orally or parenterally) or high-dose cimetidine.

SPECIAL INVESTIGATIONS

> ► CBC with differential
> ► HIV antibody test
> ► Immunoglobulins
> ► Thyroid-stimulating hormone (TSH)
> ► Fasting blood glucose
> ► Serum iron and ferritin
> ► Plasma cortisol level
> ► Parathyroid hormone
> ► Serum calcium
> ► Serum iron
> ► Chest X-ray
> ► CT scan if recommended

Fungal intracranial aneurysm in a child with familial chronic mucocutaneous candidiasis. Loeys BL, Van Coster RN, Defreyne LR, Leroy G. Eur J Pediatr 1999; 158: 650–2.

This report describes the rare association of CMC with an intracranial aneurysm, complicated by cerebral infarction, highlighting yet another risk of inadequately treated candidiasis.

New perspectives on the immunology of chronic mucocutaneous candidiasis. Lilic D. Curr Opin Infect Dis 2002; 15: 143–7.

This paper highlights the role of cell-mediated immunity in chronic mucocutaneous candidiasis. The associated abnormalities in type 1 cytokines appear to be the likely cause of predisposition to infection with *Candida* species. The respective roles of reduced type 1 cytokines and increased levels of IL-10 in CMC are reviewed.

Growth hormone deficiency in autoimmune polyglandular disease type I. Al-Herbish A, Bailey J, Kooh S. Saudi Med J 2000; 21: 765–8.

Two patients were diagnosed with autoimmune polyglandular disease type I. Both developed mucocutaneous candidiasis, hypoparathyroidism, vitiligo, and adrenocortical insufficiency. Both were noticed to have subnormal linear growth velocity and delayed bone age. Both showed subnormal stimulated serum growth hormone values, indicating growth hormone deficiency. A favorable response to growth hormone therapy was observed in one case.

Autosomal dominant familial chronic mucocutaneous candidiasis associated with acne rosacea. Ee HL, Tan HH, NS SK. Ann Acad Med Singapore 2005; 34: 571–4.

A new association is reported in a family (mother and non-identical twin sons) with distinctive acne rosacea and an autosomal dominant form of CMC lacking any clinical endocrinopathies.

FIRST-LINE THERAPIES

► Systemic azole antimycotics	C
► Systemic amphotericin	B
► Systemic echinocandins	E

Itraconazole in the treatment of two young brothers with chronic mucocutaneous candidiasis. Tosti A, Piraccini BM, Vincenzi C. Pediatr Dermatol 1997; 14: 146–8.

Two children affected by CMC involving the mouth and nails were successfully treated with itraconazole 200 mg/day for 2 months. A rapid cure rate of both infections was observed. The drug was very well tolerated.

Fluconazole in the management of patients with chronic mucocutaneous candidiasis. Hay RJ, Clayton YM. Br J Dermatol 1988; 119: 683–4.

In 13 patients with CMC and oroesophageal candidiasis who were treated with 50 or 200 mg of fluconazole daily, clinical and mycologic remissions were achieved over a mean of 10 days.

Voriconazole: a broad spectrum triazole for the treatment of serious and invasive fungal infections. Maschmeyer G, Haas A. Future Microbiol 2006; 1: 365–85.

This is an excellent review of voriconazole (a second-generation triazole) for treating life-threatening fungal infections. Voriconazole is available for intravenous or oral administration. It is effective for fluconazole-susceptible and -resistant candidiasis, invasive aspergillosis, and other serious fungal pathogens. Voriconazole is well tolerated. Although transient visual disturbances, liver enzyme abnormalities and skin rashes are the most common adverse events reported, these rarely lead to discontinuation of treatment.

Evidence Levels: **A** Double-blind study **B** Clinical trial ≥ 20 subjects **C** Clinical trial < 20 subjects **D** Series ≥ 5 subjects **E** Anecdotal case reports

Successful treatment of azole-resistant chronic mucocutaneous candidiasis with caspofungin. Jayasinghe M, Schmidt S, Walker B, Rocken M, Schaller M. Acta Dermatol Venereol 2006; 86: 563–4.

An 18-year-old woman was diagnosed with CMC caused by persistent and recurrent *C. albicans* infection of the skin, nails, and oral mucosa. At the age of 10 years, systemic treatment was started with daily fluconazole 4 mg/kg; with substantial improvement this was reduced to 2 mg/kg daily. After 3 years an azole-resistant strain of *C. albicans* was cultured from an oropharyngeal specimen. The patient was hospitalized with perioral erythematous erosive lesions, white plaques on the buccal mucosa, palate, and tongue, brownish discoloration of her finger nails, swelling, dystrophy, and periungual erythema. Following a 70 mg loading dose of intravenous caspofungin on the first day, the regimen was adjusted to 50 mg infusions four to seven times per week. Clinical improvement of oral and cutaneous candidiasis was sustained during a follow-up period of 12 months. The treatment was well tolerated and no drug-related toxicity was encountered.

Terbinafine effectiveness in ketoconazole-resistant mucocutaneous candidiasis in polyglandular autoimmune syndrome type 1. Hassan G. J Assoc Physicians India 2003; 51: 323.

Terbinafine was found to be effective in azole-resistant CMC.

SECOND-LINE THERAPIES

▶ Transfer factor	C
▶ Cimetidine	E
▶ Zinc sulphate	E

Case report: successful treatment with cimetidine and zinc sulphate in chronic mucocutaneous candidiasis. Polizzi B, Origgi L, Zuccaro G, Matti P, Scorza R. Am J Med Sci 1996; 311: 189–90.

The clinical efficacy of high-dose cimetidine, 400 mg three times daily, and zinc sulphate, 200 mg daily (subsequently adjusted to maintain blood zinc levels at the upper normal range), was evaluated in a patient with CMC for 16 months. An impressive reduction in infectious events was correlated with an increased CD4 (helper/inducer) cell count.

Transfer factor in chronic mucocutaneous candidiasis. Masi M, De Vinci C, Baricrdi OR. Biotherapy 1996; 9: 97–103.

Fifteen patients with CMC were treated with an in vitro-produced transfer factor (TF) specific for *C. albicans* antigens and/or with TF extracted from pooled buffy coats of blood donors: 400 million CEU per week for the first 2 weeks, followed by 100 million CEU per week for 6–12 months. All but one patient experienced significant improvement during treatment with specific TF.

Capillaritis (pigmented purpuric dermatoses)

Cord Sunderkötter, Thomas A Luger

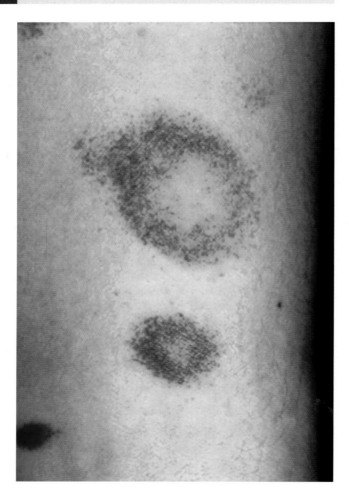

Capillaritis (a generic term for the various pigmented purpuric dermatoses) presents with the common feature of petechial macules or plaques and is characterized histologically by erythrocyte extravasation and perivascular infiltration with T lymphocytes. Lesions develop a characteristic brown to orange color due to hemosiderin deposits in macrophages. These conditions may also present with additional, distinctive, and sometimes overlapping morphological patterns, which have given rise to several descriptive or eponymous names: papules in pigmented purpuric lichenoid dermatosis of Gougerot and Blum; eczematous spongiosis with pruritus in eczematoid-like or itching purpura; annular forms with telangiectases in Majocchi's disease; and often solitary, ochre-golden plaques or patches with bandlike infiltrates including a grenz zone in lichen aureus. The etiology of capillaritis, including these variants, is not known. The reason for extravasation of erythrocytes is unclear, because inflammatory fibrinoid necrosis of vessels (vasculitis) cannot be demonstrated.

MANAGEMENT STRATEGY

Diagnostic hallmarks are the yellow-brown or orange patches with superimposed pinpoint cayenne pepper spots, which represent petechiae and persist with diascopy. The main differential diagnosis is leukocytoclastic vasculitis. The discerning criterion is the lack of a palpable infiltrate in capillaritis, but there are variants of vasculitis with petechial maculae (e.g., as part of Sjögren's syndrome). Thus, biopsies are warranted when in doubt.

In the differential diagnosis, contact allergic dermatitis may be hemorrhagic, mimicking capillaritis. Thrombocytopenia, hypergammaglobulinemic purpura of Waldenström, and rare cases of mycosis fungoides also need to be excluded. Although the majority of the cases have a completely benign course, capillaritis has recently been reported to precede cases of cutaneous T-cell lymphoma.

Usually there is no need for treatment unless the patient has pruritus or suffers from cosmetic disfigurement. Detection and avoidance of possible eliciting agents should always be attempted. Reported causes include:

- Drugs (14% in one series), e.g., thiamine, bromine-containing drugs, carbamazepine, furosemide, acetaminophen, non-steroidal anti-inflammatory drugs (NSAIDs), raloxifene (selective estrogen receptor modulator), interferon-α. As a rule, drug-induced capillaritis is more generalized and does not usually present with epidermal involvement or lichenoid infiltrate. Other reported triggers include dietary supplements (creatine) and the ingredients of an energy drink (vitamin B complex, caffeine, taurin).
- Chronic infections such as viral hepatitis B or C or odontogenic infections.

When the etiology remains obscure therapy has to be somewhat empirical. However, immunohistochemical analyses have suggested a cell-mediated immune response, so treatment with *local corticosteroids, calcineurin inhibitors, or psoralen plus UVA* (PUVA) may be rational. Increased venous pressure (particularly in the legs) or exercise are not direct causes, but can sometimes aggravate capillaritis. In these cases compression stockings may be helpful.

There is some evidence for increased vascular permeability or vascular fragility due to subtle defects in the extracellular matrix. This may explain reported responses to *bioflavonoids* (which may be due to inhibition of elastase and hyaluronase and of leukocyte activation), *ascorbic acid* (antioxidant effects and perhaps reduction of vascular permeability), and *calcium dobesilate* (reduction of microvascular permeability in part by antioxidant properties).

SPECIFIC INVESTIGATIONS

▶ C-reactive protein, differential blood count (thrombocytopenia, leukemia, chronic infections)
▶ IgG, IgM, IgA in serum (in patients with symmetrical petechial and slightly hemorrhagic macules to exclude monoclonal gammopathy; when raised → serum protein electrophoresis)
▶ Histology – whenever in doubt, to exclude vasculitis, mycosis fungoides (criteria for capillaritis are dense lichenoid infiltrate, hemosiderin deposits in the upper dermis, extravasal erythrocytes)
▶ Careful drug history
▶ Look for signs of chronic infection or rheumatoid arthritis
▶ Exclude contact eczema, chronic venous insufficiency
▶ Dermatoscopy

Purpura simplex (inflammatory purpura without vasculitis): a clinicopathologic study of 174 cases. Ratnam KV, Su WP, Peters MS. J Am Acad Dermatol 1991; 25: 642–7.

A retrospective review of 174 cases. A correlation between purpuric reaction and drugs was observed in 14%. Of the 87 patients who were followed up, 67% appeared to eventually have clearing of lesions.

Progression of pigmented purpura-like eruptions to mycosis fungoides: report of three cases. Barnhill RL, Braverman IM. J Am Acad Dermatol 1988; 19: 25–31.

CD8-positive mycosis fungoides presenting as capillaritis. Ameen M, Darva A, Black MM, McGibbon DH, Russell-Jones R. Br J Dermatol 2000; 142: 564–7.

Drug-induced chronic pigmented purpura. Nishioka K, Katayama I, Masuzawa M, Yokozeki H, Nishiyama S. J Dermatol 1989; 16: 220–2.

A close correlation between purpuric reaction and drugs was observed in seven cases of chronic pigmented purpura. The drugs included thiamine propyldisulfide and chlordiazepoxide. The purpuric lesions ceased after withdrawal of drug intake.

Drug-induced purpura simplex: clinical and histological characteristics. Pang BK, Su D, Ratnam KV. Ann Acad Med Singapore 1993; 22: 870–2.

A prospective study of 183 patients with purpura simplex was carried out. Of these, 27 cases were confirmed to be drug induced, as the purpura cleared within 4 months of withdrawal of medications – NSAIDs, diuretics, meprobamate, and ampicillin were the commonest offenders.

Acetaminophen-induced progressive pigmentary purpura (Schamberg's disease). Abeck D, Gross GE, Kuwert C, Steinkraus V, Mensing H, Ring J. J Am Acad Dermatol 1992; 27: 123–4.

Capillaritis: a manifestation of rheumatoid disease. Wilkinson SM, Smith AG, Davis M, Dawes PT. Clin Rheumatol 1993; 12: 53–6.

Seven cases of capillaritis were described in patients with rheumatoid arthritis. In the majority, the rash resolved spontaneously with the use of a topical corticosteroid to treat the symptom of itch.

Pigmented purpuric dermatosis and hepatitis profile: a report on 10 patients. Dessoukey MW, Abdel-Dayem H, Omar MF, Al-Suweidi NE. Int J Dermatol 2005; 44: 486–8.

Of 10 patients, 5 had antibodies against hepatitis C virus and two against hepatitis B virus.

Chronic pigmented purpura associated with odontogenic infection. Satoh T, Yokozeki H, Nishioka K. J Am Acad Dermatol 2002; 46: 942–4.

Five patients with chronic pigmented purpura associated with odontogenic infection were resistant to topical corticosteroid treatment, but the appearance of purpuric spots ceased after treatment for periodontitis, pulpitis, or both. No circulating immune complexes or perivascular deposits of immunoglobulins were detected.

Capillaritis associated with interferon-alfa treatment of chronic hepatitis C infection. Gupta G, Holmes SC, Spence E, Mills PR. J Am Acad Dermatol 2000; 43: 937–8.

Dermoscopy of pigmented purpuric dermatoses (*lichen aureus*): a useful tool for clinical diagnosis. Zaballos P, Puig S, Malvehy J. Arch Dermatol 2004; 140: 1290–1.

Dermatoscopy is a useful aid in diagnosis. In lichen aureus, in which the lichenoid tissue reaction is condensed, it shows coppery-red to brownish diffuse coloration of the background (this could be caused by the dermal infiltrate and extravascular or intracellular hemosiderin) as well as a partial network of interconnected pigmented lines (hyperpigmentation of the basal layer and pigment released into the dermis) and round to oval red dots, globules or patches (these could reflect dilated vessels and extravasated erythrocytes) and gray dots (probably accumulation of hemosiderin-containing macrophages). It is likely that these criteria also apply for other forms of capillaritis with different accentuations.

FIRST-LINE THERAPIES

▶ Local corticosteroids initially in cases of pruritus/ eczematoid or itching purpura	D
▶ PUVA	D
▶ Calcium dobesilate	D
▶ Oral bioflavonoids and ascorbic acid	E
▶ Compression stocking when aggravated by increased venous pressure	E

Capillaritis: a manifestation of rheumatoid disease. Wilkinson SM, Smith AG, Davis M, Dawes PT. Clin Rheumatol 1993; 12: 53–6.

Seven cases of capillaritis were described in patients with rheumatoid arthritis. In the majority, the rash resolved spontaneously with the use of a topical corticosteroid to treat the symptom of itch.

PUVA therapy in lichen aureus. Ling TC, Goulden V, Goodfield MJ. J Am Acad Dermatol 2001; 45: 145–6.

One case of lichen aureus that responded dramatically to photochemotherapy (PUVA).

A report of two cases of pigmented purpuric dermatoses treated with PUVA therapy. Wong WK, Ratnam KV. Acta Dermatol Venereol 1991; 71: 68–70.

Successful treatment of two patients with PUVA.

Calcium dobesilate (Cd) in pigmented purpuric dermatosis (PPD): a pilot evaluation. Agrawal SK, Gandhi V, Bhattacharya SN. J Dermatol 2004; 31: 98–103.

Nine male patients (seven with Schamberg's disease and one each with lichenoid dermatosis of Gougerot and Blum and lichen aureus) were given calcium dobesilate 500 mg twice daily for 2 weeks initially, and then 500 mg once daily for 3 months. No new lesions occurred within 2 weeks, and itching ceased in all patients. Follow-up continued for 1 year after cessation of therapy. The improvement of existing lesions was moderate in 11.11% and mild in 66.67% of cases; 22.22% did not show any improvement.

Treatment of progressive pigmented purpura with oral bioflavonoids and ascorbic acid: an open pilot study in 3 patients. Reinhold U, Seiter S, Ugurel S, Tilgen W. J Am Acad Dermatol 1999; 41: 207–8.

Rutoside (50 mg twice daily) (a form of bioflavonoid, often available without prescription) and ascorbic acid (500 mg twice daily) were administered orally to three patients with chronic progressive pigmented purpura in an open pilot study. Complete clearance of skin lesions was achieved after 4 weeks of treatment in all three patients, and persisted for 3 months after treatment.

Since then, more than 10 patients have been treated successfully (U. Reinhold, personal communication).

The treatment of progressive pigmented purpura with ascorbic acid and a bioflavonoid rutoside. Laufer F. J Drugs Dermatol 2006 5: 290–3.

This is only a case report, but it is consistent with the previously reported efficacy of this drug combination and with our own experience (Schneider SW, Thomas K, Sunderkötter C, Bonsmann G, unpublished). We therefore prefer this combination (rutoside 50 mg twice daily and ascorbic acid 500 mg twice daily).

SECOND-LINE THERAPIES

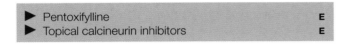

▶ Pentoxifylline	**E**
▶ Topical calcineurin inhibitors	**E**

Successful treatment of Schamberg's disease with pentoxifylline. Kano Y, Hirayama K, Orihara M, Shiohara T. J Am Acad Dermatol 1997; 36: 827–30.

Three patients with Schamberg's disease were treated with pentoxifylline 300 mg daily for 8 weeks. A significant response was observed within 2–3 weeks. One patient had recurrence after discontinuation of this treatment, but promptly responded to resumption of therapy.

Schamberg's purpura: association with persistent hepatitis B surface antigenemia and treatment with pentoxifylline. Wahba-Yahav AV. Cutis 1994; 54: 205–6.

A 54-year-old man experienced extensive Schamberg's purpura 3 months after an episode of hepatitis B. He was treated orally with pentoxifylline, 400 mg three times daily. After 3 months the purpuric elements had disappeared and pigmentation had faded.

Segmental lichen aureus: combination therapy with pentoxifylline and prostacyclin. Lee HW, Lee DK, Chang SE, Lee MW, Choi JH, Moon KC, et al. J Eur Acad Dermatol Venereol 2006 20: 1378–80.

A 17-year-old Korean girl had segmental lichen aureus that responded well to oral combination therapy with pentoxifylline and prostacyclin (PGI_2).

Resolution of lichen aureus in a 10-year-old child after topical pimecrolimus. Böhm M, Bonsmann G, Luger TA. Br J Dermatol 2004; 150: 519–20.

A 10-year-old boy presented with lichen aureus resistant to topical corticosteroids for 4 months. A significant improvement was observed within 3 weeks with pimecrolimus cream twice daily.

Unlike topical corticosteroids, topical immunomodulators do not cause fragility of blood vessels, which is an advantage when treating this group of diseases thought to be caused by vascular fragility and permeability.

THIRD-LINE THERAPIES

▶ Colchicine	**E**
▶ Griseofulvin	**E**
▶ Ciclosporin	**E**

Benefit of colchicine in the treatment of Schamberg's disease. Geller M. Ann Allergy Asthma Immunol 2000; 85: 246.

Successful treatment of pigmented purpuric dermatosis with griseofulvin. Tamaki K, Yasaka N, Osada A, Shibagaki N, Furue M. Br J Dermatol 1995; 132: 159–60.

Only a solitary case report attests to the efficacy of griseofulvin.

Purpura pigmentosa chronica successfully treated with oral cyclosporin A. Okada K, Ishikawa O, Miyachi Y. Br J Dermatol 1996; 134: 180–1.

The authors would not recommend ciclosporin because of the severity of possible side effects.

Cat scratch disease

Adam H Wiener, Bryan A Selkin, George J Murakawa

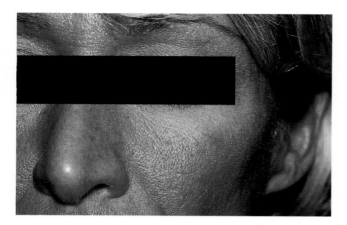

Cat scratch disease (CSD) is a benign, usually self-limited disease caused by *Bartonella henselae* (formerly *Rochalimaea henselae*), a Gram-negative pleomorphic rod. The primary lesion consists of a 0.5–1 cm papule or pustule, which may undergo ulceration, and adjacent unilateral lymphadenopathy is the hallmark of the disease. Systemic symptoms and complications include low-grade fever, malaise, nonspecific exanthem, hepatosplenomegaly, lytic bone lesions, oculoglandular syndrome of Parinaud (granulomatous conjunctivitis and preauricular adenopathy), and encephalopathy.

MANAGEMENT STRATEGY

No clear guidelines for the treatment of CSD exist. As there is a paucity of data showing a clear benefit of antimicrobial therapy in the treatment of patients with mild to moderate CSD, these patients should be managed with *conservative, symptomatic treatment*. The lymphadenopathy associated with CSD is self-limited and resolves in 2–4 months; therefore, most patients can be managed with *observation* until involution of the node.

For patients with systemic symptoms and/or complications, antibiotic therapy should be instituted. *Azithromycin* (500 mg on day 1, followed by 250 mg on days 2–5) is the only antibiotic that has been shown in a double-blind placebo-controlled evaluation to be beneficial to immunocompetent patients with CSD. In a retrospective analysis of 202 patients with CSD who had been on at least 3 days of antimicrobial therapy, only four antibiotics (*rifampin, ciprofloxacin, gentamicin,* and *trimethoprim-sulfamethoxazole*) provided clinical benefit. Presumably, it is the paucity of organisms and the host inflammatory response that result in the poor efficacy of antibiotics.

In immunosuppressed patients infection with the CSD bacillus can produce a spectrum of disease, from classic CSD to bacillary angiomatosis (BA), peliosis, or septicemia (see Bacillary angiomatosis, page 72). Antimicrobial treatment for such patients is beneficial and clearly indicated. Lesions and symptoms respond rapidly to *erythromycin* 500 mg four times daily or *doxycycline* 100 mg twice daily. Other antimicrobials used to successfully treat BA in immunocompro-mised patients include *tetracycline, minocycline, azithromycin,* and *trimethoprim-sulfamethoxazole*. A Jarisch–Herxheimer reaction frequently occurs after the first dose. Patients with AIDS should be maintained on lifelong antimicrobial therapy.

Of note, *B. henselae* has rarely been isolated from patients with CSD; however, patients who are immunosuppressed may be culture positive. A single dose of oral antibiotics will rapidly sterilize blood and lesional cultures.

SPECIFIC INVESTIGATIONS

► Histopathology
► Culture
► Serology
► Polymerase chain reaction (PCR)-based techniques

The agent of bacillary angiomatosis. Relman DA, Loutit JS, Schmidt TM, Falkow S, Tompkins LS. N Engl J Med 1990; 323: 153–80.

PCR was used to amplify, clone, and sequence a portion of eubacterial 16S rRNA gene directly from tissue infected with the presumed agent of BA. Subsequent analysis of this sequence and study of infected tissues from other patients suggested that BA is caused by a rickettsia-like organism closely related to *Rochalimaea quintana*.

Bartonella-associated infections. Spach DH, Koehler JE. Infect Dis Clin North Am 1998; 12: 137–55.

Findings on lymph node biopsy specimens from immunocompetent patients with CSD depend on the stage of the infection. Early in the course, lymphoid hyperplasia and arteriolar proliferation are prominent. Subsequently, granulomas appear. Late in the disease, multiple stellate microabscesses are prominent. Warthin–Starry stains may show clumps of pleomorphic bacilli.

Cat scratch disease in Connecticut: epidemiology, risk factors and evaluation of a new diagnostic test. Zangwill KM, Hamilton DH, Perkins BA, Regnery RL, Plikaytis BD, Hadler JL, et al. N Engl J Med 1993; 320: 8–13.

Serologic testing for the presence of antibodies to *B. henselae* is most widely used for laboratory confirmation of CSD. Indirect fluorescent antibody (IFA) assay has a sensitivity of 88% and a specificity of 97%. However, the IFA assay is not yet widely available and depends to some degree on subjective interpretation.

Cat-scratch disease. Midani S, Ayoub EM, Anderson B. Adv Pediatr 1996; 43: 397–422.

PCR is a powerful tool for the detection of *B. henselae* but is not widely available. Using PCR, *B. henselae* can be detected in aspirates from lymph nodes or cutaneous lesions within 1–2 days. Currently, serologic and PCR-based analyses are considered definitive.

Detection by immunofluorescence assay of *Bartonella henselae* in lymph nodes from patients with cat scratch disease. Rolain JM, Gouriet F, Enea M, Aboud M, Raoult D. Clin Diagn Lab Immunol 2003; 10.4: 686–91.

Immunofluorescence detection (IFD) in lymph node smears using a specific monoclonal antibody directed against *B. henselae* and a commercial serology assay (IFA) compared with PCR detection showed high specificity in diagnosis of *B. henselae*, especially when associated with histological analysis and conventional bacterial culture.

The use of *Bartonella henselae*-specific age dependent IgG and IgM in diagnostic models to discriminate diseased from non-diseased in cat scratch disease serology. Herremans M, Vermeulen MJ, Van de Kassteele J, Bakker J, Schellekens JF, Koopmans MP. J Microbiol Meth 2007; 71: 107–13.

The use of diagnostic models using the combination of both the ELISA IgM and the IgG results combined with a correcting age factor can be useful in serodiagnosis of CSD.

FIRST-LINE THERAPY

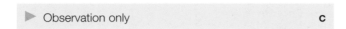

> ▶ Observation only   C

Bartonellosis. Murakawa GJ, Berger T. In: Freedberg IM, Eisen AZ, Wolff K, Austen KF, et al., eds. Dermatology in general medicine, 5th edn. New York: McGraw-Hill, 1999; 2249–56.

In the majority of patients with CSD, conservative management with careful observation over several months is sufficient. Spontaneous involution of lymphadenopathy should occur over 6 months.

SECOND-LINE THERAPIES

> ▶ Azithromycin   A

Prospective randomized double blind placebo-controlled evaluation of azithromycin for treatment of cat-scratch disease. Bass JW, Freitas BC, Freitas AD, Sisler CL, Chan DS, Vincent JM, et al. Pediatr Infect Dis J 1998; 17: 447–52.

Seven of 14 azithromycin-treated patients (500 mg on day 1, followed by 250 mg on days 2–5) showed an 80% reduction in initial lymph node volume compared to one of 15 placebo-treated controls during the first 30 days of observation.

This is the only controlled clinical trial of an antibiotic for the therapy of CSD; the use of all other antibiotics is based on anecdotal reports.

THIRD-LINE THERAPIES

> ▶ Erythromycin   C
> ▶ Doxycycline   C
> ▶ Rifampin   C
> ▶ Ciprofloxacin   C
> ▶ Gentamicin   C
> ▶ Trimethoprim-sulfamethoxazoler   C
> ▶ Surgical intervention   C

Immunocompetent individuals

Antibiotic therapy for cat-scratch disease: clinical study of therapeutic outcome in 268 patients and a review of the literature. Margileth AM. Pediatr Infect Dis J 1992; 11: 474–8.

In 60 patients with CSD with systemic symptoms, one of four antibiotics was effective at least 72% of the time. Patients who received rifampin (10–20 mg/kg daily for 7–14 days), ciprofloxacin (20–30 mg/kg daily for 7–14 days), gentamicin (5 mg/kg daily intravenously in divided doses every 8 hours for at least 3 days) or trimethoprim-sulfamethoxazole (6–8 mg/kg of trimethoprim component two to three times daily for 7 days) had a shorter mean duration of post-treatment illness

than those who received either no antibiotics or antibiotics thought to be ineffective.

Antimicrobial susceptibility of *Rochalimaea quintana*, *Rochalimaea vinsonii*, and the newly recognized *Rochalimaea henselae*. Maurin M, Raoult D. J Antimicrob Chemother 1993; 32: 587–94.

In-vitro testing revealed β-lactam drugs to be ineffective, tetracyclines to be intermediate, and erythromycin and rifampin to be most effective against *Rochalimaea* spp.

Hepatosplenic cat-scratch disease in children: selected clinical features and treatment. Arisoy ES, Correa AG, Wagner ML, Kaplan SL. Clin Infect Dis 1999; 28: 78–84.

Sixteen children with hepatosplenic CSD treated with rifampin (15–20 mg/kg daily), either alone or in combination with gentamicin (7.5 mg/kg daily) or trimethoprim-sulfamethoxazole (10–12 mg/kg daily) showed clinical improvement within 1–5 days.

Successful treatment of cat-scratch disease with ciprofloxacin. Holley HP. JAMA 1991; 265: 1563–5.

Five patients treated with oral ciprofloxacin, 500 mg twice daily, had a dramatic improvement in symptoms within a few days, with no relapse during follow-up. It should be noted that quinolones are not recommended for children or adolescents because of concerns about arthropathy. Moreover, in-vitro studies show only intermediate efficacy for ciprofloxacin.

Cat-scratch disease of the head and neck in a pediatric population: surgical indications and outcomes. Munson PD, Boyce TG, Salomao DR, Orvidas LJ. Otolaryngol Head Neck Surg 2008; 139: 358–63.

In children, failure of medical therapy in cases that presented as persistent lymphadenopathy often were accompanied by violaceous skin changes, extreme tenderness to palpation, and even chronic drainage. In this subgroup of patients the benefit of surgical intervention and concurrent tissue examination outweighed the risk.

Immunosuppressed individuals

Molecular epidemiology of *Bartonella* infections in patients with bacillary angiomatosis-peliosis. Koehler JE, Sanchez MA, Garrido CS, Whitfeld MJ, Chen FM, Berger TG, et al. N Engl J Med 1997; 337: 1876–83.

Treatment with macrolide antibiotics (e.g., erythromycin or clarithromycin) is protective for patients with *Bartonella* spp. infection.

Cat scratch disease, bacillary angiomatosis, and other infections due to *Rochalimaea*. Adal KA, Cockerell CJ, Petri WA. N Engl J Med 1994; 330: 1509–15.

For the treatment of BA, bacillary peliosis hepatis, and *Rochalimaea* spp. bacteremic syndrome, erythromycin 500 mg four times daily is the drug of choice on the basis of an excellent clinical response in virtually all patients treated to date.

Cutaneous vascular lesions and disseminated cat-scratch disease in patients with the acquired immunodeficiency syndrome (AIDS) and AIDS-related complex. Koehler JE, LeBoit PE, Egbert BM, Berger GT. Ann Intern Med 1988; 109: 449–55.

Erythromycin (500 mg four times daily), rifampin, and doxycycline (100 mg twice daily) were effective in the treatment of angiomatous skin nodules in three patients with HIV infection.

Cellulite

Bruce E Katz, Doris M Hexsel

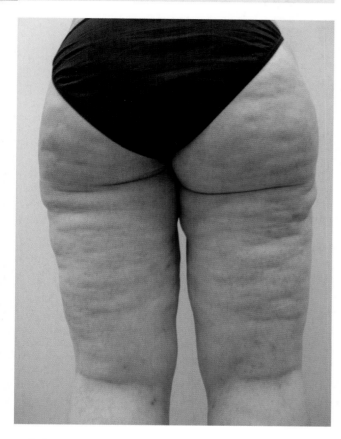

Cellulite may be defined as the surface relief alterations that give the skin an orange-peel, cottage cheese, or mattress-like appearance. The lesions tend to be asymptomatic and may be considered the anatomic expressions of the structures in the affected area, such as the fat and subcutaneous septa. Females are most frequently affected by this condition. Cellulite occurs mainly on the thighs and buttocks, but may also be found on the arms, abdomen, and legs.

MANAGEMENT STRATEGY

In managing cellulite, the aim is to obtain aesthetic improvement. This may be achieved by means of:

1. *Diet, weight control* (preferably maintaining a body mass index (BMI) between 19 and 24), and *physical exercise.*
2. Treatment of possible associated conditions, such as circulatory alterations, edema, obesity, endocrine alterations, and flaccidity.
3. Specific treatments:
   - *Subcision*
   - *Lasers, radiofrequency and ultrasound* (Triactive, Velasmooth, and Velashape, Accent, and others)
   - *Mechanical treatments* (e.g., Endermologie and massage)
   - Topical treatment (e.g., many different compounds of doubtful value).

SPECIFIC INVESTIGATIONS

▶ No investigation is routinely required

So called cellulite: an invented disease. Nurnberger F, Muller G. Dermatol Surg Oncol 1978: 4: 221–9.

This was the first study in which the anatomic basis for cellulite was demonstrated. The authors showed, by means of biopsies taken from the thighs and buttocks of 150 cadavers and 30 living women with cellulite, that the adipose tissue is projected into the dermis, forming the so-called 'papillae adipose' that are responsible for the mattress-like appearance on the skin surface.

An exploratory investigation of the morphology and biochemistry of cellulite. Rosenbaum M, Prieto V, Hellmer J, Boschmann M, Krueger J, Leibel RL, et al. Plast Reconstruct Surg 1998; 101: 1934–9.

This study evaluated cellulite by means of biopsies, sonographic examination, and physiologic examination of the thighs of seven individuals. In those with cellulite, the studies showed a diffuse pattern of extrusion of underlying adipose tissue into the reticular dermis. This study also found differences between the sexes. Women had a diffuse pattern of irregular discontinuous connective tissue immediately below the dermis, but in men this same layer was smooth and continuous.

Anatomy of subcutaneous structures in areas with and without cellulite depressions by magnetic resonance imaging. Hexsel D, Abreu M, Rodrigues TC, Soirefmann M, Lima MM, Zechmeister do Prado D. Dermatol Surg 2008; (in press).

This observational study evaluated 30 patients by magnetic resonance imaging (MRI) regarding the presence and characteristics of the fibrous septa in buttocks with and without cellulite. MRI showed fibrous septa in 96.7% of the subjects in the areas with cellulite depression; most of them were ramified (73.3%) and presented a high-intensity signal on T_2-weighted scans (70%), suggesting a liquid compound. All fibrous septa found in the examined areas were perpendicular to the skin surface. The thickness of fibrous septa in the areas with cellulite depressions varied from 0.1 to 4 mm (2.18± 0.89), whereas in the area without cellulite it varied from 0.1 to 2 mm (0.27±0.64). This was the first study to show a significant presence of thick vascular–fibrous septa in the subcutaneous areas of the great majority of cellulite depressions compared to the areas without cellulite, analyzed by MRI and special skin markers.

FIRST-LINE THERAPIES

▶ Subcision   **B**
▶ Lasers and radiofrequency devices   **C**

Subcision: a treatment for cellulite. Hexsel DM, Mazzuco R. Int J Dermatol 2000; 39: 539–44.

In this paper the authors give a description of the subcision procedure and report the results based on a sample of 232 patients. Subcision was shown to be efficient in the treatment of high-level cellulite, such as degrees II and III. This technique improves the major depressions on the skin surface of patients with cellulite through three mechanisms of action: sectioning the connective tissue septa responsible for the depressions; provoking the formation of new connective tissue from blood components; and redistributing the adipose tissue and the mechanical forces between the adipose lobules.

An innovative surgical technique that has recently generated scientific interest.

A study evaluating the safety and efficacy of the VelaSmooth system in the treatment of cellulite. Sadick N, Margo C. J Cosmet Laser Ther 2007; 9: 15–20

Sadick and Margo studied the VelaSmooth system, a combination of radiofrequency energy, infrared light, and mechanical manipulation of the skin and fat. Sixteen patients with cellulite were treated twice weekly for 6 weeks, with one thigh serving as the control and the other as the treatment site. The investigator and an independent evaluator determined the efficacy via circumference measurements of both thighs before and after treatments. Thigh circumference decreased in nearly 72% of the treated legs. The mean decrease was 0.44 cm of the lower thigh and 0.52 cm of the upper thigh. The investigators also noted significant visual improvements in cellulite and skin texture. Overall, 50% of subjects had greater than 25% improvement. The study suggested using higher energy levels and increased frequency of treatments to optimize results.

A single center randomized, comparative, prospective clinical study to determine the efficacy of VelaSmooth system versus the Triactive system for the treatment of cellulite. Nootheti PK, Magpantay A, Yosowitz G, Calderon S, Goldman M. J Cosmet Laser Ther 2006; 38: 908–12.

Nootheti and colleagues compared the TriActive (combination of low-energy diode laser, contact cooling, suction, and massage) and VelaSmooth (combination of infrared and radiofrequncy energies) systems in 20 women for the treatment of cellulite. Each patient was treated with TriActive on one leg and VelaSmooth on the other. Patients were evaluated with photographs and circumferential thigh measurement before treatment and after the final treatment. Both devices reduced the appearance of cellulite. However, no significant difference could be determined with regard to reduction in thigh circumference, photographic evaluation, or perceived change in before- and- after photographic images between the two devices.

Effect of controlled volumetric tissue heating with radiofrequency on cellulite and the subcutaneous tissue of the buttocks and thighs. Emilia del Pino M, Rosado RH, Azuela A, Graciela Guzmán M, Argüelles D, Rodríguez C, et al. J Drugs Dermatol 2006; 5: 714–22.

The authors used real-time ultrasound image scanning to evaluate the effect of non-invasive high-energy radiofrequency to the skin of the thigh and buttocks in 26 women aged 18–50. Patients were treated in two sessions 15 days apart using a unipolar RF device (Accent, Alma Lasers Inc.). The unipolar energy was delivered in three passes of 30 seconds each, and the thickness of the subcutaneous tissue on the buttocks and thighs was evaluated at baseline, before the second treatment, and 15 days after the second treatment by real-time scanning ultrasound. From the measurements of the distance between the stratum corneum to Camper's fascia and from the stratum corneum to the muscle the investigators were able to demonstrate that 68% of the patients showed a contraction in volume of approximately 20%. The investigators concluded that two RF treatments on the subcutaneous tissue of the buttocks

and thigh provided volumetric contraction in the majority of patients, and proposed that this effect should be the same on any other body part.

SECOND-LINE THERAPIES

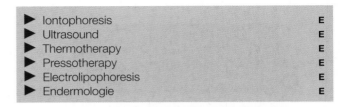

▶ Iontophoresis	E
▶ Ultrasound	E
▶ Thermotherapy	E
▶ Pressotherapy	E
▶ Electrolipophoresis	E
▶ Endermologie	E

Analysis of the effects of deep mechanical massage in the porcine model. Adcock D, Paulsen S, Jabour K, Davis S, Nanney LB, Shack RB. Plast Reconstruct Surg 2001; 108: 233–40.

This study evaluated the effects of deep mechanical massage in the dermis and hypodermis of pigs. Histologic examination of the areas submitted to the treatment showed a greater accumulation of dense longitudinal collagen.

Reductions in thigh and infraumbilical circumference following treatment with a novel device combining ultrasound, suction, and massage. Foster KW, Kouba DJ, Hayes J, Freeman V, Moy RL. J Drugs Dermatol 2008; 7: 113–15.

In this pilot study five patients were treated with a device that combines computerized massage, vacuum suction, and ultrasound with a continuous sinusoidal pulse delivered at a frequency of 3 Hz. A total of 12 treatments were performed on a semiweekly basis to two abdomens and three pairs of thighs. The treatments were well tolerated and without side effects. The results observed after 12 treatments were similar to or better than those seen with other minimally invasive body-contouring devices.

THIRD-LINE THERAPIES

▶ Topical products	C
▶ Oral supplements	C

Botanical extracts used in the treatment of cellulite. Hexsel D, Orlandi C, Zechmeister do Prado D. Dermatol Surg 2005; 31: 866–72; discussion 872.

The reduction in fat deposits through the continuous use of anti-cellulite products depends on the availability of the active ingredient at the action site, the concentration of the ingredient in the formulation, and the physiochemical characteristics particular to each active ingredient. The botanicals used in topical products must have standardized extracts, which would permit each phytomedicine to have the same effect anywhere in the world.

A randomized, placebo-controlled trial of topical retinol in the treatment of cellulite. Piérard-Franchimont CP, Piérard GE, Henry F, Vroome V, Cauwenbergh G. Am J Clin Dermatol 2000; 1: 369–74.

A controlled study in 15 women who had requested liposuction for the improvement of cellulite assessed a topical product containing retinol versus a placebo formulation. Prior to liposuction the women used topical retinol once a day on one leg and placebo on the other. After 6 months of treatment, the elasticity of the skin had increased 10.7% and the viscosity had diminished 15.8% on the side treated with the product containing retinol.

A two-center, double-blinded, randomized trial testing the tolerability and efficacy of a novel therapeutic agent for cellulite reduction. Rao J, Gold MH, Goldman MP. J Cosmet Dermatol 2005; 4: 93–102.

Forty women with a moderate degree of cellulite participated in a double-blinded, randomized trial where an anti-cellulite cream was applied nightly to the affected sites for 4 continuous weeks. Each subject was randomized to receive active cream on either the right or the left leg, with the contralateral side serving as control. Bioceramic-coated neoprene shorts were worn overnight to enhance penetration of the topical agents by occlusion. Five blinded independent physician reviewers assessed high-quality digital photographs for improvement. Subject questionnaires were completed to assess tolerability and efficacy. The authors concluded that the active topical agent used in this study was found to be effective in reducing the appearance of cellulite. All subjects tolerated the formulation well, with no adverse effects.

Modification of subcutaneous adipose tissue by a methylxanthine formulation: a double-blind controlled study. Lesser T, Ritvo E, Moy LS. Dermatol Surg 1999; 25: 455–62.

A placebo-controlled, double-blind study in 41 patients evaluated a product containing liposome-encapsulated caffeine in concentrations of 1% or 2%. The product was used daily for 2 months on the thighs, arms, buttocks, and abdomen. The final assessment of the treatment concluded that both concentrations of the cream significantly reduced the thickness of the adipose tissue in all treated areas.

Effects of caffeine and siloxanetriol alginate caffeine, as anticellulite agents, on fatty tissue: histological evaluation. Velasco MV, Tano CT, Machado-Santelli GM, Consiglieri VO, Kaneko TM, Baby AR. J Cosmet Dermatol 2008; 7: 23–9.

This study analyzed the effects of topical caffeine and siloxanetriol alginate caffeine on fatty tissue by histological evaluation on female Wistar mice. The emulsion with caffeine caused a reduction of 17% on the diameter of the fatty cells compared to the control. Emulsion with SAC was considered more indicated to promote the lipolytic action on fatty tissue,

acting as a complement to treat cellulite. When sodium benzoate was added to the preparations it inhibited the efficiency of the caffeine. Gel was not an adequate vehicle to be incorporated with caffeine and SAC.

Evaluation of the effects of caffeine in the microcirculation and edema on thighs and buttocks using the orthogonal polarization spectral imaging and clinical parameters. Lupi O, Semenovitch IJ, Treu C, Bottino D, Bouskela E. J Cosmet Dermatol 2007; 6: 102–7.

A new non-invasive method, orthogonal polarization spectral imaging, evaluated skin microvascular alterations in patients with cellulite who used an anti-cellulite drug composed mainly of 7% caffeine. The results showed that microcirculatory parameters did not change significantly after treatment. Smoking as well as alcohol consumption and regular physical activity were not significantly related to the centimetric reduction observed in treated thighs and hips.

Treating cellulite. Gasbarro V, Vettorello GF. Cosmet Toiletries 1992; 107: 64–6.

This study evaluated extract of *Aesculus hippocastanum* in the treatment of cellulite. The results showed that 80% of patients reduced by one clinical stage of cellulite, and in 4% of these there was a reduction in the circumference of the thigh.

Addition of conjugated linoleic acid to a herbal anticellulite pill. Birnbaum L. Adv Ther 2001; 18: 225–9.

The treatment of cellulite with herbal anti-cellulite pills, together with supplements of conjugated linoleic acid in 60 female volunteers, showed that 75% of the patients who used the supplement obtained a beneficial effect.

A double-blind evaluation of the activity of an anti-cellulite product containing retinol, caffeine and ruscogenine by a combination of several non-invasive methods. Bertin C, Zunino H, Pittet JC, Beau P, Pineau P, Massonneau M, et al. J Cosmet Sci 2001; 52: 199–210.

This study assessed an anti-cellulite product containing retinol microcapsules, caffeine, Asian centella, ruscus and L-carnitine. The efficacy parameters included the appearance of the cellulite after treatment, histology, cutaneous flowmetry, and the mechanical characteristics of the skin. The results showed improvement in cellulite in the treated areas.

Cellulitis and erysipelas

Adrian HM Heagerty

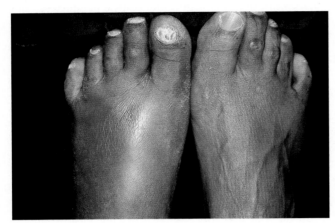

From Lebwohl MG. The Skin and Systemic Disease: A Color Atlas, 2nd edn. Churchill Livingstone 2003, with permission of Elsevier.

Cellulitis is strictly an acute, subacute, or chronic infection of the subcutaneous tissues, whereas erysipelas is an infection of the dermis and superficial subcutis. Infection of the more superficial layers gives rise to superficial edema and inflammation, with the consequent development of a palpable, often advancing edge. The causative organism is usually regarded as *Streptococcus*, though many organisms have been isolated, including *Haemophilus influenzae*, and more rarely staphylococci, *Aeromonas hydrophilia*, and *Pseudomonas aeruginosa*, as well as Gram-negative rods and fungi. Fulminating and necrotic cellulitis and fasciitis may occur rarely, usually in relation to immunosuppression or atypical organisms.

MANAGEMENT STRATEGY

The management of cellulitis and erysipelas should initially be directed to trying to *identify the organism responsible for the infection*, and then directing *appropriate antimicrobial therapy*. Any underlying and predisposing condition should be identified and treated to prevent subsequent recurrence. Perhaps the commonest condition that is not identified and treated is toe web tinea pedis, which provides a portal of entry for infection.

Uncomplicated cellulitis and erysipelas may be managed without admission if the patient does not exhibit signs of systemic toxicity. In such cases *oral broad-spectrum antibiotics*, chosen to cover group A streptococci and staphylococci, may be sufficient, supplemented with a single parenteral loading dose or long-acting preparation. The drug of choice is *oral penicillin V (phenoxymethylpenicillin) with or without flucloxacillin*, or *erythromycin*, if the patient has a known penicillin allergy. Some authorities have recommended the use of clindamycin rather than a macrolide because of apparent increased tissue penetration, but this may be associated with an increased incidence of *Clostridium difficile* superinfection. Further, although most group A β-hemolytic streptococci are sensitive to this, increasing numbers of MRSA are displaying resistance to clindamycin, and widespread use may exacerbate this resistance.

Immunocompromised patients, those with signs of systemic toxicity, and otherwise debilitated patients should be treated as inpatients with *intravenous antimicrobials* (such as penicillin G (benzylpenicillin)) or *one of the newer antibiotics* (such as ciprofloxacin, ticarcillin, teicoplanin, or imipenem/cilastatin). If there is evidence of head and neck disease or sinus infection, *amoxicillin combined with clavulanic acid* should be considered to cover *H. influenzae* infection.

Sites of entry for infection should be sought, such as excoriations in eczema or following trauma, and these should be treated.

SPECIFIC INVESTIGATIONS

- ▶ Blood cultures
- ▶ Cultures of aspirates and lesions
- ▶ Skin scrapings for mycology

Blood cultures may be positive and significant in only about 25% of cases, but should always be taken if there is any evidence of systemic toxicity. Swabs of wounds and broken skin may be helpful, but surface swabs of unbroken skin provide little or no useful information. If available, aspirate of bullae may yield positive cultures. Slightly better rates for isolation than those of needle aspirates have been achieved with punch skin biopsies. Rising titers of streptococcal antibodies may be helpful.

In the case of cellulitis or erysipelas of the lower leg, skin scrapings from toe webs should be taken for mycological examination. Facial erysipelas should warrant sinus radiographs to exclude underlying sinusitis. Crepitus should prompt the clinician to the presence of either clostridia or non-spore-forming anerobes, either alone or mixed with other bacteria such as *Pseudomonas*, *Escherichia coli*, or *Klebsiella* spp.

FIRST-LINE THERAPIES

▶ Penicillin G	B
▶ Penicillin G with flucloxacillin	B
▶ Penicillin V	B
▶ Amoxicillin with clavulanic acid	B
▶ Oral versus parenteral antibiotics	B
▶ Ceftriaxone versus flucloxacillin	A
▶ Roxithromycin	B

The course, costs and complications of oral versus intravenous penicillin therapy of erysipelas. Jorup-Ronstrum C, Britton S, Gavlevik A, Gunnarsson K, Redman AC. Infection 1984: 12; 390–4.

In this study of 60 patients there appeared to be no appreciable benefit from intravenous rather than oral therapy with penicillin for erysipelas, and so oral therapy is recommended if there are no associated complications with the infection.

Management and morbidity of cellulitis of the leg. Cox NH, Colver GB, Paterson WD. J Roy Soc Med 1998: 91; 634–7.

A case note review of 92 patients admitted for inpatient care for ascending cellulitis of the leg revealed a portal of entry, most commonly minor injury. The mean hospital stay was 10 days. Bacteriology was seldom helpful, but group G

132

streptococci were the most frequently identified pathogens. Benzylpenicillin was used in 43 cases (46%).

The authors emphasize the need for benzylpenicillin, treatment of tinea pedis, and retrospective diagnosis of streptococcal infection by serology.

Case survey of management of cellulitis in a tertiary teaching hospital. Aly AA, Roberts NM, Seipol KS, MacLellan DG. Med J Aust 1996: 165; 553–6.

This retrospective survey examined the management of 118 patients with lower limb cellulitis in a tertiary teaching hospital. In 79% of cases there was underlying disease, but only 20% were investigated. Blood cultures were taken from 55%, all with negative results. A combination of flucloxacillin and penicillin was given intravenously for a mean of 6 days to 76% of patients, and where documented 94% responded within 5 days. However, 40% of patients had intravenous therapy for longer than this, and 10% for 10 days or more. The length of inpatient stay averaged 13 days, prolonged stay being associated with surgical intervention or intercurrent problems, but 15% of patients had no clear indication for an extended stay. The authors concluded that excessive microbiological investigations, inadequate investigation, and treatment of underlying disease with prolonged use of intravenous antibiotics and questionable use of combinations of antibiotic therapy were common.

Skin concentrations of phenoxymethylpenicillin in patients with erysipelas. Sjoblom AC, Bruchfeld J, Eriksson B, Jorup-Rönström C, Karkkonen K, Malmborg AS, et al. Infection 1992; 20: 30–3.

Tissue and serum blood levels were measured in 45 patients with erysipelas after oral penicillin (phenoxymethylpenicillin), and the minimal inhibitory concentrations were exceeded for streptococci isolated, supporting the role of oral therapy.

A randomized comparative study of once-daily ceftriaxone and 6-hourly flucloxacillin in the treatment of moderate to severe cellulitis. Clinical efficacy, safety and pharmacoeconomic implications. Vinen J, Hudson B, Chan B, et al. Clin Drug Invest 1996; 12: 221–5.

A randomized comparative study in 58 patients with cellulitis; intravenous ceftriaxone cured 92%, but intravenous flucloxacillin cured only 64% after 4–6 days.

Roxithromycin versus penicillin in the treatment of erysipelas in adults: a comparative study. Bernard P, Plantin P, Roger H, Sassolas B, Villaret E, Legrain V, et al. Br J Dermatol 1992; 127: 155–9.

This prospective randomized multicenter trial compared oral roxithromycin with intravenous benzylpenicillin. Overall efficacy was similar.

Amoxicillin combined with clavulanic acid for the treatment of soft tissue infections in children. Fleischer GR, Wilmott CM, Capos JM. Antimicrob Agents Chemother 1983; 24: 679–81.

Amoxicillin with clavulanic acid was compared with cefaclor in children with impetigo and cellulitis due to staphylococci, streptococci, and *Haemophilus* sp. There was a 100% response to therapy with the combination, compared to 90% with the cephalosporin; the incidence of relapse and re-infection and side effects was small, but greater with the combination therapy.

Nurse-led management of uncomplicated cellulitis in the community: evaluation of a protocol incorporating intravenous ceftriaxone. Seaton RA, Bell E, Gourlay Y, Semple L. J Antimicrob Chemother 2005; 55: 764–7.

The safety and efficacy of a nurse-led outpatient parenteral antibiotic therapy service for cellulitis were examined in 114 patients and 230 historical controls. No alteration in outcomes, complications, or readmission rates was seen compared to the earlier physician-supervised outpatient treatment. Treatment duration was reduced from 4 to 3 days.

Prospective evaluation of the management of moderate to severe cellulitis with parenteral antibiotics at a paediatric day treatment centre. Gouin S, Chevalier I, Gautier M, Lamarre V. Paediatr Child Health 2008; 44: 214–18.

The clinical outcomes of 92 children receiving outpatient treatment in a day treatment centre were examined prospectively, and after a mean of 2.5 days of intravenous therapy 73 patients (79.3%) were switched to oral agents and discharged from the day treatment centre. There were no relapses in this group.

There is an increasing trend for the use of parenteral antibiotics given out of hospital for the treatment of cellulitis, either at home or in a day treatment centre.

SECOND-LINE THERAPIES

▶ Ciprofloxacin	**B**
▶ Teicoplanin	**B**
▶ Imipenem/cilastatin	**B**

Ciprofloxacin for soft tissue infections. Wood MJ, Logan MN. J Antimicrob Chemother 1986: 18; 159–64.

Twenty-one patients with cellulitis or other soft tissue infection were treated with oral ciprofloxacin; 19 were clinically cured or improved, and one was withdrawn from the study because of nausea and vomiting. Nine of the original 18 bacterial isolates were eradicated, but the majority of failures were due to staphylococci and streptococci.

Teicoplanin in the treatment of skin and soft tissue infections. Turpin PJ, Taylor GP, Logan MN, Wood MJ. J Antimicrob Chemother 1988: 21; 117–22.

Twenty-four patients with cellulitis or other soft tissue infection were treated with once-daily teicoplanin, resulting in clinical cure or improvement without severe adverse reactions, but with a rise in the plasma platelet count.

Twice daily intramuscular imipenem/cilastatin in the treatment of skin and soft tissue infections. Sexton DJ, Wlodaver CG, Tobey LE, Yangco BG, Graziani AL, MacGregor RR. Chemotherapy 1991: 37; 26–30.

Of 102 patients enrolled in this study with mild to moderately severe skin and soft tissue infections, 74 were evaluable, with 20 having cellulitis, 23 wound infections, and 31 abscesses. Imipenem/cilastatin was given intramuscularly using doses of 500 or 750 mg 12-hourly. In this study there was no assessment by type of infection, but 82% were cured and 16% improved. Eight patients reported minor side effects.

THIRD-LINE THERAPIES

▶ Prednisolone as an adjunct to antibiotics	A
▶ Granulocyte colony-stimulating factor (G-CSF)	A
▶ Hyperbaric oxygen	E

Antibiotic and prednisolone therapy of erysipelas: a randomized, double blind, placebo-controlled study. Bergkvist PI, Sjobeck K. Scand J Infect Dis 1997: 29; 377–82.

Although prednisolone may predispose to infection, its use in combination with intravenous antibiotics reduced the median time to cure by 1 day (5 vs 6 days); at the 90th percentile healing time was 10 days vs 14.6 days, and median hospital stay was reduced from 6 days to 5. The relapse rate within 3 weeks was approximately the same in both groups.

Randomized placebo controlled trial of granulocyte-colony stimulating factor in diabetic foot infection. Gough A, Clapperton M, Rolando N, Foster Foster A. Lancet 1997; 350: 855–9.

This randomized controlled trial compared the ability of G-CSF to improve clinical outcome in the treatment of cellulitis in diabetes mellitus, using resolution as the endpoint. The G-CSF stimulates the neutrophil response, which is impaired in diabetes mellitus, but is important for defense against infection. The risk is principally that of high white cell counts, which may predispose to coronary and cerebral vascular events.

Cellulitis owing to *Aeromonas hydrophilia*: treatment with hyperbaric oxygen. Mathur MN, Patrick WG, Unsworth IP, Bennett FM. Aust NZ J Surg 1995: 65; 367–9.

This case report of *Aeromonas hydrophilia* cellulitis, unresponsive to antibiotics and surgical debridement, responded to hyperbaric oxygen therapy. Although there are few objective reports of similar treatment in streptococcal necrotizing fasciitis, it has been suggested that in all types of necrotizing fasciitis hyperbaric oxygen reduces mortality.

PROPHYLAXIS

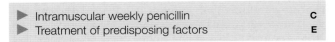

| ▶ Intramuscular weekly penicillin | C |
| ▶ Treatment of predisposing factors | E |

Prophylactic antibiotics in erysipelas. Duvanel T, Merot Y, Saurat JH. Lancet 1985; 1: 1401.

Sixteen patients who received weekly intramuscular penicillin as prophylaxis were followed and assessed at 2 years. On cessation of prophylaxis the risk of recurrence rapidly returned to the non-treatment/no prophylaxis level.

Cellulitis and erysipelas. Morris A. Clin Evid 2004; 12: 2268–74.

Although there is a consensus that successful treatment of predisposing factors such as leg edema, tinea pedis, and traumatic wounds reduces the risk of developing cellulitis, there are no randomized controlled trials or observational studies to support these.

Chancroid

Patricia A Henry, Glenn C Newell

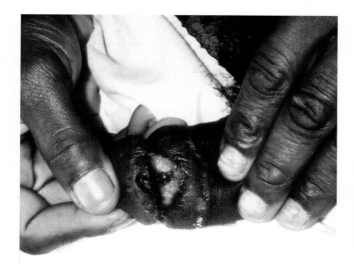

Chancroid is a genital ulcer disease caused by the Gram-negative facultative anaerobic bacillus *Haemphilus ducreyi*. It is common in many parts of the world, including Africa, the Caribbean basin, and southwest Asia. In more developed countries the incidence of chancroid appears to be decreasing. Chancroid typically is described as a painful, ragged, deep genital ulcer 3–20 mm in diameter. There may be surrounding erythema, and the base is often covered with a yellow-gray exudate. The lesion may be single, but can be multiple as a result of autoinoculation (kissing lesions). Painful lymphadenitis occurs in 30–60% of patients, and approximately one-quarter of patients with lymphadenopathy may develop a suppurating bubo. The groove sign (more typical of lymphogranuloma venereum) has been described.

MANAGEMENT STRATEGY

Diagnosis on clinical criteria alone is difficult. The painful ulcer of chancroid can easily be confused with genital herpes. Syphilis, especially if secondarily infected, can also mimic chancroid. The ulcer of chancroid may be transient and the disease may then be present as painful lymphadenopathy suggesting lymphogranuloma venereum. Co-infection with herpes simplex virus (HSV) or *Treponema pallidum* occurs in as many as 10% of patients, making the diagnosis more confusing. The combination of a painful genital ulcer with tender suppurative lymphadenopathy is the only clinical presentation that is nearly pathognomonic. Chancroid has been noted to increase the susceptibility to human immunodeficiency virus (HIV) infection, probably by disrupting mucosal integrity, thereby allowing a portal of entry for HIV.

A definitive diagnosis may be made by culturing the exudates from the ulcer base or by aspiration of a bubo. Gram stain of the ulcer base in chancroid may show Gram-negative coccobacilli in a 'school of fish' appearance. Special culture media need to be used, and the specimen should be handled by laboratories familiar with *Haemophilus ducreyi*. Polymerase chain reaction testing and indirect immunofluorescence are used as alternatives but are generally not commercially available.

HIV prolongs the incubation period of *H. ducreyi* and increases the number of genital ulcers. These tend to heal slowly and poorly. Extragenital sites are also frequently found in co-infection with HIV. Notably, there are increased treatment failures with HIV co-infection. Treatment guidelines for patients co-infected with HIV are the same as for those without HIV, but closer follow-up and potentially a longer course of therapy may be recommended.

Chancroid is usually treated on a presumptive basis in endemic areas if clinical features are suggestive. Empiric therapy is also often used if patients fail to respond to treatment of syphilis and/or herpes genitalis.

SPECIFIC INVESTIGATIONS

> ► Gram stain of ulcer base or bubo aspiration
> ► Culture of ulcer base or bubo aspirate
> ► Syphilis serology
> ► HIV serology

FIRST-LINE THERAPIES

> ► Azithromycin 1 g orally – one dose **B**
> ► Ceftriaxone 250 mg intramuscularly – one dose **B**
> ► Ciprofloxacin 500 mg twice a day for three days **B**
> ► Erythromycin 500 mg orally four times a day for 7 days **B**

Treatment of chancroid, 1997. Schmid GP. Clin Infect Dis 1999; 28: S14–20.

This source provides a comprehensive review of chancroid therapy. Single-dose quinolones may have failure rates approaching 10%. However, a regimen of azithromycin (1 g orally, once), ceftriaxone (250 mg intramuscularly, once), or erythromycin (500 mg orally, four times a day for 7 days) remains effective for the treatment of chancroid in the United States and is recommended.

Ceftriaxone no longer predictably cures chancroid in Kenya. Tyndall M, Malisa M, Plummer FA, Ombetti J, Ndinya-Achola JO, Ronald AR. J Infect Dis 1993: 167: 469–71.

Single-dose ceftriaxone has been found in some areas and with HIV co-infection to have a significant treatment failure rate. Among 133 men who had culture-proven chancroid and were treated with ceftriaxone in Nairobi, Kenya, treatment failed in 35%. Poor outcome was associated with human immunodeficiency virus type 1 seropositivity.

Sexually transmitted disease treatment guidelines. Centers for Disease Control and Prevention. Morb Mortal Wkly Rep 2006: 55: 14–30.

These guidelines agree with the above first-line therapies. They also state that ciprofloxacin is contraindicated in pregnant or lactating women. Other special considerations mentioned are increased treatment failure rates in uncircumcised men and in patients with HIV infection (see above). Patients should be tested for HIV at the time chancroid is diagnosed.

Patients should also be retested for HIV and syphilis 3 months after the diagnosis of chancroid if initial tests were negative.

A randomized, double-blind, placebo-controlled trail of single dose ciprofloxacin versus erythromycin for the treatment of chancroid in Nairobi, Kenya. Malonza IM, Tyndall MW, Ndinya-Achola JO, Maclean I, Omar S, MacDonald KS, et al. J Infect Dis 1999; 180: 1886–93.

This clinical trial compared single-dose therapy with ciprofloxacin to a 7-day course of erythromycin for the treatment of chancroid. Cure rates of 92% and 91% were reported with ciprofloxacin and erythromycin, respectively, for the 111 participants with chancroid. Failure rates were attributed to ulcer etiologies of HSV or syphilis.

SECOND-LINE THERAPIES

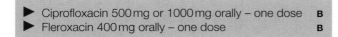

▶ Ciprofloxacin 500 mg or 1000 mg orally – one dose   **B**
▶ Fleroxacin 400 mg orally – one dose   **B**

Treatment of chancroid, 1997. Schmid GP. Clin Infect Dis 1999; 28: S14–20.

Single-dose ciprofloxacin therapy is less effective than multiple-dose therapy, probably owing to the short half-life of ciprofloxacin and inadequate peak serum levels.

Single-dose therapy is recommended only in HIV-seronegative uncircumcised men with close follow-up.

THIRD-LINE THERAPY

▶ Amoxicillin/clavulanic acid – specific dosing not defined   **E**

Comparison of the in vitro activites of various parenteral and oral antimicrobial agents against *Haemophilus ducreyi*. Aldridge KE, Cammarata C, Martin DH. Antimicrob Agents Chemother 1993; 37: 1552–5.

Although there are some in vitro data to suggest amoxicillin/clavulanic acid, there is a paucity of data in clinical practice.

Evidence Levels: **A** Double-blind study **B** Clinical trial ≥ 20 subjects **C** Clinical trial < 20 subjects **D** Series ≥ 5 subjects **E** Anecdotal case reports

Chilblains

Antonios Kanelleas, John Berth-Jones

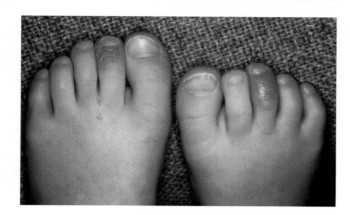

Chilblains (also called perniosis) are localized inflammatory erythematous lesions that are caused by exposure to cold ambient temperatures above freezing point. High humidity and wind, which exacerbate conductive heat loss, also play a significant part. The onset is usually in the autumn or winter. Chilblains are more common in temperate climates, when winters get rather cold and damp and people are not used to these conditions. Lesions occur acutely as single or multiple erythematous or dusky swellings that may ulcerate or blister. They are usually accompanied by a pruritic or burning sensation. Sites of predilection are the fingers, toes, heels, lower legs, thighs, nose, and ears. A specific subset occurs on the thighs of patients wearing tight-fitting, poorly insulating trousers (e.g., young horsewomen). Acral perniosis is also associated with eating disorders (anorexia or bulimia). In this case, chilblains come as a result of vigorous exercise in order to maintain a low body weight; the perniosis may persist for several years after return to an acceptable body weight.

MANAGEMENT STRATEGY

The most important thing in the management of chilblains is *prophylaxis*. This will be achieved through the use of *warm clothing and warm housing*, properly insulated. Avoidance of exposure in cold weather is, obviously, equally important. Once the chilblains occur, they usually run a self-limiting course over a period of a few weeks. Treatment includes *rest in a warm environment and possibly topical antipruritics*, if needed. *Vasodilator calcium channel blockers* (nifedipine 20–60 mg daily, diltiazem 60–120 mg three times daily) have been shown to be an effective therapy and preventative measure in patients with idiopathic acral perniosis, and in those patients with perniosis associated with low body weight. Be aware that perniosis has been associated with myeloproliferative disorders, connective tissue diseases, and eating disorders. Appropriate investigation to exclude the above is required. Particularly in children, chilblains have been linked with cryoproteins. In elderly patients and those with ulcerative lesions, peripheral vascular insufficiency must be excluded. The condition must be distinguished from chilblain lupus erythematosus, which is a different entity, precipitated by cold and damp climates.

SPECIFIC INVESTIGATIONS

- ▶ Full blood count
- ▶ Autoimmune profile
- ▶ Cryoglobulins
- ▶ Cold agglutinins
- ▶ Consider vascular imaging in elderly patients
- ▶ Histology and immunofluorescence

Chilblain lupus erythematosus – a review of literature. Hedrich CM, Fiebig B, Hauck FH, Sallmann S, Hahn G, Pfeiffer C et al. Clin Rheumatol 2008; 27: 949–54.

This article reviews the clinical presentation, pathogenesis, diagnosis, and management of chilblain lupus erythematosus.

Pernio. A possible association with chronic myelomonocytic leukaemia. Kelly JW, Dowling JP. Arch Dermatol 1985; 121: 1048–52.

A series of four elderly men has been described in whom perniosis preceded the onset of chronic myelomonocytic leukemia.

Anorexia nervosa associated with acromegaloid features, onset of acrocyanosis and Raynaud's phenomenon and worsening of chilblains. Rustin MH, Foreman JC, Dowd PM. J Roy Soc Med 1990; 83: 495–6.

Two patients are reported who developed severe perniosis in association with anorexia nervosa.

Perniosis in association with anorexia nervosa. White KP, Rothe MJ, Milanese A, Grant-Kels JM. Paediatr Dermatol 1994; 11: 1–5.

Celiac disease presenting with chilblains in an adolescent girl. St Clair NE, Kim CC, Semrin G, Woodward AL, Liang MG, Glickman JN, et al. Pediatr Dermatol 2006; 23: 451–4.

This is a case report of an adolescent girl in whom chilblains were the main presenting sign of celiac disease. A gluten-free diet resulted in both weight gain and resolution of chilblains.

Childhood pernio and cryoproteins. Weston WL, Morelli JG. Pediatr Dermatol 2000; 17: 97–9.

A 10-year retrospective study of a pediatric clinic identified eight patients with perniosis, four of whom had cryoglobulins or cold agglutinins and two had positive rheumatoid factor.

Equestrian perniosis associated with cold agglutinins: a novel finding. De Silva BD, McLaren K, Doherty VR. Clin Exp Dermatol 2000; 25: 285–8.

Two cases of equestrian perniosis associated with cold agglutinins.

FIRST-LINE THERAPIES

▶ Conservative management	
▶ Avoidance of further cold injury	
▶ Calcium channel blockers	C
▶ Topical corticosteroids	E

The treatment of chilblains with nifedipine: the results of a pilot study, a double blind placebo-controlled randomized

study and a long term open trial. Rustin MH, Newton JA, Smith NP, Dowd PM. Br J Dermatol 1989; 120: 267–75.

Ten patients with severe recurrent acral perniosis were treated with 20 mg of nifedipine retard or placebo in a double-blind crossover trial for 12 weeks in total. No patients developed new lesions while on treatment and 70% were clear after a mean of 8 days. In the open study, 34 patients received up to 60 mg of nifedipine retard for 2 months; this was shown to be effective in reducing the healing time and symptoms of lesions.

Diltiazem vs. nifedipine in chilblains: a clinical trial. Patra AK, Das AL, Ramadasan P. Indian J Dermatol Venereol Leprol 2003; 69: 209–11.

The authors compared two groups of patients with chilblains. Group A (12 patients) was treated with diltiazem 60 mg three times daily and group B (24 patients) with nifedipine 10 mg three times daily until complete relief, and then 20 mg twice daily for maintenance. They concluded that nifedipine has greater efficacy than diltiazem (80–90% of patients from group B showed relief by the 14th day of treatment).

Corticosteroid therapy for pernio. Gaynor S. J Am Acad Dermatol 1983; 8: 13.

This author reports successful treatment of patients with perniosis using topical corticosteroids (0.025% fluocinolone cream) under occlusion nightly.

Topical corticosteroids are frequently used for the treatment of chilblains, but their use is not based on controlled trials.

SECOND-LINE THERAPIES

▶ Topical 2% hexyl nicotinate cream	E
▶ Minoxidil 5% lotion	E
▶ Acidified nitrate cream	E
▶ Tamoxifen	E

Chilblains. Dowd PM, Blackwell V. In: Lebwohl M, Heymann W, Berth-Jones J, Coulson I, eds. Treatment of skin disease, comprehensive therapeutic strategies, 2nd edn. Chicago: Mosby, 2006; 39–40.

These authors reported use of 2% hexyl nicotinate in aqueous cream preparation and minoxidil 5% lotion applied three times a day, in a number of patients with chilblains and Raynaud's phenomenon, and acidified nitrite cream (3% salicylic acid and 3% potassium nitrate) three times daily in patients with chilblains intolerant of calcium channel blockers. Low-dose (5 mg daily) tamoxifen proved useful in anorexia-associated perniosis.

THIRD-LINE THERAPIES

▶ Phototherapy	E
▶ Intense pulsed light	E
▶ Oral pentoxifylline	D

A double blind study of ultraviolet phototherapy in the prophylaxis of chilblains. Langry JA, Diffey BL. Acta Dermatol Venereol 1989; 69: 320–2.

Anecdotally, UV light was used at the beginning of winter for the prophylactic treatment of chilblains, but this randomized double-blind study concluded that UV light was of no benefit.

Pernio of the hips in young girls wearing tight-fitting jeans with a low waistband. Weismann K, Grønhøj Larsen F. Acta Dermatol Venereol 2006; 86: 558–9

The authors report on two adolescent girls from Denmark who developed chilblains on their right hip. This was attributed to exposure to cold, associated with wearing tight-fitting jeans with a low waistband that left uncovered the upper part of the hip region. Both were treated with intense pulsed light (555–950 nm), 14 J/cm². After 3 monthly treatments, the redness was reduced.

Treatment of perniosis with oral pentoxyfylline in comparison with oral prednisolone plus topical clobetasol ointment in Iraqi patients. Noaimi AA, Fadheel BM. Saudi Med J 2008; 29: 1762–4.

Forty patients with chilblains were randomly divided into two equal groups. Group A received oral prednisolone 0.5 mg/kg/day, in 2 doses, and topical clobetasol ointment for 2 weeks. Patients in group B received pentoxifylline tablets 400 mg three times daily for 2 weeks. In group B, five of nine patients (55.5%) who completed the study showed a significant improvement, compared with three of 11 patients (27.2%) in group A with similar results.

Evidence Levels: **A** Double-blind study **B** Clinical trial ≥ 20 subjects **C** Clinical trial < 20 subjects **D** Series ≥ 5 subjects **E** Anecdotal case reports

Chondrodermatitis nodularis helicis chronica

Clifford Lawrence

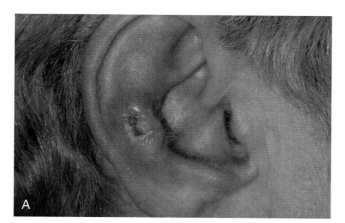

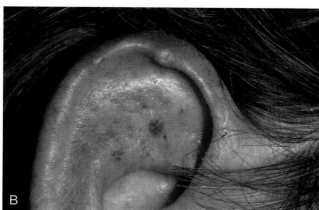

Chondrodermatitis is a benign condition; the only indication for treatment is pain causing sleep disturbance. Painless areas of chondrodermatitis can be ignored or managed conservatively. Lesions on the helix are easier to treat surgically than antihelix lesions, and give better cure results. A pressure-relieving cushion is a good first-choice alternative to surgery for antihelix lesions.

MANAGEMENT STRATEGY

Chondrodermatitis almost always occurs on the lateral portion of the ear on the preferred sleeping side. It is mainly caused by the pressure of the head crushing the ear into the pillow during sleep. Localized pressure from telephone earpieces, rigid headgear, etc. can also be a cause. Ear injury or surgery may leave an irregular ear margin which becomes a focus for sleep-related pressure. The most protuberant part of the ear is affected; this is generally the helix in men and the antihelix in women. Patients who can only adopt one sleeping position due to pain from arthritis, etc. are particularly vulnerable. Children are rarely affected. The incidence increases with age because ear cartilage becomes less flexible with time. Patients should be reassured that it is not skin cancer, advised to use a soft pillow that still has some bounce in it when the head is resting on it, and to change their sleeping position. Conservative or medical treatment, such as *lidocaine (lignocaine) gel*, a potent *topical or intralesional corticosteroid* or a *pressure-relieving cushion* can be tried in all patients. If sleep is not disturbed there is really no need for any further intervention unless cosmesis is a problem.

Numerous surgical strategies have been described to treat chondrodermatitis and most work to some degree; it is tempting to suggest that some work by making the ear so painful that the subject is forced to adapt their sleeping position until the lesion resolves spontaneously. It is generally accepted that the principle of surgical treatment is *excision* of the affected area of cartilage without the need for skin or ulcer excision. Some operators include skin excision to facilitate the procedure. Other destructive therapies have been advocated, but overall are less effective. Antihelix lesions respond so well to cartilage excision that many recommend surgery as a first-line treatment.

SPECIFIC INVESTIGATIONS

> ▶ None required
> ▶ Biopsy of a lesion only necessary if surgery is indicated. Lesions managed conservatively do not require biopsy

FIRST-LINE THERAPIES

> ▶ Reassurance that it is not cancer   **B**
> ▶ Conservative management   **B**
> ▶ Topical corticosteroids   **B**
> ▶ Intralesional corticosteroids   **B**

Treatment of chondrodermatitis nodularis helicis and conventional wisdom? Beck MH. Br J Dermatol 1985; 113: 504–5.

Topical corticosteroids (betamethasone valerate cream 0.025%) used twice a day for 6 weeks and intralesional triamcinolone (0.2–0.5 mL 10 mg/mL) are effective in almost 25% of patients.

Intralesional triamcinolone for chondrodermatitis nodularis: a follow-up study of 60 patients. Cox NH, Denham PF. Br J Dermatol. 2002; 146: 712–13.

A retrospective analysis of 60 patients with CNH treated with 0.1 mL intralesional triamcinolone acetonide 10 mg/mL or triamcinolone hexacetonide 5 mg/mL showed a good response on 43% of helix and 31% of antihelix lesions.

Reassurance that this is not a tumor puts the patient's mind at rest. In many instances the symptoms are mild and can be tolerated without any major intervention. Initially, conservative therapy should be tried. Recommend a change in sleeping position and a soft pillow that can still be further compressed when the head is resting on it. Lidocaine 2% gel applied 30 minutes before going to bed can also produce some symptomatic relief.

SECOND-LINE THERAPIES

> ► Helix lesions – excision of cartilage without skin
>   excision   **B**
> ► Antihelix lesions – pressure-relieving cushion   **B**

The treatment of chondrodermatitis nodularis with cartilage removal alone. Lawrence CM. Arch Dermatol 1991; 127: 530–5.

Topical and intralesional steroids were used in 44 patients preoperatively and were successful in 27%. Surgery was performed on symptomatic patients who did not respond to medical therapy. Surgical excision of the affected cartilage without removal of skin resulted in long-term cure rates of 84% for helix and 75% for antihelix lesions. Local anesthesia with lidocaine and epinephrine (adrenaline) reduced bleeding and improved visibility for the surgeon, and is not known to result in skin necrosis on the ear. A 3 mm punch biopsy is drilled into the lesion at the start of the procedure and this is best removed, attached to cartilage, when the sliver of cartilage is removed. On the helix an incision was made along the helix rim and the skin reflected to expose the cartilage. A sliver of cartilage approximately 20 mm long was taken to include the 3 mm punch biopsy of the skin nodule. On the antihelix a flap of skin had to be raised over the affected area and the underlying cartilage excised. Care was taken to ensure that all remaining cartilage edges were smooth and gently shelving up to the uninvolved cartilage to prevent recurrences, which occur on rough or protuberant cartilage. Cartilage excision alone is not disfiguring, and further cartilage edges can be removed if recurrences occur after surgery, without producing a deformed ear.

The long-term results of cartilage removal alone for the treatment of chondrodermatitis nodularis. Hudson-Peacock MJ, Cox NH, Lawrence CM. Br J Dermatol 1999; 141: 703–5.

Sixty-two helix lesions were followed up for a mean of 52 months (range 8–99). There was recurrence in 10 patients (all men; 16%). Twenty antihelix lesions were followed up for a mean of 55 months (range 8–93). There was recurrence in five patients (all women; 25%). This study confirms that only cartilage needs to be excised for the long-term effective treatment of chondrodermatitis nodularis.

Treatment of chondrodermatitis nodularis with removal of the underlying cartilage alone: retrospective analysis of experience in 37 lesions. de Ru JA, Lohuis PJ, Saleh HA, Vuyk HD. J Laryngol Otol 2002; 116: 677–81.

Most otolaryngologists treat patients with chondrodermatitis nodularis by wedge excision. Although the results of this technique are generally good, it can leave the patient with an asymmetric, deformed ear. The authors describe their results after changing to removal of cartilage alone. In a mean follow-up of 30 months, all 34 patients remained symptom free and only one required revision surgery.

Simplified surgical treatment of chondrodermatitis nodularis by cartilage trimming and sutureless skin closure. Hussain W, Chalmers RJG. Br J Dermatol 2009; 160: 116–8.

After skin incision mosquito forceps were used to 'nibble' away fragments of cartilage to leave a smooth contour without the need for full exposure of the cartilage edge. The final ear cartilage must be left completely smooth to palpation after trimming; if new potential pressure points are created there is a danger that chondrodermatitis may recur. Skin nodules or ulcers are not excised but are left to resolve spontaneously. Tape strips were used for skin closure. A similar procedure can be used for chondrodermatitis of the antihelix, where it is sometimes necessary to remove a full-thickness oval of cartilage to achieve the desired pressure redistribution. Of 34 (94%) patients with chondrodermatitis, 32 (seven on the antihelix and 27 on the helix) showed no discomfort or clinical recurrence 4 months after this procedure.

Chondrodermatitis nodularis chronica helicis et antihelicis. Munnoch DA, Herbert KJ, Morris AM. Br J Plast Surg 1996; 49: 473–6.

Fifty-four chondrodermatitis lesions (36 helix, 18 antihelix), including 23 recurrent after previous surgery, were treated by minimal skin excision combined with extensive cartilage resection. There were no recurrences and minimal postoperative deformity.

Narrow elliptical skin excision and cartilage shaving for chondrodermatitis nodularis. Rex J, Ribera M, Bielsa I, Mangas C, Xifra A, Ferrándiz C. Dermatol Surg 2006; 32: 400–4.

A narrow elliptical excision of the papule, followed by a slice of the underlying cartilage, was taken and trimmed carefully to remove any cartilage spikes. Good cosmetic results were obtained in all 74 patients retrospectively analyzed. The recurrence rate ranged from 10% for helical and 37% for antihelical lesions after a median follow-up of 54 and 50 months, respectively.

Modified surgical excision for the treatment of chondrodermatitis nodularis. Ormond P, Collins P. Dermatol Surg 2004; 30: 208–10.

Excision of the cartilage alone is therapeutically and cosmetically effective. To simplify the surgical procedure a narrow ellipse of skin over the nodule was excised and cold steel dissection of the adjacent skin replaced by hydrodissection to create a plane of cleavage between the skin and the cartilage. These two refinements maintained the clinical and cosmetic efficacy but simplified the surgical technique.

All the above techniques are based on removal of damaged cartilage and avoiding leaving irregular cartilage margins, as these may act as a focus for recurrence. Skin excision can be included if this makes the procedure easier to perform, but is not required for surgical success.

Auricular pressure relieving cushions for chondrodermatitis nodularis helicis. Allen DL, Swinson PA, Arnstein PM. J Maxillofac Prosthet Tech 1998; 2: 5–10.

Thirty-five of 46 patients treated in this way had complete resolution of their symptoms.

Effective treatment of chondrodermatitis nodularis chronica helicis using a conservative approach. Moncrieff M, Sassoon EM. Br J Dermatol 2004; 150: 892–4.

A simple-to-construct ear cushion was used made up of a bath sponge with the centre removed and held in place with a headband; 13 out of 15 patients followed for 1 month responded.

The bath sponge pressure-relieving device is commercially available (CNH ear protector, Delasco, Council Bluffs, Iowa).

Management of chondrodermatitis nodularis chronica helicis using a 'doughnut pillow'. Sanu A, Koppana R, Snow DG. J Laryngol Otol 2007; 121: 1096–8.

Patients used a doughnut-shaped pillow made of a modern orthopaedic 'memory foam.' This distributes the weight of the recumbent head more evenly and is designed to relieve the pressure on the affected ear. Of 23 patients treated, 13 (56%) remained pain free after a 1-year follow-up.

Management of chondrodermatitis nodularis helicis by auricular pressure-relieving device: a retrospective study. Belgi A, Logan RA. Br J Dermatol 2007; 157: 68.

Seventy-eight patients with CNH used a custom-made ear pressure-relieving device designed and built by the local maxillofacial technicians; 48 patients responded to a questionnaire examining the outcome. Only seven (15%) found it helpful, 20 (42%) reported no benefit, and 20 (42%) found some benefit.

Management of chondrodermatitis helicis by protective padding: a series of 12 cases and a review of the literature. Timoney N, Davison PM. Br J Plast Surg 2002; 55: 387–9.

Fourteen patients with CNH were prospectively enrolled and used protective padding of the ear at night. Most patients were rapidly relieved of their symptoms, although healing was frequently prolonged.

Various types of ear cushion are described. They all share the same aim, i.e. to transfer the weight of the sleeping head from the ear to the surrounding scalp. Authors report a wide range of benefit, with between 15% and 80% of patients not requiring surgery. In the hands of this writer the results are generally disappointing. This technique can be helpful for patients in whom surgery has been unsuccessful and recurrences of antihelix lesions are more common after surgery.

THIRD-LINE THERAPIES

▶ Curettage	B
▶ Incision and cartilage curettage	E
▶ CO$_2$ laser ablation	C
▶ Punch and graft	B

Chondrodermatitis nodularis chronica helicis treated with curettage and electrocauterization: follow-up of a 15-year material. Kromann N, Hoyer H, Reymann F. Acta Dermatol Venereol 1983; 63: 85–7.

One hundred and forty-two cases of chondrodermatitis were treated principally by curettage followed by electrocautery. Seventy-eight patients were re-examined after an average of 7.1 years. This simple surgical technique produced a relapse rate of 31%.

The surgical management of chondrodermatitis nodularis chronica helicis. Coldiron BM. J Dermatol Surg Oncol 1991; 17: 902–4.

An ellipse of skin is removed around the ulcerated area. The central necrotic or damaged cartilage is removed using a curette and the skin edges are sutured. A series is not reported.

Chondrodermatitis nodularis chronica helicis. Successful treatment with the carbon dioxide laser. Taylor MB. J Dermatol Surg Oncol 1991; 17: 862–4.

The CO$_2$ laser was used to vaporize the cutaneous nodules and involved cartilage. The wounds were allowed to heal with only minimal care, using hydrogen peroxide cleansing and applications of topical antibiotic ointment. Twelve lesions have been treated, with no recurrences after 2–15 months.

The punch and graft technique: a novel method of surgical treatment for chondrodermatitis nodularis helicis. Rajan N, Langtry JA. Br J Dermatol 2007; 157: 744–7.

Twenty-three lesions (15 helix, three antihelix, five not recorded) were treated by punch removal of the nodule and underlying cartilage. The small defect was closed with a full-thickness skin graft taken from behind the ear using the same punch.

This novel 'punch and graft' technique eschews all the dogma about the need to just remove cartilage and leave smooth cartilage margins, but still produces a cure rate of 83%.

Cryotherapy has been advocated, but there are no published outcomes.

Chromoblastomycosis

Wanda Sonia Robles, Mahreen Ameen

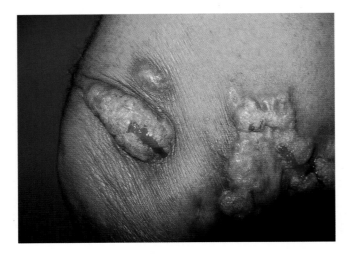

Chromoblastomycosis is a chronic fungal infection of cutaneous and subcutaneous tissues that is endemic in Central and South America, Africa, Australia, and Japan. It is caused by the traumatic implantation of pigmented (dematiaceous) fungi, which produce characteristic thick-walled sclerotic bodies in infected tissues, also known as muriform or Medlar bodies. The commonest etiologic agents are *Fonsecaea pedrosoi*, *Phialophora verrucosa*, and *Cladophialophora carrionii*. Clinically, chromoblastomycosis presents as plaques, nodules, or warty exophytic lesions that most commonly affect the feet and lower legs. Lesions are slow growing and over years extend centripetally, leaving central areas of scarring. Disease is usually localized, but can spread through autoinoculation or lymphatic dissemination, producing metastatic lesions away from the primary site. Complications include ulceration, secondary bacterial infection, and lymphedema. Rarely, malignant transformation (squamous cell carcinoma) in chronic lesions and systemic involvement has been reported.

MANAGEMENT STRATEGY

Chromoblastomycosis is a difficult-to-treat, deep mycosis characterized by low cure rates and high rates of relapse, particularly in chronic and extensive disease. Studies report highly variable rates of clinical and mycological cure, ranging from 15% to 80%. The choice of treatment and the outcome depend on the etiologic agent, the extent of the lesions, clinical topography, and the presence of complications (dermal fibrosis and edema may reduce tissue antifungal levels). *F. pedrosoi* is the most common etiologic agent, but has the lowest sensitivity to the major systemic antifungals. *C. carrionii* and *P. verrucosa* are much more sensitive and have been found to respond more favorably to treatment.

Surgical excision may be successful for small and localized lesions. It is performed with wide surgical margins and is usually accompanied by chemotherapy in order to reduce the risk of recurrence. Curettage and electrodessication is not recommended because it may promote lymphatic spread. Other physical modalities include *cryosurgery* using liquid nitrogen, and *thermotherapy*

(applying local heat to produce controlled temperatures ranging from 42° to 45°C, which inhibit fungal growth) using a variety of methods including benzene pocket warmers and pocket handkerchief-type warmers. Cryosurgery and thermotherapy have the advantage that they are relatively inexpensive.

There are no comparative trials of antifungal chemotherapy for chromoblastomycosis. *Itraconazole* (100–400 mg daily) and *terbinafine* (250–500 mg daily) are considered first-line treatments, both drugs having shown high in vitro activity against the causative agents of chromoblastomycosis. They are typically given for long periods of time at high doses. Dual therapy with itraconazole and terbinafine is recommended if it is affordable and tolerated. It is not uncommon for more than one treatment modality to be used, such as oral antifungals combined with surgery, cryotherapy, or thermotherapy. For example, itraconazole and/or terbinafine combined with cryosurgery is advocated for extensive disease. The antifungal is given first until there is a maximum reduction in lesion size, which usually requires 6–12 months of chemotherapy. The lesions then require several treatments with cryosurgery.

Of the other antifungal agents, ketoconazole is not recommended for treating chromoblastomycosis as it cannot be given at high doses for long periods because of its toxicity profile. Despite a few cases in the early literature reporting successful treatment with fluconazole, it too is not recommended as in vitro studies have shown that it has little activity against black fungi. *Flucytosine* (converted into 5-fluorouracil in fungal cells) was an early treatment that demonstrated some degree of efficacy. It is associated with a high risk of developing resistance, but this can be overcome if it is used in combination with another antifungal. It is also hepatotoxic and myelotoxic, requiring regular monitoring of serum levels. With the emergence of newer antifungals it is rarely used now except for resistant cases. Amphotericin B monotherapy is ineffective, and even in combination with other antifungals results are generally poor. However, amphotericin B and flucytosine dual therapy has demonstrated efficacy, in vitro studies having demonstrated synergistic activity between the two drugs. The new second-generation triazoles such as *posaconazole* and *voriconazole* are promising in the management of deep cutaneous mycoses, but experience to date is limited by their prohibitive high costs in endemic settings.

SPECIFIC INVESTIGATIONS

> ▶ Direct microscopy
> ▶ Culture
> ▶ Histopathology

A positive direct examination of scrapings in 10% potassium hydroxide will demonstrate the thick-walled, brown sclerotic cells that are pathognomonic of chromoblastomycosis, irrespective of the causative species. Specimens are more likely to yield a positive result if they include the 'black dots' visible on the surface of the lesion. Culture enables the identification of the causative agent. It is a slow-growing fungus and culture may be inconclusive due to poor morphological differentiation. Polymerase chain reaction (PCR) has been developed for the identification of *Fonsecaea* and *Cladophialophora carrionii*. Serological tests such as ELISA can be useful in evaluating the response to therapy, but like PCR it is not widely available in most endemic settings. A biopsy demonstrates the typical sclerotic bodies in a granulomatous lesion with transepithelial elimination.

FIRST-LINE THERAPIES

▶ Itraconazole	**B**
▶ Terbinafine	**B**
▶ Posaconazole	**D**

Treating chromoblastomycosis with systemic antifungals. Bonifaz A, Paredes-Solis V, Saul A. Exp Opin Pharmacother 2004; 5: 247–54.

A review article highlighting the difficulties in treating this condition. The authors state that the best results for therapy have been obtained with combination and high-dose itraconazole and terbinafine for a minimum of 6–12 months.

Management of chromoblastomycosis: novel perspectives. Esterre P, Queiroz-Telles F. Curr Opin Infect Dis 2006; 19: 148–52.

This review focuses on recent developments in our understanding of the etiopathogenesis of chromoblastomycosis, including mechanisms of immunity, which could lead to improvements in medical therapies. Therapy combining surgery and itraconazole or terbinafine is recommended.

Chromoblastomycosis. López Martínez R, Méndez Tovar LJ. Clin Dermatol 2007; 25: 188–94.

This is a recent and comprehensive review article. It considers itraconazole to be the treatment of choice in combination with surgery in some cases.

Chromoblastomycosis: clinical and mycologic experience of 51 cases. Bonifaz A, Carrasco-Gerard E, Saúl A. Mycoses 2001; 44: 1–7.

This is a study of 51 cases diagnosed over a 17-year period in a tertiary referral center in Mexico: 90% of the cases were caused by *Fonsecaea pedrosoi*. The overall cure rate for all treatment modalities was 31%, and a further 57% showed clinical improvement. For large lesions itraconazole proved to be the most effective treatment, and for small lesions cryosurgery. Itraconazole combined with cryosurgery was also effective.

Subcutaneous mycoses. Queiroz-Telles F, McGinnis MR, Salkin I, Graybill JR. Infect Dis Clin North Am 2003; 17: 59–85.

In this study from Brazil, 30 patients with chromoblastomycosis due mainly to *Fonsecaea pedrosoi* were treated with itraconazole 200–400 mg daily depending on their clinical severity. Nineteen patients (63%) achieved clinical and mycological cure after 12 months of treatment (range 5–31 months). Treatment success depended on lesion size and extent.

This is the largest case series of itraconazole monotherapy for chromoblastomycosis.

Itraconazole pulse therapy in chromoblastomycosis. Kumarasinghe SP, Kumarasinghe MP. Eur J Dermatol 2000; 10: 220–2.

A case report describing cure after seven pulses of itraconazole (200 mg twice daily for 1 week every month) with no recurrence at follow-up 8 months after the end of the treatment course.

Pulse itraconazole 400 mg daily in the treatment of chromoblastomycosis. Ungpakorn R, Reangchainam S. Clin Exp Dermatol 2006; 31: 245–7.

In this small study, six cases of *F. pedrosoi* infection in Thailand were treated with pulse itraconazole 400 mg daily for 1 week each month. All achieved clinical and mycological

cure. Four patients were cured after 12 pulses of treatment, and one after 15 pulses. The remaining patient required 20 pulses of itraconazole as well as cryosurgery. Disease severity and duration did not appear to be predictive of treatment response. This study demonstrated that the monthly pulse regimen is well tolerated and as effective as the conventional continuous 200–400 mg daily regimen for the treatment of *F. pedrosoi*. The authors recommend that treatment is continued until absence of organisms is proven by histology and tissue culture. Given that the total drug dosage is reduced, there is a marked reduction in cost of therapy by 50–75%. They also claim that pulse therapy is associated with higher compliance, although therapy duration remains long.

The cost of long-term itraconazole therapy is high in endemic settings, making this an important and relevant study.

Treatment of chromomycosis with terbinafine: preliminary results of an open pilot study. Esterre P, Inzan CK, Ramarcel ER, Andriantsimahavandy A, Ratsioharana M, Pecarrere JL, et al. Br J Dermatol 1996; 134: 33–6.

This multicenter study from Madagascar treated 43 patients, but only 36 (*Fonsecaea pedrosoi*, n=29; *Cladosporium carrionii*, n=7) could be completely evaluated. Approximately one-third of the patients had been resistant to previous treatment with thiabendazole. Oral terbinafine 500 mg daily was given for 6–12 months. Within 2–4 months of the start of treatment there was a marked clinical improvement, with resolution of secondary bacterial infection, edema, and elephantiasis. There was mycological cure in 83% (24/29) of patients infected with *Fonsecaea pedrosoi* at 12 months. Of those infected with *C. carrionii*, there was cure in one and clinical improvement in a further three. Total cure was observed even in imidazole-refractory patients and those with chronic disease present for over 10 years. There was a mild transient rise of hepatic enzymes in some patients, but no serious adverse effects were reported.

Treatment of chromoblastomycosis with terbinafine: experience with four cases. Bonifaz A, Saúl A, Paredes-Solis V, Araiza J, Fierro-Arias L. J Dermatol Treat 2005; 16: 47–51.

Four cases from Mexico (*Fonsecaea pedrosoi*, n=3; *Phialophora verrucosa*, n=1) were treated with oral terbinafine 500 mg daily. Three achieved clinical and mycological cure after a mean treatment period of 7 months. Treatment was well tolerated, with no abnormalities of liver enzymes.

Treatment of chromoblastomycosis with terbinafine: a report of four cases. Xibao Z, Changxing L, Quan L, Yuqing H. J Dermatol Treat 2005; 16: 121–4.

Four patients from China (*Cladosporium carrionii*, n=2; *Fonsecaea pedrosoi*, n=2) treated with terbinafine 500 mg daily for the first month followed by 250 mg daily were cured after 4–8 months of therapy, without evidence of relapse at follow-up 6 months later. The total dosage of terbinafine ranged from 37.5 g to 60 g. Treatment was very well tolerated.

Alternate week and combination itraconazole and terbinafine therapy for chromoblastomycosis caused by *Fonsecaea pedrosoi* in Brazil. Gupta AK, Taborda PR, Sanzovo AD. Med Mycol 2002; 40: 529–34.

Four patients with long-standing disease refractory to standard therapies were treated with alternate-week and combination therapy using itraconazole (200–400 mg daily) and terbinafine (250–1000 mg daily). Combination therapy proved to be more effective and was well tolerated.

The authors suggest that combination therapy with itraconazole and terbinafine may be synergistic, in vitro studies having already demonstrated this against other fungi. Larger studies are required to evaluate combination therapy with itraconazole and terbinafine. However, it must be noted that both drugs are expensive in endemic settings.

Posaconazole treatment of refractory eumycetoma and chromoblastomycosis. Negroni R, Tobon A, Bustamante B, Shikanai-Yasuda MA, Patino H, Restrepo A. Rev Inst Med Trop São Paolo 2005; 47: 339–46.

Cure was achieved in five of six patients with chromoblastomycosis refractory to standard antifungal therapies. They were treated with posaconazole 800 mg in divided doses. The maximum treatment period was 34 months, and treatment was very well tolerated.

This new triazole demonstrates high efficacy and tolerability, but its use in most endemic settings is currently restricted due to its high cost.

SECOND-LINE THERAPIES

▶ Cryosurgery	B
▶ Surgical excision	D
▶ Local heat	D

Treatment of chromoblastomycosis with itraconazole, cryosurgery, and a combination of both. Bonifaz A, Martinez-Soto E, Carrasco-Gerard E, Peniche J. Int J Dermatol 1997; 36: 542–7.

This study included 12 patients assigned to three different groups. Group 1, with small lesions, was treated with itraconazole 300 mg/day. Group 2, also with small lesions, was treated with one or more sessions of cryosurgery. Group 3, with large lesions, started treatment with itraconazole 300 mg/day until reduction of lesions was achieved, followed by one or more sessions of cryosurgery. The results showed completed clinical and mycological cure in two of four patients in both groups 1 and 3. All four patients in group 2 achieved complete cure.

Although the case numbers were small, this study suggests that cryosurgery is a more suitable treatment option than antifungal therapy for small lesions.

Treatment of chromomycosis by cryosurgery with liquid nitrogen: 15 years' experience. Castro LG, Pimentel ER, Lacaz CS. Int J Dermatol 2003; 42: 408–12.

This retrospective study included 22 patients with *Fonsecaea pedrosoi* chomoblastomycosis. Small lesions were frozen in a single session, whereas larger lesions were frozen in small parts. The average number of cryosurgery treatments that each patient received was 6.7 (range 1–22 sessions). Nine patients (40.9%) were considered cured (a clinically disease-free period of at least 3 years), and eight (36.4%) were under observation (clinically disease free but <3 years of follow-up). The rest failed to clear with treatment.

This study suggests high efficacy for cryosurgery therapy. This study, as well as others, suggests that it is a useful and inexpensive option for small lesions.

Successful treatment of chromoblastomycosis with topical heat therapy. Tagami H, Ginoza M, Imaizumi S, Urano-Suehisa S. J Am Acad Dermatol 1984; 10: 615–19.

Four patients (*Fonsecaea pedrosoi* isolated from three) were treated with topical application of tolerable heat from pocket warmers. Three responded after 2, 3, and 6 months of

treatment, respectively. The fourth patient, who received treatment in an irregular manner, cleared only after a 12-month period.

Hyperthermic treatment of chromomycosis with disposable chemical pocket warmers. Report of a successfully treated case, with a review of the literature. Hiruma M, Kawada A, Yoshida M, Kouya M. Mycopathologia 1993; 122: 107–14.

This report from Japan describes the successful treatment of a 7 × 10 cm plaque on the arm with disposable chemical pocket warmers. They were secured over the lesion with an elastic bandage in order to keep the area warm for 24 hours. Mycological cure was achieved after only 1 month, but treatment was continued for 4 months with no subsequent relapse.

There are few studies of this form of therapy. This is a case report as well as a good review article describing it.

THIRD-LINE THERAPIES

▶ Flucytosine	C
▶ Amphotericin B	D
▶ Carbon dioxide laser	E
▶ Ajoene	E

Six years' experience in treatment of chromomycosis with 5-fluorocytosine. Lopez CF, Alvarenga RJ, Cisalpino EO, Resende MA, Oliveira LG. Int J Dermatol 1978; 17: 414–18.

Twenty-three patients with chromoblastomycosis were treated with oral flucytosine for 2–67 months. Sixteen achieved clinical and mycological cure (59%). However, seven patients developed resistance and failed to respond with subsequent treatment with amphotericin B, calciferol or thiabendazole. Resistance appeared to occur particularly in those with long-standing lesions or widespread involvement.

A case of chromomycosis treated by a combination of cryotherapy, shaving, oral 5-fluorocytosine, and oral amphotericin B. Poirriez J, Breuillard F, Francois N, Fruit J, Sendid B, Gross S, et al. Am J Trop Med Hyg 2000; 63: 61–3.

A case of *Fonsecaea pedrosoi* infection which showed clinical and in vitro resistance against itraconazole. In vitro testing demonstrated sensitivity to combination 5-fluorocytosine and amphotericin B therapy, results also suggesting that these drugs have synergistic activity. The patient was given oral 5-fluorocytosine (90 mg/kg/day) combined with oral amphotericin B (30 mg/kg/day). There was very good clinical response to treatment and it was well tolerated. However, treatment was stopped after 6 months, with subsequent relapse 2 years later.

This report illustrates the need for and efficacy of alternative antifungal therapy in cases of itraconazole resistance. However, 5-FC is renally excreted, and therefore careful monitoring is required when used with other nephrotoxic drugs.

A case of chromoblastomycosis with an unusual clinical manifestation caused by *Phialophora verrucosa* on an unexposed area: treatment with a combination of amphotericin B and 5-flucytosine. Park SG, Oh SH, Suh SB, Lee KH, Chung KY. Br J Dermatol 2005; 152: 560–4.

This patient from Korea was treated with liposomal amphotericin monotherapy for 3 months, which had some effect.

144

The addition of 5-flucytosine 4g daily resulted in marked clinical improvement after only 1 month. Amphotericin was then discontinued, and dual therapy with 5-flucytosine and itraconazole 200mg daily was given for 12 months until mycological cure.

This case illustrates the low efficacy of amphotericin B monotherapy, and the synergistic activity in combination with 5-flucytosine.

Successful treatment of chromomycosis using carbon dioxide laser associated with topical heat applications. Hira K, Yamada H, Takahashi Y, Ogawa H. J Eur Acad Dermatol Venereol 2002; 16: 273–5.

This is a report of a case of *Fonsecaea pedrosoi* infection in Japan which failed on previous treatment with terbinafine. It was successfully treated with the application of topical heat, which maintained the surface temperature at 46°C for at least 5 hours a day for 2 months. This was followed by CO_2 laser therapy to any unresponsive lesions. One year after treatment there was no evidence of recurrence.

Ajoene and 5-fluorouracil in the topical treatment of *Cladophialophora carrionii* chromoblastomycosis in humans: a comparative open study. Perez-Blanco M, Valles RH, Zeppenfeldt GF, Apitz-Castro R. Med Mycol 2003; 41: 517–20.

An open comparative trial in Venezuela assessed the safety and efficacy of topical ajoene (an organosulfur compound originally derived from garlic, 0.5% gel) and 5-FU (1% cream) in the treatment of localized chromoblastomycosis. Both compounds have shown in vitro activity against *Cladophialophora carrionii*. They were applied once daily with occlusion for 12–16 weeks to either localized lesions or those <2.5cm in diameter. Complete clinical and mycological remission was achieved in 14/19 patients (74%) treated with ajoene and 14/18 patients (78%) treated with 5-FU. After a 4-year follow-up period there was only a single relapse in the 5-FU treatment group.

These are very promising results for a topical treatment. Topical ajoene has shown efficacy in the treatment of superficial mycoses, but topical treatments are not usually considered effective for most deep cutaneous mycoses.

Chronic actinic dermatitis

John LM Hawk, Sandra Albert, Roy A Palmer

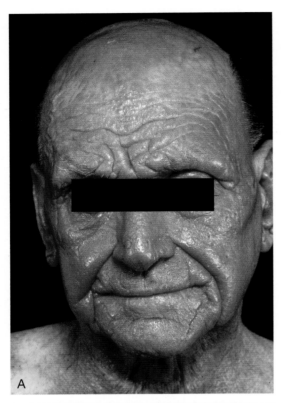

A

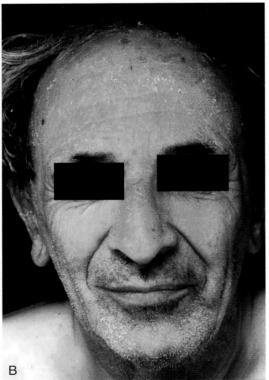

B

Chronic actinic dermatitis (CAD) is an ultraviolet (UV) (280–400 nm) and rarely visible (400–800 nm) radiation-induced eczema affecting mainly the face, upper chest, neck, and exposed areas of the limbs, with very occasional generalized spread towards erythroderma. It is frequently associated with *contact sensitivity* to airborne allergens such as fragrances, colophony, and sesquiterpene lactone from *Compositae* plants. Although it most often affects elderly men, it has of late occurred increasingly often in women, as well as at an earlier age in some patients with atopic eczema.

MANAGEMENT STRATEGY

Once fully evolved, CAD is generally extremely persistent over many years, although it not infrequently remits gradually thereafter. Treatment involves the *restriction of exposure to UV* and also, where appropriate, *visible radiation*. Patients should also be carefully advised about effective behavioral measures, namely sunlight avoidance between about 10am and 4pm, the wearing of protective clothing such as long-sleeved shirts made of closely woven material and of broad-brimmed hats, and the use of filtering window films where possible in the many patients sensitive to long-wave UV (UVA, 315–400 nm) or visible radiation. In addition, *broad-spectrum, high protection-factor sunscreens* of low allergenic potential should be used liberally on exposed sites every 2 hours; the *avoidance of relevant contact allergens* is also of major importance.

In the many patients for whom this is not enough, the use of superpotent or potent *topical steroids* on affected sites and regular application of emollients is also necessary. Intermittent *systemic steroid* courses, generally as prednis(ol)one 30–60 mg daily, tapered over weeks, may be used to control acute flares, followed by topical steroids for maintenance. If control remains poor, *azathioprine* 50–200 mg (1–2.5 mg/kg) daily may be introduced, usually in lower doses initially to avoid adverse effects. Thiopurine methyltransferase (TPMT) blood assay is a useful initial test, patients with low levels being much more prone to myelotoxicity. Possible adverse effects include occasional gastrointestinal intolerance, usually progressively worsening and immediately recurrent if the drug is given again; bone marrow suppression; and liver toxicity, such that appropriate blood tests are needed a week after any dose increase and then every month or two. *Ciclosporin* 125–400 mg (2.5–5 mg/kg) daily is probably more reliably effective but more prone to adverse effects, most commonly renal impairment or hypertension, both initially reversible. Blood and blood pressure testing are therefore necessary every month or two during therapy. Mycophenolate mofetil 1–4 g (20–50 mg/kg) daily and thioguanine 40–120 mg (1–1.5 mg/kg) may also be effective, with dose increases and careful blood testing to check particularly for myelosuppression, which is sometimes severe with thioguanine. *Psoralen and UVA (PUVA) therapy* under reducing oral steroid cover may also help, 0.6 mg/kg 8-methoxypsoralen (8-MOP) followed by an initial UVA dose 2 hours later of often only 0.1–0.2 J/cm^2, with increments of 0.1–0.2 J/cm^2 at each daily or alternate daily session thereafter generally being helpful. However, higher doses and less frequent exposures have also been used successfully. After several weeks the frequency of treatment may be reduced over weeks to once weekly, then to 3- or 4-weekly maintenance exposures, still generally at low doses, say 0.5–1 J/cm^2, according to clinical response. A potent topical steroid should be applied to all treated areas just after irradiation for the first month or so. Broadband UVB phototherapy has also been effective, such that narrowband 311 nm UVB (TL-01), now more commonly used, would be expected to help as well, though confirmatory studies remain to be undertaken. More recently, topical tacrolimus and pimecrolimus have been shown to help, but anecdotal reports of the efficacy of hydroxychloroquine, danazol, and thalidomide remain to be confirmed. Finally, dermabrasion has surprisingly been used and said to help on one occasion.

SPECIFIC INVESTIGATIONS

> ► Patch and photopatch tests
> ► Phototesting (with UVA, UVB and visible light from monochromator or broadband sources)
> ► Provocation testing (with solar simulator or other broadband source)

Contact and photocontact sensitization in chronic actinic dermatitis: sesquiterpene lactone mix is an important allergen. Menagé H du P, Ross JS, Norris PG, Hawk JLM, White IR. Br J Dermatol 1995; 132: 543–7.

Of 89 CAD patients with abnormal responses to the irradiation monochromator, 9% reacted to UVB alone, 83% to UVB and UVA, and 8% to UVB, UVA and visible light, 72% also had positive patch tests, mainly to sesquiterpene lactone (36%), fragrance (21%), and colophony (20%); 11% had positive photopatch tests, 7% to sunscreen agents.

FIRST-LINE THERAPIES

> ► Photoprotective measures   C
> ► Avoidance of relevant contact allergens   C
> ► Topical corticosteroids   C
> ► Topical emollients   C

Chronic actinic dermatitis: a retrospective analysis of 44 cases referred to an Australian photobiology clinic. Yap LM, Foley P, Crouch R, Baker C. Australas J Dermatol 2003; 44: 256–62.

Restriction of sunshine and allergen exposure, along with sunscreen and topical steroid use, gave relief in 36% of CAD patients, the rest requiring oral immunosuppressive agents or phototherapy in addition.

Photosensitivity dermatitis/actinic reticuloid syndrome in an Irish population: a review and some unusual features. Healy E, Rogers S. Acta Dermatol Venereol 1995; 75: 72–4.

Of nine CAD patients treated just with sunscreens, emollients, topical steroids, and antigen avoidance, six responded well, two achieving complete remission and four remaining controlled on topical steroids alone, although five also required oral steroids initially.

Protection against ultraviolet radiation by commercial summer clothing: need for standardised testing and labelling. Gambichler T, Rotterdam S, Altmeyer P, Hoffmann K. BMC Dermatol 2001; 1: 6.

Two hundred and thirty-six summer clothing textiles were investigated spectrophotometrically for their ultraviolet protection factors (UPF). Over 70% of wool and polyester, but less than 30% of cotton, linen and viscose fabrics, had UPFs over 30.

SECOND-LINE THERAPIES

> ► Azathioprine   A
> ► Ciclosporin   C
> ► Mycophenolate   D
> ► Thioguanine   E
> ► PUVA   D
> ► UVB   D
> ► Topical tacrolimus, pimecrolimus   D

Azathioprine treatment in chronic actinic dermatitis: a double-blind controlled trial with monitoring of exposure to ultraviolet radiation. Murphy GM, Maurice PD, Norris PG, Morris RW, Hawk JL. Br J Dermatol 1989; 121: 639–46.

Out of 18 severely affected CAD patients, with complete pruritus and eczema remission as the end-point, five of eight on azathioprine 150 mg daily cleared, one improved, one defaulted at 6 weeks with gastrointestinal side effects, and one did not improve over 8 weeks. None of 10 placebo patients improved significantly.

Azathioprine in dermatology: a survey of current practice in the UK. Tan BB, Gawkrodger DJ, English JSC. Br J Dermatol 1997; 136: 351–5.

A questionnaire survey of 253 UK dermatologists demonstrated that 68% use azathioprine in CAD, 66% alone, and the others as a steroid-sparing agent. Most used 100 mg daily, only 13% prescribing it by body weight (1–2.5 mg/kg daily). CAD had the highest proportion of perceived efficacy (62%) of all disorders treated with the drug.

Severe chronic actinic dermatitis treated with cyclosporine: 2 cases. Paquet P, Piérard GE. Ann Dermatol Venereol 2001; 128: 42–5.

Two men aged 58 and 66 years, with CAD on clinical, histologic and photobiologic grounds, were unresponsive to high-dose oral steroids over weeks but settled rapidly with 3 months each of oral ciclosporin at a maximum of 4 mg/kg daily, without significant adverse effects. One relapsed in summer off treatment, but the other remained clear for 3 years.

Chronic actinic dermatitis treated with mycophenolate mofetil. Thomson MA, Stewart DG, Lewis HM. Br J Dermatol 2005; 152: 784–6.

Two men aged 49 and 55 years with CAD, both with much reduced 24-hour minimal erythema doses on phototesting, were refractory to or developed adverse effects with topical steroids, prednisolone, PUVA, azathioprine and ciclosporin. Each then improved and cleared over weeks on mycophenolate mofetil without adverse effects, one then requiring 500 mg twice daily to prevent relapse, the other 1000 mg twice daily just during spring and summer.

PUVA therapy of chronic actinic dermatitis. Hindson C, Spiro J, Downey A. Br J Dermatol 1985; 113: 157–60.

Four patients with severe CAD were treated twice weekly with PUVA, with starting UVA doses of 0.25 J/cm^2 and increases of 0.25–1 J/cm^2 up to a maximum 10 J/cm^2. Hydrocortisone 1% to the face and betamethasone valerate to the rest of the body were applied immediately after each of the first six exposures. All patients responded well and remained controlled on twice-monthly treatments of 10 J/cm^2.

Actinic reticuloid. A clinical photobiologic, histopathologic, and follow-up study of 16 patients. Toonstra J, Henquet CJ, van Weelden H, van der Putte SC, van Vloten WA. J Am Acad Dermatol 1989; 21: 205–14.

Fifteen CAD patients were treated with broadband UVB phototherapy five times a week, starting with one-tenth of their minimal erythema dose, followed by gradual increments according to skin response. Thirteen improved well clinically, with increased sunlight tolerance. Discontinuation of therapy was followed by gradual relapse.

A case of chronic actinic dermatitis treated with topical tacrolimus. Baldo A, Prizio E, Mansueto G, Somma P, Monfrecola G. J Dermatol Treat 2005; 16: 245–8.

A 58-year-old man with CAD resistant to topical and systemic steroids, oral ciclosporin, and PUVA was treated with tacrolimus ointment 0.1% once daily, leading to significant improvement in his pruritus and severe eczema within 3 weeks.

Successful treatment of nodular actinic reticuloid with tacrolimus ointment. Grone D, Kunz M, Zimmermann R, Gross G. Dermatology 2006; 212: 377–80.

Severe recalcitrant and nodular chronic actinic dermatitis responded well to topically applied tacrolimus twice daily, continued over 2 years to prevent relapse.

Erythrodermic chronic actinic dermatitis responding only to topical tacrolimus. Evans AV, Palmer RA, Hawk JLM. Photodermatol Photoimmunol Photomed 2004; 20: 59–61.

An erythrodermic patient resistant to or failing to tolerate standard oral immunosuppressive treatments and phototherapy responded well to topical tacrolimus 0.1%.

THIRD-LINE THERAPIES

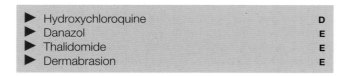

▶ Hydroxychloroquine	D
▶ Danazol	E
▶ Thalidomide	E
▶ Dermabrasion	E

Chronic actinic dermatitis. An analysis of 51 patients evaluated in the United States and Japan. Lim HW, Morison WL, Kamide R, Buchness MR, Harris R, Soter NA. Arch Dermatol 1994; 130: 1284–9.

General photoprotective measures, sunscreens, and topical steroids were used in 51 CAD patients. Azathioprine 50–200 mg daily was also commonly helpful, and PUVA and oral steroids helped seven patients, ciclosporin four, and etretinate two. Finally, hydroxychloroquine 200 mg once or twice daily was said without further qualification to give partial to good responses in nine patients

Chronic actinic dermatitis responding to danazol. Humbert P, Drobacheff C, Vigan M, Quencez E, Laurent R, Agache P. Br J Dermatol 1991; 124: 195–7.

A CAD patient with low α_1-antitrypsin levels responded dramatically to danazol 600 mg daily over 3 weeks, relapsing on stopping, improving on restarting, and remaining well 18 months later still on the drug. Danazol raises low serum α_1-antitrypsin and protease inhibitor levels, and a protease–antiprotease imbalance has been said to cause abnormal inflammatory responses in several dermatoses. There are no other reports of danazol efficacy in CAD.

Recalcitrant chronic actinic dermatitis treated with low-dose thalidomide. Safa G, Pieto-Le Corvaisier C, Hervagault B. J Am Acad Dermatol 2005; 52: E6.

A 37-year-old man with CAD for 5 years, on clinical, histologic and photobiological grounds, had reduced minimal erythema doses to UVA and -B and positive patch tests to nickel. PUVA, azathioprine, ciclosporin, and hydroxychloroquine were ineffective, but thalidomide 100 mg daily tapered gradually to 50 mg twice weekly produced a dramatic response over 5 months without adverse effect.

Surgical management of chronic actinic dermatitis. Reichenberger MA, Stoff A, Richter DF. J Plast Reconstruct Aesthet Surg 2007; Epub ahead of print.

In a 48-year-old woman with severe CAD, topical steroids and systemic immunosuppressants were unhelpful, but two manual dermabrasion sessions led to improvement.

Evidence Levels: **A** Double-blind study **B** Clinical trial ≥ 20 subjects **C** Clinical trial < 20 subjects **D** Series ≥ 5 subjects **E** Anecdotal case reports

Coccidioidomycosis

Mahreen Ameen, Wanda Sonia Robles

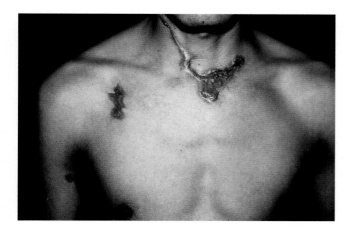

Coccidioidomycosis is an endemic systemic mycosis caused by inhalation of dimorphic fungi of the genus *Coccidioides* (*C. immitis* and *C. posadasii*). It is endemic in desert regions of the southwestern United States, Central and South America. Primary pulmonary disease is usually subacute and self-limiting. The immunocompromised are particularly susceptible to chronic pulmonary disease: 1% progress to disseminated disease, and again those with impaired cell-mediated immunity are at greater risk of this. Coccidioidomycosis is an opportunistic infection with advanced HIV infection and CD4 counts <250. Solid-organ transplant recipients, patients with hematologic malignancies, and those on long-term immunosuppressants, including corticosteroids and TNF-α antagonists, are also at risk. Extrapulmonary hematogenous dissemination can affect almost any organ, but most frequently involves the skin, lymph nodes, skeletal system, and meninges. Dissemination to the skin can give rise to ulcerative and verrucous lesions, with a predilection for the nasolabial area. Subcutaneous abscesses, sinus tracts, and fistulae can develop as a result of coccidioidal infection in neighboring lymph nodes, bones, or joints. Other dermatological manifestations include erythema nodosum and erythema multiforme associated with primary pulmonary infection. Primary infection of the skin is rare.

Dermatologists should be aware that the combination of atypical skin lesions, pulmonary infiltrates, and a history of travel to areas endemic for the disease may represent disseminated infection with coccidioidomycosis.

MANAGEMENT STRATEGY

Treatment depends on the extent of the disease and predisposing factors. Those with primary pulmonary infection and no risk factors require only periodic assessments up to 2 years to ensure that the infection is self-limiting. Some clinicians, however, prefer to treat with oral azoles to prevent any risk of progression, although there are no trial data to support this. Antifungal therapy is indicated for severe or chronic pneumonia, progressive or disseminated infection. *Itraconazole* (200–600 mg daily) and *fluconazole* (400–800 mg daily) have replaced *amphotericin B* (AmB) as the initial choice of therapy for most chronic pulmonary and disseminated infections.

Ketoconazole (400 mg daily) shows comparable efficacy to the other azoles, but is associated with a higher risk of adverse effects with long-term use. Parenteral AmB (AmB deoxycholate 0.5–1.5 mg/kg/day or lipid formulations of AmB 2.0–5.0 mg/kg/day) is now recommended for those with severely acute infection with respiratory failure, those with rapidly progressive and disseminated infection, and women during pregnancy. Published reports of its use, however, are still limited to small numbers of patients treated in open-label, non-randomized studies. There have been no clinical trials assessing the efficacy of lipid formulations of amphotericin B. Newly available antifungals which may be used for refractory infection include the triazoles *posaconazole* and *voriconazole*, in vitro studies having demonstrated their efficacy. However, there have as yet been no comparative studies evaluating their efficacy against the established azoles used for treating coccidioidomycosis. There are early reports too of the successful use of caspofungin, an echinocandin, although results of in vitro susceptibility studies have varied widely.

In addition to drug therapy, *surgery* is sometimes indicated for the removal of focal infection such as pulmonary cavities, focal osseous infection, or the debridement of soft tissue. Long-term prophylaxis with azoles is indicated for the immunocompromised, and meningeal infection requires lifelong azole therapy in order to prevent recurrence. Recovery from infection confers lifelong immunity and provides the rationale for the ongoing development of a possible vaccine.

SPECIFIC INVESTIGATIONS

- ▶ Direct microscopy
- ▶ Culture
- ▶ Serological tests
- ▶ Imaging studies (chest and bone radiography)
- ▶ Serology for HIV/AIDS infection (where relevant)

The characteristic globular spherules may be seen in potassium hydroxide mounts of infected material: sputum, cerebrospinal fluid, or pus. Culture is the definitive method of establishing the diagnosis. *Coccidioides* spp. grow rapidly on most media within 5 days. In the mycelial form the fungus is highly infectious, so cultures should be handled with care. Serological tests are useful and can be used to assess response to therapy.

FIRST-LINE THERAPIES

▶ Fluconazole	A
▶ Itraconazole	A

Fluconazole therapy for coccidioidal meningitis. Galgiani JN, Catanzaro A, Cloud GA, Higgs J, Friedman BA, Larsen RA, et al.; The NIAID Mycoses Study Group. Ann Intern Med 1993; 119: 28–35.

An uncontrolled clinical trial which included 50 patients with coccidioidal meningitis. Forty-seven patients were evaluated: 25 had received no previous treatment, and nine were HIV positive. Of the 47 patients, 37 (79%) responded to treatment. Response rates were similar in patients who had or had not received previous therapy.

Fluconazole demonstrates efficacy in the treatment of coccidioidal meningitis.

Fluconazole in the treatment of chronic pulmonary and non-meningeal disseminated coccidioidomycosis. Catanzaro A, Galgiani JN, Levine BE, Sharkey-Mathis PK, Fierer J, Stevens DA, et al.; NIAID Mycoses Study Group. Am J Med 1995; 98: 249–56.

A multicenter open-label, single-arm study. Of 78 patients enrolled, 22 had soft tissue, 42 had chronic lung, and 14 had skeletal coccidioidomycosis. Forty-nine had at least one concomitant disease, seven of whom had HIV infection. Patients were given fluconazole 200 mg daily. Non-responders were increased to 400 mg daily. Length of treatment was 4–8 months. From among 75 evaluable patients, a satisfactory response was observed in 12 (86%) of those with bone, 22 (55%) of those with lung, and 16 (76%) of those with soft tissue disease. There was a 37% relapse rate in patients whose treatment was interrupted (15/47). The study concluded that fluconazole 200–400 mg daily is well tolerated but demonstrates only moderate efficacy in the treatment of non-meningeal coccidioidomycosis.

Itraconazole treatment of coccidioidomycosis. Graybill JR, Stevens DA, Galgiani JN, Dismukes WE, Cloud GA; NIAID Mycoses Study Group. Am J Med 1990; 89: 282–90.

A multicenter study which included 51 patients with non-meningeal coccidioidomycosis who suffered with either chronic pulmonary, skin and soft tissue, or osteoarticular disease. Patients were treated with itraconazole 100–400 mg daily for periods up to 39 months. Of 44 patients who completed therapy, 25 (57%) achieved remission, but four (16%) later experienced relapse. Three patients were not able to tolerate treatment which had to be discontinued.

Itraconazole therapy for chronic coccidioidal meningitis. Tucker RM, Denning DW, Dupont B, Stevens DA. Ann Intern Med 1990; 112: 108–12.

This was a prospective, non-randomized, multicenter study. Eight patients with coccidioidal meningitis refractory to standard therapy were treated with itraconazole 300–400 mg daily for a median of 10 months. Three patients received intrathecal amphotericin B in addition, and were able to successfully discontinue amphotericin without relapse. Four of five patients on itraconazole monotherapy responded to treatment.

This small but important study demonstrates the efficacy of itraconazole for the treatment of meningeal infection.

Comparison of oral fluconazole and itraconazole for progressive, non-meningeal coccidioidomycosis. A randomized, double-blind trial. Galgiani JN, Catanzaro A, Cloud GA, Johnson RH, Williams PL, Mirels LF, et al. Ann Intern Med 2000; 133: 676–86.

In this randomized, double-blind, placebo-controlled trial, 198 patients with pulmonary and non-meningeal infection were treated with either fluconazole 400 mg daily or itraconazole 200 mg twice daily. Overall efficacy rates at 12 months were similar (itraconazole, 63%; fluconazole 50%; p=0.8). However, the response rate was higher in patients with bone disease treated with itraconazole (52% vs 26%; p=0.05). The rates of relapse were comparable (itraconazole, 18%; fluconazole, 28%; p>0.2). Both drugs were well tolerated.

This is the first prospective, randomized trial comparing two different azole drugs for the treatment of an endemic mycosis. The results demonstrate that both itraconazole and fluconazole are effective for non-meningeal coccidioidomycosis.

SECOND-LINE THERAPIES

| ▶ Amphotericin B | D |
| ▶ Ketoconazole | B |

Amphotericin B and coccidioidomycosis. Johnson RH, Einstein HE. Ann NY Acad Sci 2007; 1111: 434–41.

This article provides a comprehensive review of the use of amphotericin B in the treatment of coccidioidomycosis. The availability of effective azoles and triazoles mean that amphotericins are only used now for widely disseminated infection, in cases of azole intolerance, or when there are contraindications to azoles, such as pregnancy. In meningitis, amphotericin B is still frequently used intrathecally by some clinicians, either alone or with a triazole. The newer lipid preparations, albeit more expensive, have significantly reduced toxicity.

Given that all studies to date of amphotericin use for coccidioidomycosis are limited by small numbers, this review article provides a detailed assessment of current indications for its use.

Intrathecal amphotericin in the management of coccidioidal meningitis. Stevens DA, Shatsky SA. Semin Respir Infect 2001; 16: 263–9.

This review advocates the use of intrathecal amphotericin B as a way to avoid the toxicity of intra-cerebrospinal fluid amphotericin treatment.

A good review.

Use of liposomal amphotericin B in the treatment of disseminated coccidioidomycosis. Antony S, Dominguez DC, Sotelo E. J Natl Med Assoc 2003; 95: 982–5.

Report of an immunosuppressed patient on long-term steroid therapy successfully treated with liposomal amphotericin B (AmBisome).

Ketoconazole therapy of progressive coccidioidomycosis. Comparison of 400- and 800-mg doses and observations at higher doses. Galgiani JN, Stevens DA, Graybill JR, Dismukes WE, Cloud GA. Am J Med 1988; 84: 603–10.

A randomized clinical trial involving 112 patients with progressive pulmonary, skeletal, or soft tissue infections. Success rates were similar for the two groups (23.2% vs 32.1% for low- and high-dose therapy). Side effects were significantly higher with high-dose therapy (66% vs 38%), as were relapse rates (52% vs 11%), although this depended also on the organs involved. The study concluded little or no benefit with high-dose ketoconazole for non-meningeal infection.

THIRD-LINE THERAPIES

▶ Posaconazole	B
▶ Voriconazole	E
▶ Caspofungin	E

Safety, tolerance, and efficacy of posaconazole therapy in patients with non-meningeal disseminated or chronic pulmonary coccidioidomycosis. Catanzaro A, Cloud GA, Stevens DA, Levine BE, Williams PL, Johnson RH, et al. Clin Infect Dis 2007; 45: 562–8.

In this multicenter trial 20 patients with chronic pulmonary or non-meningeal disseminated coccidioidomycosis were treated with posaconazole 400 mg daily for up to 6 months

Evidence Levels: **A** Double-blind study **B** Clinical trial ≥ 20 subjects **C** Clinical trial < 20 subjects **D** Series ≥ 5 subjects **E** Anecdotal case reports

(median 173 days). Seventeen (85%) patients had a satisfactory response to treatment (=50% reduction in the Mycoses Study Group score from baseline). No serious adverse effects were reported. Paired baseline and end-of-treatment culture results for *Coccidioides* species were available for four patients, all of whom converted from being positive to being negative for *Coccidioides*. Relapse was experienced by three of nine patients who did not receive antifungal therapy during the follow-up period.

Posaconazole therapy for chronic refractory coccidioidomycosis. Stevens DA, Rendon A, Gaona-Flores V, Catanzaro A, Anstead GM, Pedicone L, et al. Chest 2007; 132: 952–8.

This was an open-label multinational study which included 15 patients with pulmonary (n=7) and disseminated (n=8) disease that was refractory to previous therapy, which included amphotericin B with and without an azole. They were treated with posaconazole 800 mg daily in divided doses for 34–365 days (median 306 days); 73% of patients (11/15) responded to treatment, with cure in four cases. Treatment was very well tolerated.

Successful treatment of disseminated non-meningeal coccidioidomycosis with voriconazole. Prabhu RM, Bonnell M, Currier BL, Orenstein R. Clin Infect Dis 2004; 39: e74–7.

Report of an HIV-negative man with severe disseminated non-meningeal coccidioidomycosis who had failed on treatment with both prolonged courses of amphotericin B deoxycholate and liposomal amphotericin B combined with azoles and caspofungin. He was switched to oral voriconazole 200 mg twice daily. After 10 months of treatment he showed a slow but favorable clinical response.

Successful use of voriconazole for treatment of *Coccidioides* meningitis. Proia LA, Tenorio AR. Antimicrob Agents Chemother 2004; 48: 2341.

A 32-year-old man failed therapy on sequential high-dose therapy with fluconazole, amphotericin B deoxycholate and amphotericin B lipid complex. He was switched to high-dose oral voriconazole 400 mg twice daily, which continued for 30 months with a favorable outcome. He was subsequently maintained on lifelong voriconazole therapy, 200 mg twice daily.

Voriconazole is characterized by extensive tissue distribution, including central nervous system penetration, making it an attractive option for meningeal disease refractory to other antifungals.

Combination therapy of disseminated coccidioidomycosis with caspofungin and fluconazole. Park DW, Sohn JW, Cheong HJ, Kim WJ, Kim MJ, Kim JH, et al. BMC Infect Dis 2006; 6: 26.

A case report of an immunocompetent Korean man with diffuse coccidioidal pneumonia with skin involvement, acquired on a trip to California. He failed initial therapy with amphotericin B deoxycholate 1 mg/kg for 40 days. He was switched to intravenous caspofungin (initially 70 mg and then 50 mg daily) and oral fluconazole 400 mg daily. Because of the excellent clinical response, caspofungin was discontinued after 4 months and fluconazole was continued as maintenance therapy.

In another report caspofungin monotherapy failed to treat a case of meningeal infection.

Use of the echinocandins (caspofungin) in the treatment of disseminated coccidioidomycosis in a renal transplant recipient. Antony S. Clin Infect Dis 2004; 39: 879–80.

Caspofungin monotherapy was successfully used to treat this case of disseminated infection without meningeal involvement.

Coccidioidomycosis. Infectious Diseases Society of America Guidelines. Galgiani JN, Ampel NM, Blair JE, Catanzaro A, Johnson RH, Stevens DA, et al. Clin Infect Dis 2005; 41: 1217–23.

These replace the 2000 guidelines, and the most notable difference is that itraconazole and fluconazole have replaced amphotericin B as first-line therapy for most chronic and disseminated forms of infection.

Primary self-limiting infection in an immunocompetent host usually requires no treatment. Recommended dosages of the commonly used azoles are fluconazole 400–800 mg daily, itraconazole 400–600 mg daily, and ketoconazole 400 mg daily. Amphotericin B deoxycholate dosage is 0.5–1.5 mg/kg/day, and the dosage for the lipid formulations is 2.0–5.0 mg/kg/day.

Persistent pulmonary infection

▶ Oral azole for 3–6 months, with follow-up period to ensure complete resolution.

Diffuse pneumonia

▶ This may indicate underlying immunosuppression and the patient should be investigated for extrapulmonary infection. Amphotericin B is usually given (especially if there is respiratory distress) and continued for several weeks before switching to an oral azole. One year of total treatment is recommended. In the immunosuppressed, azoles should be continued as secondary prophylaxis.

Chronic progressive pulmonary infection

▶ Oral azoles for 1 year. If there is a lack of response, higher-dose or alternative azoles, or amphotericin B can be used.

Disseminated extrapulmonary infection

▶ High-dose azoles are recommended. Treatment can be switched to amphotericin B if there is no improvement. Surgical debridement may be required for abscesses or bony sequestrations.

Meningitis

▶ Oral fluconazole (400–1000 mg daily) is favored. Itraconazole (400–600 mg daily) can also be used. Intrathecal amphotericin B (0.1–1.5 mg/dose) in addition to an azole is an alternative regimen. Patients who respond to an azole should continue with this treatment indefinitely.

Cryptococcosis

Wanda Sonia Robles, Mahreen Ameen

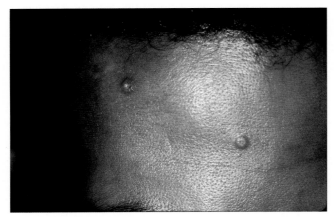

From Lebwohl MG. The Skin and Systemic Disease: A Color Atlas, 2nd edn. Churchill Livingstone 2003, with permission of Elsevier.

Cryptococcosis is a systemic mycosis acquired by the respiratory route with the primary focus of infection in the lungs. It is caused by an encapsulated yeast known as *Cryptococcus neoformans*, of which there are two variants, *C. neoformans* var. *neoformans* and *C. neoformans* var. *gattii*. The yeasts are associated with avian feces. *C. neoformans* var. *neoformans* occurs worldwide. *C. neoformans* var. *gattii* is restricted mainly to subtropical regions, and usually affects immunocompetent hosts only. Pulmonary infection is usually asymptomatic and self-limiting. Hematogenous dissemination typically involves the central nervous system (CNS), causing meningitis. Dissemination to the skin usually occurs in 10–15% of cases and produces a variety of lesions, including flesh-coloured or erythematous papules and nodules. In the immunocompromised, molluscum contagiosum-like and acneform lesions occur, particularly affecting the face. Cryptococcal cellulitis with necrotizing vasculitis can mimic bacterial cellulitis, and occurs more commonly in the immunocompromised.

With the global emergence of AIDS the incidence of cryptococcosis is increasing and it represents the most common invasive mycosis in advanced HIV infection. With HIV co-infection the disease is characteristically widespread, affecting the lungs, meninges, skin, bone marrow, and genitourinary tract, including the prostate. Other immunosuppressed patients also at risk include solid organ transplant recipients, those with hematologic malignancies, and those on long-term immunosuppressive therapy, including corticosteroids and anti-TNF-α therapies.

MANAGEMENT STRATEGY

Cryptococcal infection, if left untreated, is fatal. Treatment depends on disease extent and predisposing factors, particularly AIDS or any other immunosuppressive state. The recommended treatment in the immunocompetent with symptomatic non-meningeal infection is *fluconazole* 200–400 mg daily for 3–6 months. An alternative is *itraconazole* 200–400 mg daily for 6–12 months. More severe non-meningeal infection is treated with *amphotericin B* (AmB) 0.5–1.0 mg/kg daily for 6–10 weeks. Meningeal infection in the immunocompe-

tent or non-HIV immunocompromised is treated with AmB 0.7–1.0 mg/kg daily plus 5-flucytosine 100 mg/kg daily for 2 weeks, followed by fluconazole 400 mg daily for a minimum of 10 weeks (up to 6–12 months, depending on the clinical status of the patient).

Cryptococcal disease with HIV always requires treatment. For non-disseminated infection, *fluconazole* (200–400 mg daily) is given or *itraconazole* (200–400 mg daily) as an alternative. More severe infection is treated with a combination of fluconazole (400 mg daily) and *flucytosine* (100–150 mg daily) for 10 weeks, followed by fluconazole maintenance therapy (200 mg daily). Cryptococcal meningitis with HIV is treated with AmB (0.7–1.0 mg/kg daily) and flucytosine (100 mg/kg daily) for a 2–10-week induction period followed by fluconazole maintenance therapy, or alternatively with fluconazole (400–800 mg daily) and flucytosine (100–150 mg/kg daily) for 6 weeks. The lipid formulation of AmB can be used instead in those with impaired renal function. There are now trial data suggesting that it is safe to discontinue maintenance therapy in patients treated for cryptococcal meningitis receiving highly active antiretroviral therapy (HAART), provided the CD4 count increases to an excess of 100 cells/μL.

SPECIFIC INVESTIGATIONS

- ► Direct microscopy
- ► Culture
- ► Cryptococcal antigen test (by latex agglutination or ELISA)
- ► Histology (Mayer mucicarmine and Masson–Fontan silver stains used to identify *C. neoformans*)
- ► Pulmonary and brain imaging studies
- ► Serology for HIV

India ink examination of CSF, pus, skin scrapings, and other fluids may demonstrate the yeast. Culture of skin, CSF, blood, sputum, urine, or bone marrow enables confirmation. The cryptococcal antigen test (on CSF, blood, and urine) is sensitive and specific, and it can be used for following therapy response. In tissue specimens *C. neoformans* is difficult to visualize with routine hematoxylin and eosin stains, and requires the use of special stains.

FIRST-LINE THERAPIES

► Amphotericin B	**B**
► Amphotericin B plus flucytosine	**B**
► Fluconazole	**B**

Cryptococcosis in human immunodeficiency virus-negative patients in the era of effective azole therapy. Pappas PG, Perfect JR, Cloud GA, Larsen RA, Pankey GA, Lancaster DJ, et al. Clin Infect Dis 2001; 33: 690–9.

A multicenter case study of HIV-negative patients with cryptococcosis from 1990 to 1996. Of 306 patients, there were 109 with pulmonary involvement and 157 with CNS involvement. Patients with pulmonary disease were usually treated with fluconazole (63%) and those with CNS disease usually received amphotericin B (92%). Two-thirds of these patients also received fluconazole for consolidation therapy. Therapy was reported as successful in 74% of patients. The mortality attributable to cryptococcosis was 12%.

Clinical and epidemiological features of 123 cases of cryptococcosis in Mato Grosso do Sul, Brazil. Lindenberg Ade S, Chang MR, Paniago AM, Lazéra Mdos S, Moncada PM, Bonfim GF, et al. Rev Inst Med Trop São Paolo 2008; 50: 75–8.

In this study 84.5% (104/123) of patients had HIV infection, 4.9% (6/123) had other predisposing conditions, and 10.6% (13/123) were immunocompetent. There was CNS involvement in 83.7% (103/123); 89.6% were infected with *C. neoformans* and 10.4% with *C. gattii*. For treatment amphotericin B was the drug of choice in 86% (106/123), followed by fluconazole in 60% (57/123).

This cohort of patients typifies features of this infection found in other study cohorts.

Combination antifungal therapies for HIV-associated cryptococcal meningitis: a randomised trial. Brouwer AE, Rajanuwong A, Chierakul W, Griffin GE, Larsen RA, White NJ, et al. Lancet 2004; 363: 1764–7.

This randomized controlled trial assessed the fungicidal activity of combinations of amphotericin B, flucytosine, and fluconazole for the treatment of cryptococcal meningitis. Sixty-four patients with a first episode of HIV-associated cryptococcal meningitis were randomized to initial treatment with amphotericin B (0.7 mg/kg daily); amphotericin B plus flucytosine (100 mg/kg daily); amphotericin B plus fluconazole (400 mg daily); or triple therapy with amphotericin B, flucytosine, and fluconazole. Results demonstrated that clearance of cryptococci from the CSF was exponential and significantly faster with amphotericin B and flucytosine dual therapy than with any other drug combination.

A multicentre, randomized, double-blind, placebo-controlled trial of primary cryptococcal meningitis prophylaxis in HIV-infected patients with severe immune deficiency. Chetchotisakd P, Sungkanuparph S, Thinkhamrop B, Mootsikapun P, Boonyaprawit P. HIV Med 2004; 5: 140–3.

This study from Thailand was conducted to assess the efficacy and survival benefit of low-dose fluconazole (400 mg weekly) for primary prophylaxis for cryptococcal meningitis. It was a prospective double-blind, placebo-controlled study of HIV-infected patients with CD4 counts <100 cells/μL. On an intent-to-treat basis, 6.8% (3/44) of the fluconazole group and 15.2% (7/46) of the placebo group developed cryptocccal meningitis. The calculated survival benefit of fluconazole was greater than that of the placebo (p=0.046), and it was concluded that fluconazole 400 mg once weekly should be considered for primary prophylaxis for cryptococcal meningitis in Thailand.

High-dose amphotericin B with flucytosine for the treatment of cryptococcal meningitis in HIV-infected patients: a randomized trial. Bicanic T, Wood R, Meintjes G, Rebe K, Brouwer A, Loyse A, et al. Clin Infect Dis 2008; 47: 123–30.

In this study from South Africa, 64 HIV-seropositive, antiretroviral therapy-naive patients with a first episode of cryptococcal meningitis were randomized to receive either AmB 0.7 mg/kg/day plus flucytosine 25 mg/kg four times daily (n=30), or AmB 1 mg/kg daily plus flucytosine 25 mg/kg four times daily (n=34). Both regimens were given for 2 weeks followed by oral fluconazole. The primary outcome measure was early fungicidal activity determined by CSF cryptococcal cultures. Early fungicidal activity was significantly greater for regimen 1. The 10-week mortality rate was 24%, with no difference between groups.

Antifungal interventions for the primary prevention of cryptococcal disease in adults with HIV. Chang LW, Phipps WT, Kennedy GE, Rutherford GW. Cochrane Database Syst Rev 2005; CD004773.

The objective of this review was to assess the efficacy of antifungal interventions for the primary prevention of cryptococcal disease in adults with HIV. Five randomized controlled trials were identified. The majority of study patients had CD4 counts <150 cells/μL. Three studies used itraconazole and two used fluconazole. When all five studies were analyzed as a single group (n=1316), the incidence of cryptococcal disease was reduced in those taking primary prophylaxis compared to those taking placebo (RR 0.21, 95% CI 0.09, 0.46). However, no significant difference in overall mortality was observed (RR 1.01, 95% CI 0.71, 1.44). The report concludes that antifungal primary prophylaxis with either itraconazole or fluconazole is effective in reducing the incidence of cryptococcal disease in adults with advanced HIV disease, although neither intervention has a clear effect on overall mortality.

SECOND-LINE THERAPIES

▶ Itraconazole	B
▶ Flucytosine plus fluconazole	C
▶ Voriconazole	B

A controlled trial of itraconazole as primary prophylaxis for systemic fungal infections in patients with advanced human immunodeficiency virus infection in Thailand. Chariyalertsak S, Supparatpinyo K, Sirisanthana T, Nelso KE. Clin Infect Dis 2002; 34: 277–84.

In this prospective, double-blind trial, 129 patients with HIV infection and CD4+ lymphocyte counts of <200 cells/μL were randomized to receive either oral itraconazole 200 mg daily or a matched placebo. The study concluded that primary prophylaxis with oral itraconazole is well tolerated and prevents both cryptococcosis and *Penicillium marneffei* infection in patients with advanced HIV infection. However, it was not associated with a survival advantage in patients with advanced HIV disease.

The efficacy of fluconazole 600 mg/day versus itraconazole 600 mg/day as consolidation therapy of cryptococcal meningitis in AIDS patients. Mootsikapun P, Chetchotisakd P, Anunnatsiri S, Choksawadphinyo K. J Med Assoc Thai 2003; 86: 293–8.

In this trial, HIV-infected patients with primary cryptococcal meningitis who had been treated with amphotericin B for 2 weeks were randomized to receive either fluconazole 600 mg daily or itraconazole 600 mg daily for 10 weeks. The results demonstrated equal efficacy for both these regimens. In addition, the results suggested that the higher-dose regimens may be superior to regimens using lower doses of these medications.

Oral versus intravenous flucytosine in patients with human immunodeficiency virus-associated cryptococcal meningitis. Brouwer AE, van Kan HJ, Johnson E, Rajanuwong A, Teparrukkul P, Wuthiekanun V, et al. Antimicrob Agents Chemother 2007; 51: 1038–42.

A randomized controlled trial conducted in Thailand compared the efficacy and toxicity of oral versus intravenous flucytosine (100 mg/kg/day) for the initial 2 weeks in combination

153

with amphotericin B. Sixteen patients were randomized to each arm of the trial. Serial quantitative cultures of CSF were taken, the results indicating no difference in early fungicidal activity between oral and intravenous flucytosine.

Voriconazole treatment for less-common, emerging, or refractory fungal infections. Perfect JR, Marr KA, Walsh TJ, Greenberg RN, DuPont B, de la Torre-Cisneros J, et al. Clin Infect Dis 2003; 36: 1122–31.

A multicenter controlled clinical trial to assess the efficacy, tolerability, and safety of voriconazole as salvage treatment for patients with refractory and intolerant-to-treatment fungal infections, as well as primary treatment for patients with infections for which there is no approved treatment. The efficacy rate for voriconazole in the treatment of cryptococcosis was 38.9%. Voriconazole was reported to be well tolerated, and discontinuation of treatment was observed in less than 10% of patients.

Discontinuation of maintenance therapy for cryptococcal meningitis in patients with AIDS treated with highly active antiretroviral therapy: an international observational study. Mussini C, Pezzotti P, Miró JM, Martinez E, de Quiros JC, Cinque P, et al. Clin Infect Dis 2004; 38: 565–71.

A retrospective multicenter study evaluating the safety of discontinuing maintenance therapy for cryptococcal meningitis after immune reconstitution. Inclusion criteria included a CD4 count of >100 cells/µL while receiving HAART, and the subsequent discontinuation of maintenance therapy for cryptococcal meningitis. The primary endpoint was relapse of cryptococcal disease. One hundred patients were enrolled. During a median follow-up period of 28.4 months (range 6.7–64.5 months) there were four episodes of relapse. Three of these patients had a CD4 count of >100 cells/µL and a positive serum cryptococcal antigen test result. The study concluded that discontinuation of maintenance therapy for cryptococcal meningitis is safe if the CD4 count increases to >100 cells/µL while receiving HAART, and that recurrent cryptococcal infection should be suspected in patients whose serum cryptococcal antigen test results revert back to positive after discontinuation of maintenance therapy.

THIRD-LINE THERAPIES

▶ Recombinant interferon-gamma 1b	**B**
▶ Amphotericin B plus Fluconazole	**C**

Recombinant interferon-gamma 1b as adjunctive therapy for AIDS-related acute cryptococcal meningitis. Pappas PG, Bustamante B, Ticona E, Hamill RJ, Johnson PC, Reboli A, et al. J Infect Dis 2004; 189: 2185–91.

This was a phase 2 double-blind, placebo-controlled study to evaluate the safety and antifungal activity of adjuvant recombinant interferon (rIFN)-γ_{1b} in patients with AIDs and acute cryptococcal meningitis. Patients received 100 or 200 µg of rIFN-γ_{1b} or placebo thrice weekly for 10 weeks, plus standard therapy with AmB, with or without flucytosine, followed by fluconazole. Among 75 patients, 2-week culture conversion occurred in 13% of placebo recipients, 36% of rIFN-γ_{1b}

(100 µg) recipients, and 32% of rIFN-γ_{1b} (200 µg) recipients. There was improved combined mycological and clinical success in rIFN-γ_{1b} recipients (26% vs 8%; p=0.078), and therapy was well tolerated.

This study suggests a role for adjuvant therapies.

Epidemiology and management of cryptococcal meningitis: developments and challenges. Pukkila-Worley R, Mylonakis E. Exp Opin Pharmacother 2008; 9: 551–60.

This review article examines developments in the management of cryptococcal meningitis, including new antifungal agents and new strategies for controlling elevated intracranial pressure.

Practice guidelines for cryptococcal disease. Saag MS, Graybill RJ, Larsen RA, Pappan PG, Perfect GR, Powderloy WG, et al. Clin Infect Dis 2000; 30: 710–18.

A subcommittee of the National Institute of Allergy and Infectious Diseases (NIAID) Mycoses Study Group evaluated available data on the treatment of cryptococcal infection. The choice of treatment was based on both the anatomical site of involvement and the immune status of the host. For immunocompetent hosts with symptomatic infection, recommended treatment is fluconazole 200–400 mg daily for 3–6 months; this includes patients with non-CNS involvement, a positive serum cryptococcal antigen titer >1:8, or urinary tract or cutaneous disease. For patients unable to tolerate fluconazole, itraconazole 200–400 mg/day for 6–12 months is an alternative. For patients with more severe disease, amphotericin B 0.5–1.0 mg/kg daily for 6–10 weeks is recommended. For immunocompetent hosts with CNS disease, standard therapy comprises amphotericin B 0.7–1.0 mg/kg daily plus flucytosine 100 mg/kg daily for 6–10 weeks. An alternative regimen is amphotericin B 0.7–1.0 mg/kg plus flucytosine 100 mg/kg daily for 2 weeks, followed by fluconazole 400 mg daily for a minimum of 10 weeks. Fluconazole 'consolidation' therapy may be continued for as long as 6–12 months, depending on the clinical status of the patient. Non-HIV immunocompromised hosts should be treated in the same way as those with CNS disease, regardless of the site of involvement. For HIV patients with isolated pulmonary or urinary tract disease, fluconazole 200–400 mg daily is indicated. HIV-infected individuals should continue prophylactic treatment for life. In individuals unable to tolerate fluconazole, itraconazole 200–400 mg daily is an alternative. For patients with more severe disease, a combination of fluconazole 400 mg daily plus flucytosine 100–150 mg/kg daily may be used for 10 weeks, followed by fluconazole maintenance treatment.

The treatment of choice for patients with HIV infection and cryptococcal meningitis is induction therapy with amphotericin B 0.7–1.0 mg/kg daily plus flucytosine 100 mg/kg daily for 2 weeks, followed by fluconazole 400 mg daily for a minimum period of 10 weeks. After 10 weeks of treatment, the dose of fluconazole may be reduced to 200 mg daily.

Amphotericin B in lipid formulations can be used for patients with renal impairment. An alternative is fluconazole 400–800 mg daily plus flucytosine 100–250 mg/kg daily for 6 weeks. Toxicity with this regimen is high.

Evidence Levels: **A** Double-blind study **B** Clinical trial ≥ 20 subjects **C** Clinical trial < 20 subjects **D** Series ≥ 5 subjects **E** Anecdotal case reports

Cutaneous amyloidosis

William Y-M Tang, Loi-yuen Chan

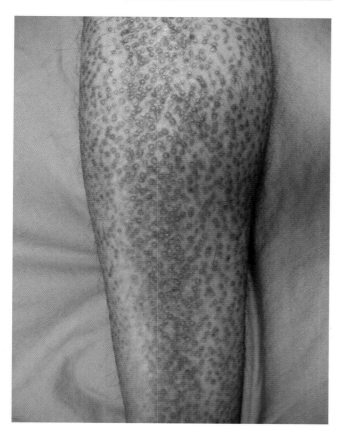

Amyloid is an altered, insoluble protein that can accumulate in one or many organs, causing dysfunction. Primary localized cutaneous amyloidosis is characterized by the deposition of amyloid in the skin without involving any internal organ. It occurs more commonly in Southeast Asians, Chinese, Middle Easterners, and South Americans. There are three clinical forms: lichen, macular, and nodular. The co-occurrence of macular and lichen amyloidosis in a patient is known as biphasic amyloidosis. The amyloid in macular and lichen amyloidosis is derived from degenerated keratinocytes, whereas in nodular amyloidosis it is derived from immunoglobulin light chains from a local plasma cell clone.

Lichen amyloidosis (see Figure) is a persistent eruption of multiple red-brown hyperkeratotic papules often affecting extensor aspects of extremities, especially the pretibial surfaces. It appears more commonly in males. Apart from its cosmetic nuisance, marked itching can occur. Although familial cases of lichen amyloidosis have been reported, most cases occur as isolated events having no association with systemic disease.

Macular amyloidosis is characterized by an eruption consisting of small, dusky-brown or grayish pigmented macules distribute symmetrically over the upper back and upper arm. It has a reticulated or rippled pattern. Itch is variable, and patients often seek medical advice for aesthetic issues and pruritus.

Nodular amyloidosis is the rarest subtype. It is characterized by single or multiple waxy, firm, brown or pink nodules involving the legs, head, trunk, arms, and genitalia. It is usually asymptomatic.

MANAGEMENT STRATEGY

Lesions of localized cutaneous amyloidosis can produce considerable pruritus. Patients seek treatment to alleviate pruritus and the undesirable appearance. Currently there are no accepted standard treatments for the various types of cutaneous amyloidosis because of a lack of good clinical trials. As pruritus is a common symptom, *antihistamines* and *topical corticosteroids* are prescribed as first-line treatments.

Phototherapy (ultraviolet B or PUVA) has been used to treat lichen amyloidosis successfully for relief of pruritus. *Acitretin* may be added for combined therapy. *Laser treatments* reported to be successful in treating cutaneous amyloidosis include *carbon dioxide, pulsed-dye and neodymium:yttrium aluminum garnet (Nd:YAG)*. Oral retinoids are another alternative treatment for lichen amyloidosis. Disappearance of pruritus has been noted after 2 weeks of acitretin 35 mg daily.

Dermabrasion has been successful in treating lichen and nodular amyloidosis. This improves cosmesis and alleviates pruritus, but brings accompanying procedural pain and the development of skin atrophy. There is an anecdotal report that dermabrasion of lichen amyloidosis under tumescent anesthesia can result in remarkable pain reduction even though the total amount of local anesthetic required is low.

Tacrolimus has been used successfully in relieving pruritus and reducing plaque thickness in lichen amyloidosis. Results were seen after 2 weeks of twice-daily application of the 0.1% ointment. *Topical dimethylsulfoxide (DMSO)* also has been reported to benefit lichen and macular amyloidosis. However, a more recent study on 25 patients reported lack of efficacy.

SPECIFIC INVESTIGATIONS

▶ Skin biopsy

All forms of amyloidosis have similar histological findings. On light microscopy, amyloid is characteristically a pink, amorphous material. Special stains, such as Congo red and crystal violet, can highlight the amyloid deposit. Amyloid can be metachromatically stained red by crystal violet staining of an aqueous mount of the specimen. Congo red staining of amyloid shows apple-green birefringence under polarized light microscopy.

FIRST-LINE THERAPIES

▶ Sedating antihistamines   E
▶ Topical high-potency or intralesional corticosteroids   E

Sedating antihistamines are commonly prescribed to relieve the pruritus. Intralesional and high-potency topical corticosteroids may provide symptom relief and thinning of lesions. Although there are no specific studies investigating the efficacy of antihistamines and intralesional or topical corticosteroids in cutaneous amyloidosis, they are the first-line treatments and some patients respond well.

SECOND-LINE THERAPIES

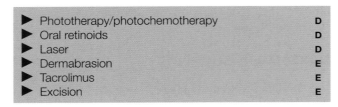

▶ Phototherapy/photochemotherapy	D
▶ Oral retinoids	D
▶ Laser	D
▶ Dermabrasion	E
▶ Tacrolimus	E
▶ Excision	E

Comparative study of phototherapy (UVB) vs. photochemotherapy (PUVA) vs. topical steroids in the treatment of primary cutaneous lichen amyloidosis. Jin AG, Por A, Wee LK, Kai CK, Leok GC. Photodermatol Photoimmunol Photomed 2001; 17: 42–3.

In this study, 14 patients with lichen amyloidosis were treated with either UVB (n=9) or PUVA (n=5) to half of the body, applying potent topical corticosteroids to the other half as a control. After 8 weeks of treatment, patients treated with phototherapy had more improvement in average roughness of lesions and itch than on the control side. Improvement of roughness in the UVB-treated lesions was significant. However, the difference in improvement in itch in the UVB- and PUVA-treated lesions compared to the control lesions was not significant.

Successful treatment of lichen amyloidosis with combined bath PUVA photo-chemotherapy and oral acitretin. Grimmer J, Weiss T, Weber L, Meixner D, Scharffetter-Kochanek K. Clin Exp Dermatol 2007; 32: 39–42.

Two male patients with lichen amyloidosis over the extensor surfaces of the lower legs were treated with bath PUVA three to four times per week for 11 weeks, plus oral administration of acitretin 0.5 mg/kg/day for 7 months. There was almost complete resolution of skin lesions in both patients. No relapse was observed for 8 months after discontinuation of treatment.

Widespread biphasic amyloidosis: response to acitretin. Hernandez-Nunez A, Dauden E, Moreno de Vega MJ, Fraga J, Aragues M, Garcia-Diez A. Clin Exp Dermatol 2001; 26: 256–9.

A 73-year-old man with a 15-year history of biphasic amyloidosis was treated with acitretin 35 mg once daily (0.5 mg/kg/day). Pruritus resolved completely after 2 weeks of treatment. Acitretin was continued for 6 months and then stopped. There was no recurrence during the subsequent 6 months of follow-up.

Excess tissue friability during CO_2 laser vaporization of nodular amyloidosis. Hamzavi I, Lui H. Dermatol Surg 1999; 25: 726–8.

A 63-year-old woman with asymptomatic nodular amyloidosis on the nose was successfully treated with CO_2 laser. Initially, the laser was set at a power of 8 W. During treatment it was noted that the tissue was highly friable, requiring an increase of the power to 15 W to achieve haemostasis. The lesion healed with an excellent cosmetic response 7 months after treatment.

The use of CO_2 laser for nodular primary localized cutaneous amyloidosis was first reported by Truhan et al. in 1986. In their report the treatment resulted in a good cosmetic result, although post-treatment biopsies showed residual amyloid.

A case of lichen amyloidosis treated with pulsed dye laser. Sawamura D, Sato-Matsumura KC, Shibaki A, Akiyama M, Kikuchi T, Shimizu H. J Eur Acad Dermatol Venereol 2005; 19: 262–3.

A 59-year-old man with lichen amyloidosis for 5 years was treated with two sessions of 585 nm pulsed-dye laser. The treatment parameters were 7 mm spot size and a fluence of 6.0 J/cm². Reassessment at 8 weeks showed great reduction of itch with decreasing size of papules, although complete clearance was not achieved. The improvement persisted for more than 15 months after treatment.

Nodular amyloidosis treated with a pulsed dye laser. Alster TS, Manaloto RM. Dermatol Surg 1999; 25: 133–5.

A 56-year-old man with nodular amyloidosis on his chin and submental area failed to improve with intralesional steroid injections. He was successfully treated with a 585 nm flashlamp-pumped long-pulse (1.5 ms) dye laser using a 10 mm spot size. A test dose was initially given at a fluence of 5.0 J/cm². Eight weeks after the test dose, the entire lesion was treated with fluences ranging from 5.0 to 5.5 J/cm² for three sessions at intervals of 6 weeks. The response included improvement in lesion color, size, and pliability, appreciated by both patient and physicians. The improvement continued for 6 months after cessation of treatment.

The mechanism of action of pulsed-dye laser on nodular amyloidosis is not known. The therapeutic effect was thought attributable to injury to cutaneous blood vessels depleting the amyloid nodule.

Treatment of lichen amyloidosis and disseminated superficial porokeratosis with frequency-doubled Q-switched Nd:YAG laser. Liu HT. Dermatol Surg 2000; 10: 958–62.

A 49-year-old woman with lichen amyloidosis received Q-switched Nd:YAG 532 nm laser treatment. The laser parameters were spot size 4 mm, fluence 1.5 J/cm², and delivery rate of 2.5 pulses per second. A total of three and two treatment sessions separated by a month were given to the forearms and legs, respectively. A biopsy of the treated area showed coalescence and homogenization of amyloid globules. Long-term response 9 months after the last treatment was noted.

In this author's experience, the procedure carries a risk of cellulitis and hyperpigmentation.

The efficacy of dermabrasion in the treatment of nodular amyloidosis. Lien MH, Railan D, Nelson BR. J Am Acad Dermatol 1997; 36: 315–6.

A 45-year-old white man with multiple nodular amyloidosis lesions on his chin for 2 years was treated by shave excision followed by superficial dermabrasion. The treatment area was first sprayed with fluoroethyl-free spray. Dermabrasion was carried out using a Bell hand engine with a regular wire brush followed by a smooth diamond fraise. There was no recurrence at 26 months of follow-up.

The largest study on efficacy of dermabrasion on nodular amyloidosis was reported by Wong CK et al. in 1982, where seven patients showed satisfactory improvement after a follow-up of at least 5 years.

Lichen amyloidosis improved by 0.1% topical tacrolimus. Castanedo-Cazares JP, Lepe V, Moncada B. Dermatology 2002; 205: 420–1.

One patient with lichen amyloidosis diagnosed clinically was treated with tacrolimus 0.1% ointment twice daily. Resolution of pruritus was noted after 2 weeks of therapy, and marked improvement of plaque thickness was observed after 2 months.

This is the only report on the treatment of lichen amyloidosis using topical tacrolimus.

Cutaneous larva migrans

Bridgette Cave, Anthony Abdullah

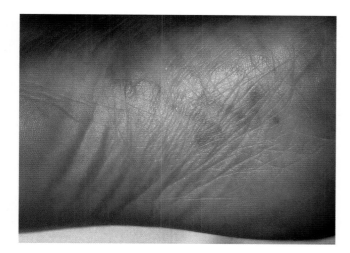

Cutaneous larva migrans (CLM) is caused by the accidental per-cutaneous penetration and migration of animal hookworm larvae in the human skin. The larvae develop from eggs released into the soil or sand from the feces of contaminated animals. CLM occurs mainly in resource-poor countries and is typically reported in returning travelers, but is also sporadically reported elsewhere. The clinical picture is that of intensely itchy lesions of characteristic erythematous serpiginous, macular, papular, or vesicular tracks which migrate daily owing to the presence of moving parasites. The exposed extremities or buttocks are most often involved, as a result of sitting on contaminated ground.

MANAGEMENT STRATEGY

Cutaneous larva migrans is self-limiting. The human is a 'dead-end host' for the parasite and the larvae usually die within 2–8 weeks. However, this length of time is quite variable, and treatment is often needed because of the severity of the symptoms. There are topical and systemic treatment options with anthelmintic agents. Topical treatment for limited disease usually takes the form of *thiabendazole* (10%) in a suitable lipophilic vehicle. The systemic treatment normally used by the authors for patients over the age of 2 years is oral *albendazole* 400 mg daily for 3 days, or as an alternative *ivermectin* given as a single dose of 12 mg or 200 µg/kg orally.

SPECIFIC INVESTIGATIONS

▶ Clinical appearance is characteristic

FIRST-LINE THERAPIES

▶ Systemic albendazole	B
▶ Topical thiabendazole in a lipophilic vehicle	D

Treatment of larva migrans cutanea (creeping eruption): a comparison between albendazole and traditional therapy. Albanese G, Venturi C, Galbiati G. Int J Dermatol 2001; 40: 67–71.

Experience of treating 56 patients, 34 of whom received oral albendazole. A prompt and definitive cure was achieved in all 56. The therapeutic effectiveness of the various methods was equivalent, but albendazole was considered the first choice because it was extremely well tolerated and patient compliance was good. Of the other patients 13 received cryotherapy, six oral thiabendazole, two cryotherapy and albendazole, and one cryotherapy and thiabendazole.

Cutaneous larva migrans: clinical features and management of 44 cases presenting in the returning traveller. Blackwell V, Vega-Lopez F. Br J Dermatol 2001; 145: 434–7.

Five patients received 10% thiabendazole cream topically for 10 days and four were cured. Thirty-one patients received oral albendazole 400 mg daily for 3–5 days and 24 were cured (77%). Four needed no treatment.

Cutaneous larva migrans of the genitalia. Rao R, Prabhu S, Sripathi H. Indian J Dermatol Venereol Leprol 2007; 73: 270–1.

A single case report of CLM of 4 months' duration in which the lesions were halted in 3 days and complete resolution was seen 1 week after treatment with oral albendazole 400 mg twice daily for 3 days

Efficacy and tolerability of thiabendazole in a lipophil vehicle for cutaneous larva migrans. Chatel G, Scolari C, Gulletta M, Casalini C, Carosi G. Arch Dermatol 2000; 136: 1174–5.

A small series of patients treated with a lipophilic formulation of thiabendazole. The treatment consisted of topical applications (twice daily for 5 days) of 15% thiabendazole (prepared by crushing the tablets of thiabendazole in the lipophilic base ointment) in a lipophilic vehicle of base fat cream (24 g) and dimethyl sulfoxide gel (35 g). All patients experienced a clinical resolution within a median of 48 hours after the start of treatment. No adverse effects and no recurrence had occurred in any patient at 3 months' follow-up.

Treatment with topical thiabendazole ointment at 10–15% concentration in a hydrophilic vehicle has shown 98% efficacy within a median of 10 days of treatment and with no contraindications.

SECOND-LINE THERAPIES

▶ Systemic ivermectin	B

A randomized trial of ivermectin versus albendazole for the treatment of cutaneous larva migrans. Caumes E, Carriere J, Datry A, Gaxotte P, Danis M, Gentilini M. Am J Trop Med Hyg 1993; 49: 641–4.

A comparison of efficacy between oral ivermectin (12 mg) and oral albendazole (400 mg). Twenty-one patients were randomly assigned to receive ivermectin (n=10) or albendazole (n=11). All patients who received ivermectin responded and none relapsed (cure rate 100%). All except one patient in the group receiving albendazole responded, but five relapsed after a mean of 11 days (cure rate 46%; p=0.017). No major adverse effects were observed. The authors suggest that a single 12 mg dose of ivermectin is more effective than a single 400 mg dose of albendazole.

Cutaneous larva migrans in travellers: a prospective study, with assessment of therapy with ivermectin. Bouchaud O, Houze S, Schiemann R, Durand R, Ralaimazava P, Ruggeri C, et al. Clin Infect Dis 2000; 31: 493–8.

An update of epidemiologic data and evaluation of therapeutic efficacy of ivermectin (a single dose of 200 μg/kg was used). Sixty-four patients were studied. The cure rate after a single dose of ivermectin was 77%. In 14 patients one or two supplementary doses were necessary, and the overall cure rate was 97%. The median times required for pruritus to disappear and lesions to resolve were 3 and 7 days, respectively. No systemic adverse effects were reported. Single-dose ivermectin therapy appears to be effective and well tolerated, although several treatments are sometimes necessary.

Cutaneous larva migrans in an unusual site. Malhotra SK, Raj RT, Pal M, Goyal V, Sethi S. Dermatol Online J 2006; 12: 11.

A single case report of CLM on the abdominal wall in a farm worker. A single dose of ivermectin 200 μg/kg resulted in remission after 1 week.

Treatment of 18 children with scabies or cutaneous larva migrans using ivermectin. Del Mar Saez-De-Ocariz M, McKinster CD, Orozco-Covarrubias L, Tamayo-Sánchez L, Ruiz-Maldonado R. Clin Exp Dermatol 2002; 27: 264–7.

Eighteen children aged 14 months to 17 years, of which seven had CLM. All seven were cured with a single dose of ivermectin, with no significant adverse effects. In the authors' experience ivermectin is a safe and effective alternative treatment for cutaneous parasitosis in children.

THIRD-LINE THERAPIES

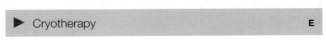

▶ Cryotherapy   E

Studies relating to creeping eruption. Hitch JM, Iralu V. South Med J 1960; 53: 447–53.

One method of treating CLM involves freezing with liquid nitrogen. This is rarely effective, however, because the larvae are ahead of the advancing track and can be missed, and because larvae may not be killed by freezing (larvae survived 5 minutes of exposure to –25°C in this study).

Darier disease

Susan M Cooper, Susan M Burge

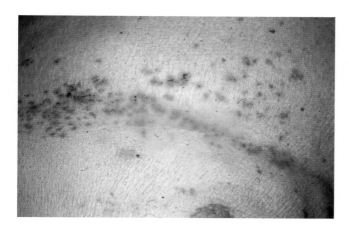

Darier disease is a dominantly inherited condition, incidence 1:25 000–1:100 000, that is characterized by persistent greasy, hyperkeratotic papules. The disease is caused by mutations in the ATP2A2 gene that encodes type 2 sarco(endo)plasmic reticulum Ca^{2+} ATPase (SERCA 2).

MANAGEMENT STRATEGY

The warty, keratotic papules, which usually appear before the age of 20, can be malodorous, irritate, and look unsightly. The flexures can be a particular problem, as plaques here are frequently hypertrophic and may smell very unpleasant. Initial treatment is aimed at controlling irritation. *Simple emollients, soap substitutes,* and *topical corticosteroid* creams are helpful. Keeping the skin cool by wearing comfortable pure cotton clothing helps. Sunblock is recommended for those with a history of photoaggravation.

In mild disease or linear disease reflecting a genetic mosaicism, *topical retinoids* may be sufficient. These include topical isotretinoin (0.05% and 0.1%), tretinoin cream, adapalene gel and tazarotene gel. Treatment is applied on alternate days to begin with, increasing to once daily if possible, as irritation is common. The addition of a topical corticosteroid (alternating with the retinoid) may alleviate some of the side effects. Superinfection with viruses and bacteria is frequent, so combined corticosteroid/antibiotic preparations are logical.

In more extensive disease, an *oral retinoid* is required. Etretinate, acitretin, and isotretinoin are effective. Teratogenicity is a problem, and pregnancy is contraindicated for 2 years after stopping treatment with etretinate or acitretin and 1 month with isotretinoin. For this reason, isotretinoin is the usual choice in women of childbearing age. Treatment may be given either long term or as intermittent short courses. The usual starting dose of acitretin is 10–25 mg daily but this can be increased gradually. Isotretinoin is usually started at 0.5–1.0 mg/kg daily. In the UK, etretinate is only available on a 'named patient' basis but may work where other retinoids have failed.

The rare vesiculobullous form of the disease may respond to *prednisolone*. Hypertrophic flexural disease, unresponsive to retinoids, may require surgery. A variety of surgical approaches have been tried, including *electrosurgery, debridement,* and *laser.* Recurrence is a problem.

Oral lithium exacerbates the disease and should be avoided if possible.

SPECIFIC INVESTIGATIONS

> ► Skin biopsy. The characteristic finding is focal acantholytic dyskeratosis. The acantholysis is suprabasal
> ► Skin swab for bacterial and viral culture if infection is suspected

Darier-White disease: a review of the clinical features in 163 patients. Burge SM, Wilkinson JD. J Am Acad Dermatol 1992; 27: 40–50.

Fourteen percent of patients in this series had herpes simplex complicating their Darier disease.

Painful blisters arising in a patient with Darier's disease are usually due to secondary infection with Staphylococcus aureus *or herpes simplex.*

FIRST-LINE THERAPIES

> ► Cool cotton clothing   E
> ► Emollients   D
> ► Topical retinoids   D

Darier's disease. Cooper SM, Burge SM. Am J Clin Dermatol 2003; 4: 97–105.

A detailed review of the current management of Darier's disease.

As in most genetic diseases, genetic counseling can be helpful. Written information is often appreciated. Patient support groups – for example, DARDIS in the UK – can provide useful information.

Linear Darier's disease successfully treated with 0.1% tazarotene gel 'short contact' therapy. Brazezelli V, Prestinari F, Barbagallo T, Vassallo C, Agozzino M, Borroni G. Eur J Dermatol 2006; 16; 59–61.

A man with linear Darier's disease affecting the trunk was treated with tazarotene for 15 minutes once a day over 6 weeks, with a good response.

Topical isotretinoin in Darier's disease. Burge SM, Buxton PK. Br J Dermatol 1995; 133: 924–8.

Six of 11 patients improved when a test patch was treated with 0.05% isotretinoin. Erythema, burning, and irritation were common.

Acral Darier's disease successfully treated with adapalene. Cianchini G, Colonna L, Camaioni D, Annessi G, Puddu P. Acta Dermatol Venereol 2001; 81: 57–8.

A single case report of acral Darier disease responding to a synthetic retinoid, adapalene 0.1% gel. Lesions cleared after 4 weeks of treatment on the hands and 6 weeks on the soles.

SECOND-LINE THERAPIES

> ► Oral retinoids   B
> ► Topical 5-fluorouracil   E

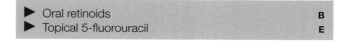

Clinical and ultrastructural effects of acitretin in Darier's disease. Lauharanta J, Kanerva L, Turjanmaa K, Geiger JM. Acta Dermatol Venereol 1988; 68: 492–8.

Thirteen patients were treated with acitretin starting at 30 mg daily. Duration of treatment was 16 weeks. All showed some improvement, but side effects included itching (five patients) and hair loss (two patients).

Isotretinoin treatment of Darier's disease. Dicken CH, Bauer EA, Hazen PG, Krueger GG, Marks JG Jr, McGuire JS, et al. J Am Acad Dermatol 1982; 6: 721–6.

This multicenter open study assessed the effect of short and longer courses of treatment. The starting dose was 0.5 mg/kg, but longer courses were adjusted according to symptoms. Isotretinoin was very effective, but did not give long-term remission. Some patients were maintained on alternate-day or alternate-week regimens.

Etretinate may work where acitretin fails. Bleiker TO, Bourke JF, Graham-Brown RA, Hutchinson PE. Br J Dermatol 1997; 136: 368–70.

Two patients with Darier's disease unresponsive to acitretin responded to etretinate.

Oral retinoid therapy for disorders of keratinisation: single-centre retrospective 25 years' experience on 23 patients. Katugampola RP, Finlay AY. Br J Dermatol 2006; 154: 267–76.

Retinoids may cause diffuse skeletal hyperostosis and extraosseous calcification. The long-term experience of 23 patients on retinoids over 25 years was reported. One patient developed diffuse skeletal hyperostosis after 21 years of retinoid therapy.

It is not clear whether X-ray screening is necessary for asymptomatic patients on long-term treatment, but it is prudent to inquire about musculoskeletal problems in these patients.

Retinoids have many side effects, including mucosal dryness and soreness, skin fragility, and itching. They may cause hepatic dysfunction and hyperlipidemia. Liver function, cholesterol, and triglycerides should be monitored during treatment.

Topical 5-fluorouracil in the treatment of Darier's disease. Knulst AC, Baart de la Faille H, Van Vloten WA. Br J Dermatol 1995; 133: 463–6.

Two cases with therapy-resistant Darier's disease responded to topical 5-fluorouracil. Both patients were also taking oral retinoids.

THIRD-LINE THERAPIES

▶ Ciclosporin	E
▶ Oral contraceptive pill	E
▶ Supplementary dietary fatty acids	E
▶ Oral prednisolone (vesiculobullous only)	E
▶ Laser (CO_2 and erbium:YAG)	E
▶ Dermabrasion	E
▶ Debridement	E
▶ Photodynamic therapy	E
▶ Botulinum toxin	E

Darier's disease: severe eczematization successfully treated with cyclosporin. Shahidullah H, Humphreys F, Beveridge GW. Br J Dermatol 1994; 131: 713–16.

Ciclosporin may be helpful in widespread eczematized Darier disease, but had no effect on the underlying disease.

Vulval Darier's disease treated successfully with ciclosporin. Stewart LC, Yell J. J Obstet Gynaecol 2008; 28: 108–9.

A previously therapy-resistant case was treated with ciclosporin (initial dose 5 mg/kg) for 6 months with good response, and was subsequently maintained on acitretin.

Oral contraceptives in the treatment of Darier-White disease – a case report and review of the literature. Oostenbrink JH, Cohen EB, Steijlen PM, Van de Kerkhof PCM. Clin Exp Dermatol 1996; 21: 442–4.

Some women report premenstrual exacerbation of their symptoms and some improve in pregnancy. The skin of a woman treated with the combined oral contraceptive pill (ethinyl estradiol 50 µg, levonorgestrel 125 µg) became less itchy and less fragile.

Essential fatty acids in the treatment of Darier's disease. du Plessis PJ, Jacyk WK. J Dermatol Treat 1998; 9: 97–101.

Fatty acid supplements helped 13 of 16 patients, but this observation needs to be confirmed.

Vesiculobullous Darier's disease responsive to oral prednisolone. Speight EL. Br J Dermatol 1998; 139: 934–5.

A patient with the vesiculobullous form of the disease responded to a short course of oral prednisolone.

Oral steroids may also be useful in the eczematized form.

Carbon dioxide laser vaporization of recalcitrant symptomatic plaques of Hailey-Hailey disease and Darier's disease. McElroy JA, Mehregan DA, Roenigk RK. J Am Acad Dermatol 1990; 23: 893–7.

In two patients, chronic localized plaques unresponsive to other treatments responded to laser vaporization.

Efficacy of erbium:YAG laser ablation in Darier disease and Hailey-Hailey disease. Beier C, Kaufmann R. Arch Dermatol 1999; 135: 423–7.

Disease cleared in two patients treated with this laser, but follow-up was less than 2 years.

Electrosurgical treatment of etretinate-resistant Darier's disease. Toombs EL, Peck GL. J Dermatol Surg Oncol 1989; 15: 1277–80.

Electrosurgery was effective in two cases unresponsive to etretinate.

Dermabrasion in Darier's disease. Zachariae H. Acta Dermatol Venereol 1979; 59: 184–5.

Five patients with severe disease were treated by dermabrasion down to and including the papillary dermis. Three-quarters of the treated skin remained disease free 6 months later. Facial treatment was less successful than treatment to the trunk area.

The surgical treatment of hypertrophic Darier's disease. Wheeland RG, Gilmore WA. J Dermatol Surg Oncol 1985; 11: 420–3.

Recalcitrant, hypertrophic lesions were debrided under local anesthesia. Symptomatic and cosmetic improvement was maintained for 2 years.

Evidence Levels: **A** Double-blind study **B** Clinical trial ≥ 20 subjects **C** Clinical trial < 20 subjects **D** Series ≥ 5 subjects **E** Anecdotal case reports

Treatment of Darier's disease with photodynamic therapy. Exadaktylou D, Kurwa HA, Calonje E, Barlow RJ. Br J Dermatol 2003; 149: 606–10.

Six patients received photodynamic therapy with topical 5-aminolaevulinic acid as a photosensitizer. One patient could not tolerate the treatment, but five experienced sustained improvement. All had an initial inflammatory response that lasted 2–3 weeks.

Botulinum toxin type A: An alternative symptomatic management of Darier's disease. Kontochristopoulos G, Katsavou AN, Kalogirou O, Agelidis S, Zakopoulou N. Dermatol Surg 2007; 33: 882–3.

Submammary disease was treated with botulinum toxin as adjuvant therapy: 100 U were injected, with improvement sustained for 4 months. Reduced sweating may alleviate maceration and reduce bacterial colonization.

Darier disease: sustained improvement following reduction mammaplasty. Cohen PR. Cutis 2003; 72: 124–6.

Recalcitrant submammary disease in a woman with large breasts improved after reduction mammaplasty.

Darier's disease, an unusual problem and solution. Sprowson AP, Jeffery SL, Black MJ. J Hand Surg 2004; 29: 293–5.

A woman with intolerable nail disease benefited from surgery to all 10 fingernails. An eponychial flap was raised and the nail complex excised. A full-thickness skin graft was obtained from the groin and sutured into place with the proximal border of the graft tucked under the eponychial fold.

Decubitus ulcers

Joseph A Witkowski, Lawrence Charles Parish, Jennifer L Parish

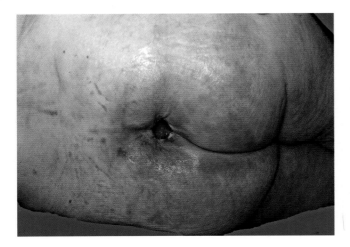

The decubitus ulcer represents a defect in the skin that can extend through the subcutaneous tissue and muscle layer onto the underlying bone.

MANAGEMENT STRATEGY

Prevention

A patient in an ordinary bed who is at risk for developing a decubitus ulcer, also referred to as pressure ulcer or bed sore, should be repositioned at frequent intervals; however, the correct timing for turning has never been established. The regularity is determined by the level of risk of developing an ulcer and the duration of blanchable erythema. Pillows and foam wedges are used to maintain position and to keep bony prominences apart. Completely immobile patients should have their heels raised from the bed by a pillow or boot and not be placed on their trochanters, unless a specialized bed is used. To avoid the latter, use a 30° position from the horizontal lying on the side. The head of the bed should not be raised more than 30° from the horizontal for an extended period. Where possible, use lifting devices or draw sheets to reposition or to transfer patients. Finally, when appropriate, the patient should be placed on a pressure-reducing device such as a foam, alternating air, gel, or water mattress.

A patient sitting in a wheelchair who is at risk for developing a decubitus ulcer should be repositioned frequently, perhaps every hour, and be taught to shift weight every 15 minutes. The chair should be adjusted appropriately for each patient. A pressure-reducing device made of foam, gel, air, or a combination of each is indicated.

Theoretically, decubitus ulcers should be preventable, but despite these measures many simply cannot be prevented. If they are associated with immobility, sustained pressure, and the loss of pain sensibility, then these problems can and should be addressed. In practice, successful prevention is often foiled by our limited understanding of the pathogenesis, as well as by complicating comorbidities. There is also some evidence that many deep ulcers are initiated by multiple microthrombosis of deep tissues. This indicates that dehydration, along with any factor that might increase blood coagulability, should be addressed.

Management

The management of skin lesions caused by pressure is based on four principles:
- Elimination of relative pressure
- Removal of necrotic debris
- Maintenance of a moist wound environment
- Correction of the underlying contributing factors.

Elimination of sustained pressure

The patient should not lie on the ulcer. A patient who is at risk for developing additional ulcers and can assume a variety of positions without lying on the ulcer should be placed on a *static support surface (i.e. air, foam, or water)*. If the patient cannot assume various positions without lying on the ulcer, or bottoms out while on a static surface, or if the ulcer does not heal after 2–4 weeks of optimal care, place the patient on a *dynamic support surface* when possible (*i.e. an alternating air overlay on the mattress, a low-air-loss bed, or an air-fluidized bed*). If a patient has large deep ulcers (stage III or IV) on multiple sleep surfaces or has excess moisture on intact skin, use a low-air-loss bed or an air-fluidized bed. A patient with an ulcer on the sitting surface should not sit, if possible.

Removal of necrotic debris

Surgical debridement is indicated for infected ulcers with necrotic debris and eschars other than those on the heel; however, the extent of tissue needed to be removed is highly variable. An eschar on the heel should be excised only if it is fluctuant, draining, or surrounded by cellulitis, and if the patient is septic.

Major debridement is performed in the operating room, but serial sharp debridement can be performed at the bedside. The use of *systemic antimicrobials* should be considered to prevent bacteremia during significant debridement. A *bone biopsy* is recommended while debriding ulcers when bone is exposed and for nonhealing deep ulcers (stage III or IV ulcers) after 2–4 weeks of optimal therapy.

Other ulcers can be *debrided by the use of saline wet-to-dry gauze* every 4–6 hours by the use of saline in a 35 mL syringe with an attached 19-gauge angiocatheter, or by whirlpool use. The use of enzymes should be reserved for ulcers that are not clinically infected. *Autolytic debridement* is indicated for noninfected ulcers that are not likely to become infected.

Debridement can also be indicated for staging of the ulcer. This assumes that staging is a requisite for treating the patient. Although debridement is a useful therapeutic tool, complete elimination of necrotic tissue is unnecessary, as is daily surgical debridement.

Maintenance of a moist wound environment

The choice of a synthetic dressing depends on the presence of infection, amount of exudate, status of the periulcer skin, and amount of pain experienced by the patient. *Saline dressings* and *alginates* are indicated for infected ulcers. *Synthetic dressings (i.e. films)* are used on ulcers with minimal exudate, *hydrocolloid wafers* for moderate exudate, and *foam wafers* and

Evidence Levels: **A** Double-blind study **B** Clinical trial ≥ 20 subjects **C** Clinical trial < 20 subjects **D** Series ≥ 5 subjects **E** Anecdotal case reports

alginates for ulcers with a large amount of exudate. Ulcers with fragile or dermatitic periulcer skin should be covered with *hydrogel wafers* or *non-adherent foam wafers*. All occlusive dressings relieve pain, when present, but the hydrogel wafers are best for this purpose.

Correction of the underlying contributing factors

Patients may have associated illnesses that interfere with wound healing. Attention to the medical status is important. For example, diabetes mellitus, malnutrition, peripheral vascular disease, cardiac disease, malignancy, and even Alzheimer's disease may prevent any ulcer healing. Unfortunately, even the best medical care may not permit healing. The clinician should bear in mind that the skin can fail, just as any other organ in the body can fail.

General measures

Treatment of the decubitus ulcer can be simplified and made more effective if the following recommendations are considered.
- Saline should be used to clean most pressure lesions; soap and disinfectants are too irritating for more than occasional use.
- When ulcers are not infected, synthetic dressings should be changed, only if they become dislodged or wound fluid escapes from under the dressing.
- Periulcer skin must be kept dry not only to avoid maceration but also to permit the dressing to adhere to the skin.
- To obliterate dead space, *fill deep ulcers loosely with a hydrocolloid, a hydrogel wound filler, or an alginate rope* before applying a synthetic dressing. This same material should be placed under the edge of the ulcer when undermining is present. Bleeding after serial surgical debridement can often be controlled with an alginate dressing; the calcium alginate assists in the clotting pathway. Moistening with saline can loosen an alginate dressing that adheres to granulation tissue.
- A clean ulcer that fails to show signs of healing, or an ulcer with persistent excessive exudate despite receiving optimal care, should be treated with an antibacterial agent (e.g., *1% silver sulfadiazine, cadexomer iodine, triple antibiotic, or retapamulin*) for 2 weeks to reduce the bacterial burden. Increased bacterial burden may impede healing before clinical signs of infection become apparent. The odor of an infected ulcer can often be eliminated by applying *metronidazole gel* to the ulcer bed. *Systemic antimicrobials* are indicated for patients with bacteremia, sepsis, advancing cellulitis, or osteomyelitis.
- Although most synthetic dressings relieve pain, treatment for moderate to severe pain can include *topical anesthetics, non-steroidal anti-inflammatory agents (NSAIDs), opiates, antidepressants,* and *sedatives*. Many patients with decubitus ulcers do not have pain.

Blanchable erythema and non-blanchable erythema

Blanchable and non-blanchable erythema represent the initial development of the decubitus ulcer. The early lesions of non-blanchable erythema are bright red; later, they become dark red to purple. Both can be treated with *adherent synthetic dressings* to protect the lesion from friction and shear, *topical corticosteroids*, or *zinc oxide paste*. The bright red lesion can also be treated with 2% *nitroglycerin ointment* –0.5–1 cm of the ointment is applied over the lesion and covered with an impermeable plastic wrap (such as Saran) for 12 hours daily.

Decubitus dermatitis

Decubitus dermatitis is treated with topical corticosteroids, Vaseline gauze, or a hydrogel wafer. Large bullae (when present) may be debrided before applying the dressing.

Superficial and deep ulcers

Superficial and deep ulcers without necrotic debris are treated with *saline wet-to-dry gauze* or an *adherent synthetic dressing*. Deep ulcers should be loosely filled with *synthetic wound filler* before applying a synthetic dressing. Ulcers that do not involve bone can also be treated with *becaplermin gel* and then packed with saline-moistened gauze once daily. The deep ulcer with necrotic debris requires debridement and is then treated as a clean ulcer.

Enzymatic debridement or the use of an *antimetabolite* can help manage the eschar. Covering the lesion with an adhesive occlusive dressing for several days will often soften the eschar before excision is undertaken. Faster softening can be accomplished by *scarifying the lesion, applying an enzyme to the surface, and covering with an impermeable plastic wrap*. The firmly adherent dry eschar that is not attached to underlying bone can often be separated from the surrounding skin with 5% *5-fluorouracil cream*. After scarification and application of zinc oxide paste to protect the surrounding skin, 5-fluorouracil is applied to the eschar, including its margin, and then covered with an impermeable plastic wrap. Application is repeated every 8 hours. When separation occurs, it can be excised.

Underlying contributing factors

Management of anemia, malnutrition, diabetes mellitus, hydration, and incontinence is essential. The patient should be ingesting approximately *30–35 calories/kg daily* and *1.25–1.50 g protein/kg daily. Ascorbic acid* 500 mg twice daily may enhance healing, but this has not been proven. Keep in mind that the patient who is debilitated and has a multitude of other conditions may have no healing capabilities (skin failure).

SPECIFIC INVESTIGATIONS

▶ Categorize patient
▶ Stage decubitus ulcer
▶ Obtain total protein, serum albumin
▶ Obtain complete blood count

Clinical observation is the key to making the diagnosis. Cutaneous biopsies will not be helpful, although biopsies for aerobic and anaerobic bacteriological cultures could be useful if infection is suspected.

Categories of patient

Patients at risk need to be considered in terms of the underlying disease process:
- Spinal cord injury in an otherwise healthy person
- Neurologic disease with no medical disease, but a devastating condition such as multiple sclerosis or a cerebral vascular accident compromising the body integrity

- Debilitation with a multitude of medical diseases affecting the patient (e.g., arteriosclerosis, diabetes mellitus, Parkinson's disease, Alzheimer's disease, malignancy, malnutrition, and peripheral vascular disease)
- Surgical procedures requiring lengthy positioning on the operating table for cardiovascular or orthopedic procedures.

Grading or evaluation

Grading or evaluation can be accomplished by dermatologic observation and staging. Bear in mind that ulcer staging is arbitrary and does not reflect the dynamics of ulcer formation.

Dermatologic observation

Observe for:
- Blanchable erythema
- Non-blanchable erythema
- Decubitus dermatitis
- Superficial ulcer
- Deep ulcer
- Eschar/gangrene.

Staging

Stages are as follows:
- Stage I – non-blanchable erythema of intact skin
- Stage II – partial-thickness skin loss involving the epidermis and/or dermis
- Stage III – full-thickness skin loss with damage to the subcutaneous tissue that may extend down to, but not through the underlying fascia
- Stage IV – full-thickness skin loss with extensive destruction, tissue necrosis, or damage to muscle, bone, or supporting structures.

Pressure sores among hospitalized patients. Allman RM, Laprade CA, Noel LB, Walker JM, Moorer CA, Dear MR, et al. Ann Intern Med 1986; 105: 337–42.

Hypoalbuminemia, fecal incontinence, and fractures may identify bedridden patients at greatest risk for developing pressure ulcers.

Anaemia and serum protein alteration in patients with pressure ulcers. Fuoco U, Scivoletto G, Pace A, Vona VU, Castellano V. Spinal Cord 1997; 35: 58–60.

All 40 patients with sacral pressure ulcers showed mild-to-moderate anemia with low serum iron and normal or increased ferritin and hypoproteinemia with albuminemia.

Pathophysiology of acute wound healing. Li J, Chen J, Kirsner R. Clin Dermatol 2007; 25: 9–18.

Pressure ulcer tissue histology: an appraisal of current knowledge. Edsberg LE. Ostomy Wound Manage 2007; 53: 40–9.

A review of scales for assessing the risk of developing a pressure ulcer in individuals with SCI. Mortenson WB, Miller WC; SCIRE Research Team. Spinal Cord 2008 46: 168–75.

FIRST-LINE THERAPIES

▶ Elimination of pressure	C
▶ Pressure-reducing and -relieving devices	C
▶ Removal of necrotic debris	C
▶ Maintenance of a moist wound environment	C
▶ Synthetic dressings	B
▶ Topical antibacterials	B
▶ Nutrition	C
▶ Dietary supplements	C

Eliminating pressure and relieving devices

An investigation of geriatric nursing problems in hospital. Norton D, McClaren R, Exton-Smith AN. London: Churchill Livingstone, 1975; 238.

Patients who developed fewer pressure sores were those who were turned every 2–3 hours.
This is based on a book published in 1916.

Shearing force as a factor in decubitus ulcers in paraplegics. Reichel SM. JAMA 1958; 166: 762–3.

As a result of shear, blood vessels in the sacral area become twisted and distorted, and the tissue may become ischemic and necrotic.

Drawsheets for prevention of decubitus ulcer. Witkowski JA, Parish LC. N Engl J Med 1981; 305: 1594.

Use of draw sheets reduces the incidence of friction burns.

Decubitus prophylaxis: a prospective trial on the efficiency of alternating-pressure air mattresses and water mattresses. Andersen KE, Jensen O, Kvorning SA, Bach E. Acta Dermatol Venereol 1983; 63: 227–30.

The incidence of pressure ulcers in patients cared for on the hospital mattress was significantly greater than in patients on alternating-pressure air mattresses.

The effectiveness of preventive management in reducing the occurrence of pressure sores. Krouskop TA, Noble PC, Garber SL, Spencer WA. J Rehab Res Dev 1983; 20: 74–83.

Weight shifting is an effective means of reducing the risk of pressure ulcer formation.

Influence of 30 degrees laterally inclined position and the supersoft 3-piece mattress on areas of maximum pressure and implications for pressure sore prevention. Seiler WO, Allen S, Stahelin NB. Gerontology 1986; 32: 158–66.

When positioned directly on their trochanters, subjects had higher interface pressures and lower transcutaneous oxygen tension than when positioned at an angle.

Air-fluidized beds or conventional therapy for pressure sores; a randomized trial. Allman RM, Walker JM, Hart MK, Laprade CA, Noel LB, Smith CR. Ann Intern Med 1987; 107: 641–8.

Patients with large pressure ulcers may benefit from the use of air-fluidized beds.

Mechanical loading and support surfaces. Agency for Health Care Policy and Research. Pressure ulcers in adults: prediction and prevention. Clinical Practice Guideline No. 3. May 1992. AHCPR Publ No. 92–0047.
An overview of pressure-relieving devices.

Evidence Levels: **A** Double-blind study **B** Clinical trial ≥ 20 subjects **C** Clinical trial < 20 subjects **D** Series ≥ 5 subjects **E** Anecdotal case reports

A clinical comparison of two pressure reducing surfaces in the management of pressure ulcers. Warner DJ. Decubitus 1992; 5: 52–5, 58–60, 62–4.

Pressure ulcers were shown to heal when a static support surface was used.

A randomized trial of low-air-loss beds for treatment of pressure ulcers. Ferrell BA, Osterweil D, Christenson PA. JAMA 1993; 269: 499–507.

Patients with pressure ulcers showed a significantly improved healing rate.

Comparison of total body tissue interface pressure of specialized pressure-relieving mattresses. Hickerson WL, Slugocki GM, Thaker RL, Dunkan R, Bishop JF, Parks JK. J Long Term Eff Med Implants 2004; 14: 81–94.

Pressure can be relieved by specialized mattresses and beds.

Lateral rotation mattresses for wound healing. Anderson C, Rappl L. Ostomy Wound Manage 2004; 50: 50–4, 56, 58.

Continuous lateral rotation therapy uses mattresses and beds that move the patient in a regular pattern around a longitudinal axis. In this study 10 patients with partial-thickness ulcers healed in an average of 9.25 weeks and full-thickness ulcers healed in an average of 11.25 weeks.

Dilemmas about the decubitus ulcer: skin-fold ulcerations and apposition lesions. Parish LC, Lowthian PT. Exp Rev Dermatol 2008; 3: 287–91.

Decubitus ulcers continue to have an uncertain etiology.

Debridement

Collagenase in the treatment of dermal and decubitus ulcers. Rao DB, Sane PG, Georgiev EL. J Am Geriatr Soc 1975; 23: 22–30.

Enzymes can be used alone or in combination with other forms of debridement.

The care of decubitus ulcers, pressure ulcers. Michocki RJ, Lamy PP. J Geriatr Soc 1976; 24; 217–24.

The benefits of sharp debridement are based on expert opinion.

Cleansing the traumatic wound by high pressure syringe irrigation. Stevenson TR, Thacker JG, Rodeheaver GT, Bacchetta C, Edgerton MT, Edlich RF. J Am Coll Emerg Phys 1976; 5: 17–21.

Cleansing provides enough force to remove bacteria and other debris, and loosen eschar.

Dissolution of wound coagulum and promotion of granulation tissue under DuoDERM. Lydon MJ, Hutchinson JJ, Rippon M. Wounds 1989; 1: 95–106.

Enzymes normally present in wound fluid digest devitalized tissue when allowed to collect under a synthetic dressing for several days.

Conservation management of chronic wounds. Feedar JA, Kloth LC. In: Kloth LC, McCulloch JM, Feedar JA, eds. Wound healing; alternatives in management. Philadelphia: FA Davis, 1990.

Debridement of cutaneous ulcer: medical and surgical aspects. Witkowski JA, Parish LC. Clin Dermatol 1991; 9: 585–93.

Debridement can be accomplished by cold steel cutting, by chemical application, or by autohemolytic destruction under an occlusive dressing.

Pressure ulcer treatment guide: quick reference guide for clinicians No. 15. Bergstrom N, Bennett MA, Carlson CE. Adv Wound Care 1995; 6: 22–44.

Histologic examination of bone biopsy specimens is the gold standard for diagnosing osteomyelitis.

More effective removal of debris can be accomplished by twice-daily wound treatment.

Maggot debridement therapy of infected ulcers: patient and wound factors influencing outcome – a study of 101 patients with 117 wounds. Steenvorde P, Jacobi CE, Van Doorn L, Oskam J. Ann Roy Coll Surg Eng 2007; 89: 596–602.

Many wounds (76%) had a successful outcome. The therapy was not so useful for the elderly who had septic arthritis, chronic ischemia of the legs, and deep wounds.

Antimicrobials

Relationship of quantitative wound bacterial counts to healing of decubiti: effect of topical gentamicin. Bendy RH Jr, Nuccio PA, Wolfe E, Collins B, Tamburro C, Glass W, et al. Antimicrob Agents Chemother 1964; 4: 147–55.

Topical metronidazole gel: the bacteriology of decubitus ulcers. Witkowski JA, Parish LC. Int J Dermatol 1991; 30: 660–1.

Metronidazole gel eliminated the odor and anaerobic organisms.

Nutrition

Ascorbic acid supplementation in the treatment of pressure sores. Taylor TV, Rimmer S, Day B, Butcher J, Dymock IW. Lancet 1974; ii: 544–6.

Healing was enhanced even in the absence of deficiency; however, in practice, this does not seem to be the case.

The importance of dietary protein in healing pressure ulcers. Breslow RA, Hallfrisch J, Guy DG, Crawley B, Goldberg AP. J Am Geriatr Soc 1993; 4: 357–62.

High protein with increased caloric contents may enhance pressure ulcer healing.

Nutritional interventions for preventing and treating pressure ulcers. Langer G, Schloemer G, Knerr A, Kuss O, Behrens J. Cochrane Database Syst Rev 2003; 4: CD003216.

There is no confirmation that enteral and/or parenteral nutrition prevents and/or promotes healing of decubitus ulcers.

Old age, malnutrition, and pressure sores: an ill-fated alliance. Mathus-Vliegen EM. J Gerontol A Biol Sci Med Sci 2004; 59: 355–60.

Although vitamins A, B, and C, proteins, and minerals such as zinc and copper promote healing in animal models, supplements of these offer disparate results in the clinic. The potential benefits of tube feeding may be lost due to diarrhea, bowel incontinence, and restricted mobility.

SECOND-LINE THERAPIES

▶ Hydrocolloid wafer dressing	C

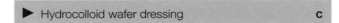

A comparison of the efficacy and cost-effectiveness of two methods of managing pressure ulcers. Colwell JC, Foreman MD, Trotter JP. Decubitus 1993; 6: 28–36.

A larger number of superficial and deep ulcers (stage II and III ulcers) healed with DuoDERM than with saline moist dressings.

Advances in wound healing. Ovington LG. Clin Dermatol 2007; 25: 33–8.

There are many occlusive dressings available which are important for accelerating wound healing.

THIRD-LINE THERAPIES

▶ Nitroglycerin ointment	D
▶ Becaplermin gel	A
▶ 5-Fluorouracil cream	D
▶ Hyperbaric oxygen	E

Pressure ulcer accelerated healing with local injections of granulocyte–macrophage colony-stimulating factor. El Saghir NS, Bizri AR, Shabb NS, Husami TW, Salem Z, Shamseddine AI. J Infect 1997; 35: 179–82.

A single report of granulocyte–macrophage colony-stimulating factor (GM-CSF) inducing accelerated healing of a sacral pressure ulcer in a bedridden patient with bilateral hemiplegia. GM-CSF was diluted and injected locally around and into the ulcer bed every 2–3 days for 2 weeks, then weekly for 4 weeks until complete healing occurred. New firm granulation tissue was noted within a few days.

The ulcer showed 85% healing within 2 weeks, and 100% by 2 months. The ulcer remained closed until the patient's sudden death 9 months later.

Becaplermin gel in the treatment of pressure ulcers: a phase II randomized, double-blind, placebo-controlled study. Rees RS, Robson MC, Smiell JM, Perry BH. Wound Repair Regen 1999; 7: 141–7.

Recombinant human platelet-derived growth factor-BB (becaplermin) the active ingredient in Regranex gel in the treatment of chronic full-thickness pressure ulcers was compared with that of placebo gel. A total of 124 adults with pressure ulcers were assigned randomly to receive topical treatment with becaplermin gel 100 μg/g (n=31) or 300 μg/g (n=32) once daily alternating with placebo gel every 12 h, becaplermin gel 100 μg/g twice daily (n=30), or placebo (n=31) twice daily until complete healing was achieved, or for 16 weeks. All treatment groups received a standardized regimen of good wound care throughout the study period. Once-daily treatment of chronic pressure ulcers with becaplermin gel 100 μg/g significantly reduced the median relative ulcer volume at endpoint compared to placebo gel (p<0.025 for all comparisons). Becaplermin gel 300 μg/g did not result in a significantly greater incidence of healing than that observed with 100 μg/g.

Hyperbaric oxygen therapy for chronic wounds. Kranke P, Bennett M, Roecki-Wiedmann I, Debus S. Cochrane Database Syst Rev 2004; 2: CD004123.

There are no satisfactory studies available to prove that hyperbaric oxygen is useful in decubitus or arterial ulcers.

Clinical aspects of full-thickness wound healing. Rivera AE, Spencer JM. Clin Dermatol 2007; 25: 39–48.

Pros and cons of various dressing materials, including vacuum-assisted closure devices are presented.

Delusions of parasitosis

Robert E. Accordino, John Koo

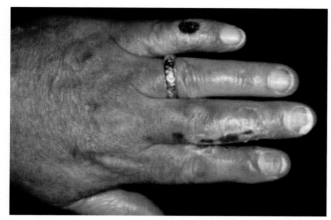

From Meehan et al. Successful Treatment of Delusions of Parasitosis with Olanzapine. Arch Dermatol 142; 352–355. Copyright 2006 American Medical Association. All rights reserved.

An uncommon primary psychiatric disorder, delusions of parasitosis is a form of delusional disorder, somatic type (known also as a monosymptomatic hypochondrial psychosis), in which patients have a cutaneous dysesthesia that causes them to pick at their skin continuously, in order to 'extract' an organism or 'foreign body' they believe is infesting their skin. The cutaneous findings that result from these attempts to dig out the suspected parasites range from normal skin to excoriations, picker's nodules, and frank ulcerations. The cutaneous symptoms may be asymmetrical owing to the effect of the dominant hand. Patients develop elaborate and complex stories associated with their condition, and their beliefs cannot be argued with reason. These patients often collect 'samples' in bottles or jars or on paper or slides of what is often lint, hair, debris, fuzz, dead skin, 'fibers,' and even bugs found in the home. Such behaviors are known as the 'matchbox sign:' patients closely document their syndrome, using these 'specimens' to provide evidence to physicians of the underlying cause of their condition. Many of these patients can have tactile hallucinatory experiences as well that are compatible with their delusion. The common characteristic hallucinatory symptom they may experience is formication, which is manifest as sensations of cutaneous crawling, biting, or stinging. The condition has a bimodal age distribution, occurring in younger adults (both men and women) and the elderly (mostly women). There can be secondary psychopathologies in delusions of parasitosis, such as depression and anxiety; these can be severe enough to cause the patient to commit suicide.

MANAGEMENT STRATEGY

The physician should first establish *good patient rapport*. This begins with a *thorough and complete skin examination*. A good skin examination sometimes entails deciding whether performing a biopsy may be worthwhile, because these patients frequently insist upon having a biopsy, if for no other reason than to estab-

lish a therapeutic alliance. To build the patient's trust, it is imperative that the dermatologist examine these patients thoroughly and carry out a detailed medical history to exclude a frank skin condition (such as scabies) or other possible organic conditions that may be the cause, such as substance abuse (such as cocaine), neurological (e.g., multiple sclerosis), endocrine (such as diabetes mellitus), hematologic/oncologic (such as lymphoma), nutritional (such as B_{12} deficiency), infectious (such as AIDS), cardiovascular (such as congestive heart failure) or renal. The condition can also develop after the patient, relative, or a pet has had a true parasitic infection, and so ruling out the presence of a real infestation may be warranted. Importantly, when patients do not know the reason why they are itching, the clinician should consider a diagnosis other than delusions of parasitosis, because patients with delusions typically 'know' that some infestation is causing their symptoms.

Examining various 'specimens' that the patient may bring to the dermatologist's office under the microscope will demonstrate to the patient that his or her concerns are being taken seriously. One should not make any comment that may reinforce their delusional ideation, such as a statement that an organism responsible for the condition was found; an agreement such as this on the part of the clinician may ultimately render the patient more difficult to deal with, by making them even more firmly fixated on their erroneous belief systems. On the other hand, by definition, rational argument or trying to talk a patient out of a delusion is also generally counterproductive. Dermatologists must acknowledge that they know the patient's sensations and suffering are real, and that they will do everything they can to help.

The most feasible way to reverse delusional ideation is to start the patient on an *antipsychotic medication*. If this is described as an antipsychotic agent, however, few, if any, patients will accept the treatment. On the other hand, if the option of this treatment is offered in a neutral way, emphasizing possible symptom reduction, such as reduced crawling, biting, or stinging sensations, while staying away from arguing over pathophysiology or the mechanism of action of these medications, patients are often eager to accept. In selected cases the physician may explain that the dysesthesia the patient is experiencing is mediated in part by neuropeptides, and that symptoms are often improved when patients go on certain, known medications that act on these neuropeptides.

The medication classically used to treat delusions of parasitosis is the traditional antipsychotic agent *pimozide*, a neuroleptic. This medication can work well, whether patients have classic delusions of parasitosis or merely formications, but are not delusional. The starting dose of pimozide is deliberately kept low at 1–2 mg/day to minimize the risk of side effects. The dose is gradually increased until the optimal clinical response is attained, as evidenced by reduced mental preoccupation, formication, and agitation. The dose of pimozide can be increased by as little as 1 mg increments, and as slowly as on a biweekly basis until significant clinical response is noted, which is usually evident by the time the dose is 4–6 mg daily. It is very rare that a patient will require a dose of more than 6 mg daily, and the use of more than 10 mg daily is almost unheard of in the treatment of delusions of parasitosis. Once the patient reaches a stable, well-tolerated dose of the medication, and agitation, mental preoccupation, and symptoms of formication have subsided, this dose can be maintained for a few months. During this time, if the patient continues to experience improvement, the dosage of pimozide can be gradually reduced by as little as 1 mg every 1–2 weeks until the minimum necessary dosage is determined or the patient is tapered off the pimozide altogether.

If the clinical state deteriorates again with a new episode of exacerbation of a delusional belief system and formication, the patient can be restarted on pimozide and again treated in a time-limited fashion to control the particular episode. Most patients with delusions of parasitosis can be treated on an episodic basis and can be tapered off pimozide after 2–3 months, but some require long-term treatment.

As pimozide blocks dopaminergic receptors, there is the possibility that extrapyramidal side effects such as stiffness in the muscles or joints or akathisia, an inner sensation of restlessness, may develop. Acute dystonic reaction and tardive dyskinesia are other potential adverse consequences associated with pimozide, although with the relatively low dosages used to treat delusions of parasitosis these side effects are rarely encountered. If they do develop, however, they can be controlled with anticholinergic agents such as benztropine 1–2 mg up to four times a day as needed, or diphenhydramine 25 mg four times a day as needed for stiffness or restlessness. Akathesia and pseudoparkinsonian side effects are not a reason for discontinuing treatment with pimozide provided they are kept under control with one of these agents.

Because pimozide can theoretically prolong the QT interval or cause ventricular arrhythmias, it is advisable to consider checking pretreatment – and, periodically, post-treatment – electrocardiograms (ECGs), especially in older patients or those with a history of cardiac arrhythmia. It should be noted that in most cases, however, the risk of ECG abnormalities, including prolongation of the QT interval, is minimal with doses at or less than 10 mg daily. Caution must also be exercised in prescribing pimozide for those with hepatic or renal dysfunction.

More recently, atypical antipsychotics, such as *risperidone*, and *olanzapine*, have been used to treat patients with delusions of parasitosis. Atypical antipsychotics block more 5HT-2 receptors than D2 receptors. Serotonin has been shown to be a key player in some states of psychosis, most cases of obsessive–compulsive disorder, and self-mutilation, which can all potentially be manifest in patients with delusions of parasitosis. Thus, atypical antipsychotics, by blocking both serotonin and dopaminergic receptors, are thought theoretically to be an effective choice for treating this condition. Furthermore, the burden of side effects with atypical antipsychotics may be reduced compared to that of typical antipsychotics. Having the patient agree to go on risperidone or olanzapine, however, may be more difficult than with pimozide, because pimozide's primary indication is Tourette's syndrome, whereas the primary indication for risperidone and olanzapine is schizophrenia. Nevertheless, over the past several years clinicians have reported many cases with good success using atypical antipsychotics. It is usually advisable to start at low doses of these agents and titrate upward as needed while avoiding side effects (starting from 0.5 mg once to twice daily to the maximum dose of 2 mg twice daily). To date, however, there have been no randomized double-blind, placebo-controlled trials comparing the efficacy of pimozide with the atypical antipsychotics, and most of the medical literature on atypical antipsychotics is limited to case reports.

At any point, if feasible, it may be beneficial to try to *refer the patient to a psychiatrist*. However, many of these patients cannot be treated by psychiatrists because of their continued refusal to believe their condition is psychiatric in nature. Therefore, for the dermatologist to understand the use of antipsychotic medication may be the only way that most of these patients will receive the treatment they need. At the same time, the most difficult aspect of managing patients with delusions of parasitosis is trying to obtain their cooperation in taking the medication. This difficulty arises as a result of the difference between the patient's belief system and the physician's understanding of how to treat the situation. Patients may be reluctant to take a psychotropic medication. It may be helpful to emphasize to them that these medications have worked well with patients with similar symptoms and that, in light of their suffering, they have nothing to lose by trying the medication empirically (i.e., trial and error). It is also important for the dermatologist to treat secondary skin changes in these patients. By doing so, the dermatologist will help to forge a therapeutic alliance with the patient by acknowledging that there are skin issues to be treated. Dermatologists should consider soothing baths and topical agents such as steroid–anesthetic combinations, creams with menthol, or other soothing agents.

SPECIFIC INVESTIGATIONS

These additional tests may be considered, depending on the patient's clinical presentation:
▶ Complete blood count
▶ Complete electrolyte panel, including serum potassium, blood urea nitrogen, creatinine, and glucose
▶ Thyroid function tests
▶ Liver function tests
▶ Serum B_{12}, ferritin
▶ ECG before initiation of pimozide
▶ Ask about recreational drug use
▶ Microscopy of specimens brought in by the patient

Delusions of parasitosis. A dermatologist's guide to diagnosis and treatment. Koo J, Lee CS. Am J Clin Dermatol 2001; 2: 285–90.

This is a good review of the diagnosis and treatment of delusions of parasitosis.

Delusions of parasitosis. Lee CS. Dermatol Ther 2008 Jan-Feb; 21: 2–7.

This is another good review of the clinical features and treatment options for this condition.

One hundred years of delusional parasitosis. Meta-analysis of 1223 case reports. Trabert W. Psychopathology 1995; 28: 238–46.

A comprehensive review of delusions of parasitosis. The delusions were present on average 3 years prior to presentation to a healthcare provider. Social isolation seemed to be present in many patients as a premorbid condition. Full remission was observed in approximately half of the patients. Short preclinical courses may indicate a better outcome. Comparing the patients of the pre-psychopharmacological era (i.e., before 1960) with those after, the rate of full remissions increased from 34% to 52%.

Diffuse pruritic lesions in a 37-year-old man after sleeping in an abandoned building. Dunn J, Murphy MB, Fox KM. Am J Psychiatry 2007; 164: 1166–72.

This is an excellent case presentation of a patient with delusions of parasitosis and contains a thorough discussion of the differential diagnosis.

Evidence Levels: **A** Double-blind study **B** Clinical trial ≥ 20 subjects **C** Clinical trial < 20 subjects **D** Series ≥ 5 subjects **E** Anecdotal case reports

FIRST-LINE THERAPIES

▶ Pimozide   B

Pimozide in dermatologic practice: a comprehensive review. Lorenzo CR, Koo J. Am J Clin Dermatol 2004; 5: 339–49.

This article reviews the utility of the use of pimozide in dermatological conditions.

Delusional parasitosis: a dermatologic, psychiatric, and pharmacologic approach. Driscoll MS, Rothe MJ, Grant-Kels JM, Hale MS. J Am Acad Dermatol 1993; 29: 1023–33.

Pimozide is suggested as the first line of therapy for this psychodermatologic condition. Relapse often occurs on discontinuation of the drug.

Neurotropic and psychotropic drugs in dermatology. Tennyson H, Levine N. Dermatol Clin 2001; 19: 179–97.

This is a review article discussing the use of psychotropic drugs for psychodermatologic conditions such as delusions of parasitosis.

Delusions of parasitosis. A psychiatric disorder to be treated by dermatologists? An analysis of 33 patients. Zomer SF, De Wit RF, Van Bronswijk JE, Nabarro G, Van Vloten WA. Br J Dermatol 1998; 138: 1030–2.

Of 33 patients with delusions of parasitosis, 24 were prescribed pimozide but only 18 took the medicine because it was difficult to convince them to do so. Of these 18 patients, five had full remission, four became less symptomatic, five were unchanged, and four died of unrelated causes.

Delusions of infestation treated with pimozide: a follow-up study. Lindskov R, Baadsgaard O. Acta Dermatol Venereol 1985; 65: 267–70.

Fourteen patients were followed up for 19–48 months after pimozide therapy was completed: seven remained in remission, three had a relapse that required repeat treatment, and four responded poorly.

SECOND-LINE THERAPIES

▶ Risperidone	E
▶ Olanzapine	E
▶ Trifluoperazine	E
▶ Haloperidol	E
▶ Sulpiride	E
▶ Fluphenazine	E
▶ Flupenthixol	E

Therapeutic update: use of risperidone for the treatment of monosymptomatic hypochondriacal psychosis. Elmer KB, George RM, Peterson K. J Am Acad Dermatol 2000; 43: 683–6.

The authors discuss risperidone as being highly effective for delusions of parasitosis while avoiding the negative long-term side effects of pimozide (as discussed above).

Risperidone in the treatment of delusions of infestation. DeLeon OA, Furmaga KM, Canterbury AL, Bailey LG. Int J Psychiatry Med 1997; 27: 403–9.

Risperidone was reported to be successful in three patients who had not responded to haloperidol or pimozide.

A case of monosymptomatic hypochondriacal psychosis treated with olanzapine. Weintraub E, Robinson C. Ann Clin Psychiatry 2000; 12: 247–9.

An elderly woman reported to have a good response with the atypical antipsychotic agent olanzapine at lower doses than those needed to treat schizophrenia (2.5 mg as a starting dose, titrated upward by 2.5 mg/week to a maximum of 10 mg daily).

Olanzapine is considered to offer considerable safety and side effect advantages over other agents in older patients.

Successful treatment of delusions of parasitosis with olanzapine. Meehan WJ, Badreshia S, Mackley CL. Arch Dermatol 2006; 142: 352–5.

Three patients (a 53- and a 54-year-old man and a 56-year-old woman) with delusions of parasitosis were reported to have had successful treatment with olanzapine.

Primary delusional parasitosis treated with olanzapine. Freudenmann RW, Schönfeldt-Lecuona C, Lepping P. Int Psychogeriatr 2007; 19: 1161–8.

Another case report of an elderly woman with delusions of parasitosis successfully treated with olanzapine monotherapy. The authors also present a review of all articles that report the use of atypical antipsychotics for delusions of parasitosis.

Atypical antipsychotics in the treatment of delusional parasitosis. Wenning MT, Davy LE, Catalano G, Catalano MG. Ann Clin Psychiatry 2003; 15: 233–9.

Favorable results were observed with the use of atypical antipsychotics in five patients with delusions of parasitosis. The rationale for this treatment choice is discussed.

Antipsychotic treatment of primary delusional parasitosis: systematic review. Lepping P, Russell I, Freudenmann RW. Br J Psychiatry 2007; 191: 198–205.

This article is the first systematic review of the use of typical and atypical antipsychotics in patients with delusions of parasitosis. Analyses showed that both typical and atypical antipsychotics were effective in the majority of patients, as described in previously published studies and case reports. Particularly effective antipsychotics to bring about full or partial remission were pimozide, trifluoperazine, haloperidol, sulpiride, fluphenazine, and flupenthixol.

Dermatitis artefacta

Robert E. Accordino, John Koo

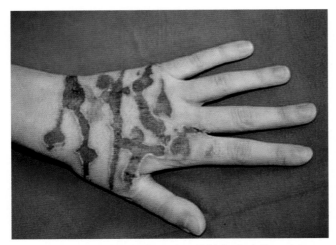

From Finore et al. Dermatitis Artefacta in a Child. Pediatric Dermatology. 2007; 24(5), E51–56.

A relatively rare disorder, dermatitis artefacta is primarily a psychiatric condition in which a patient self-induces a variety of skin lesions to satisfy a conscious or unconscious psychological need. However, the patient will invariably deny responsibility for their injuries. The method used to inflict the lesions is typically more elaborate than simple excoriations. In turn, the appearance of the lesions depends upon the manner in which they are created, and can range from minor cuts to large areas of trauma, but is usually characterized by peculiarly shaped injured areas surrounded by normal-looking skin on parts of the body easily contacted by the dominant hand. Chemical or thermal burns, injection of foreign materials, circulatory occlusion, and tampering with old lesions, such as existing scars or prior surgical incision sites, are some common methods of self-injury. More serious wounds can result in abscesses, gangrene, or other life-threatening infection. A large proportion of patients with dermatitis artefacta manifest borderline personality disorder. Interestingly, when the patient is asked about the manner in which the skin condition evolved, he or she is often vague, generally unmoved, and cannot provide sufficient detail, an unusual aspect of the illness termed the 'hollow history.'

MANAGEMENT STRATEGY

It is first important to rule out malingering as the etiology of the skin lesions. If the lesions were made deliberately for secondary gain, such as disability or insurance benefits, the case is no longer considered psychiatrically based and cases may eventually need to be dealt with legally.

Most treatment for dermatitis artefacta is symptomatic and supportive. *Protective dressings*, such as an Unna boot, can occlude the involved areas and protect against further self-injurious behavior.

Antidepressant medications, such as *selective serotonin reuptake inhibitors (SSRIs)*, may be helpful for patients with dermatitis

artefacta who have primary or secondary depression. If there is clinical evidence of a psychotic process, *pimozide* could be considered empirically in resistant cases. There have also been recent case reports of patients responding to the atypical antipsychotic *olanzapine* when all other modes of therapy, including anti-depressants and other anti-psychotics, have failed.

Importantly, physicians should be aware that patients presenting with dermatitis artefacta have a psychiatric illness, and the skin lesions are often an appeal for help. However, suggesting that the illness is psychiatrically based often has a negative effect on patient rapport. Direct confrontation should be avoided if possible, and instead, *a supportive environment* and a *stable physician–patient therapeutic alliance* should be fostered, often initially through short, frequent office visits. The clinician should be non-judgmental, empathize with the pain, discomfort, and restrictions imposed by the illness, and potentially explore events and possible stressors in the patient's life. In the case of an adolescent, the clinician should encourage the parents to become involved in identifying psychosocial stressors in the patient's life and helping to modify their environment to meet his or her needs. Importantly, most parents are resistant to this diagnosis and can be angry and critical toward the clinician, so great tact is advisable. Once the patient establishes trust in the physician by means of a stable relationship, the physician may help the patient recognize the psychosocial impact of the disorder and *recommend consultation with a psychiatrist* or *psychotherapy*. The patient, however, may still not acknowledge the psychogenic etiology of the illness.

Most patients with dermatitis artefacta have a chronic, waxing and waning course. Thus, even when the condition is under control, the physician should still follow the patient at regular intervals to ensure that the self-destructive behavior does not reinitiate. *Regular visits*, whether or not lesions are present, will help the patient feel cared for and diminish the need for self-mutilation as a call for help.

SPECIFIC INVESTIGATIONS

▶ Rule out malingering
▶ Rule out any organic dermatologic disease
▶ Assess for associated psychiatric disorders (i.e. depression)

Cutaneous manifestations of psychiatric disease that commonly present to the dermatologist – diagnosis and treatment. Koblenzer CS. Int J Psychiatry Med 1992; 22: 47–63.

This article describes common dermatological presentations of psychopathology, including dermatitis artefacta.

Self-mutilation and the borderline personality. Schaeffer CB, Carrol J, Abramowitz SI. J Nerv Ment Dis 1982; 170: 468–73.

Patients with dermatitis artefacta usually have borderline personality disorder.

Psychiatric aspects of dermatitis artefacta. Fabisch W. Br J Dermatol 1980; 102: 29–34.

Some psychiatrists believe that the patient may have an underlying immature personality, with the dermatitis artefacta being 'an appeal for help.'

Dermatitis artefacta: A review of 14 cases. Obasi OE, Naguib M. Ann Saudi Med 1999; 19: 223–7.

Evidence Levels: **A** Double-blind study **B** Clinical trial ≥ 20 subjects **C** Clinical trial < 20 subjects **D** Series ≥ 5 subjects **E** Anecdotal case reports

This is a study of the characteristics of 14 patients seen with dermatitis artefacta at the King Fahad Hospital in Al Baha, Saudi Arabia. The authors reported that 12 of the 14 were female, with a mean age of 25.9 years (range 12–71). Nine of the 12 females had identifiable severe emotional or psychiatric problems.

Dermatitis artefacta in pediatric patients: experience at the National Institute of Pediatrics. Saez-de-Ocariz M, Orozco-Covarrubias L, Mora-Magaña I, Duran-McKinster C, Tamayo-Sanchez L, Gutierrez-Castrellon P, et al. Pediatr Dermatol 2004; 21: 205–11.

In this study, the incidence of dermatitis artefacta was 1:23 000, and is considered a rarity in children; 12 of the 29 patients reported had an associated chronic illness, and seven displayed mild mental retardation.

Dermatitis artefacta in a child. Finore ED, Andreoli E, Alfani S, Palermi G, Pedicelli C, Paradisi M. Pediatr Dermatol 2007; 24: E51–6.

This article is an excellent and detailed case study of an 11-year-old girl with dermatitis artefacta that includes a thorough report of the patient's psychodiagnostic interview.

FIRST-LINE THERAPIES

▶ Occlusive dressings	D
▶ Psychotropic agents	D
▶ Psychotherapy (even if only supportive)	D
▶ Management of secondary cutaneous complications	D

Diagnostic clues to dermatitis artefacta. Joe EK, Li VW, Magro CM, Arndt KA, Bowers KE. Cutis 1999; 63: 209–14.

This is a case report of a 36-year-old man who had several of the classic features of dermatitis artefacta. The clinical and histopathologic features, diagnostic aids, approach to therapy, and prognosis for the condition are reviewed.

Self-inflicted skin diseases. A retrospective analysis of 57 patients with dermatitis artefacta seen in a dermatology department. Nielsen K, Jeppesen M, Simmelsgaard L, Rasmussen M, Thestrup-Pedersen K. Acta Dermatol Venereol 2005; 85: 512–15.

This retrospective analysis of 57 patients reports the following epidemiological findings: diagnosis was 2.8 times more likely in females than in males; symptoms were most common in patients aged 18–60 years, with a median age of 39; and 88% of patients had multiple (as opposed to single) lesions. When self-infliction was suggested as the potential cause of illness to patients (n=30), only one patient agreed to see a psychiatrist and two-thirds denied self-infliction or stopped coming for treatment. Ten patients had a psychiatric diagnosis. The most common subjective complaints were 'pain' (59%) and 'itching' (37%). The three most common lesion types were skin ulcers (72%), excoriations (46%), and erythema (30%). Of the entire group of 57 patients, 61% were treated with anxiolytic or antidepressant medications. In 32 patients occlusive dressings could be administered, and the lesions all showed improvement except in two cases. The authors strongly recommend frequent patient visits to allow for regular monitoring of lesions.

Training future dermatologists in psychodermatology. Van Moffaert M. Gen Hosp Psychiatry 1986; 8: 115–18.

Palliative dermatological measures such as occlusive bandages, ointments, or placebo drugs, as well as hospitalization that includes bathing and massaging by nurses, can have a therapeutic impact on the psychiatric problem by symbolizing the medical attention and care the patient with dermatitis artefacta is craving.

Dermatitis artefacta. Clinical features and approach to treatment. Koblenzer CS. Am J Clin Dermatol 2000; 1: 47–55.

A good review article.

SECOND-LINE THERAPIES

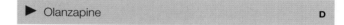

▶ Olanzapine	D

Treatment of self-mutilation with olanzapine. Garnis-Jones S, Collins S, Rosenthal D. J Cutan Med Surg 2000; 4: 161–3.

Three patients successfully treated with low-dose olanzapine when multiple other therapies (including antidepressants and other antipsychotics) failed.

Olanzapine is effective in the management of some self-induced dermatoses: case reports. Gupta MA, Gupta AK. Cutis 2000; 66: 143–6.

Three patients with acne excorié, factitious ulcers, and trichotillomania, respectively, responded to 2–4 weeks of olanzapine 2.5–5 mg/day.

Dermatitis herpetiformis

John J Zone

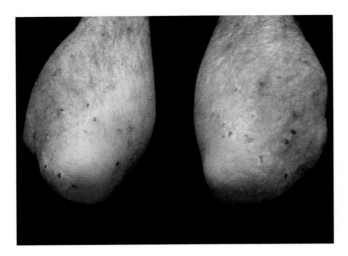

Dermatitis herpetiformis (DH) is a cutaneous manifestation of celiac disease. Virtually all patients have an associated gluten-sensitive enteropathy which varies in severity. Both the skin disease and the histological intestinal inflammatory process respond to dietary gluten restriction. DH patients present with a spectrum of severity, ranging from minimal pruritic papules on the elbows and knees to severe, intensely pruritic vesicular lesions over multiple extensor surfaces. The prevalence of DH is approximately 10–39 per 100 000 persons in the Caucasian population. DH is distinguished from other bullous diseases by characteristic histologic, immunologic, and associated gastrointestinal findings. Histologically, vesicle formation at the dermoepidermal junction, and infiltration of dermal papillary tips with neutrophils are seen. Direct immunofluorescence shows granular IgA localized in the dermal papillary tips of perilesional skin.

MANAGEMENT STRATEGY

The course of DH depends on the therapeutic choices that are made at the time of diagnosis. If patients choose a strict gluten-free diet and adopt a conscientious change in eating habits and lifestyle, they are likely to have a long-term remission and not be bothered by the skin disease. Associated intestinal symptoms are also minimized. In such situations relapses are usually associated with dietary indiscretions. Elevated levels of IgA antibodies to tissue transglutaminase are characteristic of celiac disease, correlate with the degree of intestinal inflammation, and decrease with gluten restriction. If medical therapy with dapsone or sulfapyridine is chosen, the cutaneous lesions can be well controlled. However, attention must be paid to potential side effects of medications. Intestinal symptoms, if present, will continue unabated. Occasional patients (10–20%) will enjoy a spontaneous remission without medication or dietary restriction. The reason for such remission is unclear.

Dapsone is the drug of choice and is currently the only drug approved by the United States Food and Drug Administration for use in this disease. Initial treatment with dapsone 25 mg daily will usually improve pruritus within 24–48 hours and the papulovesicular lesions within 1 week in adults. Correspondingly smaller doses (0.5–1 mg/kg) should be used in children. Maintenance therapy is then adjusted on a weekly basis to maintain adequate suppression of symptoms. The average maintenance dose is 0.5–1.0 mg/kg daily. Despite adequate dapsone dosages, outbreaks of facial and scalp lesions are common.

Adherence to a gluten-free diet (GFD) improves clinical symptoms in patients with DH. The advantages of gluten restriction include a reduction of dapsone dosage and its attendant complications, improvement of gastrointestinal symptoms (which range from cramping pain to overt diarrhea), and a therapy aimed at the cause rather than the symptoms of the disease. The increased risk of lymphoma incident to DH and celiac disease is also reduced with a GFD, but not with dapsone. Dapsone improves the cutaneous lesions, but has no effect on intestinal disease. Strict adherence to a GFD is, however, challenging, and reintroduction of gluten can exacerbate symptoms of DH. Rare patients will not respond to gluten restriction, and it is not possible to predict with certainty which patients will respond. In the author's opinion, a useful therapeutic strategy is the initial control of DH symptoms with dapsone at the same time as a GFD, with subsequent tapering of dapsone. Oats have been found to be non-toxic in most patients with DH, and may broaden the dietary options in an otherwise restrictive GFD.

Sulfapyridine is an alternative choice in patients who are intolerant to dapsone and has been shown to result in significant therapeutic efficacy. Sulfapyridine is started at 500 mg three times daily, and is usually increased to a maximum maintenance dose of 1.5 g three times daily.

Other agents that have been reported to have a therapeutic benefit in DH include *nicotinamide, tetracycline* (or a combination of the two), *heparin, ciclosporin, colchicine,* and *systemic corticosteroids. Topical corticosteroids* are generally inadequate when used alone to control DH symptoms. However, potent corticosteroids in gel form may provide relief for occasional lesions that develop on otherwise adequate dapsone or GFD therapy. This allows patients to treat lesions without increasing the dosage of dapsone.

SPECIFIC INVESTIGATIONS

> ► Biopsy for histology and direct immunofluorescence
> ► Complete blood count (CBC) and liver function tests (LFTs)
> ► Glucose-6-phosphate dehydrogenase levels
> ► IgA tissue transglutaminase antibodies

Deposition of granular IgA relative to clinical lesions in dermatitis herpetiformis. Zone JJ, Meyer LJ, Petersen MJ. Arch Dermatol 1996; 132: 912–18.

It is accepted that granular IgA deposition in clinically normal-appearing perilesional skin is the most reliable diagnostic criterion for DH. Although the combination of characteristic clinical and pathological features is highly suggestive of DH, the diagnosis should not be made without the identification of granular IgA in dermal papillae. If direct immunofluorescence is negative and histology is suggestive of DH, a repeat biopsy for direct immunofluorescence is recommended.

Evidence Levels: **A** Double-blind study **B** Clinical trial ≥ 20 subjects **C** Clinical trial < 20 subjects **D** Series ≥ 5 subjects **E** Anecdotal case reports

Celiac disease. Green PHR, Cellier C. N Engl J Med 2007; 357: 1731–43.

DH is best regarded as a cutaneous manifestation of celiac disease. Celiac disease occurs in nearly 1% of the population. The pathogenesis of both disorders involves the immune response of genetically susceptible individuals (HLA DQ2 and DQ8) to dietary gluten-containing proteins in wheat, barley, and rye. There is an association with autoimmune disorders, especially autoimmune thyroiditis. IgA tissue transglutaminase antibodies can be used as an initial diagnostic screening tool as well as an indication of intestinal disease activity and response of the intestinal inflammatory process to gluten restriction.

FIRST-LINE THERAPIES

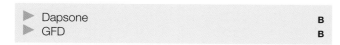

▶ Dapsone	B
▶ GFD	B

Suggested guidelines for patient monitoring: hepatic and hematologic toxicity attributable to systemic dermatologic drugs. Wolverton SE, Remlinger K. Dermatol Clin 2007; 25: 195–205.

Dapsone may produce a drug hypersensitivity syndrome with liver toxicity in the first 3–12 weeks. Monitoring of the AST and ALT and eosinophil count is indicated. Hepatocellular toxicity may also occur in a dose-related fashion, especially with doses higher than 2 mg/kg. AST and ALT should be monitored when the dosage is increased. There are three main hematologic toxicities of dapsone: hemolysis, methemoglobinemia, and agranulocytosis. Methemoglobinemia is usually mild and not problematic unless the patient has underlying cardiopulmonary problems. Agranulocytosis is rare and usually occurs in the first 3–12 weeks of therapy. Symptoms demanding attention include pharyngitis, fever, and oral ulcerations. Virtually all patients have at least some degree of hemolysis, and a fall in hemoglobin of 1–3 g/dL is to be expected. A compensatory reticulocytosis occurs and may be monitored with a reticulocyte count. Hemolysis may be severe in patients with glucose-6-phosphate dehydrogenase (G6PD) deficiency. G6PD levels should be evaluated in blacks and those of southern Mediterranean origin prior to the initiation of therapy to avoid potentially catastrophic hemolytic anemia.

Complete blood count and liver function test should be checked every 2–3 weeks for the first 3 months, and then every 3–6 months thereafter.

Advances in celiac disease and gluten free diet. Niewinski MN. J Am Dietet Assoc 2008; 108: 661–72.

This review focuses in detail on the gluten-free diet and the importance of expert dietary counseling for patients with celiac disease. Recent advances in the GFD include food allergen labeling as well as the US Food and Drug Administration's proposed definition of the term 'gluten-free.' The GFD is complex, and patients need comprehensive nutrition education from a skilled dietitian. Support groups are also helpful.

A long-term gluten-free diet as an alternative treatment in severe forms of dermatitis herpetiformis. Nino M, Ciacci C, Delfino M. J Dermatol Treat 2007; 18: 10–12.

This study evaluated the efficacy of treating severe skin manifestations of DH with a gluten-free diet alone and compared the results to treatment with GFD and dapsone. Eighty-seven percent of patients on GFD alone had a complete remission within 18 months (67% of severe patients). A total of 89% of patients on diet and dapsone had remission of skin disease (70% of severe patients) and 11% were improved.

SECOND-LINE THERAPIES

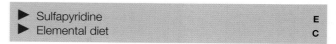

▶ Sulfapyridine	E
▶ Elemental diet	C

Sulfonamides and sulfones in dermatologic therapy. Bernstein JE, Lorincs AL. Int J Dermatol 1981; 20: 81–8.

An extensive review of sulfonamides such as sulfapyridine. Sulfapyridine has been used extensively for the treatment of DH with variable clinical efficacy, but there are no controlled clinical studies of its use. Sulfapyridine is no longer commercially available in the USA, so more recent studies are lacking. Sulfapyridine may be obtained by contacting Jacobus Pharmaceuticals, the USA manufacturer of dapsone, or it can be prepared by a compounding pharmacy.

The effect of elemental diet with and without gluten on disease activity in dermatitis herpetiformis. Kadunce DP, McMurry MP, Avots-Avontins A, Chandler JP, Meyer LJ, Zone JJ. J Invest Dermatol 1991; 97: 175–82.

In severe refractory cases of DH elemental diet therapy is effective and produces dramatic clinical improvement within 2–4 weeks. It involves the ingestion of amino acid and carbohydrate alone, and is commercially available as Vivonex. It produces rapid healing of the intestine and relief of cutaneous symptoms, but was designed for tube feeding and is considered unpalatable by many.

In this author's experience elemental diet containing short-chain polypeptides is less effective.

THIRD-LINE THERAPIES

▶ Tetracycline and nicotinamide	E
▶ Heparin	E
▶ Ciclosporin	E
▶ Colchicine	E
▶ Systemic corticosteroids	E

Dermatitis herpetiformis effectively treated with heparin, tetracycline and nicotinamide. Shah SAA, Ormerond AD. Clin Exp Dermatol 2000; 25: 204–5.

This is a case report of a patient with severe DH who was intolerant to dapsone and sulfapyridine. His DH lesions resolved with combination treatment consisting of subcutaneous low-dose heparin, nicotinamide 1.5 g daily in divided doses, and tetracycline 2 g daily. The patient was, however, on a GFD.

A rare case of dermatitis herpetiformis requiring parenteral heparin for long-term control. Tan CC, Sale JE, Brammer C, Irons RP, Freeman JG. Dermatology 1996; 192: 185–6.

A patient with severe DH who was intolerant of dapsone and sulfapyridine was treated with parenteral heparin, with complete resolution of her skin lesions within 1 week. This treatment is not practical for long-term management.

Efficacy of cyclosporine in two patients with dermatitis herpetiformis resistant to conventional therapy. Stenveld HJ,

Starink TM, van Joost T, Stoof TJ. J Am Acad Dermatol 1993; 28: 1014–15.

Two patients with severe DH who were intolerant and/or unresponsive to conventional therapy were treated with ciclosporin (5–7 mg/kg daily) with resolution of skin lesions.

Dermatitis herpetiformis responsive to systemic corticosteroids. Lang PG. J Am Acad Dermatol 1985; 13: 513–15.

A patient with DH was treated successfully with a short course of prednisone and remained clear 4 months after discontinuation. He was successfully retreated with systemic corticosteroids for recurrence of the skin lesions.

Treatment of dermatitis herpetiformis with colchicine. Silver DN, Juhlin EA, Berczeller PH, McSorley J. Arch Dermatol 1980; 116: 1373–84.

Oral colchicine resulted in significant improvement of skin lesions in three of four patients with DH. The authors suggest that colchicine may be used when dapsone or sulfapyridine are contraindicated.

Dermatologic non-disease

Richard Fried

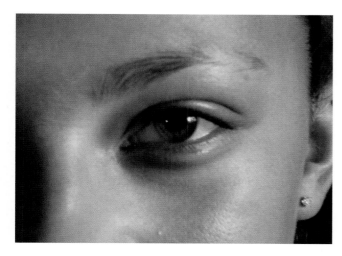

Dermatologic non-disease, also known as body dysmorphic disorder (BDD) and dysmorphophobia, is an alteration in perception of body image that causes preoccupation with minimal or imagined defects in appearance. The preoccupation can be markedly excessive, causing clinically significant distress or impairment in social, occupational, or other important areas of functioning. Preoccupations commonly involve the face and head, the skin and hair being the most frequent areas of concern. Dermatologic preoccupations are distressing, time-consuming, and difficult or impossible for patients to resist. Insight is typically poor, and alterations in perception are often to delusional proportions. Most patients have ideas of reference, thinking that others take special notice or mock them for their perceived defect. Repetitive behaviors are present in almost all patients: excessive checking or grooming, constant need for reassurance, and skin picking are common. The risk of suicide is high, with approximately one-quarter of patients attempting suicide.

MANAGEMENT STRATEGY

Dermatologic non-disease is common in dermatologic settings, with prevalence estimated at 11.9%. Recognition of these patients is extremely important, as they typically have a poor response to cosmetic dermatological treatments. Dissatisfaction, anger, and even aggression toward the treating dermatologist have been reported. Patients with dermatologic non-disease often have associated psychiatric disorders, including major depression, substance abuse and dependence, social phobia, and obsessive–compulsive disorder. The majority of these patients also have a personality disorder. Appropriate psychiatric treatment can result in a generally favorable outcome

Typical body areas of preoccupation include:

• **Face**. Preoccupation with facial itching and burning, or obsessive preoccupation with imagined acne, scars, wrinkles, pigmentation, oiliness, redness, paleness, facial vessels, and facial hair are common. Preoccupation with the nose, ears, and pore size is reported. Despite the fact that others usually do not see these minimal or non-existent flaws, patients can spend hours in front of mirrors, preventing them from working or socializing.
• **Scalp**. Dysesthesias (burning or itch) and obsession with imagined hair loss are common.
• **Genital**. Scrotal, perineal, and perianal burning as well as vulvar redness and burning are common symptoms. Preoccupation with sexually transmitted disease or neoplastic process is common. Symptoms can be incapacitating.

Patients presenting with extreme concern that appears out of proportion to their chief complaint, accompanied by a paucity of objective physical findings, should raise suspicion that dermatologic non-disease may be present. Obsession, rumination, and extreme psychological distress are striking features. These patients usually report dissatisfaction with previous physicians and describe poor outcomes from past medical and surgical interventions. Skin picking and related behaviors such as excessive tanning, excessive grooming, and relentless need for reassurance are characteristic. Attempts at reassurance are inevitably futile, as their perceptions and thinking are usually delusional, which by definition suggests that the distorted perceptions are unresponsive to logic and persuasion. The frequent presence of referential thinking further substantiates the delusional nature of the perceptions. Patients often wear heavy makeup and hats to hide their imperfections and perceived ugliness.

Patients with dermatologic non-disease make unusual and excessive requests for cosmetic procedures in the belief that they will transform or fix their lives. Poor psychosocial functioning, with difficulties in relationships, school, and work, is almost always seen. Depression is frequently evident and previous suicide attempts not infrequent. *Bear in mind that there have been instances of violent behavior toward treatment providers.*

Clinical interactions and consultations with these patients are typically long, difficult, and emotionally draining. Regardless of the actual length of time spent with them, patients often feel that they were not given adequate time and attention. It is inadvisable to perform procedures on these patients, as less than 10% will be satisfied with the results.

Serotonin reuptake inhibitors (SRIs) and cognitive–behavioral psychotherapy are the treatments of choice. *Fluoxetine, fluvoxamine,* and *citalopram* are the best-studied agents, but recent evidence suggests that all SRIs are probably effective. Higher dosing regimens than those used for depression are usually required. For example, fluoxetine and citalopram should be titrated to 60 mg/day, and fluvoxamine should be increased to 300 mg/day at monthly intervals. Patients should receive a trial of 12–16 weeks before efficacy is assessed. If one agent fails another should be substituted, as some patients idiosyncratically respond more favorably to one agent over another. Interestingly, SRIs appear to be more effective than antipsychotic agents, despite the fact that dermatologic non-disease is frequently a delusional disorder. Only about 20% of patients will become free of their delusional thinking. However, the intrusiveness of the thoughts and distress will diminish sufficiently, such that many patients will be able to resume some social and vocational functioning.

Cognitive–behavioral therapy (CBT) is a reality-based, in-the-present therapy that focuses specifically on the symptoms of dermatologic non-disease. The key elements are known as exposure, response prevention, and cognitive restructuring. Exposure consists of having patients expose the perceived defect in social situations. Response prevention consists of helping patients avoid their repetitive behaviors. Cognitive restructuring helps patients change their erroneous beliefs about their appearance and the importance they attribute to it. Ideally, treatment of dermatologic non-disease should encompass both CBT and an SRI.

To initiate treatment or referral, suggest to the patient in a gentle manner that they may have a body image disorder called body dysmorphic disorder. Convey your concern regarding the amount of their time being usurped by their preoccupation and their emotional distress. Psychiatric referral is preferable, but often not feasible. Dermatologists are encouraged to align themselves if possible with mental heath professionals who are experienced in treating this entity. Euphemisms such as skin-emotion specialist reduce the stigma of psychiatric referral and may increase patient acceptance. If referral is not possible, treatment with an SRI may be successful. If suicidal ideation or intent are present, immediate hospitalization is recommended.

INVESTIGATIONS

> ► Assess impairments in quality of life and functional status, the degree of emotional distress, and the potential suicide risk.

Depression, anxiety, anger, and somatic symptoms in patients with body dysmorphic disorder. Phillips KA, Siniscalchi JM, McElroy SL. Psychiatr Q 2004; 75: 309–20.

Seventy-five patients with BDD completed a symptom questionnaire assessing depression, anxiety, somatic/somatization, and anger–hostility. Compared to normal controls, BDD subjects had markedly elevated scores on all four scales, indicating severe distress and psychopathology. When treated with fluvoxamine, all symptoms significantly improved.

Quality of life for patients with body dysmorphic disorder. Phillips KA. J Nerv Ment Dis 2000; 188: 170–5.

This is the only published study looking at quality of life in BDD patients. These patients were found to have a poorer mental health quality of life than has been reported for patients with other severe illnesses, such as type II diabetes, recent myocardial infarction, or depression. These findings highlight the dramatic impact of a non-disease.

33 cases of body dysmorphic disorder in children and adolescents. Albertini RS, Phillips KA. J Am Acad Child Adolesc Psychiatry 1999; 38: 453–9.

Thiryt-three cases were examined. Onset was usually during adolescence, but sometimes occurred in childhood. Earlier identification and treatment may avert unnecessary cosmetic and medical interventions as well as suicide.

Gender differences in body dysmorphic disorder. Phillips KA, Diaz S. J Nerv Ment Dis 1997; 185: 570–7.

This study looked at a large series of patients with DSM-IV-defined BDD and found that one-quarter had attempted suicide. Female patients with severe symptoms are at greater risk.

Dysmorphophobia. Schwartz RA, Patterson WM, Bienvenu OJ III, Chodynicki MP, Janniger CK. emedicine May 2008.

Excellent overview of entity and treatment strategies.

Suicide in dermatological patients. Cotterill JA, Cunliffe WJ. Br J Dermatol 1997; 137: 246–50.

Sixteen patients who had committed suicide are described, most of whom had acne or body dysmorphic disorder. Females with facial complaints and men with facial scarring appeared more at risk for suicide. The authors relate these findings to the possible preventative benefits of early isotretinoin to prevent scarring in patients predisposed to dermatologic non-disease.

FIRST-LINE THERAPIES

► Serotonin reuptake inhibitors	A
► Cognitive–behavioral therapy	B

Treating body dysmorphic disorder with medication: evidence, misconceptions, and a suggested approach. Phillips KA, Hollander E. Body Image 2008; 5: 13–27.

A randomized placebo-controlled trial of fluoxetine in body dysmorphic disorder. Phillips KA, Albertini RS, Rasmussen SA. Arch Gen Psychiatry 2002; 59: 381–8.

This is the only placebo-controlled study of pharmacotherapy in BDD. In the 74 patients studied, fluoxetine was significantly more effective than placebo, with a response rate of 53% versus 18%.

An open label study of venlafaxine in body dysmorphic disorder. Allen A, Hadley SJ, Kaplan A, Simeon D, Friedberg J, Priday L, et al. CNS Spectr 2008; 13: 138–44.

Of 17 patients enrolled, 11 completed 12–16 weeks of venlafaxine minimum 150 mg qd. All 11 improved significantly.

Clomipramine versus desipramine crossover trial in body dysmorphic disorder: selective efficacy of a serotonin reuptake inhibitor in imagined ugliness. Hollander E, Allen A, Kwon J, Mosovich S, Schmeidler J, Wong C. Arch Gen Psychiatry 1999; 56: 1033–9.

This double-blind crossover study of 29 randomized patients found clomipramine (an SRI) superior to desipramine (a non-SRI tricyclic antidepressant).

Efficacy and safety of fluvoxamine in body dysmorphic disorder. Phillips KA, Dwight MM, McElroy SL. J Clin Psychiatry 1998; 59: 165–71.

This open-label study of fluvoxamine demonstrated that 19 (63%) of 30 patients with BDD responded to this SRI.

Delusionality and response to open-label fluvoxamine in body dysmorphic disorder. Phillips KA, McElroy SL, Dwight MM, Eisen JL, Rasmussen SA. J Clin Psychiatry 2001; 62: 87–91.

Thirty patients with BDD were treated with fluvoxamine for 16 weeks in this open-label trial: 63% improved significantly. Both delusional and non-delusional patients responded similarly.

Change in psychosocial functioning and quality of life of patients with body dysmorphic disorder treated with fluoxetine: a placebo-controlled study. Phillips KA, Rasmussen SA. Psychosomatics 2004; 45: 438–44.

This was a 12-week placebo-controlled study of psychosocial functioning and mental health-related quality of life in 60 patients. At baseline, the patients had impaired psychosocial functioning and markedly poor mental health-related quality of life. A significant reduction in the severity of body dysmorphic disorder was demonstrated, along with improvement in functioning and quality of life.

An open label study of citalopram in body dysmorphic disorder. Phillips KA, Najar F. J Clin Psychiatry 2003; 64: 715–20.

This open-label study found that 11 of 15 patients (73%) with DSM-IV-documented BDD demonstrated a statistically significant improvement. Psychosocial functioning and quality of life also improved.

Cognitive–behavioral body image therapy for body dysmorphic disorder. Rosen JC, Reiter J, Orosan P. J Consult Clin Psychol 1995; 63: 263–9.

Exposure and response prevention was effective in 77% of 27 women treated with cognitive–behavioral group therapy for 8 weeks. Subjects in the treatment group improved more than those in the no-treatment waiting-list control group.

Cognitive–behavioral group therapy for body dysmorphic disorder: a case series. Behav Res Ther 1999; 37: 71–5.

Thirteen BDD patients improved significantly after 12 group therapy sessions.

Body dysmorphic disorder: a cognitive behavioral model and pilot randomized controlled trial. Veale D, Gournay K, Dryden W, Boocock A, Shah F, Wilson R, et al. Behav Res Ther 1996; 34; 717–29.

Nineteen patients were randomly assigned to cognitive–behavioral therapy or a waiting-list control group. There was significantly greater improvement in BDD symptoms in the cognitive–behavioral therapy group.

SECOND-LINE THERAPIES

► Additional psychotropic agents and insight-oriented psychotherapy   **D**

Pharmacologic treatment of body dysmorphic disorder: a review of the evidence and a recommended treatment approach. Phillips KA. CNS Spectr 2002; 7: 453–60.

An open study of buspirone augmentation of serotonin-reuptake inhibitors in body dysmorphic disorder. Phillips KA. Psychopharmacol Bull 1996; 32: 175–80.

Thirteen patients with DSM-IV BDD who had not responded or had responded only partially to an SRI had buspirone added to the SRI. Six of these subjects (46%) improved. Three who reduced or discontinued buspirone experienced an increase in symptom severity.

The dysmorphic syndrome. Koblenzer CS. Fitzpatrick's J Clin Dermatol 1994; March/April: 14–19.

Dermatomyositis

Jeffrey P Callen

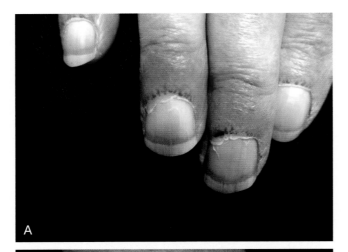

A

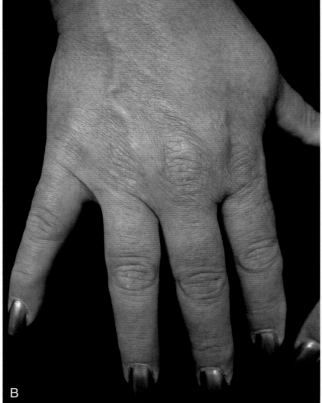

B

Dermatomyositis (DM) is one of the idiopathic inflammatory myopathies characterized by cutaneous disease, including a heliotrope rash, Gottron's papules, a violaceous erythema on extensor surfaces and in a photodistribution, and/or periungual changes. Patients with cutaneous lesions of DM often have demonstrable muscle disease, weakness of the proximal muscles, elevated enzymes such as creatine kinase or aldolase, or abnormal electromyograms or muscle biopsy findings. Some, however, have cutaneous disease that either precedes the onset of demonstrable muscle disease or occurs in its absence. DM in children and adolescents may be complicated by calcinosis, particularly when treatment is delayed. Adults with DM have a greater risk of having or developing a malignancy, usually within the first 3 years following diagnosis.

MANAGEMENT STRATEGY

Prior to treatment the patient should be thoroughly evaluated to assess the severity of the disease, the presence of systemic involvement such as pulmonary, cardiac, or gastrointestinal involvement, and the presence of malignancy.

The goal of management is to *reverse the weakness* and allow the patient to return to normal functional status. The *prevention of contractures* is also a consideration, and the *prevention or treatment of calcinosis* is usually an issue in the management of children and adolescents, but may occur rarely in adults. Patients with cutaneous disease are troubled by extreme pruritus and the appearance of their skin and therefore request management even when the muscle disease has been effectively treated or is absent.

For the myopathy, *corticosteroid with or without an immunosuppressive agent* is the standard treatment. Most patients respond to these agents, but for those who do not, *high-dose intravenous immunoglobulin* may be of benefit. Patients with cutaneous disease are photosensitive and are treated with *sunscreens, topical corticosteroids, oral antimalarials*, or an *oral immunosuppressant*. One of the problems with any of the reports published thus far is the lack of a validated measure of activity to judge the activity and response to therapy. To this end there are three measures that are currently under development: the Dermatomyositis Skin Severity Index (DSSI) (Br J Dermatol 2008; 158: 345–50), the Cutaneous Dermatomyositis Area and Severity Index (CDASI) (Arch Dermatol Res 2008; 300: 3–9) and a Cutaneous Assessment Tool in Juvenile Dermatomyositis (Arthritis Rheum 2008; 59: 352–6.). Unfortunately, none of these measures has yet to be applied to populations in whom therapeutic interventions have taken place.

SPECIFIC INVESTIGATIONS

> ► A thorough evaluation to exclude other causes of myopathy
> ► Malignancy evaluation, including CT scans of chest, abdomen, and pelvis
> ► Serum aldolase or creatine kinase
> ► Electromyogram
> ► Muscle biopsy
> ► Magnetic resonance imaging (MRI) or ultrasound of muscle
> ► Assessment for the presence of systemic involvement (e.g., pulmonary disease, esophageal dysfunction, cardiac involvement)
> ► Assessment of myositis-specific antibodies

Scalp involvement in dermatomyositis. Often overlooked or misdiagnosed. Kasteler JS, Callen JP. JAMA 1994; 272: 1939–41.

Skin lesions in patients with DM, particularly of the scalp, are often confused with psoriasis, seborrheic dermatitis, or

178

lichen planus. Often the lesions simulate cutaneous lupus erythematosus.

Idiopathic inflammatory diseases of muscle. Wortmann RL. In: Weisman M, Weinblatt M, Louie J, eds. Treatment of the rheumatic diseases, 2nd edn. Philadelphia: WB Saunders, 2001; 390–402.

This chapter details the evaluation and the types of muscle disease that need to be excluded prior to classifying patients as having an idiopathic inflammatory myopathy.

Influence of age on characteristics of polymyositis and dermatomyositis in adults. Marie I, Hatron PY, Levesque H, Hachulla E, Hellot MF, Michon-Pasturel U, et al. Medicine (Baltimore) 1999; 78: 139–47.

This group compared characteristics of younger versus older adults and found that the incidence of malignancy was much higher in the older population, and therefore the prognosis for the older population was poorer.

MR imaging in amyopathic dermatomyositis. Lam WW, Chan H, Chan YL, Fung JW, So NM, Metreweli C. Acta Radiol 1999; 40: 69–72.

These authors conducted a prospective study to investigate the role of MRI in 10 patients with amyopathic DM. Three patients demonstrated abnormal signal intensity in muscles on both T_2-weighted and fat-suppression sequences. Thus, one-third of patients with DM and clinically normal muscles may have detectable muscle inflammation on MRI, indicating that MRI has a potential role for locating the relevant biopsy site and for longitudinal follow-up. MRI is useful for demonstrating subclinical muscle involvement in patients with the clinical diagnosis of amyopathic DM.

Dermatomyositis with normal muscle enzyme concentrations. A single-blind study of the diagnostic value of magnetic resonance imaging and ultrasound. Stonecipher MR, Jorizzo JL, Monu J, Walker F, Sutej PG. Arch Dermatol 1994; 130: 1294–9.

This single-blind study evaluated the use of MRI and ultrasound in five patients with classic DM but normal levels of serum muscle enzymes. Ultrasonography revealed hyperechogenicity, and MRI revealed high signals on T_2-weighted images in several muscle groups of the patient with active myositis (positive control). Non-invasive examinations such as MRI and ultrasound are beneficial as adjunctive means of examination in the evaluation of patients with amyopathic or classic DM. Ultrasound appears to be the more cost-effective and simple test; MRI, although more expensive, may be more sensitive and specific.

The value of malignancy evaluation in patients with dermatomyositis. Callen JP. J Am Acad Dermatol 1982; 6: 253–9.

DM has been linked to internal malignancy in adults, but the value of an extensive malignancy evaluation in patients with DM is controversial. Fifty-seven patients who had DM with malignancies for whom data were available regarding the discovery of malignancy have been analyzed: 53 of these were reported previously. There were 67 malignancies in the 57 patients. The malignancy preceded (26 cases), followed (23 cases), or occurred with the DM (18 cases). A 'blind' (non-directed) malignancy search was not of value in any of the cases analyzed. Rather, the tumors were discovered in 40 cases by history (preceding tumor or abnormal symptoms),

in 14 cases by physical examination, and in 12 cases by abnormal laboratory findings (e.g. chest radiograph, urinalysis, stool guaiac). One case was not discovered until autopsy (adenocarcinoma of the broad ligament). Analysis of tumor sites further negates the value of a malignancy work-up because most tumors (>90%) occur in areas not amenable to a 'routine malignancy search.' In several instances patients had an extensive search without having a complete physical examination.

Malignancy evaluations should be directed by abnormalities found on history, physical findings, or routine laboratory testing. However, since this paper was published, new, less invasive methods of malignancy search have been developed, and therefore the initial search should include CT scans of the chest, abdomen, and pelvis in most patients, and these scans should be repeated annually for at least 3 years.

Frequency of specific cancer types in dermatomyositis and polymyositis: a population-based study. Hill CL, Zhang Y, Sigurgeirsson B, Pukkala E, Mellemkjaer L, Airio A, et al. Lancet 2001; 357: 96–100.

This study combined prior studies from Sweden, Finland, and Denmark and demonstrated that patients with dermatomyositis were at increased risk of an accompanying malignancy, whereas those with polymyositis were less clearly associated. The malignancy risk decreased with each passing year after diagnosis, and approached background levels at 3 years. Malignancy of the ovaries, pancreas, stomach, colon and rectum, and non-Hodgkin's lymphoma were overrepresented in the DM patients. The authors suggested an approach to evaluation of the patient based on these findings.

A new approach to the classification of idiopathic inflammatory myopathy: myositis-specific autoantibodies define useful homogeneous patient groups. Love LA, Leff RL, Fraser DD, Targoff IN, Dalakas M, Plotz PH, et al. Medicine (Baltimore) 1991; 70: 360–74.

This study compared the usefulness of myositis-specific autoantibodies (anti-aminoacyl-tRNA synthetases, anti-signal recognition particle [anti-SRP], anti-Mi-2 and anti-MAS) to the standard clinical categories (polymyositis, DM, overlap myositis, cancer-associated myositis, and inclusion body myositis) in predicting clinical signs and symptoms and prognosis in 212 adult patients. Compared to those without these antibodies, patients with anti-amino-acyl-tRNA synthetase autoantibodies (n=47), had significantly more frequent arthritis, fever, interstitial lung disease, and 'mechanic's hands;' higher mean prednisone dose at survey; higher proportion of patients receiving cytotoxic drugs; and higher death rates. Those with anti-SRP antibodies (n=7) had more frequent palpitations, myalgias, severe refractory disease, and higher death rates. Patients with anti-Mi-2 antibodies (n=10) had increased 'V-sign' and 'shawl-sign' rashes and cuticular overgrowth, and a good response to therapy. These findings suggest that myositis-specific autoantibody status is a more useful guide than clinical group in assessing patients with myositis. The authors proposed that myositis-specific autoantibody status be incorporated into future studies of epidemiology, etiology, and therapy of myositis.

These antibodies are less common in patients with DM than in patients with polymyositis, and thus should remain investigational at present.

FIRST-LINE THERAPIES

For cutaneous disease

▶ Sunscreens	E
▶ Topical corticosteroids	E
▶ Antimalarials – hydroxychloroquine or chloroquine	D
▶ Combination antimalarial therapy	E

For muscle disease

▶ Systemic corticosteroids	B
▶ Immunosuppressive agents – methotrexate, azathioprine	A

The use of pulse corticosteroid therapy for juvenile dermatomyositis. Paller AS. Pediatr Dermatol 1996; 13: 347–8.

This report details preliminary experience from the Children's Hospital in Chicago. It has been suggested that this method of administration might result in less toxicity from corticosteroids, and further that this therapy aids in the prevention of calcinosis.

Dermatomyositis: comparative studies of cutaneous photosensitivity in lupus erythematosus and normal subjects. Dourmishev L, Meffert H, Piazena H. Photodermatol Photoimmunol Photomed 2004; 20: 230–4.

About half of the patients with DM were found to have a reduced minimal erythema dose to UVB radiation. The action spectrum of DM remains unknown.

Cutaneous lesions of dermatomyositis are improved by hydroxychloroquine. Woo TY, Callen JP, Voorhees JJ, Bickers D, Hanno R. J Am Acad Dermatol 1984; 10: 592–600.

DM is a collagen vascular disease with prominent cutaneous findings. Although the myositis often responds to therapy with corticosteroids and/or immunosuppressants, the cutaneous disease may not respond. Seven patients with cutaneous lesions of DM that had not responded to therapy were treated with hydroxychloroquine in an open study. Three patients had idiopathic DM, one had DM without myositis, one had DM with malignancy, one had an overlap syndrome, and one had adolescent DM. The response to the addition of hydroxychloroquine was good in all patients, and three had total resolution of their skin lesions. In two patients the corticosteroid dosage could be tapered. Therapy with hydroxychloroquine did not appear to have any beneficial effect on the myositis. It was concluded that hydroxychloroquine may have a role as an adjuvant therapy for patients with cutaneous lesions of DM.

Combination antimalarials in the treatment of cutaneous dermatomyositis: a retrospective study. Ang GC, Werth VP. Arch Dermatol 2005; 141: 855–9.

This is a retrospective analysis of 17 patients who were managed at the University of Pennsylvania. Seven of 17 patients experienced at least near clearance of cutaneous symptoms with the use of antimalarial therapy alone: four of them required combination therapy (hydroxychloroquine sulfate–quinacrine hydrochloride or chloroquine phosphate–quinacrine), and three of them responded well to antimalarial monotherapy. The median time required to efficacy was 3 months.

Prednisone and azathioprine for polymyositis: long-term follow up. Bunch TW. Arthritis Rheum 1981; 24: 45–8.

This follow-up study measured outcome after a double-blind, placebo-controlled trial of azathioprine had failed to demonstrate significant improvement. Unfortunately, this report dealt with the open-label experience following the previously reported 3-month controlled trial; however, there was significant improvement in the treated group and lower corticosteroid dosage.

This study and its predecessor demonstrate that the effect of immunosuppressive therapy is often delayed.

SECOND-LINE THERAPIES

For cutaneous disease

▶ Tacrolimus or pimecrolimus	D
▶ Methotrexate	D
▶ Mycophenolate mofetil	D
▶ Intravenous immune globulin	A

For muscle disease

▶ Other immunosuppressive agents – cyclophosphamide, chlorambucil, mycophenolate mofetil, ciclosporin	D
▶ Intravenous immunoglobulin	A
▶ Rituximab	D

Topical tacrolimus 0.1% ointment for refractory skin disease in dermatomyositis: a pilot study. Hollar CB, Jorizzo JL. J Dermatol Treat 2004; 15: 35–9.

This is an open-label study of six patients with cutaneous lesions of DM who were treated with topical tacrolimus. A very good to excellent response was noted in two patients, a moderate response in one, and essentially no response in three. This agent is worthy of a trial, but does not seem to be highly effective.

Low-dose methotrexate administered weekly is an effective corticosteroid-sparing agent for the treatment of the cutaneous manifestations of dermatomyositis. Kasteler JS, Callen JP. J Am Acad Dermatol 1997; 36: 67–71.

The records of 13 patients who received oral methotrexate in doses ranging from 2.5 to 30 mg weekly were reviewed. Their skin lesions had not been completely responsive to sunscreens, topical corticosteroids, oral prednisone, oral antimalarial therapy, or, in one patient each, chlorambucil and azathioprine. At the end of the study period, four of these 13 patients were free of all cutaneous manifestations of DM, and another four had almost complete clearance. In the remaining five patients, methotrexate induced moderate clearing of their cutaneous lesions. In all patients the addition of methotrexate allowed a reduction in or discontinuation of other therapies, including prednisone.

Mycophenolate mofetil as an effective corticosteroid-sparing therapy for recalcitrant dermatomyositis. Edge JC, Outland JD, Dempsey JR, Callen JP. Arch Dermatol 2006; 142: 65–9.

Mycophenolate mofetil in dermatomyositis: is it safe? Rowin J, Amato AA, Deisher N, Cursio J, Meriggioli MN. Neurology 2006; 66: 1245–7.

These two open-label studies suggest that in 60–75% of patients with myositis, mycophenolate mofetil is an effective steroid-sparing agent for skin and muscle disease. The first

Evidence Levels: A Double-blind study   **B** Clinical trial ≥ 20 subjects   **C** Clinical trial < 20 subjects   **D** Series ≥ 5 subjects   **E** Anecdotal case reports

report dealt only with patients with DM, whereas the latter included some with PM. In addition, there was toxicity that occurred in these relatively small case series, including an Epstein–Barr virus-associated lymphoma of the central nervous system which resolved upon cessation of therapy in the former study, and opportunistic infections in the latter study, one of which was fatal.

This agent, albeit seemingly useful, needs careful monitoring for the development of neoplasia and infection.

A controlled trial of high-dose intravenous immune globulin infusions as treatment for dermatomyositis. Dalakas MC, Illa I, Dambrosia JM. N Engl J Med 1993; 329: 1993–2000.

These authors conducted a double-blind, placebo-controlled trial of intravenous immunoglobulin in 15 patients with biopsy-proven treatment-resistant DM. The patients continued to receive prednisone (mean daily dose 25 mg) and were randomly assigned to receive one infusion of immunoglobulin (2 g/kg body weight) or placebo monthly for 3 months, with the option of crossing over to the alternative therapy for 3 more months. The eight patients assigned to immunoglobulin showed a significant improvement in scores of muscle strength (p<0.018) and neuromuscular symptoms (p<0.035), whereas the seven patients assigned to placebo did not. With crossovers, a total of 12 patients received immunoglobulin. Of these, nine with severe disabilities showed a major improvement to near normal function. Of 11 placebo-treated patients, none had a major improvement, three had a mild improvement, three had no change in their condition, and the condition of five worsened. Skin disease also responded in the treated patients.

Chlorambucil. An effective corticosteroid-sparing agent for patients with recalcitrant dermatomyositis. Sinoway PA, Callen JP. Arthritis Rheum 1993; 36: 319–24.

Five patients with recalcitrant DM were treated with oral chlorambucil, 4 mg daily, after discontinuation of the other immunosuppressive agent (azathioprine or methotrexate). Three patients were treated with a combination of prednisone and chlorambucil, and two with chlorambucil alone. Beneficial effects were noted within 4–6 weeks in all five patients, and corticosteroids were eventually discontinued in four. The chlorambucil was stopped after 13–30 months of treatment in four patients, and their disease remained in remission. Minimal chlorambucil toxicity was noted, consisting of leukopenia in two patients.

Although chlorambucil was effective, its potential for subsequent malignancy makes it a less desirable choice.

Ciclosporin A and intravenous immunoglobulin treatment in polymyositis/dermatomyositis. Danieli MG, Malcangi G, Palmieri C, Logullo F, Salvi A, Piani M, et al. Ann Rheum Dis 2002; 61: 37–41.

This is a retrospective review of 20 patients, including 12 with DM. It suggests that combining prednisone, ciclosporin, and intravenous immunoglobulin was the most useful regimen.

Ciclosporin A versus methotrexate in the treatment of polymyositis and dermatomyositis. Vencovský J, Jarosová K, Machácek S, Studýnková J, Kafková J, Bartünková J, et al. Scand J Rheumatol 2000; 29: 95–102.

Patients were randomly assigned to receive either methotrexate or ciclosporin in addition to prednisone. The methotrexate dosage was 7.5–15 mg/week and that of ciclosporin

3.0–3.5 mg/kg daily. Both groups improved. This is a small study of a heterogeneous group of patients treated with adequate doses of corticosteroid, but relatively low doses of the second agent.

THIRD-LINE THERAPIES

► Dapsone for cutaneous disease	E
► Antiestrogen medication for cutaneous disease	E
► Diltiazem for calcinosis	D
► Etanercept	D
► Infliximab	D
► Total body irradiation	D
► Rituximab	D
► Sirolimus	E

Regression of calcinosis during diltiazem treatment in juvenile dermatomyositis. Oliveri MB, Palermo R, Mautalen C, Hubscher O. J Rheumatol 1996; 23: 2152–5.

An 8-year-old girl with juvenile DM developed dystrophic calcifications 26 months after diagnosis. She also had severe corticosteroid-induced bone loss (osteoporosis). Despite successful treatment of her myopathy with methylprednisolone and immunosuppressive drugs, the calcifications turned into generalized heterotopic calcinosis with an exoskeleton-like pattern. She was subsequently treated with oral diltiazem (5 mg/kg daily) to control calcinosis and oral pamidronate (4 mg/kg daily) in addition to calcium and vitamin D supplementation, which she had been taking for 3 years. After 21 months of treatment, clinical and radiological examination revealed dramatic regression of the calcinosis. Bone mass reached normal levels, as determined by bone absorptiometry. Diltiazem, alone or in combination with other drugs, could be a useful therapy in patients with juvenile DM and pronounced calcifications.

Response to total body irradiation in dermatomyositis. Kelly JJ, Madoc-Jones H, Adelman LS, Andres PL, Munsat TL. Muscle Nerve 1988; 11: 120–3.

Two patients with severe DM refractory to immunosuppressive therapy were treated with 15 Gy of total body irradiation given over a period of 5 weeks. Both patients responded promptly, with minimal side effects, and remain in partial remission respectively 42 and 18 months after completion of the treatment. Total body irradiation is effective in some patients with DM who are refractory to standard therapy.

Open-label trial of anti-TNF-alpha in dermato- and polymyositis treated concomitantly with methotrexate. Hengstman GJ, De Bleecker JL, Feist E, Vissing J, Denton CP, Manoussakis MN, et al. Eur Neurol 2008; 59: 159–63.

In the previous edition of this book a small case series by these authors suggested that infliximab might be a useful agent. In this study the authors detail the results of a trial which was stopped due to low rate of patient acquisition, as well as poor responses in many of the patients. Their conclusion is that TNF antagonists do not have a place in the therapeutic armamentarium of dermatomyositis.

Rituximab in the treatment of dermatomyositis: an open-label pilot study. Levine TD. Arthritis Rheum 2005; 52: 601–7.

This is an open-label study of seven patients. In the six evaluable patients there was an improvement in muscle disease as well as the skin disease.

A pilot trial of rituximab in the treatment of patients with dermatomyositis. Chung L, Genovese MC, Fiorentino DF. Arch Dermatol 2007; 143: 763–7.

This is an open-label pilot study in which two infusions given 2 weeks apart were given to eight patients. Of the seven evaluable patients only three had an excellent response for their muscle disease, but the response of the skin disease generally was only fair.

These two reports, along with other case reports, suggest that there might be a place for this agent eventually. Fortunately, there is an NIH-sponsored randomized, placebo-controlled trial currently enrolling patients that might answer the question of efficacy for inflammatory myopathy, including DM.

Improvement in dermatomyositis rash associated with the use of antiestrogen medication. Sereda D, Werth VP. Arch Dermatol 2006; 142: 70–2.

In this report two women experienced an improvement in their DM-associated skin eruptions while taking antiestrogen medication, either tamoxifen, a selective estrogen receptor modulator, or anastrozole, an aromatase inhibitor. When tamoxifen therapy was discontinued after 4 years of use in the first patient, her DM rash worsened and remained difficult to control with conventional immunosuppressant medication.

This observation offers a novel agent to consider for women with DM; however, no further reports of either medication have appeared in the literature.

Rapamycin (sirolimus) as a steroid-sparing agent in dermatomyositis. Nadiminti U, Arbiser JL. J Am Acad Dermatol 2005; 52: 17–19.

A single case of dermatomyositis that was recalcitrant to prior therapies responded to this anti-rejection agent.

Diaper dermatitis

Pamela Chayavichitsilp, Lawrence F Eichenfield

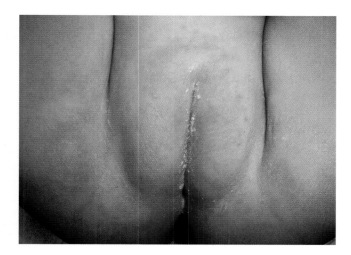

Diaper (napkin) dermatitis is a form of irritant contact dermatitis which presents as erythema and mild scaling on the convex surfaces of the inner upper thigh, lower abdomen, and buttock areas, classically sparing the inguinal folds where the skin is not in contact with irritants. It can present as early as 3 weeks of age or as late as 2 years. Many other dermatoses can affect the diaper area and may need to be excluded.

MANAGEMENT STRATEGY

Diaper dermatitis is triggered by irritants present in the area covered by the diaper, which acts as an occlusive surface. Moisture from urine and feces increases the friction coefficient of the skin, causing frictional damage. Skin integrity is further compromised by the increased pH from urine and fecal enzymes and the physical erosive effects of these activated enzymes. The reduction in skin barrier function and increase in pH contribute to the increased susceptibility to infections with microorganisms such as *Candida albicans*, which further increases the severity of diaper dermatitis. Therefore, management should aim at preventing overhydration and frictional damage in the diaper area.

Frequent diaper changes, particularly after defecation, reduce moisture and prevent the build-up of irritants. This is therefore one of the most important steps in the management of diaper dermatitis. Disposable diapers containing superabsorbent-gelling materials and breathable backsheets are preferred to those without. Cloth diapers can be avoided, as they have been shown to be associated with an increased incidence of diaper dermatitis compared to disposable diapers.

The skin in the area may be cleaned with water alone or with mild soap. Baby wipes should not contain fragrance or alcohol. Rubbing of the area can cause damage to the skin and should be avoided.

A *barrier cream* may be applied at every diaper change. This can provide a barrier between the skin and irritants in order to reduce friction and contact with stool and urine.

A *low-potency topical steroid* such as hydrocortisone 1% ointment can be used in more severe cases of diaper dermatitis, but must be used sparingly to avoid skin atrophy and systemic absorption. High-potency steroids should be avoided in diaper dermatitis, including the use of compound formulations containing potent steroids and antimicrobial agents.

Topical antifungal preparations are recommended for use in proven or suspected cases of *C. albicans* infection.

SPECIFIC INVESTIGATIONS

▶ Inquiry about recent antibiotic usage

In selected cases

▶ KOH preparation, fungal and bacterial cultures
▶ Serum zinc and biotin levels
▶ Skin biopsy
▶ Patch testing

Amoxicillin and diaper dermatitis. Honig PJ, Gribetz B, Leyden JJ, McGinley KJ, Burke LA. J Am Acad Dermatol 1988; 19: 275–9.

Skin cultures for *C. albicans* were done in 57 infants with otitis media before and after amoxicillin therapy in sites including the mouth, nose, rectum, perineum, inguinal folds, and buttocks. A twofold increase in *C. albicans* was detected after 10 days of antibiotic therapy. Infants who later developed diaper dermatitis had a significant increase in the number of *C. albicans* compared to those who did not.

Microbiological aspects of diaper dermatitis. Ferrazzini G, Kaiser RR, Hirsig Cheung SK, Wehrli M, Dela Casa V, Pohlig G, et al. Dermatology 2003; 206: 136–41.

Skin from the perianal, inguinal, and oral regions of 48 children with healthy skin and 28 children with diaper dermatitis was cultured for *C. albicans* and *S. aureus*. Colonization by *C. albicans* was significantly more frequent in children with diaper dermatitis than in healthy skin. There was also a positive correlation between the disease severity and the extent of *C. albicans* colonization.

Diaper dermatitis: a review and brief survey of eruptions of the diaper area. Scheinfeld N. Am J Clin Dermatol 2005; 6: 273–81.

This excellent review article explains the pathogenesis of diaper dermatitis. The author divided the differential diagnoses of diaper dermatitis into two categories: primary and secondary. Primary diaper dermatitis includes irritant diaper dermatitis, granuloma gluteale infantum, and perianal pseudoverrucous papules. Secondary diaper dermatitis is further divided into inflammatory (allergic contact dermatitis, miliaria rubra, seborrheic dermatitis, acrodermatitis enteropathica, pustular psoriasis, infantile granular parakeratosis, Langerhans' cell histiocytosis, child abuse, and other nutritional deficiencies) and infectious processes (most commonly caused by *C. albicans*, *S. aureus* and group A streptococci). In recalcitrant diaper dermatitis that does not improve after 2–3 weeks of treatment, further testing to rule out the above differential diagnoses is indicated.

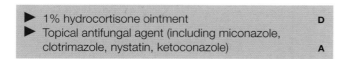

► Water-repellant barrier cream	**A**
► Frequent changing of diapers	**B**
► Superabsorbent disposable diapers	**A**

Prevention, diagnosis, and management of diaper dermatitis. Nield LS, Kamat D. Clin Pediatr (Philadelphia) 2007; 46: 480–6.

This is an excellent review article that discusses differential diagnoses, prevention and management strategies of diaper dermatitis in a stepwise, tabular format. The key prevention strategy is to keep the area dry. This can be accomplished by using superabsorbent disposable diapers, frequent diaper changes, eliminating irritants (for example, avoiding baby wipes that contain fragrance and alcohol), using a water-impermeable topical barrier, and allowing for daily diaper-free time.

Diaper dermatitis and advances in diaper technology. Odio M, Friedlander SF. Curr Opin Pediatr 2000; 12: 342–6.

This article discusses advances in diaper technology. Absorbent gelling materials (AGM) have been proved to reduce skin overhydration and reduce the frequency and severity of diaper dermatitis compared to cellulose-only disposable diapers. In a study with nearly 4000 children, a temporal association between the introduction of AGM and a reduction in the incidence of severe diaper dermatitis was found. Polymeric covers or films, commonly known as breathable backsheets, allow moisture vapor to flow out of the diaper and significantly reduce overhydration in the area. The inner lining of diapers designed to deliver a petrolatum-based formulation to the skin continuously during use has been shown to be associated with a statistically significant and sustained reduction in the severity of diaper dermatitis.

SECOND-LINE THERAPY

► 1% hydrocortisone ointment	**D**
► Topical antifungal agent (including miconazole, clotrimazole, nystatin, ketoconazole)	**A**

Absorption and efficacy of miconazole nitrate 0.25% ointment in infants with diaper dermatitis. Eichenfield LF, Bogen ML. J Drugs Dermatol 2007; 6: 522–6.

Twenty-four infants with moderate to severe diaper dermatitis were evaluated for relative safety from systemic absorption of topical miconazole. Nineteen received 0.25% miconazole nitrate ointment and five received 2% miconazole nitrate cream for 7 days. The results showed blood concentrations in the 0.25% miconazole nitrate treatment group to be minimal (undetectable in 83% and minimal in 17%), thereby demonstrating its safety as a treatment for diaper dermatitis.

Topical miconazole nitrate ointment in the treatment of diaper dermatitis complicated by candidiasis. Spraker MK,

Gisoldi EM, Siegfied EC, Fling JA, de Espinosa ZD, Quiring JN, et al. Cutis 2006; 77: 113–20.

This double-blinded, vehicle-controlled, parallel-group study compared the efficacy and safety of 0.25% miconazole nitrate in a zinc oxide/petrolatum base ointment versus zinc oxide/petrolatum vehicle control for the treatment of diaper dermatitis complicated by candidiasis in 330 patients. Results showed miconazole nitrate ointment to be well tolerated and significantly more effective than vehicle control in the treatment of diaper dermatitis complicated by *Candida* infection.

Pediatricians who prescribe clotrimazole-betamethasone diproprionate (Lotrisone) often utilize it in inappropriate settings regardless of their knowledge of the drug's potency. Railan D, Wilson JK, Feldman SR, Fleischer AB. Dermatol Online J 2002; 8: 3.

This article stresses the importance of refraining from the use of high-potency topical corticosteroid in diaper dermatitis as it can cause skin atrophy and systemic absorption. Combined topical corticosteroid and antibiotic products, such as clotrimazole–betamethasone diproprionate, often contain high-potency corticosteroids and should therefore be avoided in the diaper area.

THIRD-LINE THERAPY

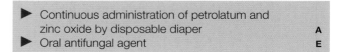

► Continuous administration of petrolatum and zinc oxide by disposable diaper	**A**
► Oral antifungal agent	**E**

Skin benefits from continuous topical administration of a zinc oxide/petrolatum formulation by a novel disposable diaper. Baldwin S, Odio MR, Haines SL, O'Connor RJ, Englehart JS, Lane AT. J Eur Acad Dermatol Venereol 2001; 1: 5–11.

This is a double-blind, randomized controlled clinical trial comparing regular diapers to diapers designed to continuously deliver zinc oxide and petrolatum in 268 infants over a 4-week period. Results showed that the ointment formulation was effectively transferred to the skin and a significant reduction in skin erythema and rash was observed.in the treatment group compared to controls.

Contact dermatitis. Friedlander SF. Pediatr Rev 1998; 19: 166–71.

Some diaper dermatitis can continue despite first- and second-line therapies. In these recalcitrant cases oral mycostatin may be beneficial. In addition, an evaluation of the mother for infections of the nipples or genital tract should be considered, as continuous reinoculation of the infant is possible. If positive, a short course of oral fluconazole (5–7 days) can help eradicate the infection.

Evidence Levels: A Double-blind study **B** Clinical trial ≥ 20 subjects **C** Clinical trial < 20 subjects **D** Series ≥ 5 subjects **E** Anecdotal case reports

Discoid eczema

Neil H Cox

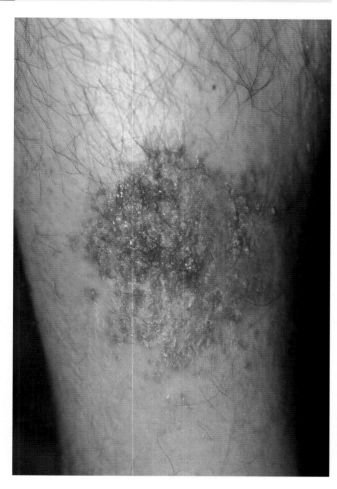

Discoid eczema comprises relatively well defined, usually multiple, coin-sized plaques with itch and weeping from acute lesions. It primarily affects the limbs (especially the legs), sometimes the trunk, and rarely the face or flexures.

MANAGEMENT STRATEGY

Eczema with a discoid morphology has many etiologies. It is usually idiopathic in older patients, but similar lesions may occur due to contact allergic reactions, drug eruptions, as a pattern of hand and foot eczema, in atopic dermatitis (AD), as an 'id' eruption related to venous eczema, or locally (e.g., insect bite reactions, 'halo eczema' around melanocytic nevi). Comparisons between studies may be limited if the site(s) and etiology are not stated, or represent a mixed spectrum.

There are few publications on the pathophysiology of discoid eczema to inform treatment. An association with dry skin (xerosis) is documented, and discoid lesions may appear during treatment with isotretinoin (which reduces sebum secretion). However, dry skin is not consistently present, and the morphology of discoid eczema differs from that of xerosis or asteatotic eczema.

One study suggested that patients with discoid eczema have a degree of xerosis similar to that of age-matched controls, but have stronger delayed hypersensitivity to allergens that permeate the skin as a result of scratching. A link with atopy has been proposed, but serum IgE levels are generally normal.

Occult infections (e.g., dental abscess) and infections causing dry skin (e.g., leprosy) have rarely been linked with discoid eczema. *Helicobacter pylori* has been implicated, but the evidence is weak.

It is difficult to provide specific therapeutic strategies because of the various different causes and the paucity of pertinent publications; most reports are retrospective from individual departments, or are anecdotal, rather than formal trials. The main therapeutic issues are:

- Other disorders may need to be excluded, especially mycoses, psoriasis, Bowen's disease, mycosis fungoides, sarcoidosis.
- A medication and alcohol history should be taken.
- Patch testing may be useful.
- The management of discoid eczema is generally similar to that of other eczemas – emollients appear to be helpful owing to the link with dry skin.
- The mainstay of treatment is topical corticosteroids – severe itch in discoid eczema usually dictates that strong agents are applied; this is safe because the individual lesions are small, rarely affect thin skin sites such as the face or flexures, and usually respond to this approach.
- If weeping is present, topical antiseptics or oral or topical antibiotics may be combined with a corticosteroid.
- Tar-based treatments and impregnated bandages may help.
- Systemic therapies are rarely required.

SPECIFIC INVESTIGATIONS

> ▶ None usually required except to exclude differential diagnoses
> ▶ Consider medications as a cause
> ▶ Consider patch testing
> ▶ Bacteriology if secondary infection likely
> ▶ Consider occult infections in resistant cases

Pityriasis rosea and discoid eczema: dose related reactions to treatment with gold. Wilkinson SM, Smith AG, Davis MJ, Mattey D, Dawes PT. Ann Rheum Dis 1992; 51: 881–4.

Discoid eczematous lesions occur in up to 30% of patients on gold therapy, and may be dose related.

Severe, generalized nummular eczema secondary to interferon alpha-2b plus ribavirin combination therapy in a patient with chronic hepatitis C virus infection. Moore MM, Elpern J, Carter DJ. Arch Dermatol 2004; 140: 215–17.

Cutaneous disease and alcohol misuse. Higgins EM, du Vivier AW. Br Med Bull 1994; 50: 85–98.

Documents a strong link between discoid eczema and alcohol consumption.

Patch testing in discoid eczema. Fleming C, Parry E, Forsyth A, Kemmett D. Contact Derm 1997; 36: 261–4.

Retrospective study of persistent and severe discoid eczema – 24 of 48 cases were positive (16 relevant) to rubber chemicals, formaldehyde, neomycin, chromate, and nickel.

Patch testing in discoid eczema. Khurana S, Jain VK, Aggarwal K, Gupta S. J Dermatol 2002; 29: 763–7.

Positive tests in 28 of 50 patients with relatively chronic discoid eczema, mainly to dichromate, nickel, cobalt, and fragrance. However, 44% had a purely hand and foot pattern, and only 12% a trunk and limb distribution.

Challenge with metal salts. (II). Various types of eczema. Veien NK, Hattel T, Justesen O, Nørholm A. Contact Derm 1983; 9: 407–10.

Patch testing can be helpful. Larger series suggest a 50% positive test rate, with clinical relevance in many. However, these are based on testing patients with chronic or therapy-resistant discoid eczema (i.e., a selected, potentially unrepresentative group); most reports are anecdotal. Implicated agents include chromate, nickel, mercury, thimerosal, rubber chemicals, formaldehyde, neomycin, fragrances, aloe, ethylene diamine, cyanoacrylate glue, textile dyes, and epoxy resin. Oral metal challenge tests rarely induce flares of discoid eczema. Irritants may also cause discoid eczema.

FIRST-LINE THERAPIES

▶ Topical corticosteroids ± antibacterial agents	C
▶ Emollients	C
▶ Tar-based preparations	C
▶ Oral antibiotics	C
▶ Oral antihistamines	C
▶ Topical doxepin	A

Most of these are standard treatments for discoid eczema; however, in terms of evidence grading, most studies include a variety of different eczemas, few specifically identify results for discoid eczema, and no comparative trials have been identified.

Successful treatment of therapy-resistant atopic dermatitis with clobetasol propionate and a hydrocolloid occlusive dressing. Volden G. Acta Dermatol Venereol (Stockh) 1992; 176: 126–8.

Nummular AD lesions cleared rapidly.

Topical corticosteroids are the usual first-line therapy. Trial evidence is limited to pharmaceutically sponsored studies that are not specific to discoid eczema.

Nummular eczema. A review, follow-up and analysis of a series of 325 cases. Cowan MA. Acta Dermatol Venereol 1961; 41: 453–60.

Tar preparations were the main treatment. Recurrent crops of lesions occurred in 25%, and relapse when treatment was discontinued in 53%, presumably representing the natural history of the disease, but possibly reflecting the limitations of therapy available at the time (other options were hydrocortisone or superficial X-ray therapy).

Tar preparations, historically used in the treatment of discoid eczema, have been superseded by potent topical corticosteroids as first-line therapy.

The antipruritic effect of 5% doxepin cream in patients with eczematous dermatitis. Drake LA, Millikan LE. Arch Dermatol 1995; 131: 1403–8.

Significant improvement in itch at 1 day, not at 7 days.

Studies suggest that doxepin has a short-term effect on itch only.

The use of antibacterial agents (e.g., clioquinol) or antibiotics is based on the fact that lesions are often moist and crusted. Secondary staphylococcal infection, as in AD, may aggravate the eczematous process.

Occlusion over a topical corticosteroid has been reported to lead to lesion clearance in previously therapy-resistant patients with discoid lesions due to AD; soaking in water for 20 minutes before treatment application has been recommended for a range of eczemas.

As with other itchy dermatoses, sedating antihistamines may help symptoms – the increase in mast cells in lesions provides the rationale for this approach. However, histamine itself has not been shown to be important.

SECOND-LINE THERAPIES

▶ Phototherapy (broadband or narrowband UVB, 311 nm)	E
▶ Photochemotherapy (psoralen plus UVA: PUVA)	E
▶ Topical immune modulators	E
▶ Ciclosporin	E
▶ Intralesional corticosteroid injection	E
▶ Oral corticosteroids	E

Formal trials of these treatments in discoid eczema are lacking and therefore the evidence gradings are weak; however, all are useful in AD or other dermatitis (see gradings in Atopic Dermatitis), and are therefore likely to be effective in discoid eczema. Personal experience is that narrowband UVB or ciclosporin are useful if required.

Photochemotherapy beyond psoriasis. Honig B, Morison WL, Karp D. J Am Acad Dermatol 1994; 31: 775–90.

Review article. Nothing specific to discoid eczema, but several eczemas respond to PUVA.

Half-side comparison study on the efficacy of 8-methoxypsoralen bath-PUVA versus narrow-band ultraviolet B phototherapy in patients with severe chronic atopic dermatitis. Der-Petrossian M, Seeber A, Honigsmann H, Tanew A. Br J Dermatol 2000; 142: 39–43.

Both were equivalent (at equi-erythemogenic doses) in AD.

Phototherapies also reduce staphylococci and superantigens, and therefore may improve eczema with weeping and infection.

Antimicrobial effects of phototherapy and photochemotherapy in vivo and in vitro. Yoshimura M, Namura S, Akamatsu H, Horio T. Br J Dermatol 1996; 135: 528–32.

Antimicrobial effects are apparent after a single exposure.

Suppressive effect of ultraviolet (UVB and PUVA) radiation on superantigen production by *Staphylococcus aureus.* Yoshimura-Mishima M, Namura S, Akamatsu H, Horio T. J Dermatol Sci 1999; 19: 31–6.

Hand dermatitis: a review of clinical features, therapeutic options, and long-term outcomes. Warshaw E, Lee G, Storrs FJ. Am J Contact Derm 2003; 14: 119–37.

One review recommends topical tacrolimus or pimecrolimus for nummular hand dermatitis. No evaluable evidence presented.

Long-term efficacy and safety of cyclosporin in severe adult atopic dermatitis. Berth-Jones J, Graham-Brown RA, Marks R, Camp RD, English JS, Freeman K, et al. Br J Dermatol 1997; 136: 76–81.

An open study of 100 patients with AD, with mostly good responses.

Side effects (drug interactions, hypertension, nephrotoxicity) limit ciclosporin therapy in older patients with discoid eczema, compared to AD. It is possibly useful for intermittent short-term treatment.

Oral corticosteroids are generally unnecessary. Intralesional corticosteroid injection is impractical, except in patients who have a small number of persistent thickened lesions.

THIRD-LINE THERAPIES

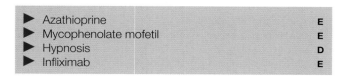

▶ Azathioprine	E
▶ Mycophenolate mofetil	E
▶ Hypnosis	D
▶ Infliximab	E

As for second-line therapies, formal trials of these treatments in discoid eczema are lacking and therefore the evidence gradings are weak; however, all are useful in AD or other dermatitis (see gradings in Atopic Dermatitis, Ch. 17), and are therefore likely to be effective in discoid eczema.

Azathioprine in dermatological practice. An overview with special emphasis on its use in non-bullous inflammatory dermatoses. Scerri L. Adv Exp Med Biol 1999; 445: 343–8.

Documents the efficacy of azathioprine in AD and pompholyx.

Azathioprine in dermatology: a survey of current practice in the UK. Tan BB, Lear JT, Gawkrodger DJ, English JSC. Br J Dermatol 1997; 136: 351–5.

A questionnaire to 248 dermatologists showed that none was using azathioprine for discoid eczema.

Azathioprine is used in the treatment of several dermatoses, including various eczemas. It is likely to be beneficial in discoid eczema, although a study of azathioprine prescribing by UK dermatologists did not identify this as a current indication.

Mycophenolate mofetil is a 'recommended treatment' for nummular hand dermatitis (in Warshaw E, et al., cited above), and there has been anecdotal response to infliximab.

Hypnosis in dermatology. Shenefelt PD. Arch Dermatol 2000; 136: 393–9.

Hypnosis as a complementary therapy may improve lesions or itch in discoid eczema.

Discoid lupus erythematosus

Bruce H Thiers, Maryanna C Ter Poorten

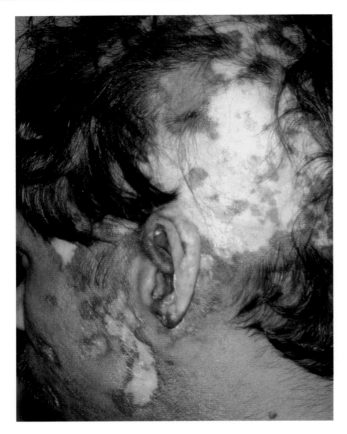

Discoid lupus erythematosus (DLE) is the most common form of chronic cutaneous lupus erythematosus. Lesions predominate in sun-exposed areas, especially the face, upper chest, and upper back. Early lesions consist of sharply demarcated, erythematous, often hyperpigmented, hyperkeratotic papules and small plaques with adherent scale; the individual lesions spread peripherally, leaving atrophic central scarring with alopecia, telangiectasia, and depigmentation.

MANAGEMENT STRATEGY

The lesions of DLE are quite characteristic, especially in their later stages. When the diagnosis is in doubt, a skin biopsy should be performed. The histologic findings are usually diagnostic, although direct immunofluorescence examination can be obtained in questionable cases. A complete history and physical examination should be performed, looking for signs of systemic disease. Laboratory examinations to be obtained include a complete blood count with differential, erythrocyte sedimentation rate, serum chemistry profile, and urinalysis. Serum should be screened for antinuclear antibodies (ANA) and Ro(SSA)/La(SSB) antibodies. It should be emphasized that although, as mentioned above, DLE is the most common form of chronic cutaneous lupus erythematosus, most

patients do not have systemic involvement. Risk factors for systemic disease include widespread skin lesions, anemia or leukopenia, and a positive ANA, especially when the titer is high. Despite the relative infrequency of internal involvement, aggressive treatment of DLE is warranted because the scarring from the disease can be devastating. The characteristic 'carpet tack' scale associated with lesions indicates follicular involvement, and the disease can result in permanent scarring alopecia. Moreover, the depigmentation in fully evolved lesions can be disfiguring, especially in dark-skinned individuals. The goal of therapy is to halt the inflammatory process quickly and effectively to prevent these changes. The predominance of lesions in exposed areas emphasizes the urgency of prompt effective therapy.

Patients should be counseled on the role of UV light in the provocation of skin lesions, and a program of *sun avoidance* and *sunscreen use* should be instituted. *Corticosteroids*, either topical or intralesional, are the cornerstone of initial therapy for patients with limited involvement. *Hydroxychloroquine* and *other antimalarial drugs* appear to afford a measure of photoprotection and are often quite effective, although their onset of action is relatively slow. *Systemic retinoids* are useful, especially for hyperkeratotic lesions. *Dapsone*, which is more commonly used for lesions of bullous lupus erythematosus, is occasionally effective for patients with DLE. Treatments reserved for refractory cases include *cytotoxic agents, gold,* and *interferon-α*. The role of *thalidomide* in the treatment of DLE is evolving. Other drugs or modalities anecdotally reported to be effective in the treatment of DLE include *clofazimine, sulfasalazine, monoclonal antibodies,* and *laser ablation* of lesions.

SPECIFIC INVESTIGATIONS

▶ Autoantibody studies
▶ Indicators of systemic disease

Cutaneous lupus erythematosus: a personal approach to management. Callen JP. Australasian J Dermatol 2006; 47: 13–27.

The author states that 5–10% of patients with DLE will have coexisting systemic lupus erythematosus (SLE). Associated findings may include widespread skin involvement, periungual telangiectasias, an elevated erythrocyte sedimentation rate, leukopenia, and ANA positivity. Although systemic disease in these patients is often diagnosed in the first few years after skin signs appear, the course is usually chronic and benign without renal involvement.

This article provides an excellent review of the cutaneous manifestations of lupus erythematosus.

FIRST-LINE THERAPIES

▶ Sunscreens	B
▶ Topical or intralesional corticosteroids	B
▶ Topical immunosuppressive agents	C

Phototesting and photoprotection in LE. Walchner M, Messer G, Kind P. Lupus 1997; 6: 167–74.

Cutaneous lupus erythematosus is a disease that is precipitated and aggravated by exposure to UV light; therefore, sun protection and sun avoidance are vital in its management. A broad-spectrum sunscreen that includes protection against both UVB (sun protection factor 15) and UVA (e.g. containing Parsol 1789) should be used. Opaque physical sunscreens such as titanium dioxide, red veterinary petrolatum, and zinc oxide can provide broad-spectrum protection and may be particularly helpful. UV-blocking filters should be considered for home and automobile windows, and diffusion shields on fluorescent lights may provide benefit. Conversely, the patient (and the referring internist) should be reminded to limit the use of potentially photosensitizing drugs.

Management of 'refractory' skin disease in patients with lupus erythematosus. Callen JP. Best Pract Res Clin Rheumatol 2005; 19: 767–84.

Topical and intralesional corticosteroids play an important role in the management of DLE; however, their use involves a delicate balancing act because the disease ultimately causes cutaneous atrophy, which is also a side effect of long-term local corticosteroid use. Potent topical corticosteroid preparations are more effective than weaker preparations, but are also more likely to cause atrophy. Only active lesions should be treated. Likewise, larger lesions, which may show residual scarring and central atrophy, and erythema, scaling and hyperkeratosis at the periphery, should only be treated in the areas of disease activity. The author points out that although topical steroids are often considered first-line therapy for DLE, many patients remain refractory to treatment and require a systemic approach.

Topical tacrolimus and pimecrolimus in the treatment of cutaneous lupus erythematosus: an evidence-based evaluation. Tzellos TG, Kouvelas D. Eur J Clin Pharmacol 2008; 64: 337–41.

The use of topical calcineurin inhibitors in lupus erythematosus: an overview. Wollina U, Hansel G. J Eur Acad Dermatol Venereol 2008; 22: 1–6.

The macrolactam immunosuppressive agents tacrolimus and pimecrolimus have been reported to be effective in the treatment of lesions of DLE, although there are few randomized controlled trials. They may be particularly useful when cutaneous atrophy, either disease or treatment-related, is a concern. Hypertrophic lesions may not respond well, presumably because of limited penetration.

SECOND-LINE THERAPIES

▶ Antimalarial drugs	B
▶ Systemic retinoids	B

Cutaneous lupus erythematosus: diagnosis and management. Fabbri P, Cardinali C, Giomi B, Caproni M. Am J Clin Dermatol 2003; 4: 449–65.

Antimalarial drugs are the favored long-term treatment for DLE and are effective in many patients for whom topical therapy alone is unsuccessful. In most patients, 6 weeks of treatment are needed before they begin to exert their effect, and therefore concomitant treatment is indicated, at least initially. Hydroxychloroquine is most often used, chloroquine being reserved for unresponsive patients. Both drugs can cause a characteristic antimalarial retinopathy, and so periodic (every 6 months) ophthalmologic examinations are necessary. Quinacrine, which is not a significant

cause of retinopathy, has become increasingly difficult to obtain. It may be used alone or in combination with other antimalarial agents.

This is a good review of treatment options for the cutaneous lesions of lupus erythematosus.

Hypertrophic lupus erythematosus treated successfully with acitretin as monotherapy. Al-Mutairi N, Rijhwani M, Nour-Eldin O. J Dermatol 2005; 32: 482–6.

Oral retinoids, either isotretinoin or acitretin, are useful in the treatment of DLE, particularly the hypertrophic variety. Their teratogenic effects must be especially respected, because patients with DLE are often women of childbearing age. The long-term adverse effects of retinoids, including hypertriglyceridemia and possible bony abnormalities, must also be considered when constructing a treatment plan. As with other treatments for DLE, the disease occasionally flares even with continued treatment.

THIRD-LINE THERAPIES

▶ Cytotoxic agents	D
▶ Thalidomide	D
▶ Antibiotics	D
▶ Biologic agents	D

Drugs for discoid lupus erythematosus. Jessop S, Whitelaw D, Jordaan F. Cochrane Database Syst Rev 2001; (1): CD002954

This review confirmed the efficacy of topical steroids, hydroxychloroquine, and acitretin for the treatment of DLE, but concluded that there is not enough reliable evidence to support the use of other drugs to treat this condition.

Theory, targets and therapy in systemic lupus erythematosus. Vasoo S, Hughes GR. Lupus 2005; 14: 181–8.

Cytotoxic agents, including azathioprine, cyclophosphamide, methotrexate, and mycophenolate mofetil, have been used in patients with SLE and in patients with DLE resistant to conservative management. However, although the scarring from the disease can be quite disfiguring, the use of cytotoxic drugs for this indication is limited by their significant toxicities. The authors speculate that new knowledge of the pathogenesis of the disease will lead to targeted, and perhaps safer, future therapeutic options.

Long-term thalidomide use in refractory cutaneous lesions of lupus erythematosus: a series of 65 Brazilian patients. Coelo A, Souto MI, Carduso CR, Salgado DR, Schmal TR, Waddington Cruz M, et al. Lupus 2005; 14: 434–9.

Thalidomide in the treatment of chronic discoid lupus erythematosus. Brocard A, Barbarot S, Milpied B, Stalder JF. Ann Dermatol Venereol 2005; 132: 853–6.

Thalidomide has been used in the treatment of patients with cutaneous lupus erythematosus refractory to other modalities. The response is variable but may be quite favorable. It must be emphasized that the disease typically affects young women of childbearing age, and the teratogenic potential of the drug should not be ignored. Sensory neuropathy and thromboembolic events are other potential complications of thalidomide administration.

A case of SLE with acute, subacute and chronic lesions successfully treated with dapsone. Neri R, Mosca M, Bernacchi E, Bombardieri S. Lupus 1999; 8: 240–3.

Dapsone is most often used in the treatment of bullous cutaneous lupus erythematosus. Occasionally, however, it has been reported to be effective in patients with DLE.

Treatment of discoid lupus erythematosus with sulfasalazine: 11 cases. Delaporte E, Catteau B, Sabbagh N, Gosselin P, Breuillard F, Doutre MS, et al. Ann Dermatol Venereol 1997; 124: 151–6.

A few DLE patients have been treated with sulfasalazine, sometimes successfully. Sulfasalazine is a potentially photosensitizing drug, and its use should be limited to patients with resistant disease that has not responded to more conventional therapy.

Dissecting cellulitis of the scalp

Andrew JG McDonagh

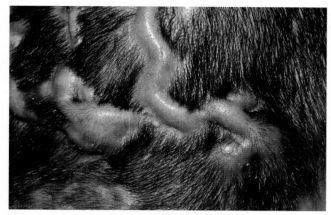

From White GM, Cox NH. Diseases of the Skin: A Color Atlas and Text, 2nd edn. Mosby Elsevier 2006, with permission of Elsevier.

Dissecting cellulitis is a rare, chronic progressive inflammatory disease of the scalp that affects predominantly the vertex and occipital scalp of men, mainly from the second to the fourth decade. Dissecting cellulitis may occur in association with hidradenitis suppurativa and acne conglobata to form the 'follicular occlusion or retention triad.' The suggested common pathogenic mechanism includes follicular retention, intense folliculitis, and granulomatous changes, leading to interconnecting sinuses along with abscess formation. Patchy alopecia is associated with extensive fibrosis and scarring, which may become keloidal.

MANAGEMENT STRATEGY

Dissecting cellulitis is characterized by a chronic, progressive course with temporary improvement on treatment followed by relapses when treatment is discontinued. There are no large therapeutic clinical trials, and recommendations for therapy are based on case reports or small series. Inflammatory tinea capitis (kerion) and the very rare case of occult squamous carcinoma should be excluded. Although no specific pathogenetic organisms have been isolated, swabs should be obtained for bacteriology and the antibiotic sensitivity of organisms reviewed.

In mild cases or when disease is limited, *improved scalp hygiene* and the use of *antiseptics, topical antibiotics* (based on bacterial culture results), *intralesional corticosteroid injections* and *aspiration of fluctuant lesions* may be adequate. At an early stage, *systemic antibiotics* such as *tetracyclines* and *clindamycin* reduce inflammation and can control disease. In more severe cases a *combination of systemic antibiotics and corticosteroids* may be effective. *Isotretinoin* has been shown to provide sustained remission if continued for at least 4 months after clinical control is achieved, at a dose of 0.75–1.0 mg/kg daily. Oral *zinc sulfate* has received anecdotal reports of success when used long term. There is a single report of success with anti-TNF therapy.

X-ray epilation of affected areas has largely been superseded by *laser epilation* before the stage of massive inflammation occurs. The most resistant cases may require *surgical excision and skin grafting*.

SPECIFIC INVESTIGATIONS

▶ Swabs for bacteriology
▶ Scrapings and plucked hair roots for mycology
▶ Scalp biopsy for histology and fungal culture

Tinea capitis mimicking dissecting cellulitis: a distinct variant. Twersky JM, Sheth AP. Int J Dermatol 2005; 44: 412–14.

Inflammatory tinea capitis (kerion) mimicking dissecting cellulitis. Sperling LC, Major MC. Int J Dermatol 1991; 30: 190–2.

Two cases of highly inflammatory tinea capitis resulting in scarring alopecia. In any case of inflammatory alopecia in adults, tinea capitis should be excluded. If scalp scrapings and plucked hair roots do not show spores, and superficial fungal culture gives negative results, a biopsy for histology and fungal culture should be performed.

Dissecting cellulitis of the scalp in 2 girls. Ramesh V. Dermatologica 1990; 180: 48–50.

Two girls with dissecting cellulitis, in one of whom *Pseudomonas aeruginosa* was isolated from a sinus discharge. The role of infection in perpetuating the condition is highlighted.

Squamous cell carcinoma arising in dissecting perifolliculitis of the scalp. Curry SS, Gaither DH, King LE. J Am Acad Dermatol 1981; 4: 673–8.

A case of squamous cell carcinoma arising in dissecting folliculitis of the scalp that was fatally aggressive. Early diagnosis and treatment are essential.

Folliculotropic mycosis fungoides with large cell transformation presenting as dissecting cellulitis of the scalp. Gillam AC, Lessin SR, Wilson DM, Salhany KE. J Cutan Pathol 1997; 24: 169–75.

A patient with follicular mycosis fungoides presenting in a manner similar to dissecting cellulitis of the scalp with non-healing, draining nodular lesions.

FIRST-LINE THERAPIES

▶ Scalp hygiene	D
▶ Topical antibiotics	D
▶ Systemic antibiotics	D
▶ Intralesional corticosteroid injection	D
▶ Incision and drainage	D

Management of primary cicatricial alopecias: options for treatment. Harries MJ, Sinclair RD, MacDonald-Hull S, Whiting DA, Griffiths CE, Paus R. Br J Dermatol 2008; 159: 1–22.

An extensive review and summary of reported treatments for disorders including dissecting cellulitis.

Perifolliculitis capitis abscedens et suffodiens successfully controlled with topical isotretinoin. Karpouzis A, Giatromanolaki A, Sivridis E, Kouskoukis C. Eur J Dermatol 2003; 13: 192–5.

Dissecting cellulitis in an 18-year-old white patient was controlled with topical isotretinoin.

Perifolliculitis capitis abscedens et suffodiens. Moyer DG, Williams RM. Arch Dermatol 1962; 85: 118–24.

A report of six cases treated with systemic antibiotics.

Perifolliculitis capitis abscedens et suffodiens (dissecting cellulitis of the scalp). Jolliffe DS, Sarkany I. Clin Exp Dermatol 1977; 2: 291.

A discussion of the therapeutic difficulties inherent in this disorder, and report of a mild case of dissecting folliculitis responding well to oral oxytetracycline 1 g daily for 2 months.

SECOND-LINE THERAPIES

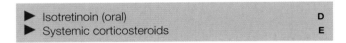

▶ Isotretinoin (oral)	**D**
▶ Systemic corticosteroids	**E**

Dissecting cellulitis of the scalp: response to isotretinoin. Scerri L, Williams HC, Allen BR. Br J Dermatol 1996; 134: 1105–8.

Three patients with dissecting cellulitis of the scalp showed a sustained therapeutic response to isotretinoin. The authors recommended that isotretinoin should be given initially at 1 mg/kg daily and maintained at a dose not less than 0.75 mg/kg daily for at least 4 months after clinical remission is achieved. Long-term post-treatment follow-up of two of the patients showed sustained benefit.

Perifolliculitis capitis: successful control with alternate day corticosteroids. Adrian RM, Arndt KA. Ann Plast Surg 1980; 4: 166–9.

The authors initially used high-dose oral prednisolone after intravenous antibiotics had failed to control dissecting cellulitis. Maintenance with 5 mg prednisolone on alternate days for 2 years is reported.

THIRD-LINE THERAPIES

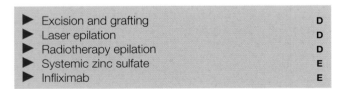

▶ Excision and grafting	**D**
▶ Laser epilation	**D**
▶ Radiotherapy epilation	**D**
▶ Systemic zinc sulfate	**E**
▶ Infliximab	**E**

Dissecting cellulitis of the scalp. Williams CN, Cohen M, Ronan SG, Lewandowski CA. Plast Reconstruct Surg 1986; 77: 378–82.

Four patients with extensive scalp disease showed a favorable response to wide excision and split-thickness skin grafting.

Dissecting cellulitis treated with the long-pulsed Nd:YAG laser. Krasner BD, Hamzavi FH, Murakawa GJ, Hamzavi IH. Dermatol Surg 2006; 32: 1039–44.

Four patients achieved sustained improvement at 1 year, with some regrowth of hair at treated sites.

Use of an 800-nm pulsed-diode laser in the treatment of recalcitrant dissecting cellulitis of the scalp. Boyd AS, Binhlam JQ. Arch Dermatol 2002; 138: 1291–3.

Complete clearance of disease poorly responsive to multiple drugs after four treatments at monthly intervals, with remission maintained 6 months after laser epilation.

Treatment of perifolliculitis capitis abscedens et suffodiens with carbon dioxide laser. Glass LF, Berman B, Laub D. J Dermatol Surg Oncol 1989; 15: 673–6.

Modern external beam radiation therapy for refractory dissecting cellulitis of the scalp. Chinnalayan P, Tena LB, Brenner MJ, Welsh JS. Br J Dermatol 2005; 152: 777–9.

Rapid improvement in four cases treated with electron beam therapy.

Successful treatment of dissecting cellulitis and acne conglobata with oral zinc. Kobayashi H, Aiba S, Tagami H. Br J Dermatol 1999; 141: 1136–8.

A case report of a patient with dissecting cellulitis and acne conglobata responding to oral zinc sulfate 135 mg tds for 12 weeks. The dose was reduced to 260 mg daily for 7 weeks, with no recurrence, but 1 week after stopping zinc therapy the scalp nodules recurred. Oral zinc was resumed and the scalp lesions diminished within 8 weeks. Afterwards, disease was well controlled for 1 year on zinc sulfate 135 mg daily.

Perifolliculitis capitis abscedens et suffodiens successfully controlled with infliximab. Brandt HRC, Malheiros APR, Teixeira MG, Machado MCR. Br J Dermatol 2008 (in press).

Case report of successful response to infliximab 8-weekly for 12 months in a case refractory to oral antibiotics and isotretinoin.

Evidence Levels: **A** Double-blind study **B** Clinical trial ≥ 20 subjects **C** Clinical trial < 20 subjects **D** Series ≥ 5 subjects **E** Anecdotal case reports

Drug eruptions

Neil H Shear, Sandra R Knowles

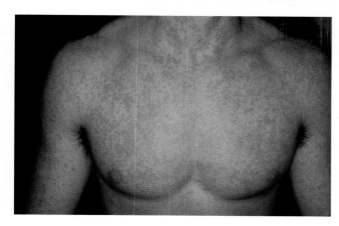

Drug eruptions are drug-induced diseases, often with a known etiology but a poorly understood pathogenesis. Drug eruptions are common adverse events. Mild eruptions may be as common as one in 10 exposures with some marketed drugs. Severe eruptions with systemic involvement occur in one in 3000 exposures, but life-threatening eruptions such as toxic epidermal necrolysis (TEN) are much less common. The image above shows a widespread exanthematous eruption. This can be localized to skin or, in the presence of fever, may be a systemic reaction.

MANAGEMENT STRATEGY

There are two steps in diagnosing drug eruptions. First, determine the morphology, e.g., exanthematous ('maculopapular eruption' – the most common), urticarial, blistering, or pustular. Second, look for signs of systemic involvement, such as fever, lymphadenopathy, or malaise. Examples of simple eruptions without systemic disease are maculopapular eruption (unfortunately the most common drug eruption has no official name), urticaria, fixed drug eruption, and drug-induced acne. Examples of complex eruptions with systemic disease are hypersensitivity drug reaction, serum sickness-like reaction, Stevens–Johnson syndrome and TEN, and acute generalized exanthematous pustulosis (AGEP).

After a diagnosis is considered, it is important to try and identify the relevant drug exposure, consider a differential diagnosis, and remember that each drug exposure has a possible etiologic role. In general, most drug eruptions occur within 3 months of starting therapy, although some eruptions can develop after 1–2 years (e.g., drug-induced lupus).

Treatment involves *stopping drugs* that have a high probability of being the cause, while providing *supportive therapy* for symptoms. Laboratory investigations may identify internal organ toxicity, and systemic therapy may be considered. The patient should be advised of the interpretation of the adverse event, what drugs were likely causes, whether tests will help confirm the cause, and what drugs should be avoided in the future. For severe reactions relatives may need to be notified by the patient, because some systemic reactions (e.g., hypersensitivity syndrome reaction, TEN) have a genetic susceptibility.

SPECIFIC INVESTIGATIONS

▶ Skin biopsy
▶ Vital signs
▶ Physical examination
▶ Hematology
▶ Liver enzymes
▶ Urinalysis
▶ Drug allergy testing
▶ Drug challenge (in carefully selected cases)

A review of drug patch testing and implications for HIV clinicians. Shear N, Milpied B, Bruynzeel DP, Phillips E. AIDS 2008; 22: 1–9.

Patch testing has been used as an adjunct for identifying patients with immunologically mediated abacavir hypersensitivity reactions. Patch testing has also been used as a research tool in pharmacogenetic studies of abacavir hypersensitivity. These studies have shown 100% sensitivity for HLA-B*5701 in patch test-confirmed abacavir HSR. Patients generally have positive patch tests for at least 6 years after experiencing an abacavir hypersensitivity reaction.

Although abacavir patch testing is helpful in identifying patients with abacavir hypersensitivity reaction, the use of patch testing with other medications may have a sensitivity of only 30%. A positive patch test may be helpful, but a negative test does not exclude the possibility of a potential reaction.

Guidelines for performing skin tests with drugs in the investigation of cutaneous adverse drug reactions. Barbaud A, Goncalo M, Bruynzeel D, Bircher A. Contact Derm 2001; 45: 321–8.

Guidelines suggest that drug skin tests should be performed 6 weeks to 6 months after complete healing of the cutaneous adverse drug reaction. Drug patch tests are performed using the commercialized form of the drug diluted to 30% with petrolatum and/or water. Drug prick and intradermal tests are performed with sequential dilutions of the commercialized form of the drug.

Drug testing is not widely available. Skin testing for penicillin allergy is very useful, but patch testing and intradermal testing may be required. Penicillin metabolites are also needed in the testing regimen (major and minor determinants). Allergists with an interest in drug reactions may have the proper reagents. Patch testing has been used and is investigational.

Allergy diagnostic testing: an updated practice parameter. Bernstein I, Li JT, Berstein DI Hamilton R, Spector SL, Tan R, et al. Ann Allergy Asthma Immunol 2008; 100: S1–S148 (see pages S109–115 for relevant drug testing guidelines).

This document provides guidelines for the management and diagnosis of patients with a history of allergic drug reactions, including cutaneous eruptions. Penicillin and cephalosporins, aspirin and NSAIDs, perioperative anaphylaxis, chemotherapeutics, local anesthetics, corticosteroids, and additives/preservatives are reviewed.

Drug provocation tests in patients with a history suggesting an immediate drug hypersensitivity reaction. Messaad D, Sahla H, Benahmed S, Godard P, Bousquet J, Demoly P. Ann Intern Med 2004; 140: 1001–6.

Eight hundred and ninety-eight patients with suspected immediate drug allergy were administered increasing doses of the suspected drug, up to the usual daily dose, in this single-blinded trial. There were 17.6% positive drug provocation results.

Oral re-challenge with the drug in question has been used, but this cannot be recommended in many cases. The clinical question should be 'What drug can the patient use in future?' not 'What drug caused the reaction?'

FIRST-LINE THERAPIES

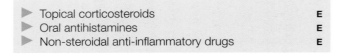

▶ Topical corticosteroids	E
▶ Oral antihistamines	E
▶ Non-steroidal anti-inflammatory drugs	E

Exanthems and urticarial eruptions are often pruritic or burning. Topical corticosteroids and oral antihistamines (either sedating or non-sedating) can reduce symptoms. Febrile symptoms may be helped by ibuprofen. Acetaminophen (paracetamol) could compromise hepatic toxicity, but is often used to treat pyrexia. Clinical trials of therapy for most simple drug eruptions have not been conducted.

Guidelines of care for cutaneous adverse drug reactions. Drake LA, Dinehart SM, Farmer ER, Goltz RW, Graham GF, Hordinsky MK, et al. J Am Acad Dermatol 1996; 35: 458–61.

Treatment for mild cutaneous eruptions includes topical corticosteroids, antihistamines, topical antipruritic agents, baths (with or without additives), and emollients.

SECOND-LINE THERAPIES

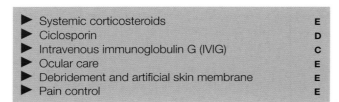

▶ Systemic corticosteroids	E
▶ Ciclosporin	D
▶ Intravenous immunoglobulin G (IVIG)	C
▶ Ocular care	E
▶ Debridement and artificial skin membrane	E
▶ Pain control	E

In complex reactions, severe discomfort or pending organ failure may require the use of oral corticosteroids. The optimal dose is unknown, but we use 1 mg/kg daily of prednisone to bring the reaction under control, usually within days, and prevent progression. If prednisone is used for complex systemic reactions, it may take months to withdraw the corticosteroid due to flares of symptoms. Without prednisone, the reaction may take weeks to settle.

Epidermal growth factor receptor inhibitors: a new era of drug reactions in a new era of cancer therapy. Cowen EW. J Am Acad Dermatol 2007; 56: 514–17.

There is a high incidence of cutaneous events following therapy with epidermal growth factor receptor inhibitors (e.g., gefitinib, erlotinib, cetuximab). A so-called acneiform rash, paronychia, dry skin, and skin fissures are most frequently reported. The offending drug is not discontinued, but treatment with topical corticosteroids, topical clindamycin, oral tetracycline, or isotretinoin is initiated.

Despite the common occurrence of drug eruptions with the epidermal growth factor receptor inhibitors, a standardized treatment approach has not been studied. The long-term skin sequelae of continued drug therapy are unknown.

Treatment of anticonvulsant hypersensitivity syndrome with intravenous immunoglobulins and corticosteroids. Prais D, Straussberg R, Amir J, Nussinovitch M, Harel L. J Child Neurol 2006; 21: 380–4.

Four adolescents with anticonvulsant hypersensitivity syndrome are described who were successfully treated with intravenous immunoglobulins and corticosteroids. IVIG 0.5–2 g/kg was administered in two divided doses. Corticosteroids were administered orally (prednisone 1 mg/kg/day) or intravenously (methylprednisolone 2 mg/kg/day). After initiation of the combination therapy, resolution was seen within 3–4 days.

Treatment of toxic epidermal necrolysis with cyclosporin A. Arevalo JM, Lorente JA, Gonzalez-Herrada C, Jimenez-Reyes J. J Trauma 2000; 48: 473–8.

A retrospective case series of 11 patients with TEN treated with ciclosporin A (3 mg/kg daily enterally every 12 hours) is reported. Treatment with ciclosporin A was associated with a rapid re-epithelialization rate and a low mortality rate compared to patients treated with cyclophosphamide and corticosteroids (0 vs 50%, respectively).

Relief is often rapid and the drug can be stopped after less than 1 week of therapy.

Effects of treatments on the mortality of Stevens-Johnson syndrome and toxic epidermal necrolysis: a retrospective study on patients included in the prospective EuroSCAR study. Schneck J, Fagot JP, Sekula P, Sassolas B, Roujeau JC, Mockenhaupt M. J Am Acad Dermatol 2008; 58: 33–40.

In this large retrospective study of 281 patients, neither intravenous immunoglobulin nor corticosteroids had any significant positive effect on mortality compared with supportive care only. However, a trend for a beneficial effect of corticosteroids was noted.

There is no standardized treatment for patients with SJS/TEN. Previous studies have shown that IVIG can significantly reduce the mortality rate compared to a SCORTEN-predicted mortality rate. However, this study suggests that IVIG may not have a beneficial effect.

Dexamethasone pulse therapy for Stevens–Johnson syndrome/toxic epidermal necrolysis. Kardaun SH, Jonkman MF. Acta Dermatol Venereol 2007; 87: 144–8.

The role of corticosteroids in the treatment of SJS/TEN is controversial. In this review of 12 patients with SJS/TEN, IV dexamethasone 1.5 mg/kg body weight for 3 consecutive days was administered. Total re-epithelialization was reached after 13.9 days, although one patient died.

Intravenous pulse therapy with corticosteroids has been used in severe, autoimmune diseases. A larger controlled trial is warranted in order to investigate the use of pulse dexamethasone in the treatment of SJS/TEN.

Erythema multiforme, Stevens–Johnson syndrome, and toxic epidermal necrolysis: acute ocular manifestations, causes and management. Chang YS, Huang FC, Tseng SH, Hsu CK, Ho CL, Sheu HM. Cornea 2007; 26: 123–9.

In this retrospective analysis, 60% of patients with SJS/TEN developed ocular manifestations. Topical antibiotic and corticosteroids and frequent lubrication were the most common treatment modalities. In patients with ocular adhesions, daily lysis, sweeping of the fornix, and debridement were necessary to prevent late complications. Therapeutic soft contact lenses can be tried in cases of persistent corneal epithelial defects.

In TEN it is important to be mindful of ocular scarring. Topical cleansing and use of a glass rod daily to prevent adhesions is very important.

OTHER THERAPIES

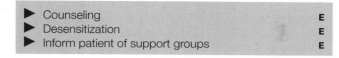

▶ Counseling	E
▶ Desensitization	E
▶ Inform patient of support groups	E

Anticonvulsant hypersensitivity syndrome: incidence, prevention and management. Knowles SR, Shapiro LE, Shear NH. Drug Safety 1999; 21: 489–501.

Patients with a history of anticonvulsant hypersensitivity syndrome should be counseled about potentially cross-reacting medications. Family counseling is a critical part of patient management in serious idiosyncratic reactions. The patient should carry a notification of the sensitivity (e.g. a MedicAlert bracelet).

Patients need to have a clear understanding that they have had a drug eruption and the risk of sequelae, the drugs that they need to avoid in future, and the risks of future exposure.

Desensitization for drug allergy. Castells M. Curr Opin Allergy Clin Immunol 2006; 6: 476–81.

Desensitization, or the gradual reintroduction of small doses of the drug at fixed intervals, has been used for various medications, including antibiotics (usually β-lactams), aspirin and non-steroidal anti-inflammatory drugs and chemotherapeutic agents. Rapid desensitization protocols have been used for anaphylactic reactions following sensitization to penicillin and cephalosporins, or for non-IgE-mediated events, as seen with aspirin, vancomycin, and taxenes.

Desensitization can be successfully employed for many different reactions. However, patients need to continue the medication for the desensitization to be effective. Once the medication is discontinued, the state of 'desensitization' is lost and the patient may react when re-exposed to the offending medication.

Eosinophilic fasciitis

Amir A Larian, Brian S Fuchs, Marsha L Gordon

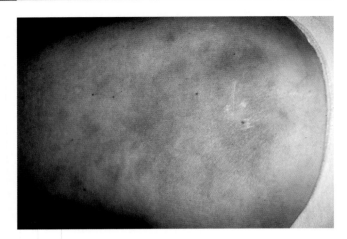

Eosinophilic fasciitis (EF) is a rare fibrosing disorder characterized by the rapid onset of symmetric woody induration of the extremities. Clinically, the progression of EF is marked by edema followed by dimpling of the skin and a *peau d'orange* appearance evolving into symmetric induration of the extremities and, less frequently, the trunk. Typically, the hands, feet, and face are spared. Although the etiology is unknown, vigorous exercise has been reported before the onset of EF in many cases.

MANAGEMENT STRATEGY

EF must be distinguished from scleroderma, from which it is differentiated by its lack of sclerodactyly, Raynaud's phenomenon, and serologic markers. EF has a more rapid onset than scleroderma, is associated with a peripheral eosinophilia, and usually responds to corticosteroid therapy. EF must also be differentiated from the eosinophilia myalgia syndrome, which is caused by the ingestion of contaminated tryptophan.

Underlying hematologic disorders such as significant cytopenias, myeloproliferative disorders, leukemias, and aplastic anemia may be associated with EF and must be checked for. Additionally, simvastatin and trichloroethylene have been associated with this disorder, and a history of their ingestion must be ruled out.

EF *may resolve spontaneously*, but treatment helps prevent the progression to flexion contractures and impaired mobility. The response may be defined by clinical improvement resulting in a softening and loosening of fibrosed skin with improvement of contractures and better mobility. Serum aldolase levels may be a useful indicator of disease activity. Magnetic resonance imaging (MRI) has been employed in diagnosing EF and in monitoring the effectiveness of treatment.

The first-line agent for EF is *prednisone*, initially at a dosage of 40–60 mg daily. A clinical response usually is noted within the first few weeks, and the dose is then tapered slowly over several months to an alternate-day regimen.

Patients who have an incomplete response or fail to respond to prednisone may benefit from the addition of *hydroxychloroquine* at a dose of 200–400 mg daily. Hydroxychloroquine has also been used successfully as monotherapy.

Clinical improvement with no recurrence after 1 year has been reported with *ciclosporin* 3.7 mg/kg daily tapered to 2.5 mg/kg. There has also been success with an aggressive course of *pulse methylprednisolone*, 1 g/day for 5 days, in conjunction with ciclosporin 150 mg twice daily.

Cimetidine 400 mg every 6–12 hours has been helpful in some cases. *Methotrexate, azathioprine, chloroquine, D-penicillamine, ketotifen, sulfasalazine, griseofulvin,* and *psoralen and UVA (PUVA)* have all been reported to have beneficial effects.

SPECIFIC INVESTIGATIONS

> ▶ Complete blood count
> ▶ Serum aldolase
> ▶ MRI
> ▶ History to exclude tryptophan, simvastatin, or trichloroethylene ingestion

Eosinophilic fasciitis. Sibrack LA, Mazur EM, Hoffman R, Bollet AJ. Clin Rheum Dis 1982; 8: 443–54.

Peripheral eosinophilia is typically present during active disease except in those patients who have an associated aplastic marrow. The eosinophilia is often transient and may precede the clinical diagnosis.

Patients with eosinophilic fasciitis should have a bone marrow examination to identify myelodysplasia. Brito-Babapulee F. Br J Dermatol 1997; 137: 316–17.

EF may be associated with significant cytopenias and myeloproliferative disorders. Therefore, those patients who have abnormal complete blood counts should have a bone marrow examination.

Serum aldolase level is a useful indicator of disease activity in eosinophilic fasciitis. Fujimoto M, Sato S, Ihn H, Kikuchi K, Yamada N, Takehara K. J Rheumatol 1995; 22: 563–5.

Three patients with EF are reported to have increased aldolase levels, which normalize with corticosteroid treatment and rise with recurrence of skin sclerosis.

Use of magnetic resonance imaging in diagnosing eosinophilic fasciitis. Report of two cases. Al-Shaikh A, Freeman C, Avruch L, McKendry RJR. Arthritis Rheum 1994; 37: 1602–8.

MRI is a useful non-invasive tool for diagnosing EF and for monitoring the effectiveness of therapy.

Eosinophilic fasciitis associated with tryptophan ingestion: a manifestation of eosinophilia myalgia syndrome. Gordon ML, Lebwohl MG, Phelps RG, Cohen SR, Fleischmajer R. Arch Dermatol 1991; 127: 217–20.

Ingestion of contaminated tryptophan is associated with a very similar clinical entity called eosinophilia myalgia syndrome.

Eosinophilic fasciitis. A pathologic study of twenty cases. Barnes L, Rodnan GP, Medsger TA, Short D. Am J Pathol 1979; 96: 493–517.

Deep fascia and subcutaneous tissue are infiltrated with lymphocytes, plasma cells, histiocytes, and eosinophils early in the course of the disease. Sclerosis of the dermis with increased collagen occurs later in the course of the disease.

FIRST-LINE THERAPIES

| ▶ Systemic corticosteroids | B |
| ▶ Pulsed methylprednisolone | E |

Eosinophilic fasciitis: clinical spectrum and therapeutic response in 52 cases. Lakhanpal S, Ginsburg WW, Michet CJ, Doyle JA, Moore SB. Semin Arthritis Rheum 1988; 17: 221–31.

Of the 52 patients, 34 were treated with prednisone dosages ranging from 40 to 60 mg daily. The remaining 18 were treated with either hydroxychloroquine, colchicine, D-penicillamine, or no medication. Twenty of the 34 patients treated with prednisone had a partial response (>25% improvement) and five had complete resolution, detected after 3–6 months. Eight of the nine patients who had a poor response were treated with the addition of hydroxychloroquine at a dose of 200–400 mg daily. Two responded completely, two had an improvement of over 50%, and three were lost to follow-up. Eight patients also responded to treatment with hydroxychloroquine alone – two had complete resolution, four had a partial response, and the others were lost to follow-up. Relapses occurred in some patients, and responses were not predictive of future recovery with the same therapy.

Diffuse fasciitis with eosinophilia: a steroid-responsive variant of scleroderma. Britt WJ, Duray PH, Dahl MV, Goltz RW. J Pediatr 1980; 97: 432–4.

A patient with EF responded completely to prednisone 40 mg/m^2 daily for 1 month, tapered to decreasing dosages every other day over 6 months.

Eosinophilic fasciitis. Helfman T, Falanga V. Clin Dermatol 1994; 12: 449–55.

Approximately 60% of patients with EF respond to prednisone at a dose of 40–60 mg daily within weeks of treatment.

A good review article.

Eosinophilic fasciitis associated with autoimmune thyroid disease and myelodysplasia treated with pulsed methylprednisolone and antihistamines. Farrell AM, Ross JS, Bunker CB. Br J Dermatol 1999; 140: 1169–99.

A 74-year-old man with EF associated with autoimmune thyroid disease and myelodysplasia responded to a combination of prednisolone, pulsed methylprednisolone, and antihistamines.

SECOND-LINE THERAPIES

▶ Hydroxychloroquine	C
▶ Ciclosporin	D
▶ Methotrexate	E
▶ Cimetidine	C

Eosinophilic rheumatic disorders. Claw DJ, Crofford LJ. Rheum Clin North Am 1995; 21: 231–46.

Hydroxychloroquine at a dose of 200–400 mg daily can be used either alone or in combination with corticosteroids.

In the series by Lakhanpal et al. (see above) hydroxychloroquine was also shown to be highly effective.

Eosinophilic fasciitis following exposure to trichloroethylene: successful treatment with cyclosporin. Hayashi N, Igarashi A, Matsuyama T, Harada S. Br J Dermatol 2000; 142: 830–2.

This case report demonstrated clinical improvement within 1 month of treatment with ciclosporin 3.7 mg/kg daily tapered to 2.5 mg/kg daily with no recurrence after 1 year.

Eosinophilic fasciitis responsive to treatment with pulsed steroids and cyclosporine. Valencia IC, Chang A, Kirsner RS, Kerdel FA. Int J Dermatol 1999; 38: 369–72.

A significant clinical response within 3 weeks was shown with pulsed methylprednisolone 1 g daily for 5 days, in conjunction with ciclosporin 150 mg twice daily.

Long-term remission by cyclosporine in a patient with eosinophilic fasciitis associated with primary biliary cirrhosis. Tahara K, Yukawa S, Shoji A, Hayashi H, Tsuboi N. Clin Rheumatol 2008; 27: 1199–201.

A 70-year-old man with eosinophilic fasciitis in association with primary biliary cirrhosis treated with ciclosporin 100 mg daily. After 4 weeks he had improvement in cutaneous induration and limited joint mobility. Treatment was discontinued after 6 months secondary to hypertension and increased serum creatinine, which were both thought to be related to ciclosporin therapy. No recurrence was noted in 12 years of follow-up.

Treatment of eosinophilic fasciitis with methotrexate. Pouplin S, Daragon A, Le Loet X. J Rheumatol 1998; 25: 606–7.

In an effort to eliminate unwanted side effects of corticosteroids, methotrexate 15 mg intramuscularly given once a week can be added to corticosteroid therapy as it is tapered.

The fasciitis–panniculitis syndromes. Clinical and pathologic features. Naschitz JE, Boss JH, Misselevich I, Yeshurun D, Rosner I. Medicine 1996; 75: 6–16.

Complete and partial remission on cimetidine 400 mg twice daily occurred in nine and five patients, respectively. Only three did not respond to cimetidine monotherapy.

The fasciitis–panniculitis syndrome: clinical spectrum and response to cimetidine. Naschitz JE, Yeshurun D, Zuckerman E, Rosner I, Shajrawi I, Missellevitch I, et al. Semin Arthritis Rheum 1992; 21: 211–20.

Six of eight patients treated with cimetidine improved significantly within 6 months. One patient's lesions remitted after 1 year, and the other patient's lesions did not respond. After 4 years therapy was discontinued and no relapses were seen.

Eosinophilic fasciitis responsive to cimetidine. Solomon G, Barland P, Rifkin H. Ann Intern Med 1982; 97: 547–9.

Cimetidine's effectiveness in treating EF may be due to its role in blocking H$_2$ receptors on suppressor T lymphocytes and other cells. In 1982, cimetidine was first described as a therapeutic option when a patient's EF lesions resolved after initiating cimetidine 400 mg every 6 hours as treatment for a presumed ulcer.

THIRD-LINE THERAPIES

▶ PUVA	E
▶ Extracorporeal photochemotherapy	D
▶ Ketotifen	E
▶ D-Penicillamine	E
▶ Azathioprine	E
▶ Chloroquine	E
▶ Griseofulvin	E
▶ Sulfasalazine	E
▶ Surgery	E
▶ Infliximab	E
▶ Hydroxyzine	E
▶ Rituximab	E
▶ Dapsone	E
▶ Combination UVA1–retinoid–corticosteroid	E

Eosinophilic fasciitis treated with psoralen-ultraviolet A bath photochemotherapy. Schiener R, Behrens-Williams SC, Gottlober P, Pillekamp H, Peter RU, Kerscher M. Br J Dermatol 2000; 142: 804–7.

PUVA had promising results within 6 months without side effects in a 56-year-old patient.

Extracorporeal photochemotherapy in the treatment of eosinophilic fasciitis. Romano C, Rubegni P, De Aloe G, Stanghellini E, D'Ascenzo G, Andreassi L, et al. J Eur Acad Dermatol Venereol 2003; 17: 10–13.

Three patients were treated with extracorporeal photochemotherapy using a UVAR XTS apparatus on 2 consecutive days at 2-week intervals for the first 3 months, followed by treatment every 4 weeks depending on response. After 1 year of therapy two patients showed a considerable improvement in clinical parameters.

Ketotifen – a therapeutic agent of eosinophilic fasciitis? Ching DWT, Leibowitz MR. J Intern Med 1992; 231: 555–9.

Ketotifen (a mast cell stabilizer) at 2 mg twice daily was effective in remitting a patient's EF lesions. There were no relapses after 4 months of no further treatment.

Eosinophilic fasciitis: review and report of six cases. Nassonova VA, Ivanova MW, Akhnazarova VD, Oskilko TG, Bjelle A, Hofer PA, et al. Scand J Rheumatol 1979; 8: 225–33.

Some patients may respond to D-penicillamine at 125–375 mg daily to a maximum of 750 mg daily, azathioprine 50 mg once or twice daily, or chloroquine.

Griseofulvin for eosinophilic fasciitis. Giordano M, Ara M, Cicala C, Valentini G, Chianese U. Arthritis Rheum 1980; 23: 1331–2.

In light of its use in progressive systemic sclerosis, griseofulvin may be useful for patients with EF through its influence on collagen metabolism.

Eosinophilic fasciitis with late onset arthritis responsive to sulfasalazine. Jones AC, Doherty M. J Rheumatol 1993; 20: 750–1.

In this patient there was a complete response to 2 g/day of sulfasalazine within 3 months.

Surgical management of eosinophilic fasciitis of the upper extremity. Suzuki G, Itoh Y, Horiuchi Y. J Hand Surg 1997; 22: 405–7.

Although one patient required a second operation for recurrence, all four patients experienced improved mobility a few weeks after fasciectomy with follow-up oral prednisolone. The recovery after surgery occurred sooner than with conservative management.

Use of infliximab, an anti-tumor necrosis alpha antibody, for inflammatory dermatoses. Drosou A, Kirsner RS, Welsh E, Sullivan TP, Kerdel FA. J Cutan Med Surg 2003; 7: 382–6.

A 69-year-old woman treated with infliximab 5 mg/kg showed marked improvement after one infusion.

Infliximab effective in steroid-dependent juvenile eosinophilic fasciitis. Tzaribachev N, Holzer U, Schedel J, Maier V, Klein R, Kuemmerle-Deschner J. Rheumatology 2008; 47: 930–2.

Report of a 12-year-old boy with debilitating progressive disease despite therapy with oral and IV steroids and methotrexate (20 mg/week) who markedly improved with initiation of infliximab. Infliximab infusions of 300 mg were given at weeks 0, 2, and every 4 weeks thereafter for 1 year. Steroids were initially continued and methotrexate was continued for 1 year after discontinuation of infliximab, at which point no residual signs of disease were noted.

Eosinophilic fasciitis successfully treated with oral hydroxyzine: a new therapeutic use of an old drug? Uckun A, Sipahi T, Akgun D, Oksal A. Eur J Pediatr 2002; 161: 118–19.

Case report of a 3-year-old boy with biopsy-proven EF successfully treated with oral hydroxyzine (2 mg/kg/day) for 15 days. He had complete clinical and laboratory improvement and showed no recurrence of disease after over 1 year of follow-up.

Rituximab in refractory autoimmune diseases: Brazilian experience with 29 patients (2002–2004). Scheinberg M, Hamerschlak N, Kutner JM, Ribiero AAF, Rerreira E, Ferreira E, et al. Clin Exp Rheumatol 2006; 24: 65–9.

Case series including a 20-year-old woman with eosinophilic fasciitis and hypergammaglobulinemia treated successfully with rituximab. (The dose was either 375 mg/m² of BSA weekly for 4 weeks, or two infusions of 1 g given 2 weeks apart. The paper does not specify which dose this patient received.)

Dapsone treatment for eosinophilic fasciitis. Smith LC, Cox NH. Arch Dermatol 2008; 144: 845–7.

Report of a 38-year-old woman with minimal improvement from oral steroids and intolerance to ciclosporin who was started on dapsone, with marked clinical improvement. She was started on 50 mg/day and increased to 100 mg within 2 weeks while reducing her prednisolone dose from 30 mg to 20 mg daily. After 2 months she was on dapsone 150 mg daily and prednisolone 10 mg daily, and at 5 months the dapsone dose was maintained while the steroid dose was reduced to 5 mg daily. This regimen was continued with maintenance of clinical improvement.

Eosinophilic fasciitis and combined UVA1-retinoid-corticosteroid treatment: two case reports. Weber HO, Schaller M, Metzler G, Rocken M, Berneburg M. Acta Dermatol Venereol 2008; 88: 304–6.

One patient, a 66-year-old man received UVA1 phototherapy (60 J/cm²) three to five times per week, isotretinoin 20 mg daily, and prednisone 75 mg daily, with marked improvement

Evidence Levels: **A** Double-blind study **B** Clinical trial ≥ 20 subjects **C** Clinical trial < 20 subjects **D** Series ≥ 5 subjects **E** Anecdotal case reports

within 3 weeks. A second patient, a 39-year-old man, was treated with UVA1 phototherapy (60 J/cm^2) three to five times per week, isotretinoin 20 mg daily, and prednisone 60 mg daily, with improvement within 2 weeks. After a few weeks the prednisone dose was reduced to 10 mg daily, and almost complete recovery was noted after 8 months of combination therapy.

Epidermal nevi

Jeffrey M Weinberg

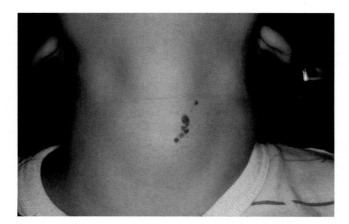

Epidermal nevi (EN) are congenital hamartomas of embryonal ectodermal origin classified on the basis of their major component. The components may be sebaceous, apocrine, eccrine, follicular, or keratinocytic. An estimated one-third of individuals with EN have involvement of other organ systems. In these cases, the condition is termed epidermal nevus syndrome (ENS).

The most common EN are verrucous epidermal nevi, which are best treated with an ablative procedure using either surgical or laser technology. Inflammatory epidermal nevi may respond to topical or systemic therapy.

MANAGEMENT STRATEGY

The pluripotential stem cell in the embryonic ectoderm can develop into any of the cell types found within the epidermis and skin adnexae. Therefore, there are many potential nevi that may develop from these cell types. Epidermal nevi may be classified according to the predominant cell type. However, there may be different cell populations, or overlap between different areas within the same nevus.

The focus of this chapter will be on nevi derived from keratinocytes. Of these, the verrucous epidermal nevus is the most common. Other forms include an inflammatory linear verrucous epidermal nevus (ILVEN), an acantholytic or Darier-like nevus, an epidermolytic form, and linear porokeratosis. Very rarely an epidermal nevus may be associated with other birth defects, and a number of epidermal nevus syndromes have been described.

Verrucous epidermal nevi may be localized, segmental, and rarely systematized. The individual lesions are verrucous papules, which may be pink, brown, or gray. These may develop as a result of mosaicism, and if there is gonadal mosaicism EN may be transmitted to future offspring.

There are very rare case reports of malignant change within epidermal nevi, including squamous cell carcinoma and basal cell carcinoma. The major focus of therapy is improved cosmesis. A possible role for the dermis in the development of epidermal nevi is suggested by the difficulty experienced in ablating such lesions surgically without destroying the underlying dermis. *Surgical management* of these lesions presents challenges. Superficial treatments, which remove only the epidermis, have a high recurrence rate, whereas excision or more aggressive ablative procedures may produce unacceptable scarring. *Laser* technology provides the surgeon with more precise tools to maximize efficacy while minimizing scarring. Alternatively, for very widespread lesions a variety of *topical regimens*, as well as *systemic retinoids*, have been reported to produce some benefit.

ILVEN presents in early childhood as a pruritic, erythematous, linear plaque. It shares many features with psoriasis, and certain cases respond to antipsoriatic therapies such as *topical vitamin D analogs*, *corticosteroids*, and *dithranol*. This has led some authors to suggest that this condition is a nevoid form of psoriasis. Epidermolytic and acantholytic nevi are more likely to respond to treatment with *retinoids*.

SPECIFIC INVESTIGATIONS

> ▶ Skin biopsy
> ▶ X-ray, imaging studies (MRI, CT scans), and ophthalmologic examinations

An epidermal nevus can most often be diagnosed solely on the clinical presentation and distribution of the lesion. A skin biopsy can be used both to confirm the diagnosis if necessary and to determine the predominant cell type and the presence of inflammatory changes, acantholysis, or dysplasia. This can be helpful in determining which therapeutic modality is most likely to succeed. If histopathology demonstrates an epidermolytic nevus, the individual should be counseled that there is a possibility that the mutation could be transmitted to offspring, with the risk that their children may have generalized cutaneous involvement. Biopsy can also indicate the rare occurrence of squamous or basal cell carcinoma, which can develop in epidermal nevi.

Epidermal nevus syndromes refer to the association of epidermal nevi with extracutaneous manifestations involving the central nervous system, eyes, or bones. The evaluation for systemic involvement should be based on the clinical extent of the epidermal nevi, and the presence of any extracutaneous signs and symptoms.

Generalized epidermolytic hyperkeratosis in two unrelated children from parents with localized linear form, and prenatal diagnosis. Chassaing N, Kanitakis J, Sportich S, Cordier-Alex MP, Titeux M, Calvas P, et al. J Invest Dermatol 2006; 126: 2715–17.

The authors report two unrelated children with epidermolytic hyperkeratosis, both born to a parent affected with epidermolyic epidermal nevi (EEN); prenatal diagnosis in two successive pregnancies of one of the patients with EEN is described.

Squamous cell carcinoma arising in a verrucous epidermal naevus. Ichikawa T, Saiki M, Kaneko M, Saida T. Dermatology 1996; 193: 135–8.

A case report of a squamous cell carcinoma arising in a 74-year-old man with an epidermal nevus, plus a review of the literature, which revealed 18 previous reports of malignant change in epidermal nevi.

Basal cell carcinoma developing in verrucous epidermal nevus. De D, Kanwar AJ, Radotra BD. Indian J Dermatol Venereol Leprol 2007; 73: 127–8.

A 58-year-old farmer with a hyperpigmented, soft verrucous plaque on the right temporoparietal region since birth presented with an ulcer of 8 months' duration. A diagnosis of basal cell carcinoma (BCC) arising in a verrucous epidermal nevus was made. Biopsy was consistent with BCC.

Epidermal nevus syndromes. Sugarman JL. Semin Cutan Med Surg 2007; 26: 221–30.

Several subsets with characteristic features have been delineated, including the nevus sebaceous syndrome, Proteus syndrome, CHILD syndrome, Becker nevus syndrome, nevus comedonicus syndrome, and phakomatosis pigmentokeratotica.

Epidermal nevus syndromes: clinical findings in 35 patients. Vidaurri-de la Cruz H, Tamayo-Sanchez L, Duran-McKinster C, de la Luz Orozco-Covarrubias M, Ruiz-Maldonado R. Pediatr Dermatol 2004; 21: 432–9.

Of patients with epidermal nevi, 10–18% may have disorders of the eye, skeletal, and nervous systems.

Does inflammatory linear verrucous epidermal nevus represent a segmental type 1/type 2 mosaic of psoriasis? Hofer T. Dermatology 2006; 212: 103–7.

The author hypothesizes that inflammatory linear verrucous eruption besides nevoid psoriasis/linear psoriasis represents a further segmental type 1/type 2 mosaic of psoriasis which, if a (verrucous) epidermal nevus exists, shows a high affinity of occurrence in close context to such a nevus. Heritability is thought to be possible.

VERRUCOUS EPIDERMAL NEVI

FIRST-LINE THERAPIES

▶ Excision under local anesthetic	D
▶ Shave or curettage under local anesthetic	D
▶ Cryotherapy	E

For small verucous epidermal nevi, excision can be performed with an acceptable cosmetic result. In these cases, this approach is the treatment of choice. However, for larger lesions, or for those in cosmetically sensitive sites, excision may not be appropriate. For larger lesions shave excision can be performed, but recurrence often occurs. Cryotherapy can be used as a destructive method for these lesions, but recurrence is frequent. All these procedures have the benefit of being cost-effective and easily performed.

Comparison of treatment modalities for epidermal nevus: a case report and review. Fox BJ, Lapins NA. J Dermatol Surg Oncol 1983; 9: 879–85.

A case report of treatment for a verrucous epidermal nevus. Review of the treatment modalities then available indicated that surgical excision was only suitable for small lesions; superficial dermabrasion often led to recurrence, and if performed more deeply, could result in hypertrophic scarring. Similar considerations applied to cryosurgery.

Epidermal nevus: surgical treatment by partial-thickness skin excision. Dellon AL, Luethke R, Wong L, Barnett N. Ann Plast Surg 1992; 28: 292–6.

A case report of treatment of a systematized epidermal nevus by partial-thickness skin excision. This cleared the nevus, but led to extensive hypertrophic and keloidal scarring.

SECOND-LINE THERAPIES

▶ Laser ablation	B
▶ Dermabrasion	E
▶ Ruby laser	E
▶ Erbium:YAG laser	C

A resurfacing procedure, either mechanically by dermabrading, or with laser technology using either the erbium:YAG or the CO_2 laser, can produce very acceptable results. However, both these techniques are operator dependent, and in the case of laser therapy access to expensive equipment is necessary. Darkly pigmented nevi may be treated using pigmented lesion lasers such as the ruby laser.

CO_2 laser therapy of verrucous epidermal nevus. Thual N, Chevallier JM, Vuillamie M, Tack B, Leroy D, Dompmartin A. Ann Dermatol Venereol 2006; 133: 131–8.

Twenty-one patients were evaluated with a 40.4-month follow-up (7 to 165 months). In 62% of cases the epidermal verrucous nevus was situated on the neck or the head. Of these 21 patients, 86% estimated their skin to be 'cured' or 'nearly normal' or 'much improved.' The dermatologist's assessment was the same.

Epidermal nevi treated by carbon dioxide laser vaporization: a series of 25 patients. Paradela S, Del Pozo J, Fernández-Jorge B, Lozano J, Martínez-González C, Fonseca E. J Dermatol Treat 2007; 18: 169–74.

A total of 25 patients were treated with the CO_2 laser in the superpulsed mode. Good results were achieved in 92% of patients with soft, flattened nevi, but in only 33% of patients with keratotic nevi. The authors concluded that the CO_2 laser in superpulsed mode is an effective and safe treatment for verrucous epidermal nevi and provides fewer recurrences than other laser therapies. They noted that the main determining factor for the cosmetic result is thickness of the nevus.

Laser therapy of verrucous epidermal naevi. Hohenleutner U, Landthaler M. Clin Exp Dermatol 1993; 18: 124–7.

A series of 43 patients (41 with verrucous epidermal nevi and two with ILVEN) were treated with either the argon laser or the CO_2 laser. Soft, papillomatous lesions responded well to the argon laser, whereas hard keratotic nevi did not. A better response was seen with the CO_2 laser, but there was a tendency to hypertrophic scarring.

Er:YAG laser treatment of verrucous epidermal nevi. Park JH, Hwang ES, Kim SN, Kye YC. Dermatol Surg 2004; 30: 378–81.

Twenty patients with verrucous epidermal nevi were treated with the erbium:YAG laser. After a single treatment, successful elimination of the verrucous epidermal nevi was observed in 15 patients. Five patients (25%) showed a relapse within the first year after treatment.

Epidermal naevi treated with pulsed erbium:YAG laser. Pearson IC, Harland CC. Clin Exp Dermatol 2004; 29: 494–6

The authors report their experience using erbium:YAG laser to treat six patients with epidermal nevi. All six had excellent cosmetic results at follow-up ranging from 6 to 60 months. The favorable results were dependent on selection of cases with superficial or small, discrete lesions which could be ablated accurately. The authors concluded that the erbium:YAG laser is an effective treatment for relatively non-verrucous or papular epidermal nevi.

Successful treatment of dark-coloured epidermal nevus with ruby laser. Baba T, Narumi H, Hanada K, Hashimoto I. J Dermatol 1995; 22: 567–70.

Five darkly pigmented epidermal nevi were successfully cleared following one to four treatments with a ruby laser in the normal mode. Two patients subsequently had hypopigmentation at the treatment site.

THIRD-LINE THERAPIES

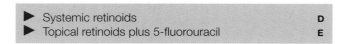

▶ Systemic retinoids	D
▶ Topical retinoids plus 5-fluorouracil	E

Systemic retinoids have been shown to reduce hyperkeratosis in very extensive and cosmetically troublesome lesions. However, long-term use is required if the benefit is to be maintained. The topical combination of tretinoin and 5-fluorouracil has also been reported to achieve a significant improvement.

A case of verrucous epidermal naevus successfully treated with acitretin. Taskapan O, Dogan B, Baloglu H, Harmanyeri Y. Acta Dermatol Venereol 1998; 78: 475–6.

Report of a case of verrucous epidermal nevus in a 20-year-old patient that responded to acitretin 75 mg daily. The nevus started to recur 6 weeks after cessation of therapy.

Management of linear verrucous epidermal naevus with topical 5-fluorouracil and tretinoin. Nelson BR, Kolansky G, Gillard M, Ratner D, Johnson TM. J Am Acad Dermatol 1994; 30: 287–8.

A case report of the use of a combination of tretinoin 0.1% cream and 5% 5-fluorouracil applied twice daily under occlusion. The lesion responded well, but was seen to recur 3–4 weeks after therapy was stopped.

Topical tretinoin and 5-fluorouracil in the treatment of linear verrucous epidermal nevus. Kim JJ, Chang MW, Shwayder T. J Am Acad Dermatol 2000; 43: 129–32.

In a 7-year-old boy with an extensive, facial epidermal nevus there was significant improvement using a combination of topical tretinoin and 5-fluorouracil.

INFLAMMATORY/DYSPLASTIC EPIDERMAL NEVI

Nevi that have inflammatory, epidermolytic, acantholytic, or dysplastic features may respond more effectively to medical therapy than to surgical treatment. Inflammatory linear verrucous epidermal nevus (ILVEN) is a relatively rare entity that presents during childhood and can be difficult to treat.

FIRST-LINE THERAPIES

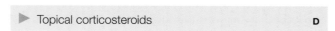

▶ Topical corticosteroids	D

Topical corticosteroids are often used as first-line therapy, but the response is often variable. There are few clinical data on the use of topical corticosteroids and their use appears to be empirical rather than evidence based; nevertheless, they are relatively cheap and safe.

Successful treatment of inflammatory linear verrucous epidermal nevus with tacrolimus and fluocinonide. Mutasim DF. J Cutan Med Surg 2006; 10: 45–7.

A report of the successful treatment of ILVEN with potent topical steroid and tacrolimus ointments.

SECOND-LINE THERAPIES

▶ Topical calcipotriol/tacalcitol	D
▶ Topical retinoids	E
▶ Systemic retinoids	E
▶ Topical dithranol	E

ILVEN have been shown to respond to a variety of antipsoriatic therapies, leading some authors to believe that it is a nevoid form of psoriasis.

Topical calcipotriol for the treatment of inflammatory linear verrucous epidermal nevus. Zvulunov A, Grunwald MH, Halvy S. Arch Dermatol 1997; 133: 567–8.

A report on the use of calcipotriol in the treatment of an ILVEN.

Successful therapy of an ILVEN in a 7-year-old girl with calcipotriol. Bohm I, Bieber T, Bauer R. Hautarzt 1999; 50: 812–14.

A report on the successful use of calcipotriol in the treatment of an ILVEN. After 8 weeks of therapy the ILVEN had almost cleared. There was no relapse 25 weeks after treatment was discontinued.

Acitretin treatment of a systematized inflammatory linear verrucous epidermal naevus. Renner R, Rytter M, Sticherling M. Acta Dermatol Venereol 2005; 85: 348–50.

In this case, treatment with oral acitretin was initiated at a dose of 25 mg daily, but had to be reduced to 20 mg daily because of increasing erythema on the face and left leg after 3 days of therapy. The dose was slowly increased to 30 mg daily. After 2 weeks at this level, the erythema had almost entirely resolved, and the hyperkeratosis was distinctly reduced. After 8 weeks on this dose the inflammatory and hyperkeratotic lesions had almost disappeared.

Dithranol in the treatment of inflammatory linear verrucous epidermal nevus. De Mare S, van de Kerkhof PC, Happle R. Acta Dermatol Venereol 1989; 69: 77–80.

Treatment with dithranol resulted in complete relief from pruritus and clearing of all linear lesions, except for a small verrucous band on the shin.

THIRD-LINE THERAPIES

▶ Pulsed-dye laser	E
▶ CO_2 laser	E
▶ Surgical excision	D
▶ Etanercept	E

Inflammatory linear verrucous epidermal nevus: successful treatment with the 585 nm flashlamp-pumped pulsed dye laser. Alster TS. J Am Acad Dermatol 1994; 31: 513–14.

The pulsed-dye laser has been reported to be successful in the treatment of ILVEN; this may be related to its effects on psoriatic lesions.

Pulsed dye laser for inflammatory linear verrucous epidermal nevus. Sidwell RU, Syed S, Harper JI. Br J Dermatol 2001; 144: 1267–9.

Evidence Levels: A Double-blind study B Clinical trial ≥ 20 subjects C Clinical trial < 20 subjects D Series ≥ 5 subjects E Anecdotal case reports

Three cases of ILVEN in children ranging in age from 2 to 8 years were treated successfully with the pulsed-dye laser. The authors surmise that the destruction of capillaries by the laser reduces the release of inflammatory mediators.

Carbon dioxide laser therapy for an inflammatory linear verrucous epidermal nevus: a case report. Ulkur E, Celikoz B, Yuksel F, Karagoz H. Aesthet Plast Surg 2004; 28: 428–30.

A case of ILVEN was treated with the CO_2 laser. All symptoms, including erythema, excoriation, granulation, and pruritus, disappeared, and a pale pigmentation remained.

Full-thickness surgical excision for the treatment of inflammatory linear verrucous epidermal nevus. Lee BJ, Mancini AJ, Renucci J, Paller AS, Bauer BS. Ann Plast Surg 2001; 47: 285–92.

The authors report four patients with extensive ILVEN treated successfully with full-thickness surgical excision.

Successful treatment of a widespread inflammatory verrucous epidermal nevus with etanercept. Bogle MA, Sobell JM, Dover JS. Arch Dermatol 2006; 142: 401–2.

A 55-year-old woman diagnosed with widespread inflammatory epidermal verrucous nevi was presented. She had a history of multiple therapies, including emollients, topical and intramuscular steroids, topical lactic acid, pimecrolimus cream, and isotretinoin. She had minimal improvement with isotretinoin and experienced the largest reduction in pruritus with IM corticosteroid injections.

Given the widespread disease and the limitations of steroids, and considering the similarities between ILVEN and psoriasis, the authors initiated subcutaneous etanercept therapy at a dose of 25 mg twice weekly. After 1 month, the patient experienced good initial improvement in pruritus and erythema. The etanercept was increased to 50 mg twice weekly, which provided nearly 50% improvement over 3 months. She continued treatment at this dose for a total of 6 months, and achieved almost complete resolution of pruritus and a significant improvement in roughness and erythema. The dose was then reduced to 25 mg twice weekly, and disease activity remained quiescent at follow-up.

Epidermodysplasia verruciformis

Slawomir Majewski, Stefania Jablonska

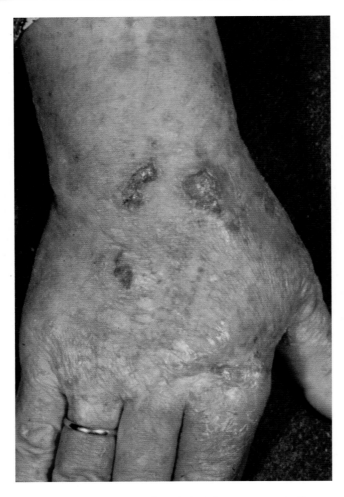

Epidermodysplasia verruciformis (EV) is a rare genetic disease characterized by an impaired immune response to human papillomavirus (HPV) and HPV-associated cutaneous oncogenesis. Chronic infection occurs with potentially oncogenic HPV types 5 and 8 as well as non-oncogenic types. Flat warts and pityriasis versicolor-like lesions begin to appear in early childhood and become widespread. In the fourth and fifth decades many patients begin to develop multiple cutaneous malignancies. It has recently been established that EV is often associated with mutations of genes EVER1 and EVER2, coding transmembrane proteins located in the endoplasmic reticulum.

MANAGEMENT STRATEGY

No compound acts directly on HPV, and no therapy produces a complete and sustained clearing of both benign wart-like and keratotic lesions associated with oncogenic EV HPVs. A most important aspect of the management of EV is protection from UVR, which is a cancer cofactor. *Light-avoiding behavior* and topical *sunblocks* (sun protection factor >50) are indicated. Other cancer cofactors (radiotherapy, immunosuppressants) must be avoided. Premalignant and troublesome benign lesions can be treated by a variety of destructive techniques: surgical (*cryotherapy, shave excision, curettage, laser, full excision*) or chemical (*trichloroacetic acid, 5% 5-fluorouracil*).

For more widespread lesions, with signs of premalignancy or malignancy, agents that modify keratinization are indicated, such as *oral or topical retinoids, vitamin D_3 analogs, interferons,* and *imiquimod. Photodynamic therapy* can be useful for early malignancy. Larger malignancies can necessitate skin autografts.

There are no good controlled trials of therapies for epidermodysplasia verruciformis. The first-line therapies listed below are drugs and procedures used for management of warts and other papillomavirus-associated proliferations. The second-line therapies are treatments found to have favorable effect in some cases, which we advise to try. As third-line therapies are listed experimental drugs and procedures and treatment for malignancies.

SPECIFIC INVESTIGATIONS

- ▶ Family history and examination of other family members
- ▶ Skin biopsy
- ▶ HPV typing to identify potentially oncogenic and non-oncogenic HPV types
- ▶ Evaluation of immune status: characteristic anergy to DNCB and other non-specific sensitizers, and the presence of factors producing or enhancing immunosuppression.
- ▶ Consider other causes of immune dysfunction:
  - ▶ Human immunodeficiency virus and other immunodeficiency syndromes
  - ▶ Iatrogenic immunosuppression

Human papillomavirus-associated tumors of the skin and mucosa. Majewski S, Jablonska S. J Am Acad Dermatol 1997; 36: 659–88.

A detailed CME article on HPV-associated tumors.

The histology of verrucous lesions demonstrates a highly characteristic cytopathic effect, with clarification of cytoplasm and nucleoplasm and prominent keratohyaline granules.

Common variable immunodeficiency syndrome associated with epidermodysplasia verruciformis. Vu J, Wallace GR, Singh R, Diwan H, Prieto V, Rady P. Am J Clin Dermatol 2007; 8: 307–10.

Epidermodysplasia verruciformis in the setting of graft-versus-host disease. Kunishige JH, Hymes SR, Madkan V, Wyatt AJ, Uptmore D, Lazar AJ. J Am Acad Dermatol 2007; 58: S78–80.

Other causes of immunosuppression may give rise to a very similar clinical picture.

FIRST-LINE THERAPIES

- ▶ Sun avoidance/protection. Sunscreens for exposed parts of at least sun protection factor 50   E
- ▶ Cryotherapy with liquid nitrogen   E
- ▶ Topical retinoic acid 0.05–0.1% for benign flat, cosmetically troublesome lesions   E

Evidence Levels: A Double-blind study **B** Clinical trial ≥ 20 subjects **C** Clinical trial < 20 subjects **D** Series ≥ 5 subjects **E** Anecdotal case reports

- ▶ Topical 5% 5-fluorouracil cream for keratotic lesions.   E
- ▶ Shave excision for flat lesions   E
- ▶ Surgical excision of premalignant and malignant lesions   E

SECOND-LINE THERAPIES

- ▶ Interferon-α with retinoids (acitretin)   E
- ▶ Systemic isotretinoin   E
- ▶ Imiquimod 5% cream   E
- ▶ Cimetidine   E

New treatments for cutaneous human papillomavirus infections. Majewski S, Jablonska S. J Eur Acad Dermatol Venereol 2004; 18: 265–6.

A helpful succinct review.

Treatment of epidermodysplasia verruciformis with a combination of acitretin and interferon alfa-2a. Anadolu R, Oskay T, Erdem C, Boyvat A, Terzi E. J Am Acad Dermatol 2001; 45: 296–9.

A report of a patient treated with oral acitretin 50 mg daily and systemic interferon-α_{2a}, 3MU subcutaneously three times weekly for 6 months. Improvement was followed by relapse after discontinuation of treatment, and the same regimen was reintroduced. The interferon was then discontinued after 4 months and the acitretin reduced to 25 mg for 3 months, then stopped. Improvement was maintained during the subsequent 12-month follow-up.

Used as monotherapy, interferon-α has only a slight effect and is not recommended.

Systemic low-dose isotretinoin maintains remission status in epidermodysplasia verruciformis. Rallis E, Papatheodorou G, Bimpakis E, Buutanska D, Menounos P, Papadakis P. J Eur Acad Dermatol Venereol 2008; 22: 523–5.

A case report in which systemic low-dose oral isotretinoin 0.8 mg/kg/day for 6 months produced complete clearance, with relapse 4 months after discontinuation of medication. Maintenance treatment with 20 mg/day sustained remission. It should be stressed that EV was associated with HPV3, hence was a more benign variant responsive to therapy.

Epidermodysplasia verruciformis, unsuccessful therapeutic approach with imiquimod. Janssen K, Lucker GP, Houwing RH, van Rijssel R. Int J Dermatol 2007; 46: 45–7.

Treatment of a patient with epidermodysplasia verruciformis carrying novel EVER2 mutation with imiquimod. Berthelot C, Dickerson MC, Rady P, He Q, Niroomand F, Tyring SK, et al. J Am Acad Dermatol 2007; 56: 882–6.

A favorable result was reported in single EV case.

Imiquimod is an immune response modifier which stimulates B cells and cytotoxic T cells, induces the production of proinflammatory cytokines, and is effective in benign HPV infections, partially preventing malignant conversion. It may reduce viral load, but does not clear EV lesions.

Cimetidine therapy for epidermodysplasia verruciformis. Micali G, Nasca MR, Dall'Oglio F, Musumeci ML. J Am Acad Dermatol 2003; 48: 9–10.

The lack of a clinical effect of cimetidine in the treatment of epidermodysplasia verruciformis. Oliveira WRP, Neto CF, Rivitti EA. J Am Acad Dermatol 2004; 50: 14.

In one patient with epidermodysplasia verruciformis with HPV5 but with no cancer a 3-month course of 40 mg/kg/day produced clearance of lesions, sustained for 6 months with no relapse. However, others reported unsuccessful results and this is also our experience.

Cimetidine may facilitate the development of cell-mediated immunity.

THIRD-LINE THERAPIES

- ▶ Photodynamic therapy   E
- ▶ CO$_2$ laser for malignant and premalignant lesions   E
- ▶ Skin autografts   D

Photodynamic therapy for human papilloma virus-related diseases in dermatology. Szeimies RM. Med Laser Appl 2003; 18: 107–16.

Topical PDT using 20% 5-aminolevulic acid (ALA) yielded excellent results in a case of epidermodysplasia verruciformis associated with HPV 5, 8, 36, and others. Twelve months after PDT the lesions started to reappear, but resolved after repeated treatments. The authors suggest that even annually repeated PDT is safe and will control EV lesions.

Skin autografts in epidermodysplasia verruciformis: human papillomavirus-associated cutaneous changes need over 20 years for malignant conversion. Majewski S, Jablonska S. Cancer Res 1997; 57: 4214–16.

In our experience in cases of very widespread, constantly developing new lesions not responding to therapy, the only effective method is removal of the most involved skin area (usually on the forehead) and its replacement with skin from non-exposed inner aspects of the arms.

Successful treatment of recalcitrant condyloma with topical cidofovir. Hengge UR, Tietze G. Sex Transm Infect 2000; 76: 143.

Cidofovir – a new antiviral compound – has more antiproliferative than antiviral activity. There are single reports of successful treatment of recalcitrant condyloma using topical cidofovir.

This agent was reported as ineffective in a single case of EV.

Epidermolysis bullosa

Ysabel M Bello, Anna F Falabella, Lawrence A Schachner

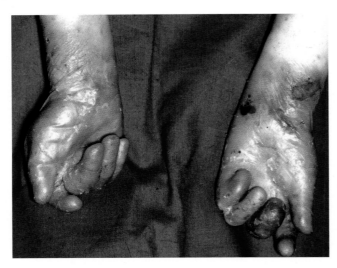

Epidermolysis bullosa is a complex group of mechanobullous disorders characterized by painful blister formation as a result of minor trauma to the skin. With the exception of the acquisita type, epidermolysis bullosa is an inherited disorder. The classification system for hereditary epidermolysis bullosa was recently revised and now includes four major types according to the level of blister formation: simplex or intraepidermal ('epidermolytic'), junctional or intralamina lucida ('lamina lucidolytic'), dystrophic or sublamina densa ('dermolytic'), and Kindler syndrome or mixed. The disease can involve the skin, mucosae, and internal organs. The severity of epidermolysis bullosa ranges from mild to severe, and skin involvement can be localized or generalized. Epidermolysis bullosa acquisita is discussed on page 209.

MANAGEMENT STRATEGY

The management of inherited epidermolysis bullosa has classically been *supportive: avoidance of trauma, treatment of infections, and nutritional support*. More recent efforts have been directed at trying to improve the ability to heal wounds and prevent new wound formation by treating the underlying disease.

Avoidance of trauma to intact skin is important but difficult. Sewing foam pads into the lining of clothing is helpful, especially over the elbows, knees, and other pressure points. Minimizing trauma to wounds is also vital. Mepilex is a non-adherent, absorbent polyurethane foam pad that can be applied, removed, and reapplied to wounds with little discomfort, no trauma to the wound bed, and no disruption of wound healing. European studies confirm that a novel contact layer dressing (Urgotul) containing petrolatum formulations and hydrocolloid is effective in the treatment of skin lesions in patients with epidermolysis bullosa. Other non-adherent dressings, such as white petrolatum-impregnated gauzes, hydrogels, and foams, can be used and held in place with soft, roller gauze bandages or elastic tube dressings.

Avoidance of wound infection is also critical to promote more rapid healing and to avoid overwhelming infections and sepsis, which are associated with an increased mortality rate. *Topical antibiotics* are routinely used, but should be rotated monthly to avoid the development of resistant organisms. Cutaneous infections unresponsive to topical measures need to be treated with *systemic antibiotics*, but the chronic use of systemic antibiotics is not recommended as a preventive measure.

Some common nutritional problems in patients with epidermolysis bullosa include chewing and swallowing difficulties, malnutrition, constipation, and vitamin and mineral deficiencies. Avoidance of malnutrition depends on *active and continuous nutritional support*. Early nutritional supplementation can promote better childhood growth rates and encourage healing of skin lesions. In patients who develop esophageal strictures, intensive nutritional support has been reported as necessary to achieve good results even associated with balloon dilatation. Daily multivitamin trace elements and zinc supplementation have been recommended. Anemia may be profound in epidermolysis bullosa, and oral iron replacement is mandatory for patients with iron deficiency. Erythropoietin has been recommended if the level is <500 mU/mL. Some have recommended intravenous iron therapy for patients resistant to oral replacement.

A variety of *skin grafts* have been used to treat the wounds of epidermolysis bullosa, including split-thickness skin grafts, allogeneic and autogeneic cultured keratinocytes, and cryopreserved acellular human dermis. A study using intradermal injections of allogeneic fibroblasts demonstrated therapeutic potential in human subjects with recessive dystrophic epidermolysis bullosa. Several trials have reported impressive results with Apligraf, a bilayered, tissue-engineered skin derived from neonatal foreskin that contains living keratinocytes and fibroblasts. Another allogeneic composite cultured skin (OrCel) has been approved by the United States Food and Drug Administration to treat hands and donor sites in patients with recessive dystrophic epidermolysis bullosa.

Many systemic therapies, such as *psoralens in combination with UVA irradiation, corticosteroids, vitamin E, ciclosporin, antimalarials, retinoids, phenytoin, tetracycline* and *cyproheptadine*, have been used, to treat epidermolysis bullosa, but their efficacy is unproven.

Current therapies are focused on gene-, protein-, and cell-based techniques. There have been improvements in genetic manipulation of keratinocytes ex vivo and of graft techniques in vivo. Gene transfer of epidermal stem cells in combination with tissue engineering procedures is promising.

SPECIFIC INVESTIGATIONS

> ► Skin biopsy for transmission electron microscopy
> ► Skin biopsy for immunofluorescence antigenic mapping
> ► Mutational analysis

The classification of inherited epidermolysis bullosa (EB): Report of the Third International Consensus Meeting on Diagnosis and Classification of EB. Fine J-D, Eady RAJ, Bauer EA, Bauer JW, Bauer JW, Bruckner-Tuderman L, et al. J Am Acad Dermatol 2008; 58: 931–50.

Both transmission electron microscopy and immunofluorescence have been successfully employed to diagnose EB. Electron

Evidence Levels: **A** Double-blind study **B** Clinical trial ≥ 20 subjects **C** Clinical trial < 20 subjects **D** Series ≥ 5 subjects **E** Anecdotal case reports

microscopy is likely to play a decreasing role in the diagnosis because there are only a few highly proficient EM laboratories, although it has an important place in research because it permits visualization and assessment of keratin filaments, hemidesmosomes, and anchoring fibrils. Immunofluorescence antigen mapping is relatively inexpensive and simple to perform, requiring immunofluorescence transport media. It can reveal the level of the split by defining its location relative to proteins expressed at various levels of the basement membrane zone. Mutational analysis remains a superb research tool that lets us determine the mode of inheritance, the precise site and the type of molecular mutation. However, it is not considered to be the first-line diagnostic test.

A comparative study between transmission electron microscopy and immunofluorescence mapping in the diagnosis of epidermolysis bullosa. Yiasemides E, Walton J, Mar P, Villanueva EV, Murrell DF. Am J Dermatopathol 2006; 28: 387–94.

Transmission electron microscopy is able to directly visualize and quantify ultrastructural features. Immunofluorescence antigenic mapping determines the precise level of skin cleavage by determining binding sites for a series of antibodies. This last method reported improving diagnosis of epidermolysis bullosa compared to electron microscopy.

FIRST-LINE THERAPIES

▶ Sterile dressing and topical antibiotics	**B**
▶ Nutritional support	**C**

Management of epidermolysis bullosa in infants and children. Bello YM, Falabella AF, Schachner LA. Clin Dermatol 2003; 21: 278–82.

Open or only partially healed erosions are best covered with polymyxin, bacitracin, or silver sulfadiazine and then covered with either petrolatum-impregnated gauze or non-adherent synthetic dressing. Such dressings are usually changed daily. Mupirocin may be substituted for those infected sites unresponsive to milder antibiotics, but is best avoided for routine use because of the potential for development of resistance.

Mupirocin-resistant *Staphylococcus aureus* after long-term treatment of patients with epidermolysis bullosa. Moy JA, Caldwell-Brown D, Lin An, Pappa KA, Carter DM. J Am Acad Dermatol 1990; 22: 893–5.

A long-term open study in 47 patients with epidermolysis bullosa who were treated with topical 2% mupirocin (Bactroban) ointment to reduce bacterial infection and promote wound healing reported evidence of the appearance of bacterial strains with reduced sensitivity to mupirocin. Clinical improvement and culture negativity were observed in four patients after treatment with oral antibiotic sensitive to *Staphylococcus aureus*.

Resistance of Staphylococcus aureus to mupirocin is a growing problem worldwide and argues against the routine use of this antibiotic for prophylaxis against cutaneous infections.

Using Urgotul dressing for the management of epidermolysis bullosa skin lesions. Blanchet-Bardon C, Bohbot S. J Wound Care 2005; 14: 490–1, 494–6.

An open-label single-center, non-randomized clinical trial was conducted on 20 patients suffering from simplex and dystrophic epidermolysis bullosa in France using Urgotul, which is a novel contact layer containing petrolatum formulation and hydrocolloid particles. The results reported that 19 of 20 wounds healed within 8.7 days and that 90% of dressing changes were reported to be pain free. This trial was not controlled and the sample was relatively small; however 19 out of 20 patients confirmed that they will treat new skin lesions with that dressing. In North America, this dressing is marketed as Restore Contact Layer Dressing.

Nutrition management of patients with epidermolysis bullosa. Birge K. J Am Diet Assoc 1995; 95: 575–9.

This report provides information based on 80 patients with epidermolysis bullosa. Estimation of protein and energy requirements should consider catch-up growth, percentage of body surface blistered, and presence of infection. Impaired nutrient intake because of chewing and swallowing problems requires more aggressive therapy, such as restorative dental therapy, dilatation of esophageal strictures, or placement of a gastrostomy tube for feeding. A high-fiber diet and adequate fluid intake may help alleviate constipation. Vitamin and mineral supplementation is recommended.

Scarring of the gastrointestinal tract may contribute to malabsorption of nutrients as well as medications.

Esophageal strictures in children with recessive dystrophic epidermolysis bullosa: experience of balloon dilatation in nine cases. Fujimoto T, Lane GJ, Miyano T, Yaguchi H, Koike M, Manabe M, et al. J Pediatr Gastroenterol Nutr 1998; 27: 524–9.

Intensive nutritional support followed by balloon dilatation is a treatment of choice for esophageal strictures complicating recessive epidermolysis bullosa.

Gastrostomy and growth in dystrophic epidermolysis bullosa. Haynes L, Atherton DJ, Ade-Ajayi N, Wheeler R, Kiely EM. Br J Dermatol 1996; 134: 872–9.

A significantly improved growth rate and improved quality of life for both child and family followed the establishment of supplementary gastrostomy feeding in 13 patients.

Correction of the anemia of epidermolysis bullosa with intravenous iron and erythropoietin. Fridge JL, Vichinsky EP. J Pediatr 1998; 132: 871–3.

A transfusion-dependent chronic anemia is seen in some types of epidermolysis bullosa. Four children whose anemia failed to respond to oral iron became transfusion independent after treatment with intravenous iron and human recombinant erythropoietin.

SECOND-LINE THERAPIES

▶ Cultured keratinocytes	**C**
▶ Skin grafts	**C**
▶ Fibroblast cell therapy	**D**

Cultured keratinocyte allografts and wound healing in severe recessive dystrophic epidermolysis bullosa. McGrath JA, Schofield OM, Ishida-Yamamoto A, O'Grady A, Mayou BJ, Navsaria H, et al. J Am Acad Dermatol 1993; 29: 407–19.

In 10 patients with recessive dystrophic epidermolysis bullosa cultured keratinocytes were applied to part of the wound, with another part left ungrafted. The only distinguishing findings were a moderate analgesic effect induced by the graft.

Tissue-engineered skin (Apligraf) in the healing of patients with epidermolysis bullosa wounds. Falabella AF, Valencia IC, Eaglstein WH, Schachner LA. Arch Dermatol 2000; 135: 1219–22.

An open-label uncontrolled study of 15 patients with 69 acute wounds and nine chronic wounds who were treated with tissue-engineered skin; a week later, 79% of the wounds were healed. The patients and their families considered that healing with the tissue-engineered skin was faster and less painful, and that quality of life was improved, compared to healing with conventional dressings.

Graftskin therapy in epidermolysis bullosa. Fivenson DP, Scherschun L, Choucair M, Kukuruga D, Young J, Shwayder T. J Am Acad Dermatol 2003; 48: 886–92.

A second series of 96 sites treated with Apligraf in nine patients reported rapid healing, with over 90% closure of 94 treated sites.

Surgical management of hands in children with recessive dystrophic epidermolysis bullosa: use of allogeneic composite cultured skin grafts. Eisenberg M, Llewelyn D. Br J Plast Surg 1998; 51: 608–13.

Composite cultured skin allografts were used as a partial substitute for autografts on digits, and were used over donor sites in the course of 16 operations performed on seven children with recessive dystrophic epidermolysis bullosa and syndactyly and flexor contracture of the fingers.

Apligraf in the treatment of severe mitten deformity associated with recessive dystrophic epidermolysis bullosa. Fivenson DP, Scherschum L, Cohen LV. Plast Reconstruct Surg 2003; 112: 584–8.

Five patients with recessive dystrophic epidermolysis bullosa were treated for mitten deformity with a bioengineered skin equivalent. These patients exhibited increased range of motion and have maintained web space separation for more than 12 months, improving the quality of their life.

Potential of fibroblast cell therapy for recessive dystrophic epidermolysis bullosa. Wong T, Gammon L, Liu L, Mellerio JE, Mellerio JE, Dopping-Hepenstal PJ, et al. J Invest Dermatol 2008; advance online publication, 3 April, 1–11.

A study using single intradermal injections of allogeneic fibroblasts to five subjects with recessive dystrophic epidermolysis bullosa demonstrated therapeutic potential. There was increased type VII collagen at the dermoepidermal junction at 2 weeks and 3 months following injection.

THIRD-LINE THERAPIES

► Phenytoin (ineffective)	A
► Tetracycline	C
► Cyproheptadine	C
► Isotretinoin	C
► Gene therapy	E

Lack of efficacy of phenytoin in recessive dystrophic epidermolysis bullosa. Epidermolysis Bullosa Study Group. Caldwell-Brown D, Stern RS, Lin AN, Carter DM. N Engl J Med 1992; 327: 163–7.

This article reports the results of a randomized, double-blind, placebo-controlled, crossover trial in 36 patients comparing phenytoin versus placebo in the treatment of dys-trophic epidermolysis bullosa. The authors reported no significant differences in disease activity (number of blisters and erosions) between the two groups.

Two familial cases of epidermolysis bullosa simplex successfully treated with tetracycline. Malkinson FD. Arch Dermatol 1999; 135: 997–8.

Suppression of the formation of new bullae was observed in two patients with epidermolysis bullosa simplex after treatment with tetracycline. Tetracycline may modulate the enzyme activity that controls matrix degradation, thereby reducing the formation of bullae.

Treatment of epidermolysis bullosa simplex with tetracycline. Veien NK, Buus SK. Arch Dermatol 2000; 136: 424–5.

A number of patients using tetracycline were observed over a 7-year period. The article reports an increase in bulla formation during the summer months, but healing was more rapid and less painful while patients took the tetracycline.

Tetracycline and epidermolysis bullosa simplex: a double-blind, placebo-controlled, crossover randomized clinical trial. Weiner M, Stein A, Cash S, de Leoz J, Fine JD. Br J Dermatol 2004; 150: 613–14.

A limited number of patients – six of 12 patients completed at least the first arm, four experienced a reduction in the total number of EB lesions; in contrast, two experienced an increased number of lesions after 4 months of active therapy (oral tetracycline administered 1000 mg every morning and 500 mg every evening). The risk of tetracycline-induced dental discoloration in children needs to be balanced against the severity and chronicity of the symptoms.

Is cyproheptadine effective in the treatment of subjects with epidermolysis bullosa simplex? Neufeld-Kaiser W, Sybert VP. Arch Dermatol 1997; 133: 251–2.

An unblinded, non-placebo-controlled study in a small cohort of patients receiving systemic cyproheptadine for 6 weeks reported a marked patient dropout (nine of 13). This prevented the authors from determining whether the reduction in blister formation and symptoms seen during the study was related to the medication.

Chemoprevention of squamous cell carcinoma in recessive dystrophic epidermolysis bullosa: results of a phase I trial of systemic isotretinoin. Fine JD, Johnson LB, Weiner M, Stein A, Suchindran C. J Am Acad Dermatol 2004; 50: 563–71.

Patients with RDEB are at high risk of developing squamous cell carcinoma. A initial study on 20 patients aged 15 years or older who were treated with isotretinoin 0.5 mg/kg/day for 8 months reported that isotretinoin may be safely used. However, a chemoprevention effect has yet to be proven.

Correction of junctional epidermolysis bullosa by transplantation of genetically modified epidermal stem cells. Mavillo F, Pellegrini G, Ferrari S, Di Nunzio F, Di Nunzio F, Di Iorio E, et al. Nature Med 2006; 12: 1397–402.

Ex vivo transduction of autologous epidermal stem cells with a normal copy of the defective gene, followed by reconstitution of the patient's skin with epithelial sheets that were grown from these genetically corrected cells, kept the epidermis firmly adherent and stable for the duration of follow-up (1 year).

Evidence Levels: A Double-blind study **B** Clinical trial ≥ 20 subjects **C** Clinical troial < 20 subjects **D** Series ≥ 5 subjects **E** Anecdotal case reports

Epidermolysis bullosa acquisita

Lawrence S Chan

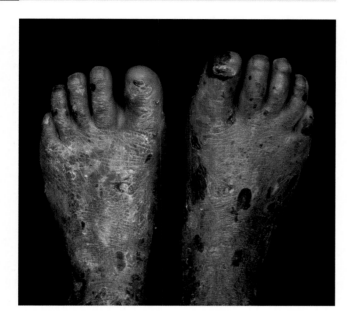

Epidermolysis bullosa acquisita is a rare, acquired, chronic, autoimmune blistering disease of the skin and mucous membranes that primarily affects elderly individuals and occurs predominantly at trauma-prone skin areas (the non-inflammatory mechanobullous scarring subset) or widespread skin areas (the generalized inflammatory non-scarring subset). IgG (or rarely IgA) autoantibodies targeting the skin basement membrane component type VII collagen (anchoring fibrils) and physical trauma are apparently the major contributing factors to the blistering process. The subset of patients with predominantly mucous membrane involvement is addressed in another chapter (Mucous membrane pemphigoidy).

MANAGEMENT STRATEGY

Epidermolysis bullosa acquisita, especially the non-inflammatory mechanobullous subset, is characteristically very resistant to medical therapies. For an immune-mediated blistering disease associated with autoantibodies that target skin components, the logical approach is to modify the immune response to reduce the production and effect of the autoantibodies to their target antigen type VII collagen. However, no target-specific treatment is currently available. Thus the currently available non-target-specific immunosuppressants not only reduce the immune responses against autoantigen, but also suppress the patient's response to pathogens, resulting in a general immunodeficiency state. Therefore, when treating patients with this disease, every effort should be made to use anti-inflammatories rather than immunosuppressants, to use the lowest possible doses of immunosuppressant for the shortest duration, and to replace immunosuppressants with other anti-inflammatory medications whenever possible. A commonly used initial regimen is *systemic corticosteroid with either*

azathioprine or dapsone or both as a corticosteroid-sparing agent. For adult patients without significant medical problems, a combination of oral prednisone (1 mg/kg daily), azathioprine (1–2 mg/kg daily), and dapsone (100–200 mg daily) can be started. Because of its rarity, no well-controlled clinical trial has been performed for epidermolysis bullosa acquisita. The following therapeutic guidelines are derived primarily from case reports of small groups or single patients.

Other therapeutic agents have been reported to be beneficial for this disease. *Colchicine* (1–2 mg daily) has been reported to significantly improve the disease. *Ciclosporin* (5–9 mg/kg daily) has been shown to be beneficial in reducing blister formation and speeding up healing. *Intravenous immunoglobulin (IVIG)* treatment (400 mg/kg daily) has also been demonstrated to reduce new blister formation and facilitate healing. In addition, *extracorporeal photochemotherapy, mycophenolate mofetil*, and *humanized anti-Tac monoclonal antibodies* have been used successfully in some patients. Most recently, a monoclonal antibody against B-cell-specific target CD20 medically termed *rituximab* (usual dose 375 mg/m^2 body surface area, multiple doses) has been shown to be quite effective in several cases of epidermolysis bullosa acquisita, considering the medication-resistant nature of the disease. At present the high cost and difficulty of obtaining insurance company approval are the major hindrances to the use of *rituximab* in epidermolysis bullosa acquisita.

In addition to medical treatments, patients with this disease should be instructed to *avoid physical trauma* as much as possible. Vigorous rubbing of their skin and the use of harsh soaps and hot water should also be avoided. Patients should be instructed to *care for open wounds promptly* and to recognize local skin infection and *seek medical attention when infection occurs*.

SPECIFIC INVESTIGATIONS

- ▶ Skin biopsy and serum for direct and indirect immunofluorescence, respectively, to detect IgG or IgA class skin basement membrane-specific autoantibodies
- ▶ Serum for enzyme-linked immunosorbent assay (ELISA) to detect IgG or IgA class type VII collagen-specific autoantibodies
- ▶ Gastrointestinal (GI) work-up for inflammatory bowel disease

Epidermolysis bullosa acquisita: ultrastructural and immunological studies. Yaoita H, Briggaman RA, Lawley TJ, Provost TT, Katz SI. J Invest Dermatol 1981; 76: 288–92.

Identification of the skin basement-membrane autoantigen in epidermolysis bullosa acquisita. Woodley DT, Briggaman RA, O'Keefe EJ, Inman AO, Queen LL, Gammon WR. N Engl J Med 1984; 310: 1007–13.

Direct immunofluorescence detects IgG deposits linearly at the dermoepidermal junction in all patients. Indirect immunofluorescence detects IgG circulating autoantibodies bound to the dermal side of salt-separated normal skin substrate in about 50% patients with this disease.

Development of an ELISA for rapid detection of anti-type VII collagen autoantibodies in epidermolysis bullosa acquisita. Chen M, Chan LS, Cai X, O'Toole EA, Sample JC, Woodley DT. J Invest Dermatol 1997; 108: 68–72.

ELISA assay using eukaryotically expressed recombinant protein of the non-collagenous (NC1) domain of type VII collagen is the most sensitive and specific method for detecting IgG class autoantibodies in patients with this disease.

IgA-mediated epidermolysis bullosa acquisita: two cases and review of the literature. Vodegel RM, de Jong MC, Pas HH, Jonkman MF. J Am Acad Dermatol 2002; 47: 919–25.

In rare cases, IgA class rather than IgG class autoantibodies were found to target the type VII collagen, resulting in a clinical phenotype indistinguishable from the classic IgG-mediated disease. However, IgA-mediated disease has a lesser tendency to form scar and is more responsive to dapsone treatment.

Epidermolysis bullosa acquisita and inflammatory bowel disease. Raab B, Fretzin DF, Bronson DM, Scott MJ, Roenigk HH Jr, Medenica M. JAMA 1983; 250: 1746–8.

Inflammatory bowel disease, particularly Crohn's disease, is strongly associated with epidermolysis bullosa acquisita. All patients should be questioned for symptoms of inflammatory bowel disease. If symptoms are present, a comprehensive GI work-up is indicated.

The epidermolysis bullosa acquisita antigen (type VII collagen) is present in human colon and patients with Crohn's disease have autoantibodies to type VII collagen. Chen M, O'Toole EA, Sanghavi J, Mahmud N, Kelleher D, Weir D, et al. J Invest Dermatol 2002; 118: 1059–64.

The presence of type VII collagen in the gut and autoantibodies to type VII collagen in patients with inflammatory bowel disease without skin manifestations supports a link between the gut and the skin.

FIRST-LINE THERAPIES

▶ Systemic corticosteroids	D
▶ Azathioprine	D
▶ Dapsone	D

Epidermolysis bullosa acquisita – a pemphigoid-like disease. Gammon WR, Briggaman RA, Woodley DT, Heald PW, Wheeler CE Jr. J Am Acad Dermatol 1984; 11: 820–32.

Five patients with the generalized inflammatory subset of disease responded at least partially to prednisone (40–120 mg daily), with or without the addition of azathioprine 100 mg daily.

Bullous pemphigoid and epidermolysis bullosa acquisita: presentation, prognosis, and immunotherapy in 11 children. Edwards S, Wakelin SH, Wojnarowska F, Marsden RA, Kirtschig G, Bhogal B, et al. Pediatr Dermatol 1998; 15: 184–90.

A survey of five childhood-onset cases showed good clinical responses to combined corticosteroids and dapsone, as well as a good long-term prognosis.

Epidermolysis bullosa acquisita responsive to dapsone therapy. Hughes AP, Callen JP. J Cutan Med Surg 2001; 5: 397–9.

One patient who failed to respond to prednisone (40 mg daily) plus tetracycline and niacinamide achieved complete control of blistering activities after 2 months on dapsone 150 mg daily.

SECOND-LINE THERAPIES

▶ IVIG	D
▶ Colchicine	D
▶ Ciclosporin	D
▶ Extracorporeal photochemotherapy	D
▶ Anti-Tac monoclonal antibody	E
▶ Mycophenolate mofetil	E

Severe, refractory epidermolysis bullosa acquisita complicated by an oesophageal stricture responding to intravenous immune globulin. Harman KE, Whittam LR, Wakelin SH, Black MM. Br J Dermatol 1998; 139: 1126–7.

The patient had the non-inflammatory mechanobullous subset of disease and esophageal stricture, and was refractory to prednisone (up to 80 mg daily), dapsone (100 mg daily), cyclophosphamide (150 mg daily), and azathioprine (3 mg/kg daily). The patient was treated with courses of IVIG (0.4 g/kg daily) on 5 consecutive days at 4–6-week intervals as a monotherapy, resulting in a dramatic fall in the circulating titers of anti-basement membrane IgG autoantibodies, reduction of new blister formation, and disappearance of dysphagia. However, not all patients reported in the literature responded to this treatment. The major disadvantage of this regimen is the extremely high cost.

Colchicine for epidermolysis bullosa acquisita. Cunningham BB, Kirchmann TT, Woodley DT. J Am Acad Dermatol 1996; 34: 781–4.

Four patients with the non-inflammatory mechanobullous subset of disease, some refractory to prednisone treatment, were treated with oral colchicine (1–2 mg daily), with or without the addition of cyclophosphamide (50 mg daily). In all patients there was substantial clinical improvement in the reduction of skin fragility and spontaneous blister formation. An initial dose of 0.4–0.6 mg daily is recommended, with an increase by 0.6 mg daily each week until diarrhea develops. The patients are instructed to take the highest tolerable doses. Other than diarrhea, the long-term administration of colchicine (up to 4 years) was well tolerated. The side effect of diarrhea, however, makes it questionably suitable for those patients who have associated inflammatory bowel disease.

Oral cyclosporine in the treatment of inflammatory and noninflammatory cases. A clinical and immunopathologic analysis. Gupta AK, Ellis CN, Nickoloff BJ, Goldfarb MT, Ho VC, Rocher LL, et al. Arch Dermatol 1990; 126: 339–50.

Two patients with epidermolysis bullosa acquisita (subset not defined) were treated with oral ciclosporin (6 mg/kg daily) for a total of 8 weeks. These patients experienced a gradual reduction in the frequency of new blister and erosion formation. The known renal toxicity of ciclosporin makes it questionable as a suitable long-term regimen and warranted only as a last-resort measure.

Treatment of refractory epidermolysis bullosa acquisita with extracorporeal photochemotherapy. Gordon KB, Chan LS, Woodley DT. Br J Dermatol 1997; 136: 415–20.

Three patients with the non-inflammatory mechanobullous subset of disease, refractory to conventional therapy (prednisone, azathioprine) and colchicine, were treated with this immunomodulatory regimen. The patients were given an oral dose of 1–1.5 mg/kg of crystalline 8-methoxypsoralen 90 minutes prior to photopheresis treatment and underwent

Evidence Levels: **A** Double-blind study **B** Clinical trial ≥ 20 subjects **C** Clinical trial < 20 subjects **D** Series ≥ 5 subjects **E** Anecdotal case reports

a discontinuous leukophoresis. The leukocyte-enriched portion of blood was passed through a photo cassette, exposing it to 2 J/cm² of UVA over 3 hours. The patients underwent a total of six to seven cycles of treatment at 3-week intervals, with each cycle consisting of treatments on two consecutive days. All three patients had improvement by objective measurement of their disease activity (increased suction blister time – an indication of increased dermoepidermal adhesion strength, and reduced titers of anti-basement membrane autoantibodies by indirect immunofluorescence). Two of these patients had significant improvement by subjective measurement (reduced frequency of new blister formation and elimination of oral mucosal lesions) during the course of treatment, and continued to improve over the 6 months following the treatment period. All patients tolerated the procedure well and none stopped because of side effects. One patient required antiemetics for nausea due to oral 8-methoxypsoralen. One patient required inhaled bronchodilator therapy for worsening of chronic obstructive pulmonary disease immediately after therapy.

The practical use of this regimen is somewhat limited by the availability of photopheresis and the high cost.

Treatment of epidermolysis bullosa acquisita with the humanized anti-Tac mAb daclizumab. Egan CA, Brown M, White JD, Yancey KB. Clin Immunol 2001; 101: 146–51.

Humanized monoclonal antibody to Tac, a fragment of IL-2 receptor (CD25) of activated T cells, at a dose of 1 mg/kg (six to 12 intravenous treatments at 2–4-week intervals), has shown effectiveness as a corticosteroid-sparing agent in one of three patients, without complications. Two other patients treated with the same medication did not have observable clinical improvement, though there was a substantial reduction in CD25+ T cells.

Mycophenolate mofetil in epidermolysis bullosa acquisita. Kowalzick L, Suckow S, Zuiegler H, Waldmann T, Pönnighaus JM, Gläser V. Dermatology 2003; 207: 332–4.

Mycophenolate mofetil (1 g twice daily) was used successfully in conjunction with plasmapheresis as a corticosteroid-sparing agent in one patient with epidermolysis bullosa acquisita not controlled by azathioprine (150 mg daily) and prednisolone (60 mg daily). The clinical improvement was associated with a reduction in autoantibody titers.

Childhood IgA-mediated epidermolysis bullosa acquisita responding to mycophenolate mofetil as a corticosteroid-sparing agent. Tran MM, Anhalt GJ, Barrett T, Cohen BA. J Am Acad Dermatol 2006; 54: 734–6.

Mycophenolate mofetil (700 mg/day) was added to the regimen of prednisolone (25 mg/day) and dapsone (25 mg/day) when the disease flared upon reduction of prednisolone dose in this 2-year-old patient affected by an IgA-mediated epidermolysis bullosa acquisita. With the addition of mycophenolate mofetil, the systemic corticosteroid was totally tapered off over a 9-month period. This case illustrates the usefulness of mycophenolate mofetil in childhood-onset disease.

THIRD-LINE THERAPIES

► Anti-CD20 antibody (Rituximab)   **D/E**

Successful adjuvant treatment of recalcitrant epidermolysis bullosa acquisita with anti-CD20 antibody rituximab.

Schmidt E, Benoit S, Brocker E-B, Zillikens D, Goebeler M. Arch Dermatol 2006; 142: 147–50.

The patient, who had both skin and oral mucosae involvement, was not controlled with prednisolone (up to 250 mg/day), dapsone (150 mg/day), and subsequently azathioprine (up to 175 mg/day), and colchicine (2.5 mg/day). The regimen was changed to rituximab 700 mg weekly infusion (375 mg/m² body surface area) for 4 consecutive weeks, with continuous use of azathioprine (175 mg/day) and colchicine (2.5 mg/day) and reducing doses of prednisolone. The patient's lesions completely healed in 11 weeks post rituximab infusion, allowing the tapering of systemic steroid, colchicine, and azathioprine. Fourteen weeks after the discontinuation of colchicine and prednisolone, the patient remained in clinical remission. No complication was reported except an event of deep vein thrombosis.

A successful therapeutic trial of rituximab in the treatment of a patient with recalcitrant, high-titre epidermolysis bullosa acquisita. Crichlow SM, Mortimer NJ, Harman KE. Br J Dermatol 2006; 156: 194–6.

A patient who has both oral mucosal and skin lesions and a high titer of IgG autoantibodies to skin basement membrane zone (indirect immunofluorescence titer up to 1:3200) was treated with conventional therapeutic agents (prednisolone up to 60 mg/day, mycophenolate mofetil 2 g/day, and subsequently IVIG infusions (2 g/kg body weight/month) without much success. Moreover, the patient could not tolerate azathioprine (due to liver toxicity) or ciclosporin (owing to nephrotoxicity and hypertension). In the mean time, the patient's conditions were worsening, with increasing autoantibody titer and involvement of the esophagus. Therefore, weekly rituximab infusions (375 mg/m² body surface area) were then given to the patient along with mycophenolate mofetil (2 g/day) and prednisolone (30 mg/day). The patient had slow but progressive improvement of the lesions and all were healed 5 months after starting rituximab. One year after the rituximab treatment the patient was still in partial remission, suffering only occasional trauma-induced blisters, and the autoantibody titer fell to 1:10.

Epidermolysis bullosa acquisita following bullous pemphigoid, successfully treated with anti-CD20 monoclonal antibody rituximab. Wallet-Faber N, Franck N, Matteux F, Mateus C, Gilbert D, Carlotti A, et al. Dermatology 2007; 215: 252–5.

An interesting patient who initially developed bullous pemphigoid, but who upon subsequent flare manifested a generalized skin and mucosal (oral and genital) blistering disease that was confirmed as epidermolysis bullosa acquisita by target antigen identification. The initial success of treatment (combined prednisone 1.5 mg/kg/day and azathioprine 100 ng/day) did not last long as the reduction of prednisone resulted in rapid worsening of the condition, further complicated by a life-threatening *Legionella pneumonophila* pneumonia infection. Furthermore, the patient could not tolerate mycophenolate mofetil. Therefore, rituximab (375 mg/m² body surface area) was initiated on a weekly interval for 4 consecutive weeks, resulting in dramatic improvement of the patient's condition. At 10 months' follow-up post rituximab initiation the patient had only a few visible blisters.

Treatment-resistant classical epidermolysis bullosa acquisita responding to rituximab. Sadler E, Schafleitner B, Lanschuetzer C, Laimer M, Pohla-Gubo G, Hametner R, et al. Br J Dermatol 2007; 157: 417–19.

A patient who has both skin and multiple mucosal (oral, esophageal, and laryngeal) lesions and failed to respond to multiple conventional immunosuppressive medications subsequently responded to rituximab. Over a 6-year period the patient failed to show complete clinical response to methylprednisolone (up to 5 mg/kg/day), azathioprine (up to 2.5 mg/kg body weight), ciclosporin (up to 9 mg/kg body weight/day), mycophenolate mofetil (up to 30 mg/kg/day), cyclophosphamide (500 mg/m² body surface area IV, followed by 1 mg/kg/day orally), colchicine (up to 1.5 mg/day), IVIG (up to 2.5 g/kg body weight/cycle), gold (1 mg/kg/week IV, followed by IM and oral preparations); daclizumab (1 mg/kg body weight, six infusions over 3 weeks). Therefore, the a regimen of reduced dose of rituximab (144 mg/m² infusion per week for 5 weeks) along with azathioprine (2 mg/kg body weight/day) was given; the patient tolerated the treatment without any side effects or infections. A remarkable improvement was noticed 4 weeks after the initiation of rituximab treatment, and all medications were subsequently discontinued. Two years after all medications were tapered off, the patient's disease activity remained at a very low level.

Clinical response of severe mechanobullous epidermolysis bullosa acquisita to combined treatment with immunoadsorption and rituximab (anti-CD20 monoclonal antibodies). Niedermeier A, Eming R, Pfutze M, Neumann CR, Happel C, Reich K, et al. Arch Dermatol 2007; 143: 192–8.

Two patients affected by the mechanobullous type of epidermolysis bullosa acquisita were treated with combined immunoadsorption (daily treatment for 8 consecutive days) and rituximab (375 mg/m² body surface area/week for total of 4 weeks). Mycophenolate mofetil (1–3 g/day) was given continuously during this period. In both patients treatment with multiple medications, including ciclosporin, azathioprine, dapsone, dexamethasone pulse, and cyclophosphamide pulse, was unsuccessful. One patient achieved near complete clinical resolution, but the other could only obtain stable disease status. This report illustrates the treatment-resistant nature of this disease.

Treatment of pemphigus vulgaris with rituximab and intravenous immune globulin. Ahmed R, Spigelman Z, Cavacini LA, Posner MR. N Engl J Med 2006; 355: 1772–9.

In this largest series of autoimmune blistering skin disease rituximab study, 11 patients affected by pemphigus vulgaris were treated with a combined regimen of rituximab and IVIG (three weekly cycles of rituximab at 375 mg/m² body surface area, followed by a dose of IVIG (2 g/kg body weight), then by four monthly cycles of (one dose rituximab and one dose of IVIG). Nine patients had rapid clearing of lesions and were subsequently in remission lasting from 22 to 37 months, and all other immunosuppressants were tapered off before the ending of rituximab treatment. No complication or infection was reported.

Although this study was not conducted for epidermolysis bullosa acquisita, it seems that combined rituximab and IVIG would give the best clinical outcomes: high remission rate and low complication rate. The high cost could be a prohibitive factor.

Erythema annulare centrifugum

Linda Y Hwang, Julia E Haimowitz

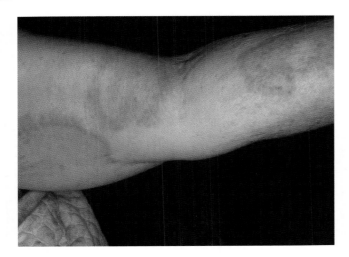

Erythema annulare centrifugum (EAC) is a gyrate erythema characterized by minimally pruritic, polycyclic, erythematous patches or plaques that may expand up to 2–3 mm/day and clear centrally. There are two forms; the more common superficial form has trailing scale at the inner borders of the erythema, whereas the deep form has erythematous induration without scale. EAC may persist for decades, with a mean duration of 2.8 years, and treatment is often difficult.

MANAGEMENT STRATEGY

EAC represents a hypersensitivity reaction to any of myriad conditions; therefore, a search for and treatment of an underlying disease is the primary management strategy. Often, an underlying cause is not found.

Concurrent infection is the most common underlying association. Fungal, bacterial, viral, mycobacterial, and parasitic pathogens have been reported. Typically, the infection is cutaneous and separate from the EAC eruption. Dermatophytosis is implicated in up to 48% of EAC patients. Thus, the skin, especially the feet, groin, and nails, should be carefully examined for tinea. Anecdotal reports of other associated skin infections include molluscum contagiosum, herpes virus infection, and *Phthirus pubis* infestation. Less commonly the infection is internal, and intestinal *Giardia* or *Candida*, latent Epstein–Barr virus infection, human immunodeficiency virus (HIV), chronic viral hepatitis, appendicitis, urinary tract *Escherichia coli*, and nematode infestations have been reported. Although EAC is typically associated with an active infection, it has also been reported to occur after reactivation of herpes zoster virus, in corresponding dermatomes.

EAC may be associated with either benign or malignant hematologic and solid neoplasms. This paraneoplastic phenomenon is thought to result from hypersensitivity to tumor proteins released by these neoplasms. However, in the absence of strong clinical suspicion, an extensive search for malignancy is not recommended. Should neoplasia be identified, EAC activity correlates with tumor response to treatment.

Ingested agents, especially medications, may be associated with EAC. Anecdotal reports of medications include acetazolamide, amitriptyline, ampicillin, cimetidine, cyclopenthiazide, co-trimoxazole, etizolam, finasteride, gold, hydrochlorothiazide, ibuprofen, iron, neutradonna (aluminum silicate and belladonna), oxprenolol, piroxicam, salicylates, spironolactone, thiacetazone, chloroquine, and hydroxychloroquine. Early reports of antimalarials as a cause of EAC may be debated: what was considered EAC in these reports may actually have been unrecognized forms of subacute cutaneous lupus erythematosus. EAC may also be caused by hypersensitivity to other ingested agents, such as blue cheese *Penicillium*.

Other conditions associated with EAC include thyroid disease, liver disease, hypereosinophilic syndrome, sarcoidosis, surgical trauma, linear IgA dermatosis, and autoimmune disease such as relapsing polychondritis, rheumatoid arthritis, and polyglandular autoimmune disease. EAC may also be seen with pregnancy and with hormonal fluctuations due to menstruation. One form of EAC, described as autoimmune progesterone dermatitis, can be reproduced by intradermal and patch testing to progesterone and may involve Th1-type cytokines. Another form of EAC may occur annually and seasonally over 2–40 years, and may be associated with hereditary lactate dehydrogenase deficiency. EAC may even be familial: there has been one report involving identical twins. Rarely, EAC may be a form of contact dermatitis: there is a single report of contact-induced EAC attributed to a hypersensitivity reaction from topical nickel and cobalt exposure.

Once the underlying condition is treated, EAC usually resolves. Frequently, however, the cause is elusive, and treatment becomes empiric and temporizing. Spontaneous remission is also possible, making assessments of therapy difficult. Topical steroids may provide symptomatic relief and may improve its appearance. In one report of EAC with unknown etiology, all lesions cleared with topical calcipotriol treatment. Topical tacrolimus can be helpful as well. In another case, EAC remitted after the patient was treated with oral metronidazole given for rosacea. A trial of empiric antimicrobials may be helpful to eradicate an underlying, clinically undetected infection. If these more conservative treatments fail, the patient's perceived need for treatment should be reassessed. Stronger treatments may be more harmful than the condition itself. Systemic glucocorticoids can usually suppress EAC, but it commonly recurs after the course is completed. If EAC is very disabling to the patient, other systemic immunomodulators may need to be considered. One patient responded very well to etanercept therapy.

EAC should be distinguished from the following clinical mimickers: tinea corporis, granuloma annulare, sarcoidosis, mycosis fungoides, psoriasis, pityriasis rosea, tinea versicolor, cutaneous lupus, annular erythema of Sjögren's syndrome, granuloma faciale, necrolytic migratory erythema, bullous pemphigoid, secondary syphilis, Hansen's disease, annular urticarial and fixed drug reactions, hypereosinophilic dermatitis, annular erythema of infancy, and other reactive erythemas such as erythema multiforme, erythema gyratum repens, erythema migrans, and erythema marginatum. Such clinical possibilities are ruled out by routine histologic examination.

SPECIFIC INVESTIGATIONS

> ▶ Punch biopsy for histologic examination
>   ▶ superficial type: focal spongiosis, superficial perivascular lymphocytic infiltrate
>   ▶ deep type: superficial and deep perivascular lymphohistiocytic infiltrate
> ▶ Full skin examination for potential skin infections
> ▶ KOH or culture of suspected EAC lesion and site of potential dermatophyte infection
> ▶ Intradermal trichophyton or candidal skin injection and tuberculin test to test for underlying infection
> ▶ Systemic work-up: CBC, LFTs, UA, CXR initial screen; if warranted, ANA, TSH, HIV, malignancy work-up including SPEP

Gyrate erythema. White JW Jr. Dermatol Clin 1985; 3: 129–39.

Allergic confirmation that some cases of erythema annulare centrifugum are dermatophytids. Jillson OF. Arch Dermatol Syphilol 1954; 70: 54–8.

Erythema annulare centrifugum and intestinal *Candida albicans* infection – coincidence or connection? [letter] Schmid MH, Wollenber A, Sander CA, Beiber T. Acta Dermatol Venereol 1997; 77: 93–4.

Intradermal trichophyton and candidal skin injection tests may demonstrate a local cutaneous hypersensitivity. These tests may help confirm this reaction pattern and support a trial of empiric antifungals despite an inability to locate the site of a pathogen.

Erythema annulare centrifugum: a review of 24 cases with special reference to its association with underlying disease. Mahood JM. Clin Exp Dermatol 1983; 8: 383–7.

A basic work-up for internal disease may include a complete blood cell count, liver function tests, urinalysis, and chest radiograph.

Erythema annulare centrifugum: results of a clinicopathologic study of 73 patients. Weyers W, Diaz-Cascajo C, Weyers I. Am J Dermatopathol 2003; 25: 451–62.

Clinicopathologic analysis of 66 cases of erythema annulare centrifugum. Kim KJ, Chang SE, Choi JH, Sng KJ, Moon KC, Koh JK. J Dermatol 2002; 29: 61–7.

Erythema annulare centrifugum induced by molluscum contagiosum. Furue M, Akasu R, Ohtake N, Tamaki K. Br J Dermatol 1993; 129: 646–7.

Erythema annular centrifugum in a HIV-positive patient. Gonzalez-Vela MC, Gonzalez-Lopez MA, Val-Bernal JF, Echevarria S, Arce F, Fernandez-Llaca H. Int J Dermatol 2006; 45: 1423–5.

Erythema annulare centrifugum induced by generalized *Phthirus pubis* infestation. Bessis D, Chraibi H, Guillot B, Guilhou J. Br J Dermatol 2003; 149: 1291.

Erythema annulare centrifugum. A case due to tuberculosis. Burkhart CG. Int J Dermatol 1982; 21: 538–9.

Recurrent acute appendicitis with erythema annulare centrifugum. Sack DM, Carle G, Shama SK. Arch Intern Med 1984; 144: 2090–2.

Erythema annulare centrifugum and *Escherichia coli* urinary infection. Borbujo J, de Miguel C, Lopez A, de Lucas R, Casado M. Lancet 1996; 347: 897–8.

Erythema annulare centrifugum associated with ascariasis. Hendricks AA, Lu C, Elfenbein GJ, Hussain R. Arch Dermatol 1981; 117: 582–5.

Erythema annulare centrifugum following herpes zoster infection: Wolf's isotopic response? Lee HW, Lee DK, Rhee DY, Chang SE, Choi JH, Moon KC, et al. Br J Dermatol 2005; 153: 1241–3.

Erythema annulare centrifugum as the presenting sign of Hodgkin's disease. Yaniv R, Shpielberg O, Shpiro D, Feinstein A, Ben-Bassat I. Int J Dermatol 1993; 32: 59–60.

Erythema annulare centrifugum associated with liver disease. Tsuji T, Kadoya A. Arch Dermatol 1986; 122: 1239–40.

Erythema annulare centrifugum and Graves' disease. Braunstein BL. Arch Dermatol 1982; 118: 623.

Erythema annulare centrifugum with autoimmune hepatitis. Gulati S, Mathur P, Saini D, Mannan R, Kalra V. Indian J Pediatr 2004; 71: 541–2.

Erythema annulare centrifugum as the presenting sign of the hypereosinophilic syndrome: observations on therapy. Shelley WB, Shelley ED. Cutis 1985; 35: 53–5.

Sarcoidosis presenting as erythema annulare centrifugum. Altomare GF, Capella GL, Frigerio E. Clin Exp Dermatol 1995; 20: 502–3.

Erythema annulare centrifugum following pancreaticobiliary surgery. Thami GP, Sachdeva A, Kaur S, Mohan H, Kanwar AJ. J Dermatol 2002; 29: 347–9.

Linear IgA dermatosis presenting with erythema annulare centrifugum lesions: report of three cases in adults. J Eur Acad Dermatol Venereol 2000; 15: 167–70.

Erythema annulare centrifugum and relapsing polychondritis. Dippel E, Orfanos CE, Zouboulis C. Ann Dermatol Venereol 2000; 127: 735–9.

Erythema annulare centrifugum in a patient with polyglandular autoimmune disease type 1. Garty B. Cutis 1998; 62: 231–2.

Erythema annulare centrifugum associated with pregnancy. Choonhakarn C, Seramethakun P. Acta Dermatol Venereol 1998; 78: 237–8.

Autoimmune progesterone dermatitis manifested as erythema annulare centrifugum: Confirmation of progesterone sensitivity by in vitro interferon-gamma release. Halevy S, Cohen AD, Lunenfeld E, Grossman N. J Am Acad Dermatol 2002; 47: 311–13.

Annually recurring erythema annulare centrifugum: a distinct entity? Garcia Muret MP, Pujol RM, Gimenez-arnau AM, Barranco C, Gallardo F, Alomar A. J Am Acad Dermatol 2006; 54: 1091–5.

Contact erythema annulare centrifugum. Sambucety PS, Agapito PG, Preto MAR. Contact Dermatitis 2006; 55: 309–10.

FIRST-LINE THERAPIES

> ▶ Treatment of underlying condition E
> ▶ Discontinue potential causative medications E
> ▶ Topical corticosteroids E

Erythema annulare centrifugum and Hodgkin's disease: association with disease activity. Arch Intern Med 1979; 139: 486–7.

Erythema annulare centrifugum associated with piroxicam. Hogan DJ, Blocka KLN. J Am Acad Dermatol 1985; 13: 840–1.

Erythema annulare centrifugum caused by aldactone. Carsuzaa F, Pierre C, Dubegny M. Ann Dermatol Venereol 1987; 114: 375–6 (in French.)

Ampicillin-induced erythema annulare centrifugum. Gupta HL, Sapra SM. J Indian Med Assoc 1975; 65: 307–8.

Etizolam-induced superficial erythema annulare centrifugum. Kuroda K, Yabunami H, Hisanaga Y. Clin Exp Dermatol 2002; 27: 34–6.

Amitriptyline-induced erythema annulare centrifugum. Garcia-Doval I, Peteiro C, Toribio J. Cutis 1999; 63: 35–6.

Erythema annulare cetrifugum secondary to treatment with finasteride. Al Hammadi A, Asai Y, Patt MI, Sasseville D. J Drugs Dermatol 2007; 6: 460–3.

Erythema annulare centrifugum associated with gold sodium thiomalate therapy. Tsuji T, Nishimura M, Kimura S. J Am Acad Dermatol 1992; 27: 284–7.

Erythema annulare centrifugum: an unusual case due to hydroxychloroquine sulfate. Hudson LD. Cutis 1985; 36: 129–30.

Erythema annulare centrifugum due to hydroxychloroquine sulfate and chloroquine sulfate. Ashurst PJ. Arch Dermatol 1967; 95: 37–9.

Erythema annulare centrifugum associated with piroxicam. Hogan DJ, Blocka KL. J Am Acad Dermatol 1985; 13: 840–1.

Erythema annulare centrifugum. A case due to hypersensitivity to blue cheese Penicillium. Shelley WB. Arch Dermatol 1964; 90: 54–8.

SECOND-LINE THERAPIES

> ▶ Empiric antimicrobials E
> ▶ Topical or systemic antipruritics E
> ▶ Topical tacrolimus E

Annular erythema responding to tacrolimus ointment. Rao NG, Pariser RJ. J Drugs Dermatol 2003; 2: 421–4.

Two patients with annular erythema of unclear etiology treated selected lesions with topical tacrolimus 0.1% ointment twice daily. Those lesions that were treated resolved within 2–6 weeks, whereas other untreated lesions did not respond until they too were treated with tacrolimus.

This suggests that tacrolimus, and not spontaneous remission, was responsible for the improvement.

THIRD-LINE THERAPIES

> ▶ Systemic corticosteroids E
> ▶ Immunomodulatory agents E
> ▶ Topical calcipotriol E
> ▶ Metronidazole E

Erythema annulare centrifugum. Seidel DR, Burgdorf WHC. In: Demis DJ, et al., eds. Clinical dermatology. Philadelphia: Lippincott Williams & Wilkins, 1999; Ch 7–5, p 1–4.

Calcipotriol for erythema annulare centrifugum. Gnaiadecki R. Br J Dermatol 2002; 146: 317–19.

A 73-year-old woman had EAC of unknown cause that was resistant to topical and systemic steroids, antifungals, and PUVA treatment. It cleared completely after 3 months of topical, once-daily calcipotriol.

Erythema annulare centrifugum successfully treated with metronidazole. De Aloe G, Rubegni P, Risulo M, Sbano P, Poggiali S, Fimiani M. Clin Exp Dermatol 2005; 30: 583–4.

A 38-year-old man with EAC failed oral antibiotics and antifungals, and topical calcipotriol. Only systemic steroids provided temporary improvement of his skin lesions. Because the patient had rosacea, oral metronidazole 400 mg daily was prescribed for 6 weeks, with resolution of EAC.

A novel therapeutic approach to erythema annulare centrifugum. Minni J, Sarro R. J Am Acad Dermatol 2006; 54: S134–5.

In a personal communication, one patient with extensive erythema annulare centrifugum was reported to clear with etanercept 25 mg twice weekly injections. After 4 weeks of treatment the patient was 95% clear, and complete remission was achieved after continued therapy. After 6 months the treatment was discontinued and EAC recurred. The lesions responded again to a repeat treatment regimen.

Erythema dyschromicum perstans

Christine Soon, John Berth-Jones

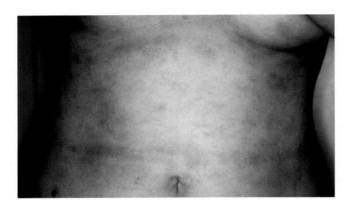

Erythema dyschronicum perstans (EDP) is an acquired, generalized dermal hypermelanosis of unknown etiology. Clinically it presents as asymptomatic, ashen-gray-blue macules of varying sizes, most commonly on the trunk and proximal extremities. Variable components include erythema and papulation. It has been reported most frequently in dark-skinned Latin-American people, although all racial groups can be affected. EDP has similarities to lichen planus pigmentosus and the 'ashy dermatosis' of Ramirez, although the precise relationship of these conditions has yet to be established.

MANAGEMENT STRATEGY

No controlled trials have been reported. Although EDP may persist for many years, there have been reports of spontaneous resolution. *Camouflage creams* can be prescribed for cosmetic purposes. The treatments discussed below have also been tried, with varying success. Treatments that are reportedly ineffective include sun protection, peeling lotions, antibiotics, topical hydroquinone, topical corticosteroid therapy, antimalarials, and griseofulvin.

SPECIFIC INVESTIGATIONS

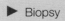 Biopsy

There is vacuolar degeneration of the basal layer associated with pigmentary incontinence. Dermal vessels are surrounded with an infiltrate of lymphocytes and histiocytes, and there are many melanophages present.

EDP may need to be differentiated from the late stage of pinta. Dark-field examination and serological tests for syphilis should be carried out to exclude this treponematosis in suspected cases.

Idiopathic eruptive macular pigmentation is a similar condition. Histology demonstrates that the pigment is located in the basal layer of the epidermis, and the lichenoid inflammation characteristic of EDP is not present.

THERAPY

▶ No therapy	D
▶ Vitamin A	D
▶ Dapsone 100 mg/day for 3 months	E
▶ Oral corticosteroid therapy	E
▶ Clofazimine 100 mg/day for 3 months	D

Erythema dyschromicum perstans. A follow-up study from Northern Finland. Palatsi R. Dermatologica 1977; 155: 40–4.

A series of four patients were followed up for 2 years. Three of the four showed spontaneous resolution.

Vitamin A in the treatment of lichen planus pigmentosus. Bhutani LK. Br J Dermatol 1979; 100: 473–4.

Lichen planus pigmentosus is considered by some to be the same entity as EDP. Vitamin A was prescribed in pulses of 100 000 units daily for 15 days. Up to 10 such pulses were given. Of the 140 patients, 28 showed a 'good' to 'excellent' response (50–100% clearance).

Erythema dyschromicum perstans: response to dapsone therapy. Kontochristopoulos G, Stavropoulos P, Panteleos D, Aroni K. Int J Dermatol 1998; 37: 796–8.

Two cases of EDP responded to dapsone 100 mg daily. The duration of therapy ranged from 8 to 12 weeks.

Erythema dyschromicum perstans: a case report and review. Osswald SS, Proffer LH, Sartori CR. Cutis 2001; 68: 25–8.

One case of EDP with active inflammatory areas responded to 3 weeks of oral corticosteroid therapy. The authors do not state the dose.

Involvement of cell adhesion and activation molecules in the pathogenesis of erythema dyschromicum perstans (ashy dermatitis). The effect of clofazimine therapy. Baranda L, Torres-Alvarez B, Cortes-Franco R, Moncada B, Potales-Perez DP, Gonzalez-Amaro R. Arch Dermatol 1997; 133: 325–9.

This was a prospective clinical and immunohistochemical study indicating that clofazimine reduces the inflammatory response in erythema dyschromicum perstans. Four out of six patients treated with clofazimine 100 mg/day showed marked improvement after 3 months of treatment.

Evedence Levels: A Double-blind study B Clinical trial ≥ 20 subjects C Clinical trial < 20 subjects D Series ≥ 5 subjects E Anecdotal case reports

Erythema elevatum diutinum

Emma C Benton, Ian Coulson

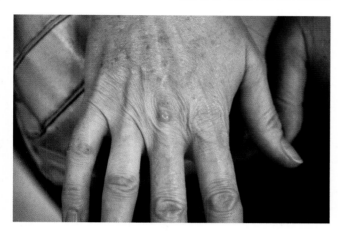

Erythema elevatum diutinum (EED) is a rare neutrophilic dermatosis consisting of violaceous, brown, or red papules, plaques and nodules over the extensor surfaces of the joints and buttocks. Cases have a female preponderance and there is a peak onset in the sixth decade, with a smaller peak in childhood. EED is thought to be a form of immune complex-mediated vasculitis, although its etiology remains unclear. Infections (including HIV and streptococcal), hematologic abnormalities, autoimmune diseases, and other conditions have been associated.

MANAGEMENT STRATEGY

EED is a chronic disease; there are only a few well-documented instances of spontaneous long-term resolution.

Dapsone 100 mg daily remains the initial treatment of choice. The response may be partial and dose dependent.

Corticosteroids have also been effective in patients with EED. Topical betamethasone and topical fluocinolone have been used under occlusion with good effect. In other patients both intralesional and systemic corticosteroids (prednisolone 30–40 mg daily) have produced favorable responses.

Sulfonamides (sulfamethoxypyridazine 500 mg once daily and sulfapyridine 0.5–1g three times daily), *nicotinamide* 100 mg three times daily, *colchicine* 0.5 mg twice daily with 0.5 mg three times daily for 3–4 days to abate minor disease flares, and *chloroquine* 300 mg daily have produced resolution of lesions.

EED has been reported in association with diseases such as HIV, hematological disorders, inflammatory bowel disease, celiac disease, and ophthalmic disorders (peripheral keratitis), and evidence of these should be sought. In these patients treatment of the associated condition has been reported as beneficial to EED resolution. There are case reports suggesting that EED may be associated with the following drug treatments: interferon-β, erythropoietin, antituberculosis chemotherapy, and cisplatin.

SPECIFIC INVESTIGATIONS

- ▶ Full blood count
- ▶ Immunoglobulins and serum electrophoresis/ immunofixation electrophoresis
- ▶ Antineutrophil cytoplasmic antibodies (ANCAs)
- ▶ Antireticulin and antigliadin antibodies
- ▶ HIV risk factors enquiry
- ▶ Histology

Erythema elevatum diutinum: a clinical and histopathologic study of 13 patients. Yiannias JA, El-Azhary RA, Gibson LE. J Am Acad Dermatol 1992; 26: 38–44.

Of 13 patients with EED, six had associated hematologic abnormalities, with IgA monoclonal gammopathy occurring most frequently.

Erythema elevatum diutinum and IgA paraproteinaemia: 'a preclinical iceberg'. Chowdhury M, Inaloz HS, Motley RJ, Knight AG. Int J Dermatol 2002; 41: 368–70.

The technique of immunofixation electrophoresis is more sensitive than immunoelectrophoresis and uses a combination of zone electrophoresis and immunoprecipitation with specific antisera to detect monoclonal immunoglobulins or light chains at very low concentrations in serum and urine. This is useful in EED because patients may have associated paraproteinemias, which in some cases may undergo malignant transformation.

The authors note that in monoclonal disorders there is extensive asymptomatic tumor proliferation and possible malignant transformation in 20% of patients during long-term follow-up. It was recommended that there should be lengthy follow-up and monitoring for patients with both EED and IgA paraproteinemia because of the risk of progression to IgA myeloma.

Antineutrophil cytoplasmic antibodies of IgA class in neutrophilic dermatoses with emphasis on erythema elevatum diutinum. Ayoub N, Charuel JL, Diemert MC, Barete S, André M, Fermand JP, et al. Arch Dermatol 2004; 140: 931–6.

In a study to evaluate the prevalence of ANCAs in EED, IgA ANCAs were present in all patients with EED (n=10). It was therefore suggested that ANCAs (particularly IgA class) may be useful.

Erythema elevatum diutinum in association with coeliac disease. Tasanen K, Raudasoja R, Kallioinen M, Ranki A. Br J Dermatol 1997; 136: 624–7.

Following the appearance of EED lesions antireticulin and antigliadin antibodies were detected.

Erythema elevatum diutinum and HIV infection: a report of five cases. Muratori S, Carrera C, Gorani A, Alessi E. Br J Dermatol 1999; 141: 335–8.

The largest case series of patients with EED and HIV infection, bringing the total number of reported cases of EED in people with HIV infection to 16. Streptococcal infection seemed to trigger exacerbations in four of five patients. EED can simulate Kaposi's sarcoma and bacillary angiomatosis, which may be particularly confusing in the context of an HIV-seropositive patient. Histopathological confirmation of the diagnosis is therefore advocated.

Erythema elevatum diutinum: clinical, histopathologic, and immunohistochemical characteristics of six patients. Wahl CE, Bouldin MB, Gibson LE. Am J Dermatopathol 2005; 27: 397–400.

The vascular endothelium of EED stains positive for CD31, CD34, VEGF, and factor VIIIa and negative for factor XIIIa, TGFB, and LANA. This pattern does not distinguish it from similar-appearing lesions. Therefore, the chronic and recurrent nature of EED is the primary means of distinguishing it from entities that are clinically and histologically similar.

Erythema elevatum diutinum: an ultrastructural case study. Lee AY, Nakagawa H, Nogita T, Ishibashi Y. J Cutan Pathol 1989; 16: 211–17.

An electron microscopic study of a patient with EED demonstrating that the characteristic histopathologic changes in early lesions include leukocytoclastic vasculitis and a massive dermal infiltrate of neutrophils, histiocytes/macrophages, and Langerhans' cells. In late lesions the inflammatory infiltrate is replaced by fibrosis, with a dermal infiltrate of lymphocytes, histiocytes/macrophages, and Langerhans' cells.

FIRST-LINE THERAPIES

▶ Dapsone	D
▶ Dapsone plus antiretroviral in HIV-associated disease	E
▶ Corticosteroids	D

Erythema elevatum diutinum: a clinicopathological study. Wilkinson SM, English JS, Smith NP, Wilson-Jones E, Winkelmann RK. Clin Exp Dermatol 1992; 17: 87–93.

Dapsone 100 mg daily was the most effective therapy in this series of 13 patients with EED. Responses were often partial and dose dependent. Other effective treatments included sulfa drugs, corticosteroids, and chloroquine.

Dapsone may be ineffective once nodules appear; treatment of associated concomitant conditions is often beneficial to EED outcome.

Nodular erythema elevatum diutinum in an HIV-1 infected woman: response to dapsone and antiretroviral therapy. [Letter] Suarez J, Miguelez M, Villalba R. Br J Dermatol 1998; 138: 706–7.

Report of a 37-year-old woman with HIV-1 infection and EED whose lesions completely resolved over 3 weeks after treatment with oral antiretroviral therapy and oral dapsone 100 mg once daily. Over 2 months her CD4 count increased and her serum P24 antigen levels diminished. The authors concluded that the therapeutic approach to patients with EED associated with HIV infection should focus on reducing circulating P24 antigen with adequate antiretroviral therapy in addition to conventional dapsone treatment.

Nodular lesions of erythema elevatum diutinum in patients infected with the human immunodeficiency virus. LeBoit PE, Cockerell CJ. J Am Acad Dermatol 1993; 28: 919–22.

A clinicopathologic study of four patients with HIV infection who had unusual nodular lesions of EED. None of the patients responded to treatment with oral dapsone, and the authors commented that this observed lack of response may reflect the preponderance of fibrosis rather than neutrophils in these advanced lesions.

Erythema elevatum diutinum with primary Sjögren syndrome associated with IgA antineutrophil cytoplasmic antibody. Shimizu S, Nakamura Y, Togawa Y, Kamada N, Kambe N, Matsue H. Br J Dermatol 2008; 159: 733–5.

Report of a 64-year-old woman with EED and Sjögren's syndrome. Administration of oral dapsone for 1 month resolved her symptoms.

Peripheral keratitis associated with erythema elevatum diutinum. Aldave AJ, Shih JL, Jovkar S, McLeod SD. Am J Ophthalmol 2003; 135: 389–90.

Report of a 25-year-old with EED who was diagnosed 15 months later with an inflammatory peripheral keratitis of the left eye. The sclerokeratitis was thought to represent an ocular extension of the patient's cutaneous vasculitis. Dapsone therapy was initiated and resulted in rapid resolution of both the cutaneous and ocular inflammation.

Although dapsone is recommended as first-line treatment for EED its use has been based solely on multiple anecdotal reports and small case series, rather than on blinded controlled clinical trials.

SECOND-LINE THERAPIES

▶ Other sulfonamides	D
▶ Chloroquine	D
▶ Nicotinamide and tetracycline	E
▶ Colchicine	E

Erythema elevatum diutinum treated with niacinamide and tetracycline. Kohler IK, Lorinez AL. Arch Dermatol 1980; 116: 693–5.

Case report of a 60-year-old woman with EED which cleared completely following 4 weeks of treatment with oral nicotinamide 100 mg three times daily and oral tetracycline hydrochloride 250 mg four times daily. Following this, oral nicotinamide alone was sufficient for disease suppression, although recurrent lesions were apparent on cessation of therapy.

Erythema elevatum diutinum – a case successfully treated with colchicine. Henriksson R, Hofer PA, Hornqvist R. Clin Exp Dermatol 1989; 14: 451–3.

A case report of a 68-year-old man with EED refractory to treatment with oral dapsone who responded well to treatment with colchicine 0.5 mg twice daily over 6 weeks. Disease flares were noted on stopping colchicine, which was maintained at a dose of 0.5 mg twice daily. Minor flares were abated by temporarily increasing colchicine to 0.5 mg three times daily for 3–4 days without provoking diarrhea.

THIRD-LINE THERAPIES

▶ Gluten-free diet	E
▶ Cyclophosphamide	E
▶ Plasma exchange	E
▶ Reduction in ciclosporin dose	E
▶ Colectomy	E
▶ Transdermal nicotine patches	E
▶ Methyl prednisolone	E

Erythema elevatum diutinum in association with coeliac disease. Tasanen K, Raudasoja R, Kallioinen M, Ranki A. Br J Dermatol 1997; 136: 624–7.

This case report describes a 47-year-old woman who presented with clinically and histologically typical EED in whom previously undiagnosed celiac disease was found. Treatment with dapsone was partially effective, but complete healing of the EED lesions was achieved only after the introduction of a strict gluten-free diet. Maintenance treatment with a gluten-free diet only was required.

Erythema elevatum diutinum in a patient with relapsing polychondritis. Bernard P, Bedane C, Delrous JL, Catanzano G, Bonnetblanc JM. J Am Acad Dermatol 1992; 26: 312–15.

A 69-year-old man with a history of relapsing polychondritis developed EED, which responded to treatment with oral cyclophosphamide 100 mg daily and prednisolone 20 mg daily. Cyclophosphamide was discontinued after 2 months and the prednisolone was subsequently tapered to 15 mg daily. This association suggests that EED may represent a cutaneous manifestation of a systemic vasculitis.

Erythema elevatum diutinum associated with IgA paraproteinemia successfully controlled with intermittent plasma exchange. Chow RK, Benny WB, Coupe RL, Dodd WA, Ongley RC. Arch Dermatol 1996; 132: 1360–4.

Intermittent plasma exchange has been reported to successfully control EED associated with IgA paraproteinemia.

Erythema elevatum diutinum after liver transplantation: disappearance of the lesions associated with a reduction in cyclosporin dosage. Hernandez-Cano N, De Lucas R, Lazaro TE, Mayor M, Burón I, Casado M. Pediatr Dermatol 1998; 15: 411–12.

Lesions of EED resolved following a reduction in ciclosporin dosage in a 10-year-old patient who had previously received a cadaveric hepatic allograft because of Alagille disease.

Erythema elevatum diutinum – an unusual association with ulcerative colitis. Buahene K, Hudson M, Mowat A, Smart L, Ormerod AD. Clin Exp Dermatol 1991; 16: 204–6.

A 58-year-old woman developed EED during a severe acute exacerbation of ulcerative colitis, which resolved following colectomy.

Erythema elevatum diutinum manifesting as a penile ulcer. Yoshii N, Kanekura T, Higashi Y, Oyama K, Azagami K, Kanzaki T. Clin Exp Dermatol 2007; 32: 211–13.

A 74-year-old man developed EED. The lesions on his limbs responded well to nicotine patches that released 6.25 mg nicotine applied once every 24 hours. The penile lesion remained recalcitrant to nicotine patches as well as dapsone, requiring treatment with methylprednisolone (40 mg/day). The ulcer stopped increasing within several days and improved thereafter. Over the course of 9 weeks the daily dose of methylprednisolone was tapered to 12.5 mg, and the ulcer was almost completely covered by regenerated epithelium.

Erythema multiforme

Jean Revuz

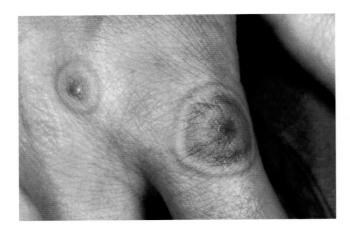

Erythema multiforme (EM) is a distinct cutaneous reaction pattern to a variety of stimuli, predominantly herpes simplex virus (HSV) infection. It usually runs a self-limiting course but has a tendency to recur. It is defined by the presence of 'typical' three-zone target lesions, with a predominantly acral distribution. The presence of mucosal involvement at more than one site distinguishes EM major from EM minor. A specific variant has only mucosal lesions without skin involvement.

EM major can be distinguished from Stevens–Johnson syndrome. EM is frequently misdiagnosed in cases of urticaria, and more rarely in cases of cutaneous lupus, vasculitis, erythema annulare, and drug eruption.

MANAGEMENT STRATEGY

In 30–50% of cases the etiology of EM is unknown. The most commonly recognized precipitant is herpes simplex virus infection, both types I and II. HSV-specific DNA has been isolated from lesional tissue in 60–70% of cases. HSV particles are found in the circulating precursors of epidermal Langerhans' cells. A variety of other viral infections – orf, VZV, EBV, CMV, HIV – bacterial infections (mainly *mycoplasma pneumoniae*), and fungal infections, mainly histoplasmosis, have been implicated. An extensive list of drugs has been reported to trigger EM but most cases if not all are the result of a confusion with Stevens–Johnson syndrome. Rare cases are attributed to contact allergy.

Acute episodes of EM need only *symptomatic treatment* in most cases. Recurrent EM which may severely affect the quality of life has a well-recognized *preventive treatment* in case of HSV infection.

There are no double-blind or open trials of treatments for acute episodes of EM. Most cases, particularly EM minor, run a self-limiting course. Symptomatic measures include *oral antihistamines* and *mild- to moderate-potency topical corticosteroids* to reduce pruritus. Underlying conditions, mainly *mycoplasma pneumoniae* infection, should be treated. Recurrent EM (>6 attacks per year) may respond to long-term *aciclovir*. In aciclovir-resistant cases a variety of other therapies can be helpful (see below).

Mucosal manifestations of EM are a source of morbidity and occur in up to 70% of cases. The commonest sites affected are the buccal mucosa and lips. Symptomatic measures include *mouthwashes*, a *soft diet*, *topical anesthetics* (lidocaine gel, benzocaine lozenges or 0.15% benzydamine hydrochloride), and *topical corticosteroids* (e.g., 0.1% triamcinolone acetonide paste). Budesonide or beclomethasone inhalers (1 puff three to four times daily) provide an alternative method of delivering local corticosteroid to the inflamed mucosal surfaces. Short courses of high-dose *oral prednisolone* may be needed for severe oral disease. Strict eye care to reduce secondary infection and scarring includes *saline washes* for removal of crusts, *local antibiotics*, and frequent *debridement of tarsal and bulbar conjunctival adherences*.

SPECIFIC INVESTIGATIONS

▶ Histology/immunofluorescence

EM is a clinical diagnosis. Histology, with direct immunofluorescence, can be useful in atypical cases to exclude other bullous diseases that present with oral manifestations, such as pemphigus vulgaris or cicatricial pemphigoid.

Investigations directed at determining the underlying trigger factors include culture or serological testing for HSV or other infections, especially *Mycoplasma pneumoniae*, as indicated by clinical findings.

Clinical characteristics of childhood erythema multiforme, Stevens–Johnson syndrome and toxic epidermal necrolysis in Taiwanese children. Lam NS, Yang YH, Wang LC, Lin YT, Chiang BL. J Microbiol Immunol Infect 2004; 37: 3667–70.

This study included 19 cases of EM, eight of Stevens–Johnson syndrome, and one of toxic epidermal necrolysis. The most common etiology in EM was infection, and the most common implicated organism was *M. pneumoniae* (42.1%).

FIRST-LINE THERAPIES

▶ Aciclovir   **A**

Recurrent erythema multiforme: clinical features and treatment in a large series of patients. Schofield JK, Tatnall FM, Leigh IM. Br J Dermatol 1993; 128: 542–5.

A review of 65 patients with recurrent EM: 71% had episodes triggered by HSV infection. In one patient, EM was related to the menstrual cycle and could be precipitated by intramuscular progesterone injection. Treatment with standard doses of aciclovir for HSV was relatively disappointing; continuous aciclovir 400 mg twice daily for 6 months was more effective, with remission in some responders. Some patients responded to dapsone, antimalarials, azathioprine, and human immunoglobulin.

A double-blind, placebo-controlled trial of continuous aciclovir therapy in recurrent erythema multiforme. Tatnall FM, Schofield JK, Leigh IM. Br J Dermatol 1995; 132: 267–70.

Aciclovir 400 mg twice daily for 6 months suppressed EM in seven of 11 patients (including one with apparently idiopathic EM). Two patients went into complete remission.

A therapeutic trial of aciclovir is justified even when clinical evidence of HSV is lacking. Aciclovir 400 mg twice daily can be administered for 6 months to 2 years because it has a good long-term safety profile. It is ineffective in an acute episode once the herpetic lesion or EM eruption has developed.

Recurrent erythema multiforme unresponsive to acyclovir prophylaxis and responsive to valacyclovir continuous therapy. Kerob D, Assier-Bonnet H, Esnault-Gelly P, Blanc F, Saiag P. Arch Dermatol 1998; 134: 876–7.

A reduced response to aciclovir may be due to the low oral bioavailability of the drug, and one of the second-generation antivirals, such as valaciclovir (500 mg daily) or famciclovir (250 mg twice daily) may need to be substituted.

SECOND-LINE THERAPIES

▶ Dapsone	C
▶ Azathioprine	C
▶ Thalidomide	B
▶ Potassium iodide	C
Oral EM	
▶ Topical corticosteroid	B
▶ Levamisole	B
▶ Systemic corticosteroid	D

Recurrent erythema multiforme: clinical features and treatment in a large series of patients. Schofield JK, Tatnall FM, Leigh IM. Br J Dermatol 1993; 128: 542–5.

Dapsone in a dose of 100–150 mg daily induced partial or complete suppression of EM in eight of nine patients. Azathioprine 100–150 mg daily was effective in 11 patients resistant to other treatments. Relapse of EM occurred on discontinuation of treatment.

Dapsone-responsive persistent erythema multiforme. Mahendran R, Grant JW, Norris PG. Dermatology 2000; 200: 281–2.

Dapsone 100 mg daily was effective in controlling EM in a patient with ovarian malignancy.

Characteristics of the oral lesions in patients with cutaneous recurrent erythema multiforme. Farthing PM, Maragou P, Coates M, Tatnall F, Leigh IM, Williams DM. J Oral Pathol Med 1995; 24: 9–13.

In this series of 82 patients with typical cutaneous EM, 70% had oral mucosal involvement. Five patients with resistant disease were controlled with azathioprine 100–150 mg daily.

Azathioprine therapy in the management of persistent erythema multiforme. Jones RR. Br J Dermatol 1981; 105: 465–7.

Azathioprine 100–150 mg daily was effective in two patients and permitted reduction of the corticosteroid dosage.

Thalidomide for recurrent erythema multiforme. Moisson YF, Janier M, Civatte J. Br J Dermatol 1992; 126: 92–3.

Recurrent EM responded to thalidomide 100–200 mg daily in two patients.

Treatment by thalidomide of chronic multiforme erythema: its recurrent and continuous variants. A retrospective study of 26 patients. Cherouati K, Claudy A, Souteyrand P, Cambazard F, Vaillant L, Moulin G, et al. Ann Dermatol Venereol 1996; 123: 375–7. (In French.)

Thalidomide reduces the duration of episodes of recurrent EM by 11 days on average; dramatically effective in the exceptional continuous variant. Remission can be maintained with low-dose (25–50 mg daily) thalidomide.

Potassium iodide in erythema nodosum and other erythematous dermatoses. Horio T, Danno K, Okamoto H, Miyachi Y, Imamura S. J Am Acad Dermatol 1983; 9: 77–81.

Fourteen of 16 subjects with EM (six related to HSV infection) responded within 1 week to 300 mg potassium iodide three times daily. Gastrointestinal and cutaneous side effects can occur with this treatment.

Erythema multiforme – response to corticosteroid. Ting HC, Adam BA. Dermatologica 1984; 169: 175–8.

Thirteen patients with EM minor treated with systemic corticosteroids were compared with 12 treated without. Apart from a shorter duration of fever, the corticosteroid-treated group did not respond better than the non-corticosteroid-treated group.

There is no reason to treat EM minor with steroids. This drug may still be useful in EM major.

Oral EM

Open preliminary clinical trial of clobetasol propionate ointment in adhesive paste for treatment of chronic oral vesiculoerosive diseases. Lozada-Nur F, Huang MZ, Zhou GA. Oral Surg Oral Med Oral Pathol 1991; 71: 283–7.

Clobetasol propionate 0.05% ointment mixed 1:1 with Orabase paste twice to three times daily was helpful in four patients with chronic oral EM.

Topically applied fluocinonide in an adhesive base in the treatment of oral vesiculoerosive diseases. Lozada F, Silverman S Jr. Arch Dermatol 1980; 116: 898–901.

Topical application of 0.05% fluocinonide in an adhesive base was used in 16 patients with oral EM. All responded to therapy, and remission was induced in some cases.

Oral erythema multiforme: clinical observations and treatment of 95 patients. Lozada-Nur F, Corsky M, Silverman S Jr. Oral Surg Oral Med Oral Pathol 1989; 67: 36–40.

As 19 of 29 patients with oral EM and oral candidiasis responded to antifungal therapy, a possible etiological role for these organisms in EM was suggested in this paper.

Only two of these 29 patients had skin lesions, the nature of which was not described. There is some doubt that it is really the same disease as the one we call EM.

Levamisole in the treatment of erythema multiforme: a double-blind trial in fourteen patients. Lozada F. Oral Surg Oral Med Oral Pathol 1982; 53: 28–31.

Fourteen patients with severe oral EM were treated in this crossover trial with levamisole 150 mg daily or placebo, 3 days a week for 4–8 weeks. Nine of 12 experienced a reduction in the severity and duration of attacks, and seven reported a reduction in disease frequency for up to 2 years after the trial.

The presence or absence of skin involvement is not mentioned in this study. Oral surgeons may have a different definition of EM.

Clinical response to levamisole in thirty-nine patients with erythema multiforme. An open prospective study. Lozada-Nur F, Cram D, Gorsky M. Oral Surg Oral Med Oral Pathol 1992; 74: 294–8.

Levamisole 150 mg daily 3 days a week was effective in 31 of 39 patients with oral EM. Nineteen patients are recorded as having skin disease, but the lesions are not described. Prednisolone 5–30 mg daily was required for 18 patients in addition to levamisole. The most common side effects from levamisole were rash, tiredness, weakness, myalgia, taste change, and insomnia. The white cell count needs to be monitored in patients on levamisole because there is a risk of drug-induced granulocytopenia.

Prednisone and azathioprine in the treatment of patients with vesiculoerosive oral diseases. Lozada F. Oral Surg Oral Med Oral Pathol 1981; 52: 257–63.

In this open trial, two patients with oral EM required lower doses of prednisolone (15–20 mg on alternate days) when treated simultaneously with azathioprine (50 mg daily).

Recurrent oral erythema multiforme. Clinical experience with 11 patients. Bean SF, Quezada RK. JAMA 1983; 249: 2810–12.

In this retrospective study, patients with severe recurrent oral EM involvement were treated with prednisolone 40–60 mg daily, subsequently tapered over 2–3 weeks. This reduced the time taken for oral erosions to heal, but did not influence recurrences.

Some authorities, however, believe that use of corticosteroids in EM increases the frequency and chronicity of attacks.

THIRD-LINE THERAPIES

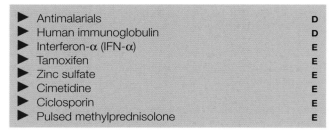

▶ Antimalarials	D
▶ Human immunoglobulin	D
▶ Interferon-α (IFN-α)	E
▶ Tamoxifen	E
▶ Zinc sulfate	E
▶ Cimetidine	E
▶ Ciclosporin	E
▶ Pulsed methylprednisolone	E

Recurrent erythema multiforme: clinical features and treatment in a large series of patients. Schofield JK, Tatnall FM, Leigh IM. Br J Dermatol 1993; 128: 542–5.

The use of normal human immunoglobulins and antimalarials was reported in a few patients in this study. Intramuscular human immunoglobulin 750 g once a month caused suppression of EM in 11 of 13 patients. One responder remained in remission after therapy was discontinued. There was a 50% success rate with antimalarials (both hydroxychloroquine and mepacrine) used in four patients.

Recurrent erythema multiforme and chronic hepatitis C: efficacy of interferon alpha. Dumas V, Thieulent N, Souillet AL, Jullien D, Faure M, Claudy A. Br J Dermatol 2000; 142: 1248–9.

One patient with recurrent EM and hepatitis C virus infection responded to two courses of IFN-α (9 MU weekly for 6 and 8 months, respectively).

Severe erythema multiforme responding to interferon alfa. Geraminejad P, Walling HW, Voigt MD, Stone MS. J Am Acad Dermatol 2006; 54: S18–21.

A patient with recurrent EM associated with hepatitis C had been in complete remission for 6 years after treatment with interferon-α. A new recurrence was successfully treated with interferon-α in the absence of recurring virus C infection.

Interferon may be a first-line treatment for patients with hepatitis C

Progesterone-induced erythema multiforme. Wojnarowska F, Greaves MW, Peachey RD, Drury PL, Besser GM. J Roy Soc Med 1985; 78: 407–8.

EM linked to the luteal phase of the menstrual cycle was controlled with tamoxifen.

Topical treatment of recurrent herpes simplex and postherpetic erythema multiforme with low concentrations of zinc sulphate solution. Brody I. Br J Dermatol 1981; 104: 191–4.

Treatment of the skin at the site of the herpetic infection with zinc sulfate solution prevented relapse of post-herpetic EM over a 2-year period of observation in one patient. For the skin, 0.025–0.05%, and for the oral mucous membrane, 0.01–0.025% zinc sulfate solution was used.

Cimetidine prevents recurrent erythema multiforme major resulting from herpes simplex virus infection. Kurkcuoglu N, Alli N. J Am Acad Dermatol 1989; 21: 814–15.

EM resistant to aciclovir responded to cimetidine 400 mg three times daily in one patient.

Cyclosporine therapy for bullous erythema multiforme. Wilkel CS, McDonald CJ. Arch Dermatol 1990; 126: 397–8.

High-dose ciclosporin (5–10 mg/kg daily) suppressed an atypical bullous eruption with histologic features of EM. The use of ciclosporin permitted tapering of the corticosteroid dosage.

High-dose systemic corticosteroids can arrest recurrences of severe mucocutaneous erythema multiforme. Martinez AE, Atherton DJ. Pediatr Dermatol 2000; 17: 87–90.

A child with recurrent EM major (associated with severe ulcerative stomatitis, conjunctival inflammation, and urethritis) responded to pulsed intravenous methylprednisolone 20 mg/kg daily for 3 consecutive days, but not to oral prednisolone 3 mg/kg daily. Intravenous methylprednisolone stopped progression of the acute attack, and repeated treatments induced remission.

Evidence Levels: **A** Double-blind study **B** Clinical trial ≥ 20 subjects **C** Clinical trial < 20 subjects **D** Series ≥ 5 subjects **E** Anecdotal case reports

Erythema nodosum

Robert A Allen, Richard L Spielvogel

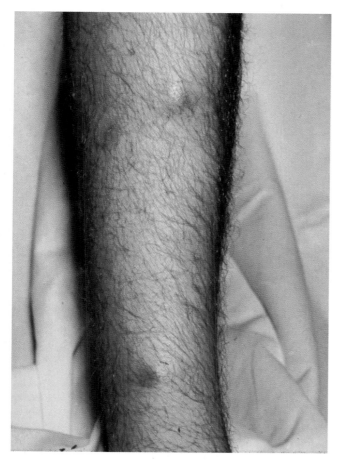

Erythema nodosum (EN) is a septal panniculitis that presents as tender, erythematous nodules and plaques located primarily on the extensor surfaces of the lower extremities. There is a predilection for females. Numerous etiologies have been implicated, including chronic inflammatory states, infections, reactions to medications, and rarely, malignancies. There is a tendency towards spontaneous regression, which usually occurs 6 months or less after the onset of the first lesions.

MANAGEMENT STRATEGIES

Treatment of EN depends on the suspected or documented etiology, if known. Common causes include infections, chronic inflammatory states, and drug reactions. Unfortunately, even after extensive evaluation many cases are classified as idiopathic.

Infectious agents include, but are not limited to, *Yersinia enterocolitica, Salmonella enteritidis, Giardia lamblia, Streptococcus, Shigella, Klebsiella* spp., and HIV. The infectious agents causing tuberculosis, brucellosis, psittacosis, cat scratch disease, chancroid, tularemia, campylobacter septicemia, nocardiosis, blastomycosis, sporotrichosis, coccidioidomycosis, histoplasmosis, and fungal kerions have also been implicated.

Patients with chronic inflammation may develop erythema nodosum. Diseases such as sarcoidosis, inflammatory bowel disease (Crohn's disease and ulcerative colitis), Behçet's syndrome, Sweet's syndrome, pyoderma faciale, and chronic abscesses have been associated.

Medications are common inciting agents. The most likely cause is oral contraceptive use, but medicines such as iodides, bromides, and sulfonamides have been implicated. Lidocaine injections, ciprofoxacin, aromatase inhibitors, ALL-*trans* retinoic acid, granulocyte colony-stimulating factor, echinacea supplements, and glatiramer acetate are thought to be causative.

Malignancies such as leukemias and lymphomas have been implicated. In cancer patients it may be difficult to determine the definitive cause of the erythema nodosum because of the multiple treatments and possible chronic inflammation that can occur.

Skin biopsy is generally not necessary if the history and physical signs are suggestive of EN. The pathology should demonstrate inflammation in the septa of the subcutis between fat lobules. Other findings can include fibrosis, increased thickness of the intralobular septa, and radial arrays of macrophages around blood vessels. A biopsy is usually helpful in ruling out other forms of panniculitis, and if an infectious cause is in the differential diagnosis, some tissue may be sent for culture and stains to look for organisms.

Treatment consists primarily of *bed rest, activity reduction, non-steroidal anti-inflammatory agents (NSAIDs)*, and *potassium iodide*. Various NSAIDs have been used successfully, including naproxen and indometacin. Potassium iodide has recently regained popularity but may be difficult to obtain because of stockpiling by national governments. We recommend a supersaturated solution of potassium iodide of five drops three times daily in orange juice. This dose is increased by one drop per dose per day until clinical effectiveness is achieved. Hypothyroidism can result from long-term use of potassium iodide. *Hydroxychloroquine* 200 mg twice a day has been used with limited success in EN. *Dapsone* was successful in a patient who developed EN after starting isotretinoin for acne fulminans. *Systemic corticosteroids* may also be helpful in refractory cases, or to 'jump start' therapy.

SPECIFIC INVESTIGATIONS

- ► Anti-streptolysin O (ASO) titer, throat culture
- ► Chest radiograph
- ► Purified protein derivative standard (PPD) tuberculosis skin test
- ► Skin biopsy

Erythema nodosum: a review. Soderstrom RM, Krull EA. Cutis 1978; 21: 806–10.

Streptococcal infection is the most common etiologic agent, and sarcoidosis is the most common disease associated with EN.

All patients should have a chest radiograph, ASO titer, throat culture, and PPD.

Erythema nodosum and associated diseases – a study of 129 cases. Cribier B, Caille A, Heid E, Grosshans E. Int J Dermatol 1998; 37: 667–72.

Streptococcal infection was the most common cause of EN and sarcoidosis the second most common.

Erythema nodosum: a study of 160 cases. Atanes A, Gomez N, de Toro J, de Toro J, Graña J, Sánchez JM, et al. Med Clin (Barc) 1996; 9: 169–72.

Of 160 cases reviewed, the majority were due to sarcoidosis, followed by drugs, streptococcal infection, and tuberculosis.

Erythema nodosum: an evaluation of 100 cases. Mert A, Kumbasar H, Ozaras R, Erten S, Tasli L, Tabak F, et al. Clin Exp Rheumatol 2007; 25: 563–70.

The results showed a 6:1 female predominance; 53% of cases were idiopathic and 11% related to streptococcal infections, 10% tuberculosis, 10% sarcoidosis, 6% Behçet's, 5% drug reactions, 3% inflammatory bowel disease, and 2% pregnancy induced.

FIRST-LINE THERAPIES

▶ NSAIDs	E
▶ Potassium iodide	B

Suppression of erythema nodosum by indomethacin. Ubogy Z, Persellin RH. Acta Dermatol Venereol 1982; 62: 265–7.

Three patients with EN secondary to streptococcal pharyngitis were treated with indometacin 100–150 mg orally for 2 weeks with excellent results, after having failed to respond to treatment with erythromycin, penicillin, and aspirin.

Chronic erythema nodosum treated with indomethacin. Barr WG, Robinson JA. Ann Intern Med 1981; 95: 659.

Idiopathic EN in a 32-year-old woman that had been unsuccessfully treated with aspirin, resolved with indometacin 25 mg three times daily for 1 month.

Control of chronic erythema nodosum with naproxen. Lehman CW. Cutis 1980; 26: 66–7.

A 28-year-old woman with recurrent EN refractory to phenylbutazone and aspirin was treated with naproxen 250 mg orally twice daily for 1 month, with cessation of symptoms within 96 hours and clearing in 14 days. Relapses occurred after stopping therapy, but cleared promptly with reinstitution of naproxen.

Potassium iodide in erythema nodosum and other erythematous dermatoses. Horio T, Danno K, Okamoto H, Miyachi Y, Imamura S. J Am Acad Dermatol 1983; 9: 77–81.

Twelve of 16 patients treated with potassium iodide experienced improvement within a few days, with complete resolution in 10–14 days. Six had recurrent attacks over 1–12 months, with resolution upon repeat dosing with potassium iodide. Of those who did not respond well, most received treatment 2–14 months after the onset of symptoms, indicating that earlier treatment is better. All patients with positive C-reactive protein responded well, and those with high fevers and arthralgias also responded well.

Potassium iodide may be a reasonable choice for those patients who cannot tolerate NSAIDs or corticosteroids. A saturated solution of potassium iodide (SSKI) may be made more palatable by adding the solution to orange juice.

Treatment of erythema nodosum and nodular vasculitis with potassium iodide. Schultz EJ, Whiting DA. Br J Dermatol 1976; 94: 75–8.

Twenty-four of 28 patients with EN experienced improvement within 48 hours, and resolution within 2 weeks with 300–900 mg daily of potassium iodide.

Potassium iodide in dermatology. A 19th century drug for the 21st century – uses, pharmacology, adverse effects, and contraindications. Sterling JB, Heymann WR. J Am Acad Dermatol 2000; 43: 691–7.

An excellent review article.

SECOND-LINE THERAPIES

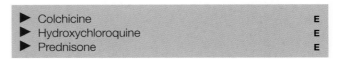

▶ Colchicine	E
▶ Hydroxychloroquine	E E
▶ Prednisone	E

Traitement de l'erythème noueux par la colchicine. De Coninck P, Baclet JL, Di Bernardo C, Büschges B, Plouvier B. Presse Med 1984; 13: 680.

Five women were treated with colchicine (2 mg daily for 3 days, then 1 mg daily for 2–4 weeks). Improvement was seen within 72 hours, with no recurrences once colchicine was stopped.

Erythema nodosum treated with colchicine. Wallace S. JAMA 1967; 202: 144.

One patient with EN was successfully treated with colchicine.

Hydroxychloroquine in the treatment of chronic erythema nodosum. Alloway JA, Franks LK. Br J Dermatol 1995; 132: 661–70.

A 38-year-old woman with a 24-year history of EN with almost monthly flares was treated with hydroxychloroquine 200 mg orally twice daily. Within 3 months she had a dramatic reduction in lesions and remained stable for at least 6 months. Previously she had occasionally responded to acetaminophen (paracetamol), but not to aspirin or indometacin. One previous flare had responded to prednisone.

Hydroxychloroquine and chronic erythema nodosum. Jarrett P, Goodfield MJD. Br J Dermatol 1996; 134: 373.

A 52-year-old with idiopathic EN was treated with hydroxychloroquine 200 mg orally twice daily and prednisone 15 mg four times daily for 8 weeks, with improvement. Prednisone was stopped and 8 weeks later the hydroxychloroquine dose was cut by half, but the patient experienced a flare and the original dose was restarted. After 3 more months the hydroxychloroquine was stopped, although intermittent dosing was required. The patient had previously been unresponsive to NSAIDs and prednisone.

THIRD-LINE THERAPIES

▶ Dapsone	E
▶ Extracorporeal monocyte granulocytapheresis	E
▶ Erythromycin	E
▶ Mycophenolate mofetil	E
▶ Etanercept	E
▶ Adalimumab	E
▶ Infliximab	E
▶ Prophylactic penicillin	E
▶ B$_{12}$ (if levels low)	E

Acne fulminans and erythema nodosum during isotretinoin therapy responding to dapsone. Tan B, Lear J, Smith A. Clin Exp Dermatol 1997; 22: 26–7.

Evidence Levels: A Double-blind study **B** Clinical trial ≥ 20 subjects **C** Clinical trial < 20 subjects **D** Series ≥ 5 subjects **E** Anecdotal case reports

Acne fulminans and EN that occurred in a patient 3 weeks after starting isotretinoin responded to dapsone without oral prednisone.

Prior to the use of isotretinoin for acne fulminans, dapsone was frequently used because it may help control both the acne and the EN. The improvement of EN may be secondary to the improvement of acne fulminans.

Extracorporeal monocyte granulocytapheresis was effective for a patient of erythema nodosum concomitant with ulcerative colitis. Fukunaga K, Sawada K, Fukuda Y, Matoba Y, Natsuaki M, Ohnishi K, et al. Ther Apher Dial 2003; 7: 122–6.

A patient with ulcerative colitis and EN that failed to respond to high-dose corticosteroids recovered from both conditions after monocyte granulocytapheresis once a week for 5 weeks. He was also on 2250 mg of 5-aminosalicylic acid daily.

Severe erythema nodosum due to Behçet's disease responsive to erythromycin. Kaya TI, Tursen U, Baz K, Ikizoglu G, Dusmez D. J Dermatol Treat 2003; 14: 124–7.

A patient with refractory Behçet's disease and EN responded to coincidental treatment with erythromycin for erythrasma.

Use of mycophenolate mofetil in erythema nodosum. Boyd AS. J Am Acad Dermatol 2002; 47: 968–9.

A patient taking estrogen replacement developed EN that was unresponsive to many treatments, including discontinuing hormone therapy and azathioprine. The EN cleared with an increasing dose of mycophenolate mofetil to 750 mg twice a day, and remained clear after a slow taper.

Dermatologic manifestations of Crohn disease in children: response to infliximab. Kugathasan S, Miranda A, Nocton J, Drolet BA, Raasch C, Binion DG. J Pediatr Gastroenterol Nutr 2003; 37: 150–4.

One child in a series of four patients with Crohn's disease had resistant concurrent EN. The patient cleared with infliximab 5 mg/kg (anti-tumor necrosis factor (TNF)-α antibody) and was maintained on 6-mercaptopurine. The conditions associated with Crohn's disease in the other children (pyoderma gangrenosum, orofacial Crohn's, and lymphedema) also cleared.

Treatment of chronic erythema nodosum with infliximab. Clayton TH, Walker BP, Stables GI. Clin Exp Dermatol 2006; 31: 823–4.

A 26-year-old woman with inflammatory bowel disease and EN was treated with infliximab as a steroid-sparing agent. She received doses at 0, 2, and 6 weeks, and then every 3 months. Both the EN and gastrointestinal symptoms improved.

Etanercept treatment of erythema nodosum. Boyd AS. SKINmed 2007; 6: 197–9.

One patient with a 5-year history of EN was treated with etanercept 25 mg subcutaneously twice weekly after failing prednisone, indometacin, SSKI, dapsone, and methotrexate. She was clear after 4 months. After 6 months the etanercept dose was reduced to 25 mg subcutaneously weekly for the rest of the year.

Prophylaxis of recurrent erythema nodosum with penicillin. Bhalla M, Thami GP. Dermatology 2007; 215: 363–4.

Three patients with recurrent EN were treated with monthly doses of IM benzathine penicillin 2.4 million units. One patient had high ASO titers, and the other two had idiopathic biopsy-proven EN. All patients were clear at 6 months' follow-up.

Refractory chronic erythema nodosum successfully treated with adalimumab. Ortego-Centeno N, Callejas-Rubio JL, Sanchez-Cano D, Caballero-Morales T. J Eur Acad Dermatol Venereol 2007; 21: 408–10.

A 79-year-old patient with EN of many years' duration was initially responsive only to steroids. She was switched to adalimumab 40 mg subcutaneously every 2 weeks, and was clear after 7 months of follow-up.

Successful treatment of chronic erythema nodosum with vitamin B$_{12}$. Volkov I, Rudoy I, Press Y. J Am Board Fam Pract 2005; 18: 567–9.

One patient had EN resolve after being treated for a low serum B$_{12}$ level. She was treated with twice-weekly injections of 1000 µg of B$_{12}$.

Erythrasma

Melissa C Barkham

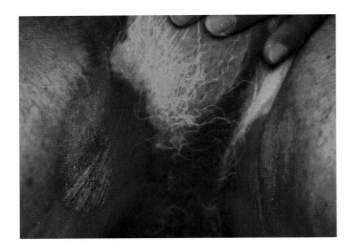

In its most typical form, erythrasma is characterized by well-defined reddish-brown flexural plaques which show fine scaling and no tendency to central clearing. It may also present with maceration of the toe webs.

The responsible organism, *Corynebacterium minutissimum*, is an inhabitant of normal human skin. Factors that predispose to clinically apparent infection include diabetes mellitus, obesity, old age, and a humid environment.

MANAGEMENT STRATEGY

Erythrasma is often a trivial infection, but therapy may be requested because of the cosmetic appearance or because of pruritus. Co-infection with dermatophyte fungi or *Candida albicans* is common and may influence the choice of treatment.

Topical antibiotics such as fusidic acid and clindamycin are effective and well tolerated.

Topical imidazoles (miconazole, clotrimazole, econazole) are well tolerated and also effective against concomitant fungal or yeast infection.

Whitfield's ointment (benzoic acid compound) is effective, but its use in the flexures is limited by a tendency to produce irritation.

Oral erythromycin is the treatment of choice in extensive disease, or when compliance with topical therapy is unlikely.

A combination of oral and topical treatment may be required for stubborn infections, particularly of the toe webs.

SPECIFIC INVESTIGATIONS

> ► Examination under Wood's light
> ► Potassium hydroxide (KOH) preparation of skin scrapings
> ► Fasting serum glucose

Rapid confirmation of the diagnosis is achieved by examination of the skin under Wood's (long-wave ultraviolet) light. The characteristic coral-red fluorescence observed is due to the production of coproporphyrin III by the organism. Fluorescence may not be seen if the patient has bathed immediately prior to examination. Culture is unreliable because the organism does not always grow satisfactorily. Microscopy of skin scrapings is performed to seek evidence of concomitant infection, such as the presence of fungal hyphae or yeasts. Consider underlying diabetes mellitus if erythrasma is severe or recurrent.

FIRST-LINE THERAPIES

► Miconazole cream	B
► Clotrimazole cream	D
► Econazole cream	E
► Fusidic acid cream	B
► Clindamycin lotion or solution	E
► Whitfield's ointment	B

Treatment of erythrasma with miconazole. Pitcher DG, Noble WC, Seville RH. Clin Exp Dermatol 1979; 4: 453–6.

Twenty-three patients were treated with miconazole cream and 25 with Whitfield's ointment twice daily for 2 weeks. In both groups a clearance rate of 88% was obtained, but irritation was a problem with Whitfield's ointment.

A clinical double-blind trial of topical miconazole and clotrimazole against superficial fungal infections and erythrasma. Clayton YM, Knight AG. Clin Exp Dermatol 1976; 1: 225–32.

This was a comparison of the two preparations in dermatophyte infection, but 11 patients with erythrasma were also studied – six treated with miconazole, five with clotrimazole, both twice daily. All patients in both groups were free of infection at 4 weeks.

Specific topical treatment for erythrasma. Macmillan AL, Sarkany I. Br J Dermatol 1970; 82: 507–9.

All eight patients treated with 2% fusidic acid ointment twice daily for 2 weeks were cured. The cream is preferable for flexural disease.

Topical treatment for erythrasma. Cochran RJ, Rosen T, Landers T. Int J Dermatol 1981; 20: 562–4.

Two cases cleared with two or three times daily application of 2% aqueous clindamycin solution for 1 week. No recurrence was noted 6 weeks later.

SECOND-LINE THERAPIES

► Erythromycin	B

Systemic or local treatment of erythrasma? A comparison between erythromycin tablets and Fucidin cream in general practice. Hamann K, Thorn P. Scand J Prim Health Care 1991; 9: 35–9

This double-blind trial compared 14 days' treatment with erythromycin 500 mg bd, 2% fusidic acid cream twice daily, and placebo. Four weeks after treatment 18 of 21 patients with erythromycin and 23 of 25 with fusidic acid cream were cured. Both were better than placebo.

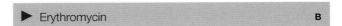

Evidence Levels: **A** Double-blind study **B** Clinical trial ≥ 20 subjects **C** Clinical trial < 20 subjects **D** Series ≥ 5 subjects **E** Anecdotal case reports

THIRD-LINE THERAPIES

▶ Clarithromycin	E
▶ Tetracycline	E
▶ Illumination with red light source	E

Erythrasma treated with single-dose clarithromycin. Wharton JR, Wilson PL, Kincannon JM. Arch Dermatol 1998; 134: 671–2.

Three patients treated with a single 1 g dose of clarithromycin showed no sign of residual disease at 2 weeks.

The treatment of erythrasma in a hospital for the mentally subnormal. Seville RH, Somerville A. Br J Dermatol 1970; 82: 502–6.

Twenty patients were treated with erythromycin 250 mg four times daily for 7 days. Nearly all cases with involvement of the axillae and groins, but only about two-thirds of toe web infections, were cured. Oral tetracycline was less effective than erythromycin, and relapse rates were high.

Photodynamic action of red light for treatment of erythrasma: preliminary results. Darras-Vercambre S, Carpentier O, Vincent P, Bonnevalle A, Thomas P. Photodermatol Photoimmunol Photomed 2006; 22: 153–6.

The aim of this trial was to harness the effect of the porphyrin produced by the organism. A red light source (635 nm) was used without a topical photosensitizer. Although this is a novel concept, complete clearance was observed in only three of 13 patients after a single treatment session.

Erythroderma

Michelle Thomson, John Berth-Jones

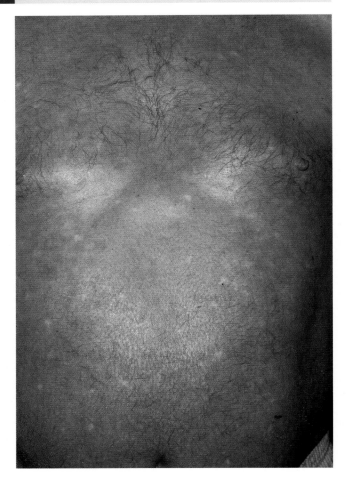

Erythroderma (exfoliative dermatitis) is persistent, severe, generalized inflammation of the skin. By convention the term tends to be reserved for cases where at least 90% of the skin is involved. Although the erythema is a constant feature, the scaling or exfoliation is highly variable. The condition arises as a 'reaction pattern' in a diverse range of circumstances (Tables 1 and 2), including genodermatoses and congenital disorders such as severe ichthyoses and ichthyosiform erythrodermas; severe cases of dermatoses such as psoriasis, atopic or seborrheic or contact allergic dermatitis; cutaneous T-cell lymphoma; allergic reactions to drugs; and reactions to internal malignancies (especially lymphoma and other lymphoreticular malignancies). In addition to this multitude of known causes, a proportion of cases develop without any apparent trigger and remain 'idiopathic.'

MANAGEMENT STRATEGY

Erythroderma, especially when fulminant, is a life-threatening state of skin failure that demonstrates vividly that the skin is as vital to life as any internal organ. The dangers arise from the loss of an effective barrier to entry of bacteria, from the loss of thermoregulation, from increased fluid loss through evaporation or exudation, from loss of protein due to the increased proliferative and metabolic activity that accompany uncontrolled desquamation, and from the risk of high-output cardiac failure. All these hazards are greatest in the very young and the elderly. Many patients who are otherwise healthy can tolerate a chronic or permanently erythrodermic state. By contrast, very young and elderly patients with fulminant disease may develop septicemia and die within a matter of hours.

Many aspects of the management of a patient with erythroderma are similar regardless of the etiology, and it is often necessary to treat a case without knowing the cause. However, for optimal longer-term management it is vital to establish a more precise diagnosis whenever possible. In many cases there has been pre-existing skin disease and the diagnosis may be quite clear from the history, but when erythroderma arises de novo establishing the cause can be difficult or impossible. A careful drug history should always be obtained and should include all over-the-counter and herbal remedies. Erythroderma has been associated with the use of St John's wort. Severe pruritus may suggest underlying lymphoma. Although findings on examination may be entirely nonspecific, there may be clues such as bullae, indicating the presence of bullous pemphigoid or pemphigus foliaceus. Severe scaling is suggestive of psoriasis. Sparing of the flexures may suggest papuloerythroderma of Ofuji. Lymphadenopathy is often present, but is more often reactive than malignant.

Histology of the skin often proves as nonspecific as the clinical features and merely shows features of dermatitis. Occasionally, however, the presence of atypical large lymphocytes will point to a diagnosis of cutaneous T-cell lymphoma, or there may be features suggestive of psoriasis, a lichenoid reaction, or pityriasis rubra pilaris. Repeated or multiple biopsies are sometimes helpful. Immunofluorescence for immunoglobulin deposition should be performed if an immunobullous disease is suspected.

Patients with acute onset of erythroderma are *usually best managed in hospital because frequent observations and intensive supportive care are required, and bed rest may be highly therapeutic.* All nonessential drugs should be withdrawn. Frequent applications of abundant quantities of *bland emollients* such as petrolatum are

Table 1 Cutaneous diseases that may present with or develop into erythroderma

Atopic dermatitis
Bullous pemphigoid
Contact allergic dermatitis
Congenital ichthyoses
Cutaneous T-cell lymphoma
Dermatomyositis
Dermatophytosis
Graft-vs-host disease
Hailey–Hailey disease
Human immununodeficieny virus
Ichthyoses
Lichen planus
Lupus erythematosus
Papuloerythroderma of Ofuji
Pemphigus foliaceus
Pityriasis rubra pilaris
Psoriasis
Reiter's syndrome
Sarcoid
Seborrheic dermatitis
Scabies
Stasis dermatitis with autosensitization

Table 2 Drugs that may induce erythroderma

Allopurinol
Amiodarone
Antimalarials
Aspirin
Captopril
Carbamazepine
Cephalosporins
Cimetidine
Codeine phosphate
Diaminodiphenyl sulfone (dapsone)
Diltiazem
Diphenylhydantoin (phenytoin)
Epoprostenol
Gold
Isoniazid
Lithium
Omeprazole
Para-aminosalicylic acid
Penicillins
Phenothiazines
Quinidine
Ranitidine
Sulfonamides
Sulfonylureas
Thiazides
Trimethoprim
Vancomycin

required to soothe the skin, and these help to partially restore the barrier. Careful attention must be paid to *hydration and nutrition*.

The use of more active pharmaceutical intervention requires careful consideration. Some patients with erythroderma have multiple drug allergies. Immunosuppressive drugs may be considered to be contraindicated if malignancy is suspected (particularly cutaneous lymphoma). Topical treatments may be far more irritant than expected, and systemic absorption will be greater than usual. *Prophylactic antibiotics* such as *erythromycin* are often given orally. *Corticosteroids* are often applied topically. *Antihistamines* are often prescribed, but act largely as sedatives.

If a diagnosis can be established, withdrawal of a causal drug or specific treatment for an underlying dermatosis, combined with the supportive measures described above, will usually produce a rapid improvement in the erythroderma. When a firm diagnosis cannot be made, treatment may have to be directed at the most likely cause, based on the clinical and histologic features.

SPECIFIC INVESTIGATIONS

▶ Hematology
▶ Urea and electrolytes
▶ Liver function tests
▶ Blood cultures
▶ Monitoring of temperature and vital signs
▶ Nasal and skin swabs
▶ Skin biopsy
▶ T-cell receptor analysis
▶ Lymph node biopsy
▶ Screening for connective tissue disease
▶ Immunodeficiency screen
▶ Potassium hydroxide (KOH) preparation and fungal culture

Diagnosing erythrodermic cutaneous T-cell lymphoma. Russell-Jones R. Br J Dermatol 2005; 153: 1–5.

A very useful review with an algorithm to help differentiate between erythroderma due to cutaneous T-cell lymphoma and 'reactive' causes of erythroderma.

T-cell receptor gene analysis in the diagnosis of Sézary syndrome. Russell-Jones R, Whittaker S. J Am Acad Dermatol 1999; 41: 254–9.

A discussion of the criteria used for diagnosis of Sézary syndrome. The demonstration of large atypical lymphocytes in peripheral blood (so-called 'Sézary cells') is not specific for this condition because these are often observed in benign reactive erythrodermas. Only when they comprise 20% or more of the circulating peripheral blood mononuclear cells do they become diagnostic of Sézary syndrome.

Diagnostic and prognostic importance of T-cell receptor gene analysis in patients with Sézary syndrome. Fraser-Andrews EA, Russell-Jones R, Woolford AJ, Wolstencroft RA, Dean AJ, Whittaker SJ. Cancer 2001; 92: 1745–52.

The definitive diagnostic criteria for patients with Sézary syndrome should include the presence of a clonal T-cell receptor gene rearrangement. Clonal patients have a poor prognosis and are likely to die from leukemia/lymphoma, whereas non-clonal patients may have a reactive, inflammatory T-cell disorder.

Mycosis fungoides and the Sézary syndrome. Kim YH, Hoppe RT. Semin Oncol 1999; 26: 276–89.

The prognosis of patients with mycosis fungoides is considered highly dependent on the initial presentation. Patients who present with limited patch/plaque disease have an overall long-term survival similar to that of a matched control population. Patients who have tumorous or erythrodermic skin involvement have a less favorable prognosis.

Bullous pemphigoid presenting as exfoliative erythroderma. Alonso-Llamazares J, Dietrich SM, Gibson LE. J Am Acad Dermatol 1998; 39: 827–30.

A patient with bullous pemphigoid presented with exfoliative erythroderma without any blistering. The diagnosis was based on the demonstration of circulating antibodies to the basement membrane zone, with an epidermal pattern on salt-split skin, and the presence of eosinophilic spongiosis in the skin biopsy.

Paraneoplastic dermatomyositis presenting as erythroderma. Nousari HC, Kimyai-Asadi A, Spegman DJ. J Am Acad Dermatol 1998; 39: 653–4.

A patient with gastric adenocarcinoma presented with erythrodermic dermatomyositis. Histology showed an interface dermatitis.

Idiopathic erythroderma: a follow-up study of 28 patients. Sigurdsson V, Toonstra J, van Vloten WA. Dermatology 1997; 194: 98–101.

During the median follow-up of 33 months, 35% of the patients went into remission and 52% improved. Three patients, all females, had persistent erythroderma. Two of these progressed to cutaneous T-cell lymphoma (one to Sézary syndrome and one to mycosis fungoides).

Inherited ichthyoses: a review of the histology of the skin. Scheimberg I, Harper JI, Malone M, Lake BD. Pediatr Pathol Lab Med 1996; 16: 359–78.

A review of the histologic features in 46 cases of congenital ichthyosis. Features of bullous ichthyosiform erythroderma, Netherton's syndrome, and neutral lipid storage disease can be recognized on routine hematoxylin and eosin staining. Electron microscopy, frozen sections, and other diagnostic techniques may also be required.

Congenital erythrodermic psoriasis: case report and literature review. Salleras M, Sanchez-Regana M, Umbert P. Pediatr Dermatol 1995; 12: 231–4.

A girl suffered from erythroderma, palmoplantar hyperkeratosis, and scalp desquamation since birth. A skin biopsy at 1 year of age showed features of psoriasis. She was successfully treated with acitretin at the age of 4. Plaque psoriasis developed at the age of 7.

Erythroderma due to dermatophyte. Gupta R, Khera V. Acta Dermatol Venereol 2001; 81: 70.

Dermatophytosis rarely presents as erythroderma. In this case, the presence of multiple mycelia without spores in KOH preparation confirmed the clinical suspicion of dermatophytosis. The scaling and erythema completely cleared with oral fluconazole 150 mg daily and miconazole nitrate cream 2% topically.

Severe subacute cutaneous lupus erythematosus presenting with generalized erythroderma and bullae. Mutasim DF. J Am Acad Dermatol 2003; 48: 947–9.

A patient presented with an erythrodermic and bullous form of subacute cutaneous lupus erythematosus. Serologic evaluation revealed a markedly elevated titer of antinuclear antibody (ANA) and La/SS-B antibodies. She later developed classic discrete lesions of subacute cutaneous lupus erythematosus. This case highlights the need to perform an autoimmune screen in cases where the etiology remains uncertain.

Papulosquamous dermatoses of AIDS. Sadick NS, McNutt NS, Kaplan MH. J Am Acad Dermatol 1990; 22: 1270–7.

This article reviews the spectrum of papulosquamous disorders in the setting of infection with the human immunodeficiency virus (HIV), including erythroderma, which can be the presenting sign of AIDS.

Neonatal and infantile erythrodermas. Pruszkowski A, Bodemer C, Fraitag S, Teillac-Hamel D, Amoric JC, de Prost Y. Arch Dermatol 2000; 136: 875–80.

The underlying cause of neonatal erythroderma is often difficult to ascertain. An immunodeficiency must be suspected in cases of severe erythroderma. The prognosis is poor in immunodeficiency disorders and severe cases of Netherton's syndrome and psoriasis.

FIRST-LINE THERAPIES

▶ Bed rest in hospital	C
▶ Emollients	C

SECOND-LINE THERAPIES

▶ Topical corticosteroids	C
▶ Psoralen and UVA (PUVA)	C
▶ Systemic corticosteroids	C
▶ PUVA with retinoid	E

Cushing's syndrome and adrenocortical insufficiency caused by topical steroids: misuse or abuse? Güven A, Gülümser O, Ozgen T. J Pediatr Endocrinol Metab 2007; 20: 1173–82.

One of many reports emphasizing that physicians should be alert to the dangerous side effects of topical steroids and avoid long-term use.

Salicylism from topical salicylates: review of the literature. Brubacher JR, Hoffman RS. J Toxicol Clin Toxicol 1996; 34: 431–6.

Hypercalcemia caused by vitamin D3 analogs in psoriasis treatment. Braun GS, Witt M, Mayer V, Schmid H. Int J Dermatol 2007; 46: 1315–17.

Low but detectable serum levels of tacrolimus seen with the use of very dilute, extemporaneously compounded formulations of tacrolimus ointment in the treatment of patients with Netherton syndrome. Shah KN, Yan AC. Arch Dermatol 2006; 142: 1362–3.

Patients with Netherton's syndrome have a skin barrier dysfunction that puts them at risk for increased percutaneous absorption. Tacrolimus levels should be carefully monitored to prevent systemic absorption and associated side effects.

Report illustrates the potential for unexpected toxicity due to systemic absorption of topical medications through erythrodermic skin. Care should be exercised with the use and quantities of topical medication.

Treatment of papuloerythroderma of Ofuji with Re-PUVA: a case report and review of the therapy. Mutluer S, Yerebakan O, Alpsoy E, Ciftcioglu MA, Yilmaz E. J Eur Acad Dermatol Venereol 2004; 18: 480–3.

Papuloerythroderma of Ofuji (PEO) is a disease of elderly men characterized by intensely pruritic and widespread red, flat-topped papules with sparing of the folds and creases. A case of PEO in a 60-year-old man who responded to retinoid plus PUVA (Re-PUVA) is discussed.

Treatment of severe erythrodermic acute graft-versus-host disease with photochemotherapy. Kunz M, Wilhelm S, Freund M, Zimmermann R, Gross G. Br J Dermatol 2001; 144: 901–22.

A 34-year-old man with grade IV graft-versus-host disease (GVHD) who did not respond to a combination of three different high-dose immunosuppressive agents.

The benefit of PUVA treatment for acute GVHD is well known, but successful treatment of severe GVHD is less common.

Ofuji's papuloerythroderma: a study of 17 cases. Bech-Thomson N, Thomsen K. Clin Exp Dermatol 1998; 23: 79–83.

In this retrospective study the clinical, laboratory and histological features, treatment methods and disease course in 17 patients with papuloerythroderma (PE) are reviewed. Psoralen photochemotherapy (PUVA) and oral prednisolone 10–20 mg daily given in combination or alone were very efficient treatments, and UVB phototherapy in combination with topical steroids was also successful.

A dermatitis–eosinophilia syndrome. Treatment with methylprednisolone pulse therapy. Dahl MV, Swanson DL, Jacob HS. Arch Dermatol 1984; 120: 1595–7.

A case in which erythroderma developed after a wasp sting and persisted for 4 months despite intensive topical therapy and oral corticosteroids. Pulsed methylprednisolone, 2 g intravenously, repeated after a week, cleared the erythroderma.

Evidence Levels: **A** Double-blind study **B** Clinical trial ≥ 20 subjects **C** Clinical trial < 20 subjects **D** Series ≥ 5 subjects **E** Anecdotal case reports

Toxic shock syndrome responsive to steroids. Vergis N, Gorard DA. J Med Case Rep 2007; 1: 5.

Toxic shock syndrome should be considered in the differential diagnosis of unexplained fever, erythroderma and features of septic shock. Systemic steroids can be life-saving.

THIRD-LINE THERAPIES

▶ Ciclosporin	D
▶ Cytotoxic drugs/antimetabolites	C
▶ Systemic retinoids	C
▶ Extracorporeal photochemotherapy	C
▶ UVA1 phototherapy	C
▶ Topical calcipotriol	E
▶ Topical tacrolimus	E
▶ Erythromycin	E
▶ Photopheresis and interferon	E
▶ Infliximab	D
▶ Etanercept	E
▶ Alefacept	E
▶ Alemtuzumab	E
▶ Daclizumab	E
▶ Bexarotene	E

Individualized short-course cyclosporin therapy in psoriasis. Finzi AF. Br J Dermatol 1996; 135 S48: 31–4.

Individualized short-course ciclosporin therapy is useful in controlling acute psoriasis flares and/or inducing remission; less potent agents can then be used for maintenance therapy. Short courses of low-dose ciclosporin may almost completely eliminate the risks of renal dysfunction from this drug.

Papuloerythroderma of Ofuji responding to treatment with ciclosporin. Sommer S, Henderson CA. Clin Exp Dermatol 2000; 25: 293–5.

A patient with papuloerythroderma of Ofuji (PE) responded to systemic steroids but remission was not maintained on reduction of the dose. Therefore, ciclosporin was added, which did lead to rapid clearing of the skin and remission was maintained after discontinuation of treatment.

Psoriatic erythroderma and bullous pemphigoid treated successfully with acitretin and azathioprine. Roeder C, Driesch PV. Eur J Dermatol 1999; 9: 537–9.

A 59-year-old man with severe psoriasis who developed bullous pemphigoid was successfully treated with a combination of acitretin and azathioprine, avoiding the use of systemic corticosteroids.

Methotrexate for psoriasis. Boffa MJ, Chalmers RJ. Clin Exp Dermatol 1996; 21: 399–408.

Methotrexate is considered especially useful in acute generalized pustular psoriasis and psoriatic erythroderma.

A useful review article.

Systemic methotrexate treatment in childhood psoriasis: further experience in 24 children from India. Kaur I, Dogra S, De D, Kanwar AJ. Pediatr Dermatol 2008; 25: 184–8.

Children with erythrodermic psoriasis were part of the study group. Response to therapy was excellent (>75% reduction in PASI) in all but two patients. This study supports the use of methotrexate in severe childhood psoriasis under expert supervision and laboratory monitoring.

An appraisal of acitretin therapy in children with inherited disorders of keratinization. Lacour M, Mehta-Nikhar B, Atherton DJ, Harper JI. Br J Dermatol 1996; 134: 1023–9.

A review of the authors' experience of using acitretin and etretinate in 46 children with severe ichthyoses and erythrodermas. Acitretin therapy is considered safe and effective provided the minimal effective dose is maintained and that side effects are carefully monitored.

Treatment of classic pityriasis rubra pilaris. Dicken CH. J Am Acad Dermatol 1994; 31: 997–9.

Classic pityriasis rubra pilaris almost always progresses to erythroderma. This is a retrospective review of 75 cases.

Retinoids are considered to offer the best chance of complete clearing. Methotrexate should be considered if retinoids fail or cannot be used.

Evidence-based practice of photopheresis 1987–2001: a report of a workshop of the British Photodermatology Group and the UK Skin Lymphoma Group. McKeena KE, Whittaker S, Rhodes LE, Taylor P, Lloyd J, Ibbotson S, et al. Br J Dermatol 2006; 154: 7–20.

Extracorporeal photopheresis in Sézary syndrome: hematologic parameters as predictors of response. Evans AV, Wood BP, Scarisbrick JJ, Fraser-Andrews EA, Chinn S, Dean A, et al. Blood 2001; 98: 1298–1301.

Data analyzed from 23 patients with Sézary syndrome undergoing monthly extracorporeal photopheresis as the sole therapy for up to 1 year showed that 57% achieved a reduction in erythema of more than 25% from baseline.

Complete remission of lichen-planus-like graft-versus-host disease (GVHD) with extracorporeal photochemotherapy (ECP). Gerber M, Gmeinhart B, Volc-Platzer B, Kalhs P, Greinix H, Knobler R. Bone Marrow Transplant 1997; 19: 517–19.

A report of a 45-year-old woman who underwent marrow transplantation for chronic myeloid leukemia and developed two episodes of acute GVHD. The first responded well to ciclosporin and corticosteroids. The second episode, which was erythrodermic, proved resistant to this regimen. Twelve cycles of extracorporeal photochemotherapy produced a lasting complete remission.

Photopheresis therapy for cutaneous T-cell lymphoma. Duvic M, Hester JP, Lemak NA. J Am Acad Dermatol 1996; 35: 573–9.

A report on 34 evaluable patients. Complete or partial remission was achieved in 50% of the patients. All responders except one had erythroderma.

'High-dose' UVA1 therapy of widespread plaque-type, nodular, and erythrodermic mycosis fungoides. Zane C, Leali C, Airò P, De Panfilis G, Pinton PC. J Am Acad Dermatol 2001; 44: 629–33.

In this series of 13 patients, 11 showed complete clinical and histological responses to 100 J/cm² UVA1 daily until remission. Unirradiated control lesions did not improve. Serious short-term side effects were not recorded. 'High-dose' UVA1 seems at least as effective as PUVA in the treatment of cutaneous mycosis fungoides.

Bullous congenital ichthyosiform erythroderma: safe and effective topical treatment with calcipotriol ointment in a

child. Bogenrieder T, Landthaler M, Stolz W. Acta Dermatol Venereol 2002; 83: 52–5.

A report of the safe and long-term (>3 years) use of topical calcipotriol ointment in a 9-year-old boy with a keratinization disorder.

Successful treatment of Netherton's syndrome with topical calcipotriol. Godic A, Dragos V. Eur J Dermatol 2004; 14: 115–17.

Efficacy and safety of tacrolimus 0.03% ointment in a 1-month-old 'red baby': a case report. Leonardi S, Rotolo N, Marchese G, La Rosa M. Allergy Asthma Proc 2006; 27: 523–6.

Successful treatment of bullous congenital ichthyosiform erythroderma with erythromycin. Freyhaus K, Kaiser HW, Proelss J, Tüting T, Bieber T, Wenzel J. Dermatol 2007; 215; 81–3.

Monitoring the decrease of circulating malignant T cells in cutaneous T-cell lymphoma during photopheresis and interferon therapy. Ferenczi K, Yawalkar N, Jones D, Kupper TS. Arch Dermatol 2003; 139: 909–13.

A patient with stage IV cutaneous T-cell lymphoma (CTCL) who was treated with photopheresis and low-dose interferon showed a dramatic reduction in the percentage of the malignant T-cell population paralleled by clinical skin improvement from initial generalized erythroderma to undetectable skin disease.

Erythrodermic cutaneous T cell lymphoma with hypereosinophilic syndrome: Treatment with interferon alfa and extracorporeal photopheresis. Int J Dermatol 2007; 46: 1198–204.

A follow-up study in 28 patients treated with infliximab for severe recalcitrant psoriasis: evidence for efficacy and high incidence of biological autoimmunity. Poulalhon N, Begon E, Lebbé C, Lioté F, Lahfa M, Bengoufa D, et al. Br J Dermatol 2007; 156: 329–36.

This group had five patients with erythrodermic psoriasis (median PASI score 54, range 48–72) treated with infliximab 5 mg/kg given at weeks 0, 2, 6, and every 8 weeks thereafter. Three of the five patients reached PASI improvement of 75% or more.

Infliximab, as sole or combined therapy, induces rapid clearing of erythrodermic psoriasis. Takahashi MD, Castro LG, Romiti R. Br J Dermatol 2007; 157: 828–31.

Efficacy of infliximab in patients with moderate and severe psoriasis treated with infliximab (Remicade). Valdés A, Mdel P, Schroeder HF, Roizen GV, Honeyman MJ, Sánchez ML. Rev Med Clin 2006; 134: 326–31.

An open prospective study including eight patients with extensive plaque or erythrodermic psoriasis who were treated with infliximab 5 mg/kg on weeks 0, 2, and 6. Evaluation with physical examination, PASI scores and photographs was done every 2 weeks. All the patients responded in the first 10 weeks. The mean reduction in PASI score was 86.6%.

Successful treatment of recalcitrant, erythroderma-associated pruritus with etanercept. Querfeld C, Guitart J, Kuzel TM, Rosen S. Arch Dermatol 2004; 140: 1539–40.

Psoriatic erythroderma treated with etanercept. Piqué-Duran E, Pérez-Cejudo JA. Actas Dermosifiliogr 2007; 98: 508–10.

Alefacept in the treatment of recalcitrant palmoplantar and erythrodermic psoriasis. Prossick TA, Belsito DV. Cutis 2006; 78: 178–80.

A report of two patients with recalcitrant psoriasis who responded completely to a course of alefacept. Alefacept provides another treatment option in the management of erythrodermic psoriasis.

Successful treatment of chemotherapy-refractory Sézary syndrome with alemtuzumab (Campath-1H). Gautschi O, Blumenthal N, Streit M, Solenthaler M, Hunziker T, Zenhausern R. Eur J Haematol 2004; 72: 61–3.

A 32-year-old man had advanced-stage extensively pre-treated Sézary syndrome with very pruritic erythroderma that had not responded to PUVA or interferon-α and which progressed on chemotherapy. Following treatment with alemtuzumab (30 mg intravenously three times weekly for 10 weeks) the itching resolved rapidly and almost complete remission was achieved within 3 months of starting this treatment.

Phase 2 study of alemtuzumab (anti-CD52 monoclonal antibody) in patients with advanced mycosis fungoides/Sézary syndrome. Lundin J, Hagberg H, Repp R, Cavallin-Stahl E, Freden S, Juliusson G, et al. Blood 2003; 101: 4267–71.

This study evaluated the efficacy and safety of alemtuzumab in 22 patients. Clinical responses were recorded in more than 50% of patients with advanced mycosis fungoides/Sézary syndrome with a preference for erythrodermic versus plaque/tumor stage of disease.

Novel treatment of Sézary-like syndrome due to adult T-cell leukaemia/lymphoma with daclizumab (humanized anti-interleukin-2 receptor alpha antibody). Osborne GE, Pagliuca A, Ho A, du Vivier AW. Br J Dermatol 2006; 15: 617–20.

A patient with erythrodermic T-cell leukaemia/lymphoma resistant to multiple therapies developed a rapid and sustained complete response to daclizumab, which suggests significant activity of anti-IL2 receptor-α antibody in this disease process.

The treatment of cutaneous T-cell lymphoma with a novel retinoid. Heald P. Clin Lymphoma 2000; 1: S45–9.

Four patients with erythrodermic CTCL were treated with high-dose oral bexarotene and all showed rapid (within 2 weeks) improvement of erythroderma.

Optimizing bexarotene therapy for cutaneous T-cell lymphoma. Talpur R, Ward S, Apisarnthanarax N, Breuer-Mcham J, Duvic M. J Am Acad Dermatol 2002; 47: 672–84.

Oral bexarotene in a therapy-resistant Sézary syndrome patient: observations on Sézary cell compartmentalization. el-Azhary RA, Bouwhuis SA. Int J Dermatol 2005; 44: 25–8.

A 63-year-old man with therapy-resistant Sézary syndrome was enrolled in a multicenter trial of oral bexarotene for advanced-stage cutaneous T-cell lymphoma (CTCL). A gradual improvement in erythema, pruritus, and scale was noted during the trial period. From weeks 20 to 40 the erythroderma continued to improve and the lymph node burden decreased, but the absolute Sézary cell count increased inversely. By week 40, intractable pruritus and erythroderma abruptly recurred. Bexarotene can be efficacious in patients with Sézary syndrome, but Sézary cells can shift between different compartments.

Evidence Levels: **A** Double-blind study **B** Clinical trial ≥ 20 subjects **C** Clinical trial < 20 subjects **D** Series ≥ 5 subjects **E** Anecdotal case reports

Erythrokeratodermas

Gabriele Richard

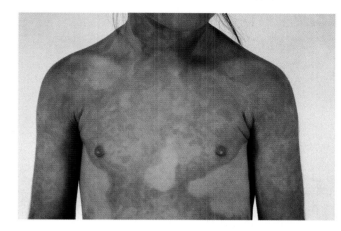

Erythrokeratodermas are a clinically and genetically hetero-geneous group of rare inherited disorders of cornification characterized by two distinct morphologic features: local-ized hyperkeratosis and erythema. The hallmark of erythro-keratodermia variabilis (EKV) is the seemingly independent occurrence of transient, figurate erythema and hyperkerato-sis, which can be localized or generalized. Progressive symmetric erythrokeratoderma (PSEK) is characterized by fixed, slowly progressive, symmetric and well-defined hyper-keratotic plaques with underlying erythema, predominantly on the extensor surface of the extremities, on the trunk, and on the face.

MANAGEMENT STRATEGY

Erythrokeratodermas are heritable, chronic disorders that often require lifelong treatment. Management depends on the severity and extent of hyperkeratosis, which may vary over time and from patient to patient. The spectrum may range from fixed hyperkeratotic plaques over the knees and elbows to generalized hyperkeratosis with accentuated skin mark-ings and peeling, or thickened plates with a spiny, hystrix-like appearance.

The *topical management* of erythrokeratodermas is often dis-appointing but remains a therapeutic cornerstone. Topical treatment of patients with mild, localized hyperkeratosis is symptomatic and focuses on hydration, lubrication, and keratolysis. Whereas in some patients *emollients* such as pet-rolatum twice daily may suffice, most patients require topi-cal treatment with *keratolytic agents*. Lactic acid (6–12%) and urea applied once or twice daily in combination with emol-lients are effective, although their use may be limited, espe-cially in children, because of irritation. Other α-hydroxy acids, salicylic acid (3–6%), propylene glycol, glycolic acid (11%), topical vitamin D analogs, or combinations of these are alter-native treatment options. Topical treatment with *retinoids* and derivatives has been successful in some patients (especially with EKV) but ineffective in others. Regimens with newer syn-thetic retinoids, such as short-contact topical tazarotene ther-apy combined with moisturizers, seems promising in EKV.

In addition, avoidance of trauma to the skin, such as sudden temperature changes, friction, and mechanical irritation, may be beneficial.

Systemic retinoids are the treatment of choice in erythroker-atodermas with extensive or generalized skin involvement. Although they are highly effective in EKV, the therapeutic response in PSEK is less satisfactory. As is the case for other disorders of cornification, the effects of acitretin or etretinate are superior to those of systemic isotretinoin. It seems advan-tageous to start at low doses of acitretin for 3–6 weeks, and then to gradually increase the dose until the desired therapeu-tic effect is achieved. The minimal effective maintenance dose for patients with EKV is usually lower than for patients with PSEK. Both morphologic components respond well to reti-noid treatment, resulting in rapid and dramatic improvement or clearing of the hyperkeratosis and significant moderation of the erythema. In some patients with EKV the erythematous component may be completely suppressed. Nevertheless, the use of retinoids should always be considered carefully, as chronic therapy is required to achieve continuing results, and long-term side effects, especially in children, may ensue. In some cases, intermittent cycles of systemic retinoid treatment may be considered to balance between beneficial therapeutic and adverse effects. Anecdotally, *PUVA therapy* has been ben-eficial in the treatment of PSEK.

The variable erythema in EKV often results in cosmetic con-cerns, which can be limited by masking uncovered skin with makeup and camouflage. Serious discomfort due to burning and pruritus, which may accompany the variable erythema in some patients, can be therapeutically challenging. If systemic aromatic retinoid therapy alone fails to reduce or suppress erythema and the associated burning and itching sensations, symptomatic relief has been achieved in anecdotal cases with systemic therapy using sedating H_1-antihistamines.

SPECIFIC INVESTIGATIONS

> ▶ Family history
> ▶ Histopathology

Family study of erythrokeratodermia figurata variabilis. Itin P, Levy CA, Sommacal-Schopf D, Schnyder UW. Hautarzt 1992; 43: 500–4.

Thorough studies in a large five-generation EKV family with 29 affected individuals revealed valuable clinical data on age of onset, relationship between erythema and hyperkeratosis, precipitating factors, frequency of palmoplantar involvement, and natural history of EKV.

Erythrokeratoderma progressiva symmetrica: report of 10 cases. Ruiz-Maldonado R, Tamayo L, del Castillo V, Lozoya I. Dermatologica 1982; 164: 133–41.

A clinical investigation of 10 patients with PSEK, six of whom belonged to three families with autosomal dominant inheritance, two were sporadic cases, and two were the product of consanguineous unions, suggesting an autosomal recessive inheritance. Eight patients were treated conventionally with topical keratolytics with moderate results, but two patients achieved complete remission with systemic retinoids.

Mutations in the human connexin gene *GJB3* cause erythro-keratodermia variabilis. Richard G, Smith LE, Bailey RA, Itin P, Hohl D, Epstein EH Jr, et al. Nature Genet 1998; 20: 366–9.

Disease-causing missense mutations in the connexin gene *GJB3*, which is localized on chromosome 1p35.1 and encodes the gap junction protein β-3 (connexin-31, Cx31), were identified in four families with EKV. The study provided evidence that intercellular communication mediated by gap junctions is crucial for epidermal differentiation and response to external factors.

Mutation in the gene for connexin 30.3 in a family with erythrokeratodermia variabilis. Macari F, Landau M, Cousin P, Mevorah B, Brenner S, Panizzon R, et al. Am J Hum Genet 2000; 67: 1296–301.

Report of a pathogenic mutation in the connexin gene *GJB4*, encoding Cx30.3, in an extended EKV family. The data suggest that EKV is genetically heterogeneous and may be caused by mutations in at least two structurally and functionally related connexin genes.

Genetic heterogeneity in erythrokeratodermia variabilis: novel mutations in the connexin gene *GJB4* (Cx30.3) and genotype–phenotype correlations. Richard G, Brown N, Rouan F, Van der Schroeff JG, Bijlsma E, Eichenfield LF, et al. J Invest Dermatol 2003; 120: 601–9.

In a large cohort of patients these authors identified six different missense mutations of *GJB4* (Cx30.3) in five families and one sporadic case of EKV. In two families these mutations were associated with the occurrence of rapidly changing erythematous patches with prominent, circinate, or gyrate borders, suggesting that this feature is specific to Cx30.3 defects.

A novel recessive connexin 31 (GJB3) mutation in a case of erythrokeratodermia variabilis. Terrinoni A, Leta A, Pedicelli C, Candi E, Ranalli M, Puddu P, et al. J Invest Dermatol 2004; 122: 837–9.

Report of a consanguineous family in which EKV is not transmitted as an autosomal dominant trait but in an unusual autosomal recessive manner. The 16-year-old proband showed almost complete remission of hyperkeratosis after 2 months of systemic acitretin therapy (20 mg/day), without improvement of erythema.

FIRST-LINE THERAPIES

▶ Emollients	E
▶ Topical keratolytics	E
▶ Topical retinoids	E
▶ Acitretin (for some patients)*	C
▶ Isotretinoin (for some patients)*	E

*Note, some patients, especially those with extensive or generalized skin involvement, have a great benefit from low doses of *systemic retinoids*, so a trial should be considered as a first line of treatment.

Other topical medications. Burkhart CN, Katz KA. In: Wolff K, Goldsmith LA, Katz SI, Gilchrest BA, Paller AS, Leffell DJ, eds. Fitzpatrick's dermatology in general medicine, 7th edn. New York: McGraw-Hill, 2008; 2130–7.

A summary of topical keratolytic agents and applications.

Topical retinoids. Kang S, Voorhees JJ. In: Wolff K, Goldsmith LA, Katz SI, Gilchrest BA, Paller AS, Leffell DJ, eds. Fitzpatrick's dermatology in general medicine, 7th edn. New York: McGraw-Hill, 2008; 2106–13.

An in-depth summary of topical retinoids, their mechanism, clinical use, dosage, and adverse effects.

Erythrokeratodermia variabilis successfully treated with topical tazarotene. Yoo S, Simzar S, Han K, Takahashi S, Cotliar R. Pediatr Dermatol 2006; 23: 382–5.

Topical short-contact (15 minutes) treatment with tazarotene gel once a day followed by the application of a topical corticosteroid (fluocinolone oil) on moist skin and hydrophilic ointments resulted in complete remission of hyperkeratotic plaques and erythematous patches in a 16-month-old child with EKV within 1 month. Emollients were continued during quiescent periods, and the above regimen during flares.

Erythrokeratodermia variabilis. Report of 3 clinical cases and evaluation of the topical retinoic acid treatment. Lacerda e Costa MH, de Brito Caldeira J. Med Cutan Ibero Lat Am 1975; 3: 281–7.

Topical retinoic acid (0.1% cream) treatment of three patients with EKV substantially reduced hyperkeratosis. Discontinuation resulted in prompt relapse.

SECOND-LINE THERAPIES

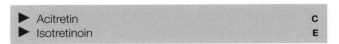

▶ Acitretin	C
▶ Isotretinoin	E

Acitretin in the treatment of erythrokeratodermia variabilis. van de Kerkhof PC, Steijlen PM, van Dooren-Greebe RJ, Happle R. Dermatologica 1990; 181: 330–3.

A patient with EKV had been successfully treated for 3 years with etretinate (on average 25 mg daily), although subsequent therapy with isotretinoin (20 mg daily) for 2 years was less efficient. Systemic therapy with acitretin at an initial dose of 35 mg daily for 8 weeks, reduced to a maintenance dose of 25–35 mg daily, resulted in a striking and sustained clinical improvement and reduced hyperkeratosis and dermal inflammation on histologic skin evaluation.

Compared to the other retinoids, acitretin was found to elicit similar effects as etretinate at lower initial doses, and thus was regarded as the first choice in treatment of EKV.

Clinical and genetic heterogeneity of erythrokeratodermia variabilis. Common JEA, O'Toole EA, Leigh IM, Thomas A, Griffiths WAD, Venning V, et al. J Invest Dermatol 2005; 125: 920–7.

Four of six EKV patients had a reportedly good to excellent response to oral acitretin when treated with 0.125–0.25 mg/kg/day. Two of these patients cleared completely, one on 20 mg acitretin daily. The remaining patients had residual hyperkeratosis, especially on the legs.

Acitretin for erythrokeratodermia variabilis in a 9-year-old girl. Graham-Brown RAC, Chave TA. Pediatr Dermatol 2002; 19: 510–12.

Oral treatment with acitretin 1 mg/kg daily resulted in complete clearing of the skin within 3 weeks. This positive therapeutic effect could be maintained with a reduced dose of 0.66 mg/kg daily.

A new type of erythrokeratoderma. van Steensel MAM, van Geel M, Steijlen PM. Br J Dermatol 2005; 152: 155–8.

A patient with static symmetrical pink keratoderma on the extremities with digital constriction bands, and palmoplantar keratoderma treated with 1 mg/kg acitretin responded with satisfactory reduction of hyperkeratosis.

Evidence Levels: **A** Double-blind study **B** Clinical trial ≥ 20 subjects **C** Clinical trial < 20 subjects **D** Series ≥ 5 subjects **E** Anecdotal case reports

[Erythrokeratodermia variabilis (EKV)-A disorder due to altered epidermal expression of gap junction proteins.] Ständer S, Stadelmann A, Traub O, Traupe H, Metze D. J Dtsch Dermatol Ges 2005; 3: 354–8. (in German)

Within 2 weeks, oral treatment with acitretin 25 mg daily combined with topical emollients and keratolytics (urea) resulted in a remarkable improvement of hyperkeratosis and erythema in a 48-year-old man. Complete clearing was achieved with 25 mg acitretin every third day for another 3 weeks. Discontinuation led to prompt relapse.

Erythrokeratodermia variabilis with adult onset: Report of a sporadic case unresponsive to systemic retinoids. Erbagci Z, Tuncel AA, Deniz H. J Dermatol Treat 2006; 17: 187–9.

An unusual case with onset of fixed erythrokeratoderma at 23 years of age. Topical steroids, topical PUVA for 3 months, and keratolytics (10% salicylic acid) did not yield satisfactory results. Subsequent systemic isotretinoin (0.7 mg/kg/day) combined with topical ointments containing 20% urea did not show improvement after 3 months. Acitretin (0.5 mg/kg/day) for 5 months also did not achieve a significant therapeutic response. However, sedating oral H_1-antihistamines were beneficial for relief of pruritus.

[Erythrokeratodermia progressiva symmetrica Darier–Gottron with generalized expression]. Emmert S, Küster W, Schauder S, Neumann C, Rünger TM. Hautarzt 1998; 49: 666–71. (In German.)

Two patients of a family with PSEK responded very well to oral treatment with acitretin. One was treated with 0.4 mg/kg daily for 3 months and showed improvement of hyperkeratosis even 3 months after discontinuation. The other patient required only intermittent therapy, twice a year, with acitretin 10 mg daily for 2 weeks.

Oral retinoid (Ro 10–9359) in children with lamellar ichthyosis, epidermolytic hyperkeratosis and symmetrical progressive erythrokeratoderma. Tamayo L, Ruiz-Maldonado R. Dermatologica 1980; 161: 305–14.

Five children with PSEK demonstrated dramatic improvement under systemic therapy with etretinate. Treatment was considered efficient and tolerable, with manageable side effects.

Etretinate is the prodrug of acitretin, which is its active metabolite.

Progressive symmetric erythrokeratodermia. Histological and ultrastructural study of patient before and after treatment with etretinate. Nazzaro V, Blanchet-Bardon C. Arch Dermatol 1986; 122: 434–40.

Treatment of a PSEK patient with etretinate diminished hyperkeratotic plaques and reduced mitochondrial swelling in granulocytes as well as the number of lipid-like vacuoles in corneocytes observed by electron microscopy.

Oral synthetic retinoid treatment in children. DiGiovanna JJ, Peck GL. Pediatr Dermatol 1983; 1: 77–88.

In one patient with EKV marked improvement was achieved with oral isotretinoin therapy. Side effects, toxicity, and therapeutic guidelines of retinoid therapy are discussed.

Retinoids. Vahlquist A, Kuenzli S, Saurat J-H. In: Wolff K, Goldsmith LA, Katz SI, Gillchrest BA, Paller AS, Leffell DJ, eds. Fitzpatrick's dermatology in general medicine, 7th edn. New York: McGraw-Hill, 2008; 2181–6.

An extensive review of the pharmacology, use, and toxicity of retinoids.

THIRD-LINE THERAPIES

▶ PUVA   E
▶ H_1-antihistamines   E

[Gottron's erythroderma congenitalis progressiva symmetrica]. Levi L, Beneggi M, Crippa D, Sala GP. Hautarzt 1982; 33: 605–8. (In German.)

In one family with PSEK an adult patient was treated with an aromatic retinoid for 8 weeks, while her child received PUVA therapy for a total of 63 J/cm² UVA. Both treatments were effective and reduced hyperkeratosis, but PUVA achieved superior results.

Erythrokeratodermia variabilis: case report and review of literature. Papadavid E, Koumantaki E, Dawber RPR. J Eur Acad Dermatol Venereol 1998; 11: 180–3.

A good therapeutic response to systemic etretinate with initial dosage of 25 mg/day and maintenance dosage of 10 mg/day. Regular use of an oral H_1-antihistamine was helpful in controlling the pruritus associated with the erythematous component of EKV.

Erythromelalgia

Cato Mørk, Knut Kvernebo

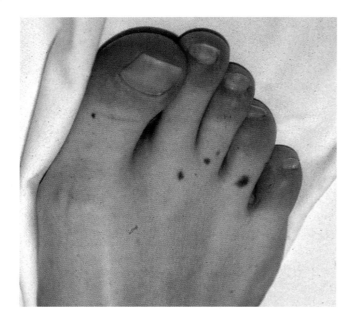

Erythromelalgia (*erythros* – redness; *melos* – extremity; *algos* – pain) is a symptom complex characterized by burning extremity pain, erythema, and increased temperature of the affected skin. Pain is aggravated by warming and relieved by cooling. The symptoms and findings are usually intermittent and often missing during examination. Between attacks acrocyanosis, pernio, and Raynaud phenomenon may occur. The severity of symptoms varies from mild discomfort (most common) to disabling pain and gangrene. In daily clinical work the terms mild, moderate, and severe may be useful. The diagnosis is often missed in cases with mild symptoms, whereas severe erythromelalgia is a rare condition.

MANAGEMENT STRATEGY

The criteria for applying the diagnosis erythromelalgia are based purely on symptoms and signs. There is growing evidence that symptoms can be triggered either by primary microvascular events, or by a primary autonomic nervous dysfunction. The final common pathway of the pathogenesis is in both cases maldistribution of skin perfusion with arteriovenous shunt flow through anatomical or functional microvascular anastomoses, leading to increased thermoregulatory perfusion and a relative lack of nutritive perfusion, with corresponding skin hypoxia.

Acute disease has a tendency to improve, whereas chronic disease tends to have a stable course. Spontaneous remissions have occurred without treatment.

The treatment strategy depends on the patient's medical history. The wide spectrum of published approaches to management reflects the heterogeneity in etiology, and there is a lack of properly documented treatment regimens. There is a marked interindividual variation in therapeutic response. Only two controlled clinical trials have been published. The main reason may be the low prevalence, the heterogeneity of patients, and the lack of laboratory diagnostic methods. Healthcare professionals and patients can obtain information about the management of erythromelalgia from The Erythromelalgia Association (TEA, www.erythromelalgia.org).

All patients benefit from *local skin cooling* (applying cold towels or wet sand, walking on cold floors or even in the snow, air-conditioned rooms, or immersion in cooled water) and from *elevation of the affected limb*. Comfortable shoes to relieve pressure over the soles can help. *Aggravating factors such as warmth, exercise, dependency of the extremity, tight shoes and gloves, and alcohol intake in some cases, should be avoided.*

Familial erythromelalgia is a rare disorder where recent studies in a few cases have demonstrated a dysfunction of sensory and sympathetic neurons, with a dominant mode of inheritance caused by a mutation in SCN9A encoding for the Nav 1.7 channel, a voltage-gated sodium channel. The mutation causes hyperexcitability in sensory neurons and hypoexcitability in sympathetic efferent neurons. *Underlying diseases (secondary erythromelalgia), such as myeloproliferative, connective tissue, cardiovascular, infectious and neurological diseases, diabetes mellitus, vasculitis, and neoplasia should be sought and optimally treated.* Drug-induced erythromelalgia has been reported secondary to substances that may alter vasomotor tone, such as calcium channel blockers, bromocriptine, norepinephrine (noradrenaline), pergolide, ticlopidine, ciclosporin, iodine contrast, mushroom, and mercury poisoning.

No single medication or treatment modality has been universally helpful. Before beginning a treatment regimen, the patient's condition should be classified according to whether it is primary or secondary, the etiology (for secondary cases), and its severity. Analgesics, including opiate analgesics, have limited effect. A few patients become free of symptoms with small doses of *acetylsalicylic acid*. Numerous drugs have been used with varying success. Case reports or series of patients have shown beneficial effect with *vasodilators* (prostaglandin E$_1$/prostacyclin or analogs, sodium nitroprusside, naftidrofuryl). Other drugs that may be of benefit are *antidepressants*, *anticonvulsants*, and *anesthetic agents*. Calcium channel blockers may help some, but exacerbate others.

Numerous treatment alternatives based on single case reports are presented in the literature. Anecdotally, nitroglycerin ointment, capsaicin cream, ketanserin, methysergide, pizotifen, β-blockers, cyproheptadine or other antihistamines, carbamazepine, clonazepam, corticosteroids or other immunosuppressants, hyperbaric oxygen treatment, pentoxifylline, phenoxybenzamine, opiates, spinal cord stimulation, thalamic stimulation, biofeedback, epidural blocks, transcutaneous electrical nerve stimulation, sympathectomy, phenoxybenzamine, prazosin, and hypnotherapy have been presented as effective. Anecdotal reports from surveys of members from TEA demonstrate more than 50 therapies. From our personal experience with 160 patients with erythromelalgia, and based on extensive studies of pathophysiology, we believe that vasoconstrictor therapy (norepinephrine, epinephrine) and sympathectomy may exacerbate symptoms and should not be given, although there are some positive reports in the literature.

Evidence Levels: **A** Double-blind study **B** Clinical trial ≥ 20 subjects **C** Clinical trial < 20 subjects **D** Series ≥ 5 subjects **E** Anecdotal case reports

SPECIFIC INVESTIGATIONS

▶ Exclude erythromelalgia secondary to hematologic, metabolic, connective tissue, cardiovascular, infectious, neurological, musculoskeletal, or neoplastic diseases
▶ Drug history of exposure to calcium channel blockers, bromocriptine, vasoconstrictors, norepinephrine, pergolide, ticlopidine, ciclosporin, iodine contrast, mushroom, mercury
▶ Full blood count with white cell differential count
▶ Serum chemistry, including blood sugar
▶ Antinuclear antibody, RA latex

Erythromelalgia: a clinical study of 87 cases. Kalgaard OM, Seem E, Kvernebo K. J Intern Med 1997; 242: 191–7.

The classification, etiology, and prognosis of erythromelalgia are presented. The findings in this paper are the main basis for the proposed investigations.

Primary erythermalgia as a sodium channelopathy: screening for SCN9A mutations: exclusion of a causal role of SCN10A and SCN11A. Drenth JP, Te Morsche RH, Mansour S, Mortimer PS. Arch Dermatol 2008; 144: 320–4.

Platelet-mediated erythromelalgic, cerebral, ocular and coronary microvascular ischemic and thrombotic manifestations in patients with essential thrombocythemia and polycythemia vera: a distinct aspirin-responsive and coumadin-resistant arterial thrombophilia. Michiels JJ, Berneman Z, Schroyens W, Koudstaal PJ, Lindemans J, Neumann HA, et al. Platelets 2006; 17: 528–44.

Erythromelalgia – a thrombotic complication in chronic myeloproliferative disorders. Tarach JS, Nowicka-Tarach BM, Matuszek B, Nowakowski A. Med Sci Monit 2000; 6: 204–8.

Erythromelalgia is seen secondary to platelet aggregation and peripheral microvascular occlusion in myeloproliferative disorders and, untreated, may progress to painful acrocyanosis and even peripheral gangrene. Remission is observed after treatment of the myeloproliferative disorder.

Verapamil-induced erythermalgia. Nanayakkara PWB, van der Veldt AAM, Simsek S, Smulders YM, Rauwerda JA. Neth J Med 2007; 65: 349–51.

FIRST-LINE THERAPIES

▶ Treatment of underlying disease   **C**
▶ Cooling   **C**
▶ Aspirin   **D**
▶ Prostaglandins/prostacyclin or oral analogs   **A**

Several accompanying diseases, conditions, and pharmacological substances have been described as associated with erythromelalgia. A beneficial effect on the symptoms of erythromelalgia after successful treatment or elimination of the primary condition indicates a causal relationship.

Immersion of an affected limb in cold water or exposure to cold air will make patients feel better for a limited time. Moderation in cooling time and temperature is important. Soak the affected extremity in cooled instead of iced water to avoid immersion foot,

frostbite, maceration and ulceration of the skin, infection, and reactive flaring. Cooling of the skin induces microvascular stasis and may in the long term increase arteriovenous shunting.

Aspirin-responsive painful red, black toe, or finger syndrome in polycythemia vera associated with thrombocythemia. Michiels JJ, Berneman Z, Schroyens W, van Urk H. Ann Hematol 2003; 82: 153–9.

Aspirin 250–500 mg daily or less may completely abolish the symptoms in erythromelalgia secondary to myeloproliferative conditions. The response is probably due to the antiplatelet effect. A reduction of platelet numbers by cytostatic treatment may also lead to relief.

The Erythromelalgia Association Survey 2003. www. erythromelalgia.org.

In a survey, 128 respondents had used aspirin (80–250 mg daily) – four reported complete, 17 moderate, and 22 minimal relief; 78 had no improvement, and six reported worsening of their symptoms.

Aspirin should be tried in all EM patients without contraindications.

Erythromelalgia – a condition caused by microvascular arteriovenous shunting. Kvernebo K. VASA 1998; 27: 3–39.

Based on the hypothesis of arteriovenous shunting, prostaglandin E_1 (PGE_1) and prostacyclin were tried as an intravenous infusion to enhance nutritive skin perfusion in severe erythromelalgia. Nine of 10 patients benefited from PGE_1 given as a continuous infusion for 3 days, starting with 6, then 10, and finally 12 ng/kg/min. Two children were cured (observation time >15 years), and the others had remission from 3 months to 2 years.

Prostacyclin reduces symptoms and sympathetic dysfunction in erythromelalgia in a double-blind randomized pilot study. Kalgaard OM, Mørk C, Kvernebo K. Acta Dermatol Venereol 2003; 83: 442–4.

For the first time in a double-blind, randomized study, reduced symptoms and sympathetic dysfunction were demonstrated. Eight patents were treated with prostacyclin infusion and four with placebo infusion.

The prostaglandin E1 analog misoprostol reduces symptoms and microvascular arteriovenous shunting in erythromelalgia – a double-blind, crossover, placebo-compared study. Mørk C, Salerud EG, Asker CL, Kvernebo K. J Invest Dermatol 2004; 122: 587–93.

This first properly designed placebo-controlled clinical trial for the treatment of erythromelalgia demonstrated that oral misoprostol (0.4–0.8 mg/day) reduced symptoms significantly more than placebo. Misoprostol is recommended as first-line treatment, although many patients do not respond.

SECOND-LINE THERAPIES

▶ Anesthetic agents (lidocaine, mexiletine, bupivacaine)   **C**
▶ Gabapentin   **D**
▶ Serotonin–noradrenalin reuptake inhibitors (venlafaxine, sertraline)   **D**
▶ Sodium nitroprusside   **D**

Primary erythromelalgia in a child responding to intravenous lidocaine and oral mexiletine treatment. Nathan A, Rose JB, Guite JW, Hehir D, Milovcich K. Pediatrics 2005; 1115: 504–7.

A single case.

Lidocaine patch for pain of erythromelalgia: Follow-up of 34 patients. Davis MD, Sandroni P. Arch Dermatol 2005; 141: 1320–1.

Anesthetic agents (lidocaine, bupivacaine, mexiletin) that block the sodium channels may be used topically, intravenously, orally, epidurally, or intrathecally. A 90% reduction in pain was demonstrated with lidocaine IV infusion, but hospitalization is required. A 5% lidocaine patch for 12 hours/day was found helpful as first-line and adjunctive treatment of severely affected patients with erythromelalgia. Sixteen patients had no improvement, but 18 patients had a 5–90% improvement in pain score.

The treatment of erythromelalgia. Cohen JS. February 2007. http://www.erythromelalgia.org/tea/skins/cms/viewarea. php?id=244.

The TEA survey report 5% complete relief and 54% moderate or minimal relief of EM symptoms with gabapentin (n=127). The treatment is safe and generally well tolerated, and can be combined with other drugs. A low starting dose increasing to 300–400 mg three times a day for 3 months is recommended. Venlafaxine may act on sympathetic fibers by inhibiting reuptake of serotoinin and norepinephrine in the brain and in the periphery. Thirteen cases with beneficial effects have been reported in the literature. A mild to moderate effect is reported in around 50% of the users in the TEA survey (n=50).

Serotonin is a vasoactive substance that may cause vasodilatation.

Gabapentin for the treatment of familial erythromelalgia pain. Pandey CK, Singh N, Singh PK. J Assoc Phys India 2002; 50; 1094.

Alleviation of erythromelalagia with venlafaxine. DiCaudio DJ, Kelley LA. Arch Dermatol 2004; 146: 621–3

Treatment of familial erythromelalgia with venlafaxine. Firmin D, Roduedas AM, Greco M, Morvan C, Legoupil D, Fleuret C, Misery L. J Eur Acad Dermatol Venereol 2007; 21: 836–7.

Combination gel of 1% amitriptyline and 0.5% ketamine to treat refractory erythromelalgia pain: a new treatment option? Sandroni P, Davis MD. Arch Dermatol 2006; 142: 283–6.

Effect reported in five patients.

Erythromelalgia – a condition caused by microvascular arteriovenous shunting. Kvernebo K. VASA 1998; 27: 3–39.

Sodium nitroprusside intravenously for 7 days in increasing doses (1, 3, and 5 μg/kg/min) was successful in two patients with severe erythromelalgia. Microvascular perfusion measurements documented the effect.

Erythromelalgia: an endothelial disorder responsive to sodium nitroprusside. Chak MK, Tucker AT, Madden S, Golding CE, Atherton DJ, Dillon MJ. Arch Dis Child 2002; 87; 229–30.

Pain relief in two children was reported.

THIRD-LINE THERAPIES

▶ Calcium antagonists	C
▶ Magnesium	C

Erythromelalgia: new theories and new therapies. Cohen JS. J Am Acad Dermatol 2000; 43: 841–7.

Various calcium channel blockers may be helpful in about 25% of patients with erythromelalgia (n=43). As they can cause or exacerbate symptoms, they should be used with caution and with the use of short-acting drugs initially. They are frequently used, but documentation for beneficial effect is sparse (six of 14 patients). Their mechanism of action may be smooth muscle relaxation and reduced vascular responses elicited by β_2-adrenoceptors.

High-dose oral magnesium treatment of chronic, intractable erythromelalgia. Cohen JS. Ann Pharmacother 2002; 36: 255–60.

Magnesium is a naturally occurring calcium channel blocker. Intravenous magnesium has also been reported to be effective in neuropathic pain. Eight of 13 patients reported improvement, four no response, and one deterioration using magnesium in various doses (up to 1000 mg/day) and forms.

The treatment of erythromelalgia. Cohen JS. February 2007. http://www.erythromelalgia.org/tea/skins/cms/viewarea. php?id=244.

Erythromelalgia. Davis MD, Rooke T. Current Treatment Opinions in Cardiovascular Medicine 2006; 8: 153–65.

Evidence Levels: **A** Double-blind study **B** Clinical trial ≥ 20 subjects **C** Clinical trial < 20 subjects **D** Series ≥ 5 subjects **E** Anecdotal case reports

Erythropoietic protoporphyria

Maureen B Poh-Fitzpatrick

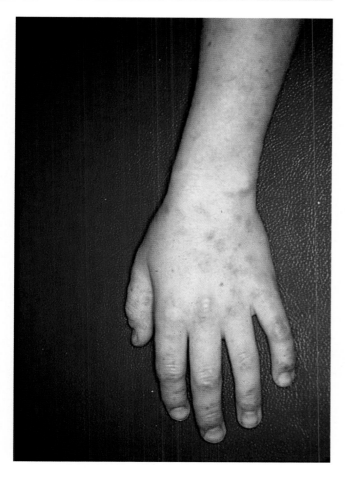

In this metabolic disorder a genetically determined deficiency of ferrochelatase enzyme activity in bone marrow erythroid cells causes abnormally high protoporphyrin levels in erythrocytes, plasma, liver, bile, and feces. Protoporphyrin is a photoactive intermediary of heme synthesis; exposure of protoporphyrin in the skin to long UV or visible light radiation can elicit oxygen-dependent acute cutaneous phototoxicity. Protoporphyrin undergoes hepatobiliary excretion, leading to cholelithiasis. Clinically evident porphyrin hepatotoxicity may develop, and may progress to irreversible liver failure. Hypochromic microcytic anemia, when present, is typically mild and rarely requires treatment.

MANAGEMENT STRATEGY

Protoporphyric photosensitivity is rarely managed adequately by *sun avoidance* alone (i.e. lifestyle changes, protective clothing, physical barriers). *Topical sunscreens* containing *titanium dioxide, zinc oxide, iron oxide,* or *dihydroxyacetone* block or filter long UV and visible light spectra, offering limited relief.

Epidermal melanization and hyperplasia achieved with *UVB* or *psoralen plus UVA (PUVA) phototherapy* increase sunlight tolerance. Oral agents believed to photoprotect by quenching excited oxygen species include *β-carotene, cysteine, vitamin E, vitamin C, flavonoids,* and possibly *pyridoxine. Antihistamines* may attenuate phototoxic flaring. Gallstones are managed *surgically.* Exacerbators of protoporphyrin-induced hepatotoxicity (alcohol, cholestatic drugs, dietary carbohydrate restriction) are best avoided. *Vaccination* against hepatitis A and B is recommended. Deteriorating liver function is only sporadically reversible by *enteric sorbents (cholestyramine, activated charcoal)* that interrupt enterohepatic porphyrin circulation, *bile acids* (to stimulate biliary protoporphyrin secretion), *blood transfusion or exchange, hematin infusion,* or *glucose loading* (to retard endogenous porphyrinogenesis), *iron* (to increase protoporphyrin conversion to heme), or various combinations thereof. It is postulated that *cimetidine* inhibits porphyrinogenesis. End-stage liver disease warrants *liver transplantation,* aided by measures to reduce pre-, intra- and postoperative porphyrin levels (*exchange transfusion, hematin infusion, plasmapheresis, vitamin E*). Operating room lamps should be filtered to exclude wavelengths that can severely damage porphyrin-photosensitized skin and internal organs. *Bone marrow transplantation* has been curative in highly selected cases, and would be optimal prophylaxis against protoporphyric hepatopathy in original or transplanted livers.

SPECIFIC INVESTIGATIONS

> ► Porphyrin analyses in erythrocytes, serum or plasma, urine, feces
> ► Hematological profile, iron studies if anemic
> ► Liver function profile, liver imaging and biopsy or non-invasive fibrosis assessment as clinically indicated

Erythropoietic protoporphyria. Todd DJ. Br J Dermatol 1994; 131: 751–66.

An excellent review of clinical, laboratory, genetic, and therapeutic aspects of the disease.

Hepatobiliary implications and complications in protoporphyria. A 20-year study. Doss MO, Frank M. Clin Biochem 1989; 22: 223–9.

Among 55 patients with protoporphyria, impaired liver function occurred in 19, cirrhosis in seven, and fatal liver failure in two. Coproporphyrinuria appeared early in the course of progressive protoporphyric hepatotoxicity.

Liver failure occurs in <5% of all cases. Because in uncomplicated protoporphyria the urine is typically free of excess porphyrins, surveillance for coproporphyrinuria may identify patients with asymptomatic hepatic dysfunction.

FIRST-LINE THERAPIES

> ► Topical sunscreens, physical barriers   **C**
> ► β-Carotene   **B**

Efficiency of opaque photoprotective agents in the visible light range. Kaye ET, Levin JA, Blank IH, Arndt KA, Anderson RR. Arch Dermatol 1991; 127: 351–5.

Iron oxide increases the light-blocking efficacy and cosmetic acceptability of 'white paste' sunscreens containing zinc oxide or titanium dioxide.

Erythropoietic protoporphyria: IV. Protection from sunlight. Fusaro RM, Runge WJ. Br Med J 1970; 1: 730–1.

Seven patients had prolonged sunlight tolerance after applying a 3% dihydroxyacetone and 0.13% lawsone skin cream causing brown coloration of the stratum corneum.

Many 'sunless tanning' formulations contain dihydroxyacetone.

Beta-carotene therapy for erythropoietic protoporphyria and other photosensitivity diseases. Mathews-Roth MM, Pathak MA, Fitzpatrick TB, Harber LH, Kass EH. Arch Dermatol 1977; 113: 1229–32.

Of 133 patients with protoporphyria, 84% had a threefold increase in sunlight tolerance after ingesting pharmaceutical-grade β-carotene.

The same efficiently absorbed β-carotene is available without prescription (Lumitene, Tischcon). Doses producing serum levels of approximately 800 μg/dL (30–120 mg/day in children, 120–300 mg/day in adults, in two to three doses with meals), should be started 4–6 weeks before seasonal symptoms are anticipated. Efficacy varies, and in some patients is nil. Increased lung cancer among heavy smokers treated with β-carotene in two cancer prevention clinical trials raises concern about its use in smokers.

SECOND-LINE THERAPIES

▶ Phototherapy (UVB, PUVA)	D

Narrow-band (TL-01) UVB phototherapy: an effective preventative treatment for the photodermatoses. Collins P, Ferguson J. Br J Dermatol 1995; 132: 956–63.

Six patients with protoporphyria had increased sunlight tolerance after serial narrowband UVB treatments.

Photo(chemo)therapy and general management of erythropoietic protoporphyria. Roelandts R. Dermatology 1995; 190: 330–1.

PUVA can increase sun tolerance in protoporphyria; other treatments are reviewed.

THIRD-LINE THERAPIES

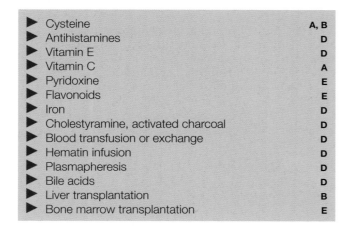

▶ Cysteine	A, B
▶ Antihistamines	D
▶ Vitamin E	D
▶ Vitamin C	A
▶ Pyridoxine	E
▶ Flavonoids	E
▶ Iron	D
▶ Cholestyramine, activated charcoal	D
▶ Blood transfusion or exchange	D
▶ Hematin infusion	D
▶ Plasmapheresis	D
▶ Bile acids	D
▶ Liver transplantation	B
▶ Bone marrow transplantation	E

Long-term treatment of erythropoietic protoporphyria with cysteine. Mathews-Roth MM, Rosner B. Photodermatol Photoimmunol Photomed 2002; 18: 307–9.

Forty-seven patients received placebo for 1 month followed by cysteine 500 mg twice daily in this phase III 3-year trial. Patient history forms and light exposure diaries were kept; some patients were phototested. Cysteine significantly increased light tolerance subjectively and objectively.

This study expanded a double-blinded smaller trial suggesting the same benefit (Mathews-Roth MM, Rosner B, Benfell K, Roberts JE. Photodermatol Photoimmunol Photomed 1994; 10: 244–8).

Inhibition of photosensitivity in erythropoietic protoporphyria with terfenadine. Farr PM, Diffey BL, Matthews JNS. Br J Dermatol 1990; 122: 809–15.

Ingestion of this H_1 receptor antagonist 60–120 mg twice daily for 48 days significantly reduced the flare surrounding, but not the erythema within, blue light phototest sites on seven subjects, compared to pretreatment reactions.

Antihistamines have not provided much relief in clinical practice.

Cimetidine reduces erythrocyte protoporphyrin in erythropoietic protoporphyria. Yamamoto S, Hirano Y, Horie Y. Am J Gastroenterol 1993; 88: 1465–6.

This H_2 receptor antagonist (800 mg four times daily orally) was given to a patient with protoporphyric liver disease. Erythrocyte protoporphyrin fell from ~16 000 to ~11 000 μg/dL during treatment. Inhibition of heme synthesis by cimetidine was postulated.

Only three porphyrin measurements were obtained: before and immediately after 2 weeks of cimetidine, and 2 weeks after discontinuation. More data are required to establish reproducibility and mechanism.

A case of erythropoietic protoporphyria with liver cirrhosis suggesting a therapeutic value of supplementation with alpha-tocopherol. Komatsu H, Ishii K, Imamura K, Maruyama K, Yonei Y, Masuda H, et al. Hepatol Res 2000; 18: 298–309.

A patient with severe protoporphyric hepatopathy received intravenous vitamin E 500 IU/day. Erythrocyte protoporphyrin decreased significantly and liver function improved. Sixteen weeks later, full clinical and biochemical recovery was noted.

Vitamin E has been used sporadically in protoporphyria, usually as adjunctive therapy, but robust data supporting efficacy are lacking.

A double-blind, placebo-controlled, crossover trial of oral vitamin C in erythropoietic protoporphyria. Boffa MJ, Ead RD, Reed P, Weinkove C. Photodermatol Photoimmunol Photomed 1996; 12: 27–30.

Vitamin C 1 g/day orally for 4 weeks was subjectively assessed by nine of 12 patients to be associated with less photosensitivity than placebo.

Antioxidants such as vitamins C and E are postulated to quench porphyrin-generated oxyradicals in vivo.

Relief of the photosensitivity of erythropoietic protoporphyria by pyridoxine. Ross JB, Moss MA. J Am Acad Dermatol 1990; 22: 340–2.

Two patients given oral pyridoxine dosages varying from 100 mg/day to 100 mg three times daily to 1 g each morning reported increased sunlight tolerance.

Treatment of erythropoietic protoporphyria with hydroxyethylrutosides. Schoemaker JH, Bousema MT, Zijlstra H, van der Horst FA. Dermatology 1995; 191: 36–8.

A flavonoid mixture was ingested by a patient for 3 months, during which time phototesting and subjective assessment indicated reduced photosensitivity.

Iron therapy for hepatic dysfunction in erythropoietic protoporphyria. Gordeuk VR, Brittenham GM, Hawkins CW, Mukhtar H, Bickers DR. Ann Intern Med 1986; 105: 27–31.

Carbonyl iron 400–4000 mg by mouth was given daily for 15 weeks to a patient with protoporphyria, iron deficiency anemia, and early liver dysfunction. Erythrocyte porphyrin fell, photosensitivity improved, and liver function normalized.

In a subsequent report on the same case, ferrous sulfate 300 mg daily by mouth was started when liver function and porphyrin levels worsened again. Liver function again normalized and remained stable for several years (Mercurio MG, Prince G, Weber FL Jr, Jacobs G, Zaim MT, Bickers DR. J Am Acad Dermatol 1993; 29: 829–33).

Symptomatic response of erythropoietic protoporphyria to iron supplementation. Holme SA, Thomas CL, Whatley SD, Bentley AV, Badminton MN. J Am Acad Dermatol 2007; 56: 1070–2.

A patient reported greater sunlight tolerance while taking oral ferrous sulfate 200 mg twice daily.

Erythropoietic protoporphyria and iron therapy. McClements BM, Bingham A, Callendar ME, Trimble ER. Br J Dermatol 1990; 122: 423–4.

Oral ferrous fumarate 580 mg/day was followed by florid photosensitivity in a patient previously tolerant of iron supplements. Abnormal liver enzymes improved and erythrocyte protoporphyrin diminished after iron discontinuation.

Iron supplementation in protoporphyria is contentious. Patients have been both better and worse after iron.

Fecal protoporphyrin excretion in erythropoietic protoporphyria: effect of cholestyramine and bile acid feeding. McCullough AJ, Barron D, Mullen KD, Petrelli M, Mukhtar H, Bickers DR. Gastroenterology 1988; 94: 177–81.

Ingesting cholestyramine 12 g, but not bile acids 300–900 mg, daily increased fecal protoporphyrin excretion threefold in one patient with hepatic dysfunction. Liver function and photosensitivity improved after 1 year of cholestyramine.

Bile acid ingestion was associated with improved liver function and erythrocyte porphyrin levels in another patient who eventually succumbed to liver failure (Doss MO, Frank M. Clin Biochem 1989; 22: 223–9). Efficacy remains uncertain, but bile acids in conjunction with an enteric sorbent in selected cases are rational therapy.

Liver failure in protoporphyria: long-term treatment with oral charcoal. Gorchein A, Foster GR. Hepatology 1999; 29: 995–6.

A patient with deteriorating hepatic function given activated charcoal 10–12.5 g orally four times a day for 2 years exhibited improved liver function, and blood porphyrin and photosensitivity diminished.

Other treatments included blood transfusions, vitamin supplements, amiloride, ranitidine and lactulose, so it is difficult to assess their relative merits.

Liver disease in erythropoietic protoporphyria: insights and implications for management. Anstey AV, Hift RJ. Gut 2007; 56: 1009–18.

A detailed review of the pathogenesis of protoporphryic hepatopathy and recommendations for its monitoring and treatment.

Liver transplantation for erythropoietic protoporphyria liver disease. Mcguire BM, Bonkovsky HL, Carithers RL, Chung RT, Goldstein LI, Lake JR, et al. Liver Transplant 2005; 11: 1590–6.

Experience with all 20 protoporphyria patients receiving liver transplants in the United States from 1999 to 2004 is reviewed, including preoperative use of hematin with or without plasmapheresis.

Perioperative measures during liver transplantation for erythropoietic protoporphyria. Meerman L, Verwer R, Sloof MJH, van Hattum J, Beukeveld GJ, Kleibeuker JH, et al. Transplantation 1994; 57: 155–8.

Protocols for exchange transfusion and shielding of operating room lamps during liver transplantation are detailed.

The value of intravenous heme-albumin and plasmapheresis in reducing postoperative complications of orthotopic liver transplantation for erythropoietic protoporphyria. Reichheld JH, Katz E, Banner BF, Szymanski IO, Saltzman JR, Bonkovsky HL. Transplantation 1999; 67: 922–8.

Three months of heme infusions (4 g daily to weekly), a high carbohydrate diet (300 mg/day), intravenous glucose, ursodeoxycholic acid (900 mg/day orally), and cholestyramine (10 g three times a day orally) initially improved severe liver dysfunction in a patient who then deteriorated and required urgent transplantation. Intensive heme infusions (daily for 18 days), plasmapheresis (twelve 1–1.5 plasma volume exchanges over 19 days) and blood transfusions (14 units packed cells over 19 days) reduced blood porphyrins prior to successful transplantation performed in illumination filtered to exclude 300–480 nm wavelengths.

A barrage of medical therapy is typical in protoporphyric crises, when it is rational to consider any treatments that might reverse deterioration or contribute to successful transplantation. Subsequently, recurrent liver dysfunction was again successfully managed with heme-albumin and plasmapheresis. (Do KD, Banner BF, Katz E, Szymanski IO, Bonkovsky HL. Transplantation 2002; 73: 469–7).

Treatment of recurrent allograft dysfunction with intravenous hematin after liver transplantation for erythropoietic protoporphyria. Dellon ES, Szczepiorkowski ZM, Dzik WH, Graeme-Cook F, Ades A, Bloomer JR, et al. Transplantation 2002; 73: 911–15.

Hematin given intermittently for 2 years after protoporphyric hepatopathy recurred 700 days after transplantation was well tolerated and aided the achievement and maintenance of disease remission in the allograft.

Erythropoietic protoporphyria: altered phenotype after bone marrow transplantation for myelogenous leukemia in a patient heteroallelic for ferrochelatase gene mutations. Poh-Fitzpatrick MB, Wang X, Anderson K, Bloomer JR, Bolwell B, Lichten AE. J Am Acad Dermatol 2002; 46: 861–6.

A symptomatic woman harboring two ferrochelatase gene mutations developed leukemia. Bone marrow transplantation from a mildly affected sibling with only one mutation and minimally elevated blood porphyrin resulted in marked reduction of the recipient's protoporphyrin levels and cutaneous photosensitivity, as well as leukemia remission.

Sequential liver and bone marrow transplantation for treatment of erythropoietic protoporphyria. Rand ER, Bunin ER, Cochran W, Ruchelli E, Olthoff KM, Bloomer JR. Pediatrics 2006; 118: e1896–9.

Bone marrow transplanted 6 months after a liver transplant corrected the severe phenotype of a 14-year-old boy and halted further protoporphyrin-induced liver graft damage.

Curative bone marrow transplantation in erythropoietic protoporphyria after reversal of severe cholestasis. Wahlin S, Aschan J, Björnstedt M, Broomé U, Harper P. J Hepatol 2007; 46: 174–9.

Eighty days of medical management normalized liver biochemistry and improved histology in a man who then received a bone marrow transplant. Ten months following the transplant, liver and porphyrin tests were normal and no photosensitivity was reported.

Extramammary Paget's disease

Lori D Prok, James E Fitzpatrick

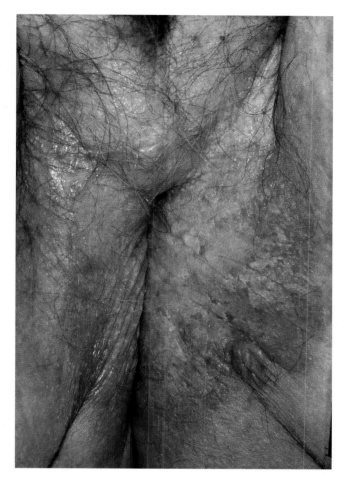

Extramammary Paget's disease (EMPD) was first described by Crocker in 1889, when he noted skin lesions affecting the penis and scrotum of a male patient that were identical to the nipple disease described by Paget in 1874. Although a rare disease, EMPD should be included in the clinical differential diagnosis of any chronic dermatitis of the groin or perineum. EMPD most commonly affects postmenopausal Caucasian women, but can also be seen in men of all ethnicities, and presents as chronic, often sharply demarcated, erythematous scaling plaques of apocrine gland-bearing skin, including the genitalia, axillae, umbilicus, and external auditory canal. Pruritus is the most common presenting symptom. Primary EMPD results from epidermal infiltration of neoplastic glandular cells. Recent evidence supports the role of Toker cells (clear cells found in 10% of normal nipples, and recently identified in tissue of the milk line and the vulva) as the pathologic cell in this disease. Approximately 25% of cases develop from secondary cutaneous extension of an underlying adenocarcinoma, most commonly of the genitourinary organs.

MANAGEMENT STRATEGY

Clinical suspicion of EMPD should prompt an immediate skin biopsy. Histologically, neoplastic cells are characterized by pale vacuolated cytoplasm and large pleomorphic nuclei, which can be seen infiltrating all levels of the epidermis. Extension into adnexal structures is common. These cells contain abundant mucin, demonstrated by positive staining with mucicarmine, colloidal iron, PAS, and Alcian blue at pH 2.5. Cells also express carcinoembryonic antigen, epithelial membrane antigen, CK7, and Ber-EP4, the latter reliably differentiating between EMPD and pagetoid variants of squamous cell carcinoma in situ and melanoma in situ. (CK7 positivity is seen in most primary EMPD, but is rarely expressed in secondary disease. CK20 positivity also suggests secondary disease.) Gross cystic disease fluid protein, traditionally thought to be a specific marker for apocrine cells, is also found in the neoplastic cells of EMPD. Tumor cells overexpress transcription factor Sp1 and vascular endothelial growth factor. Emerging research has also identified several tumor markers overexpressed in invasive disease, including Ki-67, cyclin D1, and p53. RCAS1 has been used to monitor tumor burden and therapeutic response in patients with EMPD.

A full-body skin examination and lymph node evaluation should be performed in all patients with histologic evidence of EMPD. Patients should then have appropriate evaluation for underlying malignancy, including age- and gender-appropriate screening (Papanicolaou smear, fecal occult blood, colonoscopy, cystoscopy, and prostate-specific antigen). Additional investigations (imaging, colposcopy, etc.) are guided by screening results and the anatomic location of cutaneous lesions.

EMPD is treated locally with surgical excision, with adjuvant therapies in selected cases. Mohs' micrographic surgery is the preferred technique, offering the most reliable margin control, maximal tissue preservation, and lowest recurrence rates. However, this technique is still limited by non-contiguous tumor spread and the high likelihood of EMPD involving clinically normal-appearing skin.

SPECIFIC INVESTIGATIONS

- ► Skin biopsy
- ► Full-body skin examination and lymph node evaluation
- ► Serum CEA level
- ► Cancer screening appropriate for age and gender (Papanicolaou smear, fecal occult blood, colonoscopy, cystoscopy, and prostate-specific antigen)

Extramammary Paget's disease: treatment, prognostic factors and outcome in 76 patients. Hatta N, Yamada M, Hirano T, Fujimoto A, Morita R. Br J Dermatol 2008; 158: 313–18.

Retrospective review of 76 patients with EMPD. Surgical margin was not correlated with local recurrence. Seventeen percent developed systemic metastases; 10 patients died. Nodules in the primary tumor, clinical lymph node swelling, elevated CEA levels, depth of tumor invasion, and lymph node metastasis were significant prognostic factors. Depth of tumor invasion and CEA level were associated with reduced survival.

Epidemiology and treatment of EMPD in the Netherlands. Siesling S, Elferink M, van Dijck J, Pierie JP, Blokx WA. Eur J Surg Oncol 2007; 33: 951–5.

Retrospective review of 226 cases of EMPD in the Netherlands Cancer Registry, most of which were treated with surgical excision. Five-year survival for those with invasive disease was 72%. Patients had an increased risk of developing a second primary cancer (standard incidence ratio 1.7).

FIRST-LINE THERAPIES

▶ Wide local excision, with or without lymph node dissection	**B, D**
▶ Frozen section-guided wide local excision	**D**
▶ Mohs' micrographic surgery	**D**

Indications for lymph node dissection in the treatment of EMPD. Tsutsumida A, Yamamoto Y, Minakawa H, Yoshida T, Kokubu I, Sugihara T. Dermatol Surg 2003; 29: 21–4.

A prospective study of 34 patients with genital or perineal EMPD treated with wide local excision. Patients with clinical or histologic evidence of metastatic disease underwent lymph node dissection. No patients with carcinoma in situ or microscopic papillary dermal invasion had lymph node metastasis; all had 100% 5-year survival. Tumor invasion into the reticular dermis correlated with 33% 5-year survival. Tumor invasion into the subcutaneous tissue correlated with 100% lymph node metastasis and death.

Evaluation using a combination of lymphatic invasion on D2–40 immunostain and depth of dermal invasion is a strong predictor for nodal metastasis in EMPD. Yamada, Y, Matsumoto T, Arakawa A, Ikeda S, Fujime M, Komuro Y, et al. Pathol Int 2008; 58: 114–17.

Retrospective review of 54 surgical specimens of EMPD of the external genitalia. Dermal invasion was present in 24 patients, and inguinal lymph node dissection was performed in 23. Nodal metastasis was present in seven patients with dermal tumor invasion >1 mm. Lymph node invasion according to D2–40 immunostain was present in five patients, and those that underwent node dissection all had nodal invasion. Three patients with >1 mm dermal invasion but no lymphatic invasion had positive nodes. Results suggest that the combination of depth of dermal invasion and demonstration of lymphatic invasion predicts nodal disease in EMPD.

Penile and scrotal Paget's disease: experiences from 130 Chinese patients with a long-term follow-up. Wang Z, Lu M, Dong G, Jiang YQ, Lin MS, Cai ZK, et al. BJU Int 2008; 102: 485–8.

Retrospective review of 130 Chinese patients with penoscrotal EMPD. All underwent wide local resection and reconstruction. Forty-five patients had frozen-section margin confirmation during surgery; five with positive margins required immediate extended resection. Mean follow-up was 3.2 years (81/130 patients). Tumor recurrence was documented in five of nine patients with positive margins and in three of 72 patients with negative margins. Five patients died from metastatic disease.

Frozen section-guided wide local excision in the treatment of penoscrotal EMPD. Zhu Y, Ye D, Chen Z, Zhang SL, Qin XJ. BJU Int 2007; 100: 1282–7.

Retrospective review of 38 patients with primary penoscrotal EMPD who received wide local excision with intraoperative frozen-section analysis. Thirty-two percent had positive frozen-section margins and required immediate extended excision. Forty percent of patients had positive surgical margins after traditional wide local excision with 2 cm margins. At a mean follow-up of 33 months 16% of patients had recurrent disease, and four had systemic involvement.

EMPD: surgical treatment with Mohs micrographic surgery. Hendi A, Brodland D, Zitelli J. J Am Acad Dermatol 2004; 51: 767–73.

Retrospective review of patients with EMPD treated with Mohs' micrographic surgery. Patients treated with MMS had recurrence rate of 16% for primary EMPD and 50% for recurrent disease, and 5-year tumor free rates of 80% for primary tumors and 56% for recurrent tumors. Literature review found 33–60% recurrence after non-MMS surgical excision.

Comparison of Mohs micrographic surgery and wide excision for EMPD. O'Connor W, Lim K, Zalla M. Dermatol Surg 2003; 29: 723–7.

Retrospective review of 95 patients at the Mayo Clinic comparing tumor recurrence in patients treated with Mohs' micrographic surgery (8%) compared to wide local excision (22%). Surgeons used intraoperative staining with CK7.

SECOND-LINE THERAPIES

▶ Photodynamic therapy	**D**
▶ Systemic chemotherapy	**E**
▶ Radiation therapy	**D**

Photodynamic therapy using a methyl ester of 5-aminolevulinic acid in recurrent Paget's disease of the vulva: a pilot study. Raspagliesi F, Fontanelli R, Rossi G, Ditto A, Solima E, Hanozet F, et al. Gynecol Oncol 2006; 103: 581–6.

Pilot study using photodynamic therapy and methyl 5-aminolevulinate (an ester of 5-ALA with higher efficacy and fewer side effects) to treat recurrent vulvar EMPD. Seven patients were treated weekly for 3 weeks, and follow-up biopsies were obtained 1 month after treatment. Four patients had complete clinical response; this was histologically confirmed in two cases.

5-Aminolevulinic acid-based photodynamic therapy for the treatment of two patients with extramammary Paget's disease. Mikasa K, Watanabe D, Kondo C, Kobayashi M, Nakaseko H, Yokoo K, et al. J Dermatol 2005; 32: 97–101.

Case report of two elderly patients with EMPD treated with photodynamic therapy and 5-ALA. Both patients had histologic elimination of tumor cells and clinical improvement. Case 1 had no recurrence at 3 months' follow-up. Case 2 had recurrence at the periphery of the treated field, which cleared with additional PDT.

Metastatic EMPD successfully controlled with tumour dormancy therapy using docetaxel. Fujisawa Y, Umebayashi Y, Otsuka F. Br J Dermatol 2006; 154: 375–6.

Report of a patient with EMPD with bone and lung metastases whose tumor markers and metastatic lesions decreased after treatment with intravenous docetaxel. The patient is still being treated on an outpatient basis, with good function and tumor control.

Evidence Levels: **A** Double-blind study **B** Clinical trial ≥ 20 subjects **C** Clinical trial < 20 subjects **D** Series ≥ 5 subjects **E** Anecdotal case reports

Trial of low-dose 5-fluorouracil/cisplatin therapy for advanced EMPD. Kariya K, Tsuji T, Schwartz R. Dermatol Surg 2004; 30: 341–4.

Case report of penoscrotal EMPD and multiple visceral metastases treated with intravenous 5-fluorouracil and cisplatin for 6 weeks. The patient had resolution of cutaneous disease, with a significant reduction in tumor markers and radiographic evidence of metastatic disease.

Low-dose mitomycin C, etoposide, and cisplatin for invasive vulvar Paget's disease. Watanabe Y, Hoshial H, Ueda H. Int J Gynecol Cancer 2002; 12: 304–7.

Three patients with invasive vulvar Paget's disease who declined surgery were treated with low-dose mitomycin, etoposide, and cisplatin. One achieved a complete response; two showed a partial response and ultimately underwent partial vulvectomy and inguinal lymph node dissection. No patients had recurrent disease at 10 months' follow-up.

Radiotherapy for extramammary Paget's disease: histopathologic findings after radiotherapy. Yanagi R, Kato N, Yamane N. Clin Exp Dermatol 2007; 32: 506–8.

Case reports of two patients with genital EMPD treated with radiotherapy, with clinical response confirmed by histopathologic studies.

EMPD: outcome of radiotherapy with curative intent. Luk N, Yu K, Yeung W. Clin Exp Dermatol 2003; 28: 360–3.

Case series of six patients treated with EMPD treated by radiotherapy, including two treated primarily, three treated after relapse, and one as adjuvant therapy. Five patients had a complete clinical response with follow-up ranging from 1.2 to 14.8 years. One patient treated primarily had no evidence of metastasis at 2-year follow-up. Two patients in the series had underlying adenocarcinoma, and both died of distant metastases.

THIRD-LINE THERAPIES

▶ Topical imiquimod	E
▶ Topical 5-fluorouracil and retinoic acid	E
▶ Intralesional interferon-α_{2b}	E
▶ Laser therapy	E
▶ Androgen receptor antagonist	E

Complete resolution of Paget's disease of the vulva with imiquimod cream. Hatch K, Davis J. J Low Genit Tract Dis 2008; 12: 90–4.

Two patients with vulvar EMPD achieved complete clinical clearance after application of topical imiquimod 5% cream. Histology confirmed tumor resolution.

Treatment of mammary and extramammary Paget's disease with topical imiquimod. Mirer E, Sayed F, Ammoury A, Lamant L, Messer L, Bazex J. J Dermatol Treat 2006; 17: 167–71.

Report of two cases of EMPD and Paget's disease of the breast successfully treated with topical imiquimod. The potential benefits of imiquimod, including reduction of the extent of excision when used prior to surgery, are highlighted.

EMPD resistant to surgery and imiquimod monotherapy but responsive to imiquimod combination topical chemotherapy with 5-fluorouracil and retinoic acid: a case report. Ye J, Rhew D, Yip F, Edelstein L. Cutis 2006; 7: 245–50.

Report of a patient with EMPD (recurrent after surgery and resistant to topical imiquimod alone) that resolved after treatment with combination imiquimod and topical 5-fluorouracil and retinoic acid.

Intralesional interferon alfa-2b as neoadjuvant treatment for perianal EMPD. Panasiti V, Bottoni U, Devirgilis V, Mancini M, Rossi M, Curzio M, et al. J Eur Acad Dermatol Venereol 2008; 22: 522–3.

Report of a patient with perianal EMPD who, after refusing surgical excision, was treated with intralesional IFN-α_{2b}. At 7 weeks the tumor had decreased in diameter and surgical resection was performed. Patient had no clinical disease at 108 months' follow-up.

Failure of carbon dioxide laser treatment in three patients with penoscrotal EMPD. Choi J, Yoon E, Yoon D, Kim DS, Kim JJ, Cho JH. BJU Int 2001; 88: 297–8.

Report of three patients with EMPD treated with CO_2 laser guided by Wood's lamp fluorescence to determine clinical margins. All three had disease recurrence within 6 months and required traditional surgical excision.

Estrogen-receptor-alpha-positive EMPD treated with hormonal therapy. Iijima M, Uhara H, Ide Y, Sakai S, Onuma H, Muto M, et al. Dermatology 2006; 213: 144–6.

Case report of a patient with scrotal and penile EMPD expressing estrogen receptor-α and associated prostate cancer. The patient was treated systemically with both anti-estrogen (tamoxifen) and anti-androgen (bicalutamide). The patient's performance status was well maintained at 17 months' follow-up.

Androgen-deprivation regimen for multiple bone metastases of EMPD. Yoneyama K, Kamada N, Kinoshita K. Br J Dermatol 2005; 153: 853–5.

Case report of EMPD with multiple bone metastases successfully suppressed with anti-androgen bicalutamide and LH-RH agonist leuprorelin. Tumor markers decreased and bone scintigraphy evidence of metastasis disappeared within 2 months. When tumor markers rose at day 70, other anti-androgens and systemic chemotherapy failed. Bone metastases reappeared, and the patient ultimately died 14 months after the start of anti-androgen therapy. The authors postulate that the rapid development of resistance to the androgen-deprivation therapy suggests that mutation or amplification in the androgen receptor gene occurred in this case, as seen in cases of prostate cancer.

Fabry disease

Pascal G Ferzli, Rhonda E Schnur

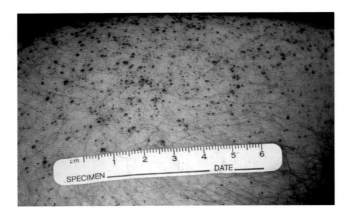

Angiokeratomas are hyperkeratotic, dark red to blue-black telangiectatic papules commonly associated with lysosomal storage diseases, including Fabry disease, fucosidosis, sialidosis, aspartylglucosaminuria and β-galactosidase deficiency. This chapter focuses specifically on the treatment of angiokeratomas in the context of Fabry disease, an X-linked disorder caused by the deficiency or absence of the lysosomal enzyme α-galactosidase A (GLA). This deficiency results in the accumulation of two neutral glycosphingolipids in major organ systems: globotriaosylceramide (Gb3) and digalactosylceramide. Systemic complications of Fabry disease include renal failure, cardiomyopathy, corneal opacities, hearing loss, gastrointestinal symptoms, and central nervous system manifestations secondary to deposition of glycosphingolipids in the vascular endothelia and perineural cells. Males are more severely affected, but female carriers may exhibit symptoms depending on the pattern of X-inactivation. About 10% of carriers develop renal failure. They may also develop cardiovascular disease. Single organ variants with more residual enzyme activity than the classic disease have also been described. To date, more than 400 *GLA* mutations have been reported. Because of the increased efficacy of treatment, neonatal screening for Fabry disease may be justifiable. The correlation between genotype and residual enzyme activity is not strong, but the correlation between enzymatic levels and clinical outcomes is unquestionable.

MANAGEMENT STRATEGY

Cutaneous manifestations of Fabry disease include angiokeratomas, hypohidrosis, pain crises, acroparesthesias, and lymphedema. Angiokeratomas increase in number and size over time. They cluster around the umbilicus, hips, thighs, buttocks and scrotum; mucosal involvement may also be seen. Lesions are usually bilateral and symmetric. The differential diagnosis of angiokeratoma includes malignant melanoma, angiokeratoma of Fordyce, angiokeratoma of Mibelli, and angiokeratoma circumscriptum. One should also consider blue rubber bleb nevus syndrome, hereditary hemorrhagic telangiectasia, cherry angiomas, and other lysosomal storage diseases.

Pain is the most debilitating cutaneous symptom of Fabry disease, typified by severe, burning, episodic pain crises of the palms and soles and acroparesthesias, a constant tingling discomfort in the extremities. Pain crises are felt to result from glycolipid accumulation in the autonomic nervous system and vascular endothelium. A similar mechanism underlies Fabry-associated hypohidrosis, which is seen early in the disease process. *Carbamazepine, gabapentin, lamotrigine, tricyclic antidepressants,* and *diphenylhydantoin* are effective for analgesia. Gastrointestinal complications (diarrhea, abdominal discomfort, nausea and vomiting) have been treated with *metoclopramide* and *pancrealipase* with some success.

Traditionally, angiokeratomas have been treated with *surgical excision, electrocoagulation,* and *cryosurgery*. These procedures can be associated with pain, bleeding, and scarring. Laser therapy is the treatment of choice for multiple angiokeratomas. Various lasers have been utilized, including the CO_2, argon, copper vapor, and flashlamp–pumped-dye lasers. Copper vapor lasers are superior to argon because of their wavelength specificity for hemoglobin. However, the flashlamp–pumped-dye laser may produce less pain and bleeding, a shorter healing time, and a reduced risk of pigment changes and scarring. Local anesthetics are used when treating sensitive areas (e.g. penile skin). Because angiokeratomas are progressive, repeated treatments are often necessary.

Renal transplantation produces marked improvement of angiokeratomas, arrests the development of new lesions, relieves acroparesthesias, and may improve sweating ability. However, the long-term improvement of cutaneous lesions in these patients is unclear.

Enzyme replacement therapy (ERT) has revolutionized the treatment of Fabry disease. In vivo, a proportion of the phosphorylated form of α-galactosidase A is secreted from the cell and is taken up by receptor-mediated endocytosis (mannose-6-phosphate receptors); this provides the rationale for ERT. Two human enzyme products have been created: agalsidase-α (Replagal, Shire Genetic Therapies, UK) and agalsidase-β (Fabrazyme, Genzyme Corp). The primary amino acid sequence is identical in both, but agalsidase-β contains a higher proportion of the mannose-6-phosphate residues for endocytosis. In 2003, the FDA approved only *recombinant human α-galactosidase A (agalsidase-β)*, although agalsidase-α is in use in many other countries. The enzymes are administered intravenously bi-weekly at a dose of 0.2 mg/kg for agalsidase-α and 1.0 mg/kg for agalsidase-β. The cost associated with treatment is very high: approximately \$250 000 per year.

ERT has been shown to improve myocardial function, reduce neuropathic pain, improve peripheral nerve function, relieve gastrointestinal symptoms, reduce cerebrovascular events, and reduce the dermatologic manifestations of angiokeratomas. It has also been shown to improve renal function in patients with mild disease and to stabilize renal function in those with advanced disease. Earlier intervention with enzyme therapy leads to a better clinical outcome, justifying neonatal screening and presymptomatic diagnosis for Fabry disease.

ERT consistently reduces Gb3 levels, but despite this some patients still show functional deterioration. Several studies have shown that Gb3 metabolites such as globotriaosylsphingosine might be contributing to the pathomechanism of disease, but more studies are needed.

Today, ERT remains the only FDA-approved medicinal therapy for the direct treatment of Fabry disease. However, new options are currently being studied, particularly for patients with more

Evidence Levels: **A** Double-blind study   **B** Clinical trial ≥ 20 subjects   **C** Clinical trial < 20 subjects   **D** Series ≥ 5 subjects   **E** Anecdotal case reports

advanced disease in whom there is less response to ERT owing to insufficient delivery of enzyme to the most affected tissues. A promising new therapeutic strategy involves the use of small molecules called 'active site-specific chaperones.' These orally active molecules act as partial competitive inhibitors of the GLA enzyme which 'rescue' misfolded, but catalytically still active enzyme from degradation, promoting its transfer to lysosomes. Chaperone therapy can only benefit patients with point mutations that result in misfolded proteins. The potential for response in a particular patient can be screened via an in-vitro transfection assay based on the specific mutation. 1-Deoxygalactonojirimycin (DGJ), also known as migalastat hydrochloride (Amigal, Amicus Therapeutics, NJ, USA), is a potent GLA inhibitor and can increase residual enzyme levels in Fabry transgenic mice, as well as in cell cultures of Fabry patients with missense mutations. Phase II trials using migalastat hydrochloride have been successfully completed in both male and female Fabry patients.

SPECIFIC INVESTIGATIONS

Diagnostic work-up

▶ Obtain family history
▶ GLA DNA analysis (nearly 100% sensitivity in affected males; can be used for both sexes)
▶ Quantitative enzyme analysis (plasma, WBCs, cultured cells) (males only; unreliable in females)
▶ Chorionic villus sampling, amniocentesis for prenatal diagnosis (enzymatic and/or molecular assay)
▶ Renal biopsy (if there is a high degree of suspicion for the disease despite normal genetic and enzymatic studies)

Systemic work-up of patients with Fabry disease (male and female)

▶ Renal function studies
▶ Cardiac evaluation, including electrocardiogram, echocardiography
▶ Audiologic testing
▶ Periodic skin biopsy to monitor clearance of globotriaosylceramide during therapy
▶ Antibody titers to agalsidase-β during therapy
▶ Ophthalmologic evaluation with slit-lamp examination (screen for corneal opacity, lenticular changes)

Alpha-galactosidase A deficiency: Fabry disease. Desnick RJ, Ioannou YA, Eng CM. In: Scriver CR, Beaudet AL, Sly WS, Valle D, Vogelstein B. The Metabolic and Molecular Basis of Inherited Disease (OMMBID). New York: McGraw-Hill, 2006; Chapter 150. Available at www.ommbid.com. Accessed July 2008.

A complete discussion of Fabry disease. Residual enzymatic activity and genotype both affect clinical outcome and may direct different diagnostic and therapeutic modalities.

Narrative review: Fabry disease. Clarke JT. Ann Intern Med 2007; 146: 425–33.

A summary of the recent advances in the diagnosis and treatment of Fabry disease patients.

The challenges of diagnosing Fabry disease. Stratta P, Quaglia M, Messina M, Cavagnino A, Ragazzoni E, Bergamo D, et al. Am J Kidney Dis 2008; 51: 860–4.

A discussion of the renal findings in patients with atypical features of Fabry disease, and/or equivocal enzymatic assays and no detectable mutation.

Elevated globotriaosylsphingosine is a hallmark of Fabry disease. Aerts JM, Groener JE, Kuiper S, Donker-Koopman WE, Strijland A, Ottenhoff R, et al. Proc Natl Acad Sci USA 2008; 105: 2812–17.

Globotriaosylsphingosine inhibits α-galactosidase A activity and may increase intima-medial thickness in Fabry patients. The authors propose that measuring circulating globotriaosylsphingosine will be a useful marker for complications of Fabry disease.

High incidence of later-onset Fabry disease revealed by newborn screening. Spada M, Pagliardini S, Yasuda M, Tukel T, Thiagarajan G, Sakuraba H, et al. Am J Hum Genet 2006; 79: 31–40.

α-gal A activity and GLA mutation analysis was performed in blood spots from 37 104 consecutive Italian male neonates. The incidence rate of Fabry disease was found to be approximately 1:3100, with an 11:1 ratio of patients having later-onset/classic phenotypes. The authors propose that the later-onset phenotype of Fabry disease may be underdiagnosed among adult males with cardiac, cerebrovascular, and/or renal disease.

Human Gene Mutation Database (HGMD): Cooper DN, Ball EV, Stenson PD, Phillips AD, Howells K, Mort ME, et al. http://www.hgmd.org. The Institute of Medical Genetics, Cardiff, United Kingdom 2008.

Over 400 mutations in the GLA gene have been identified. Mutation information is used for diagnosis, particularly in heterozygotes, prenatal testing, and correlation with clinical phenotype.

Fabry disease. Desnick RJ, Astrin KH, Hughes DA, Mehta A. Updated February 26, 2008. In: GeneReviews at GeneTests: Medical Genetics Information Resource (database online). Copyright, University of Washington, Seattle 1997–2008. Available at http://www.genetests.org. Accessed August 23, 2008

A comprehensive review of Fabry disease.

Fabry disease and the skin: data from FOS, the Fabry Outcome Survey. Orteu CH, Jansen T, Lidove O, Jaussaud R, Hughes DA, Pintos-Morell G, et al. Br J Dermatol 2007; 157: 331–7.

The authors used the Fabry Outcome Survey (FOS), a multicentre European database, to establish the prevalence of dermatologic complications of Fabry disease in 345 males and 369 females. They found a high incidence of cutaneous involvement, including angiokeratoma (66% males, 36% females), hypohidrosis (53% males, 28% females), telangiectasia (23% males, 9% females), and lymphedema (16% males, 6% females). They also found that the presence of dermatological manifestations was a marker for greater severity of systemic disease.

FIRST-LINE THERAPIES

▶ Enzyme replacement therapy	A
▶ Laser therapy	C
▶ Surgical excision	D
▶ Diphenylhydantoin	C
▶ Gabapentin	C
▶ Carbamazepine	C

Long-term safety and efficacy of enzyme replacement therapy for Fabry disease. Wilcox WR, Banikazemi M, Guffon N,

Waldek S, Lee P, Linthorst GE, et al. Am J Hum Genet 2004; 75: 65–74.

Latest data from phase III clinical trials of ERT after 30–36 months of treatment. ERT resulted in reduced GL-3 levels and sustained endothelial GL-3 clearance with few adverse reactions. ERT also stabilized renal function.

Monitoring the 3-year efficacy of enzyme replacement therapy in Fabry disease by repeated skin biopsies. Thurberg BL, Randolph Byers H, Granter SR, Phelps RG, Gordon RE, O'Callaghan M. J Invest Dermatol 2004; 122: 900–8.

Long-term treatment with recombinant enzyme replacement may halt the progression of the cutaneous lesions in patients with Fabry disease. Periodic skin biopsy to assess the clearance of globotriaosylceramide in dermal tissues may serve as a reliable indicator of the efficacy of ERT.

Enzyme replacement therapy with agalsidase beta improves cardiac involvement in Fabry's disease. Spinelli L, Pisani A, Sabbatini M, Petretta M, Andreucci MV, Procaccini D, et al. Clin Genet 2004; 66: 158–65.

A statistically significant reduction of left ventricular (LV) mass and amelioration of LV stiffness was seen in nine patients.

Sustained, long-term renal stabilization after 54 months of agalsidase beta therapy in patients with Fabry disease. Germain DP, Waldek S, Banikazemi M, Bushinsky DA, Charrow J, Desnick RJ, et al. J Am Soc Nephrol 2007; 18: 1547–57.

This was an open-label, phase III extension study of agalsidase beta in 58 patients with classic Fabry disease treated for up to 54 months. Most patients had stabilization of serum creatinine and estimated GFR at month 54 (n=41). Six patients with more severe renal disease prior to treatment had disease progression.

Angiokeratomas in Fabry's disease and Fordyce's disease: successful treatment with copper vapor laser. Lapins J, Emtestam L, Marcusson JA. Acta Dermatol Venereol 1993; 73: 133–5.

Angiokeratomas were undetected at 3-month follow-up; treated skin was smooth, with minimal pigmentary alteration.

Successful treatment of angiokeratoma with potassium titanyl phosphate laser. Gorse SJ, James W, Murison MSC. Br J Dermatol 2004; 150: 620–1.

Excellent results were seen in two subjects with angiokeratomas.

Use of gabapentin to reduce chronic neuropathic pain in Fabry disease. Ries M, Mengel E, Kutschke G, Kim KS, Birklein F, Krummenauer F, et al. J Inherit Metab Dis 2003; 26: 413–14.

Six patients with Fabry disease experienced less pain than at baseline, with few side effects after 4 weeks of treatment.

Fabry disease during childhood: clinical manifestations and treatment with agalsidase alfa. Ramaswami U. Acta Paediatr Suppl 2008; 97: 38–40.

Early therapeutic intervention in females with Fabry disease? Hughes DA. Acta Paediatr Suppl 2008; 97: 41–7.

This pair of articles reviews the indications for, and the potential benefits of, early treatment in non-traditional patient groups. They point out that it remains uncertain whether early, or even presymptomatic, treatment with ERT can fully prevent the development of severe and life-threatening complications.

Safety and efficacy of enzyme replacement therapy with agalsidase beta: an international, open-label study in pediatric patients with Fabry disease. Wraith JE, Tylki-Szymanska A, Guffon N, Lien YH, Tsimaratos M, Vellodi A, et al. J Pediatr 2008; 152: 563–70.

In this open-label study of 14 boys and two girls with Fabry disease, agalsidase beta safely and effectively reduced GL-3 accumulation in biopsied dermal endothelium.

Enzyme replacement therapy with agalsidase alfa in a cohort of Italian patients with Anderson–Fabry disease: testing the effects with the Mainz Severity Score Index. Parini R, Rigoldi M, Santus F, Furlan F, De Lorenzo P, Valsecchi G, et al. Clin Genet 2008; 74: 260–6.

The Mainz Severity Score Index (MSSI) was used as a measure of disease severity to study ERT efficacy in 30 Fabry patients treated with agalsidase alfa for a median of 2.9 years. Total MSSI scores were significantly lower after at least 1 year of ERT, suggesting significant clinical improvement.

SECOND-LINE THERAPIES

▶ Renal transplantation/dialysis   **A**

Chronic renal failure, dialysis, and renal transplantation in Anderson–Fabry disease. Sessa A, Meroni M, Battini G, Righetti M, Mignani R. Semin Nephrol 2004; 24: 532–6.

This is a review of renal involvement in Fabry disease. Patients who are treated with dialysis have a better prognosis than diabetics, but fare worse than uremic patients with other nephropathies. The outcome of renal transplantation is similar to that in other patients with end-stage renal disease. The authors also note that recurrence of glycosphingolipid deposition in newly grafted kidney can occasionally occur.

Kidney transplantation improves survival and is indicated in Fabry's disease. Inderbitzin D, Avital I, Largiadèr F, Vogt B, Candinas D. Transplant Proc 2005; 37: 4211–14.

In this study of 10 transplanted Fabry patients, overall prognosis improved in the first decade post transplant, with median survival time of 128 months after transplant. However, ERT after transplant was recommended, as there were fatalities in the second decade post transplant.

THIRD-LINE AND FUTURE THERAPIES

▶ Gene transfer   **E**
▶ Migalastat hydrochloride   **B**

Long-term correction of globotriaosylceramide storage in Fabry mice by recombinant adeno-associated virus-mediated gene transfer. Park J, Murray GJ, Limaye A, Quirk JM, Gelderman MP, Brady RO, et al. Proc Natl Acad Sci USA 2003; 100: 3450–4.

Enzyme expression, activity and levels of glycosphingolipid were measured in transgenic mice. Accumulation of globotriaosylceramide in hepatic, cardiac and splenic tissues was greatly reduced.

Mutant alpha-galactosidase A enzymes identified in Fabry disease patients with residual enzyme activity: biochemical characterization and restoration of normal intracellular processing by 1-deoxygalactonojirimycin. Ishii S, Chang HH, Kawasaki K, Yasuda K, Wu HL, Garman SC, et al. Biochem J 2007; 406: 285–95.

Enzymatic activity in cultured fibroblasts and lymphoblasts of Fabry patients with missense mutations was substantially increased by cultivation of their cells with DGJ (migalastat hydrochloride), which is similar to the natural substrate for GLA and is a competitive inhibitor of the enzyme. DGJ may prevent excessive degradation in the endoplasmic reticulum of mutant but kinetically active residual enzyme, and thus may be a useful treatment for patients with missense mutations.

Prediction of response of mutated alpha-galactosidase A to a pharmacological chaperone. Shin SH, Kluepfel-Stahl S, Cooney AM, Kaneski CR, Quirk JM, Schiffmann R, et al. Pharmacogenet Genomics 2008; 18: 773–80.

The authors developed a screening assay to test the susceptibility of specific Fabry mutations to chaperone therapy and identified types of mutations that were more likely to respond.

Amicus Therapeutics Announces Positive Results From Phase 2 Clinical Trials of Amigal (TM) for Fabry Disease. http://www.amicustherapeutics.com, Cranbury, NJ. Accessed Dec 2007.

Migalastat hydrochloride (Amigal) is a chemical chaperone that selectively binds to and stabilizes proteins in cells. In open-label phase II studies of 18 male and 7 female Fabry patients, Amigal was safe and well tolerated, with no serious adverse reactions. Patients also had in vitro lymphocyte screening for their potential response to this therapy. Most patients demonstrated increased GLA activity regardless of baseline GLA levels, as well as reduced GL-3 levels. They also showed clinical improvement in renal and cardiac function. Males had a generally greater response. Different dosing regimens have been investigated, and phase III studies are about to begin.

Flushing

Jonathan K Wilkin

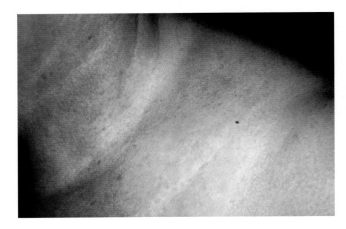

Flushing is a transient reddening of the face and frequently other areas, including the neck, upper chest, pinnae, and epigastric area. Flushing is the visible sign of a generalized increase in cutaneous blood flow despite the limited distribution of the erythema.

MANAGEMENT STRATEGY

The first step in the management of a patient with a flushing disorder is a specific diagnosis, because therapy is individualized according to the specific factors causing the flushing, and there is no broad-spectrum antiflushing treatment. The first algorithmic step is to distinguish between autonomic neural-mediated flushing, in which eccrine sweating occurs at the time of the flushing ('wet flushing'), and direct vasodilator-mediated flushing, in which there is no accompanying eccrine sweating ('dry flushing'). The 'dry flushing' reactions are further divided into those with prominent dysesthesia and those without.

Patients with dry flushing and no dysesthesia have circulating vasodilator substances that are either exogenous or endogenous. Exogenous vasodilator agents are almost always elicited from the patient's history. Patient diaries listing all foods, beverages, medications, activities, etc., can not only pinpoint the inciting agent, but also the temporal relationship can be convincing, for both patient and physician. The usual strategy for most vasodilator agents is *simple avoidance of the agent*, although *niacin (nicotinic acid) therapy for hyperlipidemia* and *tamoxifen for breast cancer* are important exceptions for which antiflushing therapies can permit continued treatment with the offending agent.

Finally, endogenous circulating vasodilator agents, typically from underlying neoplasias, are suggested by both multiple stimuli that provoke flushing (rather than one or a few provocative agents) and prominent features associated with the flushing attack. The differential diagnosis is usually generated from the prominent associated feature. Itching or urticaria with flushing suggests circulating mast cell mediators – examples include systemic mastocytosis and mast cell leukemia. Flushing following an attack of hypertension, pallor,

tachycardia, palpitations, and sweating suggests pheochromocytoma. Flushing with diarrhea can occur with cholinergic urticaria, cholinergic erythema, anxiety reactions, intolerance to foods, menopausal flushing, the dumping syndrome (a common complication of gastric surgery), diabetes mellitus, pancreatic cholera (watery diarrhea syndrome, Verner–Morrison syndrome), medullary carcinoma of the thyroid, pheochromocytoma, multiple endocrine neoplasia syndromes II and III, mastocytosis, and carcinoid syndrome.

SPECIFIC INVESTIGATIONS

> ▶ 5-Hydroxyindoleacetic acid (5-HIAA) urine test
> ▶ Histamine urine test
> ▶ Serotonin blood/platelet test
> ▶ Histamine plasma test

The red face: flushing disorders. Wilkin JK. Clin Dermatol 1993; 11: 211–23.

The first step in diagnosing a flushing reaction is to determine the mechanism: autonomic neural-mediated flushing, which includes eccrine sweating ('wet flush'), versus flushing from agents that act directly on vascular smooth muscle ('dry flush'). This review describes the three types of blushing, including the type that responds to a low-dose, long-acting non-selective β-blocker such as nadolol 40 mg every morning. The use of aspirin to block niacin-induced flushing, and amitriptyline to treat facial dysesthesia, is described.

Flushing reactions in the chemotherapy patient. Wilkin JK. Arch Dermatol 1992; 128: 1387–9.

Chemotherapy causes of flushing are reviewed, along with other drugs that cause flushing.

Flushing reactions. Wilkin JK. In: Rook AJ, Maibach H, eds. Recent advances in dermatology. New York: Churchill Livingstone, 1983; 157–87.

This reviews categories of flushing reactions with catalogs of specific causes.

Influence of a serotonin- and dopamine-rich diet on platelet serotonin content and urinary excretion of biogenic amines and their metabolites. Kema IP, Schellings AM, Meiborg G, Hoppenbrouwers CJ, Muskiet FA. Clin Chem 1992; 38: 1730–6.

Serotonin, catecholamines, histamine, and their metabolites in urine, platelets, and tumor tissue of patients with carcinoid tumors. Kema IP, de Vries EG, Slooff MJ, Biesma B, Muskiet FA. Clin Chem 1994; 40: 86–95.

The platelet serotonin level measured by high-performance liquid chromatography (HPLC) and gas chromatography/ mass spectrometry (GC/MS) has a higher sensitivity for the detection of carcinoid tumors and is more consistently elevated than urinary 5-HIAA. Carcinoid flushing may occur with foregut carcinoids, which can have a low rate of serotonin production. Also, in contrast to urinary 5-HIAA, platelet serotonin is not influenced by the consumption of a serotonin-rich diet.

The quantitative 24-hour urinary 5-HIAA level is useful in the follow-up of carcinoid tumors with a high serotonin production rate. It is also useful initially for diagnosis, but only when it is positive during a low-serotonin diet. If the urinary 5-HIAA level is not elevated in a patient with flushing and other features characteristic of carcinoid, the platelet or blood serotonin level should be obtained.

FIRST-LINE THERAPIES

▶ Ice chips	B
▶ Aspirin	B
▶ Hormone replacement	A

Oral thermal-induced flushing in erythematotelangiectatic rosacea. Wilkin J. J Invest Dermatol 1981; 76: 15–8.

It is heat, not caffeine, that causes the flushing from drinking hot coffee.

Sucking on ice chips can abort mild menopausal, thermal, or spicy food-induced flushing.

Aspirin blocks nicotinic acid-induced flushing. Wilkin JK, Wilkin O, Kapp R, Donachie R, Chernosky ME, Buckner J. Clin Pharmacol Ther 1982; 31: 478–82.

Not only does aspirin block niacin flushing, but other cyclooxygenase inhibitors (non-steroidals) also block this prostaglandin-mediated flushing reaction. Importantly, the inhibition of cyclooxygenase does not reduce the lipid-lowering effect of niacin.

Although 975 mg of aspirin 1 hour before taking the niacin will greatly suppress the flushing reaction, a substantial number of the patients taking niacin are already taking non-steroidals, mostly for rheumatologic conditions. Generally, all that is needed is to change the time of dosing to 1 hour before the niacin, rather than adding a second non-steroidal drug and risking toxicity.

Aspirin attenuation of alcohol-induced flushing and intoxication in Oriental and Occidental subjects. Truitt EB, Gaynor CR, Mehl DL. Alcohol 1987; 1: 595–9.

Eight Oriental and three Occidental subjects sensitive to alcohol manifested as facial flushing were given 0.64 mg of aspirin 1 hour before orange juice with vodka at levels known to cause flushing. Facial flushing was markedly reduced after aspirin pretreatment.

Combined versus sequential hormonal replacement therapy: a double-blind, placebo-controlled study on quality of life-related outcome measures. Bech P, Munk-Jensen N, Obel EB, Ulrich LG, Eiken P, Nielsen SP. Psychother Psychosom 1998; 67: 259–65.

In a double-blind, placebo-controlled study of 105 early postmenopausal women, hormone replacement therapy (HRT) was superior to placebo for many symptoms, including hot flushing.

Although effective for controlling hot flashes, HRT has associated risks and is contraindicated for many women.

SECOND-LINE THERAPIES

▶ H$_1$ and H$_2$ antihistamines	C
▶ Clonidine, SSRIs, SNRIs	A

Scombroid fish poisoning – Pennsylvania, 1998. Centers for Disease Control and Prevention. MMWR Morb Mortal Wkly Rep (CDC) 2000; 49: 398–400.

Four adults in Pennsylvania had facial flushing, nausea, diarrhea, sweating, headache, metallic taste, and burning sensations in the mouth occurring within 5 minutes to 2 hours after eating tuna. Scombroid fish poisoning has been associated primarily with the consumption of tuna, mahi-mahi, and bluefish. Certain bacteria on such fish can grow in warm temperatures and produce enzymes that liberate histamine and other products from precursors in fish flesh.

The association of features of histamine toxicity (flushing, itching, hives, nausea, diarrhea, etc.) and the ingestion of fish should alert the physician to the possibility of scombroid fish poisoning. Both H$_1$ and H$_2$ antihistamines may be sufficient symptomatic therapy, and epinephrine (adrenaline) and systemic corticosteroids considered for more severe cases.

Histamine receptor antagonism of intolerance to alcohol in the Oriental population. Miller NS, Goodwin DW, Jones FC, Pardo MP, Anand MM, Gabrielli WF, et al. J Nerv Mental Dis 1987; 175: 661–7.

Each of 17 subjects received placebo, diphenhydramine 50 mg, and cimetidine 300 mg, singly and in combination, 1 hour before ethanol in a soft drink at a level sufficient to produce flushing. Cimetidine given alone blocked the flushing significantly more than diphenhydramine alone or placebo, but less than the combined antihistamines.

The obvious disadvantages are that non-steroidals can worsen an alcohol-provoked gastritis, and sedating antihistamines can enhance the alcohol-induced drowsiness. Patients should be screened for alcohol abuse using the CAGE questionnaire or a similar instrument, and warned about gastritis and sedation before combination pretreatment consisting of cimetidine, a non-sedating H$_1$ antihistamine, and a non-steroidal are prescribed. The author has found that such combination pretreatment greatly reduces the flushing and headache caused by red wine in sensitive subjects.

Primary care for survivors of breast cancer. Burstein HJ, Winer EP. N Engl J Med 2000; 343: 1086–94.

Table 4 of this paper summarizes a variety of non-estrogenic agents used to ameliorate hot flushes. Selective serotonin reuptake inhibitors received the most favorable comments.

Although the focus of this article is on breast cancer survivors, the list of non-estrogenic agents is useful for all women in whom estrogenic agents are contraindicated or not desirable. Clonidine patches are frequently associated with a contact dermatitis, so the author favors oral clonidine.

Phytoestrogens for vasomotor menopausal symptoms. Lethaby AE. Brown J, Marjoribanks J, et al. Cochrane Database Syst Rev 2007; (4): CD001395.

The current evidence indicates no clinically meaningful effect for phytoestrogens.

Nonhormonal therapies for menopausal hot-flashes. Nelson HD, Vesco KK, Haney E, Fu R, Nedrow A, Miller J, et al. JAMA 2006; 295: 2057–71.

In a review of published randomized controlled trials, there was evidence for the effectiveness of selective serotonin reuptake inhibitors, serotonin norepinephrine reuptake inhibitors, clonidine and gabapentin in controlling menopausal hot flashes. However, the efficacy of these non-hormonal treatments was less than that of estrogen.

Treatment strategies for reducing the burden of menopause-associated vasomotor symptoms. Umland EM. J Manag Care Pharm 2008; 14: S14–S19.

Non-pharmacologic modalities such as relaxation techniques and ways to avoid overheating are described along with pharmacologic interventions in a review of strategies for reducing hot flashes during the menopausal transition and perimenopause.

The hope for a 'natural cure' provided by phytoestrogens is not supported by the evidence. Non-hormonal drugs do not provide the full effectiveness provided by HRT; however, non-hormonal drugs coupled with strategies to avoid overheating, sucking on ice chips, and relaxation techniques may be sufficient to avoid resorting to HRT. Clonidine 0.1 mg orally daily may be better accepted by patients than fluoxetine, paroxetine, or venlafaxine, which carry the designation of 'antidepressant.'

THIRD-LINE THERAPIES

► Somatostatin analogs	E
► Excision for carcinoid tumors	D
► Sympathectomy for severe, refractory blushing	B

Treatment of type II gastric carcinoid tumors with somatostatin analogues. Tomassetti P, Migliori M, Caletti GC, Fusaroli P, Corinaldesi R, Gullo L. N Engl J Med 2000; 343: 551–4.

This is a report of three patients with multiple type II gastric carcinoids treated with lanreotide or octreotide acetate. In all three patients there was a reduction in size and number of the carcinoid tumors after 6 months of somatostatin analog treatment, and complete disappearance of tumors after 1 year. A report of regression of a type III gastric carcinoid with octreotide is also cited.

Although all three types of gastric carcinoid tumor are usually removed surgically, somatostatin analogs, especially the longer-acting octreotide acetate (20 mg intramuscularly every 28 days), provide a successful medical option.

Management of facial flushing. Licht PB, Pilegaard HK. Thorac Surg Clin 2008; 18: 223–8.

Although the title might imply flushing disorders more generally, the specific focus is on the uncontrollable, rapid onset of blushing in response to embarrassment from the attention of others. 'The key to success in sympathetic surgery for facial blushing lies in a meticulous and critical patient selection and in ensuring that the patient is thoroughly informed about the high risk of side effects.'

The authors must be congratulated for the unvarnished presentation of side effects which may dissuade all but those with truly refractory, severe blushing from considering sympathetic surgery.

Evidence Levels: **A** Double-blind study **B** Clinical trial ≥ 20 subjects **C** Clinical trial < 20 subjects **D** Series ≥ 5 subjects **E** Anecdotal case reports

Follicular mucinosis

Sasha Dhoat, Malcolm Rustin

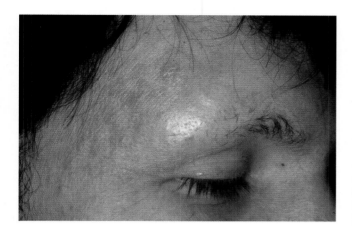

Follicular mucinosis is characterized histologically by mucinous degeneration of the follicular outer root sheaths and sebaceous glands with an inflammatory infiltrate composed of lymphocytes, histiocytes, and eosinophils. Lesions consist of erythematous, scaly, and infiltrated plaques with follicular papules or prominent follicular orifices, and may demonstrate alopecia (alopecia mucinosa). Benign follicular mucinosis tends to affect younger patients (under 40 years), with a small number of lesions, usually situated on the head and neck. Although lesions may resolve spontaneously within 2 years, a more generalized benign form, with lesions on the trunk and extremities, may run a chronic relapsing course over many years. Follicular mucinosis is associated with lymphoma, particularly mycosis fungoides, in 15–30% of cases. It is still unclear whether follicular mucinosis is a transitional state evolving into mycosis fungoides in these cases. No single clinical or histological feature predicts which patients will have a benign course, although those found to have mycosis fungoides rarely had initial lesions on the head and neck. Associated lymphoma tends (although not invariably) to be associated with age over 30 years, a wider distribution of lesions, and possibly systemic features such as night sweats, weight loss, or lymphadenopathy.

MANAGEMENT STRATEGY

There is no standard therapy for follicular mucinosis. Because spontaneous resolution occurs in the benign forms, *observation* alone is certainly justified, particularly in the younger patient with limited disease. However, the need for *follow-up and evaluation to exclude lymphoma* must be emphasized. Follicular mucinosis associated with mycosis fungoides or other neoplastic or inflammatory disorders is managed by treating the underlying associated condition.

SPECIFIC INVESTIGATIONS

▶ Skin biopsy
▶ Immunohistochemistry and T-cell gene receptor analysis may be helpful adjuncts to skin biopsy

▶ Consider investigations to rule out lymphoma or other underlying disorders, depending on the presenting clinical features (general examination, plain radiology, and CT scans)

The cutaneous mucinoses. Truhan AP, Roenigk HH. J Am Acad Dermatol 1986; 14: 1–18.

Follicular mucinosis: a critical reappraisal of clinicopathologic features and association with mycosis fungoides and Sézary syndrome. Cerroni L, Fink-Puches R, Bäck B, Helmut K. Arch Dermatol 2002; 138: 182–9.

Two excellent reviews of the follicular mucinosis literature, including histopathology and investigation.

FIRST-LINE THERAPIES

▶ Topical and intralesional corticosteroids	**D**
▶ Dapsone	**E**
▶ Mepacrine	**E**
▶ Tetracycline	**E**

Follicular mucinosis: a study of 47 patients. Emmerson RW. Br J Dermatol 1969; 81: 395–413.

Topical or intralesional corticosteroids improved surface eczematous change in eight of 22 patients with benign disease whose lesions resolved spontaneously within 2 years. Deeper follicular and dermal changes were not affected. Resolution was considered to have occurred independently of treatment. Six of 10 patients with benign chronic disease of more than 2 years' duration showed slight improvement with topical or intralesional corticosteroids.

Alopecia mucinosa: a follow-up study. Coskey RJ, Mehregan AH. Arch Dermatol 1970; 102: 193–4.

Topical or intralesional corticosteroids were applied to seven patients with one or two facial lesions. All lesions resolved, as did lesions in two untreated patients. In patients with more than two lesions, including extremity lesions, nine of 15 patients given topical corticosteroids had complete clearance.

Urticaria-like follicular mucinosis responding to dapsone. Al Harthi F, Kudwah, A, Ajlan A, Nuaim A, Shehri F. Acta Dermatol Venereol 2003; 83: 389–90.

Itchy urticaria-like papules on the face, chest, and back of a 25-year-old man for 2 years responded to dapsone 100 mg daily long term after previously failing to respond to oral prednisolone. Attempts to reduce the dosage resulted in recurrence.

Follicular mucinosis presenting as acute dermatitis and response to dapsone. Rustin MHA, Bunker C, Levene GM. Clin Exp Dermatol 1989; 14: 382–4.

Facial follicular mucinosis clinically resembling acute extensive dermatitis in a 34-year-old man rapidly responded to dapsone 100 mg daily and topical clobetasol propionate; 6 months of maintenance therapy was required.

Atypical follicular mucinosis controlled with mepacrine. Sonnex TS, Ryan T, Dawber RPR. Br J Dermatol 1981; 105: 83–4.

Facial lesions in a 39-year-old man responded to mepacrine 100 mg twice daily. Lesions redeveloped on cessation of therapy.

A case of follicular mucinosis treated successfully with minocycline. Yotsumoto S, Uchimiya H, Kanzaki T. Br J Dermatol 2000; 142: 841–2.

A 36-year-old man presented with itchy papular lesions on his head, nape, and chest. After histological confirmation of the diagnosis, indometacin was tried (no time specified), but was not effective. Minocycline 100 mg daily for 6 weeks induced complete remission.

Follicular mucinosis presenting as an acneiform eruption: report of four cases. Wittenberg GP, Gibson LE, Pittelkow MR, el-Azhary RA. J Am Acad Dermatol 1988; 38: 849–51.

Facial acneiform lesions in a 21-year-old woman responded well to tetracycline (dose not recorded) and benzoyl peroxide gel. There was a minor improvement in the facial papules of a 31-year-old man with minocycline 100 mg daily for 4 months.

SECOND-LINE THERAPIES

► Isotretinoin	E
► Psoralen and UVA (PUVA)	E
► UVA1	E
► Indometacin	E
► Interferon (IFN)	E
► Superficial radiotherapy	D
► Systemic corticosteroids	E
► Photodynamic therapy	E

Follicular mucinosis successfully treated with isotretinoin. Guerriero C, De Simone C, Guidi B, Rotoli M, Venier A. Eur J Dermatol 1999; 9: 22–4.

A 33-year-old man with facial lesions and no systemic disease was treated with isotretinoin 0.5 mg/kg daily. After 2 months remission was achieved, with tapering of the dose of isotretinoin after a further 3 weeks.

Follicular mucinosis presenting as an acneiform eruption: report of four cases. Wittenberg GP, Gibson LE, Pittelkow MR, el-Azhary RA. J Am Acad Dermatol 1998; 38: 849–51.

Two women under 40 years of age had acneiform facial lesions. One had reduced numbers and size of lesions following tretinoin gel 0.01% daily and oral pentoxifylline 400 mg three times daily, followed 2 years later by isotretinoin 40 mg daily. The second significantly improved following isotretinoin 40 mg daily and intermittent clobetasol cream.

Follicular mucinosis treated with PUVA. Kenicer KJA, Lakshmipathi T. Br J Dermatol 1982; 107: 48–9.

A 79-year-old woman with facial, truncal, and limb papules with no evidence of systemic disease failed to respond to topical corticosteroids and localized radiotherapy (100 Gy over 5 days). After a total of 98 treatments of PUVA over 5 months, with total exposure dose 45.4 J/cm^2, she remained disease free.

Treatment of idiopathic mucinosis follicularis with UVA1 cold light phototherapy. Von Kobyletzki G, Kreuter JA, Nordmeier R, Stücker M, Altmeyer P. Dermatology 2000; 201: 76–7

A 26-year-old Caucasian woman with itchy follicular papules on the trunk for 7 months was diagnosed histologically

and started on potent corticosteroids with no success. A UVA1 cold light source (340–530 nm) was used five times a week for 3 weeks and induced remission that had been sustained at 3 months.

Follicular mucinosis: response to indomethacin. Kodama H, Umemura S, Nohara N. J Dermatol 1988; 15: 72–5.

Plaques and papules on the face and back of a 48-year-old man with no signs of cutaneous lymphoma were unresponsive to topical corticosteroids, UVA, or dapsone. Indometacin 1% in white petrolatum was applied topically until the lesions disappeared. Oral indometacin 75 mg daily reduced untreated lesions, but was not tolerated. The patient was lesion free at 5-year follow-up.

Successful treatment of primary progressive follicular mucinosis with interferons. Meissner K, Weyer U, Kowalzick L, Altenhoff J. J Am Acad Dermatol 1991; 24: 848–50.

A 37-year-old man had a 5-year history of facial, truncal, and upper extremity lesions with alopecia, and no evidence of systemic disease. Isotretinoin, dapsone, and systemic corticosteroids were unhelpful. Increasing doses of recombinant IFN-α_{2b} up to 9 million IU/m^2 were administered subcutaneously three times weekly, with recombinant IFN-γ 100 mg subcutaneously daily every 4th week. For 4 months, 5 million IU of IFN-α_{2b} were injected intralesionally into the chin lesion three times weekly. Slight relapse led to an increase in the dosage to 10 million IU/m^2. Complete remission was achieved by week 46. The treatment was well tolerated.

Follicular mucinosis: a study of 47 patients. Emmerson RW. Br J Dermatol 1969; 81: 395–413.

Two patients with benign disease lasting more than 2 years were treated with 40 Gy X-rays and had complete resolution. Two patients with benign chronic disease treated with X-rays (dose not recorded) had no benefit.

Acneiform follicular mucinosis. Passaro EMC, Silveira MT, Valente NYS. Clin Exp Dermatol 2004; 29: 396–8.

A 36-year-old man presented with a 1-year history of acneiform follicular mucinosis and was commenced on 40 mg prednisolone for 20 days. His symptoms improved quickly and the prednisolone was weaned off by day 48. He had been clear for 7 months at the time of writing.

Alopecia mucinosa: a follow-up study. Coskey RJ, Mehregan AH. Arch Dermatol 1970; 102: 193–4.

Patients with one or two facial lesions were given superficial X-ray therapy in a weekly dose of 7.5 Gy for 4 weeks (three cases) or a combination of X-ray therapy and topical corticosteroid cream (six cases). In all cases lesions resolved.

Primary follicular mucinosis: excellent response to treatment with photodynamic therapy. Fernandez-Guarino M, Harto Castano A, Cariilo R. J Eur Acad Dermatol Venereol 2008; 22: 393–404.

A 74-year-old woman with a 4-year history of recalcitrant facial plaques cleared with one session of photodynamic therapy (topical methylaminolevulinic acid, red light source, 630 nm, 37 J/cm^2, 7.5 min). She had previously been recalcitrant to topical corticosteroids, narrowband UVB, and sulfone. She remained clinically clear 9 months post treatment.

Folliculitis

Rebecca Kleinerman, Robert Phelps

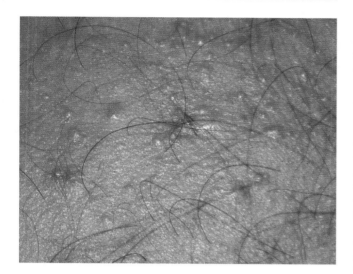

Folliculitis is a term used to describe inflammation around the pilosebaceous unit. Such inflammation may be superficial, resulting in the clinical appearance of erythematous papules and pustules, or deep, with extension into furuncles and abscesses. The etiology of folliculitis may be broadly divided into infectious and non-infectious.

Infectious folliculitis is bacterial (Gram-positive, usually *Staphylococcus aureus*, as well as Gram-negative, including *Klebsiella*, *Proteus*, *Pseudomonas* and *Enterobacter* spp.), viral (molluscum, herpetic), fungal (including yeasts such as *Candida* and *Pityrosporum* spp. and the dermatophytes), syphilitic, or parasitic (typically *Demodex* spp.). A detailed history, close physical inspection, and specific laboratory investigations may be helpful in reaching a diagnosis. For instance, patients taking retinoids and those with atopic dermatitis are susceptible to staphylococcal folliculitis; a lamellar circle of desquamation surrounding the papules or pustules may be a clue that this is the case. Patients on long-term acne treatment with antibiotics are particularly vulnerable to Gram-negative infections; these may occur in the perinasal area due to nasal carriage of coliforms. Jacuzzi bathers may develop a widespread folliculitis due to *Pseudomonas aeruginosa* soon after exposure. Immunocompromised patients, particularly those with HIV infection, develop a variety of follicular inflammatory lesions caused by bacteria and viruses, as well as a characteristic sterile eosinophilic folliculitis that is paradoxically related to both immune suppression and reconstitution. *Pityrosporum* folliculitis, often occurring in warmer climates, favors the upper trunk and is often seen in teenagers and males. Folliculitis of the beard area (also called sycosis) may be related to both *Staphylococcus* and *Candida albicans* infections. *Demodex* mites have been tied to many follicular eruptions, particularly rosacea-like lesions on the face. A series of laboratory tests (below) serves to point the clinician in the appropriate direction.

The non-infectious forms of folliculitis include those associated with sun exposure (superficial actinic folliculitis), occupational contact with oils or tars, epilation (traumatic folliculitis), or systemic diseases including rheumatologic (Behçet's disease, Reiter's syndrome, systemic lupus erythematosus, mixed connective tissue disease, and rheumatoid arthritis), renal (perforating folliculitis), gastrointestinal (inflammatory bowel disease), and blood dyscrasias. Pregnancy and drugs (e.g., corticosteroids, ciclosporin, lithium, halogens, anti-tuberculosis medications, and epidermal growth factor receptor (EGFR) inhibitors) may also cause folliculitis.

MANAGEMENT STRATEGY

Treatment for infective forms of folliculitis should be directed at the underlying infection. Preferred treatments include *topical antibiotics or antiseptics, or systemic antibiotics*. Although little evidence-based information is available on these treatments, clinical evidence supports the use of topical antibiotics and antiseptics for localized infections. The recent emergence of widespread community-acquired methicillin-resistant *Staphylococcus aureus (CA-MRSA)* infections, usually manifesting as folliculitis or as an abscess, requires the clinician to consider early coverage of *MRSA* in high-risk populations and areas. Oral antibiotics should be used if infections are widespread.

Folliculitis associated with external agents such as tar, oils or systemic corticosteroids improves when the agents are discontinued, although the improvement may be delayed for weeks to months.

New treatments for refractory folliculitis have been suggested in recent years, including intramuscular immunoglobulin and photodynamic therapy. More studies are necessary to confirm their efficacy in order to recommend them for general use.

SPECIFIC INVESTIGATIONS

▶ Complete clinical investigation: history of medications used, concurrent systemic diseases, occupational exposures, other non-occupational exposure (sun exposure, new clothing); family history
▶ Culture with sensitivity from pustules
▶ Gram stain and mycology from touch prep, Tzanck or scraping; or biopsy if necessary with Gram and fungal stains ordered
▶ Complete blood count, immunologic work-up (for immunodeficiency), routine blood chemistry, renal function, HIV status if necessary
▶ Nasal culture if carrier state is suspected in chronic cases

FIRST-LINE THERAPIES

Topical

▶ Fusidic acid, or mupirocin for *S. aureus*	A
▶ Retapamulin for *S. aureus*	B
▶ Mupirocin for eradication of *S. aureus* colonization of the nares; tea tree oil soap or body wash for body	B
▶ Povidone-iodine, acetic acid or gentamicin for *Pseudomonas aeruginosa*	A
▶ Topical corticosteroid for eosinophilic pustular folliculitis	C
▶ Pimecrolimus for eosinophilic pustular folliculitis	D
▶ Permethrin cream for *Demodex* spp.	D

Topical therapy

A comparison of sodium fusidate ointment and mupirocin ointment in superficial skin sepsis. Morley PAR, Munot LD. Curr Med Res Opin 1988; 11: 142–8.

These antibiotics were equally effective in 354 patients.

Topical retapamulin ointment, 1%, versus sodium fusidate ointment, 2%, for impetigo: A randomized, observer-blinded, noninferiority study. Oranje AP, Chosidow O, Sacchidanand S, Todd G, Singh K, Scangarella N, et al. Dermatology 2007; 215: 331–40.

Retapamulin demonstrated equal efficacy with sodium fusidate in the topical treatment of superficial skin infections. Retapamulin may be slightly more effective in treating MRSA strains.

A randomized, controlled trial regimen for the clearance of MRSA colonization. Dryden MS, Dailly S, Crouch M. J Hosp Infect 2004; 56: 283–6.

A controlled study comparing standard treatment to eradicate MRSA colonization with newer treatments; mupirocin is first-line treatment for the nares, whereas tea tree soap and body wash worked slightly better than chlorhexidine on the body.

Optimum outpatient therapy of skin and skin structure infections. Failla DM, Pankey GA. Drugs 1994; 49: 172–8.

Most cases of pseudomonal folliculitis require no treatment. If the infection is widespread, however, topical povidone-iodine, 1% acetic acid soaks, or gentamicin cream are useful.

Eosinophilic pustular folliculitis. A comprehensive review of treatment options. Ellis E, Scheinfeld N. Am J Clin Dermatol 2004; 5: 189–97.

There are no controlled trials for any of the treatment options for this condition. This review covers current treatment options.

Eosinophilic pustular folliculitis: successful treatment with topical pimecrolimus. Rho NK, Kim BJ. Clin Exp Dermatol 2007; 32: 108–9.

Significant improvement was observed after 1 week of therapy and failure of other modalities.

Recalictrant papulopustular rosacea in an immunocompetent patient responding to combination therapy with with oral ivermectin and topical permethrin. Kallen KJ, Davis CL, Billings SD, Mousdicas N. Cutis 2007; 80: 149–51.

Permethrin 5% in combination with ivermectin resulted in resolution of the folliculitis.

Systemic therapy

A comparison of fusidic acid and flucloxacillin in the treatment of skin and soft-tissue infections. Eur J Clin Res 1994; 5: 97–106.

Flucloxacillin 500 mg three times daily and 500 mg fusidic acid over 5–10 days resulted in an equal improvement in these infections.

Fusidic acid tablets in patients with skin and soft-tissue infection: a dose-finding study. Carr WD, Wall AR, Georgala-Zervogiani S, Stratigos J, Gouriotou K. Eur J Clin Res 1994; 5: 87–95.

Fusidic acid 500 mg daily was approximately as effective as 1.5 mg daily.

Skin diseases associated with *Malassezia* species. Gupta AK, Batra R, Bluhm R, Boekhout T, Dawson TL Jr. J Am Acad Dermatol 2004; 51: 785–98.

Oral itraconazole is effective for extensive pityrosporum folliculitis.

Hot tub folliculitis or hot hand–foot syndrome caused by *Pseudomonas aeruginosa*. J Am Acad Dermatol. 2007; 57: 596–600.

Ciprofloxacin was effective for acute manifestations of this syndrome, which quickly resolved following therapy.

SECOND-LINE THERAPIES

Comparison of two regimens of oral clindamycin versus dicloxacillin in the treatment of mild to moderate skin and soft tissue infections. Blaszczyk-Kostanecka M, Dobozy A, Dominguez-Soto L, Guerrero R, Hunyadi J, Lopera J. Curr Ther Res Clin Exp 1998; 59: 341–53.

In this prospective, randomized study, clindamycin 150 mg four times a day, clindamycin 300 mg twice daily, and dicloxacillin 250 mg four times a day for 7–14 days were compared in patients with skin infections including folliculitis. There was no difference in the healing or relapse rates. Patients were followed for up to 3 weeks after completing treatment.

A comparative study of the efficacy, safety and tolerance of azithromycin, dicloxacillin and flucloxacillin in the treatment of children with acute skin and skin structure infections. Rodrigues-Solares A, Pérez-Gutiérrez F, Prosperi J, Milgram E, Martin A. J Antimicrob Chemother 1993; 31: 103–9.

This was an open, randomized study to compare a 3-day regimen of azithromycin with a 7-day course of dicloxacillin and flucloxacillin in the treatment of acute skin infections in children. Bacteriological cure was similar with all treatment regimens.

Intramuscular immunoglobulin for recalcitrant suppurative diseases of the skin: a retrospective review of 63 cases. Goo B, Chung HJ, Chung WG, Chung KY. Br J Dermatol 2007; 157: 563–8.

Intramuscular human immunoglobulin injections reduced the severity and appearance of new lesions in patients with intractable suppurative skin diseases, including folliculitis, with minimal adverse effects.

Topical methyl aminolevulinate photodynamic therapy for the treatment of folliculitis. Horn M, Wolf P. Photodermatol Photoimmunol Photomed 2007; 23: 145–7.

Seven patients with recalcitrant folliculitis were treated with methyl aminolevulinate photodynamic therapy; this resulted in a significant reduction in inflammatory lesions in six of the seven patients studied.

Folliculitis decalvans

Andrew JG McDonagh

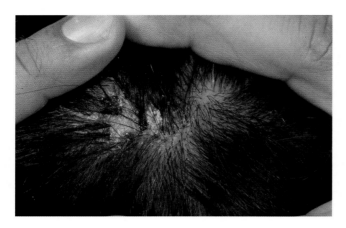

Folliculitis decalvans is a rare progressive purulent folliculitis of the scalp resulting in follicular atrophy and subsequent scarring alopecia. 'Tufted folliculitis' is a characteristic of the disorder in evolution, with multiple hair tufts emerging from inflamed and crusted follicular orifices.

The etiology is unknown. Impaired immune responses, *Staphylococcus aureus* infection, nevoid lesions, and seborrheic states have been suggested as playing a role in its pathogenesis, though much controversy surrounds the role of each factor. Gram-positive organisms are usually present during active disease phases.

Folliculitis decalvans may affect any hairbearing region – scalp, face, axillae, pubes, and inner thighs. Scalp disease affects both sexes. In other sites it is confined to adult males. It occurs predominantly in men from adolescence onwards, and in women between the third and sixth decades.

MANAGEMENT STRATEGY

Treatment of this chronic and progressive disease is notoriously difficult. *Underlying diseases such as immunodeficiency* or *fungal infection* should be sought. *Staphylococcus aureus* or other Gram-positive organisms are present in follicular pustules and sometimes also in the anterior nares. *Bacteriology swabs* should be taken for culture and to determine sensitivity.

Topical and systemic antibiotics are the mainstay of treatment. Systemic antibiotics such as *tetracycline, minocycline, flucloxacillin,* and *third-generation cephalosporins* may inhibit the extension of disease, but only for as long as they are administered. *Rifampin* has been proposed as the most beneficial therapeutic option in recalcitrant cases, but should not be used as monotherapy because of the rapid emergence of resistance. A regimen of systemic *rifampin* 300 mg twice daily and *clindamycin* 300 mg twice daily for 10 weeks has produced marked improvement, with infrequent relapse after one or more treatment courses. Prolonged courses of *dapsone* can also be beneficial.

Systemic corticosteroids suppress the inflammatory response and may provide moderate temporary improvement. There have been anecdotal reports of success using oral *zinc sulfate* (*in combination with fusidic acid*). Treatments that destroy hair follicles and prevent hair regrowth may be considered; these

include *X-ray epilation, laser epilation, cryosurgery,* and *surgical excision.* Improvement has also been reported with shaving the scalp. *Keratolytics* and *tar shampoos* may reduce the scaling and erythema that herald extension of the disease.

SPECIFIC INVESTIGATIONS

> ► Swabs for bacteriology of follicular pustules and carrier sites
> ► Fungal microscopy and culture
> ► Scalp biopsy
> ► Immunodeficiency screen

Acquired scalp alopecia. Part II: A review. Sullivan JR, Kossard S. Australas J Dermatol 1999; 40: 61–72.

A case of an individual with HIV infection who developed severe folliculitis decalvans after commencing triple antiviral therapy.

Folliculitis decalvans with hypocomplementaemia. Fraser NG, Grant PW. Br J Dermatol 1982; 107: 88 [Abstract].

A case of a 12-year-old girl with folliculitis decalvans, recurrent nasal sores, bronchitis, and secondarily infected chilblain reactions on her feet. She also had low C3 and C4 levels.

Folliculitis decalvans and cellular immunity – 2 brothers with oral candidiasis. Shitara A, Igareshi R, Morohashi M. Jpn J Dermatol 1974; 28: 133.

Severe folliculitis decalvans in two siblings who also had chronic oral candidiasis; defective cell-mediated immunity was demonstrated.

Tufted folliculitis of the scalp; a distinctive clinicohistological variant of folliculitis decalvans. Amnessi G. Br J Dermatol 1998; 138: 799–805.

Purulent material from dilated follicules was sampled in 10 patients. *S. aureus* was isolated in all cases, whereas fungal cultures were negative.

FIRST-LINE THERAPIES

Topical antibiotics	
► Fusidic acid, clindamycin	E
Systemic antibiotics	
► Rifampin and clindamycin	C
► Tetracycline, minocycline, flucloxacillin, and third-generation cephalosporins	C

Management of primary cicatricial alopecias: options for treatment. Harries MJ, Sinclair RD, MacDonald-Hull S, Whiting DA, Griffiths CE, Paus R. Br J Dermatol 2008; 159: 1–22.

An extensive review and summary of reported treatments for disorders including folliculitis decalvans.

Folliculitis decalvans including tufted folliculitis: clinical, histological and therapeutic findings. Powell JJ, Dawber RPR, Gatter K. Br J Dermatol 1999; 140: 328–33.

Eighteen patients with folliculitis decalvans treated with a combination of oral rifampin 300 mg twice daily and clindamycin 300 mg twice daily for 10 weeks. Ten of the 18 patients responded well, with no evidence of recurrence 2–22 months

Evidence Levels: **A** Double-blind study **B** Clinical trial ≥ 20 subjects **C** Clinical trial < 20 subjects **D** Series ≥ 5 subjects **E** Anecdotal case reports

after one course of treatment, and 15 of the 18 responded after two to three courses.

Tufted folliculitis of the scalp: a distinctive clinicohistological variant of folliculitis decalvans. Annessi G. Br J Dermatol 1998; 138: 799–805.

A useful review of the strengths and limitations of topical and oral antibiotics for folliculitis decalvans.

Folliculitis decalvans – response to rifampicin. Brozena SJ, Cohen LE, Fenske NA. Cutis 1988; 42: 512–15.

A recalcitrant case of folliculitis decalvans with excellent response to rifampin 600 mg daily for 10 weeks.

SECOND-LINE THERAPIES

▶ Fusidic acid and oral zinc sulfate	E
▶ Dapsone	E
▶ Prednisolone and isotretinoin	E

Folliculitis decalvans. Abeck D, Korting HC, Braun-Falco O. Acta Dermatol Venereol 1992; 72: 143–5.

Three patients with folliculitis decalvans, followed up for more than a year, responded to a combination of oral and topical fusidic acid and oral zinc sulfate. Each patient received a 3-week oral course of fusidic acid 500 mg tds and a 6-month course of zinc sulfate 200 mg bd, after which the dose was reduced to 200 mg daily. Treatment with fusidic acid and zinc sulfate was started simultaneously. In addition, 1.5% fusidic acid cream was applied for the first 2 weeks.

Dapsone treatment of folliculitis decalvans. Paquet P, Pierard GE. Ann Dermatol Venereol 2004; 131: 195–7.

Two cases of folliculitis decalvans treated with dapsone 75–100 mg daily, with clearance of pustular folliculitis after 1–2 months. Moderate relapse occurred within a few weeks of stopping dapsone; remission was sustained for 1–3 years on a maintenance dose of 25 mg daily.

Simultaneous occurrence of folliculitis decalvans capillitii in identical twins. Douwes KE, Landthaler M, Szeimies R-M. Br J Dermatol 2000; 143: 195–7.

The use of oral prednisolone with low-dose isotretinoin to control folliculitis decalvans is described.

THIRD-LINE THERAPIES

▶ Surgical excision	E
▶ Keratolytics and tar shampoo	E E
▶ X-ray epilation	E E
▶ Laser epilation	E

Tufted hair folliculitis. Tong AK, Baden HP. J Am Acad Dermatol 1989; 21: 1096–9.

Successful treatment of tufted folliculitis by surgical excision.

Tufted hair folliculitis. A study of 4 cases. Leulmo-Aguilar J, Gonzalez-Castro U, Castells-Rodelas A. Br J Dermatol 1993; 128: 454–7.

The authors consider that erythema and scaling herald extension of the disease process, and that treatment with keratolytics and tar shampoo is important.

Folliculitis decalvans treated with radiation therapy. Smith EP, Hardaway CA, Graham BS, Johnstone PA. Cutis 2006; 78: 162–4.

X-rays used as the final resort in a patient who failed to respond to other modalities.

Nd:YAG laser treatment of recalcitrant folliculitis decalvans. Parlette EC, Kroeger N, Ross EV. Dermatol Surg 2004; 30: 1152–4.

Remission achieved by laser epilation in an African-American patient.

Based on the optical properties of light in skin, the Nd:YAG laser is the best for laser depilation in dark individuals.

Fox–Fordyce disease

Ian Coulson

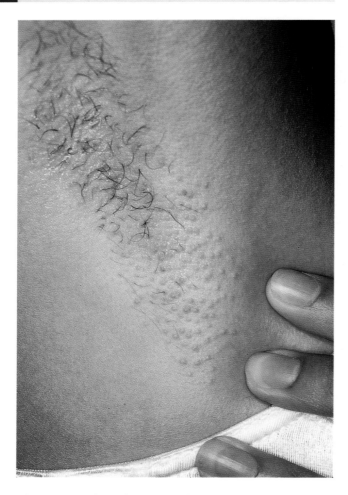

Obliteration of the follicular infundibulum with keratin in the apocrine gland-bearing skin is the cause of this rare, paroxysmally intensely itchy condition. Apocrine sweat retention and rupture of the gland duct under periods of apocrine sudomotor stimulation, particularly emotional stress, results in the development of an itchy, spongiotic intraepidermal vesicle. Itchy, dome-shaped, flesh-colored or keratotic papules that develop peripubertally in the apocrine areas of the axillae and pubic and periareolar skin characterize this condition, which predominates in women. Sparsity of axillary hair is usual. Improvement in pregnancy and during the administration of the oral contraceptive pill has led to speculation regarding an endocrine etiology, but this has been unsubstantiated by blood sex hormone investigations. It has been reported in Turner's syndrome.

MANAGEMENT STRATEGY

There are no controlled trials of any agents in Fox–Fordyce disease.

Topical and intralesional corticosteroids are frequently tried and may be of limited benefit, but atrophy in the axillary area will limit their potency and duration of use. Topical *tretinoin* has been reported to reduce itch, but its alternation with a mild corticosteroid may be needed to reduce retinoid irritancy. *Clindamycin* lotion may be of help. The *oral contraceptive pill (OCP)* may bring relief to some women. Oral *isotretinoin* may give temporary help. *Electrocautery* and *excision* of the periareolar skin may offer permanent solutions. A recent report advocates an ingenious method of removal of the apocrine glands using a microliposuction cannula.

SPECIFIC INVESTIGATIONS

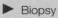 Biopsy

Fox–Fordyce disease: diagnosis by transverse histologic sections. Stashower ME, Krivda SJ, Turiansky GW. J Am Acad Dermatol 2000; 42: 89–91.

Transverse sectioning demonstrates the follicular plugging and infundibular spongiosis more readily than conventional sections.

Patterns histopathologic of Fox–Fordyce disease. Böer A. Am J Dermatopathol 2004; 26: 482–92.

An exhaustive review of the subtleties of the dermatopathology of Fox–Fordyce disease.

Axillary perifollicular xanthomatosis resembling Fox–Fordyce disease. Kossard S, Dwyer P. Australas J Dermatol 2004; 45: 146–8.

Perifollicular xanthomatosis as a key histological finding in Fox–Fordyce disease. Mataix J, Silvestre JF, Niveiro M, Lucas A, Pérez-Crespo M. Actas Dermosifiliogr 2008; 99: 145–8.

There are occasional conditions to consider in the differential diagnosis! There is even controversy as to whether perifollicular xanthomatosis is part of the spectrum of this disorder.

FIRST-LINE THERAPIES

▶ Topical and intralesional corticosteroids	**D**
▶ Topical clindamycin	**E**
▶ Oral contraceptive pill	**D**
▶ Topical retinoids	**D**
▶ UVB	**D**
▶ Topical pimecrolimus	**D**

A new treatment of Fox–Fordyce disease. Helfamn RJ. South Med J 1962; 55: 681–4.

A single report of successful symptom relief of axillary lesions with 10 mg/mL triamcinolone diluted with an equal volume of 1% lidocaine to four sites on nine occasions over 3 months.

Fox–Fordyce disease – successful treatment with topical clindamycin in alcoholic propylene glycol solution. Feldmann R, Masouye I, Chavaz P, Saurat JH. Dermatology 1992; 184: 310–13.

A single report of Fox–Fordyce disease in the axillary, pubic, and inguinal areas responding to 1% clindamycin in an alcoholic propylene glycol solution within 1 month (clindamycin 10 mg/mL; propylene glycol 50 mg/mL; isopropyl alcohol 0.5 mg/mL; water). Nine months later the treatment was stopped and no recurrence was observed. The authors speculate that the keratolytic effect of propylene glycol may have been responsible for the therapeutic effect.

Evidence Levels: A Double-blind study **B** Clinical trial ≥ 20 subjects **C** Clinical trial < 20 subjects **D** Series ≥ 5 subjects **E** Anecdotal case reports

Fox–Fordyce disease. Treatment with an oral contraceptive. Kronthal HI, Pomeranz JR, Sitomer G. Arch Dermatol 1965; 91: 243–5.

Two female patients responded to a high estrogen dose combined OCP, norethynodrel and mestranol.

Fox–Fordyce disease. Control with tretinoin cream. Giacobetti R, Caro WA, Roenigk HH Jr. Arch Dermatol 1979; 115: 1365–6.

A single report of 0.1% tretinoin cream applied to the axillae on alternate nights resulting in reduction of itch and regrowth of hair. Local retinoid irritation was controlled with 1% hydrocortisone cream.

Treatment of Fox–Fordyce disease. Pinkus H. JAMA 1973; 223: 924.

Erythemogenic doses of UVB (once weekly for 4–6 weeks) produced long-lasting relief to several patients.

Pimecrolimus is effective in Fox–Fordyce disease. Pock L, Svrcková M, Macháčková R, Hercogová J. Int J Dermatol 2006; 45: 1134–5.

A series of three patients who benefited from topical pimecrolimus.

The treatment of Fox–Fordyce disease. Shelley WB. JAMA 1972; 222: 1069.

A concise review of the therapies available to that date. The author admits that sometimes all fails and that relief may only come at the menopause.

SECOND-LINE THERAPIES

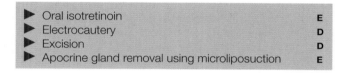

▶ Oral isotretinoin	E
▶ Electrocautery	D
▶ Excision	D
▶ Apocrine gland removal using microliposuction	E

Fox–Fordyce disease in a male patient – response to oral retinoid treatment. Effendy I, Ossowski B, Happle R. Clin Exp Dermatol 1994; 19: 67–9.

Oral treatment with isotretinoin (30 mg daily for 8 weeks then 15 mg daily for 2 months) resulted in temporary relief. Relapse occurred 3 months after discontinuation.

Fox–Fordyce disease in the post-menopausal period treated successfully with electrocoagulation. Pasricha JS, Nayyar KC. Dermatologica 1973; 147: 271–3.

Electrocoagulation to a level of 3–4 mm under local anesthetic produced a permanent resolution of symptoms in the axillae of two patients.

Surgical treatment of areolar hidradenitis suppurativa and Fox–Fordyce disease. Chavoin J-P, Charasson T, Barnard J-D. Ann Chir Plast Esthet 1994; 39: 233–8.

A simple technique involving dermal detachment of the areola, excision of the underlying apocrine glands, and reattachment of the areola with good cosmetic results.

This treatment has not proved beneficial long term.

Axillary Fox–Fordyce disease treated with liposuction-assisted curettage. Chae KM, Marschall MA, Marschall SF. Arch Dermatol 2002; 138: 452–4.

A novel technique of curettage removal of the apocrine glands using a small liposuction cannula with symptom relief, great cosmesis, and a follow-up at publication of 8 months. A liposuction cannula was introduced through a stab incision in the axilla and, with the aperture of the cannula turned up towards the underside of the dermis, the deeper dermis was curetted to create inflammation and subsequent fibrosis. The same technique can be used to treat axillary hyperhidrosis.

Furunculosis

Charles A Gropper, Karthik Krishnamurthy

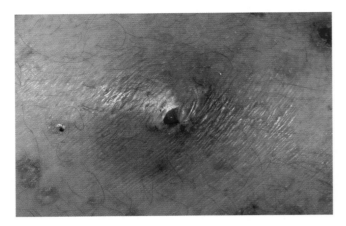

Furunculosis, commonly referred to as 'boils,' is a deep infection of the pilosebaceous unit. Lesions may occur on any hair-bearing surface, including the nares. When many hair follicles are involved, the term carbuncle is used. These large, suppurative lesions are usually very tender and may have multiple draining sites.

The infectious agent most commonly implicated is *Staphylococcus aureus*. Most patients with furunculosis are nasal carriers; community-acquired methicillin-resistant strains of *S. aureus* (CA-MRSA) are now recognized as a major concern. In cases of CA-MRSA, delay in diagnosis and inappropriate initial antibiotic therapy can lead to systemic involvement, including rare reports of epidural abscess, bacterial endocarditis, and pulmonary infection. Also, *Mycobacterium* spp., especially *M. fortuitum*, have been implicated in non-responsive furunculosis in patients using footbaths in beauty salons. Rarely, myiasis may present as furunculosis.

Many patients have recurrent disease, though the majority show no immunologic defect. In rare cases, patients with impaired neutrophil function and immunodeficiency syndromes, such as common variable immunodeficiency and hyper-IgE syndrome, present with recurrent furunculosis. Evaluation for these diseases is recommended if clinically warranted.

MANAGEMENT STRATEGY

Isolated lesions should be *incised and drained*, and oral *antistaphylococcal* antibiotics should be reserved for those with numerous lesions, substantial surrounding cellulitis, or fever. Swabs of any purulent discharge should be collected for Gram stain and bacterial culture. Acid-fast staining and culture may be warranted if a temporal relationship to a pedicure is noted. Evidence of nasal carriage of staphylococci should be sought in those with recurrent disease, and eradicated with either *oral rifampicin* or *nasal fusidic acid* or *mupirocin*. Unresponsive recurrent disease may be controlled by *azithromycin, low-dose clindamycin*, or a *fluoroquinolone* antibiotic such as *ciprofloxacin*. Predisposing factors should be eliminated if possible.

SPECIFIC INVESTIGATIONS

▶ Culture and sensitivity of pus
▶ Acid-fast stain and culture if indicated
▶ Nasal swab (moistened)
▶ Neutrophil count

Skin and skin structure infections in the patient at risk: carrier state of *Staphylococcus aureus*. Tauzon CU. Am J Med 1984; 76: 166–71.

Carriage of staphylococci in the nares may predispose to outbreaks of infection in nurseries and in postoperative patients, and may lead to more severe infections in the immunocompromised. Factors predisposing to carriage are varied and carriage rates are greater in patients with renal failure, diabetes mellitus, and a history of drug abuse. *S. aureus* may be carried in the nose, throat, umbilicus, groin, and rectum, as well as other body sites.

Recurrent staphylococcal furunculosis: bacteriology and epidemiology in 100 cases. Hedstrom SA. Scand J Infect Dis 1981; 13: 115–19.

Occasionally patients with Job's syndrome and cyclic neutropenia develop recurrent furunculosis. A white cell count should be sought. Alcoholics, diabetics, and drug abusers may be predisposed to recurrent furunculosis.

Furunculosis and IgG subclass deficiency. Mahe E, Girszin N, Descamps V, Crickx B. Dermatology 2004; 209: 189–97.

Immunodeficiency may present with furunculosis. Immunoglobulin levels may be helpful.

An outbreak of mycobacterial furunculosis associated with footbaths at a nail salon. Winthrop KL, Abrams M, Yakrus M, Schwartz I, Ely J, Gillies D, et al. N Engl J Med 2002; 346: 1366–71.

Mycobacterium fortuitum has been associated with many cases of recurrent furunculosis in patients with exposure to nail footbaths. Isolates were recovered from the both patients and the footbaths in the salons.

FIRST-LINE THERAPIES

▶ Surgery – incision and drainage	C
▶ Eradication of nasal carriage of staphylococci	B
▶ Topical antibiotics – fusidic acid	A
▶ Systemic antibiotics	
▶ Flucloxacillin	C
▶ Low-dose clindamycin	B

Treatment and prevention of recurrent staphylococcal furunculosis: clinical and bacteriological follow-up. Hedstrom SA. Scand J Infect Dis 1985; 17: 55–8.

Sodium fusidate ointment was used as a prophylactic agent to prevent nasal furunculosis. Patients used the ointment twice daily for a month, with cessation of furuncles in 10 of 20 cases. Controls took antibiotics systemically, and three of 20 had no furuncles. After a year, those who used topical therapy had fewer recurrent lesions than those who had taken systemic therapy.

Comparison of two regimens of oral clindamycin versus dicloxacillin in the treatment of mild to moderate skin and soft tissue infections. Blaszcyk-Kostanecka M, Dobozy

Evidence Levels: **A** Double-blind study **B** Clinical trial ≥ 20 subjects **C** Clinical trial < 20 subjects **D** Series ≥ 5 subjects **E** Anecdotal case reports

A, Dominguez-Soto L, Guerrero R, Hunyadi J, Lopera J. Curr Ther Res Clin Exp 1998; 59: 341–53.

A prospective, double-blind, randomized study carried out in 14 countries throughout Asia. The study included a number of infections, including furuncles (which were not incised and drained). Treatment varied between 7 and 14 days, with no difference found between the three regimens (clindamycin 150 mg four times daily, clindamycin 300 mg twice daily, or dicloxacillin 250 mg four times daily). Flucloxacillin will be the equivalent of dicloxacillin in the UK.

Successful termination of a furunculosis outbreak due to lukS-lukF-positive, methicillin-susceptible *Staphylococcus aureus* in a German village by stringent decolonization, 2002–2005. Wiese-Posselt M, Heuck D, Draeger A, Mielke M, Witte W, Ammon A, et al. Clin Infect Dis 2007; 44: e88–95.

Risk of furunculosis was associated with contact with case patients (relative risk, 6.8) and nasal colonization with a lukS-lukF-positive strain of *S. aureus* (relative risk, 3.6). This report describes a successful strategy for terminating the transmission of epidemic strains of *S. aureus* among a non-hospitalized population by stringent decolonization with nasal mupirocin.

SECOND-LINE THERAPIES

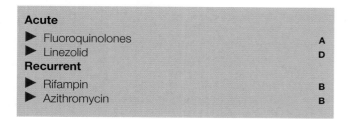

Acute	
▶ Fluoroquinolones	A
▶ Linezolid	D
Recurrent	
▶ Rifampin	B
▶ Azithromycin	B

A multicenter, double blind, double placebo comparative study of grepafloxacin versus ofloxacin in the treatment of skin and skin structure infections. Arata J, Matsuura Y, Umemura S, Nagao H, Katayama H, Miyoshi K, et al. Jpn J Chemother 1997; 45: 506–24.

Two fluoroquinolones were compared for efficacy. There were no significant differences in the improvement rates or in the side-effect profiles of the drugs. Patients were treated for 7 days and evaluated by day 7. Relapse rates (not mentioned) would have been helpful.

Treatment of bacterial skin and skin structure infections. Guay DR. Expert Opin Pharmacother 2003; 4: 1259–75.

Although most skin infections are still treated with β-lactams, macrolides, and lincosamides (clindamycin), antimicrobial resistance may lead to treatment failures. Some of the newer agents such as linezolid, quinupristin/dalfopristin, and moxifloxacin are discussed. At present these are not often used.

Efficacy of rifampicin in eradication of carrier state of *Staphylococcus aureus* in anterior nares with recurrent furunculosis. Mashhood AA, Shaikh ZI, Qureshi SM, Malik SM. J Coll Phys Surg Pakistan; 2006; 16: 396–9.

Patients with recurrent furunculosis and nasal carriage of *S. aureus* were treated with co-amoxiclav (equivalent to amoxicillin-clavulinate in the US) and then additionally randomized to receive either rifampicin 450–600 mg daily or placebo. In the rifampicin group, 77% of *S. aureus* carrier states were eliminated. Nasal swabs remained positive in all patients in the placebo group.

Prevention of chronic furunculosis with low-dose azithromycin. Aminzadeh A, Demircay Z, Ocak K, Soyletir G. J Dermatol Treat 2007; 18: 105–8.

Patients with a history of three or more episodes of furuncles were assigned to receive 12 weeks of suppressive treatment with azithromycin at a weekly dosage of 500 mg. At the end of 3 months, azithromycin was found to be effective for prevention of furunculosis 79.2% of patients; 18 of these remained in remission during the 3 months of follow-up. All of the strains were methicillin sensitive.

THIRD-LINE THERAPIES

▶ Colonization with less pathogenic staphylococci	E
▶ Retapamulin	E

Recurrent staphylococcal infection in families. Steele R. Arch Dermatol 1980; 116: 189–90.

A different, less pathogenic strain of *S. aureus* was inoculated into the nose of family members to try to prevent the spread of staphylococci in an attempt to minimize recurrent infections. A control group was inoculated with sterile broth. All patients and their family members were given oral antibiotics, nasal bacitracin, and hexachlorophene washes prior to inoculation. Fifteen of 17 families inoculated with less pathogenic strains of *S. aureus* remained disease free at 6 months, whereas only four of the 15 control families had no recurrences.

In vitro activity of retapamulin against *Staphylococcus aureus* isolates resistant to fusidic acid and mupirocin. Woodford N, Afzal-Shah M, Warner M, Livermore DM. J Antimicrob Chemother 2008; 766–8.

Retapamulin is a topical antibiotic recently approved by the FDA for the treatment of impetigo. This study evaluated the in-vitro efficacy of retapamulin against *S. aureus*. The strains of *S. aureus* were resistant to methicillin (73%), fusidic acid (51%), and mupirocin (38%), with 16% of isolates resistant to both fusidic acid and mupirocin. Retapamulin inhibited 99.9% of all *S. aureus* isolates. Further in-vivo studies are indicated to assess efficacy in the treatment of furunculosis and MRSA.

Geographic tongue

Alison J Bruce, Roy S Rogers III

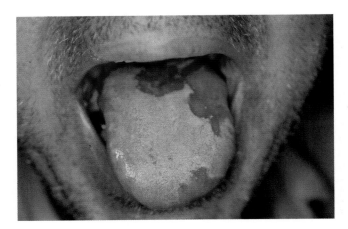

Geographic tongue is a reactive mucosal inflammatory condition characterized by arcuate or annular alternating hypertrophic or atrophic filiform papillae producing a geographic pattern. Synonyms include geographic stomatitis, benign transitory plaques of the tongue, and glossitis areata migrans. The geographic tongue may be an asymptomatic incidental finding. Some patients complain of a sore, burning sensation, particularly in atrophic areas of the tongue. Similar changes may occur in oral sites other than the tongue (geographic stomatitis).

MANAGEMENT STRATEGY

Geographic tongue is a common glossitis that affects 2% of the population. There is no racial predilection and the condition may be seen in patients of all ages, but more often in children than in adults. Because geographic tongue is usually asymptomatic, no treatment is necessary other than reassurance that the condition is benign, reactive, and self-limiting, and that it is not a sign of systemic illness. Geographic tongue often will remit spontaneously, but may persist for years. Occasional patients may be symptomatic, complaining of a burning discomfort. Effective therapy can be challenging.

The changes of geographic tongue may occur in patients with psoriasis vulgaris, pustular psoriasis, Reiter's disease, pityriasis rubra pilaris, or atopic diathesis. The clinician should also consider acute or chronic atrophic candidiasis.

For those patients whose geographic tongue is symptomatic, measures that may be considered include the avoidance of hot, spicy, or acidic foods; gentle brushing of the tongue; avoidance of harsh antibacterial mouthwashes, chewing gum, and breath mints; and soothing rinses with saline solutions. Occasionally, the topical application of *fluorinated corticosteroids* or *elixir of diphenhydramine* 12.5–25.0 mg/5 mL after meals and at bedtime may be recommended. *Topical anesthetic rinses or gels* provide temporary relief. *Anti-yeast treatments* may be palliative.

SPECIFIC INVESTIGATIONS

> ▶ Culture for candidiasis
> ▶ Medical evaluation as per burning mouth syndrome

Geographic stomatitis: A critical review. Hume WJ. J Dent 1975; 3: 25–43.

The topic and the differential diagnosis are carefully reviewed.

Culture of the tongue for yeast organisms may help direct therapy. Some patients require reassurance that they do not have a systemic illness. A laboratory evaluation along the lines discussed for burning mouth syndrome would be reasonable to exclude systemic causes.

FIRST-LINE THERAPIES

> ▶ Avoidance of spicy food, mouthwashes, chewing gum, and breath mints   **D**
> ▶ Topical fluorinated corticosteroids such as 0.05% fluocinonide gel   **C**
> ▶ Topical antihistamines   **C**
> ▶ Anti-yeast therapy   **E**

Symptomatic benign migratory glossitis: Report of two cases and literature review. Sigal MJ, Mock D. Pediatr Dent 1992; 14: 392–6.

Management with topical corticosteroids and topical antihistamines is discussed.

Glossitis and other tongue disorders. Byrd JA, Bruce AJ, Rogers RS III. Dermatol Clin 2003; 21: 123–34.

A review of geographic and other tongue disorders.

Oral psoriasis. Bruce AJ, Rogers RS III. Dermatol Clin 2003; 21: 99–104.

The concept of the geographic tongue as the mucosal equivalent of psoriasis is discussed.

Painful geographic tongue (benign migratory glossitis) in a child. [Letter] Menni S, Boccardi D, Crosti C. J Eur Acad Dermatol Venereol 2004; 18: 737–8.

The authors report a case of painful geographic tongue in a child in whom the only acceptable treatment was mometasone furoate cream. Mouth rinses and benzydamine, diphenhydramine, and betamethasone are suggested for symptomatic geographic tongue, but treatment can be challenging in children because of the unpleasant taste of creams and difficulty with using mouth washes.

SECOND-LINE THERAPIES

> ▶ Topical anesthetics   **C**
> ▶ Topical tretinoin   **E**
> ▶ Discontinue dentifrices and other oral flavoring agents   **D**
> ▶ Topical tacrolimus   **E**

Glossodynia and other disorders of the tongue. Powell FC. Dermatol Clin 1987; 5: 687–93.

A review of tongue disorders.

Despite concerns, tretinoin may be used on mucosal surfaces in a judicious manner.

The treatment of geographic tongue with topical retin-A solution. Helfman RJ. Cutis 1979; 24: 179–80.

The use of topical retin-A solution is described in three cases.

Anecdotally we have used tacrolimus 0.1% ointment for symptomatic geographic tongue, with occasional improvement.

THIRD-LINE THERAPIES

▶ 5.0% Carbolfuchsin paint	E
▶ 0.5% Gentian violet paint	E

Disorders of the oral cavity and lips. Pindborg JJ. In: Rook A, Wilkinson DS, Elbing FJG, eds. Textbook of dermatology, 3rd edn. Vol 2. Oxford: Blackwell Scientific, 1979; 1900.

Because of their color, patient compliance with the use of carbolfuchsin paint or gentian violet paint is a challenge.

Gianotti–Crosti syndrome

Carlo Gelmetti

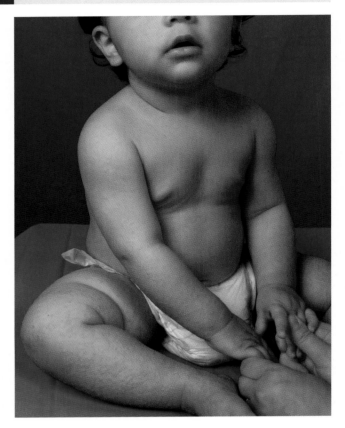

Gianotti–Crosti syndrome was originally described in three children in 1955 by Ferdinando Gianotti as a disease characterized by an erythematous papular eruption symmetrically distributed on the face, buttocks, and extremities. Besides the typical topography of the dermatosis, Gianotti also pointed out that the disease had mild, if any, constitutional symptoms, was not preceded by fever or by severe prodromes, the lesions had a simultaneous evolution, and the course of the disease was quite long (3–6 weeks). The term 'Gianotti–Crosti syndrome' is now used to include all eruptive acrolocated dermatoses clinically characterized by papular or papulovesicular lesions caused by a range of viruses. These almost always run a benign and self-healing course over a few weeks. The first virus associated with this eruption was hepatitis B, but many others have subsequently been documented.

Synonyms include papular acrodermatitis of childhood, infantile papular acrodermatitis, papulovesicular acrolocated syndrome, Crosti–Gianotti disease, Gianotti's disease, acrosyndrome de Gianotti–Crosti (France), and akrodermatitis papulosa eruptiva infantum (Germany).

MANAGEMENT STRATEGY

The diagnosis of Gianotti–Crosti syndrome is clinical. Like many other viral exanthems it mainly affects children of preschool age, though occasional adult cases have occurred. The typical eruption consists of monomorphic, flat, lentil-sized lesions symmetrically distributed on the face, buttocks, and limbs. The lesions are papular or papulovesicular, sometimes edematous, and rarely purpuric. They may coalesce over the elbows and knees. The trunk, antecubital, and popliteal surfaces are usually spared, even though a transient rash may be noted on the trunk in the early stage of the eruption. Mucous membranes are not affected. In the early eruptive phase the Koebner phenomenon may be elicited. In children below 1 year of age lesions may be edematous, whereas in adolescents and young adults they tend to be consistently papular. The eruption develops within a week, typically beginning on the thighs and buttocks, then involving the extensor aspects of the arms, and finally the face. Individual lesions look hemispherical, are a few millimeters in diameter (lesions 8–10 mm in diameter are uncommon), and vary in color from rose to red-brown. The pruritus is usually mild, and excoriation is never seen. The lesions fade in 3–4 weeks with mild desquamation, and relapse is rare. A longer course of up to 6–8 weeks is occasionally seen. Inguinal and axillary lymphadenopathy is common but not invariable. Nodes are moderately enlarged, elastic in consistency, and mobile.

In cases associated with hepatitis B the hepatitis begins at the same time as, or 1–2 weeks after, the onset of the dermatitis. The liver is usually enlarged but not tender; jaundice is exceptional. There are high serum levels of liver enzymes, and the various viral markers become detectable in the serum of all patients depending on the duration of infection. Serious complications are very rare, although some patients have developed chronic periportal hepatitis. Abnormalities in the peripheral blood are inconsistent: there may be a leukopenia or a slight leukocytosis with 2–15% of monocytes; the erythrocyte sedimentation rate is not raised.

In hepatitis B-negative cases hepatomegaly and liver function abnormalities, if present, are slight: serum transaminases rarely are higher than 100 U/mL. In these cases, the liver involvement can by explained by the fact that some viruses which are able to provoke Gianotti–Crosti syndrome are considered among the minor hepatitic viruses (e.g. Epstein–Barr virus).

There is no specific treatment for the rash. We do not recommend any topical or systemic drug; however, when itching is present oral antihistamines or various topical antipruritics can be prescribed for their symptomatic effect. Although topical and systemic corticosteroids are sometimes used, the benefit is not firmly established. Systemic absorption of superpotent topical corticosteroids could prolong or delay the recovery of the disease.

In cases associated with hepatitis B, the hepatitis must be treated with PEGylated interferon-α_{2a} and nucleoside analogs. It is also important to investigate and treat other members of the family who may be carriers of the hepatitis B virus or may benefit from vaccination. Prophylactic vaccination against hepatitis B virus, which has been introduced in the last two decades, will potentially eradicate all cases of Gianotti–Crosti syndrome due to this virus, as has happened in Italy, where such vaccination was instituted in 1983 and is routinely administered to all newborns. The present vaccine is not only effective against hepatitis but also seems effective in reducing the incidence of hepatocellular carcinoma. Other infective causes may also require treatment if identified.

SPECIFIC INVESTIGATIONS

▶ Liver enzymes
▶ Viral serology for Epstein–Barr virus, hepatitis B, hepatitis A, cytomegalovirus
▶ Total IgE (PRIST) and specific IgE (RAST)

Other possible causes include Coxsackie virus, adenovirus, enterovirus, human herpes virus 6, reovirus, varicella, roseola, rotavirus, respiratory syncytial virus, Lyme borreliosis, *Mycoplasma pneumoniae*, meningococcal infection, etc., and immunization.

Gianotti–Costi syndrome associated with transfusion acquired hepatitis B virus infection in a patient of sickle cell anemia. Pise GA, Vetrichevvel TP, Agarwal KK, Thappa DM. Indian J Dermatol Venereol Leprol 2007; 73: 123–4.

A 9-year-old boy, treated with multiple transfusions for his sickle cell disease, presented with GCS. Liver function tests showed indirect hyperbilirubinemia and mildly elevated liver enzymes. HBsAg was detected. The patient was managed with antihistamines and skin lesions cleared in 2 weeks. He had no recurrences in the subsequent 6 months of follow-up.

Gianotti–Crosti syndrome in a child following hepatitis B virus vaccination. Karakas M, Durdu M, Tuncer I, Cevlik F. J Dermatol 2007; 34: 117–20.

A 5-year-old boy presented with a 1-month history of GCS. The lesions had appeared 3 weeks after a first dose of HBV recombinant vaccine. Antibody to HBsAg was positive; other viral serologic tests, including CMV, EBC, HAV, HCV, and EBV, were negative. The patient was treated with an emollient and the eruption subsided within 4 weeks.

Skin manifestations with rotavirus infections. Di Lernia V, Ricci C. Int J Dermatol 2006; 45: 759–61.

GCS is considered a nonspecific cutaneous host response to a variety of infectious agents, particularly viruses, which have been associated with this distinctive exanthem. In 1988, the first two cases of GCS associated with rotavirus infection were reported. A new case was observed in 1998 by the author, confirming the possibility of such an association.

Gianotti–Crosti syndrome. Brandt O, Abeck D, Gianotti R, Burgdorf W. J Am Acad Dermatol 2006; 54: 136–45.

Viral infections are still the key factor. The most likely explanation for the decline of HBV is the increasing use of anti-HBV immunization around the world. Numerous studies confirm that EBV is now the most common cause of GCS. In addition, many other viruses have been connected with GCS, including HVA, CMV, HHV6, Coxsackie virus A16, B4, and B5; rotavirus; parvovirus B19; molluscum contagiosum; respiratory syncytial virus; mumps virus; and parainfluenza virus types 1 and 2. Apparently HIV can also be associated with acral papules. Bacteria (*Bartonella henselae*, *Mycoplasma pneumoniae*, β-hemolytic streptococci and *Borrelia burgdorferi*) also appear capable of triggering GCS, although it must be a rare event. The association between various immunizations and GCS has long been known. Despite the proven connection between HBV and GCS, immunization against HBV only rarely causes GCS.

Gianotti–Crosti syndrome and allergic background. Ricci G, Patrizi A, Neri I, Specchia F, Tosti G, Masi M. Acta Dermatol Venereol. 2003; 83: 202–5.

In 29 children affected by Gianotti–Crosti syndrome and 59 age- and sex-matched controls, the presence of atopic dermatitis (24.1%) was significantly higher (p<0.005) than in the control group (6.8%). In addition, the percentage of patients with total IgE >2 SD for age was higher than in controls (27.6% vs 13.7%), as was the percentage with specific IgE present (31% vs 17.2%).

FIRST-LINE THERAPIES

▶ Systemic antihistamines	E
▶ Systemic corticosteroids	E
▶ Topical corticosteroids	E
▶ Topical antiseptics	E
▶ Topical antipruritics	E
▶ Systemic steroids	E
▶ Systemic antibiotics	E
▶ Emollients	E
▶ Vitamin C	E
▶ Interferon-α	B
▶ Nucleoside analogs	B
▶ Hepatitis B vaccine	B

Gianotti–Crosti syndrome in two adult patients. Ting PT, Barankin B, Dytoc MT. J Cutan Med Surg 2008; 12: 121–5.

Two cases of GCS in a previously healthy 37-year-old Asian and a 21-year-old Caucasian woman are reported. As both patients experienced significant pruritus, patient 1 was initially treated with a high-potency topical corticosteroid followed by a 2-week course of oral prednisone, and patient 2 was treated with a potent topical corticosteroid. Both were asymptomatic at follow-up 3–4 weeks after their initial presentation.

Gianotti–Crosti syndrome: clinical, serologic and therapeutic data from nine children. Boeck K, Mempel M, Schmidt T, Abeck D. Cutis 1998; 62: 271–4.

In nine children with Gianotti–Crosti syndrome therapeutic interventions included systemic antihistamines, topical clioquinol lotion 1%, topical corticosteroids, and systemic methylprednisolone. Skin lesions resolved after 2–4 weeks in treated as well as in untreated children. Whole-body involvement seemed to correlate with severe pruritus and additional general symptoms, requiring more intensive therapy.

Infantile acrodermatitis of Gianotti–Crosti and Lyme borreliosis. Baldari U, Cattonar P, Nobile C, Celli B, Righini MG, Trevisan G. Acta Dermatol Venereol 1996; 76: 242–3.

One patient was treated with ceftriaxone (500 mg IM daily for 30 days) and the second with josamicin (250 mg/day for 14 days).

Truncal lesions do not exclude a diagnosis of Gianotti–Crosti syndrome. Chuh AA. Australas J Dermatol 2003; 44: 215–16.

Although most patients with Gianotti–Crosti syndrome only have the typical acrally distributed eruption, additional truncal lesions, if few in number, do not exclude the diagnosis. Topical calamine lotion and a sedating oral antihistamine were prescribed. The truncal lesions subsided in 3 weeks, and remission of all lesions was seen after 6 weeks.

Gonorrhea

Patrice Morel

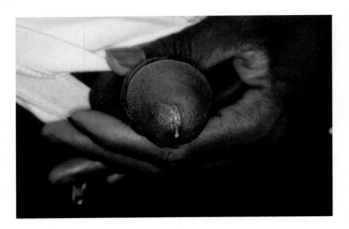

Gonorrhea is one of the commonest and most severe sexually transmitted diseases. It is caused by the Gram-negative aerobic diplococcus *Neisseria gonorrhoeae*, which primarily infects the mucous membranes of the urethra, endocervix, rectum, and pharynx. The infection may be asymptomatic.

MANAGEMENT STRATEGY

Individuals with gonorrhea should be treated as promptly as possible, (a) to prevent regional infection such as epididymitis or pelvic inflammatory disease leading to infertility or ectopic pregnancy, (b) to prevent disseminated gonococcal infection, which occurs in about 1–3% of cases, and (c) to stop transmission to sexual partners.

Urethritis is typically characterized by a discharge of mucopurulent or purulent material and by a burning sensation during urination. Dysuria may be the only symptom.

Gonococcal cervicitis is characterized by a mucopurulent or purulent endocervical exudate. However, a cervical discharge is not specific for a gonococcal infection, and gonococcal infection of the cervix is often asymptomatic.

Pharyngeal infection is asymptomatic in more than 90% of cases.

Rectal infection is prevalent in homosexual men, causing anal discharge and pain. In women, rectal infection results from spread through vaginal secretions and does not necessarily imply anal intercourse.

Patients in whom gonorrhea is suspected should be investigated for *N. gonorrhoeae* using the most sensitive and specific tests, though empiric treatment of the symptoms may be recommended for patients at high risk for infection who are unlikely to return for a follow-up evaluation. In this circumstance, the recommended antibiotic treatment must be effective against all strains of *N. gonorrhoeae*, including the penicillinase-producing and the high-level tetracycline-resistant strains.

Patients infected with *N. gonorrhoeae* are often co-infected with *Chlamydia trachomatis*. A co-treatment effective against *C. trachomatis* should therefore be considered.

Patients should be instructed (a) to return for evaluation if symptoms persist or recur after completion of therapy, and (b) to abstain from sexual intercourse until they and their sexual partners are cured.

SPECIFIC INVESTIGATIONS

Men
- ▶ Microscopy of Gram-stained urethral secretions
- ▶ Culture on Thayer–Martin medium
- ▶ Non-culture test

Women
- ▶ Culture on Thayer–Martin medium
- ▶ Non-culture test

Male urethritis with and without discharge. A clinical and microbiological study. Janier M, Lassau F, Casin I, Grillot P, Scieux C, Zavaro A, et al. Sex Transm Dis 1995; 22: 244–52.

N. gonorrhoeae was found in 21% of patients with urethral discharge and in no patient without discharge. A systemic treatment for *N. gonorrhoeae* in patients without discharge in the absence of proven contact with an infected patient is not recommended.

Sexually Transmitted Diseases Treatment Guidelines 2006. MMWR Recomm Rep 2006; 55(RR11): 1–94.

Because of its high specificity (>99%) and sensitivity (>95%), a Gram stain of a male urethral specimen that demonstrates polymorphonuclear leukocytes with intracellular Gram-negative diplococci can be considered diagnostic for infection with *N. gonorrhoeae* in symptomatic men. Culture is the most widely available option for the diagnosis of infection with *N. gonorrhoeae* in asymptomatic men, in women, and in non-genital sites (rectum and pharynx). Non-culture tests cannot provide antimicrobial susceptibility results.

Screening tests to detect *Chlamydia trachomatis* and *Neisseria gonorrhoeae* infections – 2002. MMWR 2002; 51 (RR-15): 1–48.

Non-culture tests called nucleic acid hybridization tests and nucleic acid amplification tests (NAATs) have been developed. Commercial NAATs differ in their amplification methods and their target nucleic acid sequences. The majority of commercial NAATs have been cleared by the FDA to detect *C. trachomatis* and *N. gonorrhoeae* in endocervical swabs and urethral swabs from men. The sensitivity of NAATs might be less when using urine than when using an endocervical swab specimen. Testing of rectal and oropharyngeal specimen with NAATs is not recommended.

Gonorrhea screening among men who have sex with men: value of multiple anatomic site testing, San Diego, California, 1997–2003. Gunn RA, O'Brien CJ, Lee MA, Gilchick RA. Sex Transm Dis 2008; Jul 2 (epub ahead of print).

Among 970 patients who had positive test results for gonorrhea infection, 369 (38%) had a negative result in their urethral or urine specimen. These results confirm that men who have sex with men should be screened annually for gonorrhea infection at the urethral, pharyngeal, and rectal sites.

Epidemiology and treatment of oropharyngeal gonorrhoea. Hutt DM, Judson FN. Ann Intern Med 1986; 104: 655–8.

Gonococci were grown from expectorated saliva in 34 of 51 cultures from patients with oropharyngeal gonorrhea, suggesting transmissibility and providing another reason for ensuring effective treatment.

Disseminated gonococcal infection (DGI)

DGI results from gonococcal bacteremia with the possibility of petechial or pustular acral skin lesions, arthralgia, tenosynovitis, or septic arthritis. The infection may be complicated by perihepatitis, and rarely by endocarditis and meningitis.

FIRST-LINE THERAPIES

▶ Cefixime 400 mg orally in a single dose **B**
▶ Ceftriaxone 125 mg intramuscularly in a single dose **B**

Oral cefixime versus intramuscular ceftriaxone in patients with uncomplicated gonococcal infections. Portilla I, Lutz B, Montalvo M, Mogabgab J. Sex Transm Dis 1992; 19: 94–8.

The only current CDC-recommended options for treating *N. gonorrhoeae* infections are from a single class of antibiotics, the cephalosporins. The 400 mg dose of cefixime cured 97% of uncomplicated urogenital and anorectal gonococcal infections. The advantage of cefixime is that it can be administered orally.

Drugs of choice for the treatment of uncomplicated gonococcal infections. Moran JS, Levine WC. Clin Infect Dis 1995; 20: s47–65.

Ceftriaxone in a single 125 mg injection provides sustained, high bactericidal levels in the blood. Extensive clinical experience indicates that ceftriaxone cures 99% of uncomplicated urogenital and anorectal infections and 94% of pharyngeal infections.

***Chlamydia trachomatis* among patients infected with and treated for *Neisseria gonorrhoeae* in sexually transmitted disease clinic in the United States.** Lyss SB, Kamb ML, Peterman AT, Moran JS, Newman DR, Bolan G, et al. Ann Intern Med 2003; 139: 178–95.

Patients infected with *N. gonorrhoeae* frequently are co-infected with *C. trachomatis*; this finding has led to the recommendation that patients treated for gonococcal infection also be treated with a regimen that is effective against uncomplicated *C. trachomatis* infection. Patients with a negative chlamydial NAAT result do not need to be treated for *Chlamydia* as well.

SECOND-LINE THERAPIES

▶ Ciprofloxacin 500 mg orally in a single dose **B**
▶ Ofloxacin 400 mg orally in a single dose **B**
▶ Levofloxacin 250 mg orally in a single dose **B**
▶ Spectinomycin 2 g intramuscularly in a single dose **B**

Update to CDC's sexually transmitted diseases treatment guidelines 2006: fluoroquinolones no longer recommended for treatment of gonococcal infections. MMWR Morb Mortal Wkly Rep 2007; 56: 332–6.

Since 1993, fluoroquinolones have been used frequently in the treatment of gonorrhea because of their high efficacy and convenience as a single-dose oral therapy. However, owing to the increasing prevalence of fluoroquinolone-resistant *N. gonorrhoeae*, CDC no longer recommends the use of fluoroquinolones for the treatment of gonococcal infections in patients who acquired their infection in the United States, Asia, or the Pacific Islands.

Spectinomycin resistance in *Neisseria* spp. due to mutations in IGSrRNA. Galimand M, Gerbaud G, Courvalin P. Antimicrob Agents Chemother 2000; 44: 1365–6.

It is possible, though rare, for a patient to be infected with a spectinomycin-resistant *N. gonorrhoeae* strain; spectinomycin is expensive and must be injected. Therefore, spectinomycin is useful for treatment of patients who cannot tolerate cephalosporins and quinolones.

SPECIAL CONSIDERATIONS

▶ Pharyngeal infection
▶ Disseminated gonococcal infection
▶ Pregnancy
▶ Ophthalmia neonatorum

Pharyngeal infection

Treating uncomplicated *Neisseria gonorrhoeae* infections: is the anatomic site of infection important? Moran JS. Sex Transm Dis 1995; 22: 39–47.

A systematic review of published therapeutic trials of various antimicrobial regimens for the biological cure of uncomplicated gonorrhea has shown that pharyngeal infection is more difficult to cure. A cephalosporin regimen is the best choice, as they are likely to cure at least 80% of pharyngeal infections. Spectinomycin is unreliable (i.e., only 52% effective) against pharyngeal infections.

Disseminated gonococcal infection

Sexually transmitted diseases. Treatment guidelines 2002. Centers for Disease Control and Prevention. MMWR Recomm Rep 2002; 51(RR-6): 1–78.

Hospitalization is recommended for initial therapy. The experts recommend ceftriaxone 1 g intramuscularly or intravenously every 24 hours as the initial regimen.

Pregnancy

Treatment of gonorrhoea in pregnancy. Cavenee MR, Farris JR, Spalding TR, Barnes DL, Castaneda YS, Wendel GD Jr. Obstet Gynecol 1993; 81: 33–8.

Two hundred and fifty-two pregnant women with gonorrhea were randomly assigned to receive ceftriaxone 250 mg intramuscularly, spectinomycin 2 g intramuscularly, or amoxicillin 3 g orally with probenecid 1 g orally. The overall efficacy was 95%, 95%, and 89%, respectively. There was no increased incidence of congenital malformations. Ceftriaxone and spectinomycin are the best choices. Pregnant women should not be treated with quinolones or tetracyclines.

Ophthalmia neonatorum

1998 Guidelines for treatment of sexually transmitted diseases. Centers for Disease Control and Prevention. MMWR 1998; 47(RR-1): 1–116.

Gonococcal ophthalmia is strongly suggested when typical Gram-negative diplococci are identified in conjunctival exudate, justifying presumptive treatment for gonorrhea after appropriate cultures for *N. gonorrhoeae* have been obtained. The recommended regimen is ceftriaxone 25–50 mg/kg IV or IM in a single dose, not to exceed 125 mg. Local treatment, with or without systemic antibiotics, is inappropriate.

Graft versus host disease

John Minni, Dwayne Montie, Carlos H Nousari

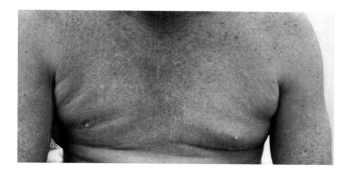

Graft versus host disease (GVHD) classically affects the skin, liver, and gastrointestinal tract and almost always occurs in the setting of allogeneic bone marrow transplants. The disease occurs as a result of interactions between the adaptive and innate immune systems of both the host and the donor.

Acute GVHD (aGVHD) occurs within 1–3 weeks after transplantation and typically presents as a maculopapular eruption which may progress to erythroderma, and less commonly to a toxic epidermal necrolysis-like eruption.

Chronic GVHD (cGVHD) is characteristically seen more than 3 months after transplantation as mucocutaneous lichenoid and/or sclerodermatous disease.

MANAGEMENT STRATEGY

Ciclosporin A and methotrexate, either alone or as combined therapy, are the most common drugs used for prophylaxis of aGVHD.

Although the combination of ciclosporin A with methotrexate has become the standard for prophylaxis, other combinations using tacrolimus and mycophenolate mofetil are also effective.

Several randomized studies in myeloablative and non-myeloablative allogenic bone marrow transplantation have shown that the combination of ciclosporin A with mycophenolate mofetil had similar incidences of aGVHD and comparable survival rates compared with the combination of ciclosporin A and methotrexate. The combination with mycophenolate mofetil was associated with faster hematopoietic engraftment and no toxicities related to the mycophenolate mofetil, thereby reducing morbidity.

Prednisone is not part of the standard regimen for prophylaxis of aGVHD. In spite of showing similar survival rates, studies have shown that the addition of prednisone may delay the onset of aGVHD but has no impact on the incidence of the disease.

The first-line therapy for aGVHD is systemic corticosteroids. A typical regimen includes the addition of prednisone at 1–2 mg/kg/day to an optimized dose of ciclosporin A. The response to first-line therapy was found to be the single most important factor predicting improved long-term survival.

If there is no response to corticosteroids, second-line therapy should be initiated; this includes mycophenolate mofetil, tacrolimus, antithymocyte globulin, and sirolimus.

In cases of refractory aGVHD, third-line therapy includes monoclonal antibodies against cytokines and their receptors. Supportive care is also critical in the management and includes cessation of oral intake, total parenteral nutrition with hyperalimentation, antibiotic and antiviral prophylaxis, and pain control. In patients with aGVHD having only cutaneous involvement, topical corticosteroids, antipruritic agents and PUVA may help to control the symptoms.

Treatment of cGVHD depends on the extent of organ involvement. Patients with localized skin disease require only topical or local therapy, whereas those with extensive disease (generalized skin disease per se or localized cutaneous disease with internal organ involvement) require systemic therapy. The standard systemic treatment is the combination of systemic corticosteroids with a calcineurin inhibitor, for example prednisone 1–2 mg/kg daily and ciclosporin 5–10 mg/kg daily or tacrolimus 0.03 mg/kg. Corticosteroid-refractory cGVHD has no standard therapy. A randomized study of antithymocyte globulin combined with ciclosporin showed a significant reduction of cGVHD. Several studies have shown that mycophenalate mofetil in combination with ciclosporin, tacrolimus, or thalidomide has been beneficial in patients with refractory disease. Unlike the lichenoid variant, which shows a high response rate to phototherapy, the sclerodermatous form seems to respond better to etretinate or extracorporeal photopheresis. PUVA therapy, topical corticosteroids, and calcineurin inhibitors are effective for localized cutaneous cGVHD. Topical calcineurin inhibitors, ciclosporin and corticosteroids are also beneficial in oral cGVHD. Successful use of extracorporeal photophoresis, hydroxychloroquine, pulse cyclophosphamide, pentostatin, and monoclonal antibodies, especially anti-TNF-α, have also recently been reported as salvage therapy.

Supportive therapy with good nutrition, physical therapy, dental hygiene and skin lubrication is also important.

SPECIFIC INVESTIGATIONS

Acute GVHD
▶ Skin biopsy
▶ Liver function tests

Acute graft versus host disease. Jacobson DA, Vogelsang GB, Orphanet J. Rare Dis 2007; 2: 35.

GVHD is a clinical diagnosis that may be supported by appropriate biopsies. The reason to pursue a tissue biopsy is to help differentiate from other diagnoses that may mimic GVHD, such as viral infection and drug reaction.

An acute graft-versus-host disease activity index to predict survival after hematopoietic cell transplantation with myeloablative conditioning regimens. Leisenring WM, Martin PJ, Petersdorf EW, Regan AE, Aboulhosn N, Stern JM, et al. Blood 2006; 108: 749–55.

A method developed to predict mortality in patients with acute GVHD. The optimal model included the total serum bilirubin concentration, oral intake, need for treatment with prednisone, and performance score.

Chronic GVHD

▶ Skin biopsy
▶ Liver function tests
▶ Schirmer's test
▶ Pulmonary function tests
▶ Complete blood count
▶ Serum immunoglobulins

National Institutes of Health consensus development project on criteria for clinical trials in chronic graft-versus-host disease: I. Diagnosis and staging working group report. Filipovich AH, Weisdorf D, Pavletic S, Socie G, Wingard JR, Lee SJ, et al. Biol Blood Marrow Transplant 2005; 11: 945–56.

Diagnosis of chronic GVHD requires the presence of at least one diagnostic clinical sign of chronic GVHD or the presence of at least one distinctive manifestation confirmed by pertinent biopsy or other relevant tests (e.g., Schirmer's test) in the same or another organ.

ACUTE GVHD

FIRST-LINE THERAPIES

▶ Corticosteroids (with optimization of ciclosporin A given for prophylaxis) **A**
▶ Ciclosporin A with mycophenolate mofetil **A**
▶ Sirolimus in combination with tacrolimus **B**

Treatment of acute graft-versus-host disease after allogenic marrow transplantation. Randomized study comparing corticosteroids and cyclosporine A. Kennedy MS, Deeg HJ, Storb R, Doney K, Sullivan KM, Witherspoon RP, et al. Am J Med 1985; 78: 978–83.

This trial comparing corticosteroids and ciclosporin A, showing response rates of respectively 41% and 60%, was done in the early days when GVHD prophylaxis consisted only of methotrexate. In the ciclosporin era, corticosteroids are now the drug of choice.

A prospective randomized trial comparing cyclosporine and short course methotrexate with cyclosporine and mycophenolae mofetil for GVHD prophylaxis in myeloablative allogenic bone marrow transplantation. Bolweel B, Sobecks R, Pohlman B, Andersen S, Rybicki L, Kuezkowski I, et al. Bone Marrow Transplant 2004; 34: 621–5.

GVHD prophylaxis with ciclosporin A and mycophenolate mofetil is associated with faster hematopoietic engraftment, a reduced incidence of mucositis, and similar incidence of aGVHD and comparable survival to treatment with ciclosporin A and methotrexate.

Extended follow-up of methotrexate-free immunosuppression using sirolimus and tacrolimus in related and unrelated donor peripheral blood stem cell transplantation. Cutler C, Li S, Ho VT, Koreth J, Alyea E, Soiffer RJ, et al. Blood 2007; 109: 3108–14.

The substitution of sirolimus for methotrexate as GVHD prophylaxis is associated with rapid engraftment, a low incidence of acute GVHD, minimal transplant-related toxicity, and excellent survival.

SECOND-LINE THERAPIES

▶ Antithymocyte globulins (ATG) **C**
▶ Monoclonal antibodies (such as anti-IL2R and anti-CD52) **B**

Protective conditioning for acute graft-versus-host disease. Lowsky R, Takahashi T, Liu YP, Dejbakhsh-Jones S, Grumet FC, Shizuru JA. N Engl J Med 2005; 353: 1321–31.

A regimen of total lymphoid irradiation plus antithymocyte globulin reduces the incidence of acute GVHD and allows graft antitumor activity.

Long-term follow-up of patients treated with daclizumab for steroid-refractory acute graft-vs-host disease. Perales MA, Ishill N, Lomazow WA, Weinstock DM, Papadopoulos EB, Dastigir H. Bone Marrow Transplant 2007; 40: 481–6.

Daclizumab has no infusion-related toxicity, is active in steroid-refractory GVHD, especially among pediatric patients, but is associated with significant morbidity and mortality due to infectious complications

Low dose almtuzumab (Campath) in myeloablative allogeneic stem cell transplantation for CD52-positive malignancies: decreased incidence of acute graft-versus-host-disease with unique pharmacokinetics. Khouri IF, Albitar M, Saliba RM, Ippoliti C, Ma YC, Keating MJ, et al. Bone Marrow Transplant 2004; 33: 833–7.

At 3 months post transplantation, 11 of 12 patients had achieved 100% donor chimerism.

THIRD-LINE THERAPIES

▶ Extracorporeal photopheresis **B**
▶ PUVA **B**
▶ Biologics (infliximab, etanercept) **B**

Extracorporeal photopheresis for acute and chronic graft-versus-host disease: does it work? Couriel D, Hosing C, Saliba R, Shpall EJ, Andelini P, Popat U, et al. Biol Blood Marrow Transplant 2006; 12: 37–40.

Sixty-three patients were treated with extracorporeal photopheresis. The overall response rate was 59% (n=37), and complete responses were seen in 13 patients

Treatment of acute graft-versus-host disease with PUVA (psoralen and ultraviolet irradiation): results of a pilot study. Wiesmann A, Weller A, Lischka G, Klingebiel T, Kanz L, Einsele H. Bone Marrow Transplant 1999; 23: 151–5.

The vast majority of 20 patients treated with PUVA for aGVHD had a good response in terms of skin improvement and reduction of corticosteroid dosage.

Tumor necrosis factor-alpha blockade for the treatment of acute GVHD. Couriel D, Saliba R, Hicks K, Ippolitti C, de Lima M, Housing C, et al. Blood 2004; 104: 649–54.

In this study including 134 patients with corticosteroid-refractory aGVHD, infliximab was well tolerated and effective, with an overall response rate of 67%.

Etanercept plus methylprednisolone as initial therapy for acute graft-versus-host disease. Levine JE, Paczesny S,

Mineishi S, Braun T, Choi SW, Hutchinson RJ, et al. Blood 2008; 111: 2470–5.

Patients treated with etanercept and corticosteroids were more likely to achieve complete response than were patients treated with steroids alone (69% vs 33%).

CHRONIC GVHD

FIRST-LINE THERAPIES

► Systemic corticosteroid and calcineurin inhibitor	A
► Combination of corticosteroids and ciclosporin	B

High-dose cyclosporine and corticosteroids for prophylaxis of acute and chronic graft-versus-host disease. Schwinghammer TL, Bloom EJ, Rosenfeld CS, Wilson JW, Przepiorka D, Shadduck RK. Bone Marrow Transplant 1995; 16: 147–54.

Ciclosporin in doses up to 15 mg/kg daily and methylprednisolone up to 1 mg/kg daily have been used for the prevention of acute and chronic graft versus host disease. Nephrotoxicity and infections are the primary side effects.

SECOND-LINE THERAPIES

Systemic	
► Thalidomide	B
► Tacrolimus and mycophenolate mofetil	B
► Tacrolimus	B
Lichenoid cutaneous GVHD	
► PUVA	B
Sclerodermatous cutaneous GVHD	
► Etretinate	B

Extended follow-up of methotrexate-free immunosuppression using sirolimus and tacrolimus in related and unrelated donor peripheral blood stem cell transplantation. Cutler C, Li S, Ho VT, Koreth J, Alyea E, Soiffer RJ, et al. Blood 2007; 109: 3108–14.

Assessment of the combination of sirolimus and tacrolimus without methotrexate after myeloablative allogeneic stem cell transplantation. The substitution of sirolimus for methotrexate as GVHD prophylaxis is associated with rapid engraftment, a low incidence of acute GVHD, minimal transplant-related toxicity, and excellent survival.

Efficacy of mycophenolate mofetil in the treatment of chronic graft-versus-host disease. Lopez F, Parker P, Nademanee A, Rodriguez R, Al-Kadhimi Z, Bhatia R. Biol Blood Marrow Transplant 2005; 11: 307–13.

Mycophenolate mofetil was added to standard ciclosporin, tacrolimus, and/or prednisone as salvage/second-line therapy in 34 patients. With a median follow-up of 24 months (range 6–28 months), 29 (85%) patients were alive.

Thalidomide after allogeneic haematopoietic stem cell transplantation: activity in chronic but not in acute graft-versus-host disease. Kulkarni S, Powles R, Sirohi B, Treleaven J, Saso R, Horton C, et al. Bone Marrow Transplant 2003; 32: 165–70.

Thalidomide was used to treat acute and chronic graft versus host disease in 80 hematopoietic stem cell allograft recipients after failure of first-line agents. For acute GVHD none of the patients responded and all died of the disease. For chronic GVHD, at a median of 53 months 19 patients were alive, 13 without evidence of chronic GVHD.

Etretinate therapy for refractory sclerodermatous chronic graft-versus-host disease. Marcellus DC, Altomonte VL, Farmer ER, Horn TD, Freemer CS, Grant J, et al. Blood 1999; 93: 66–70.

Of 27 patients who had sclerodermatous GVHD 20 showed improvement in terms of skin softening and increased range of movement.

Etretinate is converted to acitretin in the body, and similar results could be expected with the latter agent.

THIRD-LINE THERAPIES

Systemic	
► Extracorporeal photochemotherapy	C
► Mycophenolate mofetil	C
► Hydroxychloroquine	B
► Pulse cyclophosphamide	C
► Pentostatin	C
► Infliximab	B
► Etanercept	C
► Daclizumab	E
► Rituximab	D
► Antithymocyte globulin	C
Lichenoid cGVHD	
► UVB	E
► Clofazimine	B
► UVA1 and mycophenolate mofetil	E
Oral GVHD	
► Topical corticosteroids	C
► Topical ciclosporin	D
► Intraoral PUVA	E
► Oral UVB	E
► Topical calcineurin inhibitors	D

Thymoglobulin prevents chronic graft-versus-host disease, chronic lung dysfunction, and late transplant-related mortality: long-term follow-up of a randomized trial in patients undergoing unrelated donor transplantation. Bacigalupo A, Lamparelli T, Bruzzi P, Guidi S, Alessandrino PE, et al. Biol Blood Marrow Transplant 2006 May; 12: 560–5.

Update of a randomized study on antithymocyte globulin (ATG). The median follow-up for surviving patients is 5.7 years. At the last follow-up, chronic graft versus host disease was present in 60% of non-ATG and 37% of ATG patients (p=0.05), and extensive chronic GVHD was present in 41% and 15%, respectively (p=0.01). The addition of ATG to ciclosporin/methotrexate provides significant protection against extensive chronic GVHD.

Pulse cyclophosphamide for corticosteroid-refractory graft-versus-host disease. Mayer J, Krejci M, Doubek M, Pospisil Z, Brychtova Y, Tomiska M, et al. Bone Marrow Transplant 2005; 35: 699–705.

In a retrospective study of 15 patients who had not responded to corticosteroids, pulse cyclophosphamide at a median dose of 1 g/m² was very effective in the treatment of skin (100% response), liver (70% response), and oral cavity (100% response).

Influence of extracorporeal photophoresis on clinical and laboratory parameters in chronic graft versus host disease and analysis of predictors of response. Seaton ED, Szydlo RM, Kanfer E, Apperley JF, Russell-Jones R. Blood 2003; 102: 1207–23.

Of 21 patients with skin cGVHD one had a complete response and nine a partial response; of 25 patients with liver cGVHD eight had a partial response; and of six patients with oral cGVHD three had a partial response.

Hydroxychloroquine for the treatment of chronic graft-versus-host disease. Gilman AL, Chan KW, Mogul A, Morris C, Goldman FD, Boyer M, et al. Biol Blood Marrow Transplant 2000; 6: 327–34.

Three complete and 14 partial responses were seen when 32 patients were treated with hydroxychloroquine 12 mg/kg.

Treatment of chronic graft-versus-host disease with clofazime. Lee SJ, Wegner SA, McGarigle CJ, Bierer BE, Antin JH. Blood 1997; 89: 2298–302.

Over 50% of the 22 patients treated achieved a complete or a partial response.

Chronic sclerodermic graft-versus-host disease refractory to immunosuppressive treatment responds to UVA1 phototherapy. Grundmann-Kollmann M, Behrens S, Gruss C, Gottlöber P, Peter RU, Kerscher M. J Am Acad Dermatol 2000; 42: 134–6.

A patient with chronic sclerodermatous graft versus host disease improved with low-dose UVA1 therapy combined with mycophenolate mofetil.

Chronic graft-versus-host disease treated with UVB phototherapy. Enk CD, Elad S, Vexler A, Kapelushnik J, Gorodetsky R, et al. Bone Marrow Transplant 1998; 22: 1179–83.

One patient with lichenoid lesions had complete clearing.

Psoralen plus ultraviolet-A-bath photochemotherapy as an adjunct treatment modality in cutaneous chronic graft versus host disease. Leiter U, Kaskel P, Krähn G, Gottlöber P, Bunjes D, Peter RU, Kerscher M. Photodermatol Photoimmunol Photomed 2002; 18: 183–90.

After a median of 14.5 treatment sessions, skin lesions improved. Out of six patients, three showed a complete remission.

Oral graft vs. host disease in children – treatment with topical tacrolimus ointment. Albert MH, Becker B, Schuster FR, Klein B, Binder V, Adam K, et al. Pediatr Transplant 2007; 11: 306–11.

Tacrolimus ointment 0.1% was applied twice daily in six patients using sterile gauze. Two patients had a complete response, two had a partial response.

Granuloma annulare

Eanas Bader, Andrew Ilchyshyn

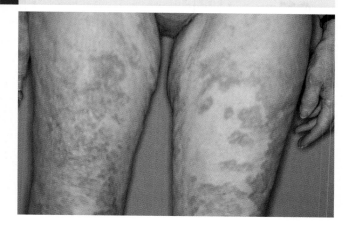

Granuloma annulare is a skin disease of unknown etiology whose four main clinical variants are localized, disseminated, subcutaneous, and perforating. It is characterized histologically by necrobiosis of collagen surrounded by a lymphohistiocytic infiltrate. The disease usually resolves spontaneously, with no long-term sequelae.

MANAGEMENT STRATEGY

In the annular, localized form of granuloma annulare the diagnosis can often be made clinically, but a skin biopsy may be required to confirm the diagnosis of the more unusual varieties (generalized, papular umbilicated, perforating, and subcutaneous). Once the diagnosis is established, it is prudent to check the urine for sugar to exclude diabetes mellitus.

Because the majority of cases of granuloma annulare do not give rise to symptoms, the need for active treatment should be considered carefully; in many cases, reassurance that the disease is benign and will resolve spontaneously is sufficient. Painful or unsightly lesions may justify more active treatment, though the evidence to support the efficacy of many of the treatments is poor.

In localized granuloma annulare, treatment with either *cryotherapy* or *topical corticosteroids* may be effective. Cryotherapy using liquid nitrogen or nitrous oxide can be repeated at intervals of 3–4 weeks. Clobetasol propionate (Dermovate) lotion, occluded with a hydrocolloid dressing changed at weekly intervals, can be used for a period of 4–6 weeks. Alternatively, 0.1 mL injections of triamcinolone acetonide (5 mg/mL) may be used, repeated, if necessary, at intervals of 6–8 weeks. Treatment of refractory lesions has included *scarification* and the use of *intralesional interferon*. Large, tumid lesions may require excision.

Generalized granuloma annulare may be persistent and its unsightly appearance causes patients to seek active treatment, though the results are often disappointing. *PUVA* with oral or topical psoralens may be used, but relapses occur and a period of maintenance photochemotherapy may be required. UVA alone has been used, with reported beneficial results. Both *etretinate* and *isotretinoin* have been associated with improvement or clearance of generalized granuloma annulare. *Topical tacrolimus* has been used, with greater success in generalized

disease than in the localized variety. Other reported treatments for this condition include *dapsone, ciclosporin, systemic corticosteroids, chlorambucil, antimalarials, potassium iodide, pentoxifylline, nicotinamide* (niacinamide), *topical vitamin E, fumaric acid esters, defibrotide, efalizumab, doxycycline, hydroxyurea,* and *pulsed dye laser.*

SPECIFIC INVESTIGATIONS

> ► Check urine for glucose

Unlike necrobiosis lipoidica, in which there is a strong association with diabetes mellitus, the relationship between granuloma annulare and diabetes is unclear. Nevertheless, it would seem sensible to use the diagnosis of granuloma annulare as a cue to exclude undiagnosed diabetes, and at least check the urine for sugar.

Carbohydrate tolerance in patients with granuloma annulare. Study of fifty-two cases. Haim S, Freidman-Birnbaum R, Haim N, Shafrir A, Ravina A. Br J Dermatol 1973; 88: 447–51.

The incidence of abnormal carbohydrate tolerance in 39 patients with localized granuloma annulare was 23.1% and similar to that of a control population, compared to an incidence of 76.9% in 13 patients with generalized disease.

Absence of carbohydrate intolerance in patients with granuloma annulare. Gannon TF, Lynch PJ. J Am Acad Dermatol 1994; 30: 662–3.

Glycosylated hemoglobin levels were found to be normal in the study population of 23 patients with granuloma annulare, 13 of whom had localized lesions and 10 the generalized form of the disease.

Localised granuloma annulare is associated with insulin-dependent diabetes mellitus. Muhlemann MF, Williams DDR. Br J Dermatol 1984; 111: 325–9.

This retrospective study looked at 557 insulin-dependent diabetics and found that 16 of them had granuloma annulare, significantly more than the 0.9 cases that might have been expected.

LOCALIZED GRANULOMA ANNULARE

FIRST-LINE THERAPIES

> ► Intralesional corticosteroids   C
> ► Topical corticosteroids   E
> ► Cryotherapy   C

Granuloma annulare and necrobiosis lipoidica treated by jet injector. Sparrow G, Abell E. Br J Dermatol 1975; 93: 85–9.

Injections of 0.1 mL of triamcinolone (5 mg/mL) into lesions of granuloma annulare produced a complete response in 68% of patients after a mean of 2.9 treatments carried out at 6–8-week intervals. About half the patients suffered recurrences, which are reported to have responded to re-treatment.

Successful treatment of chronic skin diseases with clobetasol propionate and a hydrocolloid occlusive dressing. Volden G. Acta Dermatol Venereol 1992; 72: 69–71.

In this trial, clobetasol propionate under hydrocolloid occlusion was used in a variety of chronic skin diseases. One of three cases of granuloma annulare showed a complete response after 4 weeks' treatment.

This treatment modality has the advantage of being painless, but the evidence for its efficacy is not at all strong.

A contact dermatitis reaction to clobetasol propionate cream associated with resolution of recalcitrant, generalised granuloma annulare. Agarwal S, Berth-Jones J. J Dermatol Treat 2000; 11: 279–82.

A single patient was cleared of disseminated lesions of granuloma annulare by topical clobetasol propionate; however, the patient developed contact sensitization to the medication, raising the possibility that this reaction may also have played a therapeutic role.

Successful outcome of cryosurgery in patients with granuloma annulare. Blume-Peytavi U, Zouboulis CC, Jacobi H, Scholz A, Bisson S, Orfanos CE. Br J Dermatol 1994; 130: 494–7.

Of 31 patients with granuloma annulare, 22 were treated with liquid nitrogen and nine with nitrous oxide; 81% of lesions cleared after a single freeze–thaw cycle. Four cases had persistent atrophic scars where large lesions had been treated with liquid nitrogen.

It should be possible to prevent cryoatrophy by avoiding freeze–thaw cycles of more than 10 seconds, and taking care not to overlap treatment areas.

SECOND-LINE THERAPIES

▶ Intralesional interferon	C
▶ Scarification	E
▶ Surgery	E
▶ Imiquimod	E
▶ UVA1 phototherapy	E
▶ 5 ALA photodynamic therapy	E

Treatment of granuloma annulare by local injections with low-dose recombinant human interferon gamma. Weiss JM, Muchenberger S, Schöpf E, Simon JC. J Am Acad Dermatol 1998; 39: 117–19.

Three patients with localized granuloma annulare were treated with intralesional injections of recombinant human interferon-γ (2.5×10^5 IU/lesion) on 7 consecutive days and thereafter three times weekly for a further 2 weeks. All lesions had cleared by the end of the treatment period.

Scarification treatment of granuloma annulare. Wilkin JK, DuComb D, Castrow FF. Arch Dermatol 1982; 118: 68–9.

Two patients are described in whom lesions of granuloma annulare were treated successfully by scarification, using the point of a 19-gauge injection needle drawn across the lesions to produce capillary bleeding. Treatment was carried out weekly for 8 weeks, and every 2–3 weeks thereafter.

Surgical pearl: surgical treatment of tumor-sized granuloma annulare of the fingers. Shelley WB, Shelley ED. J Am Acad Dermatol 1997; 37: 473–4.

The report is of a case of nodular granuloma annulare treated with shave excision, allowing the wound to heal by second intention.

Successful treatment of granuloma annulare with imiquimod cream 5%: A report of four cases. Badavanis G, Monastirli A, Pasmatzi E, Tsambaos D. Acta Dermatol Venereol 2005; 85: 547–8.

Four patients with multiple lesions of granuloma annulare on the extremities were treated once daily with 5% imiquimod cream. The majority of lesions cleared within 6–12 weeks and did not recur during a follow-up period of 10–18 months.

Granuloma annulare: Dramatically altered appearance after application of 5% imiquimod cream. Stephenson S, Nedorost S. Pediatr Dermatol 2008; 25: 138–9.

This letter reports the case of a child in whom granuloma annulare lesion worsened after the accidental application of 5% imiquimod being used to treat adjacent plane warts.

Multiple localized granuloma annulare: Ultraviolet A1 phototherapy. Frigerio E, Franchi C, Garutti C, Spadino S, Altomare GF. Clin Exp Dermatol 2007; 32: 762–4.

Four patients with multiple localized granuloma annulare were treated with high-dose UVA1. It was started at a dose of $60\,J/cm^2$ per half body on day 1, followed by fixed daily doses of $100\,J/cm^2$.

Successful treatment of granuloma annulare with topical 5-aminolaevulinic acid photodynamic therapy. Kim YJ, Kang HY, Lee ES, Kim YC. J Dermatol 2006; 33: 642–3.

GENERALIZED GRANULOMA ANNULARE

FIRST-LINE THERAPIES

▷ Photochemotherapy	C
▷ UVA1 phototherapy	B
▷ Systemic isotretinoin	C
▷ Dapsone	C
▷ Topical tacrolimus	E

Photochemotherapy of generalised granuloma annulare. Kerker BJ, Huang CP, Morison WL. Arch Dermatol 1990; 126: 359–61.

Five patients with diffuse granuloma annulare were treated with PUVA, using oral methoxypsoralen, two to three times weekly. All patients cleared after a period of 3–4 months, but four relapsed after PUVA was stopped. These patients responded to further treatments.

There have been similar reports with oral PUVA using 5-methoxypsoralen, and also with bath PUVA and polythene sheet bath-PUVA.

UVA1 phototherapy for disseminated granuloma annulare. Schnopp C, Tzaneva S, Mempel M, Schulmeister K, Abeck D, Tanew A. Photodermatol, Photoimmunol Photomed 2005; 21: 68–71.

Twenty patients with disseminated granuloma annulare underwent UVA1 (340–400 nm) phototherapy, which provided good or excellent results in half of them and satisfactory responses in the majority. Discontinuation of treatment was followed by early recurrence of disease.

Resolution of disseminated granuloma annulare with isotretinoin. Schleicher SM, Milstein HJ, Lim SJ. Int J Dermatol 1992; 31: 371–2.

Evidence Levels: A Double-blind study B Clinical trial ≥ 20 subjects C Clinical trial < 20 subjects D Series ≥ 5 subjects E Anecdotal case reports

Six women treated with isotretinoin showed complete or almost complete resolution of diffuse granuloma annulare.

Generalized granuloma annulare in a patient with type II diabetes mellitus: successful treatment with isotretinoin. Sahin MT, Turel-Ermertcan A, Ozturkcan S, Türkdogan P. J Eur Acad Dermatol Venereol 2006; 20: 111–14.

In the reported cases, the dose of isotretinoin used has not always been clear. In a number of reports doses tend to be about 40 mg daily, with improvement occurring after about 3 months. There is a report in which etretinate was used successfully in this condition, but none that mentions acitretin.

The response of generalised granuloma annulare to dapsone. Czarnecki DB, Gin D. Acta Dermatol Venereol 1986; 66: 82–4.

Six patients with generalized granuloma annulare were treated with dapsone at a dose of 100 mg daily. All showed a complete response, with five subjects clearing within 8 weeks, and four were documented to have remained clear for 4–20 months after stopping dapsone therapy.

Efficacy of dapsone in disseminated granuloma annulare: a case report and review of literature. Martín-Sáez E, Fernández-Guarino M, Carrillo-Gijón R, Muñoz-Zato E, Jaén-Olasolo P. Actas Dermosifiliogr 2008; 99: 64–8.

Successful treatment of disseminated granuloma annulare with topical tacrolimus. Jain S, Stephens CJM. Br J Dermatol 2004; 150: 1042–3.

Four patients were treated with tacrolimus for a period of 6 weeks: two showed complete clearance, maintained for at least 6 weeks, and two had marked improvement.

SECOND-LINE THERAPIES

▶ Ciclosporin	E
▶ Systemic corticosteroids	E
▶ Chlorambucil	D
▶ Antimalarials	D
▶ Pentoxifylline	E
▶ Topical vitamin E	E
▶ Nicotinamide	E
▶ Fumaric acid esters	D
▶ Defibrotide	E
▶ Efalizumab	E
▶ Pulsed dye laser	E
▶ Doxycycline	E
▶ Hydroxyurea	E
▶ Bath PUVA	E
▶ Potassium iodide	E
▶ Pimecrolimus	E

Disseminated granuloma annulare: efficacy of cyclosporine therapy. Spadino S, Altomare A, Cainelli C, Franchi C, Frigerio E, Garutti C, et al. Int J Immunopathol Pharmacol 2006; 19: 433–42.

Four patients with disseminated granuloma annulare were treated with ciclosporin starting at a dose of 4 mg/kg/day for 4 weeks, subsequently reduced by 0.5 mg/kg/day every 2 weeks. Lesions resolved completely within 3 weeks in all patients, with no relapses during the following 12 months.

Granuloma annulare, generalised. Larralde J. Arch Dermatol 1963; 87: 777–8.

A case report describing the use of systemic steroids in generalized granuloma annulare.

Low-dose chlorambucil in the treatment of generalised granuloma annulare. Kossard S, Winkelmann RK. Dermatologica 1979; 158: 443–50.

Chlorambucil 2 mg twice daily was used to treat six patients, five of whom showed a marked improvement by 12 weeks. The authors state that chlorambucil should only be considered in refractory cases of granuloma annulare in which there is a compelling requirement for therapy, and then only for a maximum of 12 weeks.

Antimalarials for control of disseminated granuloma annulare in children. Simon M, von den Driesch P. J Am Acad Dermatol 1994; 31: 1064–5.

Six children achieved complete clearance within 4–6 weeks of starting hydroxychloroquine, and remained clear for a mean period of 2.5 years. The dose of hydroxychloroquine was 3 mg/kg/day in four subjects and 6 mg/kg/day in the other two.

Generalised granuloma annulare successfully treated with pentoxifylline. Rubel DM, Wood G, Rosen R, Jopp-McKay A. Australas J Dermatol 1993; 34: 103–8.

Disseminated granuloma annulare: therapy with vitamin E topically. Burg G. Dermatology 1992; 184: 308–9.

Response of generalized granuloma annulare to high-dose niacinamide. Ma M, Medenica M. Arch Dermatol 1983; 119: 836–9.

Disseminated granuloma annulare – treatment with fumaric acid esters. Eberlein-König B, Mempel M, Stahlecker J, Forer I, Ring J, Abeck D. Dermatology 2005; 210: 223–6.

Eight patients with disseminated granuloma annulare were treated with fumaric acid esters, with remission in three and partial remission in four. Associated side effects led to withdrawal of treatment in half the patients.

A case of disseminated granuloma annulare treated with defibrotide: complete clinical remission and progressive hair darkening. Rubegni P, Sbano P, Fimiani M. Br J Dermatol 2003; 149: 437–8.

Disseminated granuloma annulare resolved with the T-cell modulator efalizumab. Goffe BS. Arch Dermatol 2004; 140: 1287–8.

Disseminated granuloma annulare cleared during the treatment of psoriasis with efalizumab.

Treatment of granuloma annulare with the 585 nm pulsed dye laser. Sniezek PJ, DeBloom JR 2nd, Arpey CJ. Dermatol Surg 2005; 31: 1370–3.

A successful outcome from treatment of a single plaque treated on three occasions.

Generalized granuloma annulare – response to doxycycline. Duarte AF, Mota A, Pereira M, Baudrier T, Azevedo F. J Eur Acad Dermatol Venereol 2009; 23: 84–5.

Treatment of recalcitrant disseminated granuloma annulare with hydroxyurea. Hall CS, Zone JJ, Hull CM. J Am Acad Dermatol 2008; 58: 525.

Two patients responded to hydroxyurea within 1–2 months, but one relapsed after discontinuation of treatment.

Clearance of generalized papular umbilicated granuloma annulare in a child with bath PUVA therapy. Batchelor R, Clark S. Pediatr Dermatol 2006; 23: 72–4.

Potassium iodide in the treatment of disseminated granuloma annulare. Smith JB, Hansen CD, Zone JJ. J Am Acad Dermatol 1994; 30: 791–2.

A double-blind, placebo-controlled, crossover trial of 10 patients concluded that oral potassium iodide does not show an advantage over placebo in the treatment of disseminated granuloma annulare.

Pimecrolimus 1% cream in the treatment of disseminated granuloma annulare. Rigopoulos D, Prantsidis A, Christofidou E, Ioannides D, Gregoriou S, Katsambas A. Br J Dermatol 2005; 152: 1364–5.

A case of generalized granuloma annulare with myelodysplastic syndrome: successful treatment with systemic isotretinoin and topical pimecrolimus 1% cream combination. Baskan EB, Turan A, Tunali S. J Eur Acad Dermatol Venereol 2007; 21: 693–5.

Evidence Levels: **A** Double-blind study **B** Clinical trial ≥ 20 subjects **C** Clinical trial < 20 subjects **D** Series ≥ 5 subjects **E** Anecdotal case reports

Granuloma faciale

Sue Handfield-Jones

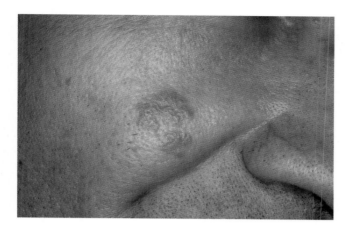

Granuloma faciale is a rare form of localized, fibrosing vasculitis that usually affects the face. Lesions are purplish-red or skin-colored plaques and nodules with accentuation of follicular openings. There are isolated reports of similar conditions affecting the eye and upper airways.

MANAGEMENT STRATEGY

Granuloma faciale is a chronic condition; spontaneous remission is unusual. Lesions are usually asymptomatic, but treatment is needed to reduce disfigurement. The condition is more common in white middle-aged men.

Clinical diagnosis is difficult. Differential diagnosis includes sarcoid, lymphocytoma cutis, persistent insect bite reactions, and lymphoma. The histological differential diagnosis includes erythema elevatum diutinum and angiolymphoid hyperplasia with eosinophilia.

Because of the rarity of the condition there are no formal trials of therapy. The optimal treatment depends on the size, site and thickness of the lesions. For small numbers of lesions intralesional steroid or destructive treatments such as cryotherapy, laser or surgical excision can be used. For multiple or widespread lesions systemic treatment, such as dapsone, can be considered. The role of topical calcineurin inhibitors is still not established.

Sun protection advice should be given to patients. Cosmetic camouflage can be helpful for some patients with flatter lesions.

SPECIFIC INVESTIGATIONS

▶ Skin biopsy
▶ Hematology (CBC)

Histological findings include a dense eosinophilic and neutrophilic infiltrate, often perivascular, affecting the upper and sometimes deep dermis. The epidermis is spared and there is a Grenz zone. Telangiectasia is common. Vasculitis with leukocytoclasis is reported. Dermal fibrosis is often seen.

Granuloma faciale: a clinicopathologic study of 66 patients. Ortonne N, Wechsler J, Bagot M, Grosshans E, Cribier B. J Am Acad Dermatol 2005; 53: 1002–9.

Peripheral blood eosinophilia is sometimes found.

FIRST-LINE THERAPIES

▶ Corticosteroids	E
▶ Cryotherapy	D
▶ Laser therapy	E
▶ Surgery	E

Granuloma faciale treated with intradermal dexamethasone. Arundell FD, Burdick KH. Arch Dermatol 1960; 82: 437–8.

This paper reports response to dexamethasone, but triamcinolone acetonide and triamcinolone hexacetonide have also been used. Patients should be warned of the risk of skin atrophy and pigment change.

Assessment of the efficacy of cryosurgery in the treatment of granuloma faciale. Panagiotopoulos A, Anyfantakis V, Rallis E, Chasapi V, Stavropoulos P, Boubouka C, et al. Br J Dermatol 2006: 154; 357–60.

Nine patients were treated with either spray or closed probe cryotherapy. The open-spray technique was given as one or two freeze–thaw cycles of 20–30 seconds. The cryoprobe was given as one to three freeze–thaw cycles of 15–20 seconds. Patients were re-treated after 1 and 3 months. All were clear of disease activity at 6 months. One patient developed severe inflammatory reaction with blistering. Two had hypopigmentation, but this resolved in 4 months. There was no recurrence within 2–4 years' follow-up.

Granuloma faciale: successful treatment of nine cases with a combination of cryotherapy and intralesional corticosteroid injection. Dowlati B, Firooz A, Dowlati Y. Int J Dermatol 1997; 36: 548–51.

Cryotherapy for 20–30 seconds was followed by triamcinolone acetonide 5 mg/mL intralesionally.

Granuloma faciale treated with pulsed-dye laser: a case series. Cheung S-T, Lanigan SW. Clin Exp Dermatol 2005: 30; 373–5.

Four patients who had all failed with cryotherapy were treated with Candela Vbeam PDL at 595 nm. In two patients the lesions resolved. Nasal lesions, especially flatter ones, seem to respond better to treatment.

New treatment modalities for granuloma faciale. Ludwig E, Allam J-P, Bieber T, Novak N. Br J Dermatol 2003; 149: 634–7.

A report of two cases of sizeable facial lesions responding rapidly to Laserscope potassium-titanyl-phosphate 532 nm laser.

Granuloma faciale: treatment with the argon laser. Apfelberg DB, Druker D, Maser MR, Lash H, Spence B, Deneau D. Arch Dermatol 1983; 119: 573–6.

A report of three cases responding to argon laser with no recurrence from 5 to 23 months. A 'white, collagenous scar' resulted.

Carbon dioxide laser treatment of granuloma faciale. Wheeland RG, Ashley JR, Smith DA, Ellis DL, Wheeland DN. J Dermatol Surg Oncol 1984; 10: 730–3.

A single treatment resulted in healing with no discernible scar. There was no recurrence at 1 year.

Recurrent facial plaques following full-thickness grafting. Phillips DK, Hymes SR. Arch Dermatol 1994; 130: 1436–7.

Although surgery is mentioned in many papers, recurrence can occur even after full-thickness excision and grafting.

Granuloma faciale: comparison of different treatment modalities. Dinehart SM, Gross DJ, Davis CM, Herzberg AJ. Arch Otolaryngol Head Neck Surg 1990; 116: 849–51.

Combined electrosurgery and dermabrasion was compared with carbon dioxide laser treatment in a patient with two similar lesions. Skin texture at 6 weeks was better on the laser-treated side, but laser treatment was more time-consuming.

SECOND-LINE THERAPIES

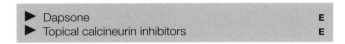

▶ Dapsone	E
▶ Topical calcineurin inhibitors	E

On the efficacy of dapsone in granuloma faciale. Van de Kerkhof PCM. Acta Dermatol Venereol 1994; 74: 61–2.

A 4 cm plaque showed 'impressive improvement' with dapsone 200 mg daily. Dapsone needs careful monitoring, and many patients would not tolerate 200 mg daily.

Many authors mention dapsone as a treatment that has been tried but failed.

Granuloma faciale: is it a new indication for pimecrolimus? A case report. Eetam I, Ertekin B, Unal I, Alper S. J Dermatol Treat 2006: 17; 238–40.

A case report of a 1 × 5 cm diameter lesion on the central face showing 'dramatic recovery' following pimecrolimus cream 1% twice daily for 2 months.

Granuloma faciale: treatment with topical tacrolimus. Marcoval J, Moreno A, Bordas X, Peyri J. J Am Acad Dermatol. 2006: 55: S110–11.

This and other papers describe response to topical tacrolimus, sometimes within a few months. In some patients lesions had previously failed to respond to other therapies. Remission for up to 2 years is described.

The possible risks of topical calcineurin inhibitors in sun-exposed sites must be considered.

THIRD-LINE THERAPIES

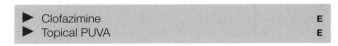

▶ Clofazimine	E
▶ Topical PUVA	E

Granuloma faciale mimicking rhinophyma: response to clofazimine. Gomez-de la Fuente E, del Rio R, Guerra A, Rodriguez-Peralto JL, Iglesias L. Acta Dermatol Venereol 2000; 80: 144.

A patient with a 10-year history of histologically proven disease on the nose was treated with 300 mg clofazimine once daily for 5 months, with 'remarkable improvement.' Two similar reports are cited.

Granuloma faciale: treatment with topical psoralen and UVA. Hudson LD. J Am Acad Dermatol 1983; 8: 559.

A 62-year-old man with a 1-month history of biopsy-proven granuloma faciale affecting the nasal alae responded to 24 J UVA given over 10 weeks, showing a very marked improvement with no evidence of residual lesion at 6 months.

There are old reports of treatment with intralesional gold and bismuth, radiotherapy, oral colchicine, isoniazid, potassium arsenite, testosterone, and antimalarials, but within the last 25 years there have been no reports of successful response to these agents.

Granuloma inguinale

Patrice Morel

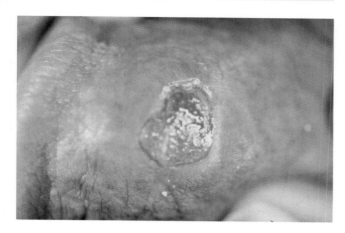

Granuloma inguinale, or donovanosis, is an infection causing granulomatous ulceration of the genital, inguinal and perineal skin. It is extremely rare in western Europe and the United States, but is still endemic or epidemic in India, South Africa, Brazil, and among aborigines in Australia. The causative organism is *Klebsiella granulomatis*, an intracellular Gram-negative bacillus.

The transmission of this infection is frequently, but not exclusively, sexual. Clinically, the disease is commonly characterized as painless, progressive ulcerative lesions without regional lymphadenopathy. The lesions are highly vascular (i.e., a beefy red appearance) and bleed easily on contact.

MANAGEMENT STRATEGY

Patients with donovanosis should be treated (a) to prevent the gradual development of the disease, which may lead to genital deformity or a life-threatening disseminated infection, (b) to prevent transmission to sexual partners, and (c) to prevent the risk of concomitant transmission of the human immunodeficiency virus.

In the absence of randomized controlled trials, antibiotic treatment of donovanosis is based on the results of clinical experience and individual reports, usually involving relatively small numbers of patients.

Trimethoprim-sulfamethoxazole or doxycycline are recommended by the Centers for Disease Control and Prevention (CDC) (2002). Azithromycin is recommended in the Australian Antibiotic Guidelines (1996–97). Many other antibiotics are also effective (e.g., ciprofloxacin, ceftriaxone, erythromycin). The addition of an aminoglycoside (gentamicin) is recommended by the CDC if lesions do not respond within the first few days.

Therapy should be continued until all lesions have healed completely (except for the 4-week azithromycin regimen). A relapse can occur 6–18 months later despite effective initial therapy. Surgical excision may be necessary for extensive disease unresponsive to medical treatment.

Sexual partners of patients who have granuloma inguinale should be examined and treated if they (a) had sexual contact with the patient during the 60 days preceding the onset of symptoms in the patient, and (b) have clinical signs and symptoms of the disease.

SPECIFIC INVESTIGATIONS

▶ Microscopic evaluation of either tissue smears or biopsy specimen stained with Wright's or Giemsa stains
▶ Culture in human peripheral blood monocytes and in Hep-2 cells
▶ Polymerase chain reaction (PCR) test

Genital ulcer disease: accuracy of clinical diagnosis and strategies to improve control in Durban, South Africa. O'Farrell N, Hoosen AA, Coetzee KD, Van den Ende J. Genitourin Med 1994; 70: 7–11.

One hundred men and 100 women with genital ulcers were recruited to investigate the accuracy of clinical diagnosis in genital ulcer disease (GUD). The clinical diagnostic accuracy for donovanosis was relatively high (63% in men, 83% in women). Compared with other causes of GUD, donovanosis ulcers bled to the touch, were larger, and were not usually associated with inguinal lymphadenopathy.

Donovanosis. Hart G. Clin Infect Dis 1997; 25: 24–32.

For laboratory confirmation of donovanosis, the preferred method involves demonstration of typical intracellular Donovan bodies within large mononuclear cells that are visualized in smears prepared from lesions or biopsy specimens. The large mononuclear cells are 25–90 μm in diameter, with a vesicular or pyknotic nucleus. There are around 20 intracytoplasmic vacuoles containing pleomorphic Donovan bodies in either young non-capsulated or mature capsulated forms.

Culture of the causative organism of donovanosis (*Calymmatobacterium granulomatis*) in Hep-2 cells. Carter J, Hutton S, Sriprakash KS, Kemp DJ, Lum G, Savage J, et al. J Clin Microbiol 1997; 35: 2915–17.

With the positive culture of *C. granulomatis* in Hep-2 cells, it is now possible to test the in-vitro susceptibility of *C. granulomatis* to antibiotics and to provide a ready source of DNA and antigenic material to enable the development of serological tests and possibly, in the future, a vaccine. Successful culture has also been reported in human peripheral blood mononuclear cells (Kharsany, 1997).

A colorimetric detection system for *Calymmatobacterium granulomatis*. Carter JS, Kemp DJ. Sex Transm Infect 2000; 76: 134–6.

A colorimetric PCR test was developed that could be used by well-equipped diagnostic laboratories. PCR tests can be performed on surface swabs of lesions and avoid the need for biopsy. Molecular techniques should help to answer some remaining questions about donovanosis (e.g., non-sexual contamination, autoinoculation).

Phylogenetic evidence for reclassification of *Calymmatobacterium granulomatis* as *Klebsiella granulomatis* comb. nov. Carter JS, Bowden FJ, Bastian I, Myers GM, Sriprakash KS, Kemp DJ. Int J Syst Bacteriol 1999; 49: 1695–700.

The new understanding of the basic molecular biology led to reclassification of the causative organism from *Calymmatobacterium granulomatis* to *Klebsiella granulomatis*.

Granuloma inguinale. Rosen T, Tschen JA, Ramsdell W, Moore J, Markham B. J Am Acad Dermatol 1984; 11: 433–7.

A report of 20 cases of granuloma inguinale in Houston, Texas. Evidence supports the venereal transmission of the infection. Three heterosexual patients had intercourse with the same prostitute during a single evening and all developed lesions 2 weeks later. The occurrence of donovanosis in young children and the low prevalence of the disease among sexual partners are cited as evidence against sexual transmission in some cases. Infants born to infected mothers may acquire the infection at birth and develop lesions of the umbilicus and sexual organs as well as disseminated infection.

Donovanosis. Seghal VN, Sharma HK. J Dermatol 1992; 19: 32–46.

Although the genitalia are the sites of primary lesions most frequently encountered, many cases report extragenital lesions due to autoinoculation, direct or contiguous spread via the bloodstream to the bones, joints, lung, liver, and spleen.

Donovanosis in Australia: going, going. Bowden FJ, on behalf of the National Donovanosis Eradication Advisory Committee. Sex Transm Infect 2005; 81: 365–6.

The donovanosis elimination program among Aboriginals in Australia appears successful and is a model that could be adopted in other donovanosis-endemic areas.

FIRST-LINE THERAPIES

▶ Azithromycin 500 mg orally daily for 7 days or 1 g orally weekly for 4 weeks	B
▶ Doxycycline 100 mg orally twice daily for at least 3 weeks	C

Donovanosis: treatment with azithromycin. Bowden FJ, Savage J. Int J STD AIDS 1998; 9: 61.

Australian authors say that they have treated over 100 patients with donovanosis using azithromycin, with no primary treatment failures. They recommend two treatment regimens: 500 mg orally daily for 7 days or 1 g orally weekly for 4 weeks. The 1996–97 edition of the Australian Antibiotic Guidelines lists azithromycin as the first-line agent for donovanosis. The drug is listed as a B1 agent in pregnancy, meaning that it can be used for the treatment of antenatal patients with the disease.

Sexually Transmitted Diseases Treatment Guidelines 2006. MMWR 2006; 55(RR11): 1–94.

Doxycycline 100 mg orally twice a day for at least 3 weeks and until all lesions have completely healed is still recommended by the CDC (2006).

SECOND-LINE THERAPIES

▶ Erythromycin 500 mg orally four times daily for at least 3 weeks	B
▶ Trimethoprim-sulfamethoxazole one double-strength tablet orally twice daily for at least 3 weeks	B
▶ Ciprofloxacin 750 mg orally twice daily for at least 3 weeks	C

Clinico-epidemiologic features of granuloma inguinale in the era of acquired immune deficiency syndrome. Jamkhedkar PP, Hira SK, Shroff HJ, Lanjewar DN. Sex Transm Dis 1998; 25: 196–200.

Indian authors treated 50 patients with granuloma inguinale (21 HIV positive and 29 HIV negative) with their 'standard treatment regimen' of erythromycin 2 g orally daily. The ulcers took longer to heal in the seropositive group (mean 25.7 vs 16.8 days). Erythromycin is less convenient to administer than azithromycin.

Granuloma inguinale. Rosen T, Tschen JA, Ramsdell W, Moore J, Markham B. J Am Acad Dermatol 1984; 11: 433–7.

Twenty patients with granuloma inguinale were treated with trimethoprim-sulfamethoxazole. The drug proved to be a safe and effective therapy. It is currently recommended for a minimum of 3 weeks by the CDC. It has been used extensively in India, with consistently good results.

Treatment of donovanosis with norfloxacin. Ramanan CR, Sarma PSA, Ghorpade A, Das M. Int J Dermatol 1990; 29: 298–9.

Ten patients with donovanosis were treated with norfloxacin in an oral dose of 400 mg twice daily. The time taken for complete healing was 2–11 days.

The CDC recommends ciprofloxacin rather than norfloxacin as an alternative regimen.

THIRD-LINE THERAPIES

▶ Ceftriaxone 1 g IM daily	C
▶ Gentamicin 1 mg/kg intravenously every 8 hours	C
▶ Surgical treatment	E

Ceftriaxone in the treatment of chronic donovanosis in Central Australia. Merianos A, Gilles M, Chuah J. Genitourin Med 1994; 70: 84–9.

Eight women and four men with chronic donovanosis (mean duration 3 years) were treated with a single daily injection of 1 g ceftriaxone diluted in 2 mL of 1% lidocaine. Clinical improvement was dramatic in most lesions, and four patients healed completely without recurrence after a total 7–10 g of ceftriaxone. The drug is safe in pregnancy.

1998 Guidelines for treatment of sexually transmitted diseases. Centers for Disease Control and Prevention. MMWR Recomm Rep 1998; 47(RR-1): 1–116.

The CDC recommends the addition of an aminoglycoside (gentamicin) if lesions do not respond within the first few days of therapy.

Surgical treatment of granuloma inguinale. Bozbora A, Erbil Y, Berber E, Ozarmagan S. Br J Dermatol 1998; 138: 1079–81.

Long-standing and complicated disease (multiple fistulas and abscesses unresponsive to antibiotics) may require surgical treatment.

SPECIAL CONSIDERATIONS

▶ Pregnancy Pregnant and lactating women should be treated with the erythromycin or azithromycin regimens
▶ HIV infection HIV-infected persons should be treated following the regimens cited previously. The addition of gentamicin should be considered

Evidence Levels: **A** Double-blind study **B** Clinical trial ≥ 20 subjects **C** Clinical trial < 20 subjects **D** Series ≥ 5 subjects **E** Anecdotal case reports

Granulomatous cheilitis

Julia E Haimowitz, Linda Y Hwang

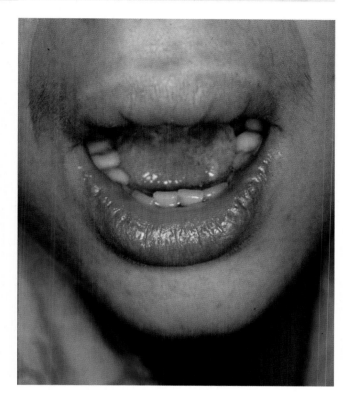

Orofacial granulomatosis describes a clinical entity of painless orofacial swelling with histologic evidence of non-caseating granulomatous inflammation. Orofacial granulomatosis encompasses the terms granulomatous cheilitis (GC), Miescher's cheilitis granulomatosa and Melkersson–Rosenthal syndrome (MRS). These terms have been used interchangeably, leading to confusion in diagnostic terminology. MRS describes the triad of recurrent orofacial edema, recurrent facial nerve palsy, and lingua plicata (fissured tongue). GC and MRS may represent separate diseases, but many investigators consider isolated GC to be a monosymptomatic form of MRS. Oligosymptomatic forms of MRS are recognized.

MANAGEMENT STRATEGY

The dermatologic treatment of MRS predominantly involves therapy for GC. Because the etiology of MRS/CG is unknown, a variety of therapeutic strategies have been attempted. No randomized clinical trials been performed. Given the waxing and waning nature of the condition, treatment outcomes are difficult to assess. Rarely, spontaneous remissions of GC may occur, further confounding assessment of therapies.

Treatment of GC is directed at preventing permanent labial deformity. Conservative measures for acute GC include *cold compresses* and *oral antihistamines* for reducing erythema, and *ointments* to protect against fissuring of the lips. Initial therapy frequently includes *corticosteroids*, either topical, intralesional or systemic. Initial topical therapy may include either triamcinolone or clobetasol (compounded into Orabase).

Intralesional steroids may be used in doses ranging from 10 to 40 mg/kg. Owing to the need for increased volumes injected at lower concentrations, nerve blocks may be needed to reduce patient discomfort. Although short courses of prednisone will frequently improve tissue swelling, flares are often noted on cessation.

Clofazamine has been reported to treat GC successfully. Response to therapy has been variable. Possible side effects include transient orange-pink discoloration of the skin, nausea, and vomiting. Fatal enteropathy may occur, but only at higher doses than those recommended for GC treatment. Thalidomide can be used safely, but is teratogenic. Patients must be monitored for the development of peripheral neuropathy. Monotherapy with *metronidazole*, penicillin, erythromycin, tetracyclines, ketotifen, *hydroxychloroquine* or sulfasalazine, although less well substantiated, may be attempted. These medications may be used with corticosteroids. The addition of *minocycline* 100 mg twice daily or *tetracycline* 500 mg daily may prevent rebound after prednisone discontinuation. The value of dapsone and topical tacrolimus in the treatment of GC is unclear.

GC may become persistent. Patients who suffer from permanent esthetic deformity or functional impairment may benefit from cheiloplasty. Surgical intervention should be performed only when more conservative approaches have failed, and when inflammation is quiescent. In the past, remission was maintained with the use of postoperative corticosteroid injections. More recent reports, however, have described long remissions after surgery, with no additional treatment needed. The newest successful therapies include *infliximab* and *adalimumab*. There has been a suggestion that infliximab is more effective than adalimumab, but too few cases have been reported to render definitive conclusions.

The differential diagnosis for GC is extensive. The clinician must be aware that, in addition to Crohn's disease, GC may be an initial presentation of sarcoidosis, and a systemic evaluation should be performed when indicated. Previous publications reported a low chance of developing Crohn's disease in GC patients. However, other series report GC preceding the diagnosis of Crohn's disease in both adults and children. The signs of symptoms of Crohn's disease may be minimal, necessitating a complete physical examination and continued observation and surveillance of the patient. A search for underlying odontogenic infections or allergenic sensitizers may be required. Other conditions, including infections (TB, leprosy, deep fungal), acquired or hereditary angioedema, and leukemic infiltrates, should be considered in the differential diagnosis.

SPECIFIC INVESTIGATIONS

▶ Biopsy for histopathologic examination: polarization and stains/cultures for fungi and acid-fast bacilli. *Initial biopsies of CG may reveal dilated lymphatic channels, nonspecific inflammatory infiltrates, and edema. In the later stages, the classic non-caseating granulomas are found. Absence of granulomata on biopsy does NOT exclude the diagnosis of GC. GC is primarily a clinical diagnosis*
▶ Complete blood count and chemistry profile, including serum calcium
▶ Angiotensin-converting enzyme level

Melkersson-Rosenthal syndrome: a review of 36 patients. Greene RM, Rogers RS III. J Am Acad Dermatol 1989; 21: 1263–70.

Cheilitis granulomatosa. van der Waal RIF, Schulten EAJM, van de Scheur MR, Wauters IM, Starink TM, van der Waal I. Eur Acad Dermatol Venereol 2001; 15: 519–23.

Orofacial granulomatosis. Armstrong DKB, Burrows D. Int J Dermatol 1995; 34: 830–3.

These articles review MRS and discuss possible etiologies and differential diagnoses.

Cheilitis granulomatosa: overview of 13 patients with long-term follow-up – results of management. van der Waal RIF, Schulten AJM, van der Meij E, van de Scheur MR, Starink TM, van der Waal I. Int J Dermatol 2002; 41: 225–9.

Is orofacial granulomatosis in children a feature of Crohn's disease? Khouri JM, Bohane TD, Say AS. Acta Paediatr 2005; 94: 501–4.

Re: Melkersson–Rosenthal syndrome as an early manifestation of Crohn's disease. Narbutt P, Dziki A. Colorectal Dis 2005; 7: 420–1.

Orofacial granulomatosis in a patient with Crohn's disease. van der Scheur MR, van der Waal RI, Völker-Dieben JH, Klinkeberg-Knol ED, Starink TM, van der Waal I. J Am Acad Dermatol 2003; 49: 952.

Cheilitis granulomatosa and Melkersson–Rosenthal syndrome: evaluation of gastrointestinal involvement and therapeutic regimens in 14 patients. Ratzinger G, Sepp N, Vogetseder W, Tilg H. J Eur Acad Dermatol Venereol 2007: 21: 1065–970.

Orofacial granlomatosis as the initial presentation of Crohn's disease in an adolescent. Bogenrieder T, Lehn N, Landthaler M, Stolz W. Dermatology 2003; 206: 273–8.

Cutaneous Crohn's disease mimicking Melkersson–Rosenthal syndrome: treatment with methotrexate. Tonkovic-Capin V, Galbraith SS, Rogers III RS, Binion DG, Yancey K. JEADV 2006: 20; 449–52.

The articles above highlight the possibility of Crohn's disease presenting with, or subsequent to, the diagnosis of GC. Narbut et al. mention the important issue that treatment for MRS/GC is mostly cosmetic, but Crohn's disease is a systemic illness with multiple potential complications.

Although it is unclear what percentage of patients with GC will develop Crohn's, it may be prudent to discuss this issue with GC patients.

Melkersson–Rosenthal syndrome and cheilitis granulomatosa. A clinicopathologic study of thirty-three patients with special reference to their oral lesions. Worsaae N, Christensen KC, Schiødt M, Reibel J. Oral Surg Oral Med Oral Pathol 1982; 54: 404–13.

The elimination of odontogenic infections led to inactivity of orofacial edema in 11 of 18 patients.

Review article: orofacial granulomatosis. Leão JC, Hodgson T, Scully C, Porter S. Aliment Pharmacol Ther 2004; 20: 1019–27.

The Melkersson–Rosenthal syndrome and food additive hypersensitivity. McKenna KE, Welsh MY, Burrows D. Br J Dermatol 1994: 131; 921–2.

Contact hypersensitivity in patients with orofacial granulomatosis. Armstrong DKB, Biagonia P, Lamey PJ, Burrows D. Am J Contact Dermatol 1997; 1: 35–8.

Ten of 48 patients showed positive reactions to an oral battery on standard patch testing. Of these 10, seven showed an improvement on an elimination diet. In most cases this was not a complete result.

FIRST-LINE THERAPIES

▶ Intralesional corticosteroids	C
▶ Oral corticosteroids	C

Management of cheilitis granulomatosa. Williams PM, Greenberg MS. Oral Surg Oral Med Oral Pathol 1991; 72: 436–9.

GC of the lower lip was successfully managed with intralesional triamcinolone hexacetonide 20 ng/mL. Doses of 2–3 mL were injected into 10–15 sites on the lower lip weekly for 4 weeks, bi-weekly for 1 month, monthly for 2 months, and bimonthly for 4 months.

Intralesional steroid injection after nerve block anesthesia in the treatment of orofacial granulomatosis. Sakuntabhai A, MacLeod RI, Lawrence CM. Arch Dermatol 1993; 129: 477–80.

Mental and infraorbital nerve blocks permitted the painless introduction of high-volume intralesional triamcinolone acetonide 10 mg/mL in five patients with GC. Three patients were available for follow-up and all experienced return to near normal lip size within 6 weeks of therapy. One patient required four treatments over a 2-year period.

No studies comparing high-dose (lower volume) intralesional corticosteroids exist.

Melkersson–Rosenthal syndrome and orofacial granulomatosis. Rogers RS III. Dermatol Clin 1996; 14: 371–9.

Oral prednisone 1–1.5 mg/kg daily tapered over 3–6 weeks may be effective for more severe and symptomatic episodes of GC.

SECOND-LINE THERAPIES

▶ Biologics, including infliximab, adalimumab	E
▶ Clofazamine	C
▶ Oral corticosteroids and minocycline/tetracycline	E
▶ Metronidazole ± corticosteroids	E

Treatment of granulomatous cheilitis with infliximab. Barry O, Barry J, Langan S, Murphy M, Fitzgibbon J. Arch Dermatol 2005; 141: 1081–3.

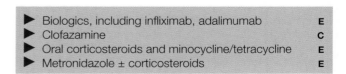

A 24-year-old woman with recalcitrant GC was treated with infliximab. In order to reduce the risk of infusion reactions, hydrocortisone (200 mg) was administered intravenously prior to treatment. The patient had restoration of normal lip architecture. Infliximab infusions were continued to maintain remission.

Melkersson–Rosenthal syndrome: a form of pseudoangio-edema. Kakimoto C, Sparks C, White AA. Ann Allergy Asthma Immunol 2007; 99: 185–9.

A 19-year-old woman with recalcitrant GC was treated with infliximab infusions. The patient improved after the second infusion and had complete resolution after the third. Because adverse effects developed, therapy was changed to adalimumab. Adalimumab 40 mg was injected subcutaneously weekly, with no evidence of relapse noted.

There is great hope that the new biologic agents will revolutionize the treatment of many inflammatory disorders, including GC.

Clofazamine as elective treatment for granulomatous cheilitis. Fdex-Freire LF, Gotarredona AS, Wittel JB, Ruis AP, Cabrera R, Ortoga MN, et al. J Drugs Dermatol 2005; 4: 374–7.

Three patients with GC treated with clofazamine 200–300 mg daily for 3–6 months obtained regression. Side effects included hyperpigmentation of the skin and elevation of liver enzymes.

Cheilitis granulomatosa Miescher: treatment with clo-fazamine and review of the literature. Ridder GJ, Fradis M, Löhle E. Ann OtoRhinol Laryngol 2001; 110: 964–7.

A 15-year-old girl's GC was treated with clofazamine 100 mg daily. Regression was noted after 30 days of treatment. Thereafter, 100 mg of clofazamine three times a week was given for 3 months. Her lip eventually returned to normal size. Follow-up for 6 years revealed no recurrence.

This article reviews several case reports and a case series of clofazamine therapy and discusses the great variability in response to therapy.

Melkersson–Rosenthal syndrome: clinical, pathological, and therapeutic considerations. Sussman GL, Yang WH, Steinberg S. Ann Allergy 1992; 69: 187–94.

Clofazamine 100 mg four times weekly for 3–11 months was used to treat 10 patients with GC/MRS. Complete remissions occurred in five, partial clinical responses occurred in three, and two patients had no clinical response.

Other studies have reported efficacy with a regimen consisting of clofazamine 100 mg daily for 10 days, followed by 200–400 mg weekly for 3–6 months.

Treatment and follow-up of persistent granulomatous cheilitis with intralesional steroid and metronidazole. Coskun B, Saral Y, Cicek D, Akpolat N. J Dermatol Treat 2004; 15: 333–5.

Melkersson–Rosenthal syndrome in childhood: successful management with combination steroid and minocycline therapy. Stein SL, Mancini AJ. J Am Acad Dermatol 1999; 41: 746–8.

THIRD-LINE THERAPIES

▶ Cheiloplasty ± postoperative intralesional cortiocosteroids	C
▶ Thalidomide	E
▶ Hydroxychloroquine	E
▶ Tranilast	E
▶ Danazol	E

Plastic surgical solutions for Melkersson–Rosenthal syndrome: facial liposuction and cheiloplasty procedures. Tan O, Atik B, Calka O. Ann Plast Surg 2006; 56: 268–73.

This article discusses surgical procedures in four patients, including reduction cheiloplasty consisting of mucosa, submucosa, and tangential muscle resection, crescent-shaped commissuroplasty, and facial liposuction. Mean follow-up duration was 13.7 months. *No postoperative steroids were given and there was no evidence of relapse in the follow-up period.*

Successful treatment of granulomatous cheilitis with thalidomide. Thomas P, Walchner M, Ghoreschi K, Rocken M. Arch Dermatol 2003; 139: 136–8.

A 39-year-old woman was treated with thalidomide 100 mg daily for 6 months. Lip swelling almost completely resolved. Thalidomide was reduced to 100 mg every other day for 2 months. Therapy was stopped. One year later, the patient's condition was stable with no signs of relapse.

Cheilitis granulomatosa: report of six cases and review of the literature. Allen CM, Camisa C, Hamzeh S. Stephens L. J Am Acad Dermatol 1990; 23: 444–50.

Hydroxychloroquine 200–400 mg daily has been reported to be efficacious in GC. Chloroquine therapy has not been successful in MRS.

Cheilitis granulomatosa: successful treatment with combined local triamcinolone injections and surgery. Krutchkoff D, James R. Arch Dermatol 1978; 114: 1203–6.

A man with GC was treated with triamcinolone injections, followed by upper and lower cheiloplasty. Four months later, repeat cheiloplasty of the upper lip revealed granulomas that were more numerous and larger than those observed initially. Postoperative corticosteroid injections maintained remission. The authors recommend postoperative corticosteroid injections to prevent exaggerated recurrences.

Long-term results after surgical reduction cheiloplasty in patients with Melkersson–Rosenthal syndrome and cheilitis granulomatosa. Ellitsgaad N, Andersson AP, Worsaaae N, Medgyesi S. Ann Plast Surg 1993; 31: 413–20.

A reduction cheiloplasty was performed on 13 patients. All were satisfied with their results, despite postoperative disease activity in six patients.

Lip reduction cheiloplasty for Miescher's granlomatous macrocheilitis (cheilitis granulomatosa) in childhood. Oliver DW, Scott MJL. Clin Exp Dermatol 2002; 27: 129–31.

Lip reduction cheiloplasty provided successful treatment of GC in an 11-year-old boy, suggesting that surgery can be safely undertaken in young children.

The surgical management of Melkersson–Rosenthal syndrome. Glickman LT, Birt BD, Kohli-Dang N. Plast Reconstruct Surg 1992; 89: 815–21.

Treatment of Miesche's cheilitis granulomatosa in Melkersson–Rosenthal syndrome. Camacho F, Garcia-Bravo B, Carrizosa A. Eur Acad Dermatol Venereol 2001; 15: 546–9.

The authors conclude that the best treatment for resistant GC is surgery with immediate injection of triamcinolone, followed by a course of oral tetracycline.

Melkersson–Rosenthal syndrome: reduction cheiloplasty utilizing a transmodiolar labial suspension suture. Cederna PS, Fiala TGS, Smith DJ, Newman MH. Aesthet Plast Surg 1998; 22: 102–5.

Cheilitis granulomatosa treated with metronidazole. Miralles J, Barnadas MA, de Moragas JM. Dermatology 1995; 191: 252–3.

A 30-year-old woman with monosymptomatic MRS was successfully treated with metronidazole 750–1000 mg daily for an 8-month tapering course.

Metronidazole has also been useful in two patients with GC associated with Crohn's disease. Treatment failures are also reported.

Successful treatment of cheilitis granulomatosa with tranilast. Kato T, Tagami H. J Dermatol 1986; 13: 402–3.

Danazol. Madanes AE, Farber M. Ann Intern Med 1982; 96: 625–30.

Hailey–Hailey disease

Susan M Burge, Robin AC Graham-Brown

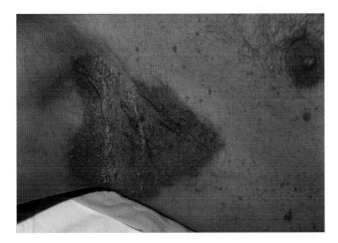

Hailey–Hailey disease is a rare blistering disorder first described by two medical brothers in 1939 and characterized by recurrent vesicles and erosions, particularly involving flexural areas. Signs may appear for the first time from the late teens to the third or fourth decades. The disease is generally of relatively limited extent, although widespread and severe involvement can occur. The most commonly affected sites are the axillae, groins, intertriginous areas such as the inframammary folds, and the neck. Lesions may also occur on the trunk and in the antecubital and popliteal fossae. A seborrheic dermatitis-like involvement of the scalp has also been described.

Hailey–Hailey disease is a dominantly inherited condition caused by a primary defect in a Ca^{2+} pump mechanism. There are clinical and histopathologic similarities with Darier's disease and Grover's disease (see relevant chapters).

MANAGEMENT STRATEGY

The lesions of Hailey–Hailey disease are frequently precipitated by friction. Infection with various bacteria, yeasts, and viruses also appears to be an aggravating factor in some patients. Thus, avoidance of precipitating trauma and skin infections can help to reduce the frequency and severity of outbreaks.

Simple anti-infective agents, topical or systemic, reduce the severity of exacerbations and remain the mainstay of treatment. Topical *tetracyclines*, *fusidic acid*, and *imidazoles* have all been recommended. *Tetracyclines* are probably the best systemic agents. If secondary infection with herpes simplex is suspected, *appropriate antiviral therapy* should be instituted.

Combining anti-infective therapy with *topical corticosteroids* seems to be particularly helpful, but corticosteroids alone may reduce the severity of lesions. Generally, moderate to potent agents are required, though some patients gain benefit from milder preparations. Caution should be exercised with long-term use because the axillae and groins are prone to atrophy. The use of the topical calcineurin inhibitor *tacrolimus*, either alone or in combination with topical

corticosteroids, has recently been reported to be effective and is certainly worth trying. Some success has also been recorded with *calcitriol*.

Patients with Hailey–Hailey disease are at high risk of developing contact allergic dermatitis, and patch testing should be performed if there is a poor response to therapy.

At one time, *superficial (Grenz) rays* were in vogue, but access is now difficult.

Patients with major exacerbations may benefit from a *short course of systemic corticosteroids*, but control seldom lasts, and there may be a rebound of the disease on withdrawal.

Systemic alternatives that have been tried in severe disease include *dapsone*, *ciclosporin*, *methotrexate*, and *retinoids*, but there is little evidence for their effectiveness beyond anecdotal case reports.

There may be a place for surgical approaches to disease of limited extent, including *excision and grafting*, *dermabrasion*, CO_2 *laser vaporization*, and the use of *botulinum toxin* to reduce sweating.

SPECIFIC INVESTIGATIONS

> ▶ Biopsy
> ▶ Microbiologic cultures for bacteria, yeast, and herpes virus
> ▶ Consider patch testing to topical medicaments

FIRST-LINE THERAPIES

▶ Anti-infectives and antibiotics	C
▶ Topical corticosteroids	C

Hailey–Hailey disease: the clinical features, response to treatment and prognosis. Burge SM. Br J Dermatol 1992; 126: 275–82.

In this series 86% of patients found combinations of topical corticosteroids and anti-infective agents helpful, especially if they were started as soon as the patient noticed the onset of discomfort.

This helpful article remains a key review of clinical and therapeutic aspects of Hailey–Hailey disease.

SECOND-LINE THERAPIES

▶ Tacrolimus	E
▶ Calcitriol	E
▶ Systemic corticosteroids	E
▶ Dapsone	E
▶ Ciclosporin	E

Topical tacrolimus ointment is an effective therapy for Hailey–Hailey disease. Sand C, Thomsen HK. Arch Dermatol 2003; 139: 1401–2.

Treatment of Hailey–Hailey disease with tacrolimus ointment and clobetasol propionate foam. Umar SA, Bhattacharjee P, Brodell RT. J Drugs Dermatol 2004; 3: 200–3.

The authors recommend alternating clobetasol and tacrolimus.

Treatment of Hailey–Hailey disease with topical calcitriol. Bianchi L, Chimenti M, Giunta A. J Am Acad Dermatol 2004; 51: 475–6.

Generalized Hailey–Hailey disease. Marsch WC, Stüttgen G. Br J Dermatol 1978; 99: 553.

The use of systemic corticosteroids was successful in controlling particularly extensive Hailey–Hailey disease, but cessation of therapy resulted in significant rebound of the disease.

Benign familial chronic pemphigus treated with dapsone. Sire DJ, Johnson BL. Arch Dermatol 1971; 103: 262.

Topical cyclosporine in chronic benign familial pemphigus (Hailey–Hailey disease). Jitsukawa K, Ring J, Weyer U, Kimmig W, Radloff H. J Am Acad Dermatol 1992; 27: 625–6.

Benign familial pemphigus responsive to cyclosporin, a possible role for cellular immunity in pathogenesis. Ormerod AD, Duncan J, Stankler L. Br J Dermatol 1991; 124: 299–300.

Benign familial chronic pemphigus (Hailey–Hailey disease) responds to cyclosporin. Berth-Jones J, Smith SG, Graham-Brown RA. Clin Exp Dermatol 1995; 20: 70–2.

These papers report small numbers or individual case reports of apparent success. Tacrolimus and calcitriol are at least safe. Dapsone is generally safe and may be worth a try. Ciclosporin has a long, daunting list of side effects, but can be used safely if doses do not exceed 5 mg/kg and patients are properly monitored.

THIRD-LINE THERAPIES

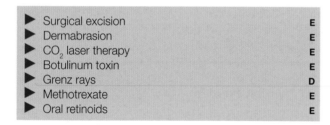

▶ Surgical excision	E
▶ Dermabrasion	E
▶ CO_2 laser therapy	E
▶ Botulinum toxin	E
▶ Grenz rays	D
▶ Methotrexate	E
▶ Oral retinoids	E

Surgical eradication of familial benign chronic pemphigus from the axillae. Shelley WB, Randall P. Arch Dermatol 1969; 100: 275.

Dermabrasion of Hailey–Hailey disease. Zachariae H. J Am Acad Dermatol 1992; 27: 136.

Familial benign chronic pemphigus (Hailey–Hailey disease): treatment with carbon dioxide laser vaporization. Kartamaa M, Reitamo S. Arch Dermatol 1992; 128: 646.

Surgery must remain a last resort in this condition, especially as the authors themselves report some recurrences, either around the edges of the treated areas or on further friction or trauma.

Intracutaneous botulinum toxin A versus ablative therapy of Hailey–Hailey disease – a case report. Konrad H, Karamfilov T, Wollina U. J Cosmet Laser Ther 2001; 3: 181–4.

A single report using intracutaneous botulinum toxin A in a standard fashion as used to treat hyperhidrosis. Remission occurred.

Botulinum toxin type A for the treatment of axillary Hailey–Hailey disease. Lapiere JC, Hirsh A, Gordon KB, Cook B, Montalvo A. Dermatol Surg 2000; 26: 371–4.

After one treatment with a low dose of botulinum toxin type A, partial improvement of the treated axilla was observed. With subsequent treatment of both axillae with the recommended dose for axillary hyperhidrosis, a sustained complete remission of the disease in the treated axillae was seen.

Grenz-ray treatment of familial benign chronic pemphigus. Sarkany I. Br J Dermatol 1959; 71: 247.

Methotrexate for intractable benign familial chronic pemphigus. Fairris GM, White JE, Leppard BJ, Goodwin PG. Br J Dermatol 1986; 115: 640.

A single report of a patient with extensive disease resistant to topical corticosteroids and antibiotics, responding to methotrexate at a dose of 15 mg/week.

Vesiculobullous Hailey–Hailey disease: successful treatment with oral retinoids. Hunt MJ, Salisbury EL, Painter DM, Lee S. Australas J Dermatol 1996; 37: 196–8.

A single case of generalized vesiculobullous Hailey–Hailey eruption. His past history revealed classic symptoms of limited Hailey–Hailey disease for 34 years. Various therapeutic modalities, including topical and oral antibiotics, oral prednisone, and dapsone, failed to achieve sustained remission. Treatment with low-dose oral etretinate (25 mg daily) produced marked clinical improvement, with complete suppression of new vesicle formation after 6 weeks.

Evidence Levels: A Double-blind study   **B** Clinical trial ≥ 20 subjects   **C** Clinical trial < 20 subjects   **D** Series ≥ 5 subjects   **E** Anecdotal case reports

Hemangiomas

Jason H Miller, Adelaide A Hebert

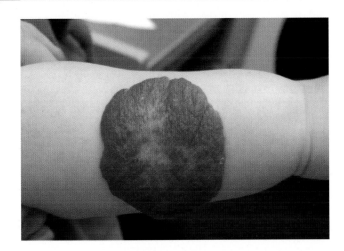

A hemangioma is a benign neoplastic proliferation of endothelial cells and is the most common soft tissue tumor of infancy. The incidence of hemangiomas in a general newborn nursery is between 1% and 2.6%, but may be as high as 10% in the Caucasian population. Hemangiomas occur four times more frequently in female infants, and also demonstrate a predilection for premature infants.

MANAGEMENT STRATEGY

Approximately 55% of hemangiomas present at birth, with the remainder arising in the first weeks of life. Initially, mature cutaneous hemangiomas grow rapidly for the first 3–9 months. After this characteristic proliferative phase, the lesions typically cease growing at 18 months of age, and subsequent spontaneous involution is the rule. Most will involve slowly over a period of 2–6 years, usually completing the process by age 7–10 years. About half of the children with hemangiomas will have normal skin after involution, but the rest may have residual changes, including telangiectasias, atrophy, fibrofatty residuum, and scarring. Therefore, for the majority of uncomplicated hemangiomas, treatment typically consists of *active non-intervention*. This involves a thorough explanation of the pathogenesis and natural history of the hemangioma to the patient and parents, and close follow-up visits.

It is important to differentiate benign, common hemangiomas from other vascular anomalies because the pathophysiology, treatment modalities, and prognoses are significantly different. Vascular malformations and tumors such as the kaposiform hemangioendothelioma (KE) and tufted angioma (TA) differ from hemangioma in both clinical and histological appearance as well as growth rate and involutional tendencies. In particular, KE and TA are associated with the Kasabach–Merritt syndrome and its accompanying coagulopathy, whereas common hemangiomas are not. Recent studies in immunoreactivity have shown that hemangiomas express high endothelial immunoreactivity for GLUT1, a glucose transporter protein present in the brain, retina, and placenta, but absent from vascular malformations. In addition, hemangiomas are highly immunoreactive for FcγRII, merosin, and Lewis Y antigens, markers present in placental chorionic villi but absent from normal skin, granulation tissue, pyogenic granulomas, and vascular malformations. The majority of common hemangiomas occur as solitary lesions, but organ system involvement or, rarely, syndromes such as diffuse neonatal hemangiomatosis and PHACES (posterior fossa malformation, hemangiomas, cardiac anomalies, eye abnormalities, and sternal cleft/supraumbilical raphe) can also occur.

Although the natural course of hemangiomas is self-limited, treatment is probably indicated for approximately 25%, including the 5% that ulcerate and the 20% that may compress, obstruct, or distort vital structures, such as the larynx, eyes, ears, and nose. Local treatment of ulcerative lesions includes gentle cleansing, application of *topical antibiotics*, and occasional *wet-to-dry dressings*. *Occlusive dressings with zinc oxide paste, hydrocolloid gels, or topical antibiotics* may be particularly useful in areas prone to trauma or superinfection, such as the anogenital region.

Medical management of low-risk hemangiomas has traditionally centered on the administration of *corticosteroids, either topically or intralesionally*. Intralesional triamcinolone acetonide, 10–40 mg/mL, in doses of 3–5 mg/kg, may be injected for small lesions (1–2 cm in diameter) on the lip, nasal tip, cheek, or ear, but must be used with caution for periocular hemangiomas. Albeit rare, serious side effects, such as central retinal artery occlusion, have been reported with intralesional injections of periocular lesions. The response rate for intralesional administration may be similar to that for systemic therapy. *Class I topical corticosteroids* may also be used, though there is a paucity of data in the medical literature regarding this modality. One group of investigators used *clobetasol propionate* cream 0.05% to treat periocular hemangiomas. Other less frequently used management options include *cryosurgery, surgical excision* (especially for pedunculated lesions), and *laser therapy*.

Systemic corticosteroids are the mainstay of therapy for larger, deforming, endangering, or life-threatening lesions, and are usually indicated during their growth phase. *Prednisone or prednisolone* can be given at doses from 2 to 4 mg/kg daily from 2–3 months, and then gradually tapered over several months. Stopping treatment before adequate therapeutic response may result in rebound growth. Approximately one-third of patients will show an accelerated rate of involution, but another one-third may have no response to this treatment modality. Therapy should be discontinued if no response is noted within 3–6 weeks. The most important side effect to consider with systemic corticosteroids is immune suppression, and the patient's pediatrician should be aware of this treatment before administering live attenuated viral vaccines. Other reported risks include hypothalamopituitary–adrenal axis suppression, growth delays, pseudotumor cerebri, and avascular bone necrosis. *Surgical excision, laser treatment* (especially flashlamp-pumped pulsed-dye laser), and *cryosurgery*, either alone or in combination with corticosteroids, may also be employed in certain cases.

For endangering or life-threatening lesions refractory to systemic corticosteroids, *interferon-α_{2a}* or *-α_{2b}* may be used. The typical delivery route is subcutaneously at a dose of 3 million units/m^2 daily for 6–12 months. Side effects include transient neutropenia, fever, elevated liver enzymes, and flu-like symptoms. In addition, there are rare reports in the literature of neurotoxicity, specifically spastic diplegia, which may develop in 5–10% of patients. For the exceptional recalcitrant hemangioma, other treatments include *cyclophosphamide, vincristine, bleomycin, propranolol*, and *embolization*. Another promising future treatment is the use of *angiogenesis inhibitors*.

SPECIFIC INVESTIGATIONS

> ▶ Ultrasound with Doppler
> ▶ MRI

The diagnosis of hemangioma is usually made clinically, and the above investigations may only be needed in atypical cases to monitor the progress of treatment, establish the extent of the vascular lesion, or screen for other complications.

Soft-tissue vascular anomalies: utility of US for diagnosis. Paltiel HJ, Burrows PE, Kozakewich HPW, Zurakowski D, Mulliken JB. Radiology 2000; 214: 747–54.

Doppler ultrasonography is an available, low-cost, non-invasive method to confirm the diagnosis of a vascular anomaly, monitor therapeutic response, or preclude the involvement of visceral organs. Hemangiomas can be differentiated from vascular malformations on ultrasonography by distinguishing features such as the presence of a solid tissue mass.

Hemangioma from head to toe: MR imaging with pathologic correlation. Vilanova JC, Barcelo J, Smirniotopoulos JG, Pérez-Andrés R, Villalón M, Miró J, et al. Radiographics 2004; 24: 367–85.

MRI is a useful non-invasive imaging technique to diagnose, characterize, and determine the extent of vascular lesions. On T_2-weighted images hemangiomas have the characteristic appearance of multiple lobules, similar to a bunch of grapes.

Although not specifically mentioned in this article, infants with large, segmental, plaque-like facial hemangiomas should have MRI head evaluation for possible posterior fossa brain abnormalities as a component of the PHACES syndrome.

FIRST-LINE THERAPIES

> ▶ Topical corticosteroids   D
> ▶ Intralesional corticosteroids   B
> ▶ Systemic corticosteroids   B

Systemic corticosteroids are the mainstay of therapy for life-threatening or endangering hemangiomas. In contrast, topical and intralesional administration remains the first-line therapy for relatively uncomplicated cases.

Ultrapotent topical corticosteroid treatment of hemangiomas of infancy. Garzon MC, Lucky AW, Hawrot A, Frieden IJ. J Am Acad Dermatol 2005; 52: 281–6.

Retrospective review of 34 charts of patients with hemangiomas treated with class I topical steroids showed good response in 35%, partial response in 38%, and no response in 27%. Treatment protocols varied between patients.

Topical treatment of periocular capillary hemangioma. Elsas F, Lewis A. J Pediatr Ophthalmol Strabismus 1994; 31: 153–6.

Five patients with sight-threatening periocular hemangiomas were treated with the ultrapotent topical corticosteroid clobetasol propionate 0.05% cream. Therapy was well tolerated, with involution proceeding at a slower rate than with intralesional therapy, but eliminating the risk of central retinal artery occlusion (Shorr N, Seiff SR. Central retinal artery occlusion associated with periocular corticosteroid injection for juvenile hemangioma. Ophthalm Surg 1986; 17: 229–31).

This may be a useful initial treatment for lesions that are not amenable to injection.

Intralesional corticosteroid therapy in proliferating head and neck hemangiomas: a review of 155 cases. Chen MT, Yeong EK, Horng SY. J Pediatr Surg 2000; 35: 420–3.

In this retrospective study, 155 hemangiomas of the head and neck region treated with intralesional corticosteroid injections (three to six injections of triamcinolone acetonide 10 mg/mL at monthly intervals, with an average of four injections per lesion) were analyzed. At the 1-month visit, 85% of hemangiomas showed greater than 50% reduction, with superficial hemangiomas showing the most improvement. Perioral hemangiomas appeared the most recalcitrant to intralesional corticosteroid treatment.

Oral corticosteroid use is effective for cutaneous hemangiomas. Bennett ML, Fleischer AB, Chamlin SL, Frieden IJ. Arch Dermatol 2001; 137: 1208–13.

This meta-analysis of 10 case series with 184 patients analyzed the efficacy of systemic corticosteroids in the treatment of cutaneous hemangiomas. The mean age of infants at the initiation of therapy was 4.5 months at an average prednisone dose equivalent to 2.9 mg/kg. The mean response rate was 84%, and the mean rate of rebound growth after treatment cessation was 36%. Treatment with higher doses of corticosteroids resulted in a higher response rate but greater adverse effects. The average incidence of side effects was 35% (behavior changes, irritability, cushingoid appearance, and transient growth delay).

SECOND-LINE THERAPIES

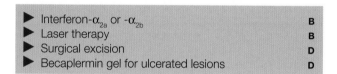

> ▶ Interferon-α_{2a} or -α_{2b} B
> ▶ Laser therapy   B
> ▶ Surgical excision   D
> ▶ Becaplermin gel for ulcerated lesions D

Interferon alfa-2a therapy for life-threatening hemangiomas of infancy. Ezekowitz RA, Mulliken JB, Folkman J. N Engl J Med 1992; 326: 1456–63.

Twenty infants with life-threatening or vision-threatening hemangiomas who failed corticosteroid therapy were treated with up to 3 million units/m² daily of interferon-α_{2a}; 90% experienced a 50% or greater regression in their lesions by 7.8 months of treatment. Side effects were transient, including fever, neutropenia, and skin necrosis. No long-term effects were documented after a mean follow-up period of 16 months.

Treatment with interferon-alpha 2b in children with life-threatening hemangiomas. Jiminez-Hernandez E, Duenas-Gonzalez MT, Quintero-Curiel JL, Velasquez-Ortega J, Magana-Perez JA, Berges-Garcia A, et al. Dermatol Surg 2008; 34: 640–7.

Of 20 patients with deforming or life-threatening hemangiomas who failed earlier treatment with interferon-α_{2b} (3 million IU/m² daily × 5 days/week) for 6 months, 85% demonstrated an excellent response, 5% a moderate response, and 10% a poor response. Toxicity was short-lived, including fever, fatigue, nausea, and hair loss. No transaminase or neurologic symptoms were reported with 7–10 year follow-up.

Although not observed in this study, spastic diplegia is a documented and potentially irreversible complication of this treatment and should be considered prior to initiation of therapy.

Flashlamp-pumped pulsed dye laser for hemangiomas in infancy: treatment of superficial vs. mixed hemangiomas. Poetke M, Philipp C, Berlien HP. Arch Dermatol 2000; 136: 628–32.

A prospective study of 165 children with 225 separate hemangiomas treated with flashlamp-pumped pulsed-dye laser demonstrated that this therapy produced excellent results in superficial hemangiomas. However, this method was less successful in treating deeper lesions because the efficacy of the laser was limited by the depth of the vascular proliferation.

Pulsed-dye laser therapy promotes epithelialization and is also a safe and effective means of treating ulcerated hemangiomas. Adverse effects more recently reported include scarring, ulceration, and pain (Witman PM, Wagner AM, Scherer K, Waner M, Frieden IJ. Complications following pulsed dye laser treatment of superficial hemangiomas. Lasers Surg Med 2006; 38: 112–15).

Surgical treatment of hemangioma in infants. Mcheik JN, Renauld V, Duport G, Vergnes P, Levard G. Br J Plast Surg 2005; 58: 1067–72.

Retrospective study of 31 patients (average age 30 months) showed very good results in 20%, good in 66%, and fair in 14%. Recommendations included consideration of surgery in lesions that had not changed in 2 years or that interfered with the child's social integration.

Response of ulcerated perineal hemangiomas of infancy to becaplermin gel, a recombinant human platelet-derived growth factor. Metz BJ, Rubenstein MC, Levy ML, Metry DW. Arch Dermatol 2004; 140: 867–70.

Eight infants were treated with becaplermin gel 0.01% for ulcerated perineal hemangiomas of infancy. Rapid ulcer healing occurred in all patients within 3–21 days (average, 10.25 days).

The rapid healing achieved with 0.01% becaplermin gel allows a reduction in the risk of secondary infection, pain, and the need for hospitalization, as well as in the costs that often accumulate from multiple follow-up visits and long-term therapy.

THIRD-LINE THERAPIES

▶ Vincristine	E
▶ Embolization	D
▶ Imiquimod	C
▶ Bleomycin	B
▶ Propranolol	C

Vincristine as a treatment for a large haemangioma threatening vital functions. Fawcett SL, Grant I, Hall PN, Kelsall AW, Nicholson JC. Br J Plast Surg 2004; 57: 168–71.

A 21-month-old infant with a large, deep hemangioma in the beard distribution, necessitating multiple hospital admissions for respiratory and feeding difficulties, was treated with vincristine after failing to respond to systemic corticosteroid therapy.

Vincristine ($1.5\,mg/m^2$) was administered in weekly doses for 1 month, with improvement in feeding, speech, and external appearance of the lesion, with no adverse effects.

Although there are literature reports of success achieved with vincristine, the data are anecdotal at best.

Embolization of hepatic hemangiomas in infants. Kullendorff CM, Cwikiel W, Sandstrom S. Eur J Pediatr Surg 2002; 12: 348–52.

Two infants with hepatic cavernous hemangiomas complicated by congestive heart failure were treated successfully by coil and glue embolization. One patient, however, continued to suffer gastrointestinal complications due to growth of the hemangioma into the intestine, and needed partial resection of the hemangioma even after embolization.

Aggressive interventions, such as embolization and resection, are viable options when there are life-threatening symptoms and medical management fails.

Topical imiquimod in the treatment of infantile hemangiomas: A retrospective study. Ho NTC, Lansang P, Pope E. J Am Acad Dermatol 2007; 56: 63–8.

Eighteen children (median age 18 weeks) with imiquimod 5% cream applied three times weekly or five times weekly for a mean of 17 weeks showed improvement in superficial hemangiomas and accelerated ulcer healing; no change was seen in deep hemangiomas. A 31% clearance rate was reported. Adverse events included crusting and inflammation. Mechanism presumably related to cytokine (such as interferon) release.

Subsequent criticisms reported control arms of earlier studies (using only observation) showing similar clearance rates those treated in this study without the use of any intervention.

Role of intralesional bleomycin in the treatment of complicated hemangiomas: prospective clinical study. Omidvari S, Nezakatgoo N, Ahmadloo N, Mohammadianpanah M, Mosalaei A. Dermatol Surg 2005; 31: 499–501.

Thirty-two patients with complicated hemangiomas (median age 45 months) were treated with intralesional bleomycin ($1–2\,mg/cm^2$ of lesion every 2 weeks for 4–6 courses). Following the initial swelling and erythema, 56% of patients had 70–100% regression; 21.9% had 50–70% regression. No severe adverse effects were reported.

Propranolol for severe hemangiomas of infancy. Leaute-Labreze C, Dumas de la Roque E, Hubiche T, Boralevi F, Thambo JB, Taieb A. N Engl J Med 2008; 358: 2649–51.

Preliminary data from 11 children treated with propranolol $2\,mg/kg/day$ showed rapid color change (intense red to purple) and softening within 24 hours. Continued treatment resulted in near flattening of lesions, with residual telangiectasia and regression in thickness on ultrasound. Proposed mechanisms include vasoconstriction, decrease in VEGF and bFGF, and endothelial apoptosis.

Hereditary angioedema

Malcolm W Greaves

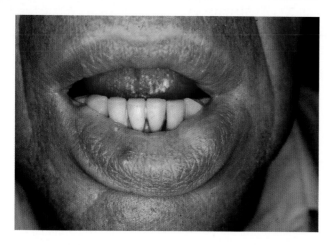

Classic hereditary angioedema (HAE) is an autosomal dominantly inherited disease with a prevalence of 1:50 000 due to mutations in the C1-esterase inhibitor (C1-INH) gene on chromosome 11 (11q12-q13.1), though de novo mutations are frequent. It is manifested by painless, non-pruritic swellings of subcutaneous and submucosal tissues, including abdominal organs and the upper airway, and is characterized by a quantitative (type 1, 85%) or functional (type 2, 15%) defect of the inhibitor of the first component of complement (C1-INH). Estrogen-dependent hereditary angioedema (type 3) has recently been reported in women with no detectable abnormality of complement components. A mutation in the gene encoding for factor 12 has been identified in some of these families. Acute abdominal pain, simulating an 'acute abdomen' is an important presentation and fatalities are possible in these hereditary angioedemas.

MANAGEMENT STRATEGY

Therapy for HAE is dependent on three considerations:
- Relief of acute angioedema, especially preservation of the airway
- Long-term prophylaxis
- Prevention of relapse due to dental and surgical interventions.

Acute angioedema

Acute presentations of HAE are treated optimally with intravenous vapor-sterilized *C1-INH concentrate*. This treatment is safe, and no proven cases of viral transmission have been reported since this sterilization process was adopted. Reduction in swelling is usually significant within minutes, and substantial within 2–3 hours. *Fresh frozen plasma (FFP)*, which contains C1-INH, can be used if concentrate is unavailable; however, FFP carries a higher risk of inadvertent viral transmission (HIV, hepatitis) and theoretically could exacerbate angioedema owing to the presence of C1 esterase substrate. Although *subcutaneous epinephrine (adrenaline)* (0.3 mg every 3 min) may be helpful due to its vasoconstrictor properties, parenterally administered corticosteroids and antihistamines are not effective for HAE. Laryngeal edema may require *tracheostomy, intubation*, and/or other life-support measures. Patients should be admitted routinely for 24 hours after acute episodes, as relapses, which may be life-threatening, are common.

Long-term prophylaxis

Generally, long-term prophylaxis is appropriate in those patients with at least one or more attacks of angioedema per month, and in those with severe symptoms. However, patients could have infrequent attacks and still present with laryngeal edema. Even first-episode angioedema can be fatal. The 17α-alkylated androgens *danazol* and *stanozolol* are first-line prophylactic medications that are extremely efficacious in preventing angioedema in types 1 and 2 HAE. The lowest possible dose of androgen should be used to obtain clinical remission, regardless of C1-INH or C4 levels. Side effects include hirsuties, deepening of voice, and menorrhagia. These attenuated androgens are unsuitable for long-term treatment of hereditary angioedema in children, in pregnant women, and for the treatment of acute attacks. However, they are safe and effective in adults, provided they are closely supervised with clinical biochemical and radiological assessments. In some patients alternate-day therapy can be achieved. Hepatocellular adenoma and hepatocellular carcinoma have been reported in patients on long-term danazol. Other prophylactic therapies include *antifibrinolytics (e.g., tranexamic acid, ε-aminocaproic acid – EACA)*, but these are of less certain value. In patients with mild infrequent attacks *avoidance of provoking factors*, including estrogens and angiotensin-converting enzyme (ACE) inhibitors, may be sufficient. For long-term management in selected cases, patients' carers can be trained to administer C1 inhibitor concentrate for occasional acute attacks if no medical facilities are at hand, thereby obviating the necessity for regular prophylaxis.

Prevention of relapse due to dental and surgical interventions

In all patients, prior to elective surgical, dental, or other invasive procedures, *higher-dose androgens can be used for 5–10 days*. If an emergency procedure is necessary, C1-INH concentrate or FFP can be administered.

Patients with HAE should all wear a *MedicAlert disc* stating the diagnosis and emergency treatment.

SPECIFIC INVESTIGATIONS

- ▶ Complement levels (C4, C2, C1q)
- ▶ C1-INH immunoreactive level
- ▶ Functional assay for C1-INH

Angioedema. (CME article) Kaplan AP, Greaves MW. J Am Acad Dermatol 2005; 53: 373–88.

Type I HAE is characterized by low antigenic and functional plasma levels of normal C1-INH. Type II HAE is characterized by normal or elevated antigenic levels of a dysfunctional mutant C1-INH together with functional C1-INH. In those patients with a low C4 but normal C1-INH levels a functional assay should be obtained to identify type II disease. A depressed C1q level in addition to low C4 and C1-INH levels is characteristic of acquired C1-INH-deficient angioedema (AAE).

Evidence Levels: A Double-blind study   B Clinical trial ≥ 20 subjects   C Clinical trial < 20 subjects   D Series ≥ 5 subjects   E Anecdotal case reports

Causes include B-cell lymphoma, cryoglobulinemia, and the presence of autoantibodies against C1-INH itself.

Hereditary and acquired C1 inhibitor deficiency: biological and clinical characteristics in 235 patients. Agostini A, Cicardi M. Medicine 1992; 71: 206–15.

C4 level is the best screening test. A reduced value is typical between attacks, and during an attack the value is almost undetectable. Rarely, the C4 level may fall within the normal range in between attacks. Therefore, if the clinical picture is highly suggestive of hereditary angioedema, the functional and quantitative C1 inhibitor levels should be determined even if the C4 level is unremarkable.

A multicentre evaluation of the diagnostic efficiency of serological investigations for C1 inhibitor deficiency. Gompels MM, Lock RJ, Morgan JE, Osborne J, Brown A, Virgo PF. J Clin Pathol 2002; 55: 145–7.

All patients with suspected C1-INH deficiency should have serum C4 measured. If C4 is normal, it is unnecessary to proceed to C1-INH analysis unless the clinical picture is highly suggestive of hereditary angioedema. If C4 is low, then C1-INH function should be analyzed. A combination of low C4 and low C1-INH function has a 98% specificity and 96% predictive value for C1-INH deficiency and is a very effective screening procedure.

ACUTE ANGIOEDEMA

FIRST-LINE THERAPIES

► C1-INH concentrate	A

Treatment of 193 episodes of laryngeal edema with C1 inhibitor concentrate in patients with hereditary angioedema. Bork K, Barnstedt S-E. Arch Intern Med 2001; 161: 714–18.

A series of 193 episodes of laryngeal edema treated with 500–1000 units (500 units initially, then repeated in 30–60 minutes if necessary) of concentrate were compared to cases that did not receive concentrate. The relief of symptoms occurred, on average, at 42 minutes after injection.

Treatment of hereditary angioedema with a vapor-heated C1 inhibitor concentrate. Waytes AT, Rosen FS, Frank MM. N Engl J Med 1996; 334: 1630–4.

Two randomized, placebo-controlled, double-blind studies evaluated the safety and efficacy of vapor-heated infusions of C1-INH concentrate in acute attacks (22 patients) and as prophylaxis (six patients). In the prophylaxis arm, concentrate was administered every third day; in the treatment arm, concentrate was begun within 5 hours of symptoms. A dose of 25 units/kg was used in both groups. Compared to placebo, significantly lower daily symptom scores were found in the prophylaxis group, and a shorter duration of symptoms was found in the treatment group (55 vs 563 minutes). No toxicity was demonstrated, and after 4 years of observation there was no evidence of seroconversion to HIV or hepatitis B or C.

Hereditary angioedema: a decade of human C1-inhibitor concentrate therapy. Farkas H, Jakab L, Temesszentandrási G, Visy B, Harmat G, Füst G, et al. J Allergy Clin Immunol 2007; 120: 941–7.

This review of 468 attacks of acute hereditary angioedema in 61 patients, including children and pregnant women, all treated with human C1-inhibitor concentrate, emphasizes the safety and efficacy of this treatment. No viral infection, antibody formation, or other adverse events were reported even after repeated administration.

C1-esterase inhibitor transfusions in patients with hereditary angioedema. Visnetin DE, Yang WH, Karsh J. Ann Allergy Asthma Immunol 1998; 80: 457–61.

C1-INH concentrate was very effective in abating attacks of HAE in seven of 13 patients. The mean duration of an attack in treated patients was 50 ± 8 minutes, compared to 1–4 days in the untreated group.

C1-INH concentrate has also been effective as short-term prophylaxis in labor induction, tonsillectomy, and maxillofacial surgery. Long-term prophylaxis has not generally been advocated owing to lack of availability, cost, and the potential for infectious transmission. However, this may be considered in children, pregnant women, and patients who do not respond to or tolerate androgens or antifibrinolytics, or if these drugs are contraindicated.

C1-INH can be obtained in Europe from Berinert HS, Aventis Behring, Liederbach, Germany. CSL Behring, King of Prussia, PA 19406, USA is also developing this product, which is currently not available in the USA.

SECOND-LINE THERAPIES

► Fresh frozen plasma	D
► Icatibant	A

Replacement therapy in hereditary angioedema: successful treatment of two patients with fresh frozen plasma. Pickering RJ, Kelley JR, Good RA, Gewurz H. Lancet 1969; 1: 326–30.

The safety of fresh frozen plasma for the treatment of hereditary angioedema. Prematta M, Thomas D, Scarupa M, Li C, Mende C, Rhoads C. J Allergy Clin Immunol 2008; 121: S99.

Fresh frozen plasma was found to be effective in 76 of 82 acute attacks of hereditary angioedema, and no patients developed significant adverse reactions.

FFP is effective and can be used if C1-INH concentrate is unavailable. It is not virally inactivated and, being larger in volume, requires a longer infusion time. Apart from the risk of virus infection, using FFP carries the **theoretical** *potential for exacerbation of attacks owing to its content of complement substrates.*

Treatment of acute edema attacks in hereditary angioedema with a bradykinin receptor-2 antagonist (Icatibant). Bork K, Frank J, Grundt B, Schlattmann P, Nussberger J, Kreuz W. J Allergy Clin Immunol 2007; 119: 1497–503.

Fifteen patients with 20 attacks were treated with icatibant, with significant improvement relative to previous episodes as assessed using visual analog scales. Symptom intensity decreased within 4 hours after administration.

European public assessment report (EPAR). EMEA/H/C/899. Firazyr. http://www.emea.europa.eu/humandocs/PDFs/EPAR/firazyr/H-899-en1.pdf.

In clinical trials Firazyr (icatibant) was more effective than tranexamic acid and placebo in controlling the symptoms of the disease. In both studies, the time it took for the patient's symptoms to improve was shorter for patients taking Firazyr than for those taking tranexamic acid or placebo. Patients experienced relief an average of 2–2.5 hours after receiving Firazyr, compared to 12.0 hours after receiving tranexamic acid and 4.6 hours after receiving placebo.

Icatibant, a synthetic decapeptide, is a bradykinin B2 receptor antagonist recently licensed in the European Union for treatment of acute episodes of hereditary angioedema. The recommended dose is one subcutaneous injection of 30 mg, preferably in the abdominal area. Mild reactions at the injection site are common.

LONG-TERM PROPHYLAXIS OF HEREDITARY ANGIOEDEMA

FIRST-LINE THERAPIES

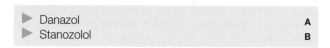

| ▶ Danazol | A |
| ▶ Stanozolol | B |

How do we treat patients with hereditary angioedema? Cicardi M, Zingale L. Transfus Apheresis Sci 2003; 29: 221–7.

In a study of 141 patients, danazol and stanozolol proved equally effective; <10% of patients failed to obtain significant remission. Normalization of C1-INH is not required. These authors start with a run-in period of 400–600 mg daily of danazol for 1 month, slowly tapering to 100–200 mg daily to determine the minimum dose that will cause remission (C1-INH level around 50% of normal; C4 within normal range; complete remission of angioedema).

Treatment of hereditary angioedema with danazol. Gelfand JA, Sherins RJ, Alling DW, Frank MM. N Engl J Med 1976; 295: 1444–8.

A randomized, placebo-controlled, double-blind trial demonstrated the effectiveness of danazol 200 mg three times daily as prophylaxis. Nine patients participated in 93 courses of therapy. The patients were crossed over after 28 days of therapy, unless an attack occurred sooner.

Long-term treatment of hereditary angioedema with attenuated androgens: a survey of a 13-year experience. Cicardi M, Bergamaschini L, Cugno M, Hack E, Agostoni G, Agostoni A. J Allergy Clin Immunol 1991; 87: 768–73.

The authors report their experience with attenuated androgens used for long-term prophylaxis. In 54 of 56 patients resolution of symptoms was achieved. The lowest effective daily dose usually did not exceed 2 mg for stanozolol and 200 mg for danazol. Twenty-four patients were observed for more than 5 years. Hepatic cell necrosis occurred in one patient treated with stanozolol 4 mg daily for 1 year.

Hereditary angioedema: safety of long-term stanozolol therapy. Sloane DE, Lee CW, Sheffer AL. J Allergy Clin Immunol 2007; 120: 654–8.

Stanozolol can safely be used in the long-term treatment of patients with hereditary angioedema, provided regular clinical biochemical and radiological assessments are carried out.

Side effects of long-term prophylaxis with attenuated androgens in hereditary angioedema: comparison of treated and untreated patients. Cicardi M, Castelli R, Zingale LC, Agostoni A. J Allergy Clin Immunol 1997; 99: 194–6.

Thirty-six patients with HAE were treated with attenuated androgens for a median of 125.5 months and compared to 34 patients with HAE who never received prophylaxis. The main side effects were menstrual irregularities (15 of 36) and weight gain (14 of 36). A statistically significant increase in arterial hypertension occurred in 25% of treated patients. No significant changes in hepatic enzymes and ultrasounds were found. Stanozolol seemed to have fewer side effects than danazol.

Side effects in female patients may be troublesome, including menstrual disturbance, deepening of the voice, and hirsuties. In males, prostate changes should be monitored. All patients should have regular liver function tests. Attenuated androgens are contraindicated in pregnancy.

SECOND-LINE THERAPIES

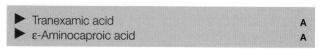

| ▶ Tranexamic acid | A |
| ▶ ε-Aminocaproic acid | A |

Hereditary and acquired C1-inhibitor deficiency: biological and clinical characteristics in 235 patients. Agostoni A, Cicardi M. Medicine (Baltimore) 1992; 71: 206–15.

Twelve of 15 patients had initially effective prophylaxis with tranexamic acid, but this agent was only effective long term in 28%, whereas danazol was effective long term in 97%.

Tranexamic acid therapy in hereditary angioneurotic edema. Sheffer AL, Austen KF, Rosen FS. N Engl J Med 1972; 287: 452–4.

A randomized, placebo-controlled, double-blind crossover trial over a 4–13-month period. Seven of 12 patients receiving tranexamic acid 1 g three times daily achieved a complete or near-complete cessation of attacks. Four additional patients experienced a moderate response.

Tranexamic acid is more potent than EACA and has been reported to cause fewer side effects.

Epsilon aminocaproic acid therapy of hereditary angioneurotic edema: a double blind study. Frank MM, Sergent JS, Kane MA, Alling DW. N Engl J Med 1972; 286: 808–12.

EACA (16 g daily) in a double-blind crossover trial prevented attacks of angioedema in four of five patients over a 2-year period. Common side effects consisted of weakness and increased fatiguability. A follow-up open trial led to control of symptoms on 7–10 g of EACA daily.

Higher-dose therapy (24–30 g) has led to elevation of creatine phosphokinase and aldolase levels and muscle necrosis.

Long-term treatment of C1 inhibitor deficiency with ε-aminocaproic acid in two patients. Van Dellen RG. Mayo Clin Proc 1996; 71: 1175–8.

Two patients were successfully treated with EACA (8–10 g daily) over a period of 12–23 years. No adverse effects were found.

EACA therapy can also be used as short-term prophylaxis for minor procedures, but because of its potential thrombotic effects it should be discontinued before major surgery.

THIRD-LINE THERAPIES

| ▶ C1-INH concentrate | C |

Long-term prophylaxis with C1 inhibitor (C1 INH) concentrate in patients with recurrent angioedema caused by hereditary and acquired C1 INH deficiency. Bork K, Witzke GL. J Allergy Clin Immunol 1989; 83: 677–82.

A report on the use of C1-INH concentrate 500 units once or twice weekly for 1 year or more.

Pharmacokinetics of pasteurised C1 inhibitor concentrate (Berinert P) in 40 patients with hereditary angioedema. Martinez-Saguer I, Rusicke E, Ayorger-Pursun E, Kreuz W. J Allergy Clin Immunol 2006; 117: S124.

C1-INH concentrate can be used for long-term prophylaxis of HAE.

Prevention of relapse due to dental and surgical interventions

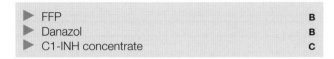

▶	FFP	B
▶	Danazol	B
▶	C1-INH concentrate	C

Hereditary angioedema: the use of fresh frozen plasma for prophylaxis in patients undergoing oral surgery. Jaffe CJ, Atkinson JP, Gelfand JA, Frank MM. J Allergy Clin Immunol 1975; 55: 386–93.

FFP (2 units) was found to be effective in six patients undergoing seven episodes of dental surgery. Two units of FFP were given 1 day prior to the surgery.

Others have effectively used danazol (600 mg daily) or stanozolol (6–8 mg daily) from 5–10 days preoperatively to 3 days postoperatively.

The efficacy of short-term danazol prophylaxis in hereditary angioedema patients undergoing maxillofacial and dental procedures. Farkas H, Gyeney L, Gidofalvy E, Füst G, Varga L. J Oral Maxillofac Surg 1999; 57: 404–8.

Twelve patients with a history of angioedema after dental procedures received danazol 600 mg daily for 4 days preoperatively and 4 days postoperatively for dental or maxillofacial procedures. None experienced angioedema.

Other preoperative options include 500–1000 units of C1-INH concentrate or antifibrinolytic agents.

Hereditary angioedema: uncomplicated faciomaxillary surgery using short term C1 inhibitor replacement therapy. Leimgruber A, Jacques WA, Spaeth PJ. Int Arch Allergy Immunol 1993; 101: 107–12.

Tranexamic acid: preoperative prophylactic therapy for patients with hereditary angioneurotic edema. Sheffer AL, Fearon DT, Austen KF, Rosen FS. J Allergy Clin Immunol 1977; 60: 38–40.

Critical role of kallikrein in hereditary angioedema pathogenesis: a clinical trial of ecallantide, a novel kallikrein inhibitor. Schneider L, Lumry W, Vegh A, Williams AH, Schmalbach T. J Allergy Clin Immunol 2007; 120: 416–22.

Bradykinin is recognized to be the principal mediator of edema in hereditary angioedema. Accordingly, icatibant, a bradykinin antagonist, and ecallantide, an inhibitor of the bradykinin-forming enzyme kallikrein, are currently undergoing phase 3 clinical trials in hereditary angioedema and the preliminary results are very encouraging.

Hereditary angioedema: treatment in children

Clinical management of hereditary angio-edema in children. Farkas H, Harmat G, Fust G, Varga L, Visy B. Pediatr Allergy Immunol 2002; 13: 153–61.

Based on data from 26 patients, these authors advise the use of C1-INH concentrate for emergency treatment of acute attacks. Tranexamic acid can be used for short- or long-term prophylaxis, provided liver function is regularly monitored. Attenuated androgens should be avoided in children and pregnant women.

Treatment of hereditary angioedema type 3

Hereditary angioedema type 3, angioedema associated with angiotensin II receptor antagonists and female sex. Bork K. Am J Med 2004; 116: 644.

The author describes two unrelated female patients who had normal C1-INH and C4 levels and who experienced severe exacerbations of hereditary angioedema following the administration of losartan and valsartan, respectively.

Acute attacks do not respond to C1-INH concentrate, and antihistamines or corticosteroids are ineffective. The value of antifibrinolytics is unproven. For prevention danazol is worth trying in non-pregnant patients, but substantiation of its value is awaited. All patients should avoid angiotensin-2-receptor antagonists (sartans) and estrogens because these are known to provoke attacks in affected women. Bradykinin antagonists such as icatibant or kallikrein inhibitors such as ecallantide, currently under development and referred to above, may possibly offer some future benefit to these patients.

Hereditary hemorrhagic telangiectasia

Mitchell S Cappell, Oscar Lebwohl

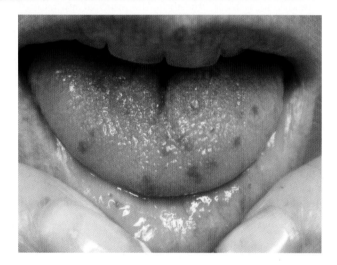

Hereditary hemorrhagic telangiectasia (HHT, or Osler–Weber–Rendu syndrome), an autosomal dominant disease, produces a syndrome of multiple orocutaneous telangiectasias, especially on the face, lips, tongue, oral mucosa, and hands, together with multiple internal telangiectasias, especially in the nose and gastrointestinal tract. Cutaneous lesions typically are 3–10 mm wide, macular, bright red, non-pulsatile, and spidery or punctate in shape with a fine reticular internal structure. They tend to blanch under pressure (with diascopy), and to slowly increase in size and number with age. Although the dermatologic lesions are usually only a minor cosmetic problem, the nasal and gastrointestinal lesions frequently bleed significantly and repeatedly. Chronic blood loss may result in iron deficiency anemia, and acute blood loss may cause hypovolemia and systemic hypotension.

The basic lesion in HHT is believed to be a defect in the wall of small vessels that leads to direct arteriovenous communications without intervening capillaries. The most common underlying genetic mutations are in the gene encoding endoglin (ENG) that causes HHT1, or in the gene encoding activin receptor-like kinase 1 (ALK-1) that causes HHT2. Underlying genetic mutations occasionally are located in the MADH4 gene that causes HHT associated with juvenile polyposis, or on chromosome 5 that causes HHT3. Shunts created by the direct arteriovenous communications in HHT can infrequently cause clinical manifestations, including hypoxia from pulmonary arteriovenous shunts; cerebral ischemia or abscesses from systemic shunts; and portal hypertension, biliary tract disease, or high-output cardiac failure from intrahepatic shunts.

MANAGEMENT STRATEGY

HHT is reliably diagnosed by the presence of three or more findings among the following clinical tetrad: recurrent, spontaneous epistaxis; mucocutaneous telangiectasias; gastrointestinal telangiectasias or visceral arteriovenous malformations; and a compatible family history (Curaçao criteria). Patients may have telangiectasias solely on the face with rosacea, or with lupus erythematosus, but lack the other manifestations of HHT. Patients with sporadic gastrointestinal angiodysplasia are differentiated from patients with HHT by clinical presentation in old age, a paucity of the characteristic lesions, a negative family history, and by exclusively gastrointestinal involvement without epistaxis.

For epistaxis, the bleeding severity is determined by inspection, vital signs, and laboratory tests. The bleeding site is precisely localized by nasal examination using bright, shadow-free illumination, with a headlight or head mirror, and spot suction, using a fine-caliber rigid tube. For gastrointestinal bleeding, the bleeding severity is indicated by patient history, vital signs, physical findings, rectal examination, nasogastric aspiration, and transfusion requirements. The bleeding site and source are conclusively diagnosed by gastrointestinal endoscopy.

Choice of therapy depends on the bleeding site, severity, and chronicity as well as individual physician expertise. Significant acute blood loss is treated with intravenous fluid resuscitation and transfusion of packed erythrocytes as needed. Chronic blood loss is treated with iron supplementation as needed. Epistaxis is initially treated by nonspecific local therapy such as nasal packing to tamponade the bleeding, and topical vasoconstrictors to reduce local blood flow. Estrogen with progesterone is used to prevent or arrest chronic epistaxis by promoting vascular integrity. Significant, refractory, chronic epistaxis is definitively treated by septal dermoplasty. Actively bleeding gastrointestinal telangiectasias are treated at endoscopy by argon plasma coagulation, thermocoagulation, electrocoagulation, or photocoagulation. Chronically bleeding gastrointestinal telangiectasias may be treated with estrogen and progesterone. Surgical resection is reserved for well localized, active bleeding from gastrointestinal telangiectasias refractory to other therapy, because patients tend to subsequently rebleed from telangiectasias at other sites. Where available, angiographic embolization can obviate the need for gastrointestinal surgery.

SPECIFIC INVESTIGATIONS

> ▶ Serial hematocrit determinations
> ▶ Serum iron, total iron binding capacity, and ferritin levels
> ▶ Esophagogastroduodenoscopy
> ▶ Colonoscopy
> ▶ Capsule endoscopy or double balloon-enteroscopy
> ▶ Angiography

Serial hematocrit determinations are important, particularly for acute bleeding, to determine the need for transfusions of packed erythrocytes. Serum levels of iron, total iron-binding capacity (TIBC), and ferritin are important, particularly for chronic bleeding, to determine the need for iron replacement therapy. Upper gastrointestinal bleeding, usually manifested by hematemesis or melena, should be investigated by esophagogastroduodenoscopy. Lower gastrointestinal bleeding, usually manifested by hematochezia or fecal occult blood, and occasionally manifested by melena, should be investigated by colonoscopy. Barium contrast radiography or virtual colonoscopy should not be performed to evaluate lower gastrointestinal bleeding in patients with HHT because the telangiectasias are mucosal and macular, and not visualized with barium contrast. Small intestinal bleeding, usually manifested by hematochezia, melena, or fecal occult blood, can be investigated by capsule endoscopy after the exclusion of upper and lower gastrointestinal bleeding by the aforementioned endoscopic tests. Double-balloon enteroscopy is being increasingly used instead of capsule endoscopy for small intestinal bleeding because of its greater diagnostic sensitivity and therapeutic capabilities despite greater costs.

At endoscopy, telangiectasias appear as intensely red maculae due to the high oxygen content in erythrocytes within vessels supplied by arteries without intervening capillaries. Telangiectasias are distinguished from lesions due to endoscopic trauma by identification during endoscopic intubation, as opposed to identification during endoscopic extubation with trauma, by a finely reticular (fern-like) internal structure due to a vascular tuft, by an irregular (fern-like) border as opposed to a round border with trauma, by an abrupt lesion margin as opposed to an indistinct margin with trauma, and by lesions lying flush (coplanar) with mucosa. Additionally, colonic lesions from endoscopic trauma usually occur at sharp colonic turns, during endoscopic looping, or after endoscopic suctioning.

Angiography is indicated for active gastrointestinal bleeding when colonoscopy and esophagogastroduodenoscopy have failed to diagnose the source of bleeding. The angiographic hallmarks of telangiectasias are a vascular tuft or tangle resulting from the local mass of irregular vessels, an early and intensely filling vein resulting from a direct arteriovenous connection without intervening capillaries, and persistent opacification beyond the normal venous phase (slowly emptying vein), attributed to vascular tortuosity. Telangiectasias bleed only intermittently, and extravasation of contrast material from telangiectasias is infrequently detected at angiography.

Clinical spectrum of hereditary hemorrhagic telangiectasia (Osler–Weber–Rendu disease). Peery WH. Am J Med 1987; 82: 989–997.

A review of the clinical manifestations and management of HHT.

Evidence of small-bowel involvement in hereditary hemorrhagic telangiectasia: a capsule-endoscopic study. Ingrosso M, Sabba C, Pisani A, Principi M, Gallitelli M, Cirulli A, et al. Endoscopy 2004; 36: 1074–9.

Recent study demonstrating a high frequency of small bowel telangiectasias in elderly patients with HHT as detected by capsule endoscopy. Chronic blood loss from these intestinal lesions may contribute to iron deficiency anemia from HHT.

Evaluation of patients with hereditary hemorrhagic telangiectasia with video capsule endoscopy: a single-center prospective study. Chamberlain SM, Patel J, Carter Balart J, Gossage JR Jr, Sridhar S. Endoscopy 2007; 39: 516–20.

A prospective study of 80 patients evaluated by capsule endoscopy for small intestinal bleeding. The 32 patients with known HHT had significantly more gastrointestinal telangiectasias than 48 control patients without HHT (75% versus 8.3% of patients had five or more telangiectasias). This study demonstrates the high sensitivity of capsule endoscopy in diagnosing small intestinal telangiectasias in patients who have HHT.

Liver disease in patients with hereditary hemorrhagic telangiectasia. Garcia-Tsao G, Korzenik JR, Young L, Henderson KJ, Jain D, Byrd B, et al. N Engl J Med 2000; 343: 931–6.

A review of the clinical findings in eight patients with high-output cardiac failure, six patients with portal hypertension, and five patients with biliary tract disease caused by intrahepatic shunts with HHT.

FIRST-LINE THERAPIES

For epistaxis

▶ Nonspecific therapy: room humidification and nasal moisteners   **A**
▶ Nasal packing   **A**
▶ Septal dermoplasty   **A**

For gastrointestinal bleeding

▶ Nonspecific therapy: avoid aspirin, non-steroidal anti-inflammatory drugs (NSAIDs), and anticoagulation; administer iron therapy for significant iron deficiency anemia   **A**
▶ Endoscopic argon plasma coagulation, thermocoagulation, electrocoagulation, or photocoagulation   **B**
▶ Angiographic embolization   **B**
▶ Segmental bowel resection   **A**

For epistaxis or gastrointestinal bleeding

▶ Oral estrogen with progesterone   **B**

Septal dermoplasty: ten years experience. Saunders WH. Trans Am Acad Ophthalmol Otol 1968; 72: 153–60.

Classic report describing a marked reduction in the frequency and severity of epistaxis in 125 patients undergoing septal dermoplasty, mostly for HHT, during a 10-year period. No significant surgical complications occurred.

Nasal moisteners and room humidification promote mucosal integrity and reduce nasal mucosal injury and epistaxis. Nasal packing often temporarily stems epistaxis by vascular tamponade. Septal dermoplasty is indicated for severe and recurrent epistaxis, especially from the anterior nasal mucosa. In this procedure, skin, removed from the upper thigh, is grafted on to the anterior nasal septum and floor to cover and protect the fragile mucosal telangiectasias from local trauma. The procedure is well tolerated using only local anesthesia, and complications, other than recurrent epistaxis, are rare. Septal dermoplasty is effective in more than 75% of cases. Failure results from inadequate graft coverage with bleeding from lesions at the border or beyond the grafted area.

Long-term outcome of argon plasma ablation therapy for bleeding in 100 consecutive patients with colonic angiodysplasia. Olmos JA, Marcolongo M, Pogorelsky V, Herrera L, Tobal F, Davalos JR. Dis Colon Rectum 2006; 49: 1507–16.

In this prospective trial, 85 of 100 patients with moderate to severe bleeding from colonic angiodysplasia treated at colonoscopy with argon plasma coagulation (mean 3.9 angiodyplasias treated per patient) had no further overt bleeding and had a stable hemoglobin level without further blood transfusions or iron therapy during a mean follow-up of 20 months. Only two minor procedure complications occurred. Although not specifically addressing argon plasma coagulation for telangiectasias in HHT, this large and prospective study demonstrated a very high efficacy of this therapy for preventing rebleeding from the similar lesions of sporadic colonic angiodysplasia.

Mucosal vascular malformations of the gastrointestinal tract: clinical observations and results of neodymium: yttrium-aluminum-garnet laser therapy. Gostout CJ, Bowyer BA, Ahlquist DA, Viggiano TR, Balm RK. Mayo Clin Proc 1988; 63: 993–1003.

Gastrointestinal bleeding from telangiectasias was successfully controlled in nine of 10 patients with HHT and in 72 of 83 patients with sporadic telangiectasias by endoscopic photocoagulation using the Nd:YAG laser. Three gastrointestinal perforations occurred in 243 treatment sessions.

Long-term results of treatment of vascular malformations of the gastrointestinal tract by neodymium YAG laser photocoagulation. Naveau S, Aubert A, Poynard T, Chaput JC. Dig Dis Sci 1990; 35: 821–6.

Thirteen patients with HHT had a reduction in transfusion requirements for 2–3 years after endoscopic photocoagulation of bleeding gastrointestinal telangiectasias. This reduction, however, was not statistically significant, and successful treatment required multiple endoscopic sessions (median of seven) owing to the large number of telangiectasias in HHT.

Nonspecific therapy for gastrointestinal bleeding from HHT includes avoidance of aspirin, NSAIDs, other antiplatelet drugs, and anticoagulants; and administration of iron for patients with significant iron-deficiency anemia. At endoscopy, isolated actively bleeding telangiectasias are treated with endoscopic argon plasma coagulation, thermocoagulation, electrocoagulation, or photocoagulation. Endoscopists increasingly prefer argon plasma coagulation because of the ease of application and the potentially greater safety due to more superficial tissue ablation. Nonetheless, all these endoscopic therapies are relatively safe and highly successful at achieving hemostasis when performed by an experienced endoscopist. However, patients with HHT often subsequently rebleed from other, untreated gastrointestinal telangiectasias, and therefore require multiple sessions of endoscopic therapy to treat those other lesions. Angiographic embolization or segmental bowel resection are reserved for active severe bleeding, localized to a single region and refractory to medical and endoscopic therapy. These therapies often provide only intermediate-term relief owing to the recurrence of telangiectasias at other gastrointestinal sites.

Diagnosis and management of gastrointestinal bleeding in patients with hereditary hemorrhagic telangiectasia. Longacre AV, Gross CP, Gallitelli M, Henderson KJ, White RI Jr, Proctor DD. Am J Gastroenterol 2003; 98: 59–65.

In a non-randomized long-term observational study, the mean hemoglobin level increased and the chronic transfusion requirements decreased in about three-quarters of 17 patients after instituting chronic estrogen hormonal therapy, either alone or with other therapies, for gastrointestinal bleeding from HHT.

Treatment of bleeding gastrointestinal vascular malformations with oestrogen-progesterone. van Custen E, Rutgeerts P, Vantrappen G. Lancet 1990; 335: 953–5.

In a double-blind, placebo-controlled crossover trial of 10 patients with frequent and severe gastrointestinal bleeding from HHT, the number of transfusions decreased significantly from 10.9 units of packed erythrocytes in controls receiving placebo to 1.1 units in patients treated with estrogen-progesterone during a 6-month period.

Use of estrogen in treatment of familial hemorrhagic telangiectasia. Harrison DFN. Laryngoscope 1982; 92: 314–20.

Report of successful control of epistaxis with estrogen therapy in 67 patients with HHT, with few complications.

Several studies have reported a markedly reduced incidence of chronic gastrointestinal or nasal bleeding from telangiectasias after instituting estrogen therapy, either alone or with progesterone, owing to the promotion of endothelial integrity. Estrogen therapy can be combined with other therapies, such as local endoscopic therapy, to increase the efficacy. Despite controversy concerning efficacy, this therapy should be considered before performing gastrointestinal or nasal surgery for chronic bleeding, because of its low risk and the risk of recurrent bleeding after surgery. Estrogen therapy is less desirable in males than in females because it can cause feminization.

SECOND-LINE OR TEMPORIZING THERAPIES

For epistaxis

▶ Arterial ligation	B
▶ Topical vasoconstrictors	B
▶ Cryosurgery/electrical cautery/argon plasma coagulation	B
▶ Unilateral or bilateral surgical closure of the nostrils	B
▶ Arterial embolization	B
▶ Submucosal resection	C
▶ Topical aminocaproic acid	D

For gastrointestinal bleeding

▶ Oral aminocaproic acid therapy	D
▶ Bevacizumab	D
▶ α-Interferon	D

Dramatic improvement in hereditary hemorrhagic telangiectasia after treatment with the vascular endothelial growth factor (VEGF) antagonist bevacizumab. Flieger D, Hainke S, Fischbach W. Ann Hematol 2006; 85: 631–2.

A dramatic single case report of a large, abrupt decline in transfusion requirements and stabilization of the hematocrit level after institution of bevacizumab, an inhibitor of vascular endothelial growth factor.

Several patients with severe bleeding from HHT responded dramatically to therapy with bevacizumab, a vascular endothelial factor inhibitor, or with α-interferon, which has known anti-angiogenic properties. These two therapies for HHT are currently experimental as there are insufficient data.

Brief report: treatment of bleeding in hereditary hemorrhagic telangiectasia with aminocaproic acid. Saba HI, Morelli GA, Logrono LA. N Engl J Med 1994; 330: 1789–90.

Case report of a rapid and sustained reduction in the frequency and severity of bleeding from the nose and gastrointestinal tract in two patients with HHT treated with aminocaproic acid.

Local nonspecific therapy of arterial ligation, cryosurgery, electrical cautery, argon plasma coagulation, or submucosal resection provides temporary relief of epistaxis from HHT. However, these treatments can cause mucosal scarring, which diminishes the efficacy of subsequent septal dermoplasty. Topical therapy with vasoconstrictors or aminocaproic acid rarely produces scarring. Nonspecific therapies are indicated only for temporary relief of acute bleeding. Life-threatening epistaxis refractory to septal dermoplasty is treated by surgical closure of one or both nostrils, depending on the bleeding source.

Aminocaproic acid promotes thrombosis and retards bleeding by inhibiting fibrinolysis. Oral aminocaproic acid therapy has had mixed success with HHT. This therapy rarely causes hypotension or rhabdomyolysis. Aminocaproic acid is a temporary and second-line therapy.

Evidence Levels: **A** Double-blind study **B** Clinical trial ≥ 20 subjects **C** Clinical trial < 20 subjects **D** Series ≥ 5 subjects **E** Anecdotal case reports

Herpes genitalis

Brenda L Bartlett, Stephen K Tyring

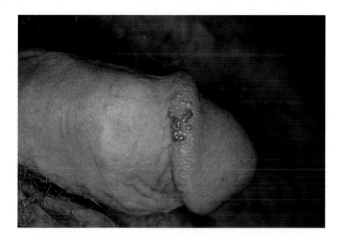

Herpes genitalis, or genital herpes, is a recurrent vesicular eruption of the skin and mucosa in the region between the navel and the buttocks, usually preceded by prodromal symptoms including itching, burning, and tingling. It is a common sexually transmitted disease caused predominantly by herpes simplex virus type 2 (HSV-2), but can also be caused by HSV-1. Primary infection may have associated influenza-like systemic signs, including fever, headache, malaise, and myalgia, which occur 2–20 days post exposure. Tender lymphadenopathy may also develop in the second and third weeks. Recurrences generally lack systemic symptoms and are less severe than the primary outbreak. Lesions of recurrences occur in the same area but are fewer in number and heal more quickly. Typical lesions of recurrent outbreaks manifest as grouped papules on an erythematous base which progress to thin-walled vesicles, ulcers, and then soft crusts. Dry crusts form in 3–4 days, allowing for healing. Residual hypopigmentation, hyperpigmentation, and scarring may occur with healing.

MANAGEMENT STRATEGY

As no cure exists for herpes genitalis, treatment is aimed at reducing the number of recurrences using suppressive therapy and at promoting rapid healing when a recurrence is present. In addition, treatment aims to reduce infectivity by reducing viral shedding, and to reduce complications such as urinary retention and aseptic meningitis. In the past, aciclovir, both topical and oral, was used as a first-line treatment for recurrences. Given aciclovir's low bioavailability, it requires frequent dosing. The standard dosing of oral aciclovir for a recurrence is 200 mg five times daily for 5 days. Alternative regimens have also been shown to be effective, including 400 mg three times daily for 5 days, 800 mg three times daily for 2 days, and 800 mg twice daily for 5 days. The frequent dosing of aciclovir led to the development of valaciclovir and famciclovir (the prodrugs of aciclovir and penciclovir, respectively) as alternative therapies with improved bioavailability. The use of topical aciclovir should be discouraged as it is less effective than oral aciclovir. Valaciclovir has been shown to be effective when dosed 500 mg twice daily for 3 days or 1000 mg once daily for

5 days. A dosing regimen of oral valaciclovir, given 2000 mg twice daily for 1 day, has been studied and shown to be more convenient; however, further comparative studies are needed. Famciclovir is effective when prescribed as 1000 mg twice daily for 1 day. It may also be taken as 125 mg twice daily for 5 days. Aciclovir, valaciclovir, and famciclovir may all be used for suppressive therapy.

Immunocompromised individuals have more frequent recurrences and can develop more severe lesions, thus requiring longer treatment periods with higher doses than those used in the immunocompetent. Severe cases may require intravenous therapy. Suppressive dosage regimens have been used in this population. Long-term therapy may lead to the selection of resistant strains of virus. In aciclovir-resistant cases, intravenous therapy with foscarnet may be required.

Another important aspect of genital herpes management is psychosocial. The recurrent nature of genital HSV infection can have severe emotional and psychological impact on patients. Counseling serves to help them cope with the infection and to prevent sexual and perinatal transmission. A physician can empower patients, allowing them to better manage the disease by educating them about the disease process.

SPECIFIC INVESTIGATIONS

> ► Viral culture
> ► PCR
> ► Serologic testing
> ► Skin biopsy of atypical lesion

Diagnosis may be made clinically when the history and presentation are consistent with HSV infection. When possible, laboratory confirmatory testing should be used. Severe or refractory cases may be due to underlying immunosuppression, which should be investigated further.

Genital herpes. Type-specific antibodies for diagnosis and management. Ashley RL. Dermatol Clin 1998; 16: 789–93.

Genital herpes: review of epidemic and potential use of type-specific serology. Ashley RL, Wald A. Clin Microbiol Rev 1999; 12: 1–8.

Using the evidence base on genital herpes: optimizing the use of diagnostic tests and information provision. Scoular A. Sex Transm Infect 2002; 78: 160–5.

Polymerase chain reaction for diagnosis of genital herpes in a genitourinary medicine clinic. Scoular A, Gillespie G, Carman WF. Sex Transm Infect 2002; 78: 21–5.

Polymerase chain reaction for detection of herpes simplex virus (HSV) DNA on mucosal surfaces: comparison with HSV isolation in cell culture. Wald A, Huang M-L, Carrell D, Selke S, Corey L. J Infect Dis 2003; 188: 1345–51.

HSV type specific serology in sexual health clinics: use, benefits, and who gets tested. Song B, Dwyer DE, Mindel A. Sex Transm Infect 2004; 80: 113–17.

Use of glycoprotein G-based type-specific assay to detect antibodies to herpes simplex virus type 2 among persons attending sexually transmitted disease clinics. Whittington WL, Celum CL, Cent A, Ashley RL. Sex Transm Dis 2001; 28: 99–104.

Factors predicting the acceptance of herpes simplex virus type 2 antibody testing among adolescents and young adults. Zimet GD, Rosenthal SL, Fortenberry JD, Brady RC, Tu W, Wu J, et al. Sex Transm Dis 2004; 31: 665–9.

FIRST LINE THERAPIES

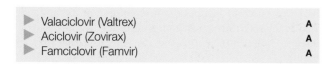

▶ Valaciclovir (Valtrex)	A
▶ Aciclovir (Zovirax)	A
▶ Famciclovir (Famvir)	A

Primary genital infection

Genital herpes. Gupta R, Warren T, Wald A. Lancet 2007; 370: 2127–37.

Antiviral treatment should be initiated promptly, even before laboratory confirmation of the diagnosis, and should be continued for 7–10 days. Treatment duration may be extended if adequate healing has not occurred. The following regimens may be used: aciclovir 400 mg three times daily or 200 mg five times daily; valaciclovir 1000 mg twice daily; or famciclovir 250 mg three times daily.

Sexually transmitted diseases treatment guidelines 2006. Centers for Disease Control and Prevention. MMWR Recomm Rep 2006; 55: 16–20.

Patients with primary genital HSV infection should receive antiviral therapy to prevent the development of severe or prolonged symptoms.

Acute reactivation episodes

One-day regimen of valaciclovir for treatment of recurrent genital herpes simplex virus 2 infection. Bavaro JB, Drolette L, Koelle DM, Almekinder J, Warren T, Tyring S, et al. Sex Transm Dis 2008; 35: 383–6.

A dosing regimen of oral valaciclovir, given 2000 mg twice daily for 1 day, may be a more convenient treatment for genital herpes recurrences but requires further comparative investigation.

Single-day therapy for recurrent genital herpes. Tyring S, Berger T, Yen-Moore A, Tharp M, Hamed K. Am J Clin Dermatol 2006; 7: 209–11.

A multicenter, randomized, double-blind placebo-controlled clinical trial found that famciclovir 1000 mg twice daily for 1 day, taken within 6 hours of prodrome onset, showed a significant reduction in lesion healing time and reduced the time of all symptom resolution compared to placebo. A greater proportion of subjects who took famciclovir did not progress to a full genital herpes outbreak compared to those taking placebo (23.3% vs 12.7%, respectively).

Sexually transmitted diseases treatment guidelines 2006. Centers for Disease Control and Prevention. MMWR Recomm Rep 2006; 55: 16–20.

Antiviral therapy should be initiated during the prodrome or within 1 day of lesion onset. Therefore, it is important that patients have a supply of drug on hand, whether aciclovir, valaciclovir or famciclovir, in order to initiate treatment immediately.

Valaciclovir for episodic treatment of genital herpes: a shorter 3-day treatment course compared with 5-day treatment. Leone PA, Trottier A, Miller JM. Clin Infect Dis 2002; 34: 958–62.

This study found that for episodic treatment of recurrent genital herpes a 3-day course of valaciclovir is as effective as a 5-day course. No significant differences in lesion healing times were noted between treatment groups, and the duration of pain and length of episodes were similar for both treatment groups.

Two-day regimen of aciclovir for treatment of recurrent genital herpes simplex virus type 2 infection. Wald A, Carrell D, Remington M, Kexel E, Zeh J, Corey L. Clin Infect Dis 2002; 34: 944–8.

This double-blind, placebo-controlled, randomized trial found a 2-day course of oral aciclovir 800 mg three times daily for 2 days to be a convenient and effective alternative treatment for recurrent genital herpes. The duration of viral shedding, lesion healing, and symptoms was reduced in the treatment group compared to placebo. The proportion of episodes with aborted lesions was significantly increased in those who received aciclovir.

Single-day patient initiated famciclovir therapy for recurrent genital herpes: a randomized, double-blind, placebo-controlled trial. Aoki FY, Tyring S, Diaz-Mitoma F, Gross G, Gao J, Hamed K. Clin Infect Dis 2006; 42: 8–13.

This study proved that in addition to being convenient (potentially a boon for increased patient compliance), single-day therapy is safe and effective for the treatment of recurrent genital herpes. Subjects receiving 1000 mg famciclovir orally twice daily for 1 day healed approximately 2 days faster than those on placebo.

A randomized, placebo-controlled comparison of oral valaciclovir and aciclovir in immunocompetent patients with recurrent genital herpes infections. Tyring SK, Douglas JM, Corey LC, Spruance SL, Esmann J. Arch Dermatol 1998; 134: 185–91.

This multicenter, double-blind, placebo-controlled, randomized parallel-design study showed that oral valaciclovir 1000 mg twice daily for 5 days was as effective and well tolerated, as was aciclovir five times daily for 5 days for the treatment of recurrent genital herpes.

Prophylactic treatment – for frequent reactivation, recurrent severe attacks, at bone marrow transplantation, or before delivery

Effect of valaciclovir on viral shedding in immunocompetent patients with recurrent herpes simplex virus 2 genital herpes: a US-based randomized, double-blind, placebo-controlled clinical trial. Fife KH, Warren TJ, Ferrera RD, Young DG, Justus SE, Heitman CK, et al. Mayo Clin Proc 2006; 81: 1321–7.

Over a 60-day period 1 g of valaciclovir daily was well tolerated and effectively reduced clinical and subclinical HSV-2 shedding compared to placebo.

Once-daily valaciclovir to reduce the risk of transmission of genital herpes. Corey L, Wald A, Patel R, Sacks SL, Tyring SK, Warren T, et al. N Engl J Med 2004; 350: 11–20.

Among heterosexual HSV-2 discordant couples, once-daily valaciclovir (500 mg) significantly reduced the risk of transmission of genital herpes. Clinically symptomatic HSV-2 infection was reduced by 75%, and acquisition of HSV-2 was reduced by 48% in the valaciclovir group versus placebo.

Evidence Levels: **A** Double-blind study **B** Clinical trial ≥ 20 subjects **C** Clinical trial < 20 subjects **D** Series ≥ 5 subjects **E** Anecdotal case reports

94

Herpes genitalis

Valaciclovir therapy to reduce recurrent genital herpes in pregnant women. Andrews WW, Kimberlin DF, Whitley R, Cliver S, Ramsey PS, Deeter R. Am J Obstet Gynecol 2006: 194: 774–81.

This double-blind, placebo-controlled, randomized trial showed that daily valaciclovir, initiated at 36 weeks' gestation in HSV-positive pregnant women with a history of recurrences, significantly reduced the number of women with subsequent clinical HSV recurrences. However, this suppressive regimen did not reduce shedding of HSV within 7 days of delivery compared to placebo. The number of women with clinical HSV lesions at delivery was similar for both the placebo and the treatment group.

Effect of serologic status and cesarean delivery on transmission rates of herpes simplex virus from mother to infant. Brown ZA, Wald A, Morrow RA, Selke S, Zeh J, Corey L. JAMA 2003; 289: 203–9.

Among women with HSV in genital secretions at the time of labor, the risk of neonatal HSV was significantly reduced in those who had a cesarean delivery.

Sexually transmitted diseases treatment guidelines 2006. Centers for Disease Control and Prevention. MMWR Recomm Rep 2006; 55: 16–20.

Severe HSV infection, or complications requiring hospitalization, such as disseminated infection, pneumonitis, hepatitis, meningitis, or encephalitis, requires intravenous antiviral therapy. A regimen of aciclovir 5–10 mg/kg IV every 8 hours for a minimum of 2 days until clinical improvement occurs is recommended. Transition to oral antiviral therapy is recommended to complete a 10-day course.

Frequent reactivation of herpes simplex virus among HIV-1-infected patients treated with highly active antiretroviral therapy. Posavad CM, Wald A, Kuntz S, Huang ML, Selke S, Krantz E, et al. J Infect Dis 2004; 190: 693–6.

In HIV-infected individuals, antiretroviral therapy reduced the frequency and severity of symptomatic genital herpes. However, frequent asymptomatic viral shedding occurred.

Sexually transmitted diseases treatment guidelines 2006. Centers for Disease Control and Prevention. MMWR Recomm Rep 2006; 55: 16–20.

Aciclovir, valaciclovir, and famciclovir are safe to use in immunocompromised patients. Treatment duration is generally for 5–10 days for the following: aciclovir 400 mg three times daily; famciclovir 500 mg twice daily; or valaciclovir 1.0 g twice daily. Intravenous therapy may be required in severe cases.

Valaciclovir prophylaxis for the prevention of herpes simplex virus reactivation in recipients of progenitor cell transplantation. Dignani MC, Mykietiuk A, Michelet M, Intile D, Mammana L, Desmery P, et al. Bone Marrow Transplant 2002; 29: 263–7.

In over 100 patients following bone marrow transplantation, equal efficacy between intravenous aciclovir and oral valaciclovir was seen when compared to no prophylaxis.

SECOND-LINE THERAPIES

▶ Foscarnet	B
▶ Cidofovir	A

A multicenter phase I/II dose escalation study of single-dose cidofovir gel for treatment of recurrent genital herpes. Sacks SL, Shafran SD, Diaz-Mitoma F, Trottier S, Sibbald RG, Hughes A, et al. Antimicrob Agents Chemother 1998; 42: 2996–9.

A randomized, double-blind, clinic-initiated, sequential dose-escalation pilot study compared the safety and efficacy of single applications of 1%, 3%, and 5% cidofovir gel with placebo in the treatment of early, lesional, recurrent genital herpes. At all strengths, cidofovir significantly reduced the median time to negative virus culture in a dose-dependent fashion. Single-dose application of cidofovir gel confers a significant antiviral effect on lesions of recurrent genital herpes.

Clinical potential of the acyclic nucleoside phosphonates cidofovir, adefovir, and tenofovir in treatment of DNA virus and retrovirus infections. De Clercq E. Clin Microbiol Rev 2003; 16: 569–96.

The acyclic nucleoside phosphonate HPMPC (cidofovir) has proved effective in vitro and in vivo against a wide variety of DNA virus and retrovirus infections, including HSV types 1 and 2.

Foscarnet treatment of aciclovir-resistant herpes simplex virus infection in patients with acquired immunodeficiency syndrome: preliminary results of a controlled, randomized, regimen-controlled trial. Hardy WD. Am J Med 1992; 92: 30s–5s.

Twenty-five patients with AIDS and aciclovir-resistant HSV infection were treated with foscarnet infusions for 2 weeks, followed by 8 more weeks with 40 mg/kg daily or without further treatment. Lesions healed most quickly in those treated for a total of 10 weeks.

THIRD-LINE THERAPIES

▶ L-Lysine	A
▶ Aspirin	B
▶ Resiquimod	A

Treatment of recurrent herpes simplex infections with L-lysine monohydrochloride. McCune MA, Perry HO, O'Fallon WM. Cutis 1984; 34: 366–73.

This double-blind, placebo-controlled, crossover trial showed significantly fewer recurrences in subjects during the 24-week period of receiving high-dose (1000 mg daily) lysine than during the 24-week placebo period. No significant difference was noted in those receiving low-dose (500 mg daily) lysine compared to placebo. All subjects were prescribed a high-lysine, low-arginine diet.

Aspirin in the management of recurrent herpes simplex virus infection. Karadi I, Karpati S, Romics L. Ann Intern Med 1998; 128: 696–7.

This study showed that patients treated with aspirin 125 mg daily had significantly fewer days of active HSV infection than controls who took no antiviral or anti-inflammatory drugs. Of the 21 subjects, only two had recurrent genital HSV; the remainder had recurrent oral HSV. All subjects who received aspirin reported milder skin involvement than before aspirin treatment. Nine of the 21 subjects took aspirin long term (several months) and had longer symptom-free periods.

Topical resiquimod 0.01% gel decreases herpes simplex virus type 2 genital shedding: a randomized, controlled trial. Mark KE, Corey L, Meng TC, Magaret AS, Huang ML, Selke S, et al. J Infect Dis 2007; 195: 1324–31.

A randomized, double-blind, vehicle-controlled trial assessed the efficacy of resiquimod 0.01% gel for reducing human anogenital HSV-2 mucosal reactivation. Adults with genital HSV-2 applied topical resiquimod or vehicle to ano-genital lesions twice weekly for 3 weeks. Daily swabs were then collected for 60 days for HSV DNA PCR. Recurrences over the next 7 months were treated with study gel. Resampling for an additional 60 days with swabs was done to assess shedding. The median lesion and shedding rates were lower for the treatment group than in the vehicle group for both sampling periods. The length of recurrence was not influenced by resiquimod treatment.

Application of a topical immune response modifier, resiquimod gel, to modify the recurrence rate of recurrent genital herpes: a pilot study. Spruance SL, Tyring SK, Smith MH, Meng T. J Infect Dis 2001; 184: 196–200.

In this pilot study in human subjects, resiquimod (a topically active immune response modifier) appeared to reduce the frequency of genital herpes recurrences. Over a 6-month observation period after treatment, the median period to first recurrence after resiquimod was 169 days, compared to 57 days for the vehicle group.

OTHER THERAPIES

> ▶ Psychosocial counseling
> ▶ Hygiene techniques: keep area clean and dry to prevent secondary infections, avoid touching lesions, and wash hands after any contact with sores
> ▶ Loose-fitting clothing and cotton underwear
> ▶ Ice pack/cool compress

Sexually transmitted diseases treatment guidelines 2006. Centers for Disease Control and Prevention. MMWR Recomm Rep 2006; 55: 16–20.

Counseling of infected individuals serves to prevent sexual and perinatal infection and to help individuals cope with infection. Education for infected individuals seems to be of benefit both at the time of diagnosis and after resolution of the acute infection, to further their understanding of the chronic nature of the disease.

Genital herpes: a review. Beauman JG, Maj MC. Am Fam Phys 2005; 72: 1527–34, 1541–2.

Prevention of secondary infection and spread of the infection can be achieved by keeping the affected area clean and dry, wearing loose-fitting clothing and cotton underwear, avoiding contact with the lesions, and by washing hands immediately should contact with any sores occur.

PREVENTION

> ▶ Condoms
> ▶ Vaccine

Glycoprotein-D adjuvant vaccine to prevent genital herpes. Stanberry LR, Spruance SL, Cunningham AL, Bernstein DI, Mindel A, Sacks S, et al.; GlaxoSmithKline Herpes Vaccine Efficacy Study Group. N Engl J Med 2002; 347: 1652–61.

Two randomized, double-blinded trials were conducted using a herpes simplex virus type 2 (HSV-2) glycoprotein-D subunit vaccine with alum and 3-O-deacylated-monophosphoryl lipid A in subjects with regular sexual partners known to have genital herpes. The vaccine was well tolerated and induced cellular and humoral immune responses. The vaccine was efficacious in women who were seronegative for both HSV-1 and HSV-2, but not in women who were seropositive for HSV-1 but seronegative for HSV-2. It has no efficacy in men, regardless of their HSV serology.

Effect of condoms on reducing the transmission of herpes simplex virus type 2 from men to women. Wald A, Langenberg AG, Link K, Izu AE, Ashley R, Warren T, et al. JAMA 2001; 285: 3100–6.

In heterosexual discordant couples in which the male is infected with herpes simplex virus type 2, the use of condoms offers significant protection against HSV-2 transmission in susceptible women. A concurrent reduction in sexual activity when the source partner had lesions also occurred as a result of counseling on sexual behavior.

Evidence Levels: **A** Double-blind study **B** Clinical trial ≥ 20 subjects **C** Clinical trial < 20 subjects **D** Series ≥ 5 subjects **E** Anecdotal case reports

Herpes labialis

Jane C Sterling

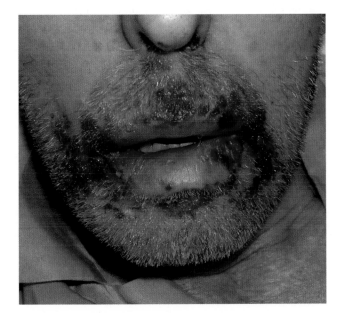

Herpes simplex virus (HSV) infects the skin and mucous membranes, damaging keratinocytes and causing intense inflammation, seen as small blisters on a background of erythema. The primary infection may be obvious or subclinical; once latency is established in sensory ganglia, the virus may reactivate at variable intervals to produce visible lesions which often recur at the same location. In immunosuppression the disease can be chronic and antiviral resistance can develop. This chapter deals with HSV infection of the non-genital skin and mucosae; genital HSV infection is discussed in Chapter 94.

MANAGEMENT STRATEGY

Both primary and reactivation episodes are usually self-limiting and may not require treatment. Antiviral therapy, in the form of *aciclovir* and related drugs, is available for topical and systemic use and is usually the most effective form of treatment. Anogenital herpes, either primary infection or a reactivation episode, will frequently respond to *topical aciclovir* applied five times daily for 5 days, the efficacy of topical aciclovir in cutaneous herpes is less certain, resulting in only marginal benefit. *Oral aciclovir*, 200 mg five times daily for 5 days, will usually reduce the time to healing and duration of virus shedding and is more effective than topical treatment. Shorter treatment courses with higher-dose aciclovir seem to produce similar effects. Topical or systemic treatment for an acute episode should be started early in the episode to have the most benefit. Pain relief may also be necessary.

A failure of response to aciclovir may be due to poor absorption and rapid clearance following ingestion, or to the emergence of aciclovir resistance. *Valaciclovir*, a prodrug of aciclovir, and *famciclovir*, a prodrug of penciclovir, have improved bioavailability and are alternatives to aciclovir, with the additional benefit of once- or twice-daily dosing. Short-course (single-day) treatment with oral famciclovir can hasten healing if

given at the start of a reactivation episode. The efficacy of oral valaciclovir can be as good as that of intravenous aciclovir.

In severe or frequently recurrent disease, or in immunosuppressed individuals, antiviral treatment is recommended and measures may be taken to avoid any precipitating factors. *UV protection* may help to reduce viral reactivation in herpes labialis. Oral aciclovir has been used extensively as prophylaxis, but needs to be taken for several weeks or months. The dose of 400 mg twice daily for aciclovir is most likely to produce a reduction in the frequency of reactivation episodes. Oral valaciclovir or famciclovir can also be used for long-term suppression of viral reactivation. There is a potential risk of selection of resistant strains of virus with long-term therapy, but this is rare even in immunosuppressed patients. The risk of herpetic reactivation at bone marrow transplantation, or mother-to-baby transmission in women with HSV infection, can be reduced by prophylactic therapy.

Topical idoxuridine and the related *trifluorothymidine* (*TFT*) have also been used.

In immunosuppressed individuals, intravenous therapy with aciclovir, or the more toxic *foscarnet* or *cidofovir*, may be necessary. Topical preparations of *cidofovir* have been shown to have an effect but are not commercially available. *Vidarabine*, *interferons*, and *interleukin-2* and other agents have also been used, but without reliable effect. Herpes simplex is a common precipitating cause of episodes of recurrent erythema multiforme (see page 220), which can be reduced in frequency by prophylactic antiviral therapy.

SPECIFIC INVESTIGATIONS

> ▶ Electron microscopy of blister fluid
> ▶ PCR of blister fluid or biopsy
> ▶ Viral culture from swab of lesion
> ▶ Immunocytology of blister floor cells
> ▶ Skin biopsy of atypical lesion
> ▶ Assessment of immune function

The diagnosis may be obvious clinically. In atypical disease, laboratory confirmation is essential. In unexplained persistent or severe disease, immunodeficiency should be excluded.

FIRST-LINE THERAPIES

> ▶ Topical aciclovir   A
> ▶ Oral aciclovir   A
> ▶ Topical idoxuridine   A
> ▶ Sunscreen   A

Primary cutaneous infection

Treatment of herpes simplex gingivostomatitis with aciclovir in children: a randomized double blind placebo controlled study. Amir J, Harel L, Smetana Z, Varsano I. Br Med J 1997; 314: 1800–3.

A total of 61 children with herpetic gingivostomatitis were treated with aciclovir suspension 15 mg/kg or placebo five times daily for 7 days. Aciclovir reduced the duration of lesions from 10 to 4 days, and reduced the period of viral shedding.

Acute reactivation episodes

Failure of aciclovir cream in treatment of recurrent herpes labialis. Shaw M, King M, Best JM, Banatvala JE, Gibson JR, Klaber MR. Br Med J 1985; 291: 7–9.

No significant benefit was obtained from topical 5% aciclovir applied five times daily in a double-blind, placebo-controlled crossover trial on 45 patients who suffered 72 episodes of recurrent herpes labialis.

Acyclovir cream for treatment of herpes simplex labialis: results of two randomized, double-blind, vehicle-controlled multicenter clinical trials. Spruance SL, Nett R, Marbury T, Wolff R, Johnson J, Spaulding T. Antimicrob Agents Chemother 2002; 46: 2238–43.

In two studies of a total of 1385 patients with recurrent herpes labialis, aciclovir 5% cream applied five times a day for 4 days reduced time to healing to an average of 4.4 days, compared to 5.0 days when placebo was used.

Recurrent herpes labialis: efficiacy of topical therapy with penciclovir compared with acyclovir. Femiano F, Gombos F, Scully C. Oral Dis 2001; 7: 31–3.

Aciclovir 5% cream or penciclovir 1% cream was applied every 2 hours during waking hours for 4 days. Penciclovir treatment reduced the duration of symptoms by 1 day.

Treatment of recurrent herpes simplex labialis with oral acyclovir. Spruance SL, Stewart JCB, Rowe NH, McKeough MB, Wenerstrom G, Freeman DJ. J Infect Dis 1990; 161: 185–90.

Herpes labialis was less painful and quicker to heal in 114 patients treated before the development of blistering with 400 mg aciclovir, five times daily for 5 days, compared to 60 patients given placebo treatment. The development of blisters and the size of the lesion were not affected by treatment.

Early application of topical 15% idoxuridine in dimethyl-sulfoxide shortens the course of herpes simplex labialis: a multicenter placebo-controlled trial. Spruance SL, Stewart CB, Freeman DJ, Brightman VJ, Cox JL, Wenerstrom G, et al. J Infect Dis 1990; 161: 191–7.

Idoxuridine 15% solution, applied six times daily for 4 days starting within 1 hour of the onset of symptoms of a recurrence, significantly reduced pain and time to healing compared to 2% idoxuridine or dimethylsulfoxide alone.

Prophylactic treatment – for frequent reactivation, recurrent severe attacks, at bone marrow transplantation, or before delivery

Prevention of ultraviolet-light-induced herpes labialis by sunscreen. Rooney JF, Bryson Y, Mannix ML, Dillon M, Wohlenberg CR, Banks S, et al. Lancet 1991; 338: 1419–22.

Using an experimental system of UV exposure to induce reactivation of herpes, 71% of 38 patients using a placebo developed lesions, whereas none developed in 35 patients using sunscreen.

Oral acyclovir to suppress frequently recurrent herpes labialis: a double-blind, placebo-controlled trial. Rooney JF, Straus SE, Mannix ML, Wohlenberg CR, Alling DW, Dumois JA, et al. Ann Intern Med 1993; 118: 268–72.

Twenty patients completed a randomized 4-month cross-over study receiving aciclovir 400 mg bd or placebo. During active treatment there were an average of 0.85 reactivation episodes, compared to 1.8 during placebo treatment.

Valacyclovir prophylaxis for the prevention of herpes simplex virus reactivation in recipients of progenitor cell transplantation. Dignani MC, Mykietiuk A, Michelet M, Intile D, Mammana L, Desmery P, et al. Bone Marrow Transplant 2002; 29: 263–7.

A comparison of intravenous aciclovir, oral valaciclovir, or no prophylaxis following bone marrow transplantation in over 100 patients showed equal efficacy of the two antivirals.

Acyclovir prophylaxis to prevent herpes simplex virus recurrence at delivery: a systematic review. Sheffield JS, Hollier LM, Hill JB, Stuart GS, Wendel GD. Obstet Gynecol 2003; 102: 1396.

A review of evidence for potential reduction of transmission from mother to baby by aciclovir suggests 200 mg four times daily or 400 mg twice daily from 36 weeks' gestation until after delivery.

SECOND-LINE THERAPIES

| ▶ Valaciclovir | A |
| ▶ Famciclovir | A |

High-dose, short-duration, early valacyclovir therapy for episodic treatment of cold sores: results of two randomized, placebo-controlled multicenter studies. Spruance S, Jones T, Blatter MM, Vargas-Cortez M, Barber J, Hill J, et al. Antimicrob Agents Chemother 2003; 47: 1072–80.

Treatment at the start of an attack with either 2 g twice daily for 1 day or 2 g twice daily for 1 day plus 1 g twice daily for 1 day reduced the duration of the episode (5–5.5 days with placebo) by 0.5–1 day. The chance of an aborted episode was increased.

Single-dose, patient-initiated famciclovir: a randomized, double-blind, placebo-controlled trial for episodic treatment of herpes labialis. Spruance SL, Bodsworth N, Resnick H, Conant M, Oeuvray C, Gao J, et al. J Am Acad Dermatol 2006; 55: 47–53.

A total of 375 patients with recurrent herpes labialis completed the study. They were randomized into three groups to self-administer placebo, famciclovir 750 mg bid for 1 day, or famciclovir 1500 mg as a single dose. Lesions healed in approximately 4 days in both groups taking famciclovir, compared to 6 days for the placebo group.

THIRD-LINE THERAPIES

▶ Vidarabine	C
▶ Foscarnet	C
▶ Cidofovir	C
▶ Trifluorothymidine	E

Foscarnet treatment of acyclovir-resistant herpes simplex virus infection in patients with acquired immunodeficiency syndrome: preliminary results of a controlled, randomized, regimen-controlled trial. Hardy WD. Am J Med 1992; 92: 30s–5s.

Evidence Levels: **A** Double-blind study **B** Clinical trial ≥ 20 subjects **C** Clinical trial < 20 subjects **D** Series ≥ 5 subjects **E** Anecdotal case reports

Twenty-five patients with AIDS and aciclovir-resistant HSV infection were treated with foscarnet infusions for 2 weeks, and then either for a further 8 weeks with 40 mg/kg daily or without further maintenance therapy. Healing of lesions was quickest in those treated for a total of 10 weeks.

A controlled trial comparing foscarnet with vidarabine for acyclovir-resistant mucocutaneous herpes simplex in the acquired immunodeficiency syndrome. Safrin S, Crumpacker C, Chatis P, Davis R, Hafner R, Rush J, et al. N Engl J Med 1991; 325: 551–5.

Foscarnet 40 mg/kg every 8 hours produced healing of aciclovir-resistant herpetic lesions within 4 weeks in eight patients with AIDS, but no improvement occurred in six similar patients treated with vidarabine 15 mg/kg daily.

Treatment with intravenous (S)-1-[hydroxy-2-(phosphonylmethoxy)propyl]-cytosine of acyclovir-resistant mucocutaneous infection with herpes simplex virus in a patient with AIDS. Lalezari JP, Drew WL, Glutzer E, Miner D, Safrin S, Owen WF, et al. J Infect Dis 1994; 170: 570–2.

Treatment with four intravenous infusions of 5 mg/kg/week of HPMPC (cidofovir) produced 95% healing in a patient with severe resistant herpetic lesions.

A randomized, double-blind, placebo-controlled trial of cidofovir gel for the treatment of acyclovir-unresponsive mucocutaneous herpes simplex virus infection in patients with AIDS. Lalezari J, Schacker T, Feinberg J, Gathe J, Lee S, Cheung T, et al. J Infect Dis 1997; 176: 892–8.

Twenty patients with AIDS applied 0.3% or 1% cidofovir gel once daily for 5 days; 50% healed or improved, compared to 0% of the 10 placebo-treated patients. Cidofovir produced local inflammation in a quarter of patients.

Trifluorothymidine 0.5% ointment in the treatment of aciclovir-resistant mucocutaneous herpes simplex in AIDS. Amin AR, Robinson MR, Smith DD, Luque AE. AIDS 1996; 10: 1051–3.

Three patients responded to topical TFT applied five times daily for 14 days and then maintenance twice daily. Healing of previously aciclovir-resistant lesions occurred within 3 weeks.

Placebo-controlled trial of topical interferon in labial and genital herpes. Glezerman M, Lunenfeld E, Cohen V, Sarov I, Movshovitz M, Doerner T, et al. Lancet Jan 23 1988; 331: 150–2.

Of 14 patients with herpes labialis, 7 applied the active interferon-ß containing gel several time a day during recurrences for at least one year. In comparison with the placebo-treated group, the attack duration reduced from 7 to 4.7 days and there was a four-fold reduction in frequency of recurrences.

Herpes zoster

Anne Marie Tremaine, Brenda Bartlett, Aron Gewirtzman, Stephen Tyring

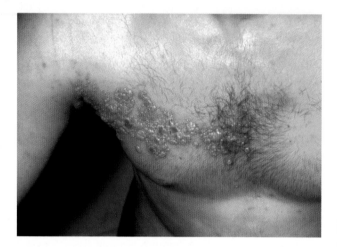

Reactivation of latent varicella zoster virus produces the clinical syndrome herpes zoster (shingles), which manifests as a unilateral eruption along a single dermatome and is usually preceded by prodromal pain and paresthesia. The eruption lasts around 7–10 days, and progresses from erythematous macules and papules to vesicles, then pustules, and finally crusts over. One of the most common complications of herpes zoster is postherpetic neuralgia (PHN), which is dermatomal pain persisting longer than 3 months.

MANAGEMENT STRATEGY

Early treatment – within the first 72 hours of vesicle formation – is important for antiviral efficacy, time to lesion healing, and minimizing zoster-associated pain (although initiating treatment after 72 hours may still be effective). *Aciclovir, valaciclovir, and famciclovir* are guanosine analogs that are phosphorylated by thymidine kinase to a triphosphate form that inhibits viral DNA polymerase. The oral bioavailability of the antivirals determines the number of daily administrations (Table 1). Patient compliance tends to decrease as the number of daily administrations increases. The most common side effects seen are nausea, headache, and GI upset, but these drugs are otherwise safe and well tolerated. Patients with renal insufficiency will need an adjusted dose, as these medications are excreted by the kidneys.

Aciclovir-resistant VZV infections have been reported in immunocompromised patients (i.e., AIDS, transplant patients) and in these cases *foscarnet* (given intravenously 40 mg/kg three times daily) can be used as an alternative.

Table 1 First-line therapy for acute herpes zoster

Medication	Dose (mg)	Number of daily doses	Duration (days)
Valacyclovir	1000	3	7
Famciclovir	500	3	7
Aciclovir	800	5	7

Acutely, *corticosteroids* may reduce zoster-associated pain, but they are associated with a risk of serious adverse events and have shown no benefit in reducing time to complete cessation of pain.

Current therapeutic options for postherpetic neuralgia include the anticonvulsants *gabapentin* and *pregabalin*, opioid analgesics, tricyclic antidepressants (Table 2), *lidocaine patch 5%*, and *capsaicin cream*. Choice of therapy should be guided by considering a patient's comorbidities, drug adverse event profiles, and preference. Combination therapy is common in clinical practice, but there is no evidence base to support this practice.

Vaccination of patients aged 60 and over with the varicella zoster virus is the most promising option for the prevention of herpes zoster. Administration of *gabapentin* in conjunction with antivirals (and analgesics) during the acute phase of zoster may offer further protection against postherpetic neuralgia. Asymptomatic reactivation of the varicella zoster virus and contact with patients with chickenpox may enhance cell-mediated immunity.

SPECIFIC INVESTIGATIONS

- ▶ Tzanck smear
- ▶ Viral culture
- ▶ Serology (acute plus chronic)
- ▶ Electron microscopy
- ▶ Polymerase chain reaction (PCR)

In most cases no investigation is required to establish the diagnosis.

FIRST-LINE THERAPIES

Antiviral agents	
▶ Aciclovir	A
▶ Famciclovir	A
▶ Valaciclovir	A

Valaciclovir compared with acyclovir for improved therapy for herpes zoster in immunocompetent adults. Beutner KR, Friedman DJ, Forszpaniak C, Andersen PL, Wood MJ. Antimicrob Agents Chemother 1995; 39: 1546–53.

Valaciclovir is comparable to aciclovir in the resolution of zoster eruption, but it accelerates the resolution of pain compared to aciclovir and is more convenient.

Antiviral therapy for herpes zoster: randomized, controlled clinical trial of valacyclovir and famciclovir therapy in immunocompetent patients 50 years and older. Tyring SK, Beutner KR, Tucker BA, Anderson WC, Crooks RJ. Arch Fam Med 2000; 9: 863–9.

Valaciclovir is comparable to famciclovir in the resolution of zoster-associated pain and PHN.

Factors influencing pain outcome in herpes zoster: an observational study with valaciclovir. Decroix J, Partsch H, Gonzalez R, Mobacken H, Goh CL, Walsh L, et al.; Valaciclovir Zoster Assessment Group (VIZA). J Eur Acad Dermatol Venereol 2000; 14: 23–33.

An open-label study using a 7-day course of valaciclovir to treat 1897 immunocompetent patients with acute herpes zoster. Valaciclovir was safe, effective (even when initiated more than 72 hours after the first vesicle), and associated with very few adverse events.

Evidence Levels: **A** Double-blind study **B** Clinical trial ≥ 20 subjects **C** Clinical trial < 20 subjects **D** Series ≥ 5 subjects **E** Anecdotal case reports

Table 2 Treatment options for postherpetic neuralgia

Drug class	Examples	Initial daily dose (mg)	Titration to maximum dose
Anticonvulsants	Gabapentin	100–300	Start qhs and increase to tid dosing; increase by 100–300 mg every 3 days to total dose of 1800–2400 mg/day
	Pregabalin	150	Titrate up to 300 or 600 mg/day
Opioids	Hydrocodone	5–10	No titration
	Oxycodone (extended-release)	20	Titrate up to 60 mg daily
Tricyclic antidepressants	Nortriptyline	10–25	Increase by 10–25 mg weekly, with a target dose of 75–150 mg
	Amitriptyline	10–25	
	Desipramine	10–25	

Famciclovir for the treatment of acute herpes zoster: effects on acute disease and postherpetic neuralgia. A randomized, double-blind, placebo controlled trial. Tyring S, Barbarash RA, Nahlik JE, Cunningham A, Marley J, Heng M, et al. Ann Intern Med 1995; 123: 89–96.

Famciclovir recipients had faster resolution of pain following an acute episode than those receiving placebo.

Double-blind, randomized, acyclovir-controlled, parallel-group trial comparing the safety and efficacy of famciclovir and acyclovir in patients with uncomplicated herpes zoster. Shen MC, Lin HH, Lee SS, Chen YS, Chiang PC, Liu YC. J Microbiol Immunol Infect 2004; 37: 75–81.

Famciclovir is comparable to aciclovir in the resolution of zoster cutaneous eruption but is more convenient.

Oral acyclovir therapy accelerates pain resolution in patients with herpes zoster: a meta-analysis of placebo-controlled trials. Wood MJ, Kay R, Dworkin RH, Soong SJ, Whitley RJ. Clin Infect Dis 1996; 22: 341–7.

In four placebo-controlled studies aciclovir was clearly shown to accelerate pain resolution.

SECOND-LINE THERAPIES

Agents to reduce postherpetic neuralgia	
▶ Anticonvulsants	A
▶ Tricyclic antidepressants	A
▶ Lidocaine patch	A
▶ Oxycodone	A

Pregabalin for the treatment of postherpetic neuralgia: a randomized, placebo-controlled trial. Dworkin RH, Corbin AE, Young JP, Sharma U, LaMoreaux L, Bockbrader H, et al. Neurology 2003; 60: 1274–83.

Pregabalin is effective in the treatment of pain and sleep interference associated with PHN. It was associated with greater global improvement than treatment with placebo.

Gabapentin for the treatment of post-herpetic neuralgia: a randomized controlled trial. Rowbotham M, Harden N, Stacey B, Bernstein P, Magnus-Miller L. JAMA 1998; 280: 1837–42.

Gabapentin is effective in the treatment of pain and sleep interference associated with PHN.

Gabapentin versus nortriptyline in post-herpetic neuralgia patients: a randomized, double blind clinical trial – the GONIP Trial. Chandra K, Shafiq N, Pandhi P, Gupta S, Malhotra S. Int J Clin Pharmacol Ther 2006; 44: 358–63.

Gabapentin and nortriptyline are equally efficacious, but gabapentin is better tolerated.

Nortriptyline versus amitriptyline in post-herpetic neuralgia: a randomized trial. Watson CP, Vernich L, Chipman M, Reed K. Neurology 1998; 51: 1166–71.

Nortriptyline is equally effective as amitriptyline but is better tolerated.

The effects of pre-emptive treatment of postherpetic neuralgia with amitriptyline: a randomized, double-blind, placebo-controlled trial. Bowsher D. J Pain Symptom Manage 1997; 13: 327–31.

Low-dose amitriptyline given at the time of the acute zoster rash may reduce the incidence of PHN.

Topical lidocaine for the treatment of postherpetic neuralgia. Khaliq W, Alam S, Puri N. Cochrane Database Syst Rev 2007; 2: CD004846.

A meta-analysis combining two studies found that lidocaine is more effective than placebo, but there is insufficient evidence to recommend it as a first-line therapy.

Efficacy of oxycodone in neuropathic pain: a randomized trial in post-herpetic neuralgia. Watson CPN, Babul N. Neurology 1998; 50: 1837–41.

Patients on slow-release oxycodone had significantly greater pain relief and reduction in allodynia and disability.

THIRD-LINE THERAPIES

▶ Vaccination of adults	A
▶ Corticosteroids	E
▶ Contact with varicella or with children	C
▶ Topical capsaicin	A
▶ Topical non-steroidal anti-inflammatory cream	C
▶ Tramadol	B
▶ Sympathetic nerve block	B
▶ Transcutaneous electrical stimulation	C

A vaccine to prevent herpes zoster and postherpetic neuralgia in older adults. Oxman MN, Levin MJ, Johnson GR, Schmader KE, Straus SE, Gelb LD, et al. N Engl J Med 2005; 352: 2271.

A randomized, double-blind, placebo-controlled trial of an investigational live attenuated Oka/Merck VZV vaccine enrolled 38 546 immunocompetent adults aged 60 or over. The vaccine significantly reduced morbidity from herpes zoster and postherpetic neuralgia. It was also shown to be safe and well tolerated.

Acyclovir with and without prednisone for the treatment of herpes zoster. A randomized placebo-controlled trial. Whitley RJ, Weiss H, Gnann JW Jr, Tyring S, Mertz GJ, Pappas PG, et al. Ann Intern Med 1996; 125: 376–83.

There was no statistical difference between aciclovir plus prednisone or aciclovir alone in the resolution of pain.

A randomized trial of acyclovir for 7 days or 21 days with and without prednisolone for treatment of acute herpes zoster. Wood MJ, Johnson RW, McKendrick MW, Taylor J, Mandal BK, Crooks J. Engl J Med 1994; 330: 896–900.

There was no statistical difference between aciclovir plus prednisolone or aciclovir alone in the resolution of pain.

Contacts with varicella or with children and protection against herpes zoster in adults: a case controlled study. Thomas SL, Wheeler JG, Hall AJ. Lancet 2002; 360: 678–82.

Social contact with many children outside the household, or occupational contacts with children ill with chickenpox, results in a graded protection against zoster.

A randomized vehicle-controlled trial of topical capsaicin in the treatment of postherpetic neuralgia. Watson CP, Tyler KL, Bickers DR, Millikan LE, Smith S, Coleman E. Clin Ther 1993; 15: 510–26.

A double-blind study with 143 patients comparing capsaicin 0.075% cream with vehicle. Capsaicin was effective. The only side effect was burning or stinging at sites of application.

Benzydamine cream for the treatment of post-herpetic neuralgia: minimum duration of treatment periods in a cross-over trial. McQuay HJ, Carroll D, Moxon A, Glynn CJ, Moore RA. Pain 1990; 40: 131–5.

Some patients benefit.

Tramadol in post-herpetic neuralgia: a randomized, double-blind, placebo-controlled trial. Boureau F, Legallicier P, Kabir-Ahmadi M. Pain 2003; 104: 323–31.

A double-blind study with 127 patients found tramadol to be an effective in reducing pain intensity and increasing the percentage of pain relief compared to placebo.

Neuraxial and sympathetic blocks in herpes zoster and postherpetic neuralgia: An appraisal of current evidence. Kumar V, Krone K, Mathieu A. Regional Anesth Pain Med 2004; 29: 454–61.

A review of the literature found that sympathetic blocks for herpes zoster and postherpetic neuralgia appear to be useful, but require randomized control trials for validation.

Transcutaneous electrical nerve stimulation for chronic pain. Bates JA, Nathan PW. Anaesthesia 1980; 35: 817–22.

One-third of patients treated were continuing to use treatment after 1 year, and one-quarter after 2 years. The rest stopped treatment because it was ineffective, made the pain worse, or the pain became worse after stopping treatment.

Evidence Levels: **A** Double-blind study **B** Clinical trial ≥ 20 subjects **C** Clinical trial < 20 subjects **D** Series ≥ 5 subjects **E** Anecdotal case reports

Hidradenitis suppurativa

Gregor BE Jemec

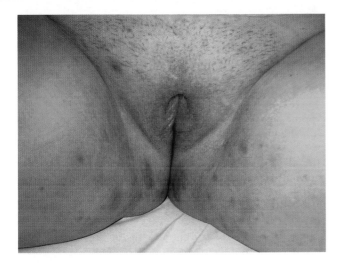

Hidradenitis suppurativa (HS) is a common chronic recurrent multifocal disease of the skin and subcutaneous tissues that affects the flexural areas, where it causes inflammation, scarring, and sinus tract formation. It is a follicular disease distinct from acne vulgaris, staphylococcosis, and furunculosis. Pain and suppuration cause considerable morbidity and significantly impair quality of life.

MANAGEMENT STRATEGY

Age of onset is usually after the teenage period. No pathognomonic test exists. Early diagnosis relies on the recognition of recurrent, multifocal, often bilateral, painful inflammatory lesions of the axillae and the anogenital region.

Early lesions are often 'blind boils' (i.e., rounded and deep). Scarring and sinus tracts gradually develop in separate areas of the affected region, and ultimately lesions coalesce to form inflamed fibrotic conglomerates of scarring, suppuration, and sinus tract formation. Early lesions are accessible to medical treatment, whereas more advanced lesions require surgical intervention for cure.

Clinically HS can be distinguished from furunculosis (often large boils not restricted to flexural areas) and epidermal cysts (often solitary lesions). Microbiology is mostly helpful in the later stages of the disease when superinfection occurs, as early lesions often are sterile on routine culture of swabs. Suspicion of mycobacterial infection, metastasis, or Crohn's disease requires specific investigations.

Current medical practice is essentially empirical. A three-stage approach gives structure to patient management. The first stage consists of topical treatment. Topical clindamycin has been shown in a double-blind, placebo-controlled study to have an effect on early lesions. Systemic tetracycline (500 mg orally twice daily) may be used as an alternative. This treatment can be supplemented with azeleic cream once daily to maintain effect, or 15% resorcinol cream twice daily for flares. Specific treatment should be directed at superinfections. Hormonal therapy with cyproterone acetate may be helpful for some women, but requires high dosage and continuous use, which raises safety concerns.

Once scarring or sinus tract formation occurs, minor excisions or CO_2 laser evaporation of lesions may be beneficial for the patient.

The third stage of treatment involves major surgery or palliative medication. Surgery should involve excision of the affected tissue, but not lancing. The recurrence rate is inversely proportional to the extent of surgery: wide extensive surgery may offer a better chance of remission. Palliative medication includes systemic anti-inflammatory drugs such as dapsone, oral corticosteroids, ciclosporin, or TNF-α inhibitors. An initial anti-inflammatory response may be followed by relapse or superinfection. HS shows little sign of improvement with isotretinoin.

General measures that reduce smoking and pressure or shearing forces at the affected sites are advisable, as is weight loss in the obese.

SPECIFIC INVESTIGATIONS

▶ Histopathology
▶ Microbiology
▶ Preoperative ultrasound scans/MRI to determine the extent of the disease

Hidradenitis suppurativa: a disease of follicular epithelium, rather than apocrine glands. Yu CC, Cook MG. Br J Dermatol 1990; 122: 763–9.

Squamous epithelium-lined structures (probably abnormal hair follicles) are a constant diagnostic feature of HS.

The bacteriology of hidradenitis suppurativa. Jemec GB, Faber M, Gutschik E, Wendelboe P. Dermatology 1996; 193: 203–6.

Bacteria are found in 50% of all lesions.

Real-time compound imaging ultrasound of hidradenitis suppurativa. Wortsman X, Jemec GB. Dermatol Surg 2007; 33: 1340–2.

High-frequency ultrasound identifies subclinical lesions.

FIRST-LINE THERAPIES

▶ Antibiotics	**B**
▶ Surgery	**B**

Topical treatment of hidradenitis suppurativa with clindamycin. Clemmensen OJ. Int J Dermatol 1983; 22: 325–8.

Topical clindamycin for 3 months was significantly more effective than placebo in early lesions.

Topical clindamycin versus systemic tetracycline in the treatment of hidradenitis suppurativa. Jemec GB, Wendelboe P. J Am Acad Dermatol 1998; 39: 971–4.

Oral tetracycline 1 g/day was not more effective than topical clindamycin for 3 months.

Clindamycin and rifampicin combination therapy for hidradenitis suppurativa. Mendonça CO, Griffiths CE. Br J Dermatol 2006; 154: 977–8.

Combination therapy with clindamycin 300 mg twice daily and rifampicin 300 mg twice daily may be effective.

Extent of surgery and recurrence rate of hidradenitis suppurativa. Ritz JP, Runkel N, Haier J, Buhr HJ. Int J Colorectal Dis 1998; 13: 164–8.

Drainage alone carried a recurrence rate of 100%; radical excision has a recurrence rate of 25% at a median observation time of 20 months.

SECOND-LINE THRAPIES

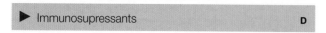

| ▶ Immunosupressants | D |

Hidradenitis suppurativa: pathogenesis and management. Slade DE, Powell BW, Mortimer PS. Br J Plast Surg 2003; 56: 451–61.

A good overview, including a mention of intralesional triamcinolone.

Cyclosporin-responsive hidradenitis suppurativa. Buckley DA, Rogers S. J Roy Soc Med 1995; 88: 289P–90P.

Immunosuppressant therapy can be helpful, but requires care in the presence of infection. The effect is unlikely to be specific for ciclosporin.

Long-term efficacy of a single course of infliximab in hidradenitis suppurativa. Mekkes JR, Bos JD. Br J Dermatol 2008; 158: 370–4.

The use of TNF-α inhibitor may induce long-lasting remission.

THIRD-LINE THERAPIES

▶ Antiandrogens	B
▶ Dapsone	D
▶ Retinoids	D

A double-blind controlled cross-over trial of cyproterone acetate in females with hidradenitis suppurativa. Mortimer PS, Dawber RP, Gales MA, Moore RA. Br J Dermatol 1986; 115: 263–8.

Some benefit may be derived from treating female patients with antiandrogens.

Hidradenitis suppurativa treated with dapsone: A case series of five patients. Kaur MR, Lewis HM. J Dermatol Treat 2006; 17: 211–13.

Dapsone may benefit some patients in long-term treatment.

Long-term results of isotretinoin in the treatment of 68 patients with hidradenitis suppurativa. Boer J, van Gemert MJ. J Am Acad Dermatol 1999; 40: 73–6.

Isotretinoin had a generally poor effect; any effect was mainly in mild disease.

Histoplasmosis

Mahreen Ameen, Wanda Sonia Robles

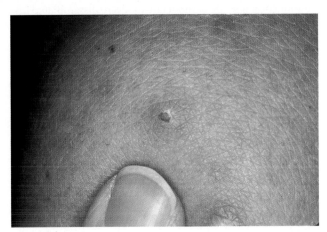

From Lebwohl MG. The Skin and Systemic Disease: A Color Atlas, 2nd edn. Churchill Livingstone 2003, with permission of Elsevier.

Histoplasmosis is an endemic mycosis caused by a dimorphic fungus, *Histoplasma capsulatum*, of which there are two varieties that are pathogenic to humans. The most common variety worldwide is *H. capsulatum* var. *capsulatum*, which is highly endemic in the USA, particularly in the Mississippi and the Ohio valleys. *H. capsulatum* var. *duboisii* is endemic only in Central and West Africa (where it coexists with *H. capsulatum* var. *capsulatum*), and it is therefore sometimes referred to as African histoplasmosis. The infection is usually contracted through inhalation of spores in dry soil or bird or bat droppings. Disease progression and severity depend on the intensity of exposure to *H. capsulatum* and host immunity. There is a wide clinical spectrum of disease. Acute pulmonary disease is the most common presentation, and most cases are either asymptomatic or mild and self-limiting. Chronic pulmonary histoplasmosis, usually occurring in patients with underlying lung disease, produces cavities and later progression to pulmonary fibrosis. Hematogenous dissemination occurs within the first few weeks, but resolves with the development of cell-mediated immunity to *H. capsulatum*. Progressive disseminated histoplasmosis occurs in the immunocompromised. Patient groups at risk include those with AIDS, hematological malignancies, those on immunosuppressive therapy (including corticosteroids and tumor necrosis factor antagonists), transplant recipients, and infants. Disseminated histoplasmosis is an AIDS-defining illness. It is usually a reactivation of prior infection and a sign of advanced immunosuppression, generally occurring in those with CD4 counts <150 cells/mm³.

Disseminated histoplasmosis can involve every organ system, most commonly presenting with hepatosplenomegaly and mucocutaneous lesions. Molluscum-like papules, nodules, or ulcerative lesions affect the skin, and are usually localized to the face, upper chest, and arms. Oropharyngeal ulcers affect the buccal mucosa, tongue, gingiva, lips, pharynx, and larynx. Histoplasmosis may also present to the dermatologist as a cause of erythema multiforme or erythema nodosum, which are thought to be a hypersensitivity response to the *H. capsulatum* antigen. Rarely, primary cutaneous lesions may arise from direct inoculation.

MANAGEMENT STRATEGY

Pulmonary forms of histoplasmosis in the acute phase usually resolve spontaneously and only require treatment if symptoms persist for more than 1 month. Oral *itraconazole* is the treatment of choice for mild to moderate disease. Severe pulmonary infection, disseminated histoplasmosis, and infection in the immunocompromised, particularly in association with AIDS, should be treated with *amphotericin B* (AmB) formulations (AmB deoxycholate, liposomal AmB or AmB lipid complex). The lipid formulations carry a lower risk of nephrotoxicity but are more expensive. Treatment is commenced with AmB until there is clinical improvement, and then stepped down to oral itraconazole. Fluconazole and ketoconazole are second-line alternatives to itraconazole. *Ketoconazole* carries higher risks of adverse effects than the other azoles. The new triazoles *voriconazole* and *posaconazole* demonstrate in vitro activity against *H. capsulatum*, and have been successfully used in individual cases for different forms of histoplasmosis infection.

Patients with AIDS-related histoplasmosis who undergo antiretroviral treatment have better outcomes than those who are not treated with antiretrovirals. Some clinicians defer commencement of antiretroviral therapy until there is a reduction in fungal burden to avoid precipitating immune reconstitution inflammatory syndrome (IRIS). However, IRIS is a rare complication of histoplasmosis and is not usually severe. Therefore, others advocate early antiretroviral therapy to improve cellular immunity, a key defense against *H. capsulatum*.

SPECIFIC INVESTIGATIONS

- ► Culture
- ► Histology
- ► Serology
- ► Serology for HIV (where relevant)
- ► Imaging studies to detect disseminated disease (CXR/CT/MRI)

The gold standard method for diagnosing histoplasmosis is the isolation of *H. capsulatum* from culture. The use of several specimens (sputum, bronchoalveolar lavage, skin lesions, blood, bone marrow, or liver) for culture will increase the yield. Culture is highly specific but limited by slow growth, and plates must be kept for as long as 12 weeks. Blood culture using the lysis–centrifugation system is more rapid and increases sensitivity. Histopathology is also more rapid, but its sensitivity is <50% in patients with disseminated disease, and even lower in pulmonary histoplasmosis. Biopsy specimens may demonstrate the distinctive 2–4 μm oval, narrow-based budding yeasts of *H. capsulatum*. Serological tests are rapid but may be falsely negative in immunosuppressed patients, and during the first 2 months following exposure while antibodies are still developing. In addition, elevated antibody titers persist for several years after the initial infection. Antigen detection is a rapid means of diagnosis in patients with disseminated disease. Sensitivity is greater with urine than with other body fluids (plasma, bronchoalveolar lavage fluid, or cerebrospinal fluid). Antigen quantification enables treatment response to be monitored.

In disseminated disease, general laboratory tests will reveal a pancytopenia, hyperbilirubinemia, elevated liver enzyme and serum lactate dehydrogenase levels.

FIRST-LINE THERAPIES

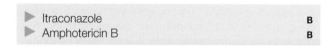

| ▶ Itraconazole | B |
| ▶ Amphotericin B | B |

Itraconazole therapy for blastomycosis and histoplasmosis. Dismukes WE, Bradsher RW Jr, Cloud GC, Kauffman CA, Chapman SW, George RB, et al.; NIAID Mycoses Study Group. Am J Med 1992; 93: 489–97.

This was a prospective, non-randomized, multicenter open trial where 37 patients with histoplasmosis received itraconazole 200–400 mg daily; 81% (n=30) were cured after a median treatment period of 9 months. Treatment failure occurred only in those patients with chronic cavitary pulmonary disease. Twenty-nine percent (n=25) experienced minor adverse effects, requiring therapy withdrawal in only one patient.

Itraconazole treatment of disseminated histoplasmosis in patients with the acquired immunodeficiency syndrome. Wheat J, Hafner R, Korzun AH, Limjoco MT, Spencer P, Larsen RA, et al. AIDS Clinical Trial Group. Am J Med 1995; 98: 336–42.

A multicenter non-randomized prospective trial in which itraconazole 300 mg twice daily for 3 days followed by 200 mg twice daily was given for 12 weeks. Evaluation of 59 patients showed that 50 (85%) responded well to therapy. Five withdrew from the study because of progressive infection. One died within the first week of therapy, and two withdrew because of itraconazole-related adverse effects. Resolution of systemic symptoms occurred after a median of 3 weeks in the less severely affected, and 6 weeks in the moderately severe cases. Fungemia cleared after a median of 1 week.

Itraconazole demonstrates efficacy in the treatment of mild disseminated histoplasmosis in patients with AIDS. For patients with moderately severe or severe histoplasmosis, amphotericin B is the drug of first choice, which can be switched to itraconazole after clinical improvement.

Clearance of fungal burden during treatment of disseminated histoplasmosis with liposomal amphotericin B versus itraconazole. Wheat LJ, Cloud G, Johnson PC, Connolly P, Goldman M, Le Monte A, et al. NIAID Mycoses Study Group. Antimicrob Agents Chemother 2001; 45: 2354–7.

Animal studies have shown that fungal burden correlates with survival during treatment with antifungal therapies for histoplasmosis. This study compared the clearance of fungal burden in patients with AIDS-related disseminated histoplasmosis treated with liposomal amphotericin B versus itraconazole. The clinical response rates were similar: 86% with liposomal amphotericin B versus 85% with itraconazole. However, there was a more rapid clearance of fungemia with liposomal amphotericin B than with itraconazole (85% vs 53%, p=0.0008). Antigen levels in serum and urine also fell more rapidly in the amphotericin B treatment group. The authors conclude that the more rapid clearance of fungemia supports the use of liposomal amphotericin B rather than itraconazole for the initial treatment of moderately severe or severe histoplasmosis.

Safety and efficacy of liposomal amphotericin B compared with conventional amphotericin B for induction therapy of histoplasmosis in patients with AIDS. Johnson PC, Wheat LJ, Cloud GA, Goldman M, Lancaster D, Bamberger DM, et al.; NIAID Mycoses Study Group. Ann Intern Med 2002; 137: 105–9.

A multicenter randomized, controlled trial compared amphotericin B deoxycholate with liposomal amphotericin B for induction therapy of moderate to severe disseminated histoplasmosis in patients with AIDS. The trial demonstrated a higher response rate (88% vs 64%) and lower mortality (2% vs 13%) in patients who were treated with liposomal amphotericin (n=51) than in those treated with amphotericin B deoxycholate (n=22). Infusion-related side effects were greater with amphotericin B deoxycholate nephrotoxicity.

This study demonstrated that liposomal amphotericin is associated with higher efficacy, lower mortality, and better tolerance during induction treatment of disseminated histoplasmosis.

Safety of discontinuation of maintenance therapy for disseminated histoplasmosis after immunologic response to antiretroviral therapy. Goldman M, Zackin R, Fichtenbaum CJ, Skiest DJ, Koletar SL, Hafner R, et al.; AIDS Clinical Trials Group A5038 Study Group. Clin Infect Dis 2004; 38: 1485–9.

Traditionally, lifelong maintenance therapy with itraconazole had been the standard of care in order to reduce the risk of relapse of histoplasmosis infection. This study concluded that discontinuation of antifungal therapy after 12 months appears to be safe in patients with previously treated disseminated histoplasmosis who have sustained immunological improvement with antiretroviral therapy.

Disseminated histoplasmosis: a comparative study between patients with acquired immunodeficiency syndrome and non-human immunodeficiency virus-infected individuals. Tobon AM, Agudelo CA, Rosero DS, Ochoa JE, De Bedout C, Zuluaga A, et al. Am J Trop Med Hyg 2005; 73: 576–82.

In this study of 52 patients with disseminated histoplasmosis, 30 had AIDS. Skin lesions were significantly more numerous in patients with AIDS. *H. capsulatum* was isolated more often in AIDS patients, but antibodies to *H. capsulatum* were detected more frequently in non-HIV patients. Itraconazole treatment was less effective in AIDS patients (p=0.012), but HAART improved the response to antifungals.

The authors emphasize that the skin constitutes a more important target organ for H. capsulatum *in HIV-infected Latin American patients than in HIV-infected North American patients.*

Literature review and case histories of *Histoplasma capsulatum* var. *duboisii* infections in HIV-infected patients. Loulergue P, Bastides F, Baudouin V, Chandenier J, Mariani-Kurkdjian P, Dupont B, et al. Emerg Infect Dis 2007; 13: 1647–52.

African histoplasmosis caused by *Histoplasma capsulatum* var. *duboisii* is much rarer than histoplasmosis caused by variety *capsulatum*, and its association with HIV infection is rarely reported. This article reports three such cases and reviews the literature on similar cases. All were successfully treated, initially with amphotericin B, which was subsequently switched to itraconazole. No clinical trials or efficacy studies have been performed for African histoplasmosis, and therefore its treatment is usually extrapolated from the guidelines of the Infectious Diseases Society of America established for histoplasmosis due to variety *capsulatum*.

Disseminated primary cutaneous histoplasmosis successfully treated with itraconazole. Singhi MK, Gupta L, Kacchawa D, Gupta D. Ind J Dermatol Venereol Leprol 2003; 69: 405–7.

Primary cutaneous histoplasmosis is rare. This is a report of a case of disseminated primary cutaneous histoplasmosis caused by *H. capsulatum* in an immunocompetent patient.

SECOND-LINE THERAPIES

▶ Ketoconazole	B
▶ Fluconazole	B
▶ Posaconazole	D
▶ Voriconazole	E

Treatment of blastomycosis and histoplasmosis with ketoconazole. Results of a prospective randomized clinical trial. Dismukes WE, Cloud G, Bowles C; NIAID Mycoses Study Group. Ann Intern Med 1985; 103: 861–72.

This was a multicentre, prospective randomized trial evaluating the efficacy and toxicity of low-dose (400 mg/day) and high-dose (800 mg/day) oral ketoconazole. The success rate for all patients treated for 6 months or more was 85%. Adverse effects occurred in 60% of patients, and were commoner with the high-dose regimen. Because of the higher frequency of side effects associated with the high dose, the authors suggested that ketoconazole therapy should be initiated at the lower dose.

With the availability of better-tolerated and new-generation azoles, there are no recent studies evaluating ketoconazole therapy for histoplasmosis. However, it is still a drug that is commonly used in endemic settings, because of its availability and low cost.

Fluconazole therapy for histoplasmosis. McKinsey DS, Kauffman CA, Pappas PG, Cloud GA, Girard WM, Sharkey PK, et al.; NIAID Mycoses Study Group. Clin Infect Dis 1996; 23: 996–1001.

Twenty-seven patients were enrolled into this trial. Two had acute pulmonary histoplasmosis, 11 had chronic pulmonary histoplasmosis, and 14 had disseminated histoplasmosis. Twenty patients received fluconazole 400–800 mg/day, and seven received fluconazole 200 mg daily. Successful treatment was reported in 17 patients (63%). There were no significant adverse effects. The authors concluded that fluconazole was only moderately effective and should be reserved for patients intolerant to itraconazole.

Treatment of histoplasmosis with fluconazole in patients with acquired immunodeficiency syndrome. Wheat J, MaWhinney S, Hafner R, McKinsey D, Chen D, Korzun A, et al.; NIAID AIDS Clinical Trials Group and Mycoses Study Group. Am J Med 1997; 103: 223–32.

Fluconazole may have a role in the treatment of non-AIDS-related histoplasmosis. However, this study of AIDS-related infection demonstrated a comparatively poor efficacy rate with even high-dose fluconazole induction therapy, and an unacceptably high relapse rate with maintenance therapy.

Salvage treatment of histoplasmosis with posaconazole. Restrepo A, Tobón A, Clark B, Graham DR, Corcoran G, Bradsher RW, Goldman M, et al. J Infect 2007; 54: 319–27.

Six patients with severe histoplasmosis infection were successfully treated with oral posaconazole (800 mg/day in divided doses) having previously failed on amphotericin B, itraconazole, fluconazole, or voriconazole.

A patient with new-onset seizure and mediastinal adenopathy. Truong MT, Sabloff BS, Munden RF, Erasmus JJ. Chest 2004; 126: 982–5.

A 41-year-old non-HIV-infected woman from Texas was diagnosed with disseminated histoplasmosis with CNS involvement. She was treated with voriconazole, with an initial loading dose followed by a maintenance dose of 200 mg twice daily. Within 1 month of treatment repeat chest radiographs showed a reduction in mediastinal and hilar adenopathy. There are no further details regarding treatment duration and follow-up period.

Clinical practice guidelines for the management of patients with histoplasmosis: 2007 update by the Infectious Diseases Society of America. Wheat LJ, Freifeld AG, Kleiman MB, Baddley JW, McKinsey DS, Loyd JE, Kauffman CA; Infectious Diseases Society of America. Clin Infect Dis 2007; 45: 807–25.

Evidence-based guidelines for the management of patients with histoplasmosis.

Mild acute pulmonary histoplasmosis

Treatment is usually unnecessary unless symptoms persist for more than 1 month, when itraconazole is given at a loading dose (200 mg three times daily for 3 days) followed by 200 mg once or twice daily for 6–12 weeks.

Severe acute pulmonary histoplasmosis

Parenteral amphotericin B (deoxycholate formulation, 0.7–1.0 mg/kg daily, or lipid formulation, 3.0–5.0 mg/kg daily) for 1–2 weeks followed by 'stepdown' itraconazole therapy, with an initial loading dose and then 200 mg twice daily for a total of 12 weeks.

Chronic cavitary pulmonary histoplasmosis

Itraconazole, initial loading dose and then 200 mg once or twice daily for at least 12 months.

Mild disseminated histoplasmosis

Itraconazole, initial loading dose and then 200 mg twice daily for at least 12 months.

Severe disseminated histoplasmosis

Amphotericin B (doses as above for severe pulmonary infection) for 1–2 weeks followed by oral itraconazole, initial loading dose and then 200 mg twice daily for at least 12 months.

CNS histoplasmosis

Liposomal amphotericin B (5.0 mg/kg daily for a total of 175 mg/kg given over 4–6 weeks) followed by itraconazole 200 mg two or three times daily for at least 1 year and until resolution of CSF abnormalities, including *Histoplasma* antigen levels.

Treatment of histoplasmosis in pregnancy

Azoles are teratogenic and therefore amphotericin B is recommended.

Hydroa vacciniforme

Herbert Hönigsmann

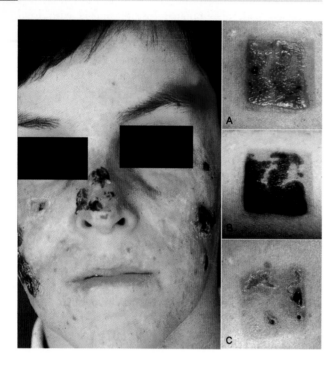

In patients with more severe disease, however, courses of *narrowband UVB phototherapy* or *psoralen with UVA (PUVA)* administered as for polymorphic light eruption may help occasionally. Both phototherapy regimens usually consist of thrice-weekly treatments for an average of 3–4 weeks. It is important to administer these therapies carefully to avoid provoking disease exacerbations.

Antimicrobial therapy has also been tried, as have antimalarials and systemic immunosuppressive therapy, including intermittent oral corticosteroids, but although occasionally helpful, none of these appear to be reliably effective. β-Carotene, used in several studies, however, was mostly shown to be ineffective.

For severe and refractory hydroa vacciniforme unresponsive to other therapies, immunosuppressive agents including *azathioprine* and *ciclosporin* may be effective, but thalidomide does not seem to be. However, the use of immunosuppressive drugs for an admittedly unpleasant, but otherwise benign, disease should be carefully considered.

In two reports, *dietary fish oil* rich in omega-3 polyunsaturated fatty acids was associated with clinical improvement in three of four patients. The mechanism may be through inhibition of prostanoid production and by their proposed buffering effect against free radical-induced damage.

The rare nature of this condition means that there are no large or randomized trials. Evidence for treatment is based on case series or single reports.

Hydroa vacciniforme is a very rare, idiopathic photodermatosis that mainly starts in childhood, frequently resolving by adolescence or young adulthood. Its prevalence is 0.1–0.5 cases per 100 000 per year. It is characterized by recurrent crops of papulovesicles or vesicles, most commonly on the face and the dorsa of the hands, but other sun-exposed areas of the skin, such as the lower lips, may also be involved. The vesicles resolve with pock-like scarring. The disease was first described by Bazin in 1862, and it is possible that before the clear definition of erythropoietic protoporphyria by Magnus et al. in 1961, some cases may have been protoporphyria rather than hydroa because of the similarity of symptoms. Several reports of an association with Epstein–Barr virus (EBV) infection are interesting, but not all these cases are typical: they are associated with NK/T-cell lymphoproliferative disorders with a frequently fatal outcome, and may not represent the usual form of hydroa vacciniforme.

MANAGEMENT STRATEGY

Hydroa vacciniforme usually presents in childhood, sometimes with spontaneous improvement during adolescence. Parents generally seek specialist advice because their children are unable to tolerate sunshine (play outdoors or travel abroad) and because the eruption can result in considerable scarring, both of which cause significant morbidity.

Hydroa vacciniforme is almost always refractory to any treatment, but *restriction of sun exposure, appropriate clothing, and regular use of broad-spectrum sunscreens with an effective UVA filter* can help in mild to moderate disease. Windows in the car and home can be covered with films that filter UV wavelengths less than 380 nm.

SPECIFIC INVESTIGATIONS

> ▶ Erythrocyte and plasma protoporphyrin levels, red cell photohemolysis, and stool analysis
> ▶ Photoprovocation testing with UVA
> ▶ Serology for antinuclear antibody and extractable nuclear antigens
> ▶ Screening for EBV infection and detection of EBV-infected cells by T-cell receptor-γ gene rearrangement with polymerase chain reaction
> ▶ A porphyrin screen will exclude erythropoietic protoporphyria.

Photoprovocation testing induces typical blisters. Light tests are abnormal in the UVA range. Photographs to the right of the figure show the result of photoprovocation with UVA (three times 30 cm² on 3 consecutive days): A. After 24 hours. B. After 48 hours. C. After 2 weeks.

Serology for antinuclear antibody and extractable nuclear antigens (anti-Ro, La, and Sm) will exclude bullous lupus erythematosus, which quite commonly can be ruled out by its clinical symptoms.

Rare cases have been associated with metabolic disorders, such as Hartnup disease, and so aminoaciduria should be ruled out.

Screening for EBV is required only if lymphoma is suspected.

Hydroa vacciniforme – Aktionsspektrum. Jaschke E, Hönigsmann H. Hautarzt 1981; 32: 350–3.

Successful photoprovocation with UVA in one case.

Hydroa vacciniforme: a review of ten cases. Sonnex TS, Hawk JLM. Br J Dermatol 1988; 118: 101–8.

Successful photoprovocation with UVA in several cases.

Hydroa vacciniforme: a clinical and follow-up study of 17 cases. Gupta G, Man I, Kemmett D. J Am Acad Dermatol 2000; 42: 208–13.

Eight of 14 patients were sensitive in the UVA spectrum. UVA provocation tests showed a papulovesicular response in six of 14 patients.

There is now strong evidence that UVA radiation is the causal factor. In addition to reduced UVA minimal erythema dose values, repetitive broad-spectrum UVA has been shown to reproduce lesions that are clinically and histologically identical to those produced by natural sunlight and which heal with scarring. All cases seen so far by this author (HH) had their action spectrum in the UVA range.

Epstein–Barr virus-associated lymphoproliferative lesions presenting as a hydroa vacciniforme-like eruption: an analysis of six cases. Cho KH, Lee SH, Kim CW, Jeon YK, Kwon IH, Cho YJ, et al. Br J Dermatol 2004; 151: 372–80.

A report of six patients and review of the literature.

This type of sunlight-induced rash may well be a different entity, but this requires further investigations.

Pathogenic link between hydroa vacciniforme and Epstein–Barr virus-associated hematologic disorders. Iwatsuki K, Satoh M, Yamamoto T, Oono T, Morizane S, Ohtsuka M, et al. Arch Dermatol 2006; 142: 587–95.

T cells positive for EBV-encoded small nuclear RNA (EBER) were detected, to various degrees, in cutaneous infiltrates in 28 (97%) of 29 patients, including all six patients with definite HV having a positive phototest reaction.

FIRST-LINE THERAPIES

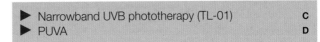

| ▶ High-factor broad-spectrum sunscreens and behavioral sunlight avoidance | C |

Hydroa vacciniforme: a clinical and follow-up study of 17 cases. Gupta G, Man I, Kemmett D. J Am Acad Dermatol 2000; 42: 208–13.

Disease in nine of 15 patients was controlled satisfactorily with high-factor broad-spectrum sunscreens and sunlight avoidance.

Hydroa vacciniforme: a review of ten cases. Sonnex TS, Hawk JLM. Br J Dermatol 1988; 118: 101–8.

Disease severity was reduced in eight of 10 patients using either Coppertone Supershade 15 or ROC Factor 10.

Most sunscreens offer good UVB but not UVA protection. The new Dundee sunscreen Reflectant Sun Screen, which is available from Tayside Pharmaceuticals, Ninewells Hospital and Medical School, Dundee DD1 9SY, UK, offers better protection in the UVA and visible spectra.

Borrowing from museums and industry: two photoprotective devices. Dawe R, Russell S, Ferguson J. Br J Dermatol 1996; 135: 1016–17.

The Museum 200 Film (manufactured by Sun Guard, Florida, USA) prevents transmission of all wavelengths less than 380 nm.

This is a clear, lightweight film that can be stuck on to any glass surface without causing visual impairment. It may be a useful adjunct in the treatment of most photodermatoses, but

in some patients with hydroa vacciniforme, particularly those who are sensitive in the 380–400 nm wavelengths, it may not be beneficial.

SECOND-LINE THERAPIES

| ▶ Narrowband UVB phototherapy (TL-01) | C |
| ▶ PUVA | D |

Narrow-band UVB (TL-01) phototherapy: an effective preventative treatment for the photodermatoses. Collins P, Ferguson J. Br J Dermatol 1995; 132: 956–63.

This was an open clinical trial in which four patients were treated on average 10 times on a daily basis. Two of these patients reported an increase in tolerance to sunshine from 1 hour to 3–6 hours.

Hydroa vacciniforme: a clinical and follow-up study of 17 cases. Gupta G, Man I, Kemmett D. J Am Acad Dermatol 2000; 42: 208–13.

Five of 15 patients who had not responded to conservative measures were treated with narrowband UVB phototherapy. In three patients there was good or moderate disease control. In the other two, narrowband UVB phototherapy was not helpful.

Narrowband ultraviolet B (UVB) phototherapy in children. Jury CS, McHenry P, Burden AD, Lever R, Bilsland D. Clin Exp Dermatol 2006; 31: 196–9.

Narrowband UVB phototherapy is a useful and well tolerated treatment for children with severe or intractable inflammatory skin disease.

Hydroa vacciniforme: a review of ten cases. Sonnex TS, Hawk JLM. Br J Dermatol 1988; 118: 101–8.

Two of 10 patients were treated with UVB and had improvement of their disease. There was a flare of hydroa vacciniforme in the one patient treated with PUVA.

It is likely that broadband UVB was used in this report, but the methodology is unclear.

Hydroa vacciniforme – Aktionsspektrum. Jaschke E, Hönigsmann H. Hautarzt 1981; 32: 350–3.

One patient received PUVA therapy and had good control of his disease.

Photosensitivity disorders: cause, effect and management. Millard TP, Hawk JL. Am J Clin Dermatol 2002; 3: 239–46.

A review of the management of various photodermatosis, with reference to the use of UVB and PUVA.

THIRD-LINE THERAPIES

▶ Antimalarials	D
▶ β-Carotene	E
▶ Azathioprine	E
▶ Ciclosporin	E
▶ Dietary fish oil	E
▶ Thalidomide	E

Hydroa vacciniforme: a review of ten cases. Sonnex TS, Hawk JLM. Br J Dermatol 1988; 118: 101–8.

Four of 10 patients were treated with either hydroxychloroquine (two patients) or chloroquine (two patients). Hydroxychloroquine 100 mg daily was ineffective, but the two patients on chloroquine (100–125 mg daily) had a reduction in the severity of their disease.

Hydroa vacciniforme: an unusual clinical manifestation. Leenutaphong V. J Am Acad Dermatol 1991; 25: 892–5.

One patient treated with chloroquine phosphate 500 mg daily did not find it beneficial.

Hydroa vacciniforme. Ketterer R, Morier P, Frenk E. Dermatology 1994; 189: 428–9.

One patient treated with chloroquine 100 mg daily and broad-spectrum sunscreens showed good disease control.

It is unclear whether the response was due to chloroquine or the sunscreen.

Hydroa vacciniforme. Bickers DR, Demar LK, DeLeo V, Poh-Fitzpatrick MB, Aronberg JM, Harber LC. Arch Dermatol 1978; 114: 1193–6.

Two patients reported an improvement of their disease with β-carotene 180 mg daily.

Hydroa vacciniforme: induction of lesions with ultraviolet A. Halasz CLG, Leach EE, Walther RR, Poh-Fitzpatrick MB. J Am Acad Dermatol 1983; 8: 171–6.

The one patient treated with β-carotene 180 mg daily reported some subjective improvement.

Hydroa vacciniforme: diagnosis and therapy. Goldgeier MH, Nordlund JJ, Lucky AW, Sibrack LA, McCarthy MJ, McGuire J. Arch Dermatol 1982; 118: 588–91.

β-Carotene 120 mg daily for 2 months in the one patient was ineffective.

Hydroa vacciniforme presenting in an adult successfully treated with cyclosporin A. Blackwell V, McGregor JM, Hawk JLM. Clin Exp Dermatol 1998; 23: 73–6.

Azathioprine 2.5–3.5 mg/kg daily was ineffective in the one patient studied.

See additional report on the use of azathioprine below.

Hydroa vacciniforme presenting in an adult successfully treated with cyclosporin A. Blackwell V, McGregor JM, Hawk JLM. Clin Exp Dermatol 1998; 23: 73–6.

There was good control of disease with ciclosporin A 3 mg/kg daily over a 2-month period.

The report does not provide details of follow-up.

Hydroa vacciniforme: traitement par huiles de poisson (Maxepa®). Modeste AB, Cordel N, Balguerie X, Leroy D, Lauret P, Joly P. Ann Dermatol Venereol 2001; 128: 247–9.

One patient was successfully treated with dietary fish oil after unsuccessful treatment with antimalarials.

Dietary fish oil as a photoprotective agent in hydroa vacciniforme. Rhodes LE, White SI. Br J Dermatol 1998; 138: 173–8.

Three patients were treated with dietary fish oil, five capsules daily for 3 months. A mild to good improvement was noted in two patients, but no improvement in the third.

The latter patient responded to azathioprine. The action of fish oils may be through inhibition of prostanoid production and by their proposed buffering effect against free radical-induced damage.

Hydroa vacciniforme: major and minor forms. Cruces MJ, de la Torre C. Photodermatology 1986; 3: 109–10.

In the one patient treated with thalidomide there was initial improvement.

Hydroa vacciniforme presenting in an adult successfully treated with cyclosporin A. Blackwell V, McGregor JM, Hawk JLM. Clin Exp Dermatol 1998; 23: 73–6.

In the one patient, thalidomide 100 mg daily was ineffective. Ciclosporin proved helpful at 3 mg/kg/day.

Hyperhidrosis

James AA Langtry

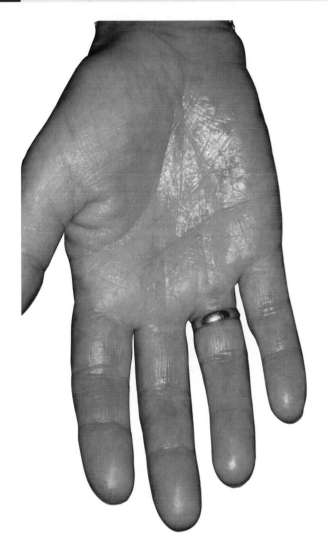

Hyperhidrosis is the result of increased secretion of eccrine sweat. This can be annoying, disabling (at work or socially), or indicative of an underlying systemic disease. The eccrine gland is unusual in that the sympathetic sudomotor fibers are cholinergic rather than adrenergic.

The classification of hyperhidrosis is variously described. Two approaches are *idiopathic/pathologic* and *neural/non-neural*.

Idiopathic hyperhidrosis is defined as excessive sweating that is symmetrical, localized to the palms, soles, or axillae (singly or in combination), and independent of thermoregulation. Craniofacial hyperhidrosis is a similar but rarer condition. The other characteristics include its episodic nature, occurrence in response to stimuli, and onset at or after puberty; there is commonly a family history. There is an absence of bromhidrosis and little or no seasonal variation. *Pathologic* hyperhidrosis may be localized or generalized. Localized hyperhidrosis may result from injury to the central or peripheral nervous systems, syringomyelia, neuritis, myelitis, tabes dorsalis, or localized vascular diseases,

including cold injury, arteriovenous malformation (AVM), and erythrocyanosis. Localized hyperhidrosis can occur as a functional nevus in which a normal number of eccrine glands are oversensitive to acetylcholine. Localized areas of hyperhidrosis can develop as a compensatory phenomenon when extensive anhidrosis develops in Ross syndrome (bilateral Holmes Adie pupils, tendon areflexia, generalized anhidrosis, and compensatory islands of hyperhidrosis). Hyperhidrosis may occur in hereditary conditions, including blue rubber bleb nevus syndrome. The causes of generalized hyperhidrosis include febrile illnesses; metabolic and endocrine diseases (diabetes, hyperthyroidism, gout, acromegaly, pregnancy, porphyria, pheochromocytoma, carcinoid syndrome, alcohol intoxication); congestive cardiac failure and shock; internal malignancy; CNS diseases (tumors and injury); and hereditary syndromes (Chediak–Higashi syndrome and phenylketonuria).

The *neural/non-neural* classification is based on the efferent sudomotor pathway, which consists of the cerebral cortex (emotional – the equivalent of idiopathic hyperhidrosis), hypothalamus (thermoregulatory, exercise, drugs, infection, metabolic, cardiovascular, vasomotor, neurologic), medulla (syringomyelia, auriculotemporal syndrome), spinal cord (syringomyelia, injury, tabes dorsalis), sympathetic ganglia, and postganglionic fibers. Facial surgery (particularly of the parotid) and trauma may result in localized gustatory sweating (Frey's syndrome). Hyperhidrosis of *non-neural* causes include local heat, local changes in blood flow (arteriovenous malformation), and drugs (cholinergic).

MANAGEMENT STRATEGY

The treatments discussed here apply primarily to the symptomatic management of idiopathic hyperhidrosis.

Local treatments, including medical, electrical, or surgical modalities, aim to stop or reduce sweating sufficiently to control symptoms. Treatments with the lowest risk should be considered first, as dictated by the severity of the condition and in discussion with the patient to assess the balance of risk and benefit.

Topical aluminum chloride hexahydrate (ACH) 20–25% solution in ethanol is the first-line treatment. The mechanism of action may result from occlusion of the intraepidermal eccrine duct below the level of the stratum corneum. Correct application technique is critical to compliance: in the axillae, the solution should be applied nightly to the unshaven skin, with or without occlusion, and washed off the following morning before daytime sweating is established. The presence of moisture results in the formation of hydrochloric acid and resultant skin irritation. Mild topical corticosteroids may be used to reduce the common problem of skin irritation, which is the usual reason for treatment failure. ACH solution should not be applied again in the morning. An oral anticholinergic (e.g., 1 mg of sodium glycopyrrolate) 45 minutes before the application of ACH may increase its efficacy by reducing sweating at the time of application, allowing the ACH to be retained on the skin and exert its effect on the sweat pores. The oral anticholinergic may be discontinued after several treatments have initiated a reduction in sweating.

Hyperhidrosis may take 2–3 weeks to be controlled with topical ACH, at which time application can be reduced to once a week, or at an interval that maintains control. Other topical therapies include formaldehyde, which is a common contact sensitizer, and glutaraldehyde, which stains the skin. *Methenamine gel* releases formaldehyde but does not appear to produce contact allergy frequently. The anticholinergic glycopyrrolate in 1.5–2% concentrations topically in an aqueous cream base or as glycopyrrolate pads may be effective.

Iontophoresis is the process of introducing salt ions in solution through the skin into the tissues, and may be effective in treating palmoplantar and axillary hyperhidrosis. Several iontophoretic devices are commercially available. Current is transmitted to electrodes in two trays filled with tap water, and the hands or feet are placed flat in the bottom of the trays. The current is increased until the patient experiences slight discomfort (average 15 mA on the palms and 20 mA on the soles). A special electrode for axillary use is available for some iontophoretic devices. The mechanism of reduction of sweating is not known. Current densities below the threshold of damage to the acrosyringium are employed, and mechanical obstruction does not occur. Iontophoresis is contraindicated in pregnancy and in patients with cardiac pacemakers and metal implants. Twenty-minute sessions three times a week are continued until sweating is sufficiently reduced; thereafter, once- or twice-monthly maintenance therapies are instituted. Anticholinergic drugs such as glycopyrridium bromide may also be introduced by electrophoresis. A recent report suggests that botulinum toxin delivered by iontophoresis to the palms may be effective in the treatment of palmar hyperhidrosis.

Oral anticholinergic drugs and *minor tranquilizers* produce a dose-related inhibition of sweating and are therefore limited by side effects. Anticholinergic effects, including dry mouth, pupillary dilatation and photophobia, glaucoma, urinary retention, constipation, vomiting, and tachycardia, may, however, occur at doses that produce satisfactory sweat inhibition, thereby limiting their use. The oral anticholinergics most commonly used are *glycopyrronium bromide* (Robinul), up to 2 mg three times daily, or *propantheline* 15 mg three times daily. Oral glycopyrronium bromide is not licensed for use in hyperhidrosis in the UK.

Other systemic drugs which have been used include the calcium channel blocker *diltiazem*, the CNS inhibitor *clonidine*, and *tricyclic antidepressants*, although these are the subject of few anecdotal reports.

Oral anticholinergic drugs, topical treatments, and iontophoresis may produce effective palliation of hyperhidrosis. More aggressive treatments may be sought, however, as a result of treatment failure, inconvenience of the treatments, or side effects.

Botulinum toxin injected intradermally produces sustained anhidrosis and has been used recently to treat axillary, palmar, facial, and other sites of focal hyperhidrosis. There are eight known serotypes of botulinum toxin, type A exotoxin (BTX-A) being the one that is commercially available as Botox and Dysport. These different commercially available BTX-A products differ in their potency and are not equivalent unit for unit. Botulinum toxin type B (BTX-B; Neurobloc) has been shown to be effective in the treatment of axillary hyperhidrosis and may be used as an alternative to BTX-A products, especially where antibody formation has resulted in a loss of clinical benefit to BTX-A. It is recommended that experience be gained with one of the products. It produces its effect by irreversibly blocking the release of acetylcholine from cholinergic junctions. Treatment of the axilla is simple and well tolerated. Multiple injections, 2 cm apart, are performed in the axillary vault corresponding to the area of maximum sweating (an area of approximately 200 cm²). Palmar skin is painful to inject (may require a regional nerve block), injection is less well tolerated, and there is a potential for producing weakness of the intrinsic hand musculature. It is not a practical treatment for plantar hyperhidrosis. Inactivation of affected cholinergic junctions is permanent, but new cholinergic junctions are produced through the natural process of tissue turnover and repair, so the effect is temporary. Onset of anhidrosis after injection occurs at 24–72 hours and lasts 3–6 months.

A number of surgical techniques have been employed in the management of axillary hyperhidrosis. These include:

- Cryotherapy (very painful and poorly tolerated).
- Methods that remove subcutaneous tissue alone. A number of skin flaps/incisions are described to gain access to the subcutaneous axillary tissues, and the deep dermis and adjacent subcutis are trimmed away. Subcutaneous curettage and axillary liposuction are other methods described for achieving this objective.
- Methods that excise skin and subcutaneous tissue.
- Methods that combine cutaneous excision and resection of subcutaneous tissue.

Selective ablation of the sympathetic innervation of the palms, axillae, and soles reduces sweating effectively. A number of side effects are associated with sympathectomy, including compensatory hyperhidrosis, Horner's syndrome, pneumothorax, and intraoperative cardiac arrest. Satisfactory long-term results are generally achieved, although recurrence of sweating usually occurs. It is best reserved for severe palmar hyperhidrosis (upper thoracic sympathectomy T2/T3 ganglia), avoiding denervation of the axillary sweat glands and thereby minimizing side effects. This is performed as an open surgical technique or endoscopically (by a transthoracic route) using electrocautery or laser. Percutaneous chemical sympathectomy with ethanol has also been used, a technique that can be employed for lumbar sympathectomy to treat plantar hyperhidrosis. Ejaculatory failure, impotence, and anorgasmia are likely sequelae, however, and it is not generally recommended.

SPECIFIC INVESTIGATIONS

Tests are not necessary for the diagnosis of idiopathic hyperhidrosis, although colorimetric sweating patterns (starch iodine) can be useful to define areas of maximum sweating, and gravimetric tests can be used for quantification.

Investigation appropriate to the clinical history and physical signs is necessary when hyperhidrosis is not idiopathic (full blood count, thyroid function, urinary metanephrines and 5-hydroxyindoleacetic acid [5-HIAA], blood glucose, chest X-ray).

FIRST-LINE THERAPIES

▶ Topical ACH solution in ethanol	B

Aluminium chloride hexahydrate versus palmar hyperhidrosis. Evaporimeter study. Goh CL. Int J Dermatol 1990; 29: 368–70.

A single-blind study of unilateral palmar treatment with 20% ACH daily for 4 weeks in 12 patients. Efficacy was reported for all patients; however, four experienced skin irritancy, three patients clearing after 1 week of stopping treatment, and one patient withdrew from the study.

Axillary hyperhidrosis. Local treatment with aluminium-chloride hexahydrate 25% in absolute ethanol with and without supplementary treatment with triethanolamine. Glent-Madsen L, Dahl JC. Acta Dermatol Venereol 1988; 68: 87–9.

318

A randomized, double-blind, half-sided experiment in 30 volunteers. Triethanolamine in 50% ethanol was applied after treatment to one axilla, to neutralize the pH and reduce skin irritation. The combined treatment was found to be less irritant, but also less effective in reducing sweating, although the reduction in efficacy was not noted by the volunteers.

SECOND-LINE THERAPIES

▶ Topical anticholinergics	B
▶ Oral anticholinergics	D
▶ Iontophoresis	B
▶ Botulinum A neurotoxin	A
▶ Botulinum A neurotoxin delivered by Dermojet	C
▶ Botulinum A neurotoxin delivered by iontophoresis	D
▶ Botulinum B neurotoxin	C
▶ Liposuction and surgical excision (axillae only)	C
▶ Sympathectomy	B
▶ CO$_2$ laser using multiple drilling method	

Topical glycopyrrolate for patients with facial hyperhidrosis. Kim WO, Kil HK, Yoon KB, Yoon DM. Br J Dermatol 2008; 158: 1094–7.

Twenty-five patients were treated with 2% topical glycopyrrolate pads to one half of the forehead; the other side was treated with a placebo. Gravimetric testing showed a reduction in sweating on the treated side in the majority of patients.

The use of topical glycopyrrolate in the treatment of hyperhidrosis. Seukeran DC, Highet AS. Clin Exp Dermatol 1998; 23: 204–5.

Topical glycopyrrolate 0.5% in aqueous solution was effective in the treatment of hyperhidrosis of the scalp and forehead after other treatments had proved ineffective.

Topical anticholinergics have been used successfully in gustatory hyperhidrosis in diabetics and in Frey's syndrome.

Propantheline bromide in the management of hyperhidrosis associated with spinal cord injury. Canaday BR, Stanford RH. Ann Pharmacother 1995; 29: 489–92.

Generalized hyperhidrosis after spinal injury was suppressed with careful titration of propantheline, starting at 15 mg daily and increasing to 15 mg three times daily.

Treating hyperhidrosis [Letter]. Klaber M, Catterall M. Br Med J 2000; 321: 703.

The authors advocate the use of oral glycopyrrolate as a safe and convenient therapy in the doses outlined in the text above.

Use of oral glycopyrronium bromide in hyperhidrosis. Baja V, Langtry JAA. Br J Dermatol 2007; 157: 118–21.

In this retrospective analysis of 19 patients with idiopathic hyperhidrosis of varying distribution, 79% reported response to treatment at a dose of 2 mg twice daily, increasing to 2 mg three times daily. In one-third of patients treatment was limited by side effects.

Iontophoresis with alternating current and direct current offset (AC/DC iontophoresis): a new approach for the treatment of hyperhidrosis. Reinauer S, Neusser A, Schauf G, Holzle E. Br J Dermatol 1993; 129: 166–9.

Palmar hyperhidrosis was controlled after an average of 11 treatments, with both the conventional DC and the AC/DC iontophoresis units studied. The AC/DC method, however, eliminated skin irritation and discomfort.

Treatment of hyperhidrosis by a battery operated iontophoretic device. Holzle E, Ruzicka T. Dermatologica 1986; 172: 41–7.

The average duration of treatment with the Hidrex device used was 14 months, without relapse (four patients were treated for more than 3 years).

Treatment of hyperhidrosis. Heymann WR. J Am Acad Dermatol 2005; 52: 509–10.

An editorial review of the treatment options available for hyperhidrosis, focusing on the current status of botulinum toxin.

Botulinum toxin A for axillary hyperhidrosis (excessive sweating). Heckmann M, Ceballos-Baumann AO, Plewig G. N Engl J Med 2001; 344: 488–93.

A multicenter trial in 145 patients with axillary hyperhidrosis, comparing 200 U and 100 U of BTX-A (Dysport) per axilla. Changes in the rates of sweat production were measured gravimetrically. Two weeks after the injections, the mean rate of sweat production was slightly less in the axilla injected with 200-U, and sweat reduction in both was significantly more than with placebo. After 24 weeks, sweat rates after 100 and 200 U were almost identical and less than half the baseline rate. Ninety-eight percent of the patients said they would recommend this therapy to others.

Botulinum toxin therapy for palmar hyperhidrosis. Shelley WB, Talanin NY, Shelley ED. J Am Acad Dermatol 1998; 38: 227–9.

Four patients with severe palmar hyperhidrosis were treated under regional nerve blocks of the median and ulnar nerve. Anhidrosis lasted for 12, 7, 7, and 4 months, respectively, and one patient experienced mild weakness of a thumb lasting 3 weeks.

Double-blind trial of botulinum A toxin for the treatment of focal hyperhidrosis of the palms. Schnider P, Binder M, Auff E, Kittler H, Berger T, Wolff K. Br J Dermatol 1997; 136: 548–52.

A significant reduction in sweating for 13 weeks is reported in this randomized, placebo-controlled, double-blind within-group study of 11 patients with palmar hyperhidrosis. Two patients reported reversible minor weakness of powerful handgrip at BTX-A injected sites.

A double-blind, randomized, comparative study of Dysport® vs. Botox® in primary palmar hyperhidrosis. Simonetta Moreau M, Cauhepe C, Magues JP, Senard JM. Br J Dermatol 2003; 149: 1041–5.

Eight patients were treated with intradermal injections of Botox in one palm and Dysport in the other (using a conversion factor of 1:4) after regional nerve blocks. Similar efficacy was reported for the two BTX-A products.

Effective treatment of frontal hyperhidrosis with botulinum toxin A. Kinkelin I, Hund M, Naumann M, Hamm H. Br J Dermatol 2000; 143: 824–7.

Ten men with focal frontal hyperhidrosis are reported to have had a good response to treatment with botulinum toxin A injections.

Treatment of plantar hyperhidrosis with botulinum toxin type A. Vadoud-Seyedi J. Int J Dermatol 2004; 43: 969–71.

Plantar hyperhidrosis in 10 patients treated with BTX-A delivered via needleless injector (Dermojet) is reported. Seven patients were symptom free for 5 months following treatment.

BOTOX® delivery by iontophoresis. Kavanagh GM, Oh C, Shams K. Br J Dermatol 2004; 151: 1093–5.

Two patients with palmar hyperhidrosis had treatment with BTX-A (Botox) delivered by iontophoresis. Control of approximately 70% was achieved for 3 months, without side effects.

Botulinum toxin type B: a new therapy for axillary hyperhidrosis. Nelson L, Bachoo P, Holmes J. Br J Plast Surg 2005; 58: 228–32.

The efficacy of BTX-B (Neurobloc) was demonstrated in the treatment of 13 patients with axillary hyperhidrosis.

Liposuction for the treatment of axillary hyperhidrosis. Lillis PJ, Coleman WP. Dermatol Clin 1990; 8: 479–82.

The authors suggest that this technique shows promise as the surgical treatment of choice for axillary hyperhidrosis resistant to other modalities.

Surgical treatment of axillary hyperhidrosis in 123 patients. Bretteville-Jensen G, Mossing N, Albrechsten R. Acta Dermatol Venereol 1975; 55: 73–8.

Excision of the axillary vault and reconstruction with a modified Z-plasty is described. Of the 123 patients studied, 57% achieved a 75–100% reduction of axillary sweating and 36% achieved a 50–75% reduction. Complications included hematomas in six patients, limited flap necrosis in five, and minor complications in 10. There were no cases of keloid formation or restricted arm movement from wound contracture.

Endoscopic thoracic sympathectomy for primary hyperhidrosis of the upper limbs: a critical analysis and longterm results of 480 operations. Herbst F, Plas EG, Fuggo R, Fritsch A. Ann Surg 1994; 220: 86–90.

Complete satisfaction was reported by 67% and partial satisfaction by 27% of patients. Patients treated for axillary hyperhidrosis alone were less satisfied. The side effects reported included compensatory hyperhidrosis in 67%, gustatory sweating in 51%, and Horner's syndrome in 2.5%.

Transthoracic endoscopic sympathectomy for palmar hyperhidrosis in children and adolescents: analysis of 350 cases. Lin TS. J Laparoendosc Adv Surg Tech A 1999; 9: 331–4.

A total of 699 sympathectomies were performed in 350 patients aged 5–17 years (mean 12.9 years). There were no surgical deaths. The mean follow-up was 25 months (range 5–44 months), with highly satisfactory results reported in 95% of patients, although compensatory hyperhidrosis (86%) affected the axillae (12%), back (86%), abdomen (48%), or lower limbs (78%). The recurrence rates of palmar hyperhidrosis were 0.6% in the first year, 1.1% in the second, and 1.7% in the third.

The treatment of syringomas by CO_2 laser using a multiple drilling method. Park HJ, Lee D-Y, Lee J-H, Yang J-M, Lee ES, Kim W-S. Dermatol Surg 2007; 33: 310–3.

The authors report good cosmetic results without complications in the treatment of eleven patients with periocular syringomas, with CO_2 laser treatment using a multiple drilling method.

THIRD-LINE THERAPIES

▶ Biofeedback and behavioral modification	D
▶ Diltiazem	E
▶ Clonazepam	E
▶ Clonidine	E
▶ Electrocoagulation	

Use of biofeedback in treating chronic hyperhidrosis. Duller P, Gentry WD. Br J Dermatol 1980; 103: 143–8.

Biofeedback and behavioral modification can be tried, but is helpful in only a small number of patients.

Emotional eccrine sweating. A heritable disorder. James WD, Schoomaker EB, Rodman OG. Arch Dermatol 1987; 123: 925–9.

Two members of a family with palmar hyperhidrosis showed reduced palmar sweat secretion during administration of diltiazem.

Unilateral localized hyperhidrosis responding to treatment with clonazepam. Takase Y, Tsushimi K, Yamamoto K, Fukusako T, Morimatsu M. Br J Dermatol 1992; 126: 416.

A single case of unilateral hyperhidrosis responding to this benzodiazepine antiepileptic agent.

Clonidine treatment in paroxysmal localized hyperhidrosis. Kuritzky A, Hering R, Goldhammer G, Bechar M. Arch Neurol 1984; 41: 1210–11.

Improvement of paroxysmal localized hyperhidrosis is described in two patients with oral clonidine hydrochloride 0.25 mg three times a day. Control of sweating was maintained with continuous treatment at 12-month follow-up.

Periorbital syringoma: A pilot study of the efficacy of low-voltage electrocoagulation. Al Aradi IK. Dermatol Surg 2006; 32: 1244–50.

Periorbital syringomas in 20 patients were treated with low-voltage electrocoagulation. Clinical improvement is reported although the clinical photographs demonstrating this do not appear to give as good results as with other reported techniques, notably when compared with published results for CO_2 laser treatment.

Hypertrichosis and hirsutism

Shannon Harrison, Najwa Somani,
Wilma F Bergfeld

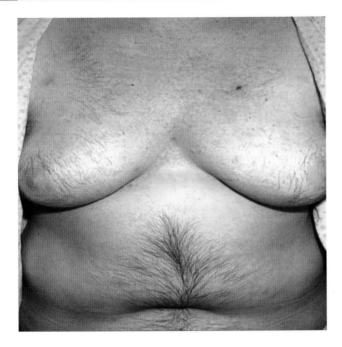

Hirsutism is a distressing symptom of excessive growth of terminal hairs in typically male androgen-dependent areas in women, such as the chin, upper lip, breasts, abdomen, and back. Hirsutism can result from endogenous sources of androgens (ovaries or adrenal glands), exogenous androgens, or from increased hair follicle sensitivity to normal androgen levels. Polycystic ovarian syndrome (PCOS) and idiopathic hirsutism are the most common causes of hirsutism. Rarer causes are endocrinopathies, non-classic congenital adrenal hyperplasia, and tumors.

Hypertrichosis is characterized by increased hair growth in an androgen-independent, non-sexual distribution. Hypertrichosis may be familial, or secondary to medications or an underlying systemic disorder.

MANAGEMENT STRATEGY

A thorough history and physical examination should identify any underlying cause of hypertrichosis and hirsutism. Drugs that cause hypertrichosis and androgenic medications known to cause hirsutism should be discontinued.

Most hirsute women will have raised circulating androgen levels. In idiopathic hirsutism, menstrual cycles appear normal and conventional testing does not detect androgen abnormalities. PCOS, HAIR-AN syndrome, and ovarian hyperthecosis present with signs of hyperandrogenism and metabolic syndrome. Weight loss can improve hirsutism and reduce cardiovascular risk.

Cushing's disease, hyperprolactinemia, and acromegaly should be recognized and treatment initiated. Acute onset or rapid progression of hirsutism or signs of virilization may indicate an adrenal or ovarian tumor. Tumor removal will reverse the hirsutism. In non-classic congenital adrenal hyperplasia, glucocorticoid therapy assists with induction of ovulation, but hirsutism may also require systemic anti-androgen therapy. Glucocorticoid therapy for classic congenital adrenal hyperplasia manages ovulation induction and hirsutism.

Mechanical hair removal is the first-line treatment choice for hirsutism and hypertrichosis. *Bleaching* with hydrogen peroxide preparations can disguise dark facial hair, but can irritate. Painless depilatory methods remove hair shafts at the skin surface. *Chemical depilatory creams* are quick to use, but can irritate. *Shaving* is inexpensive, but is time-consuming and not acceptable to most women except for the axillae and legs. Shaving does not affect the diameter or rate of growth of hair.

Epilatory hair removal methods remove the entire hair, including the root, and are painful. *Tweezing or plucking* may be used in areas with fewer hairs. *Waxing* is also useful, but more expensive. Epilation with *electrolysis* can often achieve a permanent reduction in hair growth. A fine needle is inserted into the hair follicle and an electrical current applied. It is time-consuming, requiring multiple treatments, and is operator dependent. It can be used on any skin or hair color. Side effects of all mechanical hair removal methods include erythema, folliculitis, pseudofolliculitis, infection, scarring, and dyspigmentation.

Photoepilation lasers include ruby (694 nm), alexandrite (755 nm), diode (800–810 nm), Nd:YAG (neodymium:yttrium–aluminium–garnet) laser (1064 nm) and IPL (intense pulsed light) non-coherent sources of 590–1200 nm. Lasers result in a partial short-term hair reduction for up to 6 months, and efficacy is improved with repeat treatments. Evidence supports alexandrite and diode lasers for partial hair reduction longer than 6 months after multiple treatments, but probably exists for ruby and Nd:YAG lasers also. IPL produces partial short-term hair reduction, improving with multiple sessions. No laser can achieve complete or persistent efficacy of hair removal. Ideal candidates have fair skin and dark hair. Side effects include erythema, scarring, burns, dyspigmentation, and rarely a paradoxical increase in hair growth.

Twice-daily *eflornithine* hydrochloride cream slows the rate of hair growth. Eflornithine irreversibly inhibits ornithine decarboxylase and is FDA approved to treat facial hirsutism. Benefits are reversed after 8 weeks of discontinuation. Side effects include acne, pseudofolliculitis barbae, and irritant and allergic contact dermatitis. Efficacy may be improved when combined with hair removal laser.

Evidence supporting pharmacological hirsutism treatments is limited by small numbers and limited methodology in trials. Several meta-analyses and treatment guidelines have been published.

Combined oral contraceptive pills (estrogen–progestin OCP) reduce hyperandrogenism predominantly by suppressing ovarian androgen synthesis, increasing sex hormone-binding globulin levels and suppressing free plasma testosterone levels. Androgenic progestins should be avoided. Low androgenic progestins in oral contraceptives (*cyproterone acetate, drospirenone, desogesterol* or *norgestimate*) should be used for hirsutism.

Shannon Harrison was funded in 2008 by the Australasian College of Dermatologists and the F.C. Florance Bequest.

Spironolactone is an anti-androgen that competitively inhibits 5α-reductase activity and the androgen receptor. The usual dose for hirsutism is 100–200 mg daily. Side effects include hyperkalemia, postural hypotension, and irregular menses. Tumorigenicity has been shown in animals; the significance in humans is unknown. All anti-androgens, including spironolactone, have feminizing teratogenic potential and should be used with a reliable form of contraception.

Cyproterone acetate inhibits 5α-reductase activity and the androgen receptor, and for hirsutism can be used in a sequential manner for the first 10 days of the menstrual cycle with an oral contraceptive pill, or low dose in a combined oral contraceptive pill (Diane-35). It has similar side effects to the OCP.

Flutamide and *insulin-lowering drugs* are not recommended for the routine treatment of hirsutism. Flutamide has significant risk of hepatotoxicity.

Finasteride, a type II 5α-reductase inhibitor, has been used for hirsutism. It is pregnancy category X and hepatotoxicity is a risk. No reports exist for dutasteride, a type I and II 5α-reductase inhibitor for the treatment of hirsutism.

GnRH analogs are only recommended if oral contraceptives and anti-androgen treatment fail in the setting of severe hyperandrogenism. GnRH treatment reduces estrogen to menopausal levels, causing hot flushes and osteoporosis risk. Cimetidine is ineffective in hirsutism. Ketoconazole has anti-androgenic properties, but has significant hepatotoxicity and drug interactions.

SPECIFIC INVESTIGATIONS

Screening test
▶ Testosterone level (total and free)

If testosterone level raised or underlying endocrinopathy or tumor suspected

▶ Sex hormone-binding globulin level
▶ Dehydroepiandrosterone sulfate level
▶ Androstenedione level
▶ Follicle-stimulating hormone (FSH) level
▶ Luteinizing hormone (LH) level
▶ Serum prolactin
▶ 17-hydroxyprogesterone level
▶ 24-hour urinary free cortisol
▶ Somatomedin C level (IGF-1)

Special tests
▶ Transvaginal ovarian ultrasound
▶ Dexamethasone suppression test
▶ CT/MRI abdomen or pelvis
▶ Cranial MRI

Hirsutism is graded clinically with a Ferriman–Gallwey scale. Moderate to severe hirsutism and hirsutism with signs of hyperandrogenism, such as clitoromegaly, central obesity, acanthosis nigricans, infertility, or irregular menstrual cycles, should be investigated. Acute-onset or rapidly progressing hirsutism should be investigated. Controversy exists as to whether investigating androgen levels will be helpful in mild isolated hirsutism (FG score 8–15). We suggest testosterone screening for all patients, including those with mild hirsutism.

A luteinizing and follicle-stimulating hormone (LH:FSH) ratio >2 is suggestive, but not diagnostic, of polycystic ovarian syndrome. Transvaginal ultrasound detects polycystic ovaries, which are not required for diagnosis, and their presence does not confirm the diagnosis. Metabolic screening is essential. Early morning serum 17-hydroxyprogesterone level detects non-classic congenital adrenal hyperplasia. A 24-hour urine cortisol and dexamethasone suppression test evaluates for Cushing's syndrome. Prolactin level and somatomedin-C (IGF-1) level screen for hyperprolactinemia and acromegaly, respectively. Suspicion of a pituitary tumor requires MRI scanning of the brain. Transvaginal ultrasound or abdominal CT or MRI scan can exclude an ovarian or adrenal tumor.

The evaluation and treatment of androgen excess. Practice Committee of the American Society for Reproductive Medicine. Fertil Steril 2006; 86: S241–7.

This article reviews the clinical diagnosis and laboratory testing for hirsutism.

The clinical evaluation of hirsutism. Somani N, Harrison S, Bergfeld WF. Dermatol Ther 2008; 21: 376–91.

The article has tables on history, examination templates, and diagnostic algorithms for evaluation of hirsutism.

FIRST-LINE THERAPIES

▶ Treat specific underlying pathology	
▶ Weight loss if obese with PCOS	B
▶ Electrolysis	B
▶ Temporary hair removal/camouflage	B
▶ Laser therapy and IPL	A
▶ Eflornithine	A

Treatment with flutamide, metformin, and their combination, added to a hypocaloric diet in overweight obese women with polycystic ovary syndrome: A randomized, 12 month placebo controlled study. Gambineri A, Patton L, Vaccina A, Cacciari M, Morselli-Labate AM, Cavazza C, et al. J Clin Endocrinol 2006; 91: 3970–80.

Hirsutism scores in this study decreased significantly over the first 6 months of treatment in all groups, including the hypocaloric diet group with placebo.

Hirsutism. Mofid A, Alinaghi SA, Zansieh S, Yazdani T. Int J Clin Pract 2008: 62: 433–43.

A review article discussing diagnostic strategies and user-friendly tables of hair removal methods and pharmacological therapies.

Guidance for the management of hirsutism. Dawber RPR. Curr Med Res Opin 2005; 21: 1227–34.

A review article on management, including electrolysis and mechanical hair removal methods.

A comparative study of axillary hair removal in women: plucking versus the blend method. Urushibata O, Kasa K. J Dermatol 1995; 22: 738–42.

There are no randomized controlled trials on electrolysis. This small comparative study showed that it was more effective than plucking for reduction of axillary hair.

Electrosurgery using insulated needles: epilation. Kobayahsi T. J Dermatol Surg Oncol 1985; 11: 993–1000.

A series of 39 patients, treated with three or four epilations using the thermolysis method applied to a variety of body

Evidence Levels: **A** Double-blind study **B** Clinical trial ≥ 20 subjects **C** Clinical trial < 20 subjects **D** Series ≥ 5 subjects **E** Anecdotal case reports

sites, had reduced hair growth 6–12 months after treatment, with little scarring.

Evidence based review of hair removal using lasers and light sources. Haedersdal M, Wulf HC. J Eur Acad Dermatol Venerol 2006; 20: 9–20.

A meta-analysis showed that laser and IPL hair reduction is more effective short-term than shaving, waxing, electrolysis, and epilation. The relative efficacies of different hair removal lasers and IPL have been compared in several studies, but the authors warn that small sample sizes can introduce type 2 errors.

Meta-analysis of hair removal laser trials. Sadoghha A, Mohaghegh zahed G. Lasers Med Sci 2007; (Epub ahead of print).

Hair reductions 6 months post treatment were 57.5%, 42.3%, 54.7%, and 52.8% after three treatments for diode, Nd:YAG, alexandrite, and ruby lasers, respectively.

Randomized, double blind clinical evaluation of the efficacy and safety of topical eflornithine HCl 13.9% cream in the treatment of women with facial hair. Wolf JE Jr, Shander D, Huber F, Jackson J, Lin C-S, Mathes BM, et al.; Eflornithine Study Group. Int J Dematol 2007; 46: 94–8.

At week 24, 58% of patients treated with eflornithine cream were improved or better compared to 34% of vehicle-treated patients using the physician's global assessment rating scale. The difference was negligible 8 weeks after discontinuing treatment. Acne, pseudofolliculitis barbae, and pruritus were reported side effects.

A randomized bilateral vehicle controlled study of eflornithine cream combined with laser treatment versus laser treatment alone for facial hirsutism in women. Hamzavi I, Tan E, Shapiro J, Lui H. J Am Acad Dermatol 2007; 57: 54–9.

Eflornithine cream continued for 6 months in combination with repeat long-pulse alexandrite laser treatments results in a more rapid and complete reduction in facial hair.

SECOND-LINE THERAPIES

▶ Oral contraceptives	B
▶ Spironolactone	A
▶ Cyproterone acetate	B

Evaluation and treatment of hirsutism in premenopausal women: an Endocrine Society Clinical Practice Guideline. Martin KA, Chang J, Ehrmann DA, Ibanez L, Lobo RA, Rosenfield RL, et al. J Clin Endocrinol Metab 2008; 93: 1105–20.

Combined analysis of studies showed that OCPs are associated with a reduction in hirsutism scores.

Cyproterone acetate for hirsutism. Van der Spuy ZM, le Roux PA. 2003 Cochrane Database Syst Rev 4: CD001125

There are no studies comparing cyproterone acetate alone with placebo. Only one small placebo controlled trial exists of cyproterone acetate 2 mg with the ethinyl estradiol oral contraceptive pill, showing that it was more effective than placebo in reducing hirsutism scores.

THIRD-LINE THERAPIES

▶ Finasteride	A
▶ Flutamide	A
▶ Insulin-lowering monotherapy	A
▶ Gonadotropin-releasing hormone (GnRH) agonist analogs	B

Antiandrogens for the treatment of hirsutism: a systematic review and meta-analyses of randomized controlled trials. Swiglo BA, Cosma M, Flynn DN, Kurtz DM, LaBella ML, Mullan RJ, et al. J Clin Endocrinol Metab 2008; 93: 1153–60.

Spironolactone appeared to be superior to placebo in improving hirsutism. Meta-analysis showed finasteride and flutamide to be superior to placebo in reducing Ferriman–Gallwey scores. Anti-androgens were superior to metformin, and when spironolactone or finasteride are combined with OCPs, or when flutamide is combined with metformin, these regimens are superior to monotherapy with OCPs and metformin, respectively.

Evaluation and treatment of hirsutism in premenopausal women: an Endocrine Society Clinical Practice Guideline. Martin KA, Chang J, Ehrmann DA, Ibanez L, Lobo RA, Rosenfield RL, et al. J Clin Endocrinol Metab 2008; 93: 1105–20.

Meta-analysis concluded that no therapeutic advantages exist for GnRH treatment compared to other anti-androgens and OCPs.

Insulin sensitizers for the treatment of hirsutism: a systematic review and metaanalyses of randomized controlled trials. Cosma M, Swiglo BA, Flynn DN, Kurtz DM, LaBella ML, Mullan RJ, et al. J Clin Endocrinol Metab 2008; 93: 1135–42.

Metformin provided no significant benefit to hirsutism compared to placebo.

Comparison of a gonadotrophin-releasing hormone agonist and a low dose oral contraceptive given alone or together in the treatment of hirsutism. Heiner JS, Greendale GA, Kawakami AK, Lapolt PS, Fisher M, Young D, et al. J Clin Endocrinol Metab 1995; 80: 3412–18.

A study of 64 women over 24 weeks found that combination treatment was the only group that showed a trend towards a reduction in Ferriman–Gallwey scores and a significant reduction (21%) in the clipped hair diameter.

Ichthyoses

Timothy H Clayton, Katherine Panting

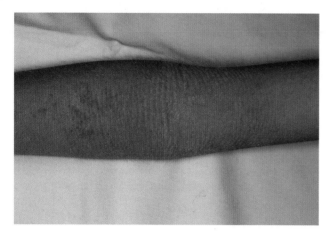

The ichthyoses represent a heterogeneous group of disorders of keratinization characterized by scaly skin. They may be inherited or acquired. Severity and extent vary widely from mild ichthyosis vulgaris (IV) to life-threatening harlequin ichthyosis. Recently, a series of exciting discoveries has led to the identification of several causative genes and molecules underlying these disorders. These studies have provided targets for future therapies. So far, however, there have been very few randomized controlled studies assessing the treatment of ichthyosis.

MANAGEMENT STRATEGY

The key to management, where possible, is to establish an exact diagnosis. This provides a platform to plan therapy, discuss prognosis, and consider genetic counseling. A simple approach to clinical diagnosis is to consider whether an ichthyosis is inherited or acquired, the age of onset, presence or absence of collodion membrane, blistering or erythroderma in the neonatal period, and the type, color, and distribution of scale. Family members should also be examined. There are a number of invaluable web resources that provide information and support for patients and families; www.scalyskin.org is a good starting place.

The genes responsible for a number of the inherited ichthyoses have recently been identified. Ichthyosis vulgaris is the most common disorder of cornification, with an incidence of 1:250 based on a survey of 6051 healthy English schoolchildren. It is usually not present at birth. Clinical features include dry skin, often with associated fine white powdery scale on extensor surfaces, palmar hyperlinearity, and keratosis pilaris. Mutations in the *filament aggregating protein (filaggrin) gene (FLG)* have recently been identified as the cause of IV. Loss-of-function mutations in FLG have also been strongly associated with atopic dermatitis. It is hoped that the discovery of FLG mutations could, in the future, provide targeted treatments that may improve and restore effective skin barrier function, with the potential to alleviate or even prevent disease in susceptible individuals.

Patients with ichthyosis have reduced epidermal barrier function, with increased transepidermal water loss, reduced pliability of the stratum corneum, and hyperkeratosis. Treatment generally involves hydration, lubrication, and keratolysis. Hydration promotes desquamation by increasing hydrolytic enzyme activity and the susceptibility to mechanical forces. In mild to moderate cases, hydration of the skin followed immediately by the application of lubricants that help retain the hydration and prevent evaporation will result in satisfactory improvement. Increasing the environmental humidity has also been shown to be beneficial. *Emollient baths* aid in softening the stratum corneum and thereby facilitate mechanical debridement of thickened hyperkeratosis.

Keratolytics such as salicylic acid, urea, lactic acid and propylene glycol reduce the adhesion of keratinocytes and aid in desquamation. However, because of the impaired barrier function, care should be taken to prevent salicylate toxicity. Cutaneous infection occurs as a result of impaired barrier function and consideration should be given to prophylactic measures, such as antiseptic soaps/baths. If skin infections do develop, topical and systemic *antibacterials* should be used, particularly *in epidermolytic hyperkeratosis (EHK)*, which often requires long-term antibiotic therapy.

Topical retinoids (e.g., tretinoin) may be beneficial. They reduce the cohesiveness of epithelial cells, stimulate mitosis and turnover, and suppress keratin synthesis. *Tazarotene*, a topical receptor-selective retinoid, was effective in one small trial.

The severe forms of ichthyosis usually respond to *systemic retinoid therapy. Acitretin* (1 mg/kg/day) and *isotretinoin* (1–2 mg/kg/day) have been shown to reduce scaling and discomfort, and improve heat tolerance and sweating. However, when retinoids are discontinued the improvement does not persist and the ichthyotic skin recurs, thereby necessitating long-term use. Long-term treatment involves a higher risk of chronic skeletal toxicity, such as calcification of tendons and ligaments, hyperostoses, and osteoporosis, which requires regular monitoring.

More recently *liarozole*, a *retinoic acid metabolism-blocking agent*, has been granted orphan drug status for congenital ichthyosis by the European Commission and the US Food and Drug Administration. This drug has been shown to inhibit the cytochrome P450-dependent 4-hydroxylation of retinoic acid, resulting in increased tissue levels of retinoic acid and a reduction in epidermal proliferation and scaling.

Acquired ichthyoses are associated with a number of systemic disorders, including HIV, malignancy, sarcoidosis, leprosy, thyroid disease, hyperparathyroidism, nutritional disorders, chronic renal failure, and autoimmune diseases. They will often improve with treatment of the underlying condition.

SPECIFIC INVESTIGATIONS

▶ Simple algorithm to aid clinical diagnosis of hereditary ichthyoses (see below)
  ▶ Genetic screening: refer to www.genetests.org
  ▶ Fatty alcohol: NAD + oxidoreductase activity (Sjögren–Larsson)
  ▶ Steroid sulfatase activity
▶ Acquired ichthyosis
  ▶ Malignancy screening
  ▶ Infection screen, including HIV
  ▶ Metabolic screening
  ▶ Skin biopsy

Molecular genetics of the inherited disorders of cornification: an update. Irvine AD, Paller AS. Adv Dermatol 2002; 18: 111–49.

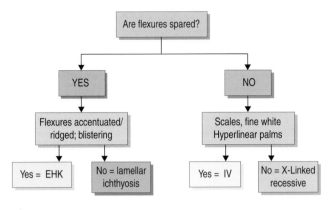

A comprehensive review of the molecular genetics of the inherited ichthyoses.

Comprehensive analysis of the gene encoding filaggrin uncovers prevalent and rare mutations in ichthyosis vulgaris and atopic eczema. Sandilands A, Terron-Kwiatkowski A, Hull PR, O'Regan GM, Clayton TH, Watson RM, et al. Nature Genet 2007; 39: 650–4.

Common filaggrin (FLG) null mutations cause ichthyosis vulgaris and predispose to eczema and secondary allergic diseases.

This paper illustrates that the common European mutations are ancestral variants carried on conserved haplotypes.

X linked ichthyosis (steroid sulphatase deficiency) is associated with increased risk of attention deficit hyperactivity disorder, autism and social communication deficits. Kent L, Emerton J, Bhadravathi V, Weisblatt E, Pasco G, Willatt LR, et al. J Med Genet 2008; 45: 519–24;. epub 2008 Apr 15.

X-linked ichthyosis is caused by deletions or point mutations of the steroid sulfatase (STS) gene on chromosome Xp22.32. Deletions of this region are associated with cognitive behavioral difficulties, including autism.

ABCA12 is the major harlequin ichthyosis gene. Thomas AC, Cullup T, Norgett EE, Hill T, Barton S, Dale BA, et al. J Invest Dermatol 2006; 126: 2408–13.

Harlequin ichthyosis (HI), the most severe and often lethal form of recessive congenital ichthyosis, is caused by functional deficiency of ABCA12, an essential lipid transporter.

Novel and recurring ABCA12 mutations associated with harlequin ichthyosis: implications for prenatal diagnosis. Thomas AC, Sinclair C, Mahmud N, Cullup T, Mellerio JE, Harper J, et al. Br J Dermatol 2008; 158: 611–13.

Prenatal DNA testing for HI is now possible.

Correlation between SPINK5 gene mutations and clinical manifestations in Netherton syndrome patients. Komatsu N, Saijoh K, Jayakumar A, Clayman GL, Tohyama M, Suga Y, et al. J Invest Dermatol 2008; 128: 1148–59.

Netherton syndrome (NS) is a congenital ichthyosis caused by serine protease inhibitor Kazal-type 5 (SPINK5) mutations. This study observed the correlation between the product of SPINK5 lymphoepithelial Kazal-type-related inhibitor (LEKTI) and tissue kallikreins (KLKs) with clinical manifestations in NS.

This study introduced possibilities for future targeted therapies.

Acquired ichthyosis. Patel N, Spencer LA, English JC 3rd, Zirwas MJ. J Am Acad Dermatol 2006; 55: 647–56.

A recent update that provides an algorithm for the evaluation of patients presenting with acquired ichthyosis.

FIRST-LINE THERAPIES

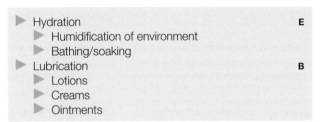

Congenital ichthyosis: an overview of current and emerging therapies. Vahlquist A, Ganemo A, Virtanen M. Acta Dermatol Venereol 2008; 88: 4–14.

A useful review providing updated information on genetic etiology, treatment strategies, and areas for future possible drug management.

Ichthyosis: etiology, diagnosis, and management. DiGiovanna JJ, Robinson-Bostom L. Am J Clin Dermatol 2003; 4: 81–95.

Review of the ichthyoses, including etiologies, approach to diagnosis, and management.

Role of topical emollients and moisturitzers in the treatment of dry skin barrier disorders. Loden M. Am J Clin Dermatol 2003; 4: 771–88.

A general review of the role of emollients, highlighting the immediate barrier-repairing effect of petrolatum; conversely, emulsifying ointment may weaken barrier function.

Efficacy of urea therapy in children with ichthyosis. A multicenter randomized, placebo-controlled, double-blind, semilateral study. Kuster W, Bohnsack K, Rippke F, Upmeyer HJ, Groll S, Traupe H. Dermatology 1998; 196: 217–22.

Sixty children aged between 1 and 16 years were treated for 8 weeks with 10% urea lotion on one side, and lotion base on the other. On each side, a control area was left untreated. Improvement was 78% after 8 weeks for 10% urea lotion and 72% for urea-free lotion base. Although urea was somewhat superior to the base, the lotion base alone was effective.

SECOND-LINE THERAPIES

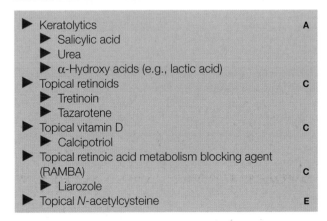

Salicylate intoxication using a skin ointment. Chiaretti A, Schembri Wismayer D, Tortorolo L, Tortorolo L, Piastra M, Polidori G. Acta Paediatr 1997; 86: 330–1.

The application of salicylic acid over large body surface areas has been associated with toxicity, especially in children. Signs and symptoms of salicylate intoxication include fever, dyspnea with respiratory alkalosis, oculogyric crisis, coma, and even death.

Propylene glycol with occlusion for treatment of ichthyosis. Goldsmith LA, Baden HP. JAMA 1972; 220: 579–80.

Aqueous propylene glycol in concentrations of 40–60% under occlusion may also be effective in softening the hyperkeratotic skin of patients with ichthyosis.

Keratolytics: Salicylic acid is the oldest keratolytic and is used in concentrations ranging from 0.5% to 60%. Urea (5–20%), lactic acid, and propylene glycol in a variety of bases are also widely used.

Effect of topical tazarotene in the treatment of congenital ichthyoses. Hofmann B, Stege H, Ruzicka T, Lehmann P. Br J Dermatol 1999; 141: 642–6.

The topical receptor-selective retinoid tazarotene 0.05% gel was evaluated, relative to 10% urea ointment, in a heterogeneous group of 12 adult patients with congenital ichthyosis. Seventy-five percent of patients responded favorably, resulting in remission lasting up to 2 months. The only side effect was local irritation.

Efficacy, tolerability, and safety of calcipotriol ointment in disorders of keratinization. Results of a randomized, double-blind, vehicle-controlled, right/left comparative study. Kragballe K, Steijlen PM, Ibsen HH, van de Kerkhof PC, Esmann J, Sorensen LH, et al. Arch Dermatol 1995; 131: 556–60.

Sixty-seven patients with disorders of keratinization were treated with calcipotriol ointment (50 µg/g) and placebo twice daily for up to 12 weeks (up to 120 g of calcipotriol ointment per week). Improvement was variable. No benefit was seen in palmoplantar keratoderma nor keratosis pilaris; eight of 12 patients with Darier's disease withdrew.

Topical treatment of Sjögren–Larsson syndrome with calcipotriol. Lucker GP, van de Kerkhof PC, Cruysberg JR, der Kinderen DJ, Steijlen PM. Dermatology 1995; 190: 292–4.

Two patients with SLS were treated with calcipotriol ointment versus ointment base for 12 weeks using a double-blind bilaterally paired comparison. Both patients had unilateral improvement on the calcipotriol-treated side.

Topical liarozole in ichthyosis: a double-blind, left-right comparative study followed by a long-term open maintenance study. Lucker GP, Verfaille CJ, Heremans AM, Vanhoutte FP, Boegheim JP, Steijlen PP. Br J Dermatol 2005; 152: 566–8.

Liarozole 5% cream, a retinoic acid metabolism-blocking agent (RAMBA), was used in 12 adult patients in a left–right comparative study, followed by a 4-week open phase. Results showed a significant reduction in the severity of skin involvement, both at the end of the double-blind treatment phase (p=0.0005; n=2) and after the 4-week open follow-up phase (p < 0.005; n=11). The severity was further reduced during the maintenance treatment of 72 weeks. Six of 12 patients experienced adverse events during the short-term trial, consisting mainly of stickiness of the skin.

Topical N-acetylcysteine treatment in neonatal ichthyosis. Sarici SU, Sahin M, Yudakok M. Turk J Pediatr 2003; 45: 245–7.

Case report comparing the simultaneous use of 10% N-acetylcysteine and 4% urea to the left and right halves of the body, respectively, for 9 days. A larger reduction in scale was seen on the N-acetylcysteine-treated side. Longer-duration double-blinded studies with larger patient numbers would be needed to further evaluate this treatment option.

THIRD-LINE THERAPIES

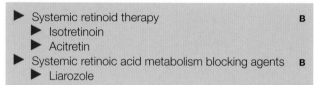

► Systemic retinoid therapy	B
► Isotretinoin	
► Acitretin	
► Systemic retinoic acid metabolism blocking agents	B
► Liarozole	

Oral retinoid therapy for disorders of keratinization: single-centre retrospective 25 years' experience on 23 patients. Katugampola RP, Finlay AY. Br J Dermatol 2006; 154: 267–76.

To date this study provides the longest available follow-up safety data on children and adults with disorders of keratinization taking oral retinoid therapy. The longest duration of retinoid treatment in this cohort was 25 years (these two patients had been switched from etretinate to acitretin after 14 years). One patient developed diffuse idiopathic skeletal hyperostosis after 21 years of retinoid therapy. Abnormalities of the fasting lipid profile and liver function were seen in small numbers.

Twenty-one years of oral retinoid therapy in siblings with nonbullous ichthyosiform erythroderma. Macbeth AE, Johnston GA. Clin Exp Dermatol 2008; 33: 190–1.

A report of long-term safety data in two male siblings with NBIE. Transient abnormalities of lipid profile were seen, but no spinal abnormalities or osteoporosis were reported.

Effective treatment of severe thermodysregulation by oral retinoids in a patient with recessive congenital lamellar ichthyosis. Haenssle HA, Finkenrath A, Hausser I, Oji V, Traupe H, Hennies HC, et al. Clin Exp Dermatol 2008 Mar 18 (Epub ahead of print).

Single case report of a 42-year-old man with autosomal lamellar ichthyosis demonstrating marked improvement in skin condition and an ability to thermoregulate by perspiration after treatment with oral retinoid.

Oral liarozole versus acitretin in the treatment of ichthyosis: a phase II/III multicentre, double-blind, randomized, active-controlled study. Verfaille CJ, Vanhoutte FP, Blanchet-Bardon C, van Steensel MA, Steijlen PM. Br J Dermatol 2007; 156: 965–73.

Thirty-two patients were randomized to either liarozole 75 mg bid or acitretin 10 mg in the morning and 25 mg at night for 12 weeks. Overall evaluation of the response to treatment at the endpoint showed that 10 of 15 patients in the liarozole group and 13 of 16 in the acitretin group were considered to be at least markedly improved.

The expected retinoic acid-related adverse events were mostly mild to moderate and tended to occur less frequently in the liarozole group.

Impetigo

Robert Burd, Michael Sladden

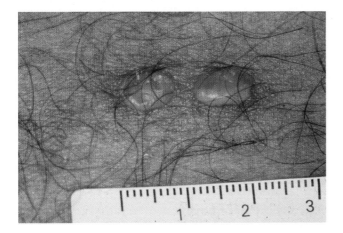

Impetigo is a superficial bacterial infection of the skin. The most common pathogen is *Staphylococcus aureus*, although β-hemolytic streptococci may also be implicated. The infection is highly contagious and can easily spread to other body sites or close contacts.

Impetigo may be primary, with direct bacterial invasion of previously normal skin, or secondary, where infection develops due to an underlying skin disease, such as scabies or eczema, disrupting the skin barrier.

Impetigo is classified as bullous or non-bullous. In the more common non-bullous form, thin-walled vesicles rupture to form superficial erosions with yellowish-brown crusts, which eventually heal without scarring. Bullous impetigo is characterized by larger bullae or blisters, which may continue to develop for several days.

MANAGEMENT STRATEGY

The main aim of treatment is to eradicate the infecting bacteria to allow rapid healing of skin lesions and control the spread of infection. This requires the use of an appropriate antimicrobial delivered in an effective manner. Antibiotics may be administered either orally or topically. The choice between topical or oral therapy depends on:

- The experience of the practitioner
- The preference of the patient
- The extent and severity of the disease
- The local bacterial resistance patterns
- The cost and availability of local resources.

In Europe *Staphylococcus aureus* has been recognized as the major pathogen in both bullous and non-bullous impetigo. Traditionally, in the United States, non-bullous impetigo was considered to be caused primarily by streptococci, but recent evidence indicates that *S. aureus* is now the most common pathogen in both forms of impetigo in the United States as well.

Oral or topical antibiotics with proven efficacy against *S. aureus* are the first choice of therapy. It is reasonable to use short courses of topical antibiotics for mild, limited impetigo, while reserving oral antibiotics for recalcitrant, extensive, systemic disease.

Globally, the majority of isolates of *S. aureus* are resistant to penicillin. Erythromycin resistance is also becoming more prevalent.

In developing countries, where impetigo causes a significant burden of disease, streptococcus is often the predominant pathogen. In these countries, topical agents are expensive and may be unavailable. Treatment strategies have to be sufficiently flexible to meet local needs.

Historically, topical treatment of impetigo was ineffective due to the emergence of bacterial resistance to tetracyclines and gentamicin, and problematic because of contact sensitivity to topical antimicrobials. More recently introduced *topical antibiotics* are as effective as traditional *oral antibiotics*. When used in courses of less than 2 weeks, bacterial resistance does not appear to be a major problem. However, bacterial resistance patterns vary with geographical location, and treatment should be influenced by local data and expertise.

Recent studies of retapamulin, a pleuromutilin antibacterial developed for topical use, indicate that it is effective and safe in the treatment of primary impetigo.

Strains of bacteria causing impetigo are often extremely virulent. Patients therefore need to be educated on personal hygiene methods to avoid the spread of infection. The use of topical antiseptics and soaks to remove dried exudate and crusts has not been shown to be of benefit. Evidence regarding the value of disinfecting measures is limited. However, common sense would indicate that cleaning lesional skin with soap and water or a mild, non-irritant antiseptic will aid the application of topical antibiotics and reduce the spread of infection.

Nasal carriage of *S. aureus* occurs in a high proportion of both patients and asymptomatic family members. Therefore, in recurrent cases or multiple familial cases, *treatment of nasal and pharyngeal carriage* may be necessary.

SPECIFIC INVESTIGATIONS

- ▶ Gram stain
- ▶ Bacterial culture and sensitivity

A Gram stain of a swab from the lesion or exudate will reveal Gram-positive cocci, confirming the clinical diagnosis. Bacterial culture and sensitivity from a pretreatment swab is useful to assess suitable alternative antibiotics in cases that do not respond to conventional treatment.

Impetigo in epidemic and nonepidemic phases: an incidence study over 4½ years in a general population. Rortveit S, Rortveit G. Br J Dermatol 2007; 157: 100–5.

In this population-based study of impetigo, *S. aureus* was the causal bacterium in 89% (117/132) and 68% (84/123) of cases during epidemic and non-epidemic periods, respectively (p<0.01). *S. aureus* was resistant to fusidic acid in 84% (98/117) and 64% (54/84) of cases in epidemic and non-epidemic periods, respectively (p<0.01).

Interventions for impetigo (Cochrane Review). Koning S, Verhagen AP, van Suijlekom-Smit LWA, et al. In: The Cochrane Library, Issue 2. Chichester, UK: John Wiley & Sons, 2004.

S. aureus is considered to be the main bacterium that causes non-bullous impetigo. However, *S. pyogenes,* or both *S. pyogenes* and *S. aureus,* are sometimes isolated. In moderate climates, staphylococcal impetigo is more common, whereas in warmer and more humid climates the streptococcal form predominates.

Impetigo: etiology and therapy. Hirschmann JV. Curr Clin Top Infect Dis 2002; 22: 42–51.

Describes the changing epidemiology of causative agents of impetigo.

DNA heterogeneity of *Staphylococcus aureus* strains evaluated by Sma1 and SgrA1 pulsed field gel electrophoresis in patients with impetigo. Capoluongo E, Giglio A, Leonetti F, Belardi M, Giannetti A, Caprilli F, et al. Res Microbiol 2000; 151: 53–61.

Samples from lesional skin, nose, and pharynx were taken from 26 patients and their families and the strain of *S. aureus* was typed; 54% of the patients had the same strain in both the nose and the lesion. In over half the families at least one other family member was found to be carrying the same strain as the patient's lesion.

FIRST-LINE THERAPIES

▶ Topical mupirocin or fusidic acid	A
▶ Topical retapamulin	A
▶ Oral flucloxacillin, cloxacillin, erythromycin, fusidic acid	A
▶ Other oral antibiotic, depending on sensitivity	B
▶ Topical antiseptics	B

Efficacy and safety of retapamulin ointment as treatment of impetigo: randomized double-blind multicentre placebo-controlled trial. Koning S, van der Wouden JC, Chosidow O, Twynholm M, Singh KP, Scangarella N, et al. Br J Dermatol 2008; 158: 1077–82.

Two hundred and thirteen patients were randomized to receive either topical retapamulin ointment 1% twice daily for 5 days or topical placebo. Retapamulin ointment was superior to placebo (clinical response after 7 days 85.6% vs 52.1%; p<0.0001) (intention to treat analysis). This suggests that topical retapamulin is effective and safe in the treatment of primary impetigo.

Topical retapamulin ointment, 1%, versus sodium fusidate ointment, 2%, for impetigo: a randomized, observer-blinded, noninferiority study. Oranje AP, Chosidow O, Sacchidanand S, Todd G, Singh K, Scangarella N, et al; TOC100224 Study Team. Dermatology 2007; 215: 331–40.

Retapamulin and sodium fusidate had comparable clinical efficacies (intention-to-treat population: 94.8 and 90.1%, respectively; p=0.062). Success rates in the small numbers of sodium fusidate-, methicillin- and mupirocin-resistant *S. aureus* were good for retapamulin (9/9, 8/8, and 6/6, respectively). Both drugs were well tolerated. The authors concluded that retapamulin is a highly effective and convenient new treatment option for impetigo, with efficacy against isolates resistant to existing therapies.

Topical retapamulin ointment (1%, wt/wt) twice daily for 5 days versus oral cephalexin twice daily for 10 days in the treatment of secondarily infected dermatitis: results of a randomized controlled trial. Parish LC, Jorizzo JL, Breton JJ, Hirman JW, Scangarella NE, Shawar RM, et al; SB275833/032 Study Team. J Am Acad Dermatol 2006; 55: 1003–13.

Retapamulin was as effective as cephalexin (clinical success rates: 85.9% and 89.7%, respectively) in the treatment of patients with secondarily infected dermatitis. Microbiologic success rates were 87.2% for retapamulin and 91.8% for cephalexin. Retapamulin was well tolerated and the topical formulation was preferred over the oral drug.

Interventions for impetigo (Cochrane Review). Koning S, Verhagen AP, van Suijlekom-Smit LWA, et al. In: The Cochrane Library, Issue 2. Chichester, UK: John Wiley & Sons, 2004.

A systematic review of 57 trials including 3533 participants. There is good evidence that topical mupirocin and topical fusidic acid are equally as or more effective than oral antibiotics for people with limited impetigo. Topical antibiotics may be more effective, for example, than erythromycin because erythromycin resistance is becoming more common.

A systematic review and meta-analysis of treatments for impetigo. George A, Rubin G. Br J Gen Pract 2003; 53: 480–7.

A review of 16 trials concluding that both topical and oral antibiotics are effective treatments for impetigo.

Topical mupirocin treatment of impetigo is equal to oral erythromycin therapy. Mertz PM, Marshall DA, Eaglstein WH, Piovanetti Y, Montalvo J. Arch Dermatol 1989; 125: 1069–73.

Seventy-five patients were treated in an investigator-blinded study comparing topical mupirocin applied three times daily with oral erythromycin 30–50 mg/kg daily. The mupirocin treated patients experienced similar clinical results to those treated with oral erythromycin, although mupirocin was superior in the microbiological eradication of *S. aureus*.

Common skin infections in children. Sladden MJ, Johnston GA. Br Med J 2004; 329: 95–9.

In this evidence-based review, the authors suggest using topical mupirocin or fusidic acid for 7 days in mild impetigo. They advise that oral antibiotics are reserved for recalcitrant, extensive, systemic disease.

Fusidic acid tablets in patients with skin and soft-tissue infection: a dose-finding study. Carr WD, Wall AR, Georgala-Zervogiani S, Stratigos J, Gouriotou K. Eur J Clin Res 1994; 5: 87–95.

Fusidic acid tablets, 250 mg twice daily, 500 mg twice daily, and the standard regimen of 500mg three times daily, were compared in a randomized, double-blind study in 617 patients with skin and soft tissue infections. Each treatment was given for 5–10 days. Cure rates after 5 days of treatment were 34.7%, 37.8%, and 37.2%, respectively. End of treatment cure rates were 75.5%, 81.1%, and 74.0%, respectively.

Impetigo. Current etiology and comparison of penicillin, erythromycin and cephalexin therapies. Demidovich CW, Wittler RR, Ruff ME, Bass JW, Browning WC. Am J Dis Child 1990; 144: 1313–15.

A randomized trial of 73 children with impetigo treated with either penicillin V, erythromycin, or cefalexin. *S. aureus* was the most common pathogen and cefalexin the most effective treatment, although erythromycin may be preferred on grounds of cost-effectiveness.

Topical 2% mupirocin versus 2% fusidic acid ointment in the treatment of primary and secondary skin infections. Gilbert M. J Am Acad Dermatol 1989; 20: 1083–7.

A double-blind randomized trial of 70 patients with primary or secondary skin infections. In those with impetigo the degree of effectiveness favored mupirocin, although both treatments were very efficacious.

Cost-effectiveness of erythromycin versus mupirocin for the treatment of impetigo in children. Rice TD, Duggan AK, DeAngelis C. Pediatrics 1992; 89: 210–14.

A controlled clinical trial of topical mupirocin or oral erythromycin in 93 children with impetigo. Both treatments were highly effective. Mupirocin was more expensive, but caused significantly fewer side effects than erythromycin.

The frequency of erythromycin-resistant *Staphylococcus aureus* in impetiginized dermatoses. Misko ML, Terracina JR, Diven DG. Pediatr Dermatol 1995; 12: 12–15.

Despite significant in-vitro erythromycin resistance in a series of 98 outpatients, there was still a low frequency of treatment failure in this group. This suggested that erythromycin may still be a reasonable agent in the treatment of uncomplicated superficial skin infections in that community at that time.

The emergence of resistance to penicillin and erythromycin is so common in isolates of S. aureus *that alternative antibiotics should be considered.*

Hydrogen peroxide cream: an alternative to topical antibiotics in the treatment of impetigo contagiosa. Christensen OB, Anehus S. Acta Dermatol Venereol 1994; 74: 460–2.

A prospective comparison of hydrogen peroxide cream with fusidic acid cream in 256 patients with impetigo. Over a 3-week treatment period, 92 patients of 128 (72%) in the hydrogen peroxide group were classified as healed, compared to 105 of 128 (82%) in the fusidic acid group. This difference was not statistically significant.

Observations on high levels of fusidic acid resistant *Staphylococcus aureus* in Harrogate, North Yorkshire, UK. Ravenscroft JC, Layton A, Barnham M. Clin Exp Dermatol 2000; 25: 327–30.

A retrospective study demonstrated a marked increase in fusidic acid-resistant (FusR) *S. aureus*, possibly owing to high usage of fusidic acid. The total number of prescriptions for these preparations was higher in the area of study than in five other local areas where increases in (FusR) *S. aureus* had not been observed.

Effect of handwashing on child health: a randomised controlled trial. Luby SP, Agboatwalla M, Feikin DR, Painter J, Billhimer W, Altaf A, et al. Lancet 2005; 366: 225–33.

In squatter settlements in Karachi, children younger than 15 years in households that received plain soap and handwashing promotion had a 34% lower incidence of impetigo than controls (95% CI, –52% to –16%).

The effect of antibacterial soap on impetigo incidence, Karachi, Pakistan. Luby S, Agboatwalla M, Schnell BM, Hoekstra RM, Rahbar MH, Keswick BH. Am J Trop Med Hyg 2002; 67: 430–5.

Routine use of antibacterial soap by children living in a community with a high incidence of impetigo was associated with a reduced incidence of the disease. The incidence among children living in households receiving soap containing 1.2% triclocarban (1.10 episodes per 100 person-weeks) was 23% lower than in households receiving placebo soap (p = 0.28) and 43% lower than the standard habit and practice controls (p = 0.02).

SECOND-LINE THERAPIES

▶ Intravenous antibiotics plus topical antibiotic	**C**
▶ Rifampin (rifampicin)	**D**

Addition of rifampin to cephalexin therapy for recalcitrant staphylococcal skin infections – an observation. Feder Jr HM, Pond KE. Clin Pediatr 1996; 35: 205–8.

Two children with staphylococcal infections failing to respond to standard antibiotics responded when rifampin was added.

THIRD-LINE THERAPIES

▶ Systemic antibiotic, topical antibiotic plus a formal antistaphylococcal regimen to reduce nasal and pharyngeal carriage	**E**

Use of 0.3% triclosan (Bacti-Stat) to eradicate an outbreak of methicillin-resistant *Staphylococcus aureus* in a neonatal nursery. Zafar AB, Butler RC, Reese DJ, Gaydos LA, Mennonna PA. Am J Infect Control 1995; 23: 200–8.

A nosocomial outbreak of infection with methicillin-resistant *S. aureus* (MRSA) in a neonatal nursery proved difficult to control even with aggressive conventional measures. The additional use of a handwashing and bathing soap containing 0.3% triclosan immediately ended the outbreak.

Prevention and control of nosocomial infection caused by methicillin-resistant *Staphylococcus aureus* in a premature infant ward: preventive effect of a povidone-iodine wipe of neonatal skin. Aihara M, Sakai M, Iwasaki M, Shimakawa K, Kozaki S, Kubo M, et al. Postgrad Med J 1993; 69: S117–21.

An outbreak of MRSA causing impetigo was halted by wiping the body surface of the infants with a diluted povidone-iodine solution (10% povidone-iodine; 1:100 dilution) to prevent colonization.

Failure of first-line therapy may indicate the presence of a resistant organism or poor patient compliance. The choice of antibiotic should be based on the sensitivities of organisms cultured from the pretreatment swab. In recurrent cases, consider the possibility of nasal or pharyngeal colonization with pathogenic S. aureus *in either the patient or a close family member. This may require eradication by the use of a systemic antibiotic in conjunction with the nasal application of a topical antibiotic and an antiseptic skin cleanser. Topical antiseptics have also proved useful in nosocomial outbreaks.*

Irritant contact dermatitis

Nathaniel K Wilkin

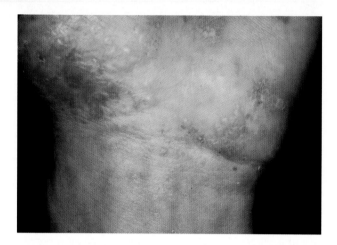

Irritant contact dermatitis (ICD) is the most common form of contact dermatitis and is defined as the reaction to an exogenous substance – the irritant – that damages the epidermis through physical or chemical mechanisms without triggering an immunological response. Acute ICD is usually attributable to a single irritant. Chronic ICD usually results from exposure to multiple irritants, often in association with endogenous factors such as atopy or stress. Chronic cumulative ICD usually involves the hands. ICD is common, often has a poor prognosis, has a significant economic impact on society, and seriously degrades the quality of life of affected individuals beyond the ability to work.

MANAGEMENT STRATEGY

The first step in any management strategy is *prevention*. Patients should be educated about proper skin care and protection, including handwashing, the use of moisturizers, avoidance of common irritants, and the use of protective clothing such as gloves and aprons when handling potentially irritating substances. Dermatologists can encourage primary prevention by counseling patients at higher risk because of endogenous factors (e.g., atopy) or exogenous factors (e.g., frequent occupational exposures, such as in hairdressing). Secondary prevention includes measures that enable patients to remain employed without interfering with the resolution of the ICD. Chronic hand dermatitis is a common presentation of ICD, and patient education can be facilitated with a handout on lifestyle management principles directed at handwashing and moisturizing, occlusive moisturizing therapy at night, special protective modalities (such as type of glove to exclude specific irritants), and specific agents to avoid.

Azathioprine, ciclosporin, oral retinoids, psoralen and UVA (PUVA), Grenz ray therapy, and *superficial radiotherapy* may be justified for short-term control in patients who are compliant with moisturizing, use of protective modalities (gloves), and application of topical corticosteroids, and still have a severe disruption of their quality of life due to active ICD. Because the goal of these second- and third-line therapies is to reduce the severity such that first-line therapies may become sufficient, patient selection is critical.

SPECIFIC INVESTIGATIONS

> ▶ Patch testing to environmentally relevant allergens
> ▶ Detailed case history of patient's work, habits, and hobbies

Irritant contact dermatitis: a review. Slodownik D, Lee A, Nixon R. Australas J Dermatol 2008; 49: 1–11.

Treatment of ICD is based on determining all contributing factors to the patient's dermatitis and prevention of contact with the causative agents where possible.

Clues to an accurate diagnosis of contact dermatitis. Rietschel RL. Dermatol Ther 2004; 17: 224–30.

Patch testing, with known environmentally relevant allergens, that is negative and sufficiently comprehensive would point to ICD, especially in patients without atopy, dyshidrosis, or psoriasis. A careful history and documentation of specific morphological changes on physical examination are essential when pursuing the presumptive diagnosis of ICD after negative patch testing.

Patch testing, a detailed history, and assessment of specific morphological changes provide for an accurate diagnosis and can identify specific environmental factors the patient should avoid. Such documentation is also useful should medicolegal questions arise regarding impairment and job placement.

FIRST-LINE THERAPIES

> ▶ Physical skin protection   C
> ▶ Emollients   C
> ▶ Barrier creams   C
> ▶ Topical corticosteroids   C
> ▶ Topical calcineurin inhibitors   C

Current concepts of irritant contact dermatitis. English JS. Occup Environ Med 2004; 61: 722–6.

Avoiding exposure to irritants, relying on the use of personal protective equipment and the use of moisturizing creams, is the basis of the treatment of ICD.

A review of the management of ICD cases from an occupational medicine perspective which includes an excellent guide to various gloves that provide protection for specific types of hazard.

Therapeutic options for chronic hand dermatitis. Warshaw EM. Dermatol Ther 2004; 17: 240–50.

A review of the therapeutic alternatives for patients with recalcitrant hand dermatitis.

Effect of glove-occlusion on human skin (II). Ramsing DW, Agner T. Contact Dermatitis 1996; 34: 258–62.

Occlusive gloves worn for prolonged periods may impair skin barrier function. Wearing cotton gloves under the occlusive gloves can prevent this negative effect.

High-fat petrolatum-based moisturizers and prevention of work-related skin problems in wet-work occupations. Mygind K, Sell L, Flyvholm MA, Jepsen KF. Contact Dermatitis 2006; 54: 35–41.

Evidence Levels: **A** Double-blind study   **B** Clinical trial ≥ 20 subjects   **C** Clinical trial < 20 subjects   **D** Series ≥ 5 subjects   **E** Anecdotal case reports

Detailed analyses revealed that protective gloves are the overall most effective protection, and did not indicate that a high-fat moisturizer could successfully replace gloves.

Protective gloves should be used for as short a time as possible, and with cotton gloves under the occlusive gloves. Gloves provide better protection than, and should not be replaced by, moisturizers or barrier creams.

A randomized comparison of an emollient containing skin-related lipids with a petrolatum-based emollient as adjunct in the treatment of chronic hand dermatitis. Kucharekova M, Van de Kerkhof PCM, Van der Valk PGM. Contact Dermatitis 2003; 48: 293–9.

The frequent use of emollients is associated with significant improvement in hand dermatitis. No significant difference in the improvement was demonstrated for the emollient containing skin-related lipids.

The frequent use of emollients is an essential component of therapy. Traditional petrolatum-based emollients are accessible, inexpensive, and just as effective as an emollient containing skin-related lipids.

Double-blind, randomized trial of scheduled use of a novel barrier cream and an oil-containing lotion for protecting the hands of health care workers. McCormick RD, Buchman TL, Maki DG. Am J Infect Control 2000; 28: 302–10.

The scheduled use of petrolatum oil-containing lotion or a barrier cream was associated with a marked improvement (69% and 52%, respectively) in chronic hand irritant dermatitis.

It is debatable whether the distinction between 'skin care' and 'skin protection' is real. Side effects in using emollients and barrier creams are irritation and sensitization to their ingredients. A useful procedure is to include patch tests of those emollients and barrier creams anticipated to be used by the patient in the initial comprehensive patch testing evaluation of the chronic contact dermatitis.

Do topical corticosteroids modulate skin irritation in human beings? Assessment by transepidermal water loss and visual scoring. Van der Valk PGM, Maibach HI. J Am Acad Dermatol 1989; 21: 519–22.

Neither the corticosteroid products nor the vehicle significantly influenced barrier function during repeated application of an irritant, sodium lauryl sulfate, in low concentration.

The first step must be the elimination, to the fullest extent possible, of exposure to irritants. Until proven otherwise, no therapy should be considered sufficiently potent as to overcome the effects of continuing exposure to irritants.

Short-term glucocorticoid treatment compromises both permeability barrier homeostasis and stratum corneum integrity: inhibition of epidermal lipid synthesis accounts for functional abnormalities. Kao JS, Fluhr JW, Man MQ, Fowler AJ, Hachem JP, Crimrine D, et al. J Invest Dermatol 2003; 120: 456–64.

ICD can be treated with glucocorticoids; however, there may be a secondary compromise in barrier function which might be correctable with topical application of lipids.

An open-label pilot study to evaluate the safety and efficacy of topically applied tacrolimus ointment for the treatment of hand and/or foot eczema. Thelmo MC, Lang W, Brooke E, Osborne BE, McCarty MA, Jorizzo JL, et al. J Dermatol Treat 2003; 14: 136–40.

Pimecrolimus cream 1%: a potential new treatment for chronic hand dermatitis. Belsito DV, Fowler JF, Marks JG, Pariser DM, Hanifin J, Duarte IA, et al. Cutis 2004; 73: 31–8.

The topical calcineurin inhibitor led to improvements over baseline in the open-label study, and there was a trend toward greater clearance than with vehicle in the pimecrolimus study.

Topical calcineurin inhibitors may have a role as an alternative to low-potency topical corticosteroids in chronic irritant dermatitis in patients with mild inflammatory changes who do not experience a burning sensation when the product is applied.

SECOND-LINE THERAPIES

▶ Ciclosporin	C
▶ UVB therapy	C
▶ PUVA therapy	C
▶ Bexarotene gel	C

Novel treatment of chronic severe hand dermatitis with bexarotene gel. Hanifin JM, Stevens V, Sheth P, Breneman D. Br J Dermatol. 2004; 150: 545–53.

A phase 1–2 open-label randomized clinical study of bexarotene gel, alone and in combination with a low- and a mid-potency steroid, was conducted in 55 patients with chronic severe hand dermatitis at two academic clinics. Patients using bexarotene gel monotherapy reached a 79% response rate for at least 50% clinical improvement and a 39% response rate for at least 90% clearance of hand dermatitis. Adverse events possibly related to treatment in all patients were stinging or burning (15%), flare of dermatitis (16%), and irritation (29%). Bexarotene gel appears to be safe, tolerated by most patients, with useful therapeutic activity in chronic severe hand dermatitis.

Comparison of cyclosporine and topical betamethasone 17,21-dipropionate in the treatment of severe chronic hand eczema. Granlund H, Erkko P, Eriksson E, Reitamo S. Acta Dermatol Venereol 1996; 76: 371–6.

Low-dose oral ciclosporin at 3 mg/kg daily was compared with topical 0.05% betamethasone dipropionate in a randomized, double-blind study of 41 patients with chronic hand dermatitis and an inadequate response to treatment with topical halogenated corticosteroids for at least 3–4 weeks, and/or PUVA and avoidance of relevant contact allergens. Both treatment groups had similar improvement and similar relapse rates after successful treatment. Adverse events were slightly more common in patients treated with ciclosporin.

Low-dose ciclosporin may be a useful alternative treatment, although very high-potency topical corticosteroids can be effective in patients who do not have an adequate response to other mid- to high-potency topical corticosteroids.

PUVA-gel vs. PUVA-bath therapy for severe recalcitrant palmoplantar dermatoses. A randomized, single-blinded prospective study. Schiener R, Gottlöber P, Müller B, Williams S, Pillekamp H, Peter RU, et al. Photodermatol Photoimmunol Photomed 2005; 21: 62–7.

PUVA-gel therapy can be an effective therapeutic alternative to conventional PUVA-bath therapy in treating localized dermatoses of the palms and soles. The advantages of PUVA-gel therapy are simplicity of use and low cost.

Local narrowband UVB phototherapy vs. local PUVA in the treatment of chronic hand eczema. Sezer E, Etikan I. Photodermatol Photoimmunol Photomed. 2007; 23: 10–14.

There was a statistically significant improvement with both treatment modalities; however, the difference in clinical response between the two was not statistically significant. Local narrowband UVB phototherapy regimen is as effective as paint-PUVA therapy in patients with chronic hand eczema of both dry and dyshidrotic types.

Given the similar improvement in chronic hand dermatitis and the increased side effects with paint-PUVA therapy, it would be prudent to begin treatment with local narrowband UVB therapy and only use paint-PUVA therapy if the response is inadequate.

THIRD-LINE THERAPIES

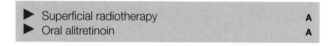

| ▶ Superficial radiotherapy | A |
| ▶ Oral alitretinoin | A |

Oral alitretinoin (9-cis-retinoic acid) therapy for chronic hand dermatitis in patients refractory to standard therapy: results of a randomized, double-blind, placebo-controlled, multicenter trial. Ruzicka T, Larsen FG, Galewicz D, Horváth A, Coenraads PJ, Thestrup-Pedersen K, et al. Arch Dermatol 2004; 140: 1453–9.

Alitretinoin given at well-tolerated doses induced substantial clearing of chronic hand dermatitis in patients refractory to conventional therapy.

Alitretinoin is not currently approved for use in the USA. Although teratogenicity might occur at any clinically relevant dose, most other side effects are dose dependent. This drug should be reserved for patients whose chronic hand dermatitis is refractory to conventional therapies, and prescribed for only as long as it takes to achieve control, which can be maintained with safer therapies.

Efficacy and patient perception of Grenz ray therapy in the treatment of dermatoses refractory to other medical therapy. Schalock PC, Zug KA, Carter JC, Dhar D, MacKenzie T. Dermatitis 2008; 19: 90–4.

Many patients treated with Grenz ray therapy (GRT) for recalcitrant dermatitis reported that this was an effective therapy in reducing the discomfort and severity of their skin condition. Overall, slightly more than half of treated patients believed GRT was a worthwhile therapy that they would use again.

Grenz ray therapy in the new millennium: still a valid treatment option? Warner JA, Cruz PD Jr. Dermatitis 2008; 19: 73–80.

Grenz ray or superficial radiotherapy is not an obvious 'go to' treatment when one second-line treatment does not provide a sufficient response, but it may be tried for some additional advantage as an adjunct to intensive first-line treatment with or without low-dose ciclosporin.

Jessner's lymphocytic infiltrate

Joanna E Gach

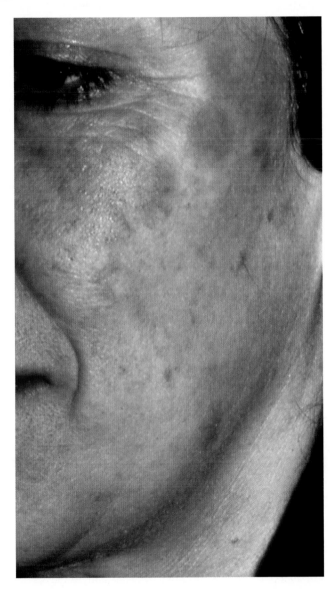

Jessner's lymphocytic infiltrate (JLI) is a chronic inflammatory condition presenting with erythematous or reddish brown papules, annular or arciform plaques which can expand peripherally and sometimes develop central healing. The lesions are usually seen in adults and affect the face, neck, or upper trunk. Although they are frequently asymptomatic, some patients report itch or burning. The lesions can persist from weeks to years and disappear without sequelae, but may recur.

MANAGEMENT STRATEGY

JLI runs a waxing and waning course marked by intermittent improvement and subsequent exacerbations, which makes the evaluations of therapeutic effectiveness difficult. Patients demand treatment because they find the lesions disfiguring or itchy.

Potent topical steroids applied once or twice daily for 4 weeks are the first-line treatment for many dermatologists. Unfortunately, the results of treatment are variable, and most importantly, only short-lasting. If the response is inadequate, injection of *intralesional corticosteroids* into localized lesions or the use of *potent topical steroid under occlusive dressing* may be beneficial, but is associated with a greater risk of skin atrophy. *Topical tacrolimus* may be a safer alternative.

In cases where ultraviolet exposure has been reported to induce or exacerbate lesions, additional therapy with sunscreens may be needed. This group of patients may respond to *antimalarials,* in particular hydroxychloroquine.

A variety of other therapies have been reported to be effective in the management of JLI. *Thalidomide, oral gold,* and *retinoids* proved to be helpful in some cases, but their use may be limited by the adverse effects, which may be difficult for the patient and physician to accept, especially as JLI is harmless.

Many other treatments, including bismuth subsalicylate injections, nicotinamide, vitamin E, phenindamine, para-aminobenzoic acid, penicillin, chlortetracycline, minocycline, dapsone, quinacrine (mepacrine), and radiotherapy, have been tried unsuccessfully.

SPECIFIC INVESTIGATIONS

> ▶ Skin biopsy
> ▶ Lesional skin for direct immunofluorescence
> ▶ Antinuclear antibodies/extractable nuclear antigen

The diagnosis can be made on clinical grounds. The investigations are helpful in differentiating the condition from discoid lupus erythematosus, lupus erythematous tumidus, and cutaneous lymphoma.

The heterogeneity of Jessner's lymphocytic infiltration of the skin. Immunohistochemical studies suggesting one form of perivascular lymphocytoma. Cerio R, Oliver GF, Jones EW, Winkelmann RK. J Am Acad Dermatol 1990; 23: 63–7.

Skin biopsy of the lesion shows normal epidermis and a moderate, dense sleeve-like perivascular and periadnexal infiltrate in the middle dermis. This consists of normal-looking lymphocytes with the B cells grouped in close proximity to the superficial vessels and T cells at the periphery, and occasional plasma cells.

Could Jessner's lymphocytic infiltrate of the skin be a dermal variant of lupus erythematosus? An analysis of 210 cases. Lipsker D, Mitschler A, Grosshans E, Cribier B. Dermatology 2006; 213: 15–22.

Immunofluorescence studies of lesional skin showed lupus band with IgG, IgM ± C3 in 9.5% of cases of JLI. Antinuclear antibodies were present in 45% of cases.

Jessner's lymphocytic infiltration of the skin. A clinical study of 100 patients. Toonstra J, Wildschut A, Boer J, Smeenk G, Willemze R, van der Putte SC, et al. Arch Dermatol 1989; 125: 1525–30.

JLI can coexist with polymorphic light eruption, and can evolve into discoid lupus erythematosus.

FIRST-LINE THERAPIES

> ▶ Potent topical/intralesional corticosteroids   C
> ▶ Topical immunomodulators   E

Jessner's lymphocytic infiltration of the skin. A clinical study of 100 patients. Toonstra J, Wildschut A, Boer J, Smeenk G, Willemze R, van der Putte SC, et al. Arch Dermatol 1989; 125: 1525–30.

A series of 100 patients with JLI assessing clinical manifestations, duration, clinical course, and treatments. Forty-three of 91 patients treated with topical steroids had an excellent (13) or good (30) response, with temporary regression of the lesions. Many patients had no response.

Childhood Jessner's lymphocytic infiltrate of the skin. Higgins CR, Wakeel RA, Cerio R. Br J Dermatol 1994; 131: 99–101.

A case report of an 11-year-old boy with JLI responding to intralesional corticosteroids.

Effective treatment of chronic inflammatory skin diseases. Once a week occlusion therapy with clobetasol propionate and Duoderm. Volden G. Tidsskr Nor Laegeforen 1992; 112: 1272–4.

JLI was among other chronic skin diseases that were treated once a week with clobetasol propionate lotion left under the completely occlusive hydrocolloid dressing Duoderm. The lesions cleared within a few weeks.

Topical calcineurin inhibitors in treating Jessner's lymphocytic infiltration of the skin: report of a case. Tzung TY, Wu JC. Br J Dermatol 2005; 152: 383–4.

Tacrolimus 0.1% ointment twice daily produced an improvement after 2 weeks but had to be withdrawn because of diffuse erythema and desquamation that occurred 2 weeks later. The same effect occurred on rechallenge and settled with a single 5 mg dose of dexamethasone IM. Subsequently, pimecrolimus 1% cream cleared the rash within 6 weeks, with no relapse 2 months later.

SECOND-LINE THERAPIES

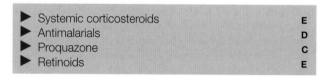

▶ Systemic corticosteroids	E
▶ Antimalarials	D
▶ Proquazone	C
▶ Retinoids	E

Jessner's lymphocytic infiltrate treated with auranofin. Farrell AM, McGregor JM, Staughton RC, Bunker CB. Clin Exp Dermatol 1999; 24: 500.

Intramuscular injection of 40 mg kenalog led to temporary improvement in this patient before oral gold was used successfully.

Jessner's lymphocytic infiltration of the skin. A clinical study of 100 patients. Toonstra J, Wildschut A, Boer J, Smeenk G, Willemze R, van der Putte SC, et al. Arch Dermatol 1989; 125: 1525–30.

Antimalarial drugs (chloroquine sulfate and hydroxychloroquine sulfate) were used in 15 patients, with a good response in six. There were no details given regarding doses or treatment regimens.

Hydroxychloroquine 200 mg once or twice a day, or chloroquine 200 mg daily were used in other case reports.

Proquazone: a treatment for lymphocytic infiltration of the skin. Comparative study with 2 other nonsteroid anti-inflammatory drugs. Johansson EA. Dermatologica 1987; 174: 117–21.

Eight of the 15 patients treated with the non-steroidal anti-inflammatory drug proquazone [1-isopropyl-4-phenyl-7-methyl-2(IH)] at a dose of 600 mg daily healed completely after 1–2 months of treatment. Two of these patients had recurrence of the rash, which was brought under control with small maintenance doses (600 mg daily for 3–4 days, alternate months) of proquazone. Two further patients from among the initial responders showed a partial remission. Indometacin (50–75 mg daily) and ibuprofen (1200 mg daily) were tried, without effect.

Satisfactory resolution of Jessner's lymphocytic infiltration of the skin following treatment with etretinate. Morgan J, Adams J. Br J Dermatol 1990; 122: 570.

One case of JLI was treated with etretinate 50 mg daily for 3 months and 25 mg daily for another 3 months. The rash subsided within 4 weeks of treatment and did not recur for 9 months after stopping treatment.

Isotretinoin 20 mg daily was used in other case reports, but was not helpful.

THIRD-LINE THERAPY

▶ Auranofin	E
▶ Thalidomide	A

Jessner's lymphocytic infiltrate treated with auranofin. Farrell AM, McGregor JM, Staughton RC, Bunker CB. Clin Exp Dermatol 1999; 24: 500.

A marked improvement was seen within 3 weeks of starting auranofin 3 mg bid in a case that was unresponsive to chloroquine, hydroxychloroquine, minocycline, dapsone, and isotretinoin.

Jessner's lymphocytic infiltrate responding to oral auranofin. Hafejee A, Winhoven S, Coulson IH. J Dermatol Treat 2004; 15: 331–2.

Oral auranofin 3 mg twice daily produced complete clearance of the plaques within 3 days of starting treatment. After 3 months of auranofin treatment, JLI recurred 2 weeks of stopping the drug. Monitoring of the therapy includes monthly full blood count for thrombocytopenia and urinalysis to detect nephritis.

Crossover study of thalidomide vs placebo in Jessner's lymphocytic infiltration of the skin. Guillaume JC, Moulin G, Dieng MT, Poli F, Morel P, Souteyrand P, et al. Arch Dermatol 1995; 131: 1032–5.

Twenty of 27 patients achieved complete remission after 2 months of therapy with thalidomide 100 mg daily. Sixteen (59%) patients were in complete remission 1 month after stopping therapy. Side effects included sleepiness, constipation, dry mouth, and sensorimotor neuropathy in two patients.

Juvenile plantar dermatosis

Stephen K Jones

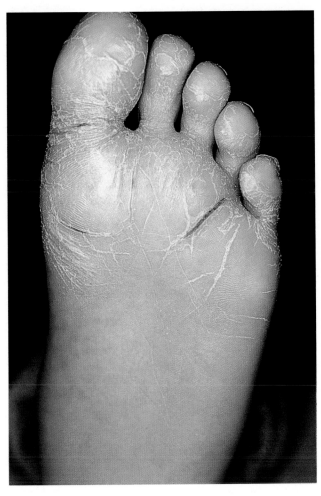

Juvenile plantar dermatosis is a specific condition comprising symmetrical erythema (sometimes with a polished 'billiard ball' appearance), scaling, and fissuring, primarily of the pressure areas of the foot. Vesiculation is never found. The commonest sites involved are the plantar aspects of the great toe, forefoot, heel, and very occasionally the fingertips and palms. The instep and the interdigital skin are rarely affected. The condition occurs almost exclusively in children, and clears around puberty.

MANAGEMENT STRATEGY

Juvenile plantar dermatosis usually presents in children between 4 and 7 years of age, although occasionally it presents before this. Most series suggest that it is a 'disease of the school years,' with clearing in most patients by puberty. It is uncommon in adults. Spontaneous resolution can be expected in the majority of patients.

The main etiologic factor is thought to be the occlusive effect of 'trainer' sports shoes and manmade fibers in hosiery, resulting in hyperhidrosis. This, some suggest, washes away surface lipids, which are already reduced because of the relative lack of sebaceous glands on the plantar surface of the foot. This hyperhidrosis is therefore followed by rapid dehydration of the skin on removal of footwear. It is proposed that this maceration/dehydration renders the skin susceptible to trauma, for example from sport. Avoidance of vigorous exercise may therefore be helpful in these patients.

The role of atopy is debated. Some series have found an increased incidence of atopy in patients and their families and, indeed, this condition was first referred to as 'atopic winter feet.' It has been argued that the atopic diathesis predisposes the skin of the foot to the traumatic effects of sport and vigorous activity, and the effects of alternating hyperhidrosis and dehydration (see below). Other series, however, have found no increased incidence of atopy.

Investigations are unlikely to be helpful. Although some series have found positive patch tests in about 10% of cases, these are often irrelevant. Indeed, even when these are to footwear-related allergens, allergen avoidance rarely affects the clinical outcome. Increased numbers of bacteria have been suggested to cause inflammation of the sweat ducts and thereby inhibit sweat secretion, but this has not been a consistent finding.

Changing to non-occlusive footwear along with cotton socks or 'open' footwear has, therefore, been proposed as a therapeutic maneuver. *Emollients*, both to reduce fissuring and to reduce the dehydration that is said to occur on removing occlusive footwear, are reported to be helpful. *Topical corticosteroids* may be beneficial if there is an inflammatory component. *Occlusive bandages* containing zinc ointment, ichthammol, or tar may help if hyperkeratosis and fissuring are a prominent feature. All the above often only help temporarily, and regular rotation of emollients may be required.

It is the impression of the author that this condition has become less common in recent years, possibly related to further changes in teenage 'fashion' and footwear materials.

SPECIFIC INVESTIGATIONS

▶ Patch tests

Juvenile plantar dermatosis; a new entity. Mackie RM, Hussain SL. Clin Exp Dermatol 1976; 1: 253–60.

Thirteen of 102 patients showed a positive patch test. Eight were considered relevant, with reactions to footwear constituents. In none did subsequent changes in footwear affect the clinical outcome.

Common pediatric foot dermatoses. Guenst BJ. J Pediatr Health Care 1999; 13: 68–71.

A practical review differentiating the various forms of tinea pedis and shoe dermatitis from juvenile plantar dermatosis. Therapeutic suggestions are offered for these entities.

FIRST-LINE THERAPIES

▶ Await spontaneous resolution   C

Juvenile plantar dermatosis – an 8 year follow-up of 102 patients. Jones SK, English JSC, Forsyth A, Mackie RM. Clin Exp Dermatol 1987; 12: 5–7.

Of 50 patients traced, the condition had resolved in 38. The mean age of remission was 14 years.

SECOND-LINE THERAPIES

▶ Change to non-occlusive footwear	C
▶ Sport avoidance	C
▶ Emollients	C
▶ Topical corticosteroids	C
▶ Rotation of topical agents	C
▶ Topical tacrolimus	C

Juvenile plantar dermatosis. Can sweat cause foot rash and peeling? Gibbs NF. Postgrad Med 2004; 115: 73–5.

A review of the disease, its etiology, and its treatment.

Juvenile plantar dermatosis. Graham RM, Verbov JL, Vickers CFH. Br J Dermatol 1987; 12: 468–70.

Although there was no association with any particular sport, intensive exercise causing skin cracking, soreness, and bleeding was a common complaint; 75% of parents said that a change in footwear had not been helpful.

In contrast to Jones et al. above, only 30% of cases in this series had resolved (mean age 11.8 years), though the ages of the remaining 70% were not stated.

Juvenile plantar dermatosis responding to topical tacrolimus. Shipley DR, Kennedy CTC. Clin Exp Dermatol 2005; 31: 453–4.

Topical tacrolimus twice daily in conjunction with a regular emollient produced improvement within 4 weeks with the feet appearing almost normal after 2 months. Intermittent tacrolimus was useful for relapses.

THIRD-LINE THERAPIES

▶ Zinc oxide/impregnated bandages	C
▶ Bed rest/footwear avoidance	E

Juvenile plantar dermatosis. Graham RM, Verbov JL, Vickers CFH. Br J Dermatol 1987; 12: 468–70.

Occlusion with zinc paste or ichthammol-impregnated bandages was among the most beneficial of treatments.

The aetiology of juvenile plantar dermatosis. Shrank AB. Br J Dermatol 1979; 100: 641–8.

Bed rest or avoidance of shoes and hosiery for 3 weeks resulted in disease clearance (said to approximate to the time taken to regrow the sweat duct apparatus in the horny layer of the foot).

Juvenile xanthogranuloma

Megan Mowbray, Olivia MV Schofield

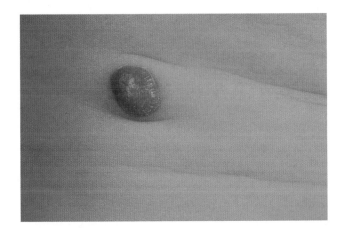

Juvenile xanthogranuloma (JXG) is a benign disorder characterized by solitary or multiple yellow-red nodules in the skin, and, occasionally, in other organs. The lesions regress spontaneously by age 6 months to 3 years. It occurs most commonly in infancy and early childhood, but adults may also be affected. Treatment is only recommended for systemic lesions if their location interferes with organ function.

MANAGEMENT STRATEGY

JXG is classified as a 'non-Langerhans' cell histiocytosis.' The diagnosis is usually made clinically, but a biopsy is required for atypical clinical variants (giant, plaque-like, paired, clustered, infiltrative, lichenoid, linear, subcutaneous, and intramuscular) and if multiple lesions are present. Unusual histological variants require further examination by immunohistochemistry and electron microscopy. JXG is characterized histologically by foamy histiocytes and multinucleated Touton-type giant cells. Immunohistochemical staining of JXG lesions shows expression of factor XIIIa, CD68, CD163, fascin, HLA-DR, and CD14, but not S100 or CD1a. This pattern of expression suggests deviation from the dermal dendrocyte.

The 'JXG family' can be divided into three groups:

1. Cutaneous – JXG, benign cephalic histiocytosis, generalized eruptive histiocytosis, adult xanthogranuloma, progressive nodular histiocytosis
2. Cutaneous with a major systemic component – xanthoma disseminatum
3. Systemic – Erdheim–Chester disease, usually seen in adults.

In the most common solitary type of JXG (60–89.5% of all cases) there is a male:female preponderance of 1.5:1 and the usual affected sites are the head, neck, and upper trunk. In young infants with multiple lesions the male:female ratio increases to 12:1. In the majority of cases no further investigation is required. The lesions will resolve spontaneously within months or years, and no follow-up is necessary. As involvement of other organs can occasionally occur in the cutaneous group, a review of systems and general examination is recommended to look for involvement of other sites and to examine for *café au lait* macules (see below).

Eye involvement

The eye is the most commonly affected extracutaneous site of JXG. Uveal lesions are the most frequently reported ophthalmologic findings, but lesions affecting the eyelid, orbit, conjunctiva, cornea, and optic nerve have also been described. Ocular symptoms and signs include unilateral redness and tearing, hyphema (hemorrhage into the anterior chamber), and/or visible lesions of the corneal limbus, eyelids, optic nerve, or papilla. Iris lesions may lead to hyphema and glaucoma. The incidence of eye involvement in cutaneous JXG is only 0.2–0.4%, but intraocular JXG can occur without cutaneous disease and can be locally aggressive.

Systemic JXG

Systemic JXG is classically defined as involvement of two or more visceral organs in addition to multiple cutaneous and subcutaneous lesions. However, there are many reports of extracutaneous involvement occurring both with and without cutaneous lesions. After the eye, the subcutis, CNS, lung, liver, and spleen are the commonest sites, but there are reports of every organ system in the body being affected. *As the differential diagnosis is usually neoplasia, it is imperative to determine an accurate diagnosis.* Lesions in extracutaneous sites, like those in the skin, regress spontaneously and therefore *treatment is only indicated in cases of compromised organ function.*

Triple association of JXG, NF-1, and JMML

The triple association of JXG, neurofibromatosis-1 (NF-1), and juvenile myelomonocytic leukemia (JMML), an aggressive myeloproliferative disorder of childhood, has been reported. There is an increased risk of JMML in children with NF-1. In a population of children with NF-1 the incidence of JMML is 5:10 000 per year. *It is likely that there is an association of JXG with NF-1, but at present there is no evidence to support an increased risk of JMML in individuals with both JXG and NF-1 compared to those with NF-1 alone.*

SPECIFIC INVESTIGATIONS

> ► In most cases, no specific investigations are required
> ► Ophthalmologic assessment in children under the age of 2 years with multiple lesions
> ► Full blood count and/or pediatric referral in children with JXG and *café au lait* macules, NF-1, or a family history of NF-1
> ► Biopsy in cases with systemic manifestations to confirm diagnosis and avoid unnecessary invasive diagnostic procedures

Radiological and clinicopathological features of orbital xanthogranuloma. Miszkiel KA, Sohaib SA, Rose GE, Cree IA, Moseley IF. Br J Ophthalmol 2000; 84: 251–8.

Of 150 cases of intraocular JXG, none was identified on routine screening of individuals with cutaneous JXG. Of those children with eye involvement, 92% are under the age of 2 years, and if they have cutaneous lesions these tend to be multiple.

Juvenile xanthogranuloma. Hernandez-Martin A, Baselga E, Drolet BA, Esterley NB. J Am Acad Dermatol 1997; 36: 355–67.

Recommendations are made in this review article following assessments of previously reported cutaneous and extracutaneous cases. In general, an awareness of the possibility of extracutaneous involvement is important.

The risk of intraocular juvenile xanthogranuloma: survey of current practices and assessment of risk. Wu Chang M, Frieden IJ, Good W. J Am Acad Dermatol 1996; 34: 445–9.

A postal survey of pediatric dermatologists (27% response rate) and ophthalmologists (44% response rate) revealed the different incidence of ocular xanthogranuloma presenting to these two groups.

Those children under the age of 2 years with multiple skin lesions have the highest risk of intraocular involvement and should be screened by an ophthalmologist.

Juvenile xanthogranuloma associated with neurofibromatosis-1: 14 patients without evidence of hematologic malignancies. Cambhiangi SD, Restano L, Caputo R. Pediatr Dermatol 2004; 21: 97–101.

A retrospective review of 14 individuals affected by JXG and NF-1. The onset of JXG was within the first 2 years of life in 13 patients. Mean follow-up was for 4.3 years (range 1–10 years) in 11 patients, and none of these children developed hematologic malignancy during this period.

JXG, NF-1 and JMML: alphabet soup or a clinical issue? Burgdorf WH, Zelger B. Pediatr Dermatol 2004; 21: 174–6.

An editorial comment and review on this triple association which concludes that there is no evidence to support an increased risk of JMML in children with the combination of JXG and NF-1 compared to those children with NF-1 alone.

FIRST-LINE THERAPIES

▶ None	E
▶ Surgical resection for symptomatic extracutaneous lesions	D
▶ Ocular lesions treated with topical or intralesional corticosteroid	D

Juvenile xanthogranuloma: forms of systemic disease and their clinical implications. Freyer DR, Kennedy R, Bostrom BC, Kohut G, Dehner LP. J Pediatr 1996; 129: 227–37.

Surgery can be an effective cure for symptomatic extracutaneous lesions of JXG.

Update on juvenile xanthogranuloma: unusual cutaneous and systemic variants. Wu Chang M. Semin Cutan Med Surg 1999; 18: 195–205.

In adults the lesions tend not to resolve spontaneously and can last up to 7 years; excision may therefore be considered appropriate.

Juvenile xanthogranuloma of the oral mucosa. Cohen DM, Brannon RB, Davis LD, Miller AS. Oral Surg 1981; 52: 513–23.

Excision can be undertaken for cosmetic and diagnostic reasons, but there have been reports of recurrences after complete excisions in both cutaneous and extracutaneous sites.

Early treatment of juvenile xanthogranuloma of the iris with subconjunctival steroids. Casteels I, Olver J, Malone M, Taylor D. Br J Ophthalmol 1993; 77: 57–60.

Ocular lesions have been successfully treated with topical and intralesional corticosteroids.

SECOND-LINE THERAPIES

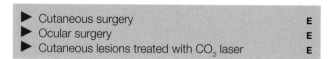

▶ Cutaneous surgery	E
▶ Ocular surgery	E
▶ Cutaneous lesions treated with CO_2 laser	E

Juvenile xanthogranuloma of the corneoscleral limbus. Lim-I-Linn Z, Li L. Cornea 2005; 24: 745–7.

Case report of successful surgical excision and grafting of a limbal juvenile xanthogranuloma in a child with no cutaneous lesions.

Multiple juvenile xanthogranulomas successfully treated with CO_2 laser. Klemcke CD, Held B, Dippel E, Goerdt S. J Deutsch Dermatol Ges 2007; 144: 481–2.

Case report describing successful treatment of cutaneous JXG with CO_2 laser; there was no recurrence at 5-year follow-up.

THIRD-LINE THERAPIES

▶ Radiotherapy	D
▶ Chemotherapy	D
▶ Pulsed methylprednisolone	E

Juvenile xanthogranuloma of the iris in an adult. Parmley VC, George DP, Fannin LA. Arch Ophthalmol 1998; 116: 377–9.

A case report of radiotherapy and methotrexate use in a young man with a lesion on his iris.

Treatment of severe disseminated juvenile systemic xanthogranuloma with multiple lesions in the CNS. Dölken R, Weigel S, Schröder H, Hartwig M, Harms D, Beck JF. J Pediatr Hematol Oncol 2006: 28: 95–7.

A case report of a patient with systemic JXG involving the lungs, liver, kidneys, ribs, scalp, and CNS. Remission of 5 years was achieved with multiagent chemotherapy based on the LCH II treatment protocol using intrathecal methotrexate and prednisolone to control CNS lesions.

Prolonged severe pancytopenia preceding the cutaneous lesions of JXG. Hara T, Hattori S, Hatano M, Kaku N, Nomura A, Takada H, et al. Pediatr Blood Cancer 2006: 47: 103–6.

A case report of a 2-month-old infant with systemic JXG: clinical improvement occurred with etoposide followed by vinblastine and prednisolone.

Successful therapy of systemic JXG in a child. Unuvar E, Devecioglu O, Akcay A, Gulluoglu M, Uysal V, Oguz F, et al. J Pediatr Hematol Oncol 2007; 29: 425–7.

A case report of systemic JXG in a 10-year-old boy. Regression of renal and liver lesions occurred with six courses of pulsed high-dose methylprednisolone 10 mg/kg/day for 3 days.

Treatment of JXG. Stover DG, Alapati S, Regueira O, Turner C, Whitlock JA. Pediatr Blood Cancer 2008; epub ahead of print.

Two case reports of multisystem JXG treated with LCH-based chemotherapy regimens which resulted in prompt resolution of symptoms. This paper includes a literature review of all reported multisystem JXG cases treated with chemotherapy. Ten earlier studies described 15 cases (29 chemotherapeutic regimens of multisystem JXG): 12 of the 15 patients received some form of corticosteroid; nine of the 12 receiving corticosteroid had stable disease (SD), a partial response (PR), or complete resolution (CR). Regimens that included corticosteroids and a vinca alkaloid had the highest rates of CR, PR, or SD. Regimens that did not include corticosteroids had the lowest rates of CR, PR, or SD.

Subdural effusion in a CNS involvement of systemic juvenile xanthogranuloma: A case report treated with vinblastin. Auvin S, Cuvellier J-C, Vinchon M, Defoort-Dhellemes S, Soto-Ares G, Nelken B, et al. Brain Dev 2008; 30: 164–8.

A case report of a 7-month-old infant with JXG affecting the skin, eyes, brain, lungs, and CNS. A treatment regimen consisting of vinblastine 6 mg/m^2/week and prednisolone 1 mg/kg/day for 1 month, with gradual tapering over 6 months, and ocular topical dexamethasone resulted in regression of skin, lung, eye, and CNS lesions.

Kaposi sarcoma

Carrie Wood Cobb, Steven M Manders

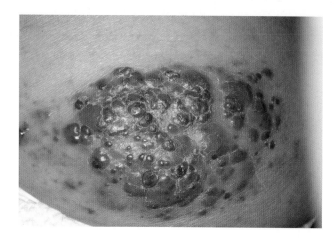

Kaposi sarcoma (KS) is a distinct, often multifocal endothelial neoplasm etiologically linked to human herpesvirus-8 (HHV-8). In the USA, epidemic or AIDS-associated KS is the most common presentation; however, transplant or iatrogenic immunosuppression-related KS is on the increase. In clinical practice, classic and endemic KS are also encountered. Therapy is similar for each type.

MANAGEMENT STRATEGY

Generally, the goals of therapy target cosmetic improvement, palliation, or cessation of progression. For treatment purposes, patients can be divided into several groups. Dermatologists most often encounter limited cutaneous KS, defined as fewer than 10 skin lesions, a lack of oral or visceral involvement, and the absence of tumor-associated lymphedema. Treatment options include *cryotherapy, intralesional vinblastine, radiotherapy,* and *alitretinoin gel*. Because treatment is essentially for cosmesis, side effects such as pigmentary changes and pain become important in therapeutic decisions.

For patients with resistant limited disease, extensive cutaneous involvement, systemic KS, or tumor-associated lymphedema, treatment modalities include liposomal anthracyclines (PEGylated liposomal doxorubicin or liposomal daunorubicin), taxanes (paclitaxel), and interferon-α. For epidemic KS, effective antiretroviral therapy can by itself be sufficient to halt disease progression, and has been found to have a synergistic effect with the *liposomal anthracyclines, paclitaxel,* and *interferon-α*. However, several cases of worsening of KS with the initiation of HAART have been reported, as part of an immune reconstitution syndrome. Iatrogenic immunosuppression-associated KS can respond to a reduction in treatment doses or change in immunosuppressive regimen, especially to sirolimus. *Radiotherapy* remains an alternative treatment option for this group of patients.

Treatment of oral lesions is problematic because of inaccessibility to cryotherapy and radiation-induced mucositis. Options include *intralesional vinblastine,* sclerosing agents such as *sodium tetradecyl sulfate,* or systemic treatments.

An increasing number of investigational therapeutics are being explored for the treatment and prevention of KS, including antiangiogenic agents, mTOR inhibitors (rapamycin, temsirolimus), orally active matrix metalloproteinase inhibitors, tyrosine kinase inhibitors, and agents targeting interleukin (IL)-12.

SPECIFIC INVESTIGATIONS

- ► Serology for HIV, CD4+ T-lymphocyte counts, viral load (if HIV positive)
- ► Complete blood count, renal and hepatic function
- ► Chest radiograph
- ► Stool for occult blood

Kaposi's sarcoma. Antman K, Chang Y. N Engl J Med 2000; 342: 1027–38.

KS remains the most common AIDS-associated cancer in the USA.

Management of AIDS-related Kaposi's sarcoma. Di Lorenzo G, Konstantinopoulos PA, Pantanowitz L, Di Trolio R, De Placido S, Dezube BJ. Lancet Oncol 2007; 8: 167–76.

Review of current treatment strategies and ongoing investigations.

Epidemic Kaposi's sarcoma. Cianfrocca M, Von Roenn JH. Oncology 1998; 12: 1375–81.

Review of appropriate patient evaluation, including thorough history and physical examination and relevant laboratory and imaging studies.

FIRST-LINE THERAPIES

▷ Cryotherapy	**B**
▷ Intralesional vinblastine	**C**
▷ Radiotherapy	**B**
▷ Alitretinoin gel	**A**
▷ PEGylated liposomal doxorubicin plus HAART	**B**
▷ Paclitaxel	**B**

Cryotherapy for cutaneous Kaposi's sarcoma (KS) associated with acquired immune deficiency syndrome (AIDS): a phase II trial. Tappero JW, Berger TG, Kaplan LD, Volberding PA, Kahn JO. J AIDS 1991; 4: 839–46.

Treatment was repeated at 3-week intervals, allowing adequate healing time. On average, subjects received three treatments per lesion, with a mean follow-up time of 11 weeks (range 6–25 weeks). One treatment consisted of two freeze–thaw cycles, with thaw times ranging from 11 to 60 per cycle. A 70% cosmetic response rate, with duration up to 6 months.

Hypopigmentation and scarring are potential problems in skin types III–VI.

Intralesional vinblastine for cutaneous Kaposi's sarcoma associated with acquired immunodeficiency syndrome. Boudreaux AA, Smith LL, Cosby CD, Bason MM, Tappero JW, Berger TG. J Am Acad Dermatol 1993; 28: 61–5.

Responses were achieved in 88% of treated lesions, but pain and hyperpigmentation are common. Pain was minimized by the addition of bicarbonate-buffered lidocaine to the diluent.

Evidence Levels: **A** Double-blind study **B** Clinical trial ≥ 20 subjects **C** Clinical trial < 20 subjects **D** Series ≥ 5 subjects **E** Anecdotal case reports

Radiotherapy of classic and human immunodeficiency virus-related Kaposi's sarcoma: results in 1482 lesions. Caccialanza M, Marca S, Piccinno R, Eulisse G. J Eur Acad Dermatol Venereol 2008; 22: 297–302.

A 98% clearance rate was reported in classic lesions, and a 91% clearance rate in HIV-associated lesions, with good overall tolerability.

Phase III vehicle-controlled, multi-centered study of topical alitretinoin gel 0.1% in cutaneous AIDS-related Kaposi's sarcoma. Bodsworth NJ, Bloch M, Bower M, Donnell D, Yocum R, International Panretin Gel KS Study Group. Am J Clin Dermatol 2001; 2: 77–87.

Response rate was 37% (compared to 7% treated with vehicle).

Marginal response rate and exorbitant cost make the usefulness of this modality questionable. Tretinoin gel may be a reasonable alternative topical retinoid option (Topical treatment of epidemic Kaposi's sarcoma with all-trans-retinoic acid. Bonhomme L, Fredj G, Averous S, Szekely AM, Ecstein E, Trumbic B, et al. Ann Oncol 1991; 2: 234–5).

Pegylated liposomal doxorubicin plus highly active antiretroviral therapy versus highly active antiretroviral therapy alone in HIV patients with Kaposi's sarcoma. Martin-Carbonero L, Barrios A, Saballs P, Sirera G, Santos J, Palacios R, et al.; Caelyx/KS Spanish Group. AIDS 2004; 18: 1737–40.

Randomized study comparing PEGylated liposomal doxorubicin plus HAART vs HAART alone showed a greater response rate (76% vs 20%, respectively, in the intent-to-treat analysis) in the former group.

These results differ from previous studies showing HAART therapy alone to be effective in regression of KS lesions.

Multicenter trial of low-dose paclitaxel in patients with advanced AIDS-related Kaposi sarcoma. Tulpule A, Groopman J, Saville MW, Harrington W Jr, Friedman-Kien A, Espina BM, et al. Cancer 2002; 95: 147–54.

Phase II trial of 107 patients showed a complete or partial response with or without concomitant protease inhibitor of 59% and 54%, respectively. Grade IV neutropenia was the most common adverse effect (35% of patients).

Two case reports of potentially serious drug–drug interactions occurring in patients on HAART and paclitaxel concomitantly (Potential drug interaction with paclitaxel and highly active antiretroviral therapy in two patients with AIDS-associated Kaposi sarcoma. Bundow D, Aboulafia DM. Am J Clin Oncol 2004; 27: 81–4).

SECOND-LINE THERAPIES

▶ Intralesional interferon	C
▶ Subcutaneous or intramuscular interferon	B
▶ Interferon plus antiretroviral therapy	B
▶ Liposomal anthracyclines as monotherapy	B

Intralesional interferon-alpha and zidovudine in epidemic Kaposi's sarcoma. Dupuy J, Prize M, Lynch G, Bruce S, Schwartz M. J Am Acad Dermatol 1993; 28: 966–72.

Intralesional interferon-α (1 million units three times weekly for 6 weeks) showed a response rate of 85%, but this was not statistically significant.

Interferon-alpha2b with protease inhibitor-based antiretroviral therapy in patients with AIDS-associated Kaposi sarcoma: an AIDS malignancy consortium phase I trial. Krown SE, Lee JY, Lin L, Fischl MA Ambinder R, Von Roenn JH. AIDS 2006; 41: 149–53.

The authors observed that the administration of interferon-α_{2b} (5 million units/day) led to a limited improvement in Kaposi sarcoma lesions.

Pegylated-liposomal doxorubicin versus doxorubicin, bleomycin, and vincristine in the treatment of AIDS-related Kaposi's sarcoma: results of a randomized phase III clinical trial. Northfelt DW, Dezube BJ, Thommes JA, Miller BJ, Fischl MA, Friedman-Kien A, et al. J Clin Oncol 1998; 16: 2445–51.

Liposomal doxorubicin was not only significantly more effective, but had less toxicity than the standard triple chemotherapeutic regimen.

Pegylated liposomal doxorubicin as second-line therapy in the treatment of patients with advanced classic Kaposi sarcoma: a retrospective study. Di Lorenzo G, Di Trolio R, Montesarchio V, Palmieri G, Palmieri G, Nappa P, et al. Cancer 2008; 112: 1147–52.

Fourteen of 20 patients achieved remission with a median duration of 9 months. The most common limiting side effect was neutropenia.

THIRD-LINE THERAPIES

▶ Thalidomide	B
▶ Liposomal ALL-*trans* retinoic acid, intravenous	B
▶ Photodynamic therapy	B
▶ Foscarnet	B
▶ 9-*cis* retinoic acid	B
▶ Etoposide	B
▶ Sirolimus	C
▶ PEGylated liposomal doxorubicin with IL-12	C
▶ IL-12	C
▶ Imiquimod 5% cream	C
▶ Sodium tetradecyl sulfate 3%	C
▶ Matrix metalloproteinase inhibitor COL-3	C
▶ Surgical excision	E

A retrospective analysis of thalidomide therapy in non-HIV-related Kaposi's sarcoma. Ben M'barek L, Fardet L, Mebazaa A, Thervet E, Biet I, Kérob D, et al. Dermatology 2007; 215: 202–5.

Only three of 11 patients achieved remission, with sensory neuropathy and vertigo limiting therapy in 27%.

A multicenter phase II study of the intravenous administration of liposomal tretinoin in patients with acquired immunodeficiency syndrome-associated Kaposi's sarcoma. Bernstein ZP, Chanan-Khan A, Miller KC, Northfelt DW, Lopez-Berestein G, Gill PS. Cancer 2002; 95: 2555–61.

A thrice-weekly dosing schedule (60 mg/m^2 escalating to 120/m^2) was more effective than once a week, without any significant difference in toxicity.

New photodynamic therapy protocol to treat AIDS-related Kaposi's sarcoma. Tardivo JP, Del Giglio A, Paschoal LH, Baptista MS. Photomed Laser Surg 2006; 24: 528–31.

Case report describing successful treatment of a solitary patient with epidemic KS.

Effect of antiviral drugs used to treat cytomegalovirus end-organ disease on subsequent course of previously diagnosed Kaposi's sarcoma in patients with AIDS. Robles R, Lugo D, Gee L, Jacobson MA. J AIDS Hum Retrovirol 1999; 20: 34–8.

In patients being treated for cytomegalovirus with foscarnet, progression of KS was markedly delayed.

9-cis-retinoic acid capsules in the treatment of AIDS-related Kaposi sarcoma: results of a phase 2 multicenter clinical trial. Aboulafia DM, Norris D, Henry D, Grossman RJ, Thommes J, Bundow D, et al. Arch Dermatol 2003; 139: 178–86.

Overall response was 19%. Moderate efficacy and substantial toxicity at higher doses limit use.

Phase II evaluation of low-dose oral etoposide for the treatment of relapsed or progressive AIDS-related Kaposi's sarcoma: an AIDS Clinical Trials Group clinical study. Evans SR, Krown SE, Testa MA, Cooley TP, Von Roenn JH. J Clin Oncol 2002; 20: 3236–41.

Overall response rate was 36.1%; neutropenia and opportunistic infections were the most common side effects.

Sirolimus for Kaposi's sarcoma in renal-transplant recipients. Stallone G, Schena A, Infante B, Di Paolo S, Di Paolo S, Loverre A, Maggio G, et al. N Engl J Med 2005; 352: 1317–23.

All of 15 transplant patients achieved total remission when switched from ciclosporin to sirolimus for immunosuppression.

Phase 2 study of pegylated liposomal doxorubicin in combination with interleukin-12 for AIDS-related Kaposi sarcoma. Little RF, Aleman K, Kumar P, Wyvill KM, Pluda JM, Read-Connole E, et al. Blood 2007; 110: 4165–71.

Thirty of 36 patients had a good response to liposomal doxorubicin with IL-12 for six 3 week cycles followed by twice-weekly IL-12 for maintenance for 3 years. No control group was included and patients received HAART in addition to the experimental regimen.

Activity of subcutaneous interleukin-12 in AIDS-related Kaposi sarcoma. Little RF, Pluda JM, Wyvill KM, Rodriguez-Chavez IR, Tosato G, Catanzaro AT, et al. Blood 2006; 107: 4650–7.

IL-12 was administered twice weekly at varying doses. Significant results were observed at doses >100 ng/mg, and side effects limited dosing above 500 ng/kg.

Imiquimod 5% cream for treatment of HIV-negative Kaposi's sarcoma skin lesions: A phase I to II, open-label trial in 17 patients. Célestin Schartz NE, Chevret S, Paz C, Kerob D, Verola O, Morel P, et al. J Am Acad Dermatol 2008: 585–91.

Imiquimod was applied under occlusion twice daily for 24 weeks. Eight of 17 patients showed some response, with six of 17 demonstrating tumor progression.

Intralesional vinblastine vs. 3% sodium tetradecyl sulfate for the treatment of oral Kaposi's sarcoma. A double blind, randomized clinical trial. Ramírez-Amador V, Esquivel-Pedraza L, Lozada-Nur F, De la Rosa-García E, Volkow-Fernández P, Súchil-Bernal L, et al. Oral Oncol 2002; 38: 460–7.

Sixteen patients were randomized to each arm. Results were equivocal, but suggested a possibly greater tolerability of sodium tetradecyl sulfate.

Randomized phase II trial of matrix metalloproteinase inhibitor COL-3 in AIDS-related Kaposi's sarcoma: an AIDS Malignancy Consortium Study. Dezube BJ, Krown SE, Lee JY, Bauer KS, Aboulafia DM. J Clin Oncol 2006; 24: 1389–94.

A response rate of 41% was observed at a dose of 50 mg/day. The medication was well tolerated overall.

Local therapy for mucocutaneous Kaposi's sarcoma in patients with acquired immunodeficiency syndrome. Webster GF. Dermatol Surg 1995; 21: 205–8.

Surgery can occasionally be helpful for isolated lesions, but recurrence is frequent; therefore this modality is of limited value.

Evidence Levels: **A** Double-blind study **B** Clinical trial ≥ 20 subjects **C** Clinical trial < 20 subjects **D** Series ≥ 5 subjects **E** Anecdotal case reports

Kawasaki disease

Adam Friedman, Ranon Mann

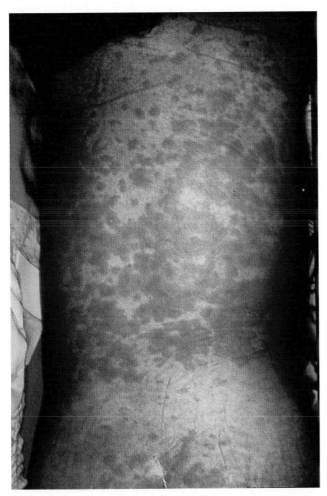

From Lebwohl MG. The Skin and Systemic Disease: A Color Atlas, 2nd edn. Churchill Livingstone 2003, with permission of Elsevier.

Kawasaki disease (KD), seen primarily in infants and children, is an acute febrile multiorgan vasculitic process well known for its mucocutaneous and nodal involvement. Although KD was described in Japan nearly 50 years ago, its pathogenesis has yet to be clarified. Increasing evidence supports an infectious etiology.

MANAGEMENT STRATEGIES

The primary goal when treating a patient with KD is the prevention of cardiac complications, including coronary artery disease, aneurysm formation, myocardial infarction, and even sudden death. The mainstay of therapy has for years been the use of high-dose salicylates (e.g., aspirin) and intravenous γ-globulin (IVIG) in order to manage the acute, intense, inflammatory characteristics of this condition and to prevent the aforementioned cardiovascular sequelae.

In the acute inflammatory phase, aspirin, a potent inhibitor of prostaglandin synthesis, is initially dosed at 80–100 mg/kg/day orally, divided four times/day for 2

weeks. After the patient is afebrile for 48 hours, the dose is reduced to 3–5 mg/kg orally daily and continued for 6–8 weeks until the sedimentation rate and platelet count normalize. Baumer et al. (2006) recently concluded that no significant randomized clinical trials have been performed to date, and therefore current evidence is insufficient to support the use of salicylates as an integral component of first-line therapy in KD.

IVIG is a known first-line therapy in the treatment of KD. IVIG, which can lead to rapid defervescence, is able to neutralize circulating myelin antibodies and to downregulate proinflammatory cytokines, including INF-γ. The pediatric dosing, which is equivalent to the adult dosing, is 400 mg/kg/day IV over 2 hours as a single daily infusion for 4 consecutive days, or alternatively – and apparently more efficaciously – a single dose of 2 g/kg IV infused over 12 hours. Failure of IVIG has been linked to a gene polymorphism in the plasma platelet-activating factor acetylhydrolase. No specific regimen has been assigned for these non-responding cases.

SPECIFIC INVESTIGATIONS

- ▶ Laboratory examination: ESR, CBC + platelet count, LDH
- ▶ Multidetector CT
- ▶ Echocardiography

Kawasaki disease: an overview. Pinna GS, Kafetzis D, Tselkas O, Skevaki CL. Curr Opin Infect Dis 2008; 21: 263–70.

Echocardiography, stress imaging, angiography, MRI, and ultrafast computed tomography (CT) scans have been useful in the diagnosis of coronary aneurysms, occlusions, and stenosis. Echocardiography is recommended both at the time of diagnosis and after 2–6 weeks. It has recently been demonstrated that multidetector CT is preferable to transthoracic echocardiography or MRI. CT can detect calcification and estimate soft plaques, offer rapid data collection and simple interpretation of images, all of which serve as an advantage over other diagnostic modalities. Conversely, MRI cannot offer rapid capture of images, thus prolonging the time under anesthesia and its associated risks. Transthoracic echocardiography can only image the proximal arteries and therefore cannot reliably detect stenosis.

The diagnosis and treatment of Kawasaki disease. Royle J, Burgner D, Curtis NJ. Pediatr Child Health 2005: 41: 87–93.

These guidelines highlight the difficulties in the diagnosis of KD. A meta-analysis of recent data offers insight that may assist in the early recognition of this important pediatric disease. The clinical features of KD are common to many other childhood illnesses, and therefore the diagnostic criteria are not highly sensitive. Blood serologies and chemistries may be helpful, but none is diagnostic and most have a low specificity. The echocardiogram should not be used as a diagnostic test. A normal echo does not exclude KD, as coronary lesions generally occur in the convalescent phase and may develop as late as 6–8 weeks after the onset of fever. Because there is no specific diagnostic test for KD, increased awareness of the epidemiology and the spectrum of clinical presentation is essential for early recognition and optimal management.

FIRST-LINE THERAPIES

▶ Aspirin (acetylsalicylic acid)	B
▶ Immunoglobulin	B

Resistance to intravenous immunoglobulin in children with Kawasaki disease. Tremoulet AH, Best BM, Song S, Wang S, Corinaldesi E, Eichenfield JR, et al. J Pediatr 2008; 153: 117–21.

IVIG treatment for the acute stage of KD has shown to be effective and safe. However, it is known that 10–20% of patients are resistant to initial therapy. These patients are at increased risk for the development of coronary artery abnormalities. Using demographic and laboratory information on IVIG-resistant cases, this retrospective study attempted to develop a scoring system to help identify future resistant cases among patients in San Diego County. This would perhaps indicate the need for secondary therapies early in the treatment of these patients. Unfortunately, the diversity of the patient population did not allow for the development of an accurate and clinically useful scoring system.

Analysis of potential risk factors associated with nonresponse to initial intravenous immunoglobulin treatment among Kawasaki disease patients in Japan. Uehara R, Belay ED, Maddox RA, Holman RC, Nakamura Y, Yashiro M, et al. Pediatr Infect Dis J 2008; 27: 155–60.

Some KD patients do not respond to initial treatment with IVIG. The purpose of this study was to determine potential risk factors associated with IVIG non-response among KD patients in Japan. The results emphasize that physicians should consider IVIG non-response in patients with recurrent KD, as well as in KD patients diagnosed and treated before the fifth day of illness who continue to have laboratory values associated with non-response, such as low platelet count, elevated alanine aminotransferase and C-reactive protein. These patients may benefit from the administration of a second-line treatment early during the illness in addition to the initial IVIG treatment.

Treatment of acute Kawasaki disease: aspirin's role in the febrile stage revisited. Hsieh KS, Weng KP, Lin CC, Huang TC, Lee CL, Huang SM. Pediatrics 2004; 114: 689–93.

In North America, high-dose aspirin is widely used during the acute phase of KD. However, the necessity of this therapy has yet to be elucidated. This study indicated that treatment in the acute stage of KD without aspirin had no effect on the response rate of IVIG therapy, duration of fever, or incidence of coronary abnormalities. This response was seen when children were treated with high-dose (2 g/kg) IVIG as a single infusion, regardless of whether treatment was commenced before or after day 5 of illness. Therefore, the available data show no appreciable benefit of aspirin in preventing IVIG non-response, aneurysm formation, or shortening of fever duration.

SECOND-LINE THERAPIES

▶ Corticosteroids	B
▶ Retreatment with immunoglobulin	D

Effects of steroid pulse therapy on immunoglobulin-resistant Kawasaki disease. Furukawa T, Kishiro M, Akimoto K, Nagata S, Shimizu T, Yamashiro Y. Arch Dis Child 2008; 93: 142–6.

In this non-randomized study the effectiveness of intravenous methylprednisone (IVMP) was compared with that of additional IVIG as second-line therapy for KD. Fever was rapidly alleviated after IVMP administration in all IVIG-resistant patients in the study; 77% recovered without recurrence of KD, and did not develop coronary artery aneurysms. The findings suggested that early IVMP treatment in IVIG-resistant patients is as effective as treatment with additional IVIG as second-line therapy.

Risk factors associated with the need for additional intravenous gamma-globulin therapy for Kawasaki disease. Muta H, Ishii M, Furui J, Nakamura Y, Matsuishi T. Acta Paediatr 2006; 95: 189.

The goal of this study, using data from a nationwide survey in Japan, was to identify the characteristics of patients who needed retreatment with IVIG. Elevated sedimentation rate, anemia, and high lactate dehydrogenase are known predictive values for necessitating IVIG retreatment. In this study, male gender, incomplete and recurrent cases of KD, and treatment with IVIG at a dose of 1 g/kg or less within 4 days of illness onset, were identified as independent risk factors associated with the need for retreatment. Identification of these risk factors would be beneficial to predict which patients might need IVIG retreatment. This could help physicians to initially create a strategy to prevent cardiovascular complications in these patients.

THIRD-LINE THERAPIES

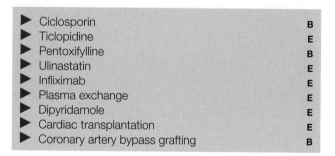

▶ Ciclosporin	B
▶ Ticlopidine	E
▶ Pentoxifylline	B
▶ Ulinastatin	E
▶ Infliximab	E
▶ Plasma exchange	E
▶ Dipyridamole	E
▶ Cardiac transplantation	E
▶ Coronary artery bypass grafting	B

Response of refractory Kawasaki disease to pulse steroid and cyclosporin A therapy. Raman V, Kim J, Sharkey A. Pediatr Infect Dis J 2001; 20: 635–7.

A case of aggressive and protracted KD with coronary aneurysms, myocarditis, pericarditis and valvular insufficiency, despite repeated administration of intravenous immunoglobulin, responded to combination therapy with pulse and high-dose corticosteroids and ciclosporin A.

Clinical utility of ulinastatin, urinary protease inhibitor in acute Kawasaki disease. Saji T. Nippon Rinsho 2008; 66: 343–8.

This review discusses the utility of ulinastatin, a trypsin inhibitor, as part of a first- or second-line treatment regimen for IVIG-resistant KD.

Incomplete and atypical Kawasaki disease in a young infant: Severe, recalcitrant disease responsive to infliximab. O'Connor MJ, Saulsbury FT. Clin Pediatr 200; 46: 345.

Evidence Levels: A Double-blind study **B** Clinical trial ≥ 20 subjects **C** Clinical trial < 20 subjects **D** Series ≥ 5 subjects **E** Anecdotal case reports

A 7-week-old infant with incomplete and atypical KD refractory to two doses of IVIG and IVMP became afebrile after two doses of infliximab 5 mg/kg.

A report of two cases of Kawasaki disease treated with plasma exchange. Harada T, Ito S, Shiga K, Inaba A, Machida H, Aihara Y, et al. Ther Apher Dial 2008; 12: 176–9.

Two cases of refractory KD are reported in which plasma exchange may have reduced the risk of coronary artery lesions and proved effective against acute heart failure with catecholamine-refractory shock. The mechanism of this improvement remains unclear.

Prevention of thrombosis of coronary aneurysms in patients with a history of Kawasaki disease. Suda K, Kudo Y, Sugawara Y. Nippon Rinsho 2008; 66: 355–9.

To prevent coronary thrombosis in KD, long-term anti-thrombotic therapy using antiplatelet drugs such as aspirin, dipyridamole, ticlopidine, clopidogrel, and abciximab, with or without warfarin, is recommended by official guidelines.

Optimal time of surgical treatment for Kawasaki coronary artery disease. Yamauchi H, Ochi M, Fujii M, Hinokiyama K, Ohmori H, Sasaki T, et al. J Nippon Med Sch 2004; 71: 279–86.

The authors studied 21 patients with Kawasaki disease and coronary complications who underwent coronary artery bypass grafting (CABG) over a 12-year period. They conclude that CABG is successful when completed shortly after the acute onset of disease.

Keloid scarring

Brian Berman, Martha Viera, Ran Huo

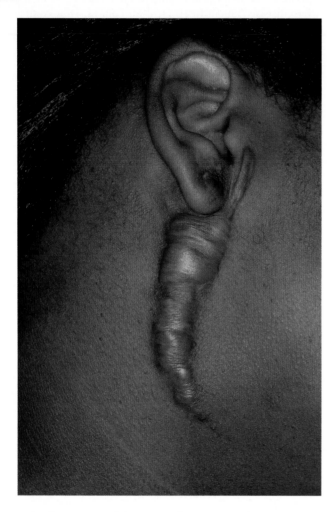

Keloids are dermal hyperproliferative growths with excessive accumulation of dense fibrous tissue that may appear in areas of trauma. By definition, keloids are scars that extend beyond the borders of the original wound and do not regress spontaneously. In addition to the cosmetic disfigurement and negative psychological impact that keloids may cause the patient, these scars can often present with intense pain and pruritus.

MANAGEMENT STRATEGY

The therapeutic options for keloids are numerous; however, there is no one modality that is considered to be universally safe and effective. Prevention of recurrence should be the main determinant in treatment selection. The initial rule of treatment involves *prevention* and *patient education*. It is of the utmost importance to close wounds with minimal tension and inflammation. Non-essential cosmetic surgery should be avoided in patients predisposed to developing keloids. These scars commonly develop in high-tension areas of the body. Incision sites in the skin of the mid-chest and skin overlying joints should be avoided, and surgical wounds should parallel skin creases.

Common therapeutic modalities include occlusive dressings, compression therapy, intralesional corticosteroid injections, intralesional interferon injections, cryosurgery, surgical excision, radiation therapy, and laser therapy. As no single therapy is vastly superior or universally efficacious, combinational therapies have led to the best success rates.

Intralesional corticosteroids have been the mainstay of treatment for keloids. The most commonly used is triamcinolone acetonide in concentrations of 10–40 mg/mL administered intralesionally with a 25–27-gauge needle at 4–6-week intervals. Topical corticosteroids and topically applied corticosteroid-impregnated tape are also used frequently; the basis for the latter involves recent data demonstrating that occlusion enhances percutaneous penetration of steroid by the formation of a drug reservoir within the stratum corneum. Silicone gel sheets and silicone occlusive dressings have anti-keloidal effects, which appear to be a result of hydration. Pressure devices are thought to induce local tissue hypoxia and have been shown to have a thinning effect on keloids. A novel idea in the treatment of keloids and hypertrophic scars is the use of intralesional interferon-α_{2b}, which has been used successfully to reduce scar height and postoperative recurrences, via a mechanism of collagen synthesis inhibition. Interferon-γ has also been evaluated in the treatment of keloids, with modest results. Cryotherapy can be used as monotherapy or in conjunction with other treatment modalities, most commonly triamcinolone, with reported efficacy. Its mechanism of action involves the induction of vascular damage and tissue anoxia that ultimately leads to necrosis. However, some reported side effects have included hypopigmentation and postoperative pain. A specialized intralesional needle cryoprobe method has been recently reported to result in better efficacy and fewer side effects. Radiation therapy has been used as monotherapy or as an adjuvant to surgical excision. The carcinogenesis risks of radiotherapy are extremely small; however, the concept of using potentially harmful radiation to treat benign lesions is a persistent and important issue. Surgical excision alone yields widely varying results with high (55–100%) recurrence rates. The combination of surgical excision with other modalities, such as intralesional corticosteroids or with pressure dressing, X-ray therapy, interstitial radiation and brachytherapy, reduces recurrence rates to a range of 10–50%. CO_2 and argon lasers have been used in the past in the treatment of keloids, but have recently been replaced by the Nd:YAG and 585 nm pulsed dye laser because of their better efficacy and fewer adverse effects. Intralesional injection of 5-fluorouracil (5-FU) has been beneficial for hypertrophic scars and, to a lesser extent, for keloids. Bleomycin, retinoic acid, and intralesional verapamil have all been reported to have good efficacy in small clinical trials, but more clinical experience with these agents is needed.

SPECIFIC INVESTIGATIONS

▶ Skin biopsy

Dermatofibrosarcoma protuberans is a unique fibrohistiocytic tumour expressing CD34. Aiba S, Tabata N, Ishii H, Ootani H, Tagami H. Br J Dermatol 1992; 127: 79–84.

Dermatofibrosarcoma protuberans can be easily misdiagnosed as a keloid. Histopathology may help differentiate the two, but expression of CD34 by tumor cells occurs only in dermatofibrosarcoma protuberans.

Evidence Levels: **A** Double-blind study **B** Clinical trial ≥ 20 subjects **C** Clinical trial < 20 subjects **D** Series ≥ 5 subjects **E** Anecdotal case reports

FIRST-LINE THERAPIES

▶ Intralesional corticosteroids	B
▶ Compression	B
▶ Occlusive dressing	B
▶ Intralesional interferon-α_{2b}	B

Keloids treated with topical injections of triamcinolone acetonide. Immediate and long term results. Kiil J. Scand J Plast Reconstruct Surg 1977; 11: 169–72.

In a prospective clinical trial of 52 patients, intralesional injections of triamcinolone acetonide alone resulted in significant flattening and reduction of pruritus in 93% of the keloids. One-third had partial recurrence at 1 year, and at 5 years more than 50% had recurred. All recurrences were successfully treated with further triamcinolone acetonide injections.

Experience with difficult keloids. Lahiri A, Tsiliboti D, Gaze NR. Br J Plast Surg 2001; 54: 633–5.

A retrospective clinical trial of 43 patients (62 keloids) treated with intralesional injections of triamcinolone acetate, cryotherapy, and another intralesional injection of triamcinolone acetate resulted in 12 patients with complete remission, 19 patients with good improvement, and 10 with some improvement.

A prospective, randomized, single-blind, comparative study evaluating the tolerability and efficacy of intralesional etanercept compared to intralesional triamcinolone acetonide for the treatment of keloids. Berman B, Perez O, Patel J, Viera M, Amini S, Block S. J Drugs Dermatol 2008; 7: 757–61.

Twenty subjects were randomly treated with 25 mg etanercept or 20 mg TAC monthly injections for 2 months. Both etanercept and TAC were safe and well tolerated. TAC improved 11 of 12 parameters, confirming its mainstay use for the treatment of keloids. Etanercept improved five of 12 parameters.

An inexpensive self fabricated pressure clip for the ear lobe. Agrawal K, Panda KN, Arumugam A. Br J Plast Surg 1998; 51: 122–3.

In 26 patients (41 earlobe keloids), self-fabricated and inexpensive pressure clips were used for a minimum of 6 months with concomitant intralesionally injected triamcinolone acetonide, resulting in 34 earlobes that underwent boring in follow-up.

Comparison of a silicone gel-filled cushion and silicon gel sheeting for the treatment of hypertrophic or keloid scars. Berman B, Flores F. Dermatol Surg 1999; 25: 484–6.

In this study of 32 keloid patients, 53% treated with silicone gel cushion and 36.3% treated with silicone gel sheeting had a reduction in keloid volume.

Clinical evaluation of a new self-drying silicone gel in the treatment of scars: a preliminary report. Signorini M, Clementoni MT. Aesthet Plast Surg 2007; 31: 183–7.

A prospective trial involving 160 patients that compared postoperative treatment with a self-drying transparent silicone gel with no treatment. Sixty-seven percent of patients in the treatment group had a significant improvement in scar quality.

Combination of different techniques for the treatment of earlobe keloids. Akoz T, Gideroglu K, Akan M. Aesthet Plast Surg 2002; 26: 184.

Nine patients were treated with surgical excision of their earlobe keloids, followed by triamcinolone acetonide injection and silicone gel sheets. No recurrences occurred in eight of the nine patients.

Effects of a water-impermeable, non-silicone-based occlusive dressing on keloids. Bieley HC, Berman B. J Am Acad Dermatol 1996; 35: 113–14.

A water-impermeable, non-silicone-based occlusive dressing worn continuously for 2 months brought about an average keloid height reduction of 35% in 19 of 21 patients, and the majority of patients had reduction in pain, pruritus, and erythema.

Recurrence rates of excised keloids treated with postoperative triamcinolone acetonide injections or interferon alfa-2b injections. Berman B, Flores F. J Am Acad Dermatol 1997; 37: 755–7.

There was a statistically significant reduction in the recurrence of 124 excised keloids with post-excision interferon-α_{2b} (18.7% recurrence) versus excision alone (51.1%), and versus treatment with postoperative intralesional triamcinolone (58.4%).

Effects of interferon-a2b on keloid treatment with triamcinolone acetonide intralesional injection. Lee JH, Kim SE, Lee A-Y. Int J Dermatol 2008; 47: 183–6.

Forty keloid lesions from 19 patients were treated either with triamcinolone acetonide intralesional (TAIL) combined with interferon-α_{2b} or with TAIL alone. Superior results were obtained with combination therapy, with more than 80% improvement in lesion depth and volume in most patients.

SECOND-LINE THERAPIES

▶ Cryosurgery	A
▶ Radiation	B

Intralesional cryotherapy for enhancing the involution of hypertrophic scars and keloids. Har-Shai Y, Amar M, Sabo E. Plast Reconstruct Surg 2003; 111: 1841–52.

Ten patients with 12 hypertrophic scars and keloids were treated with one session of intralesional cryosurgery, with an average of 51.4% scar volume reduction and no recurrence after 18 months.

Use of cryosurgery in the treatment of keloids. Rusciani L, Rossi G, Bono R. J Dermatol Surg Oncol 1993; 19: 529–34.

Sixty-five lesions were treated with cryosurgery, resulting in complete resolution with no recurrence in 73% of patients after 17–42 months of follow-up.

Cryotherapy in the treatment of keloids. Rusciani L, Paradisi A, Alfano C, Chiummariello S, Rusciani A. J Drugs Dermatol 2006; 5: 591–5.

Of 135 patients with 166 keloids treated with cryotherapy between 1990 and 2004, 79.5% responded very well with a volume reduction of 80% or more after three treatments.

Median follow-up time was 4 years. The most common adverse effects included atrophic depressed scars and, in 75% of cases, residual hypopigmentation.

A comparison of the combined effect of cryotherapy and corticosteroid injections versus corticosteroids and cryotherapy alone on keloids: a controlled study. Yosipovitch G, Widijanti Sugeng M, Goon A, Chan YH, Goh CL. J Dermatol Treat 2001; 12: 87–90.

Ten patients with 28 keloids were treated with cryotherapy alone, steroid injection alone, or cryotherapy and steroid injection. At eight months' follow-up the combination therapy was significantly better at reducing keloid thickness and pruritus than either treatment alone. None of the keloids treated with combination therapy recurred. No significant side effects were noted.

Treatment of earlobe keloids using the cobalt 60 teletherapy unit. Malaker K, Zaidi M, Franka MR. Ann Plast Surg 2003; 52: 602–4.

Forty-seven patients were treated with postoperative telecobalt external beam radiation and 87.2% had no recurrence at the 6-month follow-up visit.

Treatment of keloids by surgical excision and immediate postoperative single-fraction radiotherapy. Ragoowansi R, Cornes PG, Moss AL, Glees JP. Plast Reconstruct Surg 2003; 111: 1853–9.

In a retrospective study of 80 patients treated with postoperative single-fraction radiotherapy, 9% of keloids relapsed after 1 year and 16% relapsed after 5 years.

The treatment of 783 keloid scars by iridium 192 interstitial irradiation after surgical excision. Escarmant P, Zimmermann S, Amar A, Ratoanina JL, Moris A, Azaloux H, et al. Int J Radiat Oncol Biol Phys 1993; 26: 245–51.

There was a recurrence rate of 21% after at least 1 year follow-up in 783 treated keloids.

Biologically effective doses of postoperative radiotherapy in the prevention of keloids. Dose–effect relationship. Kal HB, Veen RE. Strahlenther Onkol 2005; 181: 717–23.

In this review, a radiotherapy regimen resulting in a biologically effective dose of at least 30 Gy is recommended to be administered, starting within 2 days after surgery, to minimize keloid recurrence rates to less than 10%.

Retrospective analysis of treatment of unresectable keloids with primary radiation over 25 years. Malaker K, Vijayraghavan K, Hodson I, Al Yafi T. Clin Oncol J Roy Coll Radiol 2004; 16: 290–8.

In this retrospective study involving 86 keloids in 64 patients, 97% of keloids showed significant regression after completing radiotherapy with either kilovoltage X-rays or electron beams, without significant side effects. The patients were treated with a total of 3750 cGy administered in five once-weekly fractions.

Postoperative high-dose-rate brachytherapy in the prevention of keloids. Veen RE, Kal HB. Int J Radiat Oncol Biol Phys 2007; 69: 1205–8.

Postoperative ^{192}Ir brachytherapy showed better cosmetic results at higher dosages, with only one keloid recurrence out of 38 observed after a once-administered 6 Gy and twice-administered 4 Gy regimen.

THIRD-LINE THERAPIES

► Laser surgery	C
► Imiquimod	A
► Intralesional 5-FU	B
► Intralesional interferon-γ	C
► Topical retinoic acid	B
► Intralesional bleomycin	B
► Verapamil	B
► Surgery	B

Treatment of keloid sternotomy scars with 585 nm flash-lamp-pumped pulsed-dye-laser. Alster TS, Williams CM. Lancet 1995; 345: 1198–200.

The 585 pulsed dye laser was used to treat 16 patients with sternotomy scars. There was a significant reduction in pruritus, erythema, and scar height in most patients. These results persisted for at least 6 months after treatment.

Effect of pulse width of a 595-nm flashlamp-pumped pulsed dye laser on the treatment response of keloidal and hypertrophic sternotomy scars. Manuskiatti W, Wanitphakdeedecha R, Fitzpatrick RE. Dermatol Surg 2007; 33: 152–61.

In 19 patients with keloidal or hypertrophic median sternotomy scars, pulsed dye laser with pulse width of 0.45 ms was significantly effective in reducing scar volume and improving elasticity. However, the reported reduction in scar volume was only 24.4% after three treatments.

The effect of carbon dioxide laser surgery on the recurrence of keloids. Norris JEC. Plast Reconstruct Surg 1991; 87: 44–9.

In this retrospective study, 23 patients had adequate follow-up. One had no recurrence, nine required corticosteroids to suppress recurrence, and 13 were considered to be treatment failures.

Pilot study of the effect of postoperative imiquimod 5% cream on the recurrence rate of excised keloids. Berman B, Kaufman J. J Am Acad Dermatol 2002; 47: S209–11.

Thirteen keloids were treated with excision and imiquimod 5% cream every night for 8 weeks. Ten patients with 11 keloids completed the 6-month study, and there were no recurrences.

Intralesional 5-fluorouracil in the treatment of keloids: an open clinical and histopathologic study. Kontochristopoulos G, Stefanaki C, Panagiotopoulos A, Stefanaki K, Argyrakos T, Petridis A, et al. J Am Acad Dermatol 2005; 52: 474–9.

Treatment with once-weekly intralesional 5-FU (average of seven treatments) resulted in a more than 50% improvement in 17 of 20 patients. However, there was a 47% keloid recurrence rate within 1 year. Average injection volumes were 0.2–0.4 mL/cm^2 at 50 mg/mL.

Treatment of inflamed hypertrophic scars using intralesional 5-FU. Fitzpatrick RE. Dermatol Surg 1999; 25: 224–32.

In a retrospective study of 1000 patients with hypertrophic scars and keloids over a 9-year period, the most effective regimen was found to be 0.1 mg of triamcinolone acetonide (10 mg/mL) and 0.9 mL 5-FU (50 mg/mL) injections up to three times a week.

Evidence Levels: **A** Double-blind study **B** Clinical trial ≥ 20 subjects **C** Clinical trial < 20 subjects **D** Series ≥ 5 subjects **E** Anecdotal case reports

Intralesional interferon gamma treatment for keloids and hypertrophic scars. Larrabee WF, East CA, Jaffe HS, Stephenson C, Peterson KE. Arch Otolaryngol Head Neck Surg 1990; 116: 1159–62.

Five of the 10 study patients had a reduction in their scar size by at least 50% in linear dimensions. The treatment protocol was one treatment per week for 10 weeks. Up to 0.05 mg of interferon-γ was injected weekly.

The local treatment of hypertrophic scars and keloids with topical retinoic acid. Janssen de Limpens AMP. Br J Dermatol 1980; 103: 319–23.

There was a reduction in keloid size and symptoms in 77% of 28 intractable keloids treated with topical retinoic acid.

Treatment of keloids and hypertrophic scars using bleomycin. Aggarwal H, Saxena A, Lubana PS, Mathur RK, Jain DK. J Cosmet Dermatol 2008; 7: 43–9.

Over 3 months, four courses of bleomycin were administered through a multiple superficial puncture technique in 50 patients with keloids and hypertrophic scars. Forty-four percent of patients experienced complete flattening of lesions, and 22% showed more than 75% lesion regression.

Prevention and treatment of keloids with intralesional verapamil. D'Andrea F, Brongo S, Ferraro G, Baroni A. Dermatology 2002; 204: 60–2.

Twenty-two patients with keloids were treated with either surgical excision plus topical silicone plus 2.5 mg/mL intralesional verapamil hydrochloride injection, or with just surgical excision plus topical silicone. Of the patients in the group with verapamil injection 54% did not have keloid recurrence, compared to 18% in the group without verapamil injection.

Keratoacanthoma

Caroline M Owen, Nicholas R Telfer

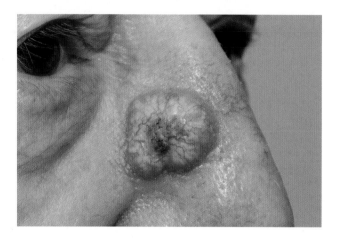

Keratoacanthoma (KA) is a distinctive tumor with characteristic histopathologic and clinical features. Classically it presents as a rapidly proliferating, firm, dome-shaped, crateriform nodule. It shares many features of a squamous cell carcinoma (SCC), but is self-healing and can be considered a form of aborted malignancy. Although eventually self-limiting, its growth can be unpredictable and locally destructive, causing problems in management. Lesions are usually solitary and mainly affect sun-exposed sites in patients of middle age and older. Less commonly, lesions may be large (giant KA), progressive with central clearing (KA centrifugum), or multiple (e.g., multiple KA of Ferguson-Smith type, generalized eruptive KA of Grzybowski).

MANAGEMENT STRATEGY

Initial management is directed at making an accurate diagnosis of KA, in particular differentiating it from SCC. Although much research has been directed at the investigation of the differential cytokine profile or ultrastructure of KA and SCC, in practice the diagnosis of KA relies on the correlation between clinical and histopathologic criteria as follows.

A KA classically has three clinical stages:
- Proliferative – early rapid growth to form a crateriform nodule;
- Fully developed – no growth;
- Involutional – the lesion regresses, usually within 4–8 months.

The five most relevant histopathologic criteria when differentiating KA from SCC have been shown to be:
- Epithelial lip (in favor of KA);
- Sharp outline between tumor and stroma (in favor of KA);
- Ulceration (in favor of SCC);
- Numerous mitoses (in favor of SCC);
- Marked pleomorphism (in favor of SCC).

Accurate assessment of these histopathologic criteria relies on the provision of an adequate histologic specimen. This should be deep enough to include subcutaneous fat, either by total excision or by transverse biopsy through the center of the lesion.

Once the diagnosis of KA has been established, the aims of treatment are to hasten resolution, prevent destruction of important structures, prevent recurrence, and obtain as favorable a cosmetic outcome as possible. Management therefore depends on the type of KA, its site, its rate of growth, and whether or not it has previously been treated.

In general, *excision* is the treatment of choice for a small solitary KA because this will remove the lesion, provide an adequate specimen for histologic examination, and generally give a good cosmetic result. An alternative to this is *transverse biopsy* to provide an adequate histologic specimen, followed by *curettage or blunt dissection* of the residual lesion.

If one is confident of the diagnosis and the lesion has been documented as being static or already starting to involute, then observation is an option. Obviously, any concern that the lesion is not following an involutional pattern makes treatment mandatory.

Recently, *topical imiquimod* has been used with success. *Intralesional methotrexate, topical 5-fluorouracil* and *argon laser ablation* have also been shown to be effective.

Large proliferating lesions for which surgical management is not possible or is likely to result in a poor cosmetic outcome can be treated with *radiotherapy, intralesional methotrexate,* or *intralesional 5-fluorouracil.*

Multiple KAs have been successfully treated with *oral retinoids* and *intralesional 5-fluorouracil.* Recurrent KA has been shown to respond well to *radiotherapy,* but oral retinoids have also been used with success. The level of evidence in the literature for the treatment of KA is poor, consisting mainly of small case series. Without a control group it is very difficult to be sure of the success of any intervention, particularly with a lesion that has a natural history of spontaneous involution.

SPECIFIC INVESTIGATIONS

▶ Skin biopsy

Keratoacanthoma: a clinico-pathologic enigma. Schwartz RA. Dermatol Surg 2004; 30: 326–33.

A review of KA with an emphasis on clinical and histologic features and a broad overview of management options.

Keratoacanthoma: a tumor in search of a classification. Karaa A, Khachemoune A. Int J Dermatol 2007; 46: 671–8.

A review of KA, including a debate on whether this tumor should be considered benign or malignant, and a further discussion of treatment options.

Differentiating squamous cell carcinoma from keratoacanthoma using histopathological criteria. Is it possible? A study of 296 cases. Cribier B, Asch P, Grosshans E. Dermatology 1999; 199: 208–12.

A study evaluating the reliability of histologic criteria used to distinguish between KA and SCC.

MANAGEMENT OF SMALL, SOLITARY KERATOACANTHOMA

FIRST-LINE THERAPIES

▶ Curettage	C
▶ Excision	D
▶ Observation	D

Evidence Levels: **A** Double-blind study   **B** Clinical trial ≥ 20 subjects   **C** Clinical trial < 20 subjects   **D** Series ≥ 5 subjects   **E** Anecdotal case reports

Evaluation of curettage and electrodesiccation in the treatment of keratoacanthoma. Nedwich JA. Australas J Dermatol 1991; 32: 137–41.

A retrospective case series of 111 KAs in 106 patients treated with curettage and electrodesiccation. There were four recurrences after a mean follow-up of 28.5 months.

Treatment of keratoacanthomas with curettage. Reymann F. Dermatologica 1977; 155: 90–6.

A case series of 47 non-biopsy-proven KAs treated with curettage; there was recurrence in one case during follow-up ranging from 4 months to 5 years (average 32 months).

Keratoacanthomas treated with Mohs' micrographic surgery (chemosurgery). A review of forty-three cases. Larson PO. J Am Acad Dermatol 1987; 16: 1040–4.

A case series of 43 biopsy-proven KAs in 42 patients treated with Mohs' micrographic surgery. There was one recurrence during a 6–24-month follow-up period.

Keratoacanthoma observed. Griffiths RW. Br J Plast Surg 2004; 57: 485–501.

Fourteen patients with a clinical diagnosis of KA were observed with serial photographs every 2 weeks. Mean time to resolution was 27 weeks (range 12–64 weeks). No recurrences occurred during a mean follow-up of 3 years and 5 months (range from 9 months to 8 years), and all scars were acceptable to the patients. Four further patients were excluded from observational follow-up when there was concern about the growth pattern of the lesions.

SECOND-LINE THERAPIES

▶ Topical imiquimod	D
▶ Intralesional methotrexate	D
▶ Topical 5-fluorouracil	E
▶ Argon laser	D

Topical treatment with imiquimod may induce regression of facial keratoacanthoma. Dendorfer M, Oppel T, Wollenberg A, Prinz JC. Eur J Dermatol 2003; 13: 80–2

Four patients with facial KA (biopsy proven in three) were treated with imiquimod cream 5% on alternate days for 4–12 weeks. Complete regression was seen in all four patients (within 4–6 weeks in three of them). No recurrences occurred during the follow-up of 4–6 months.

Spontaneous regression of keratoacanthoma can be promoted by topical treatment with imiquimod cream. Di Lernia V, Ricci C, Albertini G. J Eur Acad Dermatol Venereol 2004; 18: 626–9.

Two biopsy-proven facial KAs were treated with imiquimod cream 5% three times per week for one patient and five times per week for the other for 8 weeks. Both resolved completely and remained clear after 1 year of follow-up. Both needed a 1-week rest period off treatment because of erythema, erosion, and crusting at the treatment site.

Intralesional methotrexate treatment for keratoacanthoma tumours: A retrospective study and review of the literature. Annest NM, VanBeek MJ, Arpey CJ, Whitaker DC. J Am Acad Dermatol 2007; 56: 989–93

Thirty-eight cases of KA treated with methotrexate, identified from the authors' institution and from a literature review.

Biopsy proven in 25 cases. Complete response rate of 92% reported; no significant adverse incidents reported, but regular blood monitoring as for systemic methotrexate recommended. Useful description of authors' standard practice detailing concentration/site/injection intervals and frequency.

Topical 5-fluorouracil as primary therapy for keratoacanthoma. Grey RJ, Meland NB. Ann Plast Surg 2000; 44: 82–5.

Two clinically diagnosed KAs in two patients were treated with 5-fluorouracil 5% once daily for 4 weeks in one and 8 weeks in the other. A rapid response was noted within 3 weeks.

Argon laser treatment of small keratoacanthomas in difficult locations. Neumann RA, Knobler RM. Pharmacol Ther 1990; 29: 733–6.

Case series of 17 small histologically proven solitary KAs on the head and neck. These were treated once with argon laser. There was resolution with no scarring in 65% and slight scarring in 35%. There were no recurrences after 2 years of follow-up.

MANAGEMENT OF LARGE, RAPIDLY PROLIFERATING KERATOACANTHOMA

FIRST-LINE THERAPIES

▶ Radiotherapy	D
▶ Intralesional 5-fluorouracil	D
▶ Intralesional methotrexate	D

Treatment of aggressive keratoacanthomas by radiotherapy. Donahue B, Cooper JS, Rush S. J Am Acad Dermatol 1990; 23: 489–93.

Case series of 29 KAs (eight recurrent after attempted surgical ablation) in 18 patients treated with radiotherapy in doses ranging from 3500 cGy in 15 fractions to 5600 cGy in 28 fractions. All lesions regressed completely. Good cosmetic results were reported in 14 patients.

Treatment of keratoacanthomas with intralesional fluorouracil. Odom RB, Goette DK. Arch Dermatol 1978; 114: 1779–83.

Case series of 14 patients with 26 KAs (12 single and rapidly growing, 14 multiple, none biopsy proven). Two to five doses of 0.2–0.5 5-fluorouracil 50 mg/mL were injected intralesionally at weekly intervals. Resolution took place with excellent cosmetic results in all but one case. There were no recurrences during a follow-up period of 3–17 months.

Large keratoacanthomas in difficult locations treated with intralesional 5-fluorouracil. Parker CM, Hanke CW. J Am Acad Dermatol 1986; 14: 770–7.

Case series of five large, facial, biopsy-proven KAs. Two to six intralesional injections of 1–3 mg of 50 mg/mL 5-fluorouracil were given at 1–4-week intervals. Resolution was reported in all five, with no recurrence during follow-up of 18–43 months, but the authors describe a further KA (that had been present for 16 weeks and static for 10) that did not respond, suggesting that intralesional therapy is most appropriate for KAs in the proliferative growth phase.

Treatment of keratoacanthomas with intralesional methotrexate. Melton JL, Nelson BR, Stogh DB, Brown MD, Swanson NA, Johnson TM. J Am Acad Dermatol 1991; 23: 1017–23.

Case series of nine solitary KAs, biopsy proven in six. One or two intralesional injections of 0.4–1.5 mg methotrexate (12.5 or 25 mg/mL) resulted in complete resolution with minimal scarring.

Intralesional methotrexate in solitary keratoacanthoma. Cuesta-Romero C, de Grado-Pena J. Arch Dermatol 1998; 134: 513–14.

Case series of six solitary KAs (four biopsy proven). Between one and four intralesional injections of 0.5–1 mg methotrexate (25 mg/mL) resulted in complete regression with no recurrence during a follow-up period of 10–20 months.

MANAGEMENT OF MULTIPLE KERATOACANTHOMAS

FIRST-LINE THERAPIES

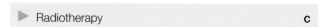

▶ Oral etretinate	E
▶ Oral isotretinoin	E
▶ Intralesional fluorouracil	E

Multiple persistent keratoacanthomas: treatment with oral etretinate. Benoldi D, Alinovi A. J Am Acad Dermatol 1984; 10: 1035–8.

Two cases of multiple KAs of the Ferguson-Smith type were treated with oral etretinate 1 mg/kg daily, reducing after 8 weeks to a maintenance dose of 0.5–0.75 mg/kg daily. Total clearance was experienced by one patient with follow-up of 1 year; there was partial clearance in the second patient, with follow-up of 6 months.

Etretinate is no longer available. It is anticipated, albeit not yet proven, that acitretin would have a similar result.

Treatment of multiple keratoacanthomas with oral isotretinoin. Shaw JC, White CR. J Am Acad Dermatol 1986; 15: 1079–82.

Report of one patient with multiple KAs who was treated with isotretinoin (induction dose 1.5 mg/kg daily). This treatment cleared existing lesions and appeared to prevent recurrences.

Treatment of multiple keratoacanthomas with intralesional fluorouracil. Eubanks SW, Gentry RH, Patterson JW, May DL. J Am Acad Dermatol 1982; 7: 126–9.

Report of one patient with multiple KAs of the Ferguson-Smith type successfully treated with intralesional 5-fluorouracil.

MANAGEMENT OF RECURRENT KERATOACANTHOMA

FIRST-LINE THERAPIES

| ▶ Radiotherapy | C |

Radiation therapy of giant aggressive keratoacanthomas. Goldschmidt H, Sherwin WK. Arch Dermatol 1993; 129: 1162–5.

Retrospective case series of 16 large or rapidly growing KAs, 14 of which were recurrent following surgery. They were treated five times weekly with individual doses ranging from 2.5 to 5 Gy (total dose 45–60 Gy). All tumors resolved, with satisfactory cosmetic results.

SECOND-LINE THERAPIES

| ▶ Oral isotretinoin | D |

Treatment of solitary keratoacanthomas with oral isotretinoin. Goldberg LH, Rosen T, Becker J, Knauss A. J Am Acad Dermatol 1990; 23: 934–6.

Case series of 12 biopsy-proven solitary KAs, six primary, six recurrent. Treatment with oral isotretinoin 0.5–1 mg/kg resulted in resolution in nine (four primary, five recurrent) of the 12 cases, with a good cosmetic result. None of these lesions recurred during an average follow-up of 12 months.

Keratosis pilaris and variants

Nisha Patel, Robert Silverman

Keratosis pilaris is a common inherited disorder of unknown etiology characterized by tenacious keratin plugging of follicular orifices in specific locations on the body. It typically becomes apparent during childhood on the extensor aspect of the upper arms, anterior surface of the thighs, and lateral aspects of the cheeks. In severe cases it may extend onto the distal extremities, shoulders, and buttocks. Perifollicular erythema and a background ruddy hue of the cheeks are common (keratosis pilaris rubra). Variants of keratosis pilaris include keratosis pilaris atrophicans (ulerythema ophryogenes), keratosis follicularis spinulosa decalvans (KFSD), folliculitis spinulosa decalvans (FSD), and atrophoderma vermiculatum; these are also addressed in this chapter.

MANAGEMENT STRATEGY

Keratosis pilaris is usually asymptomatic and often does not require treatment. In most cases it is a cosmetic nuisance. This is especially true in pre-teens and teenagers. Young children are mostly unaware of and unbothered by the condition. Teenagers and adults will complain of skin roughness, an unsightly cosmetic appearance, or an occasional secondary, painful folliculitis. Parents will mistakenly complain that their children with KP have early acne, or they will be concerned about the intense facial redness that occurs after exercise or exposure to cold. Those with extensive or symptomatic involvement often desire treatment, although even without therapy the condition often becomes less prominent with increasing age.

Initial treatment involves measures to reduce excessive skin roughness and follicular accentuation that often waxes and wanes over a period of months. Harsh soaps are to be avoided, but cleansers containing 2% salicylic acid or glycolic acid may be helpful. Bathing should be followed by the application of an emollient to damp skin. Keratolytic agents such as lactic acid, ammonium lactate, salicylic acid, glycolic acid and urea-containing humectants are the mainstays of treatment used to soften the keratotic papules. Salicylic acid 2%

in 20% urea cream, or salicylic acid 6% in propylene glycol, combines the properties of an emollient with a keratolytic agent. Twice-daily application of one of these compounds for at least a 3-week trial is recommended. Products composed of higher concentrations of α-hydroxy acids, or those that are not neutralized, may sting on application and reduce compliance, especially in children. Some patients may find that the addition of gentle massage with a polyester sponge such as a Buf-Puf during a shower or bath is particularly helpful. Vigorous scouring, though, can lead to irritation. Once adequate relief of symptoms has been achieved, maintenance therapy of weekly or twice-weekly application of 20–40% urea cream is recommended.

Topical retinoids may be tried in some cases but can be irritating and expensive if large areas are treated. The lowest concentrations of topical tretinoin, such as 0.025% cream, can be used at first. If there is no significant irritation, higher concentrations can be used. In a recent placebo-controlled trial tazarotene 0.05% cream was also shown to reduce the pruritus, erythema, and roughness of keratosis pilaris.

If a significant inflammatory component is present, it can be reduced for defined, short periods with a medium potency topical corticosteroid in an emollient base. Once inflammation has abated, corticosteroids are discontinued and keratolytics are introduced. The presence of pustules suggests a bacterial infection, and topical antibiotics, such as clindamycin lotion or mupirocin, can be used in those circumstances. A 3-month course of oral vitamin A, 50 000 units three times a day, has been advocated for some patients. Oral isotretinoin has been helpful in some patients with ulerythema ophryogenes and atrophoderma vermiculatum. In the author's experience, calcipotriol and calcineurin inhibitors have not been helpful.

Laser therapy has been used for several variants of keratosis pilaris. Pulsed tunable dye laser (PDL) treatment has recently been demonstrated to be a safe treatment for the erythema associated with keratosis pilaris atrophicans and keratosis pilaris rubra (KPR). Potassium titanyl phosphate (KTP) laser has also cleared the keratotic papules and reduced the erythema of KPR lesions. However, reports involved only a few cases, and no mention of sustained long-term effectiveness is documented for the authors to recommend laser therapy for most patients. Keratosis pilaris spinulosa decalvans has been treated with laser-assisted hair removal using a normal-mode, non-Q-switched, high-energy pulsed ruby laser at fluences of 19–21 J/cm² at 6-week intervals. This mode of treatment has been effective in producing persistent reductions of inflammation in this keratosis pilaris variant, albeit at the expense of permanent hair loss in treated areas.

SPECIFIC INVESTIGATIONS

Laboratory studies may uncover conditions associated with KP or its variants, but their presence does not alter the basic therapeutic approach.

> ► Serum testosterone levels (in obese females)
> ► Complete physical examination (for atopic diseases)
> ► Ophthalmologic examination (cataracts, keratitis in KPA)
> ► Urinary hCG (if pregnancy is suspected)
> ► Hemoglobin A₁C (if type 1 diabetes is suspected)

The prevalence of cutaneous manifestations in young patients with type 1 diabetes. Pavlovic MD, Milenkovic T, Dinic M, Misovic M, Dakovic D, Todorovic S, et al. Diabetes Care 2007; 30: 1964–7. Epub 2007 May 22.

The presence and frequency of skin manifestations were examined and compared in 212 unselected type 1 diabetic patients and 196 healthy sex- and age-matched controls. Keratosis pilaris affected 12% of the diabetic patients versus 1.5% of controls. A significant association was also found between acquired ichthyosis and keratosis pilaris.

High body mass index, dry scaly leg skin and atopic conditions are highly associated with keratosis pilaris. Yosipovitch G, Mevorah B, Mashiach J, Chan YH, David M. Dermatology 2000; 201: 34–6.

Keratosis pilaris is associated with multiple factors, including high BMI, leg skin dryness, and atopic conditions.

Keratosis pilaris in pregnancy: an unrecognized dermatosis of pregnancy? Jackson JB, Touma SC, Norton AB. WV Med J 2004; 100: 26–8.

Five cases presented in this study demonstrate keratosis pilaris as a condition in which the onset or severity of the dermatosis may be linked to the hormonal changes of pregnancy.

Is keratosis pilaris another androgen-dependent dermatosis? Barth JH, Wojnarowska F, Dawber RPR. Clin Exp Dermatol 1988; 13: 240–1.

In this study of serum testosterone level and body mass index in 78 premenopausal women with hirsutism, hyperandrogenism in the presence of obesity was associated with an increased prevalence and severity of keratosis pilaris.

FIRST-LINE THERAPIES

▶ Sodium lactate and urea cream	B
▶ Polyester sponge	D
▶ Salicylic acid in urea	D
▶ Topical corticosteroids	D
▶ Glycolic acid	D

Evaluation of a sodium lactate and urea crème to ameliorate keratosis pilaris. Weber TM, Kowcz A, Rizer R. J Am Acad Dermatol 2004; 50: 47 [Abstract].

A formulation containing sodium lactate and urea was tested on 32 subjects with mild to severe keratosis pilaris. The authors reported progressive, statistically significant improvements in overall condition, skin roughness, and skin tone, at 3, 6, and 12 weeks of use.

Polyester sponge adjunct in acne management. Diamant F. Clin Ther 1980; 3: 250–3.

Seven patients who used polyester sponges from three times per week to once daily for their keratosis pilaris improved after a mean treatment duration of 7.4 weeks.

Practical management of widespread, atypical keratosis pilaris. Novick NL. J Am Acad Dermatol 1984; 11: 305–6.

Thirty patients with widespread, atypical or psychologically troubling keratosis pilaris were treated according to a protocol that included prevention of excessive skin drying, application of salicylic acid 2–3% in 20% urea cream using a polyester sponge, and use of emollient-based topical corticosteroids if a prominent inflammatory component was present. All patients reported satisfaction with cosmetic results. Clearing of lesions was noted in 75–100% of cases, with elimination of most lesions achieved within 2–3 weeks of daily therapy.

Keratosis pilaris decalvans non-atrophicans. Drago F, Maietta G, Parodi A, Rebora A. Clin Exp Dermatol 1993; 18: 45–6.

Case report of a patient with keratosis pilaris decalvans non-atrophicans with follicular keratotic papules on the limbs and trunk accompanied by loss of body hair. The patient was successfully treated over the course of 3 months with topical emollients and multivitamins. The keratosis pilaris completely disappeared, leaving no scars, and there was complete regrowth of hair.

Traditional methods of treating uncomplicated keratosis pilaris seem to be effective in treating cases of keratosis pilaris decalvans non-atrophicans.

SECOND-LINE THERAPIES

▶ Topical tazarotene	A
▶ Topical tretinoin	D
▶ Isotretinoin	E

Efficacy, tolerability, and safety of calcipotriol ointment in disorders of keratinization. Results of a randomized, double-blind, vehicle-controlled, right/left comparative study. Kragballe K, Steijlen PM, Ibsen HH, van de Kerkhof PC, Esmann J, Sorensen LH, et al. Arch Dermatol 1995; 131: 556–60.

A randomized, double-blind, vehicle-controlled study of calcipotriol ointment for the treatment of disorders of keratinization included nine patients with keratosis pilaris. No therapeutic effect was detected in keratosis pilaris.

Folliculitis spinulosa decalvans: successful therapy with dapsone. Kunte C, Loeser C, Wolff H. J Am Acad Dermatol 1998; 39: 891–3.

Case report of a patient with folliculitis spinulosa decalvans with keratotic follicular papules on the trunk, the extremities, and the lateral, alopecic part of the eyebrows, and erythema, scaling, and follicular hyperkeratoses on the scalp. Isotretinoin and topical corticosteroids were ineffective. Dapsone 100 mg/day led to the resolution of inflammation and pustulation on the scalp within 1 month. The scarring alopecia did not expand after the dapsone therapy. No improvement of the follicular roughness was reported.

Tazarotene 0.05% cream for the treatment of keratosis pilaris. Bogle MA, Ali A, Bartel H. J Am Acad Dermatol 2004; 50: 39 [Abstract].

A randomized, placebo-controlled, double-blind prospective study of tazarotene 0.05% cream for the treatment of keratosis pilaris on the posterior arms of 33 patients reportedly resulted in statistically significant improvement in pruritus, erythema, and roughness of keratosis pilaris lesions.

Natural history of keratosis pilaris. Poskitt L, Wilkinson JD. Br J Dermatol 1994; 130: 711–13.

This retrospective questionnaire study of 49 patients with keratosis pilaris yielded 14 who had benefited from a variety of treatments for keratosis pilaris. Of these patients, eight reported therapy with topical tretinoin cream to be helpful.

Clinical findings, cutaneous pathology, and response to therapy in 21 patients with keratosis pilaris atrophicans. Baden HP, Byers HR. Arch Dermatol 1994; 130: 469–75.

Twenty-one patients with keratosis pilaris atrophicans were treated with various agents and combinations of agents, including keratolytics, antibiotics, topical corticosteroids, and retinoids, all with very limited response. Treatment of four patients with isotretinoin 1 mg/kg resulted in little or no improvement in three patients and exacerbation of the condition in one.

A case of atrophoderma vermiculatum responding to isotretinoin. Weightman W. Clin Exp Dermatol 1998; 23: 89–91.

Atrophoderma vermiculatum is a rare variant of keratosis pilaris that results in reticular or honeycomb scarring of the face. In this case report, isotretinoin induced a remission in the inflammatory component of the disease, which was maintained after cessation of treatment.

In severe cases of atrophoderma vermiculatum with significant scarring, a trial of isotretinoin therapy is worthwhile to halt progression of the disease.

Atrophoderma vermiculatum. Case reports and review. Frosch PJ, Brumage MR, Schuster-Pavlovic C, Bersch A. J Am Acad Dermatol 1988; 18: 538–42.

In this variant of keratosis pilaris a symmetric worm-eaten or reticular atrophy may result. Dermabrasion may be used to reduce the eventual scarring.

A case of ulerythema ophryogenes responding to isotretinoin. Layton AM, Cunliffe WJ. Br J Dermatol 1993; 129: 645–6.

Ulerythema ophryogenes, a variant of keratosis pilaris, begins in the eyebrows as small, discrete, horny, pinhead-sized papules at the hair follicle orifices that spread to the forehead and scalp. Atrophy and alopecia of the eyebrows and scalp may result. There is a variable response to isotretinoin.

THIRD-LINE THERAPIES

▶ Tetracyclines: oxytetracycline, minocycline	E
▶ Long-pulse, non-Q-switched, ruby laser (for keratosis pilaris spinulosa decalvans)	E
▶ Pulsed tunable dye laser (for keratosis pilaris atrophicans and keratosis pilaris rubra)	C
▶ Potassium titanyl phosphate laser (for keratosis pilaris rubra)	E

Keratosis pilaris rubra: a common but underrecognized condition. Marqueling AL, Gilliam AE, Prendiville J, Zvulunov A, Antaya RJ, Sugarman J, et al. Arch Dermatol 2006; 142: 1611–16.

In this case series from dermatology practices in the United States, Canada, Israel, and Australia, the clinical characteristics of 27 patients with keratosis pilaris rubra are described. Treatments given for KPR in these patients included emollients; emollients containing urea, lactic acid, topical corticosteroids, or a combination of these ingredients; topical agents containing cholecalciferol, topical or systemic retinoid agents;

topical corticosteroids; and topical salicylic acid. One patient had an excellent response with pulsed-dye laser. No single agent or combination of products was felt to be uniformly effective.

Natural history of keratosis pilaris. Poskitt L, Wilkinson JD. Br J Dermatol 1994; 130: 711–13.

Two patients responding to a retrospective questionnaire stated that treatment with tetracyclines had 'dramatically' improved their keratosis pilaris. The authors warned that the questionnaire did not permit the exclusion of possible coincidental acne in these patients, and that their reported improvement may have been secondary to the known therapeutic effects of tetracycline on acne. However, tetracyclines are recognized anti-inflammatory agents, and this may explain the improvements in keratosis pilaris that are sometimes noted with their use.

Recalcitrant scarring follicular disorders treated by laser-assisted hair removal: a preliminary report. Chui CT, Berger TG, Price VH, Zachary CB. Dermatol Surg 1999; 25: 34–7.

A patient with keratosis pilaris spinulosa decalvans of the scalp complicated by recurrent secondary infection was treated with a variety of oral antibiotics and topical corticosteroids, with limited success. The patient subsequently underwent five treatments with a normal-mode, non-Q-switched, high-energy, pulsed ruby laser at fluences of 19–21 J/cm^2 at 6-week intervals. Eight months after the initiation of treatment a significant reduction of inflammation occurred in the treated areas, at the expense of a persistent diminution of hair growth.

This is a promising mode of therapy for patients with severe or symptomatic conditions who have not responded to other modes of therapy and are willing to accept permanent hair loss on treated areas as a side effect.

Treatment of keratosis pilaris atrophicans with the pulsed tunable dye laser. Clark SM, Mills CM, Lanigan SW. J Cutan Laser Ther 2000; 2: 151–6.

All facial areas involved with keratotis pilaris atrophicans in 12 patients were treated with the pulsed dye laser at 585 nm. Patients received two to eight treatments with the laser, with energies ranging from 6.0 to 7.5 J/cm^2. The authors reported clinical improvement in all patients, with a significant reduction in erythema scores. A significant improvement was not achieved in skin roughness. Treatment was generally well tolerated, with side effects mostly limited to local pain during treatment.

Keratosis rubra pilaris responding to potassium titanyl phosphate laser. Dawn G, Urcelay M, Patel M, Strong AMM. Br J Dermatol 2002; 147: 822–4.

A 15-year-old girl with erythematous papules on her cheeks, eyebrows, and chin was treated with a potassium titanyl phosphate laser (532 nm) with energy fluence of 12–14 J/cm^2 and pulse width of 510 ms. Both cheeks were treated seven times at 6–8-week intervals, resulting in good cosmetic clearance of keratotic papules and gradual reduction of erythema on her face. During a follow-up period the patient required two treatments at 4-month intervals, and was happy with her cosmetic result.

Langerhans' cell histiocytosis

Rakesh Patalay, Tony Chu

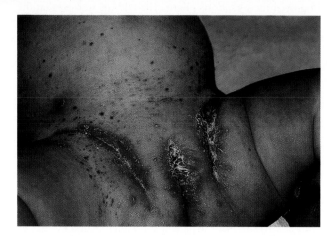

Langerhans' cell histiocytosis (LCH) is a reactive condition defined by the accumulation/proliferation of a clonal population of epidermal Langerhans' cells. Patients can have either single or multiple organ involvement. Children tend to have more aggressive disease than adults, yet most evidence is based on case reports and small case series in children.

MANAGEMENT STRATEGY

LCH encompasses the diseases previously known as histiocytosis X, eosinophilic granuloma, Hand–Schuller–Christian disease, Letterer–Siwe disease, congenital self-healing reticulohistiocytosis (Hashimoto–Pritzker), Langerhans' cell granulomatosis, and non-lipid reticuloendotheliosis.

A definitive diagnosis can be made histologically by identification of Langerhans' cells that express CD1a by immunohistochemistry, and the finding of Birbeck granules by electron microscopy.

Prior to institution of therapy a full investigation must be completed.

Treatment depends on the organ(s) involved and the severity of the disease, and therefore should be tailored to the individual patient. Most published data concern childhood disease and may not always be directly applicable to adults. Patients are staged as single-system disease (with bone involvement this is further stratified into mono-ostotic and polyostotic bone disease), multisystem disease, and multisystem disease with evidence of organ dysfunction. Although some patients with LCH may undergo spontaneous remission, the disease is unpredictable and many patients progress from single-system to multisystem disease. Organs most commonly involved include bone, skin, lymph nodes, pituitary, liver, lungs, central nervous system, gastrointestinal tract, spleen, bone marrow, and endocrine system.

Single-system bone or skin disease has a good prognosis and may not require treatment. Curettage or intralesional steroid injections can also be used in single-system bone disease. Single-system skin disease may respond to local measures with topical steroids, topical nitrogen mustard, or phototherapy.

Single-system lung disease may respond to prednisolone at 2 mg/kg/day. In single-system disease that does not respond to these measures, single-system lymph node disease, and multisystem disease without organ dysfunction, systemic treatment with azathioprine (2 mg/kg/day) with or without low-dose weekly methotrexate (5–10 mg/week) may lead to resolution.

In recalcitrant disease or in multisystem disease with evidence of organ dysfunction, treatment will depend on the age of the patient. Dysfunction of key organs – liver, lungs, spleen, and bone marrow – carries the worst prognosis. Trials have demonstrated that in children, prednisolone with vinblastine is the treatment of choice. This combination is less effective in adults, who are also more sensitive to the side effects of these drugs. In adults the first-line treatment is etoposide.

In pediatric studies the use of maintenance therapy has been shown to reduce the overall morbidity of the disease. Adults often have a more chronic and relapsing course to their disease, and maintenance therapy with azathioprine for 1 year should be considered in all patients with multisystem disease.

In both children and adults with multisystem disease with organ dysfunction, there remains a small group who do not respond to conventional therapy. In these patients 2-chlorodeoxyadenosine has proved useful, and in severe disease bone marrow transplantation has been successful. A number of drugs have been used in various stages of the disease, but most are anecdotal case reports. Long-term morbidity can be correlated to organ involvement or may occur as a direct consequence of treatment, and includes skeletal deformities, risk of secondary malignancies (particularly with the use of alkylating agents and radiotherapy), endocrine dysfunction, and infertility.

SPECIFIC INVESTIGATIONS

Routine investigations
▶ Biopsy of organ involved for staining for S100 and CD1a, or electromicroscopy for Birbeck granules
▶ Full blood count with differential
▶ Coagulation tests (PT, APTT)
▶ ESR
▶ Liver function tests
▶ CRP
▶ Chest X-ray
▶ Whole-body MRI is the most effective way to identify both skeletal and non-skeletal disease

In selected cases
▶ Lung function tests in patients with lung disease
▶ CT chest scan for all adult smokers or children with chest signs or symptoms
▶ Bronchoalveolar lavage for CD1a+ cells, or open lung biopsy if evidence of lung involvement
▶ CT scan of brain and pituitary fossa if signs of diabetes insipidus
▶ Plasma and urinary osmolality if signs of diabetes insipidus. A water deprivation test, if required
▶ Full hormone screen if diabetes insipidus confirmed
▶ MRI brain scan if lytic skull lesions, diabetes insipidus, or symptoms suggestive of CNS involvement
▶ Panorthogram if gum involvement
▶ Bone marrow biopsy if hematological abnormalities
▶ Abdominal ultrasound and liver biopsy if abnormal liver function
▶ Multiple bowel biopsies if evidence of malabsorption or failure to thrive in an infant

Histiocytosis syndromes in children: Approach to the clinical and laboratory evaluation of children with Langerhans' cell histiocytosis. Broadbent V, Gadner H, Komp DM, Ladisch S. Med Pediatr Oncol 1989; 17: 492–5.

Multiple organ systems may be affected in patients with LCH. Therefore, the following studies are recommended for all patients at diagnosis: a complete blood count with white blood cell differential, liver function tests, coagulation times (PT and PTT), chest radiograph, and radiographic skeletal survey (more sensitive than a radionuclide bone scan for detecting bone lesions). A measurement of urine osmolality after overnight water deprivation should also be obtained. Further evaluations should be tailored to patients based on specific presenting signs and symptoms.

FIRST-LINE THERAPIES

Skin disease	
▷ Topical nitrogen mustard	C
▷ Phototherapy (PUVA, narrowband UVB)	E
Multisystem disease	
▷ Vinblastine	B
▷ Etoposide (VP16)	B

Topical nitrogen mustard: an effective treatment for cutaneous Langerhans' cell histiocytosis. Sheehan MP, Atherton DJ, Broadbent V, Pritchard J. J Pediatr 1991; 119: 317–21.

Sixteen children with multisystem LCH and severe skin involvement were treated with topical nitrogen mustard, with rapid clinical improvement. One child developed a contact allergy after use.

Long term follow up of topical mustine treatment for cutaneous Langerhans' cell histiocytosis. Hoeger PH, Nanduri VR, Harper JI, Atherton DA, Pritchard J. Arch Dis Child 2000; 82: 483–7.

Topical nitrogen mustard (0.02% mechlorethamine hydrochloride mustard) was found to be safe in cutaneous disease. Follow-up in this study was an average of 8.3 years.

Topical nitrogen mustard ointment with occlusion for Langerhans' cell histiocytosis of the scalp. Treat JR, Suchin KR, James WD. J Dermatol Treat 2003; 14: 46–7.

Topical nitrogen mustard ointment 0.01% under occlusion cleared a patient with scalp LCH in 3 weeks without irritation.

Topical nitrogen mustard is the best-studied and most effective topical therapy. Contact allergy and risk of cutaneous carcinogenicity limit its use.

Satisfactory remission achieved by PUVA therapy in Langerhans' cell histiocytosis in an elderly patient. Sakai H, Ibe M, Takaahashi H, Matsuo S, Okamoto K, Makino I, et al. J Dermatol 1996; 23: 42–6.

Case report of a 74-year-old man with cutaneous LCH and diabetes insipidus. Five weeks of PUVA therapy led to complete clearance of skin lesions. The endocrinopathy persisted.

Cutaneous Langerhans' cell histiocytosis in an elderly man successfully treated with narrowband ultraviolet B. Imafuku S, Shibata S, Tashiro A, Furue M. Br J Dermatol 2007; 157: 1277–9.

Eleven sessions of narrowband UVB led to almost complete resolution in a 72-year-old Japanese man which persisted at least 12 months after therapy was discontinued. He was given 0.4–1.0 J/cm² irradiation incrementally (total irradiation of 9.3 J/cm²).

Etoposide in recurrent childhood Langerhans' cell histiocytosis: an Italian cooperative study. Ceci A, De Terlizzi M, Colella R, Balducci D, Toma MG, Zurlo MG, et al. Cancer 1988; 62: 2528–31.

Twelve of 18 patients with recurrent LCH had a complete and three had a partial response after treatment with etoposide (200 mg/m²/day given 3 days every 3 weeks).

Langerhans' cell histiocytosis in childhood: results from the Italian Cooperative AIEOP-CNR-H.X. '83 study. Ceci A, de Terlizzi M, Colella R, Loiacono G, Balducci D, Surico G, et al. Med Pediatr Oncol 1993; 21: 259–64.

Ninety patients were divided into those with and those without organ dysfunction. Monotherapy with either vinblastine or etoposide was an effective treatment in patients without organ dysfunction.

A randomised trial of treatment for multisystem Langerhans' cell histiocytosis. Gadner H, Grois N, Arico M, Broadbent V, Ceci A, Jakobson A, et al. J Pediatr 2001; 138: 728–34.

This randomized controlled trial of 24 weeks of vinblastine (6 mg/m², IV weekly) or etoposide (150 mg/m²/day for 3 days every 3 weeks) and an initial dose of methylprednisolone (30 mg/kg/day for 3 days) recruited 143 untreated children with multisystem Langerhans' cell histiocytosis. The two treatments were found to be equally effective, with response rates of 58% for vinblastine, and 69% for etoposide. Vinblastine is considered safer for use in children

Etoposide has been consistently shown to be effective in multifocal LCH. However, the small risk of secondary leukemia following treatment of children with etoposide limits its use to the most high-risk pediatric patients.

SECOND-LINE THERAPIES

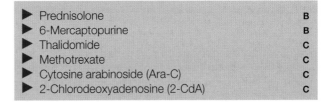

▷ Prednisolone	B
▷ 6-Mercaptopurine	B
▷ Thalidomide	C
▷ Methotrexate	C
▷ Cytosine arabinoside (Ara-C)	C
▷ 2-Chlorodeoxyadenosine (2-CdA)	C

Improved outcome in multisystem Langerhans' cell histiocytosis is associated with therapy intensification. Gadner H, Grois N, Pötschger U, Minkov M, Aricò M, Braier J, et al. Blood 2008; 111: 2556–62.

This randomized controlled trial had 193 patients with multisystem disease. Arm A consisted of 4 weeks' prednisone 40 mg/m² once daily, tapering over 2 weeks, vinblastine 6 mg/m² IV weekly for 6 weeks, followed by 18 weeks of 6-mercaptopurine 50 mg/m² daily with vinblastine (6 mg/m²) and prednisolone (40 mg/m² for 5 days) pulses every 3 weeks; etoposide 150 mg/m² weekly for the first 6 weeks followed by pulsed therapy every 3 weeks were added in arm B. Both regimens had similar response rates (63% vs 71%), 5-year survival probability (74% vs 79%), relapse rate (46% vs 46%).

The more intense chemotherapy regimen with etoposide was better in patients with liver, lung, spleen, and hematopoietic system involvement.

Treatment strategy for disseminated Langerhans' cell histiocytosis. Gadner H, Heitger A, Grois N, Gatterer-Menz I, Ladisch S. Med Pediatr Oncol 1994; 23: 72–80.

One hundred and six patients with disseminated LCH were divided into three groups: group A (multifocal bone disease); group B (soft-tissue disease without organ dysfunction); and group C (patients with organ dysfunction). All patients received 6 weeks of etoposide, vinblastine, and prednisone, followed by continuation therapy with 1 year of 6-mercaptopurine, vinblastine, and prednisone. Patients in group B also received etoposide during continuation therapy, and group C received both etoposide and methotrexate. A complete response was seen in 89% of group A, 91% of group B, and 67% of group C patients.

This study treated patients with 1 year of 'maintenance' chemotherapy, which has not been shown to be superior to the use of intermittent treatment for disease exacerbations.

A case of adult Langerhans' cell histiocytosis showing successfully regenerated osseous tissue of the skull after chemotherapy. Suzuki T, Izutsu K, Kako S, Ohta S, Hangaishi A, Kanda Y, et al. Int J Hematol 2008; 87: 284–8.

A case report of an adult with large osteolytic lesions in the skull that successfully responded to 6 weeks of prednisolone and vinblastine, followed by the addition of 6-mercaptopurine for a further 12 months. After-treatment X-ray examination confirmed bone regeneration.

Successful treatment of cutaneous Langerhans' cell histiocytosis with thalidomide. Sander CS, Kaatz M, Elsner P. Dermatology 2004; 208: 149–52.

Thalidomide 200 mg once daily was given to a 38-year-old man with recurrent mucocutaneous LCH. He had significant improvement within 4 weeks and complete healing after 3 months. Treatment was continued at 100 mg daily without relapse.

A phase II trial using thalidomide for Langerhans' cell histiocytosis. McClain KL, Kozinetz CA. Pediatr Blood Cancer 2007; 48: 44–9.

Sixteen patients with LCH who had relapsed once or twice despite treatment were included in the trial. Six were considered high risk. The rest consisted of patients with skin and/or bone and/or brain involvement. The doses commenced at 100 mg (adults) or 50 mg (children) daily, which was increased by 50 mg per month until efficacy or toxicity was achieved. No high-risk patient responded to treatment. Four low-risk patients had a complete response, three had a partial response, and two did not respond.

Oral methotrexate and alternate-day prednisone for low-risk Langerhans' cell histiocytosis. Womer RB, Anunciato KR, Chehrenama M. Med Pediatr Oncol 1995; 25: 70–3.

Thirteen low-risk children were treated successfully with prednisone 40 mg/m²/day on alternate days and weekly methotrexate 20 g/m² for a minimum of 3 months. Toxicity was minimal, and recurrences were treated with the same regimen.

Cytosine-arabinoside, vincristine, and prednisolone in the treatment of children with disseminated Langerhans' cell

histiocytosis with organ dysfunction: experience at a single institution. Egeler RM, de Kraker J, Voûte PA. Med Pediatr Oncol 1993; 21: 265–70.

Eighteen patients with multiorgan involvement (eight with organ dysfunction and 10 without) received chemotherapy containing cytosine-arabinoside, vincristine, and prednisolone; 63% with organ dysfunction and 80% without had sustained remission.

This regimen is well tolerated, results compare satisfactorily with other chemotherapeutic regimens, and it avoids the risk of secondary malignancies associated with etoposide.

Successful treatment of Langerhans' cell histiocytosis with 2-chlorodeoxyadenosine. Goh NS, McDonald CE, MacGregor DP, Pretto JJ, Brodie GN. Respirology. 2003; 8: 91–4.

A young man with LCH involving the lungs and bone who had previously failed to respond to two chemotherapy regimens was treated with 2CdA. A complete symptomatic remission was achieved following five cycles of 0.1 mg/kg/day for 7 days per cycle, with no evidence of recurrence 5 years after completion of chemotherapy.

Efficacy of continuous infusion 2-CDA (cladribine) in pediatric patients with Langerhans' cell histiocytosis. Stine KC, Saylors RL, Saccente S, McClaine KL, Becton DL. Pediatr Blood Cancer 2004; 43: 81–4.

Ten children with reactivated LCH or high-risk disease were treated with 2CdA (initially 5 mg/m²/day for 3 days, increasing to 6.5 mg/m²/day for 3 days). All 10 had clinical responses. Seven patients remained disease free for a median of 50 months. Three patients needed further drug therapy, but were clinically in remission.

This confirms the efficacy of 2-CdA in LCH, particularly in patients who have failed on other forms of treatment.

THIRD-LINE THERAPIES

▶ Radiotherapy	**B**
▶ Ciclosporin	**B**
▶ Bone marrow transplantation	**C**
▶ Trimethoprim/sulfamethoxazole	**C**
▶ Interferon-α	**D**
▶ 2-Deoxycoformycin	**E**
▶ Interleukin-2	**E**
▶ Isotretinoin	**E**
▶ Clofarabine	**E**
▶ Mistletoe	**E**

Results of treatment of 127 patients with systemic histiocytosis (Letterer–Siwe syndrome, Schüller–Christian syndrome, and multifocal eosinophilic granuloma). Greenberger JS, Crocker AC, Vawter G, Jaffe N, Cassady JR. Medicine 1981; 60: 311–38.

Many patients discussed in this retrospective study achieved remission from local radiation therapy for bone and soft tissue lesions.

Chemotherapy is now generally preferred because of the slight risk of secondary malignancy, but also the fact that LCH is often a generalized disease and local treatment is therefore limited.

Cyclosporine A therapy for multisystem Langerhans' cell histiocytosis. Minkov M, Grois N, Broadbent V, Ceci A, Jakobson A, Ladisch S. Med Pediatr Oncol 1999; 33: 482–5.

Twenty-six patients with refractory LCH were treated with ciclosporin alone or combined with prednisolone, vinblastine, or etoposide and/or antithymocyte globulin. The median dose was 6 mg/kg/day (range 2–12 mg/kg/day) for a median of 4.5 months. One patient had a complete response and three had a partial response.

Ciclosporin has been effective in only a small number of patients with LCH, and remissions tend to be short.

Hematopoietic stem cell transplantation in patients with severe Langerhans' cell histiocytosis and hematological dysfunction: experience of the French Langerhans' Cell Study Group. Akkari V, Donadieu J, Piguet C, Bordigoni P, Michel G, Blanche S, et al. Bone Marrow Transplant 2003; 31: 1097–103.

Eight patients with LCH and hematologic dysfunction received a hematopoietic stem cell transplant (three autologous and five allogeneic). All patients had responded poorly to initial chemotherapy. Autologous transplant failed in all patients. Three patients had a complete response and two died from toxicity after the allogeneic transplant. Ultimately only two patients had no recurrences after 21 months and 7 years of follow-up, respectively.

Improved outcome of treatment-resistant high-risk Langerhans' cell histiocytosis after allogeneic stem cell transplantation with reduced-intensity conditioning. Steiner M, Matthes-Martin S, Attarbaschi A, Minkov M, Grois N, Unger E, et al. Bone Marrow Transplant 2005; 36: 215–25.

Nine patients received an allogeneic stem cell transplant followed by a reduced-intensity conditioning regimen after failing to respond to conventional chemotherapy. Two patients died and seven survived, remaining disease free after a median follow up of 390 days.

Stem cell transplant for refractory LCH can be highly toxic but can achieve sustained disease control. Several other case reports have documented long-term remissions following bone marrow transplantation. This approach is generally reserved for patients with fulminant disease not responding to chemotherapy.

Effect of trimethoprim-sulphamethoxazole in Langerhans' cell histiocytosis: preliminary observations. Tzortzatou-Stathopoulou F, Xaidara A, Mikraki V, Moschovi M, Arvantis D, Ageloyianni P, et al. Med Pediatr Oncol 1995; 25: 74–8.

Twenty-three children with both single- and multisystem disease were treated for 4 weeks to 3 months. Patients with single-system disease responded well, whereas those with multisystem disease had a more limited response.

Widespread skin-limited Langerhans' cell histiocytosis: complete remission with interferon alpha. Kwong YL, Chan ACL, Chan TK. J Am Acad Dermatol 1997; 36: 628–9.

Subcutaneous interferon-α at 6 MU daily for 9 months followed by 3 MU for 9 months led to complete resolution in a patient with extensive single-system cutaneous disease.

Intralesional interferon-α has also been used for localized cutaneous disease.

Successful treatment of two children with Langerhans' cell histiocytosis with 2′-deoxycoformycin. McCowage GB, Frush DP, Kurtzberg J. J Pediatr Hematol Oncol 1996; 18: 154–8.

Two patients (aged 3 and 5) who were refractory to multiple chemotherapeutic agents were treated with 2′-dCF 4 mg/m^2 IV weekly for 8 weeks, then every 2 weeks for at least 16 months. Both achieved a sustained remission with continued treatment. Toxicity was limited to asymptomatic grade III-IV lymphopenia and abnormalities of lymphocyte mitogen responses.

Interleukin-2 therapy of Langerhans' cell histiocytosis. Hirose M, Saito S, Yoshimoto T, Kuroda Y. Acta Pediatr 1995; 84: 1204–6.

A 20-month-old girl with disseminated LCH who had failed chemotherapy achieved a transient remission with intravenous IL-2.

Langerhans' cell histiocytosis: complete remission after oral isotretinoin therapy. Tsambaos D, Georgiou S, Kapranos N, Monastirli A, Stratigos A, Berger H. Acta Dermatol Venereol 1995; 75: 62–4.

A patient with single-system cutaneous disease achieved a complete response to oral isotretinoin at 1.5 mg/kg/day for 9 months, with no relapse at 5 years.

Clofarabine in refractory Langerhans' cell histiocytosis. Rodriguez-Galindo C, Jeng M, Khuu P, McCarville MB, Jeha S. Pediatr Blood Cancer 2008; in press. [Epub ahead of print]

Two children with LCH refractory to treatment (including 2-CdA) were treated with five or six cycles of clofarabine (optimized to 25 mg/m^2/day for 5 days), which induced remission in both patients.

Response to subcutaneous therapy with mistletoe in recurrent multisystem Langerhans' cell histiocytosis. Seifert G, Laengler A, Tautz C, Seeger K, Henze G. Pediatr Blood Cancer 2007; 48: 591–2.

A patient with multisystem disease, recurrent relapses, and persistent cutaneous lesions despite chemotherapy was treated with an aqueous extract of mistletoe (*Helixor*) subcutaneously three times a week, alternating doses weekly between 1 mg, 2.5 mg, and 5 mg. Cutaneous lesions cleared after 4 weeks of treatment and the patient remains in remission after 5 years of continuous treatment.

Leg ulcers

David J Margolis

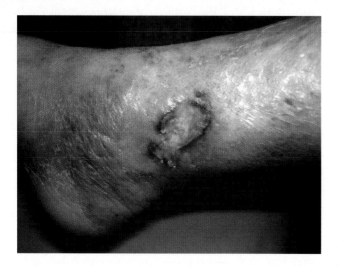

Leg ulcers are a common problem, affecting millions of individuals worldwide. The term leg ulcer can be used to include many different types of chronic wound, including those also called pressure ulcers, venous leg ulcers, and diabetic foot ulcers, and those due to atherosclerosis. Venous leg ulcers are probably the most common and most likely to be treated by a dermatologist. Leg ulcers caused by infection, basal or squamous cell cancer, or pyoderma gangrenosum are discussed elsewhere.

MANAGEMENT STRATEGY

Accurate diagnosis is key in the management of these wounds. For healthcare providers who are not primarily surgeons it is especially important to determine that a patient has adequate arterial flow for a lower extremity wound to heal. In general, therapy is aimed at both altering any anatomic impediment to healing and optimizing the healing environment. When approaching a leg ulcer it is important to keep a broad differential diagnosis in mind, as although the majority will ultimately be classified as venous leg ulcers, wounds due to arterial insufficiency, pressure ulcers, or diabetic neuropathic foot ulcers must be considered. Patients who have wounds that are primarily due to arterial insufficiency should seek surgical advice.

Venous ulcers are caused indirectly by ambulatory venous hypertension, most often due to the failure of the calf muscle pump system. Therefore, management hinges on *lower limb compression* and *good wound care*. *Good wound care* includes debridement and/or cleansing, management of exudate, and the use of a moist dressing. Elevation of the legs at night and, when necessary, weight reduction may also reduce the impact of any venous abnormalities. In the setting of lower limb compression, exercise of the lower extremity may be of benefit. Other approaches to management include the use of *topical recombinant growth factors*, *skin equivalents* (or cell-based therapies), and *oral pentoxifylline*. Most patients will improve with conservative management (compression and dressings), although compliance with compression therapy (e.g., compression

stockings, compression bandages, etc.) may be a challenge. Most of these wounds heal in less than 6 months. The likelihood that a wound will heal is often related to how it responds to therapy with in the first 4 weeks of care, and based on the size and age of the wound when first examined.

Patients with diabetes mellitus may develop venous leg ulcers and wounds due to arterial insufficiency. However, diabetics may also develop neuropathic foot ulcers, which stem from the neuropathy associated with diabetes. As a result, at least in part, the unperceived repetitive trauma and pressure from walking leads to the ulcer. Management hinges on optimal control of diabetes, offloading of the affected limb, and good wound care. Other treatment options include recombinant growth factors such as recombinant human platelet-derived growth factor (rh-PDGF), and skin equivalents, which may be necessary in order to achieve optimal results. Finally, individuals with diabetes may commonly have a wounds owing to a combination neuropathy and lower extremity ischemia. Recurrent ulcerations and lower extremity amputations are a real and serious problem for those with diabetes.

SPECIFIC INVESTIGATIONS

▶ Hemoglobin A1c (glycosylated hemoglobin) measurement for those with diabetes
▶ Clinical testing for neuropathy (e.g., monofilament testing) for those with diabetes
▶ Lower extremity vascular studies, including ankle–brachial index (ABI) and potentially duplex ultrasound
▶ Skin biopsy may be considered

Effectiveness of Semmes–Weinstein monofilament examination for diabetic peripheral neuropathy screening. Kamei N, Yamane K, Nakanishi S, Yamashita Y, Tamura T, Ohshita K, et al. J Diabetes Complications 2005; 19: 47–53.

Sensory evaluation using a Semmes–Weinstein filament that provides 2 g of pressure at the great toe or the plantar aspect of the fifth metatarsal was the most useful diagnostic test for diabetic peripheral neuropathy, providing 60.0% sensitivity and 73.8% specificity.

Early healing rates and wound are measurements are reliable predictors of later complete wound closure. Cardinal M, Eisenbud DE, Phillips DE, Harding K. Wound Repair Regen 2008; 16: 19–22.

Surrogate endpoints for the treatment of diabetic neuropathic foot ulcers. Margolis DJ, Gelfand JM, Hoffstad O, Berlin JA. Diabetes Care 2003: 26: 1696–1700

Surrogate endpoints for the treatment of venous leg ulcers. Gelfand JM, Hoffstad O, Margolis DJ. J Invest Dermatol 2002; 119: 1420–5.

A series of three studies of several thousand patients in different settings demonstrating that the changes in the size of a wound during the first 4 weeks of care for those with either diabetic neuropathic foot ulcers or venous leg ulcers is correlated with ultimate healing.

The accuracy of venous leg ulcer prognostic models in a wound care system. Margolis DJ, Taylor LA, Hoffstad O, Berlin JA. Wound Repair Regen 2004; 12: 163–8.

Diabetic Neuropathic Foot Ulcers: Predicting Who Will Not Heal. Margolis DJ, Taylor LA, Hoffstad O, Berlin JA. American Journal of Medicine 2003; 115: 627–631.

Two studies of several thousand patients showing that the size and age of the wound, and for those with diabetes the anatomic depth of the wound when the patient is first examined, are predictive of a wound healing.

FIRST-LINE THERAPIES

▶ Compression for venous ulcers   A
▶ Offloading for diabetic neuropathic ulcers   A

A factorial, randomized trial of pentoxifylline or placebo, four-layer or single-layer compression, and knitted viscose or hydrocolloid dressing for venous leg ulcer. Nelson EA, Prescott RJ, Harper DR, Gibson B, Brown D, Ruckley CV. J Vasc Surg 2007; 45: 134–41.

A large clinical trial that demonstrates the superiority of four-layer compression over single-layer, as well as the potential benefit associated with the use of pentoxifylline.

A randomized trial of two irremovable off-loading devices in the management of plantar neuropathic foot ulcers. Katz IA, Harlan A, Miranda-Palma B, Prieto-Sanchex L, Armstrong D, Mizel JH, et al. Diabetes Care 2005; 28: 555–9.

A randomized trial demonstrating the importance of properly and continuously offloading a wound in a patient with a diabetic neuropathic foot ulcer. A removable cast walker made irremovable may be as effective as a contact cast with respect to successful healing.

SECOND-LINE THERAPIES

▶ Topical rh-PDGF (becaplermin)   A
▶ Skin equivalent dressings (Graftskin, Apligraf)   A
▶ Oral pentoxifylline   A
▶ Skin grafting (autograft)   A

Skin grafting for venous leg ulcers. Jones JE, Nelson EA. Cochrane Database Syst Rev 2007; CDE001737.

A comprehensive review of studies of autografts, xenografts, and allografts used to treat venous leg ulcers. The conclusion was that bilayer artificial skin (skin equivalents)

used with compression did increase the chance of healing. A request was made for more research into the other forms of skin grafting.

THIRD-LINE THERAPIES

▶ Intermittent pneumatic compression   C
▶ Oral antibiotic therapy   E
▶ Laser   B
▶ Therapeutic ultrasound   B
▶ Vitamins and minerals   E
▶ Maggots   D
▶ Electromagnetic   B
▶ Stem cells   D

Therapeutic ultrasound for venous leg ulcers. Al-Kurdi D, Bell-Syer SE, Flemming K. Cochrane Database Syst Rev 2008; CD001180.

This review showed that evidence may indicate an increased rate of healing associated with the use of ultrasound, but this conclusion is based on small studies of generally poor quality.

Electromagnetic therapy for treating venous leg ulcers. Ravaghi H, Flemming K, Cullum N, Olyaee M. Cochrane Database Syst Rev 2006; CD002933.

A total of three randomized trials have been reported for this modality. Only one has shown a benefit with respect to healing. However, electromagnetic therapy may reduce pain.

Maggot debridement therapy of infected ulcers: patient and wound factors influencing outcome – a study of 101 patients with 117 wounds. Steenvoorde P, Jacobi CE, Van Doorn L, Oskam J. Ann Roy Coll Surg Engl 2007; 89: 596–602.

The majority of patients who received maggot therapy had beneficial results with respect to debridement and wound healing. Older patients with limb ischemia and deeper wounds were less likely to benefit.

The use of marrow-derived stem cells to accelerate healing in chronic wounds. Rogers LC, Bevilacqua NJ, Armstrong DG. Int Wound J 2008; 5: 20–5.

One of now several case series demonstrating that bone marrow-derived stem cells taken from a bone marrow aspirate may aid the healing of chronic wounds. This is a developing therapy and technology.

Leiomyoma

Loma S Gardner, Ian Coulson

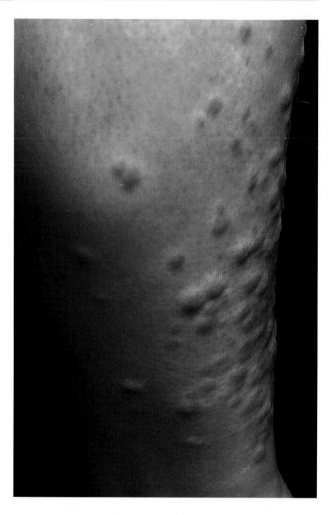

Cutaneous leiomyomas are rare benign neoplasms originating from smooth muscle that are frequently not recognized by clinicians. Three types exist: (1) piloleiomyoma, the most common type, arising from the arrectores pilorum muscle; (2) dartoic myoma or genital leiomyoma, arising from scrotal/labial dartos muscle or smooth muscle of the nipple; and (3) angioleiomyoma, arising from vascular wall muscle. Piloleiomyoma frequently occurs as multiple lesions (80%). Multiple leiomyomas can be inherited in an autosomal dominant fashion in association with uterine leiomyoma (Reed's syndrome, *multiple cutaneous and uterine leiomyomata* [MCUL1; OMIM 150800]). Familial multiple leiomyomata can rarely be associated with renal cell cancer (*hereditary leiomyomatosis and renal cell cancer* [HLRCC; OMIM 605839]). Both familial forms are caused by mutations in the fumarate hydratase gene (coding for an enzyme in the tricarboxylic acid cycle) on 1q42.1, which is hypothesized to act as a tumor suppressor gene through an unknown mechanism. Clinically, cutaneous leiomyomas present as flesh-colored or brownish-red dermal papules or nodules up to 2 cm in diameter, typically distributed on the trunk and extensor surfaces of extremities. They often appear from the second to fourth decade and gradually increase in number and size. Paroxysmal pain, described as stabbing, burning, or pinching, may be triggered by cold or mechanical stimulation and is possibly due to muscle contraction or compression of entrapped nerves. Angioleiomyomas are less frequently symptomatic, and genital leiomyomas are asymptomatic.

MANAGEMENT STRATEGY

Symptomatic solitary lesions are best *excised*. Symptomatic multiple leiomyomas are therapeutically challenging because they involve a large area and recur after excision in 50% of cases. Selective excision of larger painful lesions may be considered. CO_2 *laser ablation* of symptomatic lesions may be successful. Other therapeutic methods aim to inhibit smooth muscle contraction by interfering with local tissue mediators, e.g., norepinephrine, epinephrine, and acetylcholine. There are reports of success with oral *doxazosin* (a selective α_1 blocker) 1–4 mg daily, oral *nifedipine* (calcium channel blocker) 10 mg three times daily, *phenoxybenzamine* (non-selective α blocker) 10 mg twice daily, topical 9% *hyoscine hydrobromide* (anticholinergic) and oral *nitroglycerine* 0.8–1.6 mg prn. Analgesics that target neuropathic pain, e.g., oral *gabapentin* 300 mg three times daily, have been beneficial. Potential triggers should be avoided.

Women, particularly those with a family history, should undergo gynecologic review to exclude possible uterine involvement ('fibroids'). Menorrhagia may necessitate hysterectomy, and leiomyosarcoma, although rare, should be excluded. Potential familial forms require referral to a clinical geneticist with informed consent for mutational analysis of the fumarate hydratase gene.

SPECIFIC INVESTIGATIONS

> ▶ Biopsy
> ▶ Biochemical assay of fumarate hydratase – for low/absent activity
> ▶ Genetic analysis – for fumarate hydratase gene mutations

Cutaneous smooth muscle neoplasms: clinical features, histological findings and treatment options. Holst VA, Junkins-Hopkins JM, Elenitas R. J Am Acad Dermatol 2002; 46: 477–90.

A well-referenced review covering leiomyoma and angioleiomyoma. On histologic examination, leiomyomas stained with special stains such as Masson trichrome reveal brick-red smooth muscle fibers. Immunohistochemical techniques demonstrating desmin, smooth-muscle actin, or muscle-specific actin confirm tumor origin.

Germline mutations in FH predispose to dominantly inherited uterine fibroids, skin leiomyomata and papillary renal cell cancer. Tomlinson IP, Alam NA, Rowan AJ, Barclay E, Jaeger EE, Kelsell D, et al.; Multiple Leiomyoma Consortium. Nature Genet 2002; 30: 406–10.

The authors demonstrate that the gene predisposing to uterine fibroids, cutaneous leiomyoma, and renal cell carcinoma encodes fumarate hydratase. This enzyme acts as a tumor suppressor in familial leiomyomas, and its measured activity in the tumor is very low or absent. Mutations of the fumarate hydratase gene are found in individuals with dominantly inherited susceptibilities to multiple cutaneous and uterine leiomyomatosis and renal cancer.

Evidence Levels: **A** Double-blind study **B** Clinical trial ≥ 20 subjects **C** Clinical trial < 20 subjects **D** Series ≥ 5 subjects **E** Anecdotal case reports

FIRST-LINE THERAPY

▶ Surgical excision   **D**

Leiomyomas of the skin. Fisher WC, Helwig EB. Arch Dermatol 1963; 88: 510–20.

The clinical findings and natural course of 54 cutaneous leiomyomas from 38 patients are described. Surgically excised leiomyomas were found to have a high recurrence rate of 50%.

SECOND-LINE THERAPIES

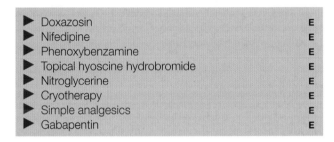

▶ Doxazosin   E
▶ Nifedipine   E
▶ Phenoxybenzamine   E
▶ Topical hyoscine hydrobromide   E
▶ Nitroglycerine   E
▶ Cryotherapy   E
▶ Simple analgesics   E
▶ Gabapentin   E

The rarity of the condition means that most publications on therapy are case reports. The therapeutic agents are not consistently effective.

Successful treatment of pain in two patients with cutaneous leiomyomata with the oral alpha-1 adrenoceptor antagonist, doxazosin. Batchelor RJ, Lyon CC, Highet AS. Br J Dermatol 2004; 150: 775–6.

Two women aged respectively 35 and 52 years, who had a long history of symptomatic cutaneous leiomyoma, were treated with oral doxazosin 1–4 mg daily, a reversible α_1 blocker which, unlike phenoxybenzamine, is selective. Doxazosin was well tolerated and patients experienced 'dramatic improvement'/complete relief of symptoms. The improvement was sustained for 6 months in the 52-year-old patient.

Pharmacological modulation of cold-induced pain in cutaneous leiomyomata. Archer CB, Whittaker S, Greaves MW. Br J Dermatol 1988; 118: 255–60.

Two cases of cutaneous leiomyoma were treated and assessed using a novel pain assessment method involving cold induction (with an ice cube). Several drugs were assessed in both patients: topical 1% phentolamine solution, 9% hyoscine hydrobromide solution, nitroglycerine paste and 2% lidocaine (lignocaine) gel, sublingual glyceryl trinitrate, and oral phenoxybenzamine, nifedipine and acetaminophen (paracetamol). One patient responded only to phenoxybenzamine 10 mg twice daily and the other responded to

hyoscine hydrobromide (the response lasted only 6 hours). The latter patient also improved with cryotherapy.

Multiple cutaneous leiomyomata and erythrocytosis with demonstration of erythropoietic activity in the cutaneous leiomyomata. Venencie PY, Puissant A, Boffa GA, Sohier J, Duperrat B. Br J Dermatol 1982; 107: 483–6.

Case report of a 41-year-old woman with leiomyomas who had complete pain relief 10 days after commencing phenoxybenzamine 10 mg twice daily, sustained throughout 7 months of follow-up.

Therapy for painful cutaneous leiomyomas. Thompson JA. J Am Acad Dermatol 1985; 13: 865–7.

Report of a 24-year-old man with multiple painful leiomyomas treated successfully with nifedipine 10 mg three times daily for 8 months. The dosage was increased to 10 mg four times daily following the onset of cool weather and increased pain. The initial side effect of headache was tolerated, but subsequent gum hypertrophy prompted a change of therapy to verapamil.

Muscle relaxing agent in cutaneous leiomyoma. Abraham Z, Cohen A, Haim S. Dermatologica 1983; 166: 255–6.

Case report of a 21-year-old man with multiple cutaneous leiomyomas who had a 'dramatic and immediate response' to nifedipine 10 mg three times daily, including complete pain relief and partial involution of the lesions, during 5 months of follow-up.

Leiomyomatosis cutis et uteri. Engelke H, Christophers E. Acta Dermatol Venereol (Stockh) 1979; 59: 51–4.

Case report of a woman with associated uterine leiomyoma. Skin symptoms responded to oral nitroglycerine 0.8–1.6 mg for acute attacks, with maintenance nifedipine 20 mg and phenoxybenzamine 60 mg administered during 2 years of follow-up.

Gabapentin treatment of multiple piloleiomyoma-related pain. Alam M, Rabinowitz AD, Engler DE. J Am Acad Dermatol 2002; 46: S27–9.

Case report of a 54-year-old woman with numerous histologically confirmed cutaneous leiomyomas who experienced pain relief ('near complete resolution') with gabapentin 300 mg three times daily introduced gradually.

Treatment of multiple cutaneous leiomyomas with CO_2 laser ablation. Christenson LJ, Smith K, Arpey CJ. Dermatol Surg 2000; 26: 319–22.

Case report of a 73-year-old woman not eligible for pharmacologic therapy who had multiple cutaneous leiomyomas. CO_2 laser ablation of six symptomatic cutaneous leiomyomas induced complete pain relief that was sustained during 9 months of follow-up.

Leishmaniasis

Suhail M Hadi, Hanadi Abdallah Al Quran

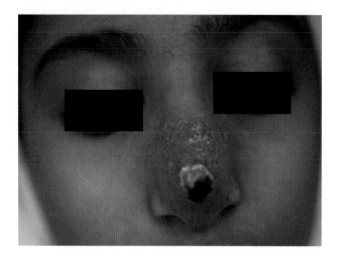

Leishmaniasis is a flagellate protozoan disease caused by many species of the genus *Leishmania*. It can be classified into three clinical forms: visceral (kala azar), which is the most severe, mucocutanous (espundia), which can lead to extensive destruction of the mucous membranes, and cutaneous (Old and New World), which involves mainly the exposed body parts, causing ulcers and scarring. Generalized, disseminated, cutaneous erysipeloid-like, and mucosal leishmaniasis may be seen in HIV infection and AIDS. Leishmaniasis is transmitted mainly by the bite of the infected female phlebotomine sandfly. However, other possible routes of transmission exist and include transfusion, congenital, needle sharing, sexual, and person-to-person contact. Only the management of cutaneous leishmaniasis is addressed here.

MANAGEMENT STRATEGY

The diagnosis of cutaneous leishmaniasis starts with the finding of a typical lesion and a history of exposure. A skin scraping for microscopic analysis is the simplest test. Cultures from an exudate or scraping show good results. Where available, polymerase chain reaction (PCR) offers a rapid, highly sensitive, and specific modality of diagnosis. Serological tests can be used and include the indirect immunofluorescent antibody test (IFAT), direct agglutination test (DAT), fast agglutination screening test (FAST), and enzyme-linked immunosorbent assay (ELISA).

A new vaccine has been recently studied for its protection against cutaneous leishmaniasis. Results showed durable protective immunity. It has the advantages of a non-invasive nasal route of vaccination and reduced cost.

Treatment is needed to improve the cosmetic outcome, as spontaneous healing may leave scarring.

Pentavalent antimonials are the first-line therapy. *Meglumine antimoniate* is the drug of choice. It can be given intralesionally with local anesthetic (particularly in children, because of pain) or systemically 10 mg/kg daily for 2 weeks. Leishmania recidivans requires higher doses for longer periods. *Sodium stibogluconate* can be infiltrated into individual lesions 1–2 mL/week.

In widespread, severe cases it can be given intramuscularly or intravenously in a dose of 10 mg/kg/day for 2 weeks.

Pentavalent antimoniate use is complicated by its high incidence of side effects, including arthralgia, fatigue, gastrointestinal upset, elevation of amylase, lipase and liver enzymes, leukopenia, anemia, and ECG abnormalities. Side effects appear to be dose related, and are more common in patients with renal and liver impairment and those with cardiac arrhythmias. Amphotericin B has been used in antimony-resistant cases.

Pentamidine isethionate (aromatic diamidine) is effective for diffuse cutaneous leishmaniasis. Side effects of pentamidine include hypoglycemia, diabetes mellitus, hypotension (if administered too rapidly), nausea, abdominal pain, vomiting, and headache.

Allopurinol has antileishmanial activity, and other oral drugs such as miltefosine, zinc sulphate, and itraconazole are also beneficial. γ-Interferon was shown to be effective as monotherapy treatment for leishmaniasis. Topical preparations such as *paramomycin* ointment and 5% imiquimod also show considerable therapeutic potential.

Good cure rates have been achieved with both thermotherapy and cryotherapy. Lasers have been used, but further studies are needed to support their role in the treatment of leishmaniasis. Additional treatment methods are presented below.

SPECIFIC INVESTIGATIONS

- ▶ Skin biopsy
- ▶ Fine needle aspiration
- ▶ Slit-skin smear
- ▶ Culture
- ▶ Leishmanin (Montenegro) skin test
- ▶ Serology
- ▶ PCR for leishmanial DNA

The margin of leishmania lesions contains amastigotes, whereas the center has dead skin and debris. Accordingly, the margin is addressed when performing a slit-skin smear. The aspirate can then be sent for culture, or for histology that shows Leishman–Donovan bodies inside macrophages using Giemsa stain.

In papular and nodular lesions the margin of the lesion is punctured with a hypodermic needle and a syringe that contains 0.1 mL saline. The aspirate is drawn up into the needle and is examined microscopically and/or cultured.

The gold standard medium for culture is Novy–MacNeal–Nicolle (NNN) with positive results in 1–3 weeks, or Schneider *Drosophila* medium, which gives positive results in 1 week. In the culture medium the amastigote stage converts to the promastigote stage.

Microculture is a new culture medium that has higher carbon dioxide concentrations and lower oxygen and pH, which encourages more rapid amastigote to promastigote differentiation. Culture is not a reliable method in older lesions as the organisms become scarce and difficult to isolate.

Serological tests aim to detect the presence of antibodies against leishmania. They are particularly valuable in visceral and mucocutaneous leishmaniasis.

PCR is a sensitive and powerful method of diagnosis of cutaneous leishmaniasis, which depends on gene amplification techniques.

Evidence Levels: **A** Double-blind study **B** Clinical trial ≥ 20 subjects **C** Clinical trial < 20 subjects **D** Series ≥ 5 subjects **E** Anecdotal case reports

Epidemic of cutaneous leishmaniasis: 109 cases in a population of 500. Anwar M, Hussain MA, Ur-Rehman H, Khan I, Sheikh RA. East Mediterr Health J 2007, 13: 1212–15.

Fine needle aspiration cytology was used to diagnose 109 cases with non-healing cutaneous ulcers.

Value of diagnostic techniques for cutaneous leishmaniasis. Faber WR, Oskam L, van Gool T, Kroon NC, Knegt-Junk KJ, Hofwegen H, et al. J Am Acad Dermatol 2003; 49: 70–4.

PCR appears to be the single most sensitive diagnostic test. The second most sensitive test for cutaneous leishmaniasis is culture.

A sensitive new microculture method for diagnosis of cutaneous leishmaniasis. Allahverdiyev AM, Uzun S, Bagirova M, Durdu M, Memisoglu HR. Am J Trop Med Hyg 2004; 70: 294–7.

This microcapillary culture method was developed for rapid diagnosis of cutaneous leishmaniasis. It was found to be superior to the traditional culture method. It needs a smaller inoculum size, has higher sensitivity for detection of promastigotes, and is more rapid (three to four times faster) with regard to the emergence of promastigotes.

Sensitivity of leishmanin skin test in patients of acute cutaneous leishmaniasis. Manzur A, Bari A. Dermatol Online J 2006; 12: 2.

One hundred patients with parasitologically proven cutaneous leishmaniasis were enrolled in the study. The leishmanin test was found to be sensitive even in cutaneous leishmaniasis of recent onset.

Enzyme-linked immunosorbent assay based on soluble promastigote antigen detects immunoglobulin M (IgM) and IgG antibodies in sera from cases of visceral and cutaneous leishmaniasis. Ryan JR, Smithyman AM, Rajasekariah GH, Hochberg L, Stiteler JM, Martin SK. J Clin Microbiol 2002; 40: 3110.

An ELISA that can detect IgM and IgG antileishmanial antibodies was developed and tested on 129 visceral and 143 cutaneous leishmaniasis patients with controls. The test showed an overall sensitivity of 95.1%.

Diagnosis of cutaneous leishmaniasis in Guatemala using a real-time polymerase chain reaction assay and the Smartcycler. Wortmann G, Hochberg LP, Arana BA, Rizzo NR, Arana F, Ryan JR. Am J Trop Med Hyg 2007; 76: 906–8.

When tested on 43 patients with cutaneous leishmaniasis, real-time PCR was found to be positive in 86% of cases. It offers many advantages over traditional PCR, including enhanced portability, faster processing time, and reduced risk of contamination.

Comparison of PCR assays for diagnosis of cutaneous leishmaniasis. Bensoussan E, Nasereddin A, Jonas F, Schnur LF, Jaffe CL. J Clin Microbiol 2006; 44: 1435–9.

This study compared three PCR assays to parasitic cultures and microscopic diagnosis in 92 specimens from suspected cases of cutaneous leishmaniasis (CL). The kinetoplast DNA (kDNA) PCR showed the highest sensitivity (98.7%), making this a very valuable test for the diagnosis of CL.

FIRST-LINE THERAPIES

Pentavalent antimonials
▶ Meglumine antimoniate — B
▶ Sodium stibogluconate antimony — B

Clinical features, epidemiology, and efficacy and safety of intralesional antimony treatment of cutaneous leishmaniasis: recent experience in Turkey. Uzun S, Durdu M, Culha G, Allahverdiyev AM, Memisoglu HR. J Parasitol 2004; 90: 853–9.

Intralesional meglumine antimoniate was given as first-line therapy for 890 patients with cutaneous leishmaniasis. A weekly dose of 0.2–1 mL was given for up to 20 weeks or until complete cure. It was found to have an efficacy of 97.2%, with a low relapse rate (3.9%) and no serious side effects.

Clinical efficacy of intramuscular meglumine antimoniate alone and in combination with intralesional meglumine antimoniate in the treatment of old world cutaneous leishmaniasis. Munir A, Janjua SA, Hussain I. Acta Dermatovenerol Croat 2008; 16: 60–4.

Sixty patients were studied. A combination of intramuscular meglumine antimoniate 20 mg/kg/day plus intralesional meglumine antimoniate 0.5 mL daily for 21 days was superior to intralesional treatment alone, with 75% complete cure for the former.

Comparative efficacy of intralesional sodium stibogluconate (SSG) alone and its combination with intramuscular SSG to treat localized cutaneous leishmaniasis: Results of a pilot study. Negi AK, Sharma NL, Mahajan VK, Ranjan N, Kanga AK. Indian J Dermatol Venereol Leprol 2007; 73: 280.

This study was performed on 32 patients with localized cutaneous leishmaniasis. One group received intralesional SSG (100 mg/mL), repeated on days 3 and 5. The second group was given the same treatment as the first, in addition to the remainder of a calculated dose of 20 mg/kg/day given intramuscularly on the same day. Intralesional combined with intramuscular SSG achieved 80–90% response after one treatment cycle, whereas intralesional SSG given alone needed two to four cycles to achieve the same response.

SECOND-LINE THERAPIES

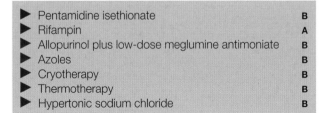

▶ Pentamidine isethionate — B
▶ Rifampin — A
▶ Allopurinol plus low-dose meglumine antimoniate — B
▶ Azoles — B
▶ Cryotherapy — B
▶ Thermotherapy — B
▶ Hypertonic sodium chloride — B

Recurrent American cutaneous leishmaniasis. Gangneux JP, Sauzet S, Donnard S, Meyer N, Cornillet A, Pratlong F, et al. Emerg Infect Dis 2007; 13: 1436–8.

Twenty-one patients with recurrent cutaneous leishmaniasis were enrolled in the study. They were given one or two courses of either three intravenous or two intramuscular pentamidine isethionate treatments (4 mg/kg) on alternate days. All were cured within 1–3 months.

The role of rifampicin in the management of cutaneous leishmaniasis. Kochar DK, Aseri S, Sharma BV, Bumb RA, Mehta RD, Purohit SK. QJ Med 2000; 93: 733–7.

Forty-six patients with cutaneous leishmaniasis were enrolled in this double-blind study: 32 received rifampin 600 mg twice daily for 4 weeks and 32 received placebo for 4 weeks. Of the rifampin group 73.9% had complete healing of their lesions, compared to 4.3% of the placebo group. The difference was statistically significant. Rifampin is well tolerated with no side effects, and is suitable for multiple lesions or if the injectable treatment is not feasible.

Treatment of cutaneous leishmaniasis with a combination of allopurinol and low-dose meglumine antimoniate. Momeni AZ, Reiszadae MR, Aminjavaheri M. Int J Dermatol 2002; 41: 441–3.

A treatment of either daily allopurinol (20 mg/kg) plus low-dose meglumine antimoniate 30 mg/kg), or meglumine antimoniate (60 mg/kg/day) alone was given for 20 days. Of 72 patients with cutaneous leishmaniasis, complete healing occurred in 80.6% of those on allopurinol and low-dose meglumine antimoniate, compared to 74.2% of those on high-dose meglumine antimoniate alone. No difference was found between the two groups with respect to side effects.

Fluconazole for the treatment of cutaneous leishmaniasis caused by *Leishmania major*. Alrajhi AA, Ibrahim EA, De Vol EB, Khairat M, Faris RM, Maguire JH. N Engl J Med 2002; 346: 891–5

A total of 106 patients received fluconazole 200 mg daily and 103 received placebo for 6 weeks. Follow-up data were available for 80 and 65 patients, respectively. Healing of lesions was complete in 79% of the fluconazole group and 34% of the placebo group at 3-month follow-up.

Comparison of oral itraconazole and intramuscular meglumine antimoniate in the treatment of cutaneous leishmaniasis. Saleem K, Rahman A. J Coll Phys Surg Pak 2007; 17: 713–16.

Two hundred patients with wet and dry cutaneous leishmaniasis were studied. Itraconazole (100 mg) twice daily for 6–8 weeks) was superior to meglumine antimoniate in achieving complete clinical and parasitological cure (75% compared to 65%), with fewer side effects.

Efficacy of a weekly cryotherapy regimen to treat *Leishmania major* cutaneous leishmaniasis. Mosleh IM, Geith E, Natsheh L, Schönian G, Abotteen N, Kharabsheh S. J Am Acad Dermatol 2008; 58: 617–24.

One hundred and twenty patients with 375 lesions of cutaneous leishmaniasis were treated with cryotherapy performed once weekly over one to seven sessions; 84% of lesions were cured after one to four sessions. The remaining lesions were cured after an additional one to three sessions. Scarring was negligible and side effects were minimal.

Efficacy of thermotherapy to treat cutaneous leishmaniasis caused by *Leishmania tropica* in Kabul, Afghanistan: a randomized, controlled trial. Reithinger R, Mohsen M, Wahid M, Bismullah M, Quinnell RJ, Davies CR, et al. Clin Infect Dis 2005; 40: 1148–55.

Four hundred and one patients with cutaneous leishmaniasis were enrolled in the study. They were given either radiofrequency waves (application at 50°C for 30 s) or sodium stibogluconate (SSG), administered either intralesionally (a total of five injections of 2–5 mL every 5–7 days, depending on lesion size) or intramuscularly (20 mg/kg daily for 21 days). At 100 days after treatment, cure (defined as complete re-epithelialization) was achieved in 69.4% of patients who received thermotherapy. Cure time was significantly shorter with thermotherapy, and treatment was well tolerated.

A new intralesional therapy of cutaneous leishmaniasis with hypertonic sodium chloride solution. Sharquie KE. J Dermatol 1995; 22: 732–7.

Hypertonic sodium chloride solution injections were given at 7–10-day intervals, with a 96% cure rates within 2–6 weeks (comparable to sodium stibogluconate). The treatment is safe, cheap, and effective.

THIRD-LINE THERAPIES

▶ γ-Interferon	E
▶ Miltefosine (hexadecylphosphocholine)	B
▶ Imiquimod 5%	D
▶ Paromomycin (aminosidine) ointment	A
▶ Photodynamic therapy (PDT)	B
▶ Direct current electrotherapy	B
▶ CO₂ laser	B
▶ Oral zinc sulphate	B
▶ Pentoxiphylline	A

Successful treatment of cutaneous leishmaniasis using systemic interferon-gamma. Kolde G, Luger T, Sorg C, Sunderkotter C. Dermatology 1996; 192: 56–60.

Systemic monotherapy with γ-interferon (100 μg/m² of body surface daily) given subcutaneously for 28 days can be effective for complicated cases of human cutaneous leishmaniasis.

Comparison of miltefosine and meglumine antimoniate for the treatment of zoonotic cutaneous leishmaniasis (ZCL) by a randomized clinical trial in Iran. Mohebalia M, Fotouhia A, Hooshmandb B, Zareia Z, Akhoundia B, Rahnema A, et al. Acta Trop 2007; 103: 33–40.

Of 32 patients enrolled for miltefosine treatment, 28 completed therapy. They were given miltefosine 2.5 mg/kg/day orally for 28 days. Assessment of cure was based on both clinical and parasitological criteria. A cure rate of 92.9% was achieved at 3 months after treatment. Miltefosine was found to be at least as good as meglumine for *Leishmania major*.

Role of imiquimod and parenteral meglumine antimoniate in the initial treatment of cutaneous leishmaniasis. Arevalo I, Tulliano G, Quispe A, Spaeth G, Matlashewski G, Llanos-Cuentas A, et al. Clin Infect Dis 2007; 44: 1549–54.

Combination treatment with imiquimod and meglumine antimoniate gave superior results, with rapid healing and better cosmetic outcome.

Imiquimod kills the intracellular leishmania amastigotes in vitro by activating macrophages to release nitric oxide.

Comparison of the effectiveness of two topical paromomycin treatments versus meglumine antimoniate for New World cutaneous leishmaniasis. Armijos RX, Weigel MM,

Calvopiña M, Mancheno M, Rodriguez R. Acta Trop 2004; 91: 153–60.

A randomized, controlled study involving 120 patients with ulcerated lesions compared the therapeutic efficacy and safety of two paromomycin-containing topical preparations with meglumine antimoniate. Paromomycin preparations were applied twice daily for 30 days. By 12 weeks 70% and 79.3% of the subjects in the two different paromomycin groups achieved cure, making it an acceptable therapeutic alternative in endemic areas where meglumine antimoniate is not available, is too costly, or is medically contraindicated.

Comparison between the efficacy of photodynamic therapy and topical paromomycin in the treatment of Old World cutaneous leishmaniasis: a placebo-controlled, randomized clinical trial. Asilian A, Davami M. Clin Exp Dermatol 2006; 31: 634–7.

A study designed to compare the parasitological and clinical efficacy of photodynamic therapy (PDT) versus topical paromomycin in 60 patients with cutaneous leishmaniasis. Topical PDT was given weekly for 4 weeks. At the end of the study complete improvement was seen in 93.5% of patients treated with topical PDT, versus 41.2% in the topical paromomycin group, making PDT a safe, rapid, and effective treatment option for cutaneous leishmaniasis.

Treatment of cutaneous leishmaniasis by direct current electrotherapy: the Baghdadin device. Sharquie KE, al-Hamamy H, el-Yassin D. J Dermatol 1998; 25: 234–7.

One hundred and forty-six lesions from 54 patients were treated with weekly sessions of direct current stimulation (5–15 mA for 10 minutes). This produced total clearance in 95.5% of treated lesions within 4–6 weeks, whereas none of the 21 control lesions showed any sign of improvement.

Evaluation of CO_2 laser efficacy in the treatment of cutaneous leishmaniasis. Asilian A, Sharif A, Faghihi G, Enshaeieh SH, Shariati F, Siadat AH. Int J Dermatol 2004; 43: 736–8.

One hundred and eighty-three lesions from 123 patients were treated with CO_2 laser with a maximum power of 100 W and a pulse width of 0.5–5 s, and 250 lesions from 110 patients were treated with glucantime (meglumine antimoniate) 50 mg/kg daily for 15 days. The CO_2 laser was 1.12 times more effective than glucantime, with shorter healing time (1 month vs 3 months) and fewer side effects (4.5% vs 24%).

Oral zinc sulphate in the treatment of acute cutaneous leishmaniasis. Sharquie KE, Najim RA, Farjou IB, Al-Timimi DJ. Clin Exp Dermatol 2001; 26: 21–6.

One hundred and four patients with cutaneous leishmaniasis were involved in the study. They were randomly assigned to receive 2.5, 5, or 10 mg/kg zinc sulphate orally. A control group received no treatment. At the end of a 45-day follow-up an 83.9% cure rate was achieved for the 2.5 mg/kg treatment group, 93.1% for the 5 mg/kg treatment group, and a 96.9% cure rate was seen in the 10 mg/kg treatment group. No healing signs were observed in the control group.

Effect of combination therapy with systemic glucantime and pentoxifylline in the treatment of cutaneous leishmaniasis. Sadeghian G, Nilforoushzadeh MA. Int J Dermatol 2006; 45: 819–21.

Sixty-four patients were studied. Systemic glucantime 20 mg/kg/day combined with pentoxifylline 400 mg three times daily for 20 days is more effective than glucantime alone.

Lentigo maligna

Ellen S Marmur, John A Carucci, Darrell S Rigel

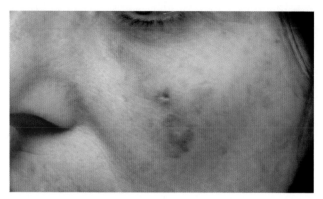

Photo courtesy of Ellen Marmur, MD

Lentigo maligna (LM) is a type of melanoma in situ that classically presents as irregular pigmented patches on sun-exposed areas of the face and neck in older individuals. If left untreated, its risk of progression to invasive melanoma (lentigo maligna melanoma, LMM) has been reported to range between 2% and 50%. LM and LMM are the most common forms of melanoma on the head and neck, are commonly found on the cheek, often present as a cosmetic concern, and their incidence is increasing. Treatment has been difficult owing to high recurrence rates, which are attributed to subclinical extension. Combination therapy with both surgical and non-surgical modalities, and surgery with wider margins are at the forefront of research in the field of LM/LMM.

MANAGEMENT STRATEGY

Successful management of LM depends on early diagnosis and definitive removal. The differential diagnosis includes lentigo, macular seborrheic keratosis, pigmented actinic keratosis, pigmented squamous cell carcinoma in situ, and pigmented superficial basal cell carcinoma. Confirmatory biopsy is necessary prior to definitive treatment. The use of a Wood's lamp may help to determine the perimeter of the lesion. Dermoscopy may also be helpful. Biopsy of the entire lesion is ideal in order to ascertain its maximum depth. However, the lesion tends to be large (>1 cm) owing to its propensity for extensive radial growth prior to vertical growth into the dermis. Therefore, biopsy of part of the lesion is often performed. Treatment is primarily surgical, although eradication by other methods may be considered. Patients with a history of LM should have periodic full-body skin examinations by a dermatologist to allow for early detection of recurrence, progression, or a second primary skin cancer. Patients with LM also require a consultation about sun protection behaviors.

SPECIFIC INVESTIGATIONS

▶ Skin biopsy and patient evaluation

Diagnosis and treatment of early melanoma. NIH Consensus Statement 1992; 10: 1–26.

Biopsy of sufficient depth is critical for diagnosis and management of pigmented lesions. Punch, saucerization, excision, or incisional biopsy may be acceptable. On microscopic examination LM is characterized by increased numbers of atypical melanocytes, which may be solitary or arranged in nests, but do not invade the dermis. Evaluation should include a personal and family history, complete skin examination, and palpation of regional lymph nodes. Blood tests or imaging studies are not indicated.

FIRST-LINE THERAPIES

▶ Excision	A
▶ Mohs' micrographic surgery (MMS)	D
▶ Modified Mohs' surgery	D
▶ Staged excision	D

Diagnosis and treatment of early melanoma. NIH Consensus Statement 1992; 10: 1–26.

Current recommendations are based on the NIH consensus for melanoma in situ, which suggests excision of the lesion or biopsy site with a margin of 0.5 cm of clinically normal skin and layer of subcutaneous tissue. In general, margins of 0.5–1.0 cm are suggested for LM where feasible. Difficulties may arise in determination of clinical margins due to diffuse background sun damage. A Wood's lamp may be useful in defining subclinical extension. Accurate determination of margins is key, because LM is likely to recur after inadequate excision.

Usefulness of the staged excision for lentigo maligna and lentigo maligna melanoma: the 'square' procedure. Johnson TM, Headington JT, Baker SR, Lowe L. J Am Acad Dermatol 1997; 37: 758–64.

With this technique, a margin of 0.5–1.0 cm is outlined with angled corners to facilitate processing. A peripheral strip of tissue 2–4 cm wide is excised and processed for evaluation of permanent sections. Residual tumor is subsequently excised in directed fashion based on mapping. There were no recurrences in 35 patients at 2 years.

Mohs' micrographic surgery for lentigo maligna and lentigo maligna melanoma. A follow-up study. Cohen LM, McCall MW, Zax RH. Dermatol Surg 1998; 24: 673–7.

A report of successful treatment at 29.2 months in 45 patients with LM and LMM with MMS aided by rush permanent sections. There was one recurrence at 50 months (97% cure rate).

Mohs' micrographic excision of melanoma using immunostains. Zalla MJ, Lim KK, Dicaudo DJ, Gagnot MM. Dermatol Surg 2000; 26: 771–84.

This modification to Mohs' technique was developed because difficulties may arise in distinguishing sun-damaged melanocytes from residual LM on frozen sections. Special histologic stains have been used to enhance sensitivity. Zalla et al. reported successful treatment of melanoma by MMS using Melan-A, HMB-45, Mel-5, and S100. There were no recurrences in 68 patients after a mean follow-up of 16 months.

Utility of rush paraffin-embedded tangential sections in the management of cutaneous neoplasms. Clayton BD, Leshin B, Hitchcock MG, Marks M, White WL. Dermatol Surg 2000; 26: 671–8.

Evidence Levels: A Double-blind study B Clinical trial ≥ 20 subjects C Clinical trial < 20 subjects D Series ≥ 5 subjects E Anecdotal case reports

The authors report treatment of 100 patients with melanoma (77 with LM/melanoma in situ, 23 with LMM), with margin control by rush permanent sections to enhance sensitivity. Recurrent LM was noted in one patient, and satellite metastasis was noted in one patient with LMM.

A potential disadvantage of relying on 'rush' permanent sections is the amount of time added to each procedure. In addition, the technique depends on off-site tissue processing and interpretation, thereby magnifying the possibility of error.

Management of lentigo maligna and lentigo maligna melanoma with staged excision: a follow up. Bub JL, Berg D, Slee A, Odland PB. Arch Dermatol 2004; 140: 552–8.

The authors report a staged, margin-controlled, vertical-edged excision technique followed by radial sectioning and preparation of paraffin sections. After a mean follow-up of 57 months, 95% of the 59 patients treated were disease free. The average excision margin was 0.55 cm. The use of radial sectioning allowed for more thorough specimen evaluation with relatively narrow margins.

Staged excision for lentigo maligna and lentigo maligna melanoma: A retrospective analysis of 117 cases. Hazan C, Dusza SW, Delgado R, Busam KJ, Halpern AC, Nehal KS. J Am Acad Dermatol 2008; 58: 142–8.

The authors conducted a retrospective study of 117 LM and LMM cases treated with a staged margin-controlled excision technique with rush paraffin-embedded sections. The mean total surgical margin required for excision of LM was 0.71 cm and was 1.03 cm for LMM. The study concluded that the standard excision margins for LM and LMM are often inadequate, and occult invasive melanoma occurs in LM.

SECOND-LINE THERAPIES

▶ Radiation therapy	D

A retrospective study of 150 patients with lentigo maligna and lentigo maligna melanoma and the efficacy of radiotherapy using Grenz or soft X-rays. Farshad A, Burg G, Pannizon R, Dummer R. Br J Dermatol 2002; 146: 1042–6.

Ninety-six patients with LM were treated with Grenz rays. Disease recurred in five of 96 patients after an average of 46 months. Four patients with recurrent LM were treated with subsequent surgery and one with radiotherapy. No patient with recurrent LM progressed to nodal or distant metastatic disease.

Fractionated radiotherapy of lentigo maligna and lentigo maligna melanoma in 64 patients. Schmid-Wendtner MH, Brunner B, Konz B, Kaudewitz P, Wendtner CM, Peter RU, et al. J Am Acad Dermatol 2000; 43: 477–82.

Sixty-four patients with LM (42) and LMM (22) were treated with fractionated radiotherapy. There was no recurrence in any of the patients with LM over a mean follow-up of 23 months (range 1–96 months).

One of the advantages of this soft X-ray or Miescher's technique is exclusion of underlying bone and minimization of risk of bony necrosis. The potential disadvantage is inadequate depth of penetration.

THIRD-LINE THERAPIES

▶ Q-switched ruby laser	E
▶ Q-switched Nd:YAG laser	D
▶ Interferon-α	D, E
▶ Imiquimod	D
▶ Tazarotene	E

Treatment of lentigo maligna with the Q-switched ruby laser. Kauvar ANB, Geronemus R. Lasers Surg Med 1995; 48.

Tumor eradication was achieved in three of four patients during a 6–24-month follow-up. The fourth patient developed amelanotic LM at 1 month. Q-switched ruby laser may be prone to failure due to inadequate depth of penetration.

Q-switched neodymium:yttrium-aluminum-garnet laser treatment of lentigo maligna. Orten SS, Waner M, Dinehart SM, Bardales RH, Flock ST. Otolaryngol Head Neck Surg 1999; 120: 296–302.

Eight patients with LM were treated with the Nd:YAG laser. Three patients were treated with both 532 and 1064 nm. Two of these had complete eradication without recurrence at 3.5 years. The other showed a partial response, but died of unrelated causes prior to completion of therapy.

The Nd:YAG laser emits energy at 532 and 1064 nm, which may be especially suited to LM. Melanin has greater absorption at 532 nm, whereas the longer wavelength, 1064 nm, may provide deeper penetration.

Intralesional interferon treatment of lentigo maligna. Cornejo P, Vanaclocha F, Polimon I, Del Rio R. Arch Dermatol 2000; 136: 428–30.

Interferon-α is a biological response modifier indicated for adjunctive treatment of high-risk melanoma. The mechanism involves both immunomodulation and direct antiproliferative effects. Successful treatment of 11 LM lesions in 10 patients at doses of $3–6 \times 10^6$ IU administered three times weekly is reported, with clearance in all patients after between 12 and 29 doses.

Intralesional interferon for treatment of recurrent lentigo maligna of the eyelid in a patient with primary acquired melanosis. Carucci JA, Leffell DJ. Arch Dermatol 2000; 136: 1415–16.

In this case report, clinical and histologic clearance was achieved after a total dose of 39 million units. Toxic effects included fever, chills, and flu-like symptoms, and were transient when interferon-α was used intralesionally.

Treatment of lentigo maligna with topical imiquimod. Naylor MF, Crowson N, Kuwahara R, Teague K, Garcia C, Mackinnis C, et al. Br J Dermatol 2003; 149: 66–9.

In this study, 30 patients with LM were enrolled in an open-labeled efficacy trial of daily application of imiquimod 5% cream for 3 months. Following treatment, 26 of 28 (93%) evaluable patients showed a 'complete response' based on four-quadrant biopsy. No recurrences were seen in 80% of the 26 patients that were followed for 1 year.

Treatment of lentigo maligna with tazarotene 0.1% gel. Chimenti S, Carrozzo AM, Citarella L, De Felice C, Peris K. J Am Acad Dermatol 2004; 50: 101–3.

In this series, two elderly patients with facial LM were treated with daily application of tazarotene gel 0.1% for 6–8 months. No recurrence in either patient was observed after follow-up periods of 18 and 30 months, respectively. These results should be interpreted with caution, considering the relatively short follow-up.

Treatment of lentigo maligna with imiquimod before staged excision. Cotter MA, McKenna JK, Bowen GM. Dermatol Surg 2008; 34: 147–51.

The authors treated 40 patients with biopsy-confirmed LM with topical 5% imiquimod cream five times a week for 3 months before staged excision. In 10 patients no erythema occurred after 1 month, and tazarotene gel 0.1% was added. A total of 33 of 40 patients were clinically clear on physical examination. Histologically, 30 of 40 patients had no residual disease; 10 of 40 had residual LM. One of 40 had invasive disease. After a mean follow-up of 18 months post excision, no patients had evidence of recurrence.

The authors conclude that 5% imiquimod may be an effective adjuvant therapy for LM but does not replace surgery.

Cryosurgery during topical imiquimod: a successful combination modality for lentigo maligna. Bassukas ID, Gamvroulia C, Zioga A, Nomikos K, Fotika C. Int J Dermatol 2008; 47: 519–21.

This is a case report of one patient treated with a combination of topical imiquimod daily to a 3 × 2 cm LM for 3 weeks. The area was then was treated with cryosurgery for 20 seconds for two cycles to a 4 × 3 cm area, followed by topical imiquimod daily for another 6 months without interruption. The authors report a sustained clearance of the LM at 26 months post treatment. They conclude that aggressive combination therapy with cryosurgery and topical imiquimod is a promising alternative in patients who refuse surgery.

Leprosy
(including reactions)

Anne E Burdick, Ivan D Camacho

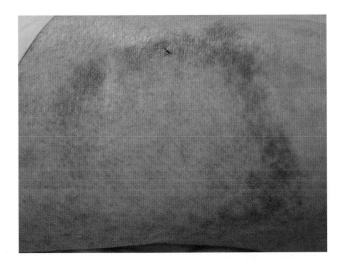

Leprosy, or Hansen's disease, is an infection caused by *Mycobacterium leprae (M. leprae)*, affecting the skin, peripheral nerves, respiratory mucosa, and other organs. It is diagnosed clinically by anesthetic skin lesions, enlarged peripheral nerves, and peripheral neuropathy, and confirmed by the presence of acid-fast bacilli in skin smears or tissue biopsies. Lesions present as anesthetic hypopigmented macules or erythematous plaques and nodules. Cell-mediated immunity against *M. leprae* determines the presentation of leprosy in the Ridley–Jopling spectrum: tuberculoid (TT), borderline tuberculoid (BT), mid-borderline (BB), borderline lepromatous (BL) and lepromatous (LL). The number of lesions varies from a few in TT leprosy to numerous in LL leprosy.

Leprosy reactions may occur before, during, and after treatment and affect 25–50% of patients. Type 1 or reversal reactions (RR) occur in borderline patients (BT, BB, BL) and are characterized by the reappearance of resolved lesions, acute peripheral neuritis, and often edema of the hands and feet or face.

Leprosy and RR may develop as an immune reconstitution inflammatory syndrome after certain drugs, including antiretroviral therapy. Type 2 reactions or erythema nodosum leprosum (ENL) occur in lepromatous patients (BL, LL) and are characterized by new tender nodules, fever, malaise, and arthralgias. A vasculitic reaction, Lucio's phenomenon, manifests with purpuric, tender lesions on the extremities that become necrotic and ulcerated.

MANAGEMENT STRATEGY

For treatment purposes TT and BT cases are classified as paucibacillary (PB), and BB, BL, and LL cases are multibacillary (MB). The US National Hansen's Disease Program (NHDP) recommends multidrug therapy (MDT) with two antibiotics (rifampin 600 mg daily and dapsone 100 mg daily) for 1 year for PB patients, and three antibiotics (rifampin, dapsone, and clofazimine 50 mg daily) for 2 years for MB patients. The

World Health Organization (WHO) recommends that PB cases receive two antibiotics for 6 months and MB cases three antibiotics for 1 year. Second-line antibiotics include minocycline 100 mg daily, ofloxacin 400 mg daily, ciprofloxacin 500 mg daily, and clarithromycin 500 mg daily. Multibacillary patients who have taken dapsone monotherapy for 5 or more years may discontinue dapsone if a biopsy and slit smears are negative. Rifampin is given once a month if a patient is taking prednisone. Pregnant patients can be treated with dapsone and clofazimine.

The NHDP recommends annual follow-up after treatment: 5 years for PB patients and 8 years for MB patients. Household contacts who lived with leprosy patients during the 3 years prior to treatment should be screened once for PB cases and annually for 5 years for MB cases.

A RR is treated with non-steroidal anti-inflammatory drugs if mild, and with prednisone 0.5–1 mg/kg/daily if severe. ENL is treated with prednisone 0.5–1 mg/kg/daily and/or thalidomide 100–400 mg daily. Various steroid-sparing agents have been reported, with mixed results. Thalidomide is tapered gradually over several months and maintained at 50–100 mg daily. Gabapentin 300–900 mg three times daily or pregabalin 50–100 mg daily may alleviate neuropathic pain. Lucio's phenomenon is treated with supportive care.

SPECIFIC INVESTIGATIONS

> ▶ Skin biopsy
> ▶ Slit smears
> ▶ Neurosensory testing
> ▶ Ophthalmologic examination (lepromatous)
> ▶ Glucose-6-phosphate dehydrogenase level prior to dapsone
> ▶ Liver function tests (rifampin or dapsone)
> ▶ Complete blood count
> ▶ Urinalysis (ENL)
> ▶ Pregnancy (thalidomide)
> ▶ Complement, cryoglobulins (Lucio's phenomenon)
> ▶ Bacterial culture (infected ulcers)

PCR based diagnosis of leprosy in the United States. Williams DL, Scollard DM, Gillis TP. Clin Microbiol Newsl 2003; 25: 57–61.

PCR is only recommended for patients who demonstrate acid-fast bacilli on pathology and have atypical clinical features of leprosy.

Hansen's disease in a patient with a history of sarcoidosis. Burdick AE, Hendi A, Elgart GW, Barquin L, Scollard DM. Int J Leprosy Other Mycobact Dis 2000; 68: 307–11.

Usefulness of the reticulum stain in distinguishing between non-infectious conditions (sarcoidosis) that preserve the reticulum network of type III collagen and infections, including leprosy, that do not.

FIRST-LINE THERAPIES

▷ Antibiotics	D
▷ Non-steroidal anti-inflammatory drugs (RR and ENL)	E
▷ Prednisone (RR and ENL)	D
▷ Thalidomide (ENL)	D

National Hansen's Disease Program website. www.bphc.hrsa.gov/nhdp

Provides the latest US diagnostic and treatment guidelines.

World Health Organization website. www.who.int/lep

Provides the latest WHO diagnostic and treatment guidelines.

Leprosy. Walker SL, Lockwood DN. Clin Dermatol 2007; 25: 165–72.

A comprehensive review.

The continuing challenges of leprosy. Scollard DM, Adams LB, Gillis TP, Krahenbuhl JL, Truman RW, Williams DL. Clin Microbiol Rev 2006; 19: 338–81.

Review of the genetics, immunology, and molecular biology of leprosy infection, reactions, mechanisms of nerve injury, and drug resistance.

Leprosy reversal reaction as immune reconstitution inflammatory syndrome in patients with AIDS. Batista MD, Porro AM, Maeda SM, Gomes EE, Yoshioka MC, Enokihara MM, et al. Clin Infect Dis 2008; 46: e56–60.

Two HIV-positive patients with undiagnosed TT and BT leprosy developed a RR2 months after the initiation of antiretroviral therapy as an immune reconstitution inflammatory syndrome (IRIS). Cases of IRIS leprosy in the literature are reviewed. Fifteen of the 16 cases presented with a RR within 2–6 months after the initiation of antiretroviral therapy.

The role of thalidomide in the management of erythema nodosum leprosum. Walker SL, Waters MF, Lockwood DN. Leprosy Rev 2007; 78: 197–215.

A review of thalidomide as an effective adjuvant and alternative to steroid therapy for ENL.

SECOND-LINE THERAPIES

▶ Minocycline	B
▶ Ofloxacin	B
▶ Levofloxacin	B
▶ Clarithromycin	B

Leprosy. Britton WJ, Lockwood DN. Lancet 2004; 363: 1209–19.

A review of clinical features, diagnostic criteria and treatment approaches to leprosy and its reactions.

THIRD-LINE THERAPIES (FOR REACTIONS)

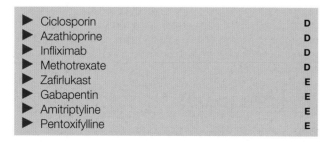

▶ Ciclosporin	D
▶ Azathioprine	D
▶ Infliximab	D
▶ Methotrexate	D
▶ Zafirlukast	E
▶ Gabapentin	E
▶ Amitriptyline	E
▶ Pentoxifylline	E

Response to cyclosporine treatment in Ethiopian and Nepali patients with severe leprosy type 1 reactions. Marlowe SN, Leekassa R, Bizuneh E, Knuutila J, Ale P, Bhattarai B, et al. Trans Roy Soc Trop Med Hyg 2007; 101: 1004–12.

Forty-one patients with RR treated with ciclosporin 5–7.5 mg/kg/day for 12 weeks and followed up for 24 weeks had 67–100% improvement. Patients with acute sensory neuritis (50–67%) relapsed after treatment was discontinued.

Treatment of recurrent erythema nodosum leprosum with infliximab. Faber WR, Jensema AJ, Goldschmidt WF. N Engl J Med 2006; 355: 739.

A BL patient on MDT developed ENL refractory to daily prednisolone 40 mg and thalidomide 300 mg. The patient responded promptly to three doses of infliximab 5 mg/kg every other week. No recurrences of ENL occurred 1 year after the last dose.

Development of leprosy and type 1 leprosy reactions after treatment with infliximab: a report of 2 cases. Scollard DM, Joyce MP, Gillis TP. Clin Infect Dis 2006; 43: e19–22.

Two patients manifested BL leprosy 1 and 3 months after treatment with infliximab for arthritis and later developed an RR 1 month after discontinuing this medication.

Type 1 leprosy reaction manifesting after discontinuation of adalimumab therapy. Camacho ID, Valencia I, Rivas MP, Burdick AE. Arch Dermatol 2009; 145: 349–351.

An undiagnosed BT patient presented with a RR 5 weeks after discontinuation of adalimumab treatment for presumed seronegative arthritis.

Azathioprine in controlling type 2 reactions in leprosy: a case report. Athreya SP. Leprosy Rev 2007; 78: 290–2.

A treated LL patient with persistent ENL for 2 years despite repeated courses of prednisolone 40 mg/daily responded when azathioprine 50 mg/daily was added, with resolution of ENL and discontinuation of prednisolone after 10 months. No ENL recurrence was observed during 2 years of follow-up.

Role of azathioprine in preventing recurrences in a patient of recurrent erythema nodosum leprosum. Verma KK, Srivastava P, Minz A, Verma K. Leprosy Rev 2006; 77: 225–9.

A patient with recurrent ENL on thalidomide 100 mg daily and prednisolone 10 mg daily was treated with azathioprine for 8 months at 2 mg/kg/day, allowing for the discontinuation of thalidomide and prednisolone with no relapses on follow-up of 1 year.

Clinical outcomes in a randomized controlled study comparing azathioprine and prednisolone versus prednisolone alone in the treatment of severe leprosy type 1 reactions in Nepal. Marlowe SN, Hawksworth RA, Butlin CR, Nicholls PG, Lockwood DN. Trans Roy Soc Trop Med Hyg 2004; 98: 602–9.

Forty patients with RR were randomly treated with prednisolone 40 mg/daily versus prednisolone 40 mg/daily together with azathioprine 3 mg/kg/daily for 12 weeks, with no difference in outcomes.

Pulse dexamethasone, oral steroids and azathioprine in the management of erythema nodosum leprosum. Mahajan VK, Sharma NL, Sharma RC, Sharma A. Leprosy Rev 2003; 74: 171–4.

Three patients with recurrent ENL unresponsive to prednisolone 80 mg daily responded to intravenous dexamethasone pulse therapy given at 4-week intervals and azathioprine 50 mg daily. The patients were able to reduce prednisolone to 10–20 mg daily.

Evidence Levels: **A** Double-blind study **B** Clinical trial ≥ 20 subjects **C** Clinical trial < 20 subjects **D** Series ≥ 5 subjects **E** Anecdotal case reports

Methotrexate treatment for type 1 (reversal) leprosy reactions. Biosca G, Casallo S, López-Vélez R. Clin Infect Dis 2007; 45: e7–9.

A BL patient with a RR and poor tolerance of corticosteroids responded to methotrexate 7.5 mg weekly, with discontinuation of prednisone after 2 months and resolution of lesions after 6 months.

Methotrexate in resistant ENL. Kar BR, Babu R. Int J Leprosy Other Mycobact Dis 2004; 72: 480–2.

An ENL patient, unresponsive to prednisolone 50 mg daily received methotrexate 15 mg weekly for 2 weeks followed by 7.5 mg weekly with a good response. Prednisolone was reduced to 20 mg daily after 2 weeks.

The role of mycophenolate mofetil in the treatment of leprosy reactions. Burdick AE, Ramirez CC. Int J Leprosy Other Mycobact Dis 2005; 73: 127–8.

Mycophenolate mofetil 2 g/day was not effective as a steroid-sparing agent in three patients.

Effect of zafirlukast on leprosy reactions. Vides EA, Cabrera A, Ahern KP, Levis WR. Int J Leprosy Other Mycobact Dis 1999; 67: 71–5.

Zafirlukast 20–40 mg twice daily for 3–5 months was an effective adjuvant to prednisone in 92% of 25 steroid-dependent patients with reactional states.

Pentoxifylline in the treatment of erythema nodosum leprosum. De Carsalade GY, Achirafi A, Flageul B. Acta Leprol 2003; 12: 117–22.

Ten of 11 patients with first episodes of ENL had complete resolution of symptoms within 7 days of pentoxifylline 400–800 mg three times daily. Relapses occurred with abrupt cessation of pentoxifylline, but not with a slow taper.

Leukocytoclastic vasculitis

Jeffrey P Callen

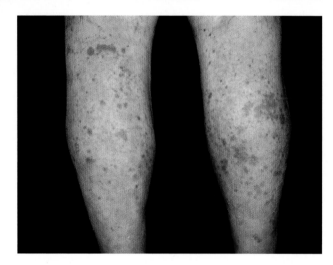

Leukocytoclastic vasculitis (LCV) is a term that defines a histopathological pattern. The clinical disease 'small vessel vasculitis' usually reflects LCV on biopsy examination. LCV is a heterogeneous group of disorders, most often represented clinically by palpable purpura or urticaria-like lesions.

MANAGEMENT STRATEGY

Therapy of cutaneous vasculitis depends on whether or not there is clinical or laboratory evidence of internal involvement, the severity of cutaneous disease, and the severity of the systemic disease. Patients with severe systemic necrotizing vasculitis are generally treated with moderate to high doses of *systemic corticosteroids, often with the addition of a cytotoxic agent.*

Patients with acute cutaneous vasculitis in whom there is an identifiable cause, such as a drug, are treated symptomatically in addition to removing the presumed causative agent. Similarly, patients with Henoch–Schönlein purpura usually have self-limiting disease and are often not given specific treatment. Symptomatic measures include *rest, elevation, gradient support stockings,* and *antihistamines.*

The challenge is to treat the patient who has chronic cutaneous vasculitis where there is no easily identifiable cause and who does not have significant systemic involvement. The need for therapy is often questioned because these patients do not have life-threatening disease; however, many patients have disease that alters their ability to function normally. Patients may develop small ulcers that can become secondarily infected or may be painful. Patients may not leave their homes because of the psychological distress caused by the presence of purpura. Lastly, patients with urticarial vasculitis complain of itching and burning of their lesions that may result in sleep disturbance. If systemic therapy is considered for disease confined to the skin, then *colchicine* and *dapsone* are often used. *Systemic corticosteroids, methotrexate,* and *azathioprine* have been used in patients who are refractory to less toxic therapies.

SPECIFIC INVESTIGATIONS

For all patients
- Careful history for drugs and other ingestants
- Skin biopsy for routine microscopy
- Serologic tests for collagen vascular diseases (ANA, rheumatoid factor, anti-Ro/SS-A, etc.)
- Serologic tests for infectious diseases (hepatitis C antibody, parvovirus, hepatitis B, etc.)
- Chest radiograph

For selected patients
- Skin biopsy for direct immunofluorescence microscopy
- Echocardiography
- Visceral angiography
- Malignancy screening tests

The purpose of evaluating the patient with cutaneous vasculitis is to identify a cause of the process and assess for the presence of systemic involvement. The evaluation begins with a careful history and physical examination, followed by selected testing based on the acuteness of the process and the findings from the history and physical examination.

Cutaneous vasculitis in children and adults: associated diseases and etiologic factors in 303 patients. Blanco R, Martinez-Taboada VM, Rodriguez-Valverde V, Garcia-Fuentes M. Medicine 1998; 77: 403–18.

These authors proposed an algorithm for evaluation that differs for children and adults. In children they do not require a skin biopsy for 'humanitarian' reasons. For children, the evaluation includes a blood count, erythrocyte sedimentation rate, urinalysis, stool hematest, and biochemistry profile. For adults, the authors suggest that additional testing include antinuclear antibodies, antineutrophil cytoplasmic antibody, chest radiograph, rheumatoid factor, cryoglobulins, complement levels, hepatitis B surface antigen, and hepatitis C antibody. Subsequent evaluation is directed by additional findings. In children with frequent relapses, suspicion of collagen vascular disease, severe vasculitic syndromes, or hepatic involvement, evaluation should be the same as for adults. Adults with persistent fever, abnormal blood smears, risk of HIV infection, or severe vasculitis should have cultures, echocardiography, hematological evaluation, HIV testing, and, when appropriate, visceral angiography and/or biopsy of involved organs.

Clinical approaches to cutaneous vasculitis. Gonzalez-Gay MA, Garcia-Porrua C, Pujol RM. Curr Opin Rheumatol 2005; 17: 56–61.

This review details an approach to the patient with small vessel vasculitis and provides a very useful algorithm.

FIRST-LINE THERAPIES

Observation	D
Removal or withdrawal of the causative agent (e.g., drug)	D
Colchicine	C
Dapsone	E

Evidence Levels: **A** Double-blind study **B** Clinical trial ≥ 20 subjects **C** Clinical trial < 20 subjects **D** Series ≥ 5 subjects **E** Anecdotal case reports

Management of necrotizing vasculitis with colchicine. Improvement in patients with cutaneous lesions and Behçet's syndrome. Hazen PG, Michel B. Arch Dermatol 1979; 115: 1303–6.

These authors were the first to note that vasculitis might respond to oral colchicine in an open-label observation of six patients.

Colchicine is effective in controlling chronic cutaneous leukocytoclastic vasculitis. Callen JP. J Am Acad Dermatol 1985; 13: 193–200.

This open-label study involved 13 patients.

Subsequent work, published only in abstract form, confirmed these initial observations.

Colchicine in the treatment of cutaneous leukocytoclastic vasculitis: results of a prospective, randomized controlled trial. Sais G, Vidaller A, Jucgla A, Gallardo F, Peyri J. Arch Dermatol 1995; 131: 1399–402.

This double-blind, placebo-controlled trial of colchicine failed to demonstrate a positive benefit; however, the colchicine-treated group included all patients who had been previously treated with dapsone and had failed to respond. In addition, there were unequal numbers of patients with hepatitis C-associated disease in each group. Thus the study population included patients with more recalcitrant disease, and there was an inadvertent bias that occurred during the process of randomization.

Sulfone therapy in the treatment of leukocytoclastic vasculitis. Report of three cases. Fredenberg MF, Malkinson FD. J Am Acad Dermatol 1987; 16: 772–8.

Three patients with LCV limited to their skin were successfully treated with moderate doses of dapsone (100–150 mg daily).

SECOND-LINE THERAPIES

▶ Systemic corticosteroids	D
▶ Immunosuppressive/cytotoxic agents – azathioprine, methotrexate, cyclophosphamide, ciclosporin, mycophenolate mofetil	D
▶ Rituximab	D

Azathioprine. An effective, corticosteroid-sparing therapy for patients with recalcitrant cutaneous lupus erythematosus or with recalcitrant cutaneous leukocytoclastic vasculitis. Callen JP, Spencer LV, Burruss JB, Holtman J. Arch Dermatol 1991; 127: 515–22.

Open-label trial involving six patients who had failed to respond to 'less toxic' therapies.

Prednisone plus azathioprine treatment in patients with rheumatoid arthritis complicated by vasculitis. Heurkens AH, Westedt ML, Breedveld FC. Arch Intern Med 1991; 151: 2249–54.

These authors studied 28 patients with rheumatoid arthritis-associated vasculitis. Nine patients with severe systemic vasculitis improved with 60 mg of prednisone and 2 mg/kg body weight of azathioprine daily. Nineteen patients with only cutaneous vasculitis entered a randomized controlled study comparing prednisone plus azathioprine treatment versus continuation of a previous regimen. Although measures of both vasculitis and arthritis activity improved to a greater degree in the patients treated with prednisone plus azathioprine in the first 3 months of therapy, and this therapy was associated with a low incidence of relapse of vasculitis, there was no significant difference between the results of the two treatment protocols at the end of the follow-up period.

The authors concluded that the combination was useful only for those patients with severe vasculitis. However, close analysis of their data suggests that there were lower corticosteroid doses in the azathioprine-treated group.

Low-dose methotrexate therapy for cutaneous vasculitis of rheumatoid arthritis. Upchurch KS, Heller K, Bress NM. J Am Acad Dermatol 1987; 17: 355–9.

A patient with classic rheumatoid arthritis who developed LCV is described. Low-dose methotrexate produced prompt healing of the skin lesions. After discontinuation of methotrexate the lesions recurred, with resolution after a second course of the drug.

This is a single case that responded; however, although there are other cases that have responded, there are many examples of patients with vasculitis which was initiated by or worsened by methotrexate, particularly patients with rheumatoid arthritis.

Chronic, recurrent small-vessel cutaneous vasculitis. Clinical experience in 13 patients. Cupps TR, Springer RM, Fauci AS. JAMA 1982; 247: 1994–8.

The clinical experience in 13 patients with small vessel cutaneous vasculitis limited to the skin is presented. This group of patients is represented by chronic and recurrent isolated cutaneous vasculitis eruptions, absence of disease progression to systemic involvement during long-term follow-up, and relative unresponsiveness to immunosuppressive therapy, including treatment with corticosteroid (prednisone) and cyclophosphamide.

This study suggests that cyclophosphamide therapy is poorly effective and, because of its potential toxicity, should be avoided. Other studies have documented individuals who have responded and individual patients whose disease was presumably induced by cyclophosphamide. However, patients with severe necrotizing vasculitis, Wegener's granulomatosis, or polyarteritis nodosa should be treated with cyclophosphamide.

Successful use of rituximab for cutaneous vasculitis. Chung L, Funke AA, Chakravarty EF, Callen JP, Fiorentino DF. Arch Dermatol 2006; 142: 1407–10.

Two women with recalcitrant LCV, one of whom with a history of non-Hodgkin's lymphoma, responded to infusions of rituximab.

Rituximab has been used in a variety of immunologically mediated disorders, including lupus erythematosus, autoimmune cytopenias, rheumatoid arthritis, dermatomyositis, and pemphigus vulgaris, in addition to its main indication, the treatment of lymphoma.

Successful treatment of rheumatoid vasculitis-associated cutaneous ulcers using rituximab in two patients with rheumatoid arthritis. Hellmann M, Jung N, Owczarczyk K, Hallek M, Rubbert A. Rheumatology (Oxford) 2008; 47: 929–30.

These two reports document improvement with rituximab in a total of four patients, two with RA and two with a history of lymphoma.

Nine patients with anti-neutrophil cytoplasmic antibody-positive vasculitis successfully treated with rituximab. Eriksson P. J Intern Med 2005; 257: 540–8.

This open-label study detailed the author's experience with rituximab, a chimeric monoclonal antibody that depletes CD20+ B cells, in patients with ANCA+ vasculitis. Several of the patients had cutaneous disease, which also improved with this therapy.

THIRD-LINE THERAPIES

▶ Antihistamines	E
▶ Non-steroidal anti-inflammatory drugs	D
▶ Dietary restriction	D
▶ Pentoxifylline (oxpentifylline)	E
▶ Interferon-α	A

Elimination diet in the treatment of selected patients with hypersensitivity vasculitis. Lunardi C, Bambara LM, Biasi D, Zagni P, Caramaschi P, Pacor ML. Clin Exp Rheumatol 1992; 10: 131–5.

Five patients with hypersensitivity vasculitis were treated with a 3-week elimination diet, followed by open and double-blind challenge tests with specific foods and additives. Four patients achieved a complete remission and one experienced great improvement on the elimination diet. In three cases the vasculitis relapsed following the introduction of food additives, in one case with the addition of potatoes and green vegetables (i.e., beans and green peas), and in the last case with the addition of eggs to the diet. The offending foods and additives were subsequently eliminated from the usual diet and no relapses were observed in 2 years of follow-up.

These results show that, in some patients, hypersensitivity vasculitis can be triggered and sustained by food antigens or additives, and possibly treated with an elimination diet.

Leukocytoclastic vasculitis caused by drug additives. Lowry MD, Hudson CF, Callen JP. J Am Acad Dermatol 1994; 30: 854–5.

A patient with chronic cutaneous LCV in whom the presumed cause was an excipient (a dye) used in the capsule form of lithium carbonate was reported. Elimination of this dye from the patient's diet led to control of her chronic cutaneous vasculitis.

Interferon alfa-2a therapy in cryoglobulinemia associated with hepatitis C virus. Misiani R, Bellavita P, Fenili D, Vicari O, Marchesi D, Sironi PL, et al. N Engl J Med 1994; 330: 751–6.

In a prospective, randomized, controlled trial, 53 patients with hepatitis C virus (HCV)-associated type II cryoglobulinemia were studied. A group of 27 patients received recombinant interferon-α_{2a} three times weekly at a dose of 1.5 million units for a week and then 3 million units three times weekly for the following 23 weeks. The 26 control patients did not receive anything apart from previously prescribed treatments. All patients were then followed for an additional 24–48 weeks. After the treatment period, serum HCV RNA was undetectable in 15 of the remaining 25 patients who received interferon-α_{2a}, but in none of the controls. Compared to the control group, the 15 patients with undetectable levels of HCV RNA in serum had a significant improvement in cutaneous vasculitis (p=0.04) and significant reductions in serum

levels of anti-HCV antibody activity (p=0.007), cryoglobulins (p=0.002), IgM (p=0.002), rheumatoid factor (p=0.001), and creatinine (p=0.006). After treatment with interferon-α_{2a} was discontinued, viremia and cryoglobulinemia recurred in all 15 HCV RNA-negative patients. On resumption of treatment, three of four patients had a virologic, clinical, and biochemical response.

In patients with HCV-associated small vessel vasculitis, interferon-α may be of benefit.

Synergistic effects of pentoxifylline and dapsone in leucocytoclastic vasculitis. Nurnberg W, Grabbe J, Czarnetzki BM. Lancet 1994; 343: 491.

A single case is reported.

Chronic leukocytoclastic vasculitis associated with polycythemia vera: effective control with pentoxifylline. Wahba-Yahav AV. J Am Acad Dermatol 1992; 26: 1006–7.

OTHER THERAPIES

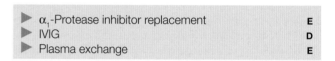

▶ α₁-Protease inhibitor replacement	E
▶ IVIG	D
▶ Plasma exchange	E

Effective treatment with alpha 1-protease inhibitor of chronic cutaneous vasculitis associated with alpha 1-antitrypsin deficiency. Dowd SK, Rodgers GC, Callen JP. J Am Acad Dermatol 1995; 33: 913–16.

A 49-year-old man with cutaneous vasculitis and α_1-antitrypsin deficiency failed to respond to colchicine, prednisone, and antibiotics, but was controlled by the intermittent administration of α_1-protease inhibitor.

Case report: steroid sparing effect of intravenous gamma globulin in a child with necrotizing vasculitis. Gedalia A, Correa H, Kaiser M, Sorensen R. Am J Med Sci 1995; 309: 226–8.

A 2½-year-old boy with fever, arthritis, and necrotizing cutaneous vasculitis improved significantly with the administration of prednisone; however, several attempts to reduce the prednisone dose resulted in relapses. The prednisone was successfully tapered and discontinued after intravenous γ-globulin administration.

Plasma exchange in refractory cutaneous vasculitis. Turner AN, Whittaker S, Banks I, Jones RR, Pusey CD. Br J Dermatol 1990; 122: 411–15.

Eight patients with intractable cutaneous LCV were treated with plasma-exchange therapy. Seven improved, five substantially. Four continued to be treated by intermittent plasma exchange for periods of 5–12 years. Apart from one episode of hepatitis B, possibly related to the administration of fresh frozen plasma, no major adverse effects have occurred.

Plasma exchange may be useful via the delivery of intravenous immunoglobulin within the fresh frozen plasma. If it were merely 'cleaning' the blood of antigen–antibody complexes, one would presumably require the addition of an immunosuppressive agent.

Lichen myxedematosus

Joslyn Sciacca Kirby

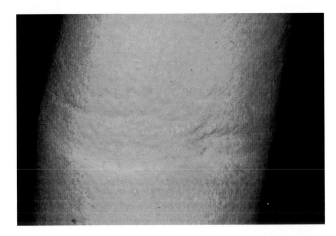

Lichen myxedematosus (LM) is a rare, chronic disease characterized by infiltration of the skin with mucin-producing fibroblasts. Typical examination findings include shiny, flesh-colored to erythematous papules, nodules, and plaques. More extensive cutaneous disease can cause widespread thickening and hardening of the skin, with large, raised folds. The disease favors the face and extremities. Localized and systemic subtypes of the disease are now recognized. The systemic form, scleromyxedema, is associated with a monoclonal IgG-λ gammopathy. Localized forms of the disease, such as acral persistent papular mucinosis, discrete LM, nodular LM, self-healing papular mucinosis, and cutaneous mucinosis of infancy, are limited to the skin and have a better prognosis. The cause of the disease is unknown.

MANAGEMENT STRATEGY

The treatment of LM remains a challenge. The absence of any controlled studies makes comparison of different drugs or drug regimens difficult. The localized form may be observed or treated with topical medications or destructive therapies such as *cryotherapy, dermabrasion*, or *hyaluronidase*. The systemic form is treated more aggressively, and patients may require treatment with multiple medications either serially or in combination before a successful therapy is found.

Given the association between scleromyxedema and monoclonal gammopathy, some of the therapies for systemic LM are taken from treatment of multiple myeloma, particularly *melphalan*. Melphalan is an alkylating agent generally prescribed as a pulse regimen of four times daily for 4 days every 4–6 weeks, or four times daily until symptoms resolve; however, its use in localized disease is limited by secondary adverse effects, including malignancy and sepsis. Melphalan has also shown beneficial results when used in combination with other therapies, including *plasmapheresis, oral prednisone*, or *autologous stem cell transplant*.

Several other agents, including *2-chlorodeoxyadenosine (cladribine), cyclophosphamide, ciclosporin, methotrexate*, and *thalidomide*, have demonstrated some efficacy.

Alternatives to immunosuppressive agents include *isotretinoin, interferon-α$_{2b}$, intravenous immunoglobulin, intralesional triamcinolone acetonide, psoralen with UVA (PUVA)*, and *extracorporeal photochemotherapy*.

SPECIFIC INVESTIGATIONS

- ▶ Serum protein electrophoresis
- ▶ Tests for HIV infection
- ▶ Thyroid function testing
- ▶ Tests for hepatitis C infection

Lichen myxedematosus (papular mucinosis): new concepts and perspectives for an old disease. Rongioletti F. Semin Cutan Med Surg 2006; 25: 100–4.

An abnormal paraprotein, most commonly a monoclonal IgG λ, is found in most patients (>80%) with scleromyxedema. Myeloma develops in fewer than 10%. It does not appear to represent a primary plasma cell dyscrasia, nor is there a consistent association with multiple myeloma. Fourteen cases of localized lichen myxedematosus in HIV-positive patients have been reported. Thyroid disease-associated mucinoses must be distinguished.

Lichen myxedematosus associated with chronic hepatitis C. Banno H, Takama H, Nitta Y, Ikeya T, Hirooka Y. Int J Dermatol 2000; 39: 212–14.

Eight of 16 Japanese patients displayed liver dysfunction with anti-HCV antibodies in association with LM. Only two cases outside Japan have been reported.

FIRST-LINE THERAPIES

▶ Melphalan	C
▶ Systemic corticosteroids	D
▶ Plasmapheresis	D

Scleromyxedema. Dinneen AM, Dicken CH. J Am Acad Dermatol 1995; 33: 37–43.

A review of 17 patients treated with melphalan revealed improvement of cutaneous symptoms in 12. Eight of the 12 had only temporary improvement. Ten of the treated patients died from complications of the disease or treatment.

Scleromyxedema: An experience using treatment with systemic corticosteroid and review of the published work. Lin YC, Wang HC, Shen JL. J Dermatol 2006; 33: 207–10.

A case report of successful treatment with prednisolone 0.3 mg/kg/day divided four times daily for 1 week and tapered for 3 more weeks, with improvement in cutaneous disease. Other studies have successfully used prednisone 60 mg four times daily for 4–6 weeks with gradual taper or pulse dexamethasone.

Scleromyxedema: successful treatment of cutaneous and neurologic symptoms. Nieves DS, Bondi EE, Wallmark J, Raps EC, Seykora JT. Cutis 2000; 65: 89–92.

A man with cutaneous and central nervous system disease had a very good response after treatment with plasmapheresis and melphalan. There is a mixed success rate, as many reports use this as an early therapy.

SECOND-LINE THERAPIES

▶ Isotretinoin/etretinate	D
▶ Intravenous immunoglobulin	D
▶ Thalidomide	D
▶ Topical or intralesional corticosteroids	E
▶ Topical calcineurin inhibitors	E

Improvement of scleromyxedema associated with isotretinoin therapy. Hisler BM, Savoy LB, Hashimoto K. J Am Acad Dermatol 1991; 24: 854–7.

A report of scleromyxedema with myopathy showing improvement after treatment with isotretinoin 40 mg twice daily for 3 months.

Scleromyxedema: a case series highlighting long-term outcomes of treatment with intravenous immunoglobulin (IVIG). Blum M, Wigley FM, Hummers LK. Medicine 2008; 87: 10–20.

Eight patients had dramatic improvement of their cutaneous and visceral disease and were subsequently maintained with IVIG.

Treatment of recalcitrant scleromyxedema with thalidomide in 3 patients. Sansbury J, Cocuroccia B, Jorizzo J, Gubinelli E, Gisondi P, Girolomoni G. J Am Acad Dermatol 2004; 51: 126–31.

Within 2 months of starting thalidomide treatment, three patients with recalcitrant scleromyxedema displayed marked improvement of cutaneous lesions, joint mobility, and reduction of paraprotein levels. Several case reports reported the use of thalidomide in doses of 50–400 mg/day for several months.

Discrete papular mucinosis responding to intralesional and topical steroids. Reynolds NJ, Collins CM, Burton JL. Arch Dermatol 1992; 128: 857–8.

A case of complete response to intralesional triamcinolone acetonide and Haelan, an adhesive polyethylene tape impregnated with flurandrenolide. Multiple case reports mention the use of topical or intralesional steroids in addition to other therapies, with mixed results.

Treatment of localized lichen myxedematosus of discrete type with tacrolimus ointment. Rongioletti F, Zaccaria E, Cozzani E, Parodi A. J Am Acad Dermatol 2008; 58: 530–2.

Near complete resolution with twice-daily application for 8 weeks. One patient previously did not respond to topical steroids.

In another report, pimecrolimus resulted in symptomatic relief.

THIRD-LINE THERAPIES

▶ Autologous stem cell transplantation	D
▶ 2-Chlorodeoxyadenosine	E
▶ Cyclophosphamide	E
▶ Ciclosporin	E
▶ Methotrexate	E
▶ Chlorambucil	E
▶ Interferon-α_{2b}	E
▶ Extracorporeal photopheresis	E
▶ PUVA	E
▶ Radiation	E

Scleromyxedema: role of high-dose melphalan with autologous stem cell transplantation. Donato ML, Feasel AM, Weber DM, Prieto VG, Giralt SA, Champlin RE, et al. Blood 2006; 107: 463–6.

Seven patients were treated; all survived, and five had complete remission of the skin disease. Visceral disease also greatly improved.

Treatment of scleromyxedema with 2-chlorodeoxyadenosine. Davis LS, Sanal S, Sangueza OP. J Am Acad Dermatol 1996; 35: 288–90.

Case report of a patient treated with 2-chlorodeoxyadenosine, a purine analog used mainly in the treatment of lymphoproliferative disorders, 0.1 mg/kg for 5 days, resulting in marked cutaneous improvement.

Scleromyxedema with subclinical myositis. Prasad PV, Joseph JM, Kaviarasan PK, Viswanathan P. Indian J Dermatol Venereol Leprol 2004; 70: 36–8.

A case report of a patient with scleromyxedema and myositis treated with cyclophosphamide 50 mg twice a day with prednisolone 40 mg a day, with 75% improvement at 1 month and without relapse.

Successful treatment of intractable scleromyxedema with cyclosporine A. Saigoh S, Tashiro A, Fujita S, Matsui M, Shibata S, Takeshita H, et al. Dermatol 2003; 207: 410–11.

After failing PUVA, oral prednisone, and plasmapheresis, a patient's condition improved with ciclosporin A at doses of 50–100 mg/day. There was a 50% improvement at 4 months and near resolution at 18 months.

Scleromyxedema myopathy: case report and review of the literature. Helfrich DJ, Walker ER, Martinez AJ, Meedsgar TA. Arthritis Rheum 1988; 31: 1437–41.

Oral prednisone and intravenous methotrexate resulted in improvement of cutaneous and systemic symptoms in one patient.

Lichen myxedematosus treated with chlorambucil. Wieder JM, Barton KL, Baron JM, Soltani K. J Dermatol Surg Oncol 1993; 19: 475–6.

One patient was treated with chlorambucil 4 mg to 4 or 6 mg alternating daily for 18 months, with improvement of her cutaneous symptoms. Her paraproteinemia was unchanged. The authors feel this medication is less immunosuppressive and causes fewer secondary malignancies than melphalan or cyclophosphamide.

Scleromyxedema: treatment with interferon alfa. Tschen JA, Chang JR. J Am Acad Dermatol 1999; 40: 303–7.

One patient who failed to respond to chlorambucil and isotretinoin improved with interferon-α_{2b} 6–10 mU three times weekly over more than 3 months. Her visceral symptoms did not improve. A couple of reports have remarked on exacerbation of scleromyxedema during interferon treatment for hepatitis C or multiple sclerosis.

Cutaneo-systemic papulosclerotic mucinosis (scleromyxedema): remission after extracorporeal photochemotherapy and corticoid bolus. D'Incan M, Franck F, Kanold J, Bacin F, Achin R, Beyvin AJ, et al. Ann Dermatol Venereol 2001; 128: 38–41.

A complete cutaneous therapeutic response was obtained in one patient after 12 extracorporeal photopheresis courses and four pulse treatments of prednisolone.

Successful treatment of lichen myxoedematosus with PUVA photochemotherapy. Adachi Y, Iba S, Horio T. Photodermatol Photoimmunol Photomed 2000; 16: 229–31.

A patient received PUVA treatments three times a week and showed improvement after only seven treatments. He had near resolution after 35 treatments and only a minor recurrence at 2 years.

Scleromyxedema: treatment of widespread cutaneous involvement by total skin electron-beam therapy. Rampino M, Garibaldi E, Ragona R, Ricardi U. Int J Dermatol 2007; 46: 864–7.

The report of one patient successfully treated with radiation therapy, and a review of previous reports.

Evidence Levels: **A** Double-blind study **B** Clinical trial ≥ 20 subjects **C** Clinical trial < 20 subjects **D** Series ≥ 5 subjects **E** Anecdotal case reports

Lichen nitidus

Andrew L Wright

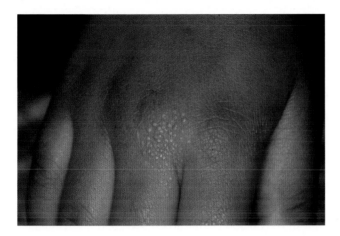

Lichen nitidus is an uncommon idiopathic condition composed of 1–2 mm diameter flat-topped or domed papules. They usually remain discrete, but may be grouped. They can occur on any part of the body, but mainly affect the forearms, penis, abdomen, chest, and buttocks. Palmar lesions may be hemorrhagic.

MANAGEMENT STRATEGY

Lichen nitidus persists for long periods of time, but is generally asymptomatic and *treatment may not be necessary*. No large controlled clinical trials have been reported; most treatments are based on anecdotal reports.

In patients with localized disease, *potent topical corticosteroids and topical tacrolimus* can be successful in clearing lesions. For more extensive disease *phototherapy* (psoralen plus UVA (PUVA) and UVB) has been reported to be successful. *Antihistamines*, including *astemizole* and *cetirizine*, are reported to have cleared lesions. Generalized lesions have cleared with *PUVA*, *UVB*, and *acitretin*.

SPECIFIC INVESTIGATIONS

- ▶ Biopsy

FIRST-LINE THERAPIES

▶ Topical corticosteroids	E
▶ UVB	D

Successful treatment of lichen nitidus. Wright S. Arch Dermatol 1984; 120: 155–6.

A 24-year-old woman with a 12-year history of extensive lesions cleared with 1 month's treatment using 0.05% fluocinonide cream twice daily. No recurrence was noted at 12-month follow-up.

Treatment of generalized lichen nitidus with narrow band ultraviolet light. Park JH, Choi YL, Kim WS, Lee DY, Yang JM, Lee ES, et al. J Am Acad Dermatol 2006; 54: 545–6.

A 33-year-old man with a 3-year history of generalized disease was reported as almost clear after 28 treatments, and remained clear 11 months after cessation of therapy. A 10-year-old with generalized disease was reported as completely clear after 41 treatments, and was clear at the 6-month follow-up.

Two cases of generalized lichen nitidus treated successfully with narrow band UVB phototherapy. Kim YC, Shim SD. Int J Dermatol 2006; 45: 615–17.

A 7-year-old girl and a 10-year-old boy, both with generalized lichen nitidus, were treated with narrowband UVB phototherapy, receiving between 17 and 30 treatments maximum 9.5 J/cm². Both were reported as almost clear at the end of treatment and remained clear for at least 11 months.

SECOND-LINE THERAPIES

▶ Topical tacrolimus	E
▶ Antihistamines	D
▶ PUVA	E
▶ Oral retinoids	E

Lichen nitidus treated with topical tacrolimus. Dobbs CR, Murphy SJ. J Drugs Dermatol 2004; 3: 683–4.

A 32-year-old man with lichen nitidus confined to the penis was treated with twice-daily tacrolimus 0.1%. The lesion was reported to be clear after 4 weeks' treatment, and had not relapsed after 4 months.

Generalised lichen nitidus – a report of two cases treated with astemizole. Ocampo J, Torne R. Int J Dermatol 1989; 28: 49–51.

Two patients treated with astemizole, a 65-year-old man with a 3-month history and a 48-year-old woman with a 4-month history, were either cleared or dramatically improved with 6–12 days of astemizole 10 mg daily.

Lichen nitidus treated with astemizole. Thio HB. Br J Dermatol 1993; 129: 342.

A 20-year-old woman with widespread disease responded to astemizole 10 mg daily, after relapsing following a successful course of PUVA. There was no recurrence of lesions at 2-year follow-up.

It should be noted that astemizole has been discontinued because of cardiotoxicity noted with certain drug interactions. It is presumed that safer antihistamines might also be valuable.

Treatment of generalized lichen nitidus with PUVA. Randle HW, Sander HM. Int J Dermatol 1986; 25: 330–1.

A 29-year-old woman with an 8-month history of a generalized eruption was treated with PUVA three times weekly. Lesions cleared after 46 treatments (290 J) and remained clear 5 years later.

Association of lichen planus and lichen nitidus – treatment with etretinate. Aram H. Int J Dermatol 1988; 27: 117.

A 35-year-old woman with a 4-month history cleared with 8 weeks of etretinate 25 mg/50 mg on alternate days. Treatment was stopped 1 month later. There was no recurrence 5 months after completing the treatment.

Treatment of palmoplantar lichen nitidus with acitretin.
Lucker GPH, Koopman RJJ, Steijlen PM, Van der Valk PG. Br J Dermatol 1994; 130: 791–3.

A 23-year-old man had a 14-month history of hand and foot involvement that failed to clear with acitretin 50 mg daily, but was reported to have improved significantly on 75 mg daily.

THIRD-LINE THERAPIES

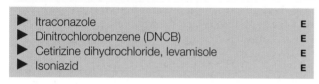

▶ Itraconazole	E
▶ Dinitrochlorobenzene (DNCB)	E
▶ Cetirizine dihydrochloride, levamisole	E
▶ Isoniazid	E

Treatment of lichen planus and lichen nitidus with itraconazole: reports of six cases. Libow LF, Coots NV. Cutis 1998; 62: 247–8.

A report of two cases showing partial clearance of lichen nitidus after 2 weeks of itraconazole 200 mg twice daily.

Improvement of lichen nitidus after topical dinitrochlorobenzene application. Kano Y, Otake Y, Shiohara T. J Am Acad Dermatol 1998; 39: 305–8.

This paper reports a patient treated with 0.1% DNCB applied at 2-weekly intervals, following sensitization with 1% DNCB. The lesions were said to have cleared after 7 months of treatment, compared to a control area. Six months after cessation of treatment lesions were said to be recurring in the treated area.

Generalised lichen nitidus in a child – response to cetirizine dihydrochloride/levamisol. Sehgal VN, Jain S, Kumar S, Bhattacharya SN, Singh N. Australas J Dermatol 1998; 39: 60.

A 6-year-old boy with a 6-month history of generalized involvement showed complete regression/healing of lesions over a 4-week period of treatment with cetirizine dihydrochloride 5 mg daily and levamisole 50 mg on alternate days for 4 weeks.

Generalised lichen nitidus is successfully treated with an antituberculous agent. Kubota Y, Kirya H, Nakayama J. Br J Dermatol 2002; 146: 1081–3.

A 10-year-old Japanese girl with a 2-year history of lichen nitidus showed almost complete clearance following a 6-month course of oral isoniazid.

Lichen planopilaris

Anwar Al Hammadi, Eric Berkowitz, Mark Lebwohl

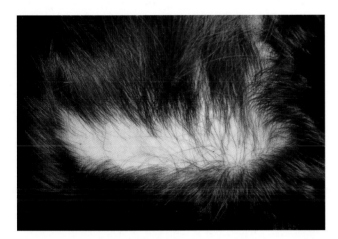

Lichen planopilaris (LPP), also known as follicular lichen planus, is a clinical syndrome consisting of lichen planus (LP) associated with cicatricial scalp alopecia. The condition is more common in women, and presents with perifollicular erythema and keratotic plugs at the margins of the expanding alopecia. The follicular involvement is limited to the infundibulum and the isthmus, both demonstrating lichenoid inflammation. The main complications of follicular lichen planus are atrophy and scarring, with permanent hair loss. Three forms of lichen planopilaris are recognized, including classic lichen planopilaris; Graham-Little syndrome, characterized by the triad of multifocal scalp cicatricial alopecia, non-scarring alopecia of the axilla and/or groin, and keratotic follicular papules; and frontal fibrosing alopecia that affects mainly postmenopausal women and appears as cicatricial alopecia of the frontoparietal hairline and is associated with non-scarring alopecia of the eyebrows.

MANAGEMENT STRATEGY

Therapeutic management for lichen planopilaris is difficult and challenging. However, if the associated inflammation can be controlled in its early stages, follicular units may be preserved and hair regrowth may be possible. A good therapeutic response would include a reduction in associated symptoms along with stabilization of the disease and some regrowth of hair in the active perimeter of the alopecic patch. For the most part, therapeutic reports are anecdotal. *Oral antihistamines* may be used to control pruritus, and *high-potency topical corticosteroids* are used to control the inflammation in early lesions. *Intralesional injections of 3–5 mg/mL of triamcinolone acetonide* are effective in well-developed lesions. *Retinoids* have demonstrated some effect in the treatment of lichen planus and therefore provide a possible alternative to corticosteroid treatment. Additional treatment modalities include the *antimalarials*, in particular hydroxychloroquine. Other agents that have been reported to be of use are *ciclosporin* and *mycophenolate mofetil*. There is some rationale for trying biologic agents such as the tumor necrosis factor (TNF)-blocking agents for this condition.

SPECIFIC INVESTIGATIONS

> ▶ Skin biopsy
> ▶ Immunofluorescence studies

A histologic review of 27 patients with lichen planopilaris. Tandon YK, Somani N, Bergfeld WF. J Am Acad Dermatol 2008; 59: 91–8.

Characteristic features of lichen planopilaris include the absence of arrector pili muscles and sebaceous glands; a perivascular and perifollicular lymphocytic infiltrate; mucinous perifollicular fibroplasia with absence of interfollicular mucin; and superficial perifollicular wedge-shaped scarring.

Elastic tissue in scars and alopecia. Elston DM, McCollough ML, Warschaw KE, Bergfeld WF. J Cutan Pathol 2000; 27: 147–52.

This investigation determined that the Verhoeff–van Gieson elastic stain can reliably differentiate scarred from non-scarred dermis, and is reliable in distinguishing lichen planopilaris from lupus erythematosus.

Immunofluorescence abnormalities in lichen planopilaris. Ioannides D, Bystryn JC. Arch Dermatol 1992; 128: 214–16.

Direct immunofluorescence studies were performed on biopsied lesions of patients with lichen planopilaris and lichen planus. All of the lichen planopilaris studies demonstrated abnormal linear deposits of immunoglobulin, consisting of IgG or IgA restricted to the basement membrane. The biopsies from those with lichen planus demonstrated fibrillar deposits.

These different appearances suggest different disease processes for LPP and LP.

FIRST-LINE THERAPIES

> ▶ High-potency corticosteroids   **D**
> ▶ Intralesional corticosteroids   **C**

Lichen planopilaris: report of 30 cases and review of the literature. Chieregato C, Zini A, Barba A, Magannini M, Rosina P. Int J Dermatol 2003; 42: 342–5.

This clinical trial reports good therapeutic benefit from early treatment with high-potency topical steroids. Only four patients did not respond to the therapy and needed other treatments.

Scarring alopecia. Newton RC, Hebert AA, Freese TW, Solomon AR. Dermatol Clin 1987; 5: 603–18.

High-potency topical corticosteroids may be used to control inflammation in early scalp lesions. Intralesional injections with triamcinolone acetonide at concentrations of 3–5 mg/mL are more effective in well-developed lesions. Additionally, oral corticosteroids have been used in short tapering dosages to control severe disease.

SECOND-LINE THERAPIES

> ▶ Oral corticosteroids   **C**
> ▶ Retinoids   **C**
> ▶ Antimalarials   **C**
> ▶ Tetracycline   **D**

Postmenopausal frontal fibrosing alopecia: a frontal variant of lichen planopilaris. Kossard S, Lee MS, Wilkinson B. J Am Acad Dermatol 1997; 36: 59–66.

Oral corticosteroids and antimalarials were found to slow the course of lichen planopilaris.

Lichen planopilaris: clinical and pathologic study of forty-five patients. Mehregan DA, Van Hale HM, Muller SA. J Am Acad Dermatol 1992; 27: 935–42.

This large study of 45 patients involved multiple different therapeutic modalities. High-potency topical steroids and oral steroids (30–40 mg daily) for 3 months demonstrated the highest success rates.

Oral treatment of keratinizing disorders of skin and mucous membranes with etretinate. Comparative study of 113 patients. Mahrle G, Meyer-Hamme S, Ippen H. Arch Dermatol 1982; 118: 97–100.

This paper reports the comparative results of the effects of the aromatic retinoid etretinate on various skin disorders.

Retinoids have been found to have a significant impact in cases of lichen planus and have therefore been tried with some success in cases of lichen planopilaris. Isotretinoin may be preferred over acitretin, as the latter agent has been associated with hair loss, but long-term therapy with low-dose acitretin has been well studied in psoriasis and is well tolerated.

A case-series of 29 patients with lichen planopilaris: The Cleveland Clinic Foundation experience on evaluation, diagnosis, and treatment. Cevasco NC, Bergfeld WF, Remzi BK, de Knott HR. J Am Acad Dermatol 2007; 57: 47–53.

In this retrospective study of 29 patients, researchers found that the most commonly prescribed treatments for the reduction of primary symptoms associated with LPP were ketoconazole shampoo (86%), topical steroids (83%), multivitamins with minerals (76%), intralesional steroids (69%), topical minoxidil (41%), and tetracycline (38%). The most common treatment combination was topical steroid, ketoconazole shampoo, tetracycline, and multivitamins with minerals (14%).

Although patient response to any of these therapies was minimal, tetracycline (1 g/day) was the only treatment associated with a significant number of positive responses (six of 11 patients).

THIRD-LINE THERAPIES

▶ Mycophenolate mofetil		E
▶ Griseofulvin		E
▶ Ciclosporin		D
▶ Tacrolimus		E
▶ Thalidomide		E
▶ TNF-blocking drugs		E

Treatment of lichen planopilaris with mycophenolate mofetil. Tursen U, Api H, Kaya Y, Ikizoglu G. Dermatol Online J 2004; 10: 24.

The authors report a case of lichen planopilaris that was successfully treated with mycophenolate mofetil.

Lichen planopilaris [cicatricial (scarring) alopecia] in a child. Sehgal VN, Bajaj P, Srivastva G. Int J Dermatol 2001; 40: 461–3.

This case report describes the successful treatment of lichen planopilaris using combination therapy with griseofulvin, prednisolone, and topical betamethasone diproprionate lotion.

Short course of oral cyclosporine in lichen planopilaris. Mirmirani P, Willey A, Price V. J Am Acad Dermatol 2003; 49: 667–71.

The authors present three patients with recalcitrant lichen planopilaris, unresponsive to hydroxychloroquine, high-potency topical steroids, and intralesional steroids, who were treated with ciclosporin. The duration of treatment ranged from 3 to 5 months, with resolution of symptoms, no progression of hair loss, and no evidence of disease activity. One of the patients had a mild recurrence, which resolved with topical 0.1% tacrolimus in Cetaphil lotion.

Thalidomide-induced remission of lichen planopilaris. Boyd AS, King LE Jr. J Am Acad Dermatol 2002; 47: 967–8.

The authors describe the case of a patient who was diagnosed with lichen planopilaris and treated with hydroxychloroquine, azathioprine, isotretinoin, cyclophosphamide, dapsone, ciclosporin, levamisole, chloroquine, acitretin, methotrexate, clofazamine, and enoxaparin, all without any benefit. The patient was then started on thalidomide 50 mg orally twice a day, with resolution of the symptoms. Side effects limited the ability to continue the medication. Initially, the patient only complained of fatigue and constipation; however, at 4 months, mild numbness and tingling of the fingers and toes developed and the patient experienced significant depression, necessitating discontinuation of the medication.

Thalidomide's mechanism of action in this disorder may involve TNF inhibition, suggesting that medications such as adalimumab, etanercept, or infliximab may be beneficial. There has, however, been a case report of LPP developing in a patient treated with etanercept.

Evidence Levels: A Double-blind study **B** Clinical trial ≥ 20 subjects **C** Clinical trial < 20 subjects **D** Series ≥ 5 subjects **E** Anecdotal case reports

Lichen planus

Mark G Lebwohl

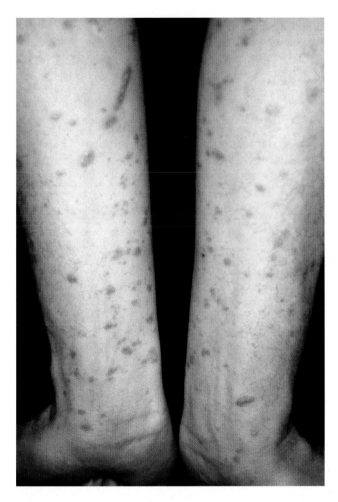

Lichen planus is a pruritic papulosquamous disease with characteristic histopathologic and clinical features. Oral erosive lichen planus, a painful erosive condition that can affect mucous membranes, is addressed in a separate chapter.

MANAGEMENT STRATEGY

Although lichen planus can resolve spontaneously, treatment is usually demanded by patients, who can be severely symptomatic. Underlying diseases such as hepatitis C or associated drugs should be sought.

In patients with localized disease, *superpotent corticosteroids* should be applied twice daily for 2–4 weeks. If the response is inadequate, *intralesional injection of corticosteroids* into localized lesions may be beneficial. Topical antipruritic agents containing *menthol, phenol, camphor, lidocaine, pramoxine* or *doxepin hydrochloride* can be useful. *Oral antihistamines* may offer limited benefit in severely pruritic patients. Sedating antihistamines are helpful at bedtime.

Traditionally, patients with extensive lichen planus have been treated with systemic corticosteroids. In recent years *oral metronidazole* has emerged as a safe and effective alternative to systemic corticosteroids: 500 mg twice daily for 20–60 days has proved effective in many patients. In patients who do not respond, *oral prednisone* 30–60 mg daily for 2–6 weeks, or its equivalent, tapered over the ensuing 2–6 weeks, is often effective. Unfortunately, even in patients who clear with systemic corticosteroids, relapses are frequent. If patients require more than two courses of high-dose systemic corticosteroids over the span of a few months, alternative treatments should be sought.

Isotretinoin in doses of 10 mg orally twice daily for 2 months has been reported to clear lichen planus in several patients, and *acitretin* 30 mg has also resulted in marked improvement or remission. In refractory cases, *psoralen and UVA (PUVA)* or narrowband UVB has demonstrated efficacy in the treatment of lichen planus. PUVA has been particularly beneficial in the lichen planus-like eruption associated with graft-versus-host disease. For severe and refractory lichen planus unresponsive to other therapies, immunosuppressive agents, including *ciclosporin, mycophenolate mofetil,* or *azathioprine,* are often effective.

SPECIFIC INVESTIGATIONS

- ▶ Serology for hepatitis B and C
- ▶ Liver function tests
- ▶ Drug history

Lichen planus and other cutaneous manifestations in chronic hepatitis C: pre- and post-interferon-based treatment prevalence vary in a cohort of patients from low hepatitis C virus endemic area. Maticic M, Poljak M, Lunder T, Rener-Sitar K, Stojanovic L. J Eur Acad Dermatol Venereol 2008; 22: 779–88.

Lichen planus was found in 2.3% of 171 hepatitis C virus-seropositive patients, compared to no cases in 171 age- and gender-matched controls.

The association between hepatitis C virus and lichen planus has been controversial, with an association reported in some studied populations but not others.

Lichen planus and chronic active hepatitis. A retrospective survey. Rebora A, Rongioletti F. Acta Dermatol Venereol 1984; 64: 52–6.

Six of 44 patients with lichen planus had abnormal liver function tests, and five of the six were found to have chronic active hepatitis on liver biopsy.

Drug-induced lichen planus. Thompson DF, Skaehill PA. Pharmacotherapy 1994; 14: 561–71.

β-Blockers, methyldopa, penicillamine, quinidine, quinine, and non-steroidal anti-inflammatory agents play a role in the development of lichen planus. There is insufficient evidence to implicate angiotensin-converting enzyme inhibitors, sulfonylurea agents, carbamazepine, gold, lithium, and other drugs.

Many drugs and chemicals have been associated with lichenoid drug eruptions, which can be difficult to distinguish from true lichen planus. In addition to those mentioned above, hepatitis B and influenza vaccinations, allopurinol, tetracyclines, furosemide, hydrochlorothiazide, isoniazid, phenytoin,, and etanercept are reported to cause lichenoid eruptions.

FIRST-LINE THERAPIES

▶ Topical corticosteroids	C
▶ Intralesional corticosteroids	D
▶ Antihistamines	C

Betamethasone-17,21-dipropionate ointment: an effective topical preparation in lichen rubra planus. Bjornberg A, Hellgren L. Curr Med Res Opin 1976; 4: 212–17.

Patients with lichen planus that had become resistant to betamethasone valerate ointment were treated with betamethasone dipropionate ointment once or twice daily for 2–3 weeks. Fourteen of 19 patients achieved better improvement with betamethasone dipropionate ointment.

A randomized controlled trial to compare calcipotriol with betamethasone valerate for the treatment of cutaneous lichen planus. Theng CT, Tan SH, Goh CL, Suresh S, Wong HB, Machin D; Singapore Lichen Planus Study Group. J Dermatol Treat 2004; 15: 141–5.

Fifteen patients were treated with calcipotriol and 16 with betamethasone valerate ointments twice daily for 12 weeks in this randomized open-label trial. Flattening occurred in half the patients, with slightly better improvement that was not statistically significant in the betamethasone-treated patients. There were more cases of local side effects in the calcipotriol-treated patients.

Although topical and intralesional corticosteroids are first-line treatments for lichen planus, their use has been based on anecdotal reports rather than on controlled clinical trials. This is one of very few comparative trials of topical therapies for lichen planus.

SECOND-LINE THERAPIES

▶ Metronidazole	C
▶ Systemic corticosteroids	B
▶ Isotretinoin, acitretin	A
▶ Narrowband or broadband UVB	C
▶ PUVA	C

Oral metronidazole treatment of lichen planus. Büyük AY, Kavala M. J Am Acad Dermatol 2000; 43: 260–2.

Nineteen patients with lichen planus were treated twice daily with 500 mg oral metronidazole for 20–60 days. Thirteen patients had 80–100% improvement and two additional patients had a 50–80% reduction in lichen planus lesions. Only four patients failed to respond.

The safety of oral metronidazole has led many dermatologists to use this treatment as first-line therapy for lichen planus.

Treatment of generalized cutaneous lichen planus with dipropionate and betamethasone disodium phosphate: an open study of 73 cases. Pitche P, Saka B, Kombate K, Tchangai-Walla K. Ann Dermatol Venereol 2007; 134: 237–40.

Injections of systemic corticosteroids performed at 2-week intervals resulted in complete remission in 61 of 73 (83.6%) patients with lichen planus; 8.2% of patients experienced partial remission, and another 8.2% failed this therapy. At 3 months, the relapse rate of initial responders was 23.3% and at 6 months 31.5% had relapsed.

Treatment of lichen planus with acitretin. A double-blind, placebo-controlled study in 65 patients. Laurberg G, Geiger JM, Hjorth N, Holm P, Hou-Jensen K, Jacobsen KU, et al. J Am Acad Dermatol 1991; 24: 434–7.

Acitretin resulted in marked improvement or remission in 64% of patients compared to 13% of placebo-treated patients in a double-blind trial in 65 subjects. Acitretin doses of 30 mg daily were used, leading to mucocutaneous side effects and hyperlipidemia.

Isotretinoin in doses of 10 mg orally twice daily has been effective in the treatment of oral lichen planus, and anecdotal use suggests efficacy in generalized lichen planus as well. The latter regimen has fewer mucocutaneous side effects than higher doses of acitretin. Restrictions on the use of isotretinoin in the US may make this less practical.

Ultraviolet-B treatment for cutaneous lichen planus: our experience with 50 patients. Pavlotsky F, Nathansohn N, Kriger G, Shpiro D, Trau H. Photodermatol Photoimmunol Photomed 2008; 24: 83–6.

This retrospective analysis reported the results of narrowband UVB in 43 patients with lichen planus and broadband UVB in another seven. Seventy percent achieved complete remission and, at a median of 34.7 months of follow-up, 85% were still in remission.

UVB, and particularly narrowband UVB, has emerged as an effective durable therapy for lichen planus.

Psoralen plus UVA vs. UVB-311 nm for the treatment of lichen planus Wackernagel A, Legat FJ, Hofer A, Quehenberger F, Kerl H, Wolf P. Photodermatol Photoimmunol Photomed 2007; 23: 15–19.

This retrospective chart review compared 15 patients treated with PUVA to 13 patients treated with narrowband UVB. Sixty-seven percent of the PUVA-treated patients achieved complete remission, and 33% achieved a partial clinical response. Thirty-one percent of patients treated with narrowband UVB achieved complete remission and 46% a partial response. The mean duration of therapy was 10.5 weeks for PUVA and 8.2 weeks for narrowband UVB, and the mean number of treatments was 25.9 PUVA treatments compared to 22.5 narrowband UVB treatments. Lichen planus recurred in 47% of PUVA-treated patients but only 30% of narrowband UVB-treated patients.

Long-term efficacy of PUVA treatment in lichen planus: comparison of oral and external methoxsalen regimens. Helander I, Jansen CT, Meurman L. Photodermatology 1987; 4: 265–8.

Good or excellent clearing occurred in 10 of 13 patients after eight to 46 bath-PUVA treatments, compared to five of 10 patients after eight to 30 oral PUVA treatments. However, examination of patients' months after PUVA suggested that treatment might prolong the duration of lichen planus.

THIRD-LINE THERAPIES

▶ Trimethoprim-sulfamethoxazole	E
▶ Griseofulvin	E
▶ Itraconazole	C
▶ Tetracycline or doxycycline	C
▶ Ciclosporin, FK 506	E

Evidence Levels: **A** Double-blind study **B** Clinical trial ≥ 20 subjects **C** Clinical trial < 20 subjects **D** Series ≥ 5 subjects **E** Anecdotal case reports

▶ Mycophenolate mofetil	E
▶ Azathioprine	E
▶ Photodynamic therapy	E
▶ Interferon	E
▶ 0.1% tacrolimus ointment	E
▶ Pimecrolimus cream	E
▶ Calcipotriol ointment	C
▶ Thalidomide	E
▶ UVA1	D
▶ Low molecular weight heparin	E

Antimicrobials

Treatment of lichen planus with Bactrim. Abdel-Aal H, Abdel-Aal MA. J Egypt Med Assoc 1976; 59: 547–9.

Oral trimethoprim-sulfamethoxazole, two tablets twice daily for 5 days, cleared lichen planus within 2 weeks only to have the skin lesions relapse 2 months later. The trimethoprim-sulfamethoxazole was again effective when readministered to patients who experienced relapse.

Histopathological evaluation of griseofulvin therapy in lichen planus: a double-blind controlled study. Sehgal VN, Bikhchandani R, Koranne RV, Nayar M, Saxena HM. Dermatologica 1980; 161: 22–7.

Griseofulvin 500 mg/day for 2 months was effective in 18 of 22 patients.

Griseofulvin therapy of lichen planus. Massa MC, Rogers RS III. Acta Dermatol Venereol 1981; 61: 547–50.

Griseofulvin was effective for lichen planus in only three of 15 patients.

Pulsed itraconazole therapy in eruptive lichen planus. Khandpur S, Sugandhan S, Sharma VK. J Eur Acad Dermatol Venereol 2008, Apr 21. [Epub ahead of print]

Sixteen patients with eruptive lichen planus were treated with itraconazole 200 mg twice daily pulsed for 1 week each month for 3 months. By the end of the first month, nine of 16 patients (56.25%) stopped developing new lesions. Only nine of the patients were followed for 3 months, and seven of the nine (77.7%) stopped developing new lesions. All of the nine patients reported improvement of pruritus, and five of the nine had complete relief of pruritus. By the end of 3 months, partial flattening was present in six of nine patients (66.66%) and complete flattening in three (33.33%).

Given the partial response seen at 3 months, longer therapy may be warranted.

Immunosuppressive agents

Successful treatment of resistant hypertrophic and bullous lichen planus with mycophenolate mofetil. Nousari HC, Goyal S, Anhalt GJ. Arch Dermatol 1999; 135: 1420–1.

Mycophenolate mofetil was reported to successfully treat resistant hypertrophic and bullous lichen planus.

Generalized severe lichen planus treated with azathioprine. Verma KK, Sirka CS, Khaitan BK. Acta Dermatol Venereol 1999; 79: 493.

Generalized severe lichen planus has been successfully treated with azathioprine.

Palmoplantar lichen planus with umbilicated papules: an atypical case with rapid therapeutic response to cyclosporin. Karakatsanis G, Patsatsi A, Kastoridou C, Sotiriadis D. J Eur Acad Dermatol Venereol 2007; 21: 1006–7.

A 63-year-old woman with lichen planus of the palms, forearms, soles, and feet was treated with ciclosporin 3.5 mg/kg daily. Pruritus improved within 2 weeks and clinical improvement occurred within 4 weeks, at which point ciclosporin was tapered over the next 4 weeks.

Other

Treatment of lichen planus of the penis with photodynamic therapy. Kirby B, Whitehurst C, Moore JV, Yates VM. Br J Dermatol 1999; 141: 765–6.

Photodynamic therapy with δ-aminolevulinic acid resulted in clearing of isolated lesions of lichen planus.

Successful interferon treatment for lichen planus associated with hepatitis due to hepatitis C virus infection. Lapidoth M, Arber N, Ben-Amitai D, Hagler J. Acta Dermatol Venereol 1997; 77: 171–2.

Lichen planus and chronic hepatitis C: exacerbation of the lichen under interferon therapy. Areias J, Velho GC, Cerqueira R, Barbêdo C, Amaral B, Sanches M, et al. Eur J Gastroenterol Hepatol 1996; 8: 825–8.

Given the association between lichen planus and hepatitis C, one might expect interferon to benefit both diseases. There are reports of interferon benefiting patients with lichen planus and exacerbating the condition in others.

Recalcitrant erosive flexural lichen planus: successful treatment with a combination of thalidomide and 0.1% tacrolimus ointment. Eisman S, Orteu CH. Clin Exp Dermatol 2004; 29: 268–70.

A patient with a 12-year history of ulcerated flexural lichen planus refractory to many treatments responded to a combination of topical 0.1% tacrolimus ointment and oral thalidomide followed by tacrolimus ointment alone.

Ultraviolet A1 in the treatment of generalized lichen planus: a report of 4 cases. Polderman MC, Wintzen M, van Leeuwen RL, de Winter S, Pavel S. J Am Acad Dermatol 2004; 50: 646–7.

Four patients with refractory generalized lichen planus were treated with UVA1 45 J/cm² 5 days per week for two 4-week treatment periods with a 3-week rest in between. All four improved, with one patient achieving 98% clearance.

Ulcerative lichen planus of the sole: excellent response to topical tacrolimus. Al-Khenaizan S, Al Mubarak L. Int J Dermatol 2008; 47: 626–8.

Ulcerated lichen planus of the soles healed completely with a few weeks of topical application of tacrolimus 0.1% ointment. The improvement was maintained for the follow-up period of more than 2 years.

Limited benefit of topical calcipotriol in lichen planus treatment: a preliminary study. Bayramgürler D, Apaydin R, Bilen N. J Dermatol Treat 2002; 13: 129–32.

For up to 3 months, patients with lichen planus were treated with calcipotriol ointment twice daily to all affected areas except the genitals. Five of 16 (31.25%) experienced complete clearing of lesions, leaving only postinflammatory hyperpigmentation. Partial improvement occurred in four of 16 (25%) of the patients. Seven of 16 (43.75%) did not improve.

Use of pimecrolimus cream in disorders other than atopic dermatitis. Day I, Lin AN. J Cutan Med Surg 2008; 12: 17–26.

Case reports indicate successful use of topical pimecrolimus cream for cutaneous lichen planus.

Treatment of severe cutaneous ulcerative lichen planus with low molecular weight heparin in a patient with hepatitis C. Neville JA, Hancox JG, Williford PM, Yosipovitch G. Cutis 2007; 79: 37–40.

A 50-year-old man with hepatitis C presented with unusual ulcerative lichen planus involving the palms and scrotum. Conventional therapy was ineffective, but low molecular weight heparin resulted in clearance.

Lichen sclerosus

Nuala O'Donoghue, Sallie Neill

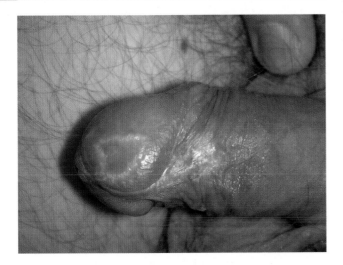

Lichen sclerosus et atrophicus (LSA) was first described as a variant of lichen planus. Some cases are not histologically atrophic, and so the term LSA has now been replaced by lichen sclerosus (LS) alone. LS is a chronic, scarring, lymphocyte-mediated dermatosis that has a predilection for the genital skin. It occurs predominantly in females, and has two peak ages of incidence: one in the prepubertal child and the other in the postmenopausal woman. In women LS is associated with the presence of circulating serum IgG autoantibodies to extracellular matrix protein 1 and other autoimmune diseases, which may support an autoimmune etiology. Fewer than 5% of cases of anogenital LS may be associated with squamous cell carcinoma (SCC).

MANAGEMENT STRATEGY

The aims of managing LS are to treat the symptoms of itch, burning, and pain, heal the cutaneous lesions, reduce further scarring, and to prevent or detect malignant change. The scarring associated with LS in females may cause loss of the labia minora, sealing over of the clitoral hood, and burying of the clitoris. Less commonly there may be introital narrowing (possibly resulting in dyspareunia, and/or difficulties micturating), and the clitoral hood adhesions can result in pseudocyst formation. In young girls constipation is a common presenting symptom and *stool softeners* may be required. Scarring in males may result in phimosis and meatal stenosis, which rarely progresses to frank obstruction to urinary flow. Both sexes may develop postinflammatory pain syndromes after clinical improvement of the skin lesions (i.e., vulvodynia/vestibulodynia), and penile dysesthesia. The sensory disorder will not respond to topical corticosteroids, so treatment needs to include *topical 5% lidocaine ointment*. Any patient with a chronic genital disorder may develop psychosexual problems, and these will need to be addressed.

An *ultrapotent topical corticosteroid* is the first line of treatment for LS at any site in either sex, although there have been no randomized controlled trials comparing potency, frequency of application, and duration of treatment. The regi-

men recommended by the authors for a newly diagnosed case is clobetasol propionate 0.05% ointment, initially once a night for 4 weeks, then on alternate nights for 4 weeks, and then twice weekly for the final third month. If the symptoms return with a drop in the schedule the patient is advised to go back up to the frequency that was effective. A 30 g tube should last 12 weeks, at which point the patient is reviewed. If the treatment has been successful, the ecchymosis, fissuring, and erosions should have resolved, but the scarring and some of the hypopigmentation may remain. LS is a disease of relapses and remissions, and topical clobetasol dipropionate is used as required; most patients with active disease seem to require 30–60 g annually. Although topical corticosteroids have been demonstrated to improve the symptoms and clinical signs in LS and obviate the need for a curative *circumcision*, to date there is no evidence to show that their use reduces the risk of developing SCC. Given the small but significant risk of malignant change, current guidelines recommend that patients with ongoing disease requiring a topical steroid should be examined annually by their primary healthcare physician. Patients who have gone into remission and have very little scarring do not need long-term follow-up.

A *soap substitute* is also recommended, alongside *bland barrier ointments*, particularly if there is urinary incontinence.

SPECIFIC INVESTIGATIONS

- ▶ Biopsy
- ▶ Thyroid function tests and organ-specific autoantibodies if clinically indicated

The diagnosis can often be made on clinical grounds particularly if there is ecchymosis. Classically there are white plaques with 'cigarette paper' atrophy in association with purpura, blisters, and erosions. In females the distribution is a figure-of-eight configuration around the vulva and anus. In males the glans penis and foreskin are usually affected, with sparing of the perianal area.

Light microscopic criteria for the diagnosis of early vulvar lichen sclerosus: a comparison with lichen planus. Fung MA, LeBoit PE. Am J Surg Pathol 1998; 22: 473–8.

A review of the light microscopic features of 68 cases of vulvar LS demonstrated the classic features: a thinned epidermis with hyperkeratosis, a wide band of homogenized collagen below the dermoepidermal junction (DEJ), and a lymphocytic infiltrate beneath this. In early lesions the inflammatory infiltrate could be close to the DEJ, so a comparison with cases of genital lichen planus was made: the presence of a psoriasiform lichenoid pattern, epidermotropism, decreased elastic fibers, follicular plugging, a thickened basement membrane, and epidermal atrophy were more suggestive of LS.

Early vulvar lichen sclerosus: a histopathological challenge. Regauer S, Liegl B, Reich O. Histopathology 2005; 47: 340–7.

In this review article the use of the periodic acid–Schiff (PAS) reaction is suggested to help to identify, where present, focal thickening of the basement membrane, which is one of the typically subtle histopathologic features of early LS.

A comparative analysis of lichen sclerosus of the vulva and lichen sclerosus that evolves to vulvar squamous cell

carcinoma. Raspollini MR, Asirelli G, Moncini D, Taddei GL. Am J Obstet Gynecol 2007; 197: 592: 592.e1–5.

A retrospective study comparing the histopathologic features of eight cases of histologically diagnosed vulvar LS in which SCC had subsequently developed with eight cases of vulvar LS which had been followed up for at least 9 years without malignant change. Labeling for MIB1 and p53 was increased in those cases that went on to develop SCC.

This was a small study that needs to be confirmed by a larger one.

FIRST-LINE THERAPIES

▶ Ultrapotent topical corticosteroids	A
▶ Emollients	E
▶ Avoidance of local irritants, including soap substitution	E

Vulvar lichen sclerosus: effect of long-term topical application of a potent steroid on the course of the disease. Renaud-Vilmer C, Cavelier-Balloy B, Porcher R, Dubertret L. Arch Dermatol 2004; 140: 709–12.

A prospective study of 83 women treated with 0.05% clobetasol propionate ointment who were followed for a median of 4.7 years. After 3 years 72% of those younger than 50 years, 23% of those aged 50–70, and none of those over 70 had gone into complete clinical and histologic remission.

Clinical and histologic effects of topical treatments of vulval lichen sclerosus. A critical evaluation. Bracco GL, Carli P, Sonni L, Maestrini G, De Marco A, Taddei GL, et al. J Reprod Med 1993; 38: 37–40.

A randomized study of 79 adults treated for 3 months. Remission of symptoms occurred in 75% of patients treated with 0.05% clobetasol, 20% treated with 2% testosterone, 10% treated with 2% progesterone, and 10% treated with placebo cream.

Clinical features of lichen sclerosus in men attending a department of genitourinary medicine. Riddell L, Edwards A, Sherrard J. J Sex Transm Infect 2000; 76: 311–13.

A case note review of 66 men with LS who were all treated with clobetasol propionate 0.05% cream. Although 12% underwent circumcision and 8% required urethral dilatation, surgery was avoided in the remainder.

Treatment of phimosis with topical steroids in 194 children. Ashfield JE, Nickel KR, Siemens DR, Macneily AE, Nickel JC. J Urol 2003; 169: 1106–8.

On referral for circumcision 194 boys with phimosis of unknown cause were treated with a 6-week course of 0.1% betamethasone ointment twice daily to the prepuce. Circumcision was avoided in 87%.

Topical corticosteroids are the standard conservative measure for treating phimosis, and up to 40% of these boys have undiagnosed LS.

Treatment of childhood vulvar lichen sclerosus with potent topical corticosteroid. Fischer G, Rogers M. Pediatr Dermatol 1997; 14: 235–8.

A case series of 11 girls treated with betamethasone dipropionate 0.05%. Eight experienced complete remission after 3 months, and three required maintenance therapy with a mild topical corticosteroid.

SECOND-LINE THERAPIES

▶ Circumcision	B
▶ Topical tacrolimus	B
▶ Topical pimecrolimus	C

High incidence of balanitis xerotica obliterans in boys with phimosis: prospective 10-year study. Kiss A, Király L, Kutasy B, Merksz M. Pediatr Dermatol 2005; 4: 305–8.

A prospective study of 1178 boys presenting consecutively with phimosis treated by circumcision: 40% had histologically confirmed LS. Of the 231 who had persistent glandular lesions postoperatively, all but two resolved spontaneously within 6 months.

Surgical treatment of balanitis xerotica obliterans. Campus GV, Ena P, Scuderi N. Plast Reconstruct Surg 1984; 73: 652–7.

Of 32 symptomatic patients, 13 required circumcision, and six either meatotomy, meatoplasty, or excision and skin grafting. All responded well to surgery, without progression of the disease.

Multicentre, phase II trial on the safety and efficacy of topical tacrolimus ointment for the treatment of lichen sclerosus. Hengge UR, Krause W, Hofmann H, Stadler R, Gross G, Meurer M, et al. Br J Dermatol 2006; 155: 1021–8.

A prospective study of 49 women, 32 men and three girls treated with tacrolimus 0.1% ointment twice daily for up to 6 months; of these, 36% had a complete and 29% a partial clinical response.

This was a drug company-supported trial; although 80% of patients had previously been treated with a topical corticosteroid the potency of this was not recorded, and the follow-up period was relatively short at 18 months. Tacrolimus has the theoretical advantage of causing less atrophy than steroids, but may reduce immune surveillance, which is of potential concern in a condition associated with SCC. The UK Medicines and Healthcare Products Regulatory Agency recommended in 2006 that tacrolimus and pimecrolimus should not be applied to premalignant conditions.

Pimecrolimus 1% cream in the treatment of vulvar lichen sclerosus in postmenopausal women. Oskay T, Sezer HK, Genç C, Kutluay L. Int J Dermatol 2007; 46: 527–32.

A case series of 16 patients treated with pimecrolimus 1% cream twice daily for 3 months: 11 achieved a significant and four a partial improvement in symptoms. Four patients relapsed over the subsequent 12 months.

See note above about the use of calcineurin inhibitors in this condition.

THIRD-LINE THERAPIES

| ▶ CO₂ laser therapy | B |

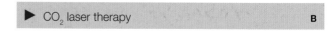

Is carbon dioxide laser treatment of lichen sclerosus effective in the long run? Windahl T. Scand J Urol Nephrol 2006; 40: 208–11.

A retrospective review of 62 men, most of whom had failed to respond to a topical steroid (potency not stated). They were treated with CO_2 laser vaporization (defocused beam, 15–20 W) to the macroscopically affected area of the glans penis. Of the 50 patients contactable a median of 14 years later, 80% judged themselves to be in complete remission. Two patients in this cohort developed penile SCC.

Evidence Levels: **A** Double-blind study **B** Clinical trial ≥ 20 subjects **C** Clinical trial < 20 subjects **D** Series ≥ 5 subjects **E** Anecdotal case reports

The risks of the Koebner phenomenon appear to be low with this treatment.

OTHER THERAPIES

▶ Intralesional triamcinolone	D
▶ Surgery for clitoral phimosis	D
▶ Buccal mucosa urethroplasty	D
▶ Tangential excision	E
▶ Cryosurgery	C
▶ Low-dose UVA1 phototherapy	C
▶ Photodynamic therapy with 5-aminolevulinic acid	C
▶ Narrowband UVB	E
▶ Ciclosporin	D
▶ Hydroxycarbamide (hydroxyurea)	E
▶ Methotrexate	E
▶ Antibiotics	D
▶ Acitretin	C
▶ Topical calcipotriol	B
▶ Topical tretinoin	B
▶ Oxatomide gel	B
▶ Oral calcitriol	E
▶ Potassium para-aminobenzoate	D
▶ Topical estrogens	E
▶ Topical testosterone	B
▶ Oral stanozolol	D

Surgical treatment of clitoral phimosis caused by lichen sclerosus. Goldstein AT, Burrows LJ. Am J Obstet Gynecol 2007; 196: 126.

A case series of 11 women whose LS was in remission and who had scarring around the clitoris. Postoperatively, clobetasol 0.05% ointment was used. Four women who had reduced clitoral sensation before surgery reported an improvement.

UVA1 phototherapy for genital lichen sclerosus. Beattie PE, Dawe RS, Ferguson J, Ibbotson SH. Clin Exp Dermatol 2006; 31: 343–7

Three out of seven women in this series with severe genital disease had moderate and two had minimal improvement in the symptoms and signs of LS after at least 15 treatments with UVA1 three to five times per week.

Extragenital lesions of LS appear to respond better to UVA1. The risk of SCC may theoretically be increased by the use of phototherapy treatment in genital LS.

Open-label trial of cyclosporine for vulvar lichen sclerosus. Bulbul Baskan E, Turan H, Tunali S, Toker SC, Saricaoglu H. J Am Acad Dermatol 2007; 57: 276–8.

A retrospective study of five women treated with ciclosporin 3–4 mg/kg/day for 3 months, resulting in improvement in symptoms in all patients, without any rebound flare on discontinuation.

There is a potentially increased risk of SCC when using an immunosuppressant as treatment in genital LS.

Treatment of lichen sclerosus with antibiotics. Shelley WB, Shelley ED, Amurao CV. Int J Dermatol 2006; 45: 1104–6.

A retrospective review of 15 patients treated with intramuscular or oral antibiotics (penicillin or a cephalosporin) for 2–20 months; four achieved clearance of symptoms and signs, the rest described an improvement in symptoms.

The use of antibiotics was suggested because of the debatable association of LS and Borrelia borgdorferi.

Topical testosterone for lichen sclerosus. Ayhan A, Urman B, Yüce K, Ayhan A, Gököz A. Int J Gynecol Obstet 1989; 30: 253–5.

An uncontrolled study of 23 patients showing a remission rate of 88% after 6 weeks' treatment with 2% testosterone.

Topical testosterone was used in the treatment of LS prior to the introduction of clobetasol propionate. Since then, multiple comparative studies (including Bracco et al.; see First-Line Therapies) have not supported its use in LS. Topical testosterone can cause virilization and is no longer recommended in the treatment of LS.

Lichen simplex chronicus

Christian Millett, Donald J Baker

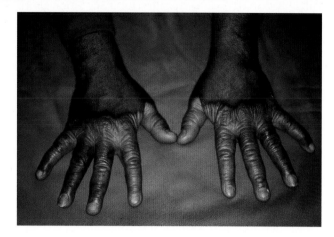

Lichen simplex chronicus (LSC; or neurodermatitis circumscripta) is characterized by pruritic, lichenified plaques that most often occur on the neck, anterior tibiae, ankles, wrists, and anogenital region in response to chronic localized scratching or rubbing. Primary LSC evolves on apparently normal skin, whereas secondary LSC is superimposed upon pre-existing dermatoses, especially atopic dermatitis, psoriasis, or dermatophytosis.

MANAGEMENT STRATEGY

The objective of treatment is to remove environmental trigger factors, break the itch–scratch cycle, and treat any underlying cutaneous or systemic disease. Patients' understanding of their role in the itch–scratch cycle is essential if their cooperation in avoiding scratching is to be enlisted, thereby facilitating a more complete and permanent recovery. However, recurrences are frequent, and complete resolution often requires multiple approaches to therapy. Environmental trigger factors, such as harsh skincare products or bathing regimens, friction, and excessive moisture or dryness, should be minimized or eliminated. High-potency *topical corticosteroids*, such as clobetasol, diflorasone, and betamethasone, as creams or ointments, are the initial treatments of choice. The potency and/or frequency of application of topical corticosteroids should be reduced as the lesion resolves to avoid atrophy associated with their long-term use. Adjunctive therapies such as *doxepin cream* may be introduced if topical corticosteroids are not easily tapered. Occlusion has been found to be a successful aid to therapy because it provides a physical barrier to prevent scratching, and permits enhanced and prolonged application of topical medications. *Occlusive plastic film* or hydrocolloid dressings has been used alone or over mid-potency corticosteroids. *Flurandrenolide tape* is very effective as both an occlusive and an anti-inflammatory measure and is usually changed once daily, although a short occlusion-free period each day will help minimize the side effects of occlusion therapy. In chronic, difficult cases on the lower leg, an Unna boot

(a gauze roll impregnated with zinc oxide) may be applied for up to 1 week, provided there is no concomitant infection of the occluded area. *Calcineurin inhibitors* such as *tacrolimus and pimecrolimus* also have been successfully used as monotherapy to treat LSC, and offer a good alternative for treatment in steroid-sensitive areas such as the genitalia.

Intralesional injections of triamcinolone at weekly intervals can rapidly induce involution. Although often highly effective, repeated injections may cause depigmentation or thinning of the epidermis. Therefore, other therapies should be used if several treatments with intralesional corticosteroids do not clear LSC. Infected areas should not be injected with corticosteroids because of the risk of abscess formation. Secondary infections should be treated with appropriate topical or systemic antibiotics. Intralesional *botulinum toxin* has been reported to offer lasting relief in patients with recalcitrant LSC.

A variety of other therapies have been reported to be effective in the management of LSC. Doxepin cream, *capsaicin cream*, or *aspirin/dichloromethane solution* are occasionally of value alone, but are probably best used as adjunctive therapy when LSC does not quickly clear with topical or intralesional corticosteroids. *Oral antihistamines* may be useful for their sedative effect on patients who scratch during their sleep. *Cryosurgery* and *surgical excision* have been reported to help some patients with nodular neurodermatitis. In more severe or recalcitrant conditions, *psychotherapy* and/or the use of *psychopharmacologic agents* may be needed for sustained improvement. *Benzodiazepines, amitriptyline, pimozide,* and *doxepin* have been used to treat neurotic excoriations and severe neurodermatitis. In certain individuals neurodermatitis has improved with habit-reversal *behavioral therapy* and *hypnotherapy*. Acupuncture and *electroacupuncture* are labor intensive, but have been effective in treating some cases of LSC. *Thuja and Graphites* are homeopathic remedies that have led to a significant improvement in the small number of patients who received them as individual therapies.

SPECIFIC INVESTIGATIONS

> ▶ Skin biopsy with periodic acid–Schiff (PAS) stain

LSC that is atypical in appearance or poorly responsive to therapy should be biopsied and cultured to look for pre-existing dermatoses and underlying cutaneous malignancy or infection. The presence of lice or scabies infestation should be excluded. Patch testing may be useful, especially in patients whose biopsy is suggestive of allergic contact dermatitis. In particularly refractory or unusual cases, systemic disease and malignancy should be ruled out.

FIRST-LINE THERAPIES

> ▶ Topical corticosteroids   **A**
> ▶ Occlusion – flurandrenolide tape   **C**
> ▶ Intralesional corticosteroids   **C**

A double-blind, multicenter trial of 0.05% halobetasol propionate ointment and 0.05% clobetasol 17-propionate ointment in the treatment of patients with chronic, localized atopic dermatitis or lichen simplex chronicus. Datz B, Yawalkar S. J Am Acad Dermatol 1991; 25: 1157–60.

In 127 patients with chronic, localized atopic dermatitis or LSC, healing was reported in 65.1% of those treated with halobetasol propionate ointment (a superpotent group I topical corticosteroid) compared to 54.7% of those treated with clobetasol propionate (a weaker group I topical corticosteroid). Success rates, early onset of therapeutic effect, and adverse effects were similar in the two treatment groups.

A review of two controlled multicenter trials comparing 0.05% halobetasol propionate ointment to its vehicle in the treatment of chronic eczematous dermatoses. Guzzo CA, Weiss JS, Mogavero HS, Ellis CN, Zaias N, Lowe NJ, et al. J Am Acad Dermatol 1991; 25: 1179–83.

Two vehicle-controlled, double-blind studies were performed: a paired comparison study in 124 patients and a parallel group study in 100 patients. In both studies, treatments were applied twice daily for 2 weeks. Severity scores and patient ratings favored halobetasol propionate over the vehicle treatment. Global assessments showed complete resolution or marked improvement in 83% of patients using halobetasol propionate versus 28% using vehicle. The study concluded that 0.05% halobetasol propionate is highly effective and well tolerated, with rapid action and a high degree of clearing.

Group I topical corticosteroids should not be used for more than 2 weeks. They are therefore best combined with adjuvant therapies such as topical doxepin cream.

A double-blind, multicenter, parallel-group trial with 0.05% halobetasol propionate ointment versus 0.1% diflucortolone valerate ointment in patients with severe, chronic atopic dermatitis or lichen simplex chronicus. Brunner N, Yawalkar S. J Am Acad Dermatol 1991; 25: 1160–3.

One hundred and twenty patients with chronic, localized atopic dermatitis or LSC were studied. Success rates and early onset of therapeutic effect were reported in a higher percentage of patients treated with halobetasol propionate ointment versus diflucortolone valerate ointment.

Flurandrenolone tape in the treatment of lichen simplex chronicus. Bard JW. J Ky Med Assoc 1969; 67: 668–70.

Of the 18 patients in the study, 10 used flurandrenolone tape and eight used a topical corticosteroid preparation without occlusion. Lasting remissions were seen in 70% of those using the tape, versus 25% of those using topical corticosteroids without occlusion. Duration of therapy is not mentioned.

The use of occlusion with topical corticosteroids is considered a treatment of choice for LSC despite the lack of adequate clinical trials.

Local infiltration of triamcinolone acetonide suspension in various skin conditions. Shah CF, Pandit DM. Indian J Dermatol Venereol 1971; 37: 231–4.

Fifteen of 17 patients with LSC experienced fair to complete improvement with up to three injections of triamcinolone acetonide suspension (10/mL).

Corticosteroid injections are considered first-line therapy despite the lack of adequate controlled clinical trials.

SECOND-LINE THERAPIES

▶ Doxepin cream	B
▶ Pimecrolimus cream	C
▶ Capsaicin cream	E
▶ Cryosurgery	E
▶ Tacrolimus ointment	E

The antipruritic effect of 5% doxepin cream in patients with eczematous dermatitis. Doxepin Study Group. Drake LA, Millikan LE. Arch Dermatol 1995; 131: 1403–8.

A multicenter double-blind trial conducted to evaluate the safety and antipruritic efficacy of 5% doxepin cream in patients with LSC (n=136), nummular eczema (n=87), or contact dermatitis (n=86). Patients treated with doxepin had significantly greater pruritus relief than those treated with vehicle. Of doxepin-treated patients, 60% experienced relief from pruritus within 24 hours, with a response rate of 84% by the end of the study.

Pimecrolimus cream 1% for treatment of vulvar lichen simplex chronicus: an open-label, preliminary trial. Goldstein AT, Parneix-Spake A, McCormick CL, Burrows LJ. Gynecol Obstet Invest 2007; 64: 180–6.

An open-label study of 12 women with biopsy-proven vulvar LSC who were treated with pimecrolimus cream 1% twice daily for 12 weeks. The median pruritus score (VAS-PR) decreased from 6 to 0, and erythema, excoriation, and lichenification improved for all patients. No adverse events were reported.

Treatment of prurigo nodularis, chronic prurigo and neurodermatitis circumscripta with topical capsaicin. Tupker RA, Coenraads PJ, van der Meer JB. Acta Dermatol Venereol 1992; 72: 463.

In this small, open study, two patients with corticosteroid-unresponsive neurodermatitis circumscripta were treated with 0.25% capsaicin applied five times daily, resulting in flatter lesions and marked relief of itching.

Cryosurgical treatment of nodular neurodermatitis with Refrigerant 12. McDow RA, Wester MM. J Dermatol Surg Oncol 1989; 15: 621–3.

This case report presents a 42-year-old man with an 8-month history of a persistent nodular, pruritic lesion, diagnosed clinically as neurodermatitis. Cryosurgery with Refrigerant 12 yielded successful clinical and esthetic results.

Topical tacrolimus for the treatment of lichen simplex chronicus. Aschoff R, Wozel G. J Dermatol Treat 2007; 18: 115–17.

This case report describes a 13-year-old boy with LSC on the face who was treated with tacrolimus 0.1% ointment for 9 months. His lesions healed completely during that time, and he was symptom free 3 years after treatment cessation.

THIRD-LINE THERAPIES

▶ Plum-blossom needle with Chinese herbal medicines	B
▶ Ketotifen	C
▶ Acupuncture	C
▶ Electroacupuncture	C
▶ Botulinum toxin	D
▶ Aspirin	A
▶ Psychotherapy	D
▶ Hypnosis	E
▶ Psychopharmacotherapy	E
▶ Surgical excision	E
▶ Homeopathy	E

Treatment of localized neurodermatitis by plum-blossom needle tapping and with the modified Yangxue Dingfeng Tang – a clinical observation of 47 cases. Weiying L, Yuanjiang D, Baolian L. J Trad Chin Med 2006; 26: 181–3.

One hundred and forty-one cases of localized neurodermatitis were randomly divided into three groups. The treatment group received local plum-blossom needle tapping and oral Chinese herbal medications. One control group was given herbal therapy alone, and the other control group received oral benadryl and vitamin C along with 10% urea cream. The short- and long-term effects for the treatment group were significantly better than those of the two control groups.

Plum-blossom needling uses a small hammer with multiple fine needles, which are lightly tapped against the skin to produce the desired effects.

Effectiveness of ketotifen in the treatment of neurodermatitis in childhood. Kikindjanin V, Vukaviic T, Stevanocvic V. Dermatol Monatsschr 1990; 176: 741–4.

Seventeen children with neurodermatitis were treated with ketotifen, a mast cell stabilizer, at a dosage of 1 mg twice daily. Alleviation of the itching occurred within 2 weeks, and the patients became itch free after an average of 20 days. Skin lesions cleared between 7 and 9 months of treatment.

Acupuncture treatment of 139 cases of neurodermatitis. Yang Q. J Trad Chin Med 1997; 17: 57–8.

Acupuncture was used to treat 96 patients with localized neurodermatitis and 43 patients with generalized neurodermatitis. A course of treatment was 10 days, and 3–5-day rest periods were given in between multiple courses of therapy. An 81% cure rate and a 14% improvement rate were reported, but the number of courses of therapy and long-term follow-up were not specified.

Acupuncture and electroacupuncture (where acupuncture needles are stimulated with low-voltage, high-frequency stimulation) may be used to reduce the proinflammatory neuropeptide state in pruritic and inflamed skin, and thereby promote a more normal state of neuropeptide homeostasis.

Treatment of 86 cases of local neurodermatitis by electroacupunture (with needles inserted around diseased areas). Liu JX. J Trad Chin Med 1987; 7: 67.

Electroacupuncture was used to treat 86 cases of localized neurodermatitis. Patients received multiple courses of daily therapy for 10 days, with 3–5-day rest periods in between courses; 88% of patients were cured and 11% were improved. However, the number of courses of therapy and long-term follow-up were not specified.

Botulinum toxin type A injection in the treatment of lichen simplex: An open pilot study. Heckmann M, Heyer G, Brunner B, Plewig G. J Am Acad Dermatol 2002; 46: 617–19.

Four patients received 20 units of botulinum toxin type A (100 units/mL) per 2 × 2 cm² area of LSC plaque; 1 week after the injection there was a noticeable reduction in pruritus levels.

Three patients were free of itching and one had over 50% reduction in itching. After 12 weeks, three patients remained asymptomatic.

The effect of topically applied aspirin on localized circumscribed neurodermatosis. Yosipovitch G, Sugeng M, Chan YH, Goon A, Ngim S, Goh CL. J Am Acad Dermatol 2001; 45: 910–13.

In this double-blind, crossover, placebo-controlled study, 29 patients with LSC were randomized to receive aspirin/dichloromethane solution treatment followed by placebo, or vice versa. In the aspirin/dichloromethane treatment group 46% achieved a significant response; 12% of the placebo group achieved a comparable improvement.

The behavioral treatment of neurodermatitis through habit-reversal. Rosenbaum MS, Ayllon T. Behav Res Ther 1981; 19: 313–18.

Four patients with neurodermatitis received a single treatment session in which they learned to substitute a competing response for their urges to scratch. There was a rapid reduction in scratching in all patients. At 6 months, scratching had been eliminated in one patient and markedly reduced in three.

Brief hypnotherapy of neurodermatitis: a case with 4-year followup. Lehman RE. Am J Clin Hypn 1978; 21: 48–51.

One patient with extensive neurodermatitis was treated with eight sessions of hypnotherapy. She was clear within 2 weeks after her last session, and remained clear at 4-year follow-up.

Improvement of chronic neurotic excoriations with oral doxepin therapy. Harris BA, Sherertz EF, Flowers FP. Int J Dermatol 1987; 26: 541–3.

Two patients with chronic neurotic excoriations had improvement in symptoms and in clinical signs of their skin condition within several weeks of oral doxepin (30–75 mg daily).

Nodular lichen simplex of the scrotum treated by surgical excision. Porter WM, Bewley A, Dinneen M, Walker CC, Fallowfield M, Francis N, et al. Br J Dermatol 2001; 144: 343–6.

Two patients with nodular LSC of the scrotum were treated by surgical excision of LSC plaques with remission lasting over 12 months.

Homoeopathy for the treatment of lichen simplex chronicus: A case series. Gupta R, Manchanda RK, Arya BS. Homeopathy 2006; 95: 245–7.

Twenty-seven patients with chronic LSC were treated using one of five different homeopathic remedies, based on their presenting symptoms. Response was measured by improvement in itching, thickening, and hyperpigmentation. Thuja lead to clearing or significant improvement in all three patients treated, and Graphites lead to near complete resolution in the one patient who received it. A modest improvement in itching alone was noted in the one patient treated with Sulfur and the one patient who received Kali bich. Hydrocotyle was not found to be useful.

Evidence Levels: **A** Double-blind study **B** Clinical trial ≥ 20 subjects **C** Clinical trial < 20 subjects **D** Series ≥ 5 subjects **E** Anecdotal case reports

Linear IgA bullous dermatosis

Neil J Korman

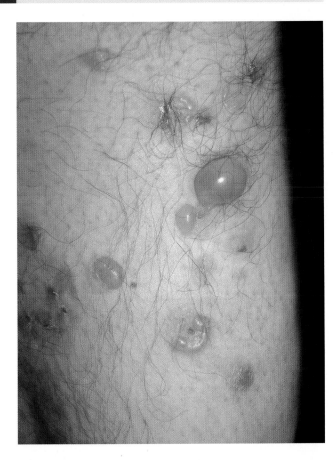

Linear IgA bullous dermatosis is an acquired autoimmune blistering disease of the skin and mucous membranes. The skin lesions consist of papulovesicles or blisters that may have an arcuate pattern, with a 'cluster of jewels' grouping of blisters along with urticarial plaques. Involvement of the oral mucous membranes is common and ocular involvement, with subsequent scarring of the conjunctiva, may uncommonly occur. Although originally believed to be a distinct entity, it is now clear that chronic bullous disease of childhood is the childhood counterpart of adult linear IgA bullous dermatosis. Direct immunofluorescence studies demonstrate that all patients have linear IgA deposits at the epidermal basement membrane zone, and the diagnosis of linear IgA bullous dermatosis is dependent upon this finding. The target antigens involved are 97 kDa and, less commonly, 290 kDa. The 97 kDa antigen is an anchoring filament protein that is part of the 180 kDa bullous pemphigoid antigen-2, and antibodies directed against the 290 kDa protein represent an IgA response directed against type VII collagen. Several reports stress the association with ulcerative colitis. Drug-induced disease is a well-recognized entity, and vancomycin is the most commonly implicated agent.

MANAGEMENT STRATEGY

If drug-induced disease is considered, the suspect trigger drug must be withdrawn. Treatment of linear IgA bullous dermatosis is dictated by the severity of disease and the areas of involvement. All patients should be evaluated by an ophthalmologist to ensure the absence of ocular disease. Because linear IgA bullous dermatosis tends to be chronic it is important to be aware of the potential not only for short-term, but also long-term toxicities in any treatment used. In addition, treatment of children with chronic bullous disease of childhood (the childhood counterpart of linear IgA bullous dermatosis of adults) requires special consideration to ensure that any medications used have no specific contraindications in children.

The majority of patients with disease limited to the skin will respond well to treatment with *dapsone*, and this is the first-line therapy for patients with linear IgA bullous dermatosis. Dapsone generally works quite rapidly, with responses often occurring in the first few days of starting the drug. It is most effective for the skin lesions of linear IgA bullous dermatosis, with the mucous membrane lesions being more resistant.

Because of a dose-related oxidant stress on normal aging red blood cells, all patients treated with dapsone will experience some degree of hemolysis that is usually dosage dependent. A reduction of approximately 2–3 g of hemoglobin is often observed. As long as this decrease is relatively gradual and patients have no history of cardiovascular disease or anemia, this is usually well tolerated. It is important to measure levels of glucose-6-phosphate dehydrogenase (G6PD) in patients to be treated with dapsone because those with a deficiency in this enzyme can develop severe hemolysis. Methemoglobinemia, which is also dosage dependent, occurs in most patients but is usually asymptomatic. More worrisome toxicities include bone marrow suppression and even agranulocytosis, which usually occurs early in the course of therapy, and a dapsone-induced neuropathy, which occurs more commonly in patients treated for several years with more than 200 mg of dapsone daily. Less commonly, hepatitis, nephritis, pneumonitis, erythema multiforme, and the dapsone hypersensitivity syndrome have all been reported.

For those patients who fail to achieve satisfactory control of their disease with dapsone as first-line therapy, it is often of value to add *systemic corticosteroids*. This combination is considered second-line therapy. The dosage of prednisone required is often in the 20–40 mg daily range. Often the addition of prednisone will not only cause significant clinical improvement, but it may also allow the dosage of dapsone to be reduced, thereby minimizing its potential toxicity.

Other viable second-line therapies include *colchicine, sulfapyridine,* and the combination of *tetracycline* and *niacinamide: sulfapyridine* at doses of approximately 1–3 g daily, and colchicine has been reported to be beneficial at doses of 1.0–1.5 mg daily. The combination of tetracycline and niacinamide, usually at doses of 1.5 g of niacinamide and 2 g of tetracycline, has been used with success. Tetracycline should not be used in children under 9 years of age because it can permanently stain teeth.

Third-line therapies include *sulfamethoxypyridazine, dicloxacillin, erythromycin, mycophenolate mofetil, azathioprine, ciclosporin, methotrexate, interferon-α,* and *intravenous immunoglobulin (IVIG)*. Toxicity profiles and financial considerations favor using either erythromycin, dicloxacillin, or sulfamethoxypyridazine prior to treatment with the immunosuppressive agents or IVIG.

SPECIFIC INVESTIGATIONS

- ▶ Skin biopsy of blister for histology
- ▶ Perilesional skin biopsy for direct immunofluorescence
- ▶ Indirect immunofluorescence
- ▶ Consider G6PD level before dapsone use
- ▶ Consider thiopurine methyl transferase estimation before azathioprine use
- ▶ Ophthalmology consult

Linear IgA disease in adults. Leonard JN, Haffenden GP, Ring NP, McMinn RM, Sidgwick A, Mowbray JF, et al. Br J Dermatol 1982; 107: 301–16.

A clinicopathological study of mucosal involvement in linear IgA disease. Kelly SE, Frith PA, Millard PR, Wojnarowska F, Black MM. Br J Dermatol 1988; 119: 161–70.

Cicatrizing conjunctivitis as predominant manifestation of linear IgA bullous dermatosis. Webster GF, Raber I, Penne R, Jacoby RA, Beutner EH. J Am Acad Dermatol 1994; 30: 355–7.

Chronic bullous disease of childhood, childhood cicatricial pemphigoid, and linear IgA disease of adults. A comparative study demonstrating clinical and immunopathologic overlap. Wojnarowska F, Marsden RA, Bhogal B, Black MM. J Am Acad Dermatol 1988; 19: 792–805.

The above are excellent reviews of the clinical and immunological features of linear IgA bullous dermatosis.

Vancomycin-induced linear IgA bullous dermatosis. Baden LA, Apovian C, Imber MJ, Dover JS. Arch Dermatol 1988; 124: 1186–8.

Litt's Drug Eruption Reference Manual, 10th edn (New York: Taylor and Francis, 2004) implicates acetaminophen, aldesleukin, amiodarone, ampicillin, atorvastatin, candesartan, captopril, carbamazepine, cefamandole, ceftriaxone, co-trimoxazole, ciclosporin, diclofenac, furosemide, glyburide, granulocyte–macrophage colony-stimulating factor (GM-CSF), ibuprofen, interferon-α, lithium, metronidazole, naproxen, penicillins, phenytoin, piroxicam, rifampin, sulfamethoxazole, and vancomycin as drug triggers for linear IgA disease. The extent of disease may sometimes simulate toxic epidermal necrolysis.

The diagnosis of linear IgA bullous dermatosis requires routine histologic studies as well as direct and indirect immunofluorescence studies. Once the diagnosis is confirmed, laboratory studies to be obtained will depend upon the specific treatment anticipated.

FIRST-LINE THERAPIES

▶ Dapsone	C

Linear IgA dapsone responsive bullous dermatosis. Wojnarowska F. J Roy Soc Med 1980; 73: 371–3.

One of the first reports of this condition and response to dapsone. Since then, most series have demonstrated dapsone to be the most effective first-line monotherapy.

SECOND-LINE THERAPIES

▶ Dapsone and prednisone	D
▶ Sulfapyridine	C
▶ Colchicine	D
▶ Tetracycline and niacinamide	E

Colchicine as a novel therapeutic agent in chronic bullous dermatosis of childhood. Banodkar DD, Al-Suwaid AR. Int J Dermatol 1997; 36: 213–16.

Eight patients were given colchicine, five of whom showed complete remission within 4–6 weeks. The remaining three also responded but required concurrent steroids to maintain remission.

Treatment of pemphigus and linear IgA dermatosis with nicotinamide and tetracycline. Chaffins ML, Collison D, Fivenson DP. J Am Acad Dermatol 1993; 28: 998–1001.

Sublamina densa-type linear IgA bullous dermatosis successfully treated with oral tetracycline and niacinamide. Yomoda M, Komani A, Hashimoto T. Br J Dermatol 1999; 141: 608–9.

There are four reports of successful use of 2 g of tetracycline and 1.5 g of nicotinamide daily in adults only.

THIRD-LINE THERAPIES

▶ Sulfamethoxypyridazine	E
▶ Dicloxacillin	E
▶ Flucloxacillin	E
▶ Erythromycin	E
▶ Trimethoprim-sulfamethoxazole	E
▶ Methotrexate	E
▶ Interferon-α	E
▶ Mycophenolate mofetil	E
▶ Azathioprine	E
▶ Ciclosporin	E
▶ IVIG	E

Sulphamethoxypridazine for dermatitis herpetiformis, linear IgA disease, and cicatricial pemphigoid. McFadden JP, Leonard JN, Powles AV, Rutman AJ, Fry L. Br J Dermatol 1989; 121: 759–62.

Reports of sulfamethoxypyridazine (0.25–1.5 g daily) use as monotherapy in four patients with linear IgA disease who were intolerant of dapsone.

Treatment of chronic bullous dermatosis of childhood with oral dicloxacillin. Skinner RB, Totondo CK, Schneider MA, Raby L, Rosenberg EW. Pediatr Dermatol 1995; 12: 65–6.

Chronic bullous disease of childhood: successful treatment with dicloxacillin. Siegfried EC, Sirawan S. J Am Acad Dermatol 1998; 39: 797–800.

Mixed immunobullous disease of childhood: a good response to antimicrobials. Powell J, Kirtschig G, Allen J, Dean D, Wojnarowska F. Br J Dermatol 2001; 144: 769–74.

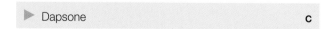

Linear IgA bullous dermatosis responsive to trimethoprim-sulfamethoxazole. Peterson JD, Chan LS. Clin Exp Dermatol 2007; 32: 756–8.

Linear IgA disease: successful treatment with erythromycin. Cooper SM, Powell J, Wojnarowska F. Clin Exp Dermatol 2002; 27: 677–9.

Antibiotics have been used largely in childhood disease and are a reasonable option because of their low toxicity.

Treatment of linear IgA bullous dermatosis of childhood with flucloxacillin Alajlan A, Al-Khawajah M, Al-Sheikh O, Al-Saif F, Al-Rasheed S, Al-Hoqail I, et al. J Am Acad Dermatol 2006; 54: 652–6.

Treatment of linear IgA bullous dermatosis of childhood with mycophenolate mofetil. Farley-Li J, Mancini AJ. Arch Dermatol 2003; 139: 1121–4.

Successful treatment of oral linear IgA disease using mycophenolate. Lewis MA, Yaqoob NA, Emanuel C, Potts AJ. Oral Surg Oral Med Oral Pathol Oral Radiol Endod 2007; 103: 483–6.

The adult dose is usually 35–45 mg/kg, which is about 1.5 g twice daily for a 75 kg adult.

Methotrexate and cyclosporine are of value in the treatment of adult linear IgA disease. Burrows NP, Jones RR. J Dermatol Treat 1992; 3: 31–3.

Linear IgA disease: successful treatment with cyclosporine. Young HS, Coulson IH. Br J Dermatol 2000; 143: 204–5.

Therapy-resistant blistering responding to ciclosporin 4 mg/kg daily.

Interferon alpha for linear IgA bullous dermatosis. Chan LS, Cooper KD. Lancet 1992; 340: 425.

High-dose intravenous immune globulin is also effective in linear IgA disease. Kroiss MM, Vogtt T, Landthaler M, Stolz W. Br J Dermatol 2000; 142: 582–4.

Successful treatment of linear IgA disease with salazosulphapyridine and intravenous immunoglobulins. Goebeler M, Seitz C, Rose C, Sitaru C, Jeschke R, Marx A, et al. Br J Dermatol 2003; 149: 912–14.

Upper aerodigestive tract complications in a neonate with linear IgA bullous dermatosis. Gluth MB, Witman PM, Thompson DM. Int J Pediatr Otorhinolaryngol 2004; 68: 965–70.

A newborn with skin involvement had life-threatening respiratory compromise from disease affecting the larynx, subglottis, trachea, and esophagus. Management with both tracheostomy and gastrostomy tube placement was necessary. Treatment included systemic corticosteroids, dapsone, and IVIG.

High-dose intravenous immunoglobulins for the treatment of autoimmune mucocutaneous blistering diseases: evaluation of its use in 19 cases. Segura S, Iranzo P, Martínez-de Pablo I, Mascaró JM Jr, Alsina M, Herrero J, et al. J Am Acad Dermatol 2007; 56: 960–7.

As the use of intravenous immunoglobulin (IVIG) therapy for autoimmune blistering diseases has evolved, it has become clear that to obtain optimal results patients should receive treatment with high-dose IVIG, defined as 2 g/kg per cycle, typically given at 4-week intervals.

Lipodermatosclerosis

Tania J Phillips, Bahar Dasgeb, Yuval Bibi

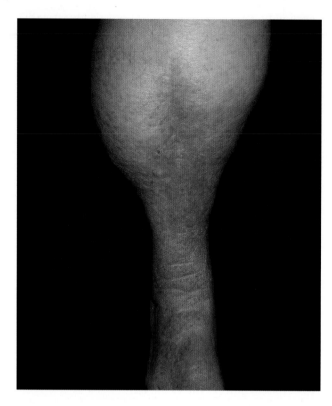

Lipodermatosclerosis (LDS) consists of a progressive fibrotic process of the skin and subcutaneous fat induced by chronic venous insufficiency. It usually presents as an indurated fibrotic region surrounding venous ulcers above the medial malleolus on the lower leg. The diagnosis is based on clinical findings. LDS more often affects elderly women who have a high body mass index and venous insufficiency. Pain is the most consistent presenting symptom. Two stages of LDS have been described: acute and chronic. The acute form is usually painful, tender, and slightly indurated. Often clinicians mistake the acute form for cellulitis, phlebitis, erythema nodosum, inflammatory morphea, or panniculitis. The chronic variant, which is strongly associated with venous insufficiency, is densely indurated and less painful than the acute form. In its late stages, chronic LDS alters the shape of the leg, making it look like an inverted bottle or bowling pin, with extreme fibrosis and sclerosis in the dermis and subcutaneous tissue. It may be associated with hyperpigmentation.

MANAGEMENT STRATEGY

The current treatment of choice is the *combination of stanozolol and compression therapy*. Compression helps increase venous return. Often patients with acute LDS find compression therapy painful: in this case stanozolol is used alone. Stanozolol is contraindicated in patients with uncontrolled hypertension and heart failure. *Pentoxifylline* is a helpful alternative that stimulates fibrinolysis, but may adversely affect the gastrointestinal tract. *Niacin* has some fibrinolytic properties and has been used for the disorder. Other treatments, such as *antibiotics, anti-inflammatory agents, antimetabolites, and long-term cimetidine*, have been proposed. Intralesional triamcinolone injections show promise, but require controlled studies. *Surgical approaches* include *subfascial perforator endoscopic surgery (SEPS), surgical correction of superficial venous reflux, ultrasound therapy*, and *complete excision of LDS followed by split-thickness skin graft repair*. Perforator vein sclerotherapy using polidocanol foam might offer a safer alternative to surgery.

SPECIFIC INVESTIGATIONS

- ▶ Biopsy
- ▶ Duplex ultrasound
- ▶ Laser Doppler scanning
- ▶ Ultrasound indentometry
- ▶ Capillary microscopy
- ▶ Magnetic resonance imaging

The clinical spectrum of lipodermatosclerosis. Kirsner RS, Pardes JB, Eaglstein WH, Falanga V. J Am Acad Dermatol 1993; 28: 623–7.

In most cases biopsy is not warranted because the diagnosis of LDS is based on clinical findings; 50% of biopsy sites do not heal, and may become chronically ulcerated.

Lipodermatosclerosis: the histologic spectrum with clinical correlation to the acute and chronic forms. Hurwitz D, Kirsner RS, Falanga V, Elgard GW. J Clin Pathol 1996; 23: 78.

If necessary, an incisional biopsy should be taken at the edges of the lesion with primary wound closure. Biopsy specimens from patients with acute LDS showed little epidermal change or capillary proliferation in papillary dermis. However, there were significant changes in the subcutis, where there was lobular and septal panniculitis. In addition, eosinophils, fibrin thrombi, and purpura were seen. Biopsy specimens from patients with chronic LDS showed significant dermal changes, which are often associated with venous insufficiency. These included capillary proliferation, hemosiderin deposition, and fibrosis. Epidermal hypertrophy and fibrosis were also detected in subcutaneous tissue in chronic disease. Patients who had both chronic and acute LDS showed overlap of the above features.

Duplex venous imaging: role for a comprehensive lower extremity examination. Badgett DK, Comerota MC, Khan MN, Eid IG, Kerr RP, Comerota AJ. Ann Vasc Surg 2000; 14: 73–6.

Results of duplex scanning of 205 lower extremities with varices: 106 not previously operated and 99 previously operated for varicose veins. Egeblad K, Baekgaard N. Ugeskr Laeger 2003; 3016–18.

Color Duplex ultrasound scanning has been shown to accurately detect the specific location of lower-extremity venous insufficiency that often leads to LDS.

Quantifying fibrosis in venous disease: mechanical properties of lipodermatosclerosis and healthy tissue. Geyer MJ, Brienza DM, Chib V, Wang J. Adv Skin Wound Care 2004; 17: 131–42.

A novel ultrasound indentometry method was used to quantify fibrotic tissue in LDS. This non-invasive technique can be used to quantify fibrosis in venous disease.

Excision of lipodermatosclerotic tissue: an effective treatment for non-healing venous ulcer. Ahnlide I, Bjellerup M, Akesson H. Acta Dermatol Venereol 2000; 80: 28–30.

In this study of seven cases, laser Doppler scanning showed that there is an increase in blood flow in lipodermatosclerotic skin. This increased flow decreased after operation and removal of the affected area.

Microangiopathy in chronic venous insufficiency: quantitative assessment by capillary microscopy. Howlader MH, Smith PD. Eur J Vasc Endovasc Surg 2003; 26: 325–31.

Capillary microscopy was used to assess patients with chronic venous disease and normal controls. Advanced venous disease (LDS and healed ulcer) was associated with a reduced number of capillaries and increased capillary convolution compared to healthy control subjects.

Magnetic resonance imaging as a diagnostic tool for extensive lipodermatosclerosis. Chan CC, Yang CY, Chu CY. J Am Acad Dermatol 2008; 58: 525–7.

In a single case report high-resolution MRI was in agreement with histopathological findings. Additional studies are necessary to validate this technique. MRI remains costly and would probably be reserved for ambiguous presentations, as in the case reported.

FIRST-LINE THERAPIES

▶ Compression therapy	A
▶ Stanozolol	B
▶ Compression therapy plus stanozolol	B
▶ HR (*O*-[betahydroxymethyl]-rutosides)	B

The clinical spectrum of lipodermatosclerosis. Kirsner RS, Pardes J, Eaglstein WH, Falanga VJ. Am Acad Dermatol 1993; 28: 623–7.

Traditionally LDS has been treated with compression therapy using graded stockings or elastic bandages. The authors suggest open-toe and below-the-knee graded stockings, with 30–40 mmHg pressure around the ankle. Some stockings come with a zipper in the back, which makes them easier for elderly patients to use. Patients with acute LDS, however, often have too much pain to be able to use compression stockings; in these patients, stanozolol, at a dose of 2 mg twice daily, was found to dramatically reduce pain and tenderness.

Graduated compression stockings reduce lipodermatosclerosis and ulcer recurrence. Vandongen YK, Stacey MC. Phlebology 2000; 25: 33–7.

A randomized controlled trial of 150 patients showed that elastic stockings alone can improve the skin changes of LDS and reduce the rate of ulcer recurrence.

Removal of dermal edema with class I and II compression stockings in patients with lipodermatosclerosis. Gniadecka M, Karlsmark T, Bertram A. J Am Acad Dermatol 1998; 39: 966–70.

In this study, high-frequency ultrasonography demonstrated that low levels of compression, class I (18–26 mmHg) in LDS are as effective as class II (26–36 mmHg) in the removal of dermal edema.

Light compression may be a useful modality for patients with chronic venous insufficiency and LDS who are not candidates for high-compression therapy.

Venous lipodermatosclerosis: treatment by fibrinolytic enhancement and elastic compression. Burnand K, Clemenson G, Morland M, Jarrett PE, Browse NL. Br Med J 1980; 280: 7–11.

From this study of 23 patients, Burnand et al. suggest that stanozolol (5 mg twice a day) and elastic stockings be used together. Stanozolol has been shown to reduce extravascular fibrin and induration, and relieve the pain, tenderness, and hyperpigmentation associated with LDS.

Patients taking stanozolol should be carefully monitored for excessive fluid retention, hirsutism, acne, liver function, and plasma fibrinogen concentration. Stanozolol is contraindicated in patients with uncontrolled hypertension or congestive heart failure.

HR (Paroven, Venoruton; *O*-(beta-hydroxyethyl)-rutosides) in venous hypertensive microangiopathy. Incandela L, Belacaro G, Renton S, DeSanctis MT, Cesarone MR, Bavera P, et al. J Cardiovasc Pharmacol Ther 2002; 7: S7–10.

HR (Paroven-Venoruton; *O*-[betahydroxyethyl]-rutosides) reduced signs and symptoms of chronic venous insufficiency and LDS.

SECOND-LINE THERAPIES

▶ Pentoxifylline	C
▶ Superficial venous surgery	B

Pentoxifylline for treating venous leg ulcer. Jull AB, Waters J, Arroll B. Cochrane Database Syst Rev 2002(1): CD001733.

Pentoxifylline is a dimethylxanthine derivative that increases red blood cell flexibility and alters fibroblast physiology. In addition, it stimulates fibrinolysis and changes fibroblast activity. The dose of 400 mg of oral pentoxifylline taken three times daily may be increased to 800 mg three times daily if no improvement occurs.

Pentoxifylline is a good alternative in those intolerant to stanozolol. Side effects include nausea, dizziness, heartburn, and, occasionally, vomiting.

Comparison of surgery and compression with compression alone in chronic venous ulceration (ESCHAR study): randomized controlled trial. Barwell JR, Davis CE, Deacon J, Harvey K, Minor J, Sassano A, et al. Lancet 2004; 363: 1854–9.

Surgical correction of superficial venous reflux reduced 12-month ulcer recurrence compared to treatment with compression alone.

The effects on LDS were not specifically mentioned in this study, but it might reasonably be expected to improve with correction of reflux.

THIRD-LINE THERAPIES

▶ Niacin	E
▶ Subfascial perforator endoscopic surgery (SEPS)	E
▶ Ultrasound	E
▶ Excision of lipodermatosclerotic tissue	E
▶ Antibiotics	E
▶ Intralesional triamcinolone injections	E
▶ Foam sclerotherapy	E

Lipid lowering and enhancement of fibrinolysis with niacin. Holvoet P, Collen D. Circulation 1995; 92: 698–9.

Niacin, taken at a dose of 100–150 mg three to five times a day, has been shown to help treat the hyperlipidemia that is often associated with LDS. In large doses it causes vasodilation and stimulates fibrinolysis. It also reduces uric acid excretion and alters glucose tolerance.

Niacin is another alternative for patients who cannot tolerate stanozolol.

Early benefit of subfascial endoscopic perforator surgery (SEPS) in healing venous ulcer. Sparks SR, Ballard JL, Bergan JJ, Killeen JD. Ann Vasc Surg 1997; 11: 367–73.

SEPS can be helpful in treating LDS in patients who do not heal with traditional methods. The perforating veins are ligated to ameliorate venous hypertension, which usually perpetuates the LDS.

No other data have been published.

The effect of ultrasound-guided sclerotherapy (UGS) of incompetent perforator veins on venous clinical severity and disability scores. Masuda EM, Kessler DM, Lurie F, Puggioni A, Kistner RL, Eklof B. J Vasc Surg 2006; 43: 551–6.

In this 68-patient (80 limb) series UGS was shown to be an effective modality in the treatments of incompetent perforator veins and the resultant venous hypertension.

Hypodermatitis sclerodermiformis. Rowe L, Cantwell A. Arch Dermatol 1982; 118: 312–14.

The authors used ultrasound to treat six patients and found promising results in four. Treatments were given two to three times weekly for a month or two, and were repeated after rest for a month or more.

This study was not randomized, blinded, or placebo controlled. No confirmatory studies have been published.

Excision of lipodermatosclerotic tissue: an effective treatment for non-healing venous ulcer. Ahnlide I, Bjellerup M, Akesson H. Acta Dermatol Venereol 2000; 80: 28–30.

From this small, uncontrolled study, Ahnlide et al. suggest that excision of lipodermatosclerotic tissue can help heal venous ulcers, because the lipodermatosclerotic area impedes the healing process. Laser Doppler scanning showed increased basal blood flow in lipodermatosclerotic skin, which normalized after surgery.

Local microcirculation in chronic venous incompetence and leg ulcer. Fagrell B. Vasc Surg 1979; 13: 217–25.

Although the number of capillaries is reduced in venous incompetence, those remaining are dilated and tortuous, causing increased blood flow to the region. This impairs healing. Thus removal of the lipodermatosclerotic tissue, together with skin grafting, can help the healing process in recalcitrant venous ulcers.

Hypodermatitis sclerodermiformis and unusual acid-fast bacteria. Cantwell A, Kelso D, Rowe L. Arch Dermatol 1979; 115: 449–52.

There is little evidence to support the use of antibiotics, antiinflammatory agents, or antimetabolites.

Severe chronic venous insufficiency treated by foamed sclerosant. Pascarella L, Bergan JJ, Mekenas LV. Ann Vasc Surg 2006; 20: 83–91.

In this prospective study sclerotherapy with 1–3% polidocanol foam combined with compression is superior to compression alone in facilitating venous ulcer healing and improving venous scores. Lipodermatosclerosis is not specifically addressed.

Intralesional triamcinolone in the management of lipodermatosclerosis. Campbell LB, Miller OF 3rd. J Am Acad Dermatol 2006; 55: 166–8.

A retrospective chart review of 28 patients (23 females, five males) 20–77 years old shows improvement in pain, erythema, edema, and induration after one to three intralesional injections of 5–10 mg/mL triamcinolone.

This study is age and gender biased, and lacks standardization with respect to timelines of treatment and follow-up, dosages, and data pooling. Moreover, adjunct therapies were used in the majority of the patients concurrently with steroid injections. Complications are not mentioned. Statistical analysis is not applicable.

Livedo reticularis

Ruwani P Katugampola, Andrew Y Finlay

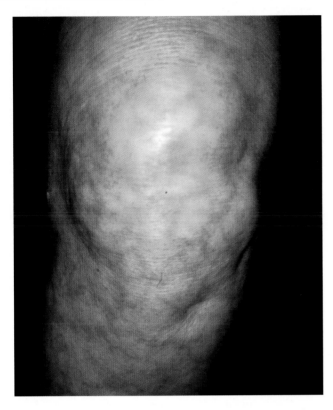

Livedo reticularis (LR) is the net-like mottled violaceous discoloration of the skin secondary to dilatation and stagnation of blood in the dermal capillaries. The unaffected normal-colored islands of skin are the areas where blood supply is sufficient; in the network areas the supply is reduced. This commonly occurs on the legs, arms, and trunk, but can be diffuse, and is more pronounced following exposure to cold. LR can be physiological (cutis marmorata), or can occur as a primary phenomenon (idiopathic LR) or secondary to a number of diseases that cause dermal vessel wall thickening and/or luminal occlusion, such as systemic lupus erythematosus, polyarteritis nodosa, antiphospholipid syndrome (page 47), cryoglobulinemia, cholesterol emboli, and drugs (minocycline and interferon). Idiopathic LR may be congenital (cutis marmorata telangiectatica congenita), or associated with painful ulcers (livedoid vasculopathy – page 401) or with cerebrovascular involvement (Sneddon's syndrome).

MANAGEMENT STRATEGY

The etiology of physiological and primary LR is unknown and there is no definitive treatment. The management of primary LR depends on the presence of associated ulcers, anomalies (congenital form), and systemic involvement (Sneddon's syndrome). In secondary LR the underlying cause needs to be identified and treated.

Physiological LR, which occurs in healthy children and adults in response to cold weather, is diffuse, mild, temporary, and usually asymptomatic. No specific treatment is required for this condition except *avoidance of cold exposure*, protection from cold exposure with *warm clothing*, and *rewarming* of the affected area.

Cutis marmorata telangiectatica congenita is rare and presents at or soon after birth. A small proportion of affected children have associated congenital anomalies such as hemangiomas, glaucoma, limb atrophy, cardiac malformation, or psychomotor retardation that need to be identified and referred for appropriate specialist care. The LR in these children usually disappears spontaneously or improves markedly with age.

Patients with Sneddon's syndrome are at risk of cerebrovascular disease and may benefit from *antithrombotic treatment*. The timing of such treatment is debated, as LR may precede the neurological events by up to 10 or more years. Advice regarding other risk factors predisposing to cerebrovascular events, such as smoking, obesity, hypertension, and oral contraceptives, is important.

Although a number of agents, including *antiplatelet therapy, danazol, pentoxifylline, and systemic steroids*, have been used to treat ulcers associated with LR, no single agent has been shown to completely resolve the LR itself.

Several medications, including those used by dermatologists, have been associated with LR. The decision to withdraw the suspected medication should be based on clinical judgment, alternative treatments, and other side effects, rather than the appearance of LR per se.

SPECIFIC INVESTIGATIONS

▶ Skin biopsies for microscopy and direct immunofluorescence (adults)
▶ Full blood count and renal function
▶ Rheumatologic serologic tests (rheumatoid factor, ANF, ANCA)
▶ Cryoglobulin level
▶ Anticardiolipin antibodies
▶ Thrombophilia screen
▶ Serum lipid profile

A detailed clinical history followed by physical examination is essential, especially in diagnosing Sneddon's syndrome, identifying congenital anomalies in infants, and excluding secondary causes of LR. The histology of LR is non-inflammatory thickening of dermal vessel walls, with eventual occlusion of the lumen.

Livedo reticularis: an update. Gibbs MM, English JC, Zirwas MJ. J Am Acad Dermatol 2005; 52: 1009–19.

This is a comprehensive review of the different causes of LR. The authors conclude that management of secondary LR should be directed at identifying and treating the underlying cause. Several deep punch biopsies, at least one from the central normal skin and one from the peripheral violaceous skin, are suggested to identify causes of secondary LR. In addition to cold avoidance, limb elevation and compression stockings are suggested for symptomatic patients based on the authors' clinical experience.

Diagnostic impact and sensitivity of skin biopsies in Sneddon's syndrome. A report of 15 cases. Wohlrab J, Fisher M, Wolter M, Marsch WC. Br J Dermatol 2001; 145: 285–8.

Deep 4 mm punch biopsies from the central white part of the LR demonstrated a sensitivity of 27% with one biopsy,

53% with two biopsies, and 80% with three biopsies of diagnosing Sneddon's syndrome in clinically suspected cases. The authors concluded that positive histology was important for commencing prophylaxis of cerebrovascular events in patients initially presenting with LR.

Livedo reticularis: an underutilized diagnostic clue in cholesterol embolization syndrome. Chaudhary K, Wall BM, Rasberry RD. Am J Med Sci 2001; 321: 348–51.

Six of eight patients with unexplained acute renal failure due to suspected cholesterol emboli syndrome (CES) demonstrated cholesterol emboli in skin biopsies of LR. Deep skin biopsy of LR is proposed as a safe diagnostic procedure to confirm CES, thereby avoiding the increased morbidity associated with biopsy of visceral organs.

The spectrum of livedo reticularis and anticardiolipin antibodies. Asherson RA, Mayou SC, Merry P, Black MM, Hughes GRV. Br J Dermatol 1989; 120: 215–21.

In this retrospective study of 65 patients with LR (idiopathic and secondary), 28 anticardiolipin antibody-positive patients were compared with 37 anticardiolipin-negative patients. There was a statistically significant increase in the incidence of strokes, transient ischemic attacks, venous thrombosis, fetal loss, and valvular heart disease in the anticardiolipin-positive patients compared to the anticardiolipin-negative patients.

FIRST-LINE THERAPY

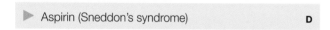

▶ Aspirin (Sneddon's syndrome)	D

Sneddon's syndrome: Generalized livedo reticularis and cerebrovascular disease – importance of hemostatic screening. Devos J, Bulcke J, Degreef H, Michielsen B. Dermatology 1992; 185: 296–9.

Two cases of Sneddon's syndrome are described, one of which was shown to have twice the normal level of tissue plasminogen activator antigen, four times the normal level of plasminogen activator inhibitor, abnormal thrombin times, and elevated levels of factor XII during a neurological event. Aspirin was commenced at 300 mg daily, with normalization of the hemostatic parameters after 4 months of treatment and freedom from neurological symptoms at 10 months. There was no change to the patient's LR with aspirin treatment.

SECOND-LINE THERAPIES

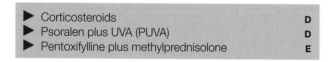

▶ Corticosteroids	D
▶ Psoralen plus UVA (PUVA)	D
▶ Pentoxifylline plus methylprednisolone	E

Cholesterol emboli syndrome in type 2 diabetes: the disease history of a case evaluated with renal scintigraphy. Piccoli GB, Sargiotto A, Burdese M, Colla L, Bilucaglia D, Magnano A, et al. Rev Diabetic Stud 2005; 2: 92–6.

A 75-year-old obese, diabetic, hypertensive man with moderate dyslipidemia developed CES following endovascular intervention, manifesting as acute renal failure and LR of both feet. Methylprednisolone 300 mg intravenously for 3 days followed by oral prednisolone 25 mg daily and tapered over 2 months, commenced because of deteriorating renal function, resulted in improvement in serum creatinine. There was disappearance of LR within 2 days of starting treatment.

Livedo reticularis and livedoid vasculitis responding to PUVA therapy. Choi HJ, Hann SK. J Am Acad Dermatol 1999; 40: 204–7.

Two patients with ulcers due to livedoid vasculitis of the lower legs resistant to treatment with other systemic treatment, including aspirin, prednisolone, and pentoxifylline, were treated with systemic PUVA using methoxsalen. Only the lower legs were exposed to UVA initially, with 4 J/cm² three times a week and subsequent 1 J/cm² increments. No significant ulcers had recurred at 3 and 6 months' follow-up of the two patients after the last treatment.

Improvement in the discoloration of the skin affected by LR was noted in one of the patients at completion of PUVA treatment.

Widespread livedoid vasculopathy. Marzano AV, Vanotti M, Alessi E. Acta Dermatol Venereol 2003; 83: 457–60.

A 37-year-old woman with widespread LR and recurrent painful ulcers on all limbs, trunk, and scalp was treated with both intravenous methylprednisolone 80 mg/day for 5 days, followed by intramuscular and subsequent tapering oral dose to 32 mg/day, and with pentoxifylline 400 mg twice daily for 2 months. There was a marked clinical improvement of the ulcers within 2 weeks of treatment.

The intensity of the LR faded but did not completely resolve.

THIRD-LINE THERAPIES

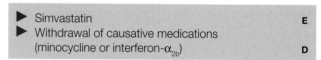

▶ Simvastatin	E
▶ Withdrawal of causative medications (minocycline or interferon-α₂b)	D

Livedo reticularis caused by cholesterol embolization may improve with simvastatin. Finch TM, Ryatt KS. Br J Dermatol 2000; 143: 1319–20.

A 69-year-old man with LR without ulceration of the legs extending to the lower abdomen due to cholesterol embolization failed to respond to low-dose aspirin and low-fat diet. Fasting serum cholesterol was 6.9 mmol/L and serum triglyceride was normal. Three months after initiation of simvastatin 10 mg daily the serum cholesterol decreased to 4.9 mmol/L, with associated reduction in extent and prominence of the LR.

Minocycline induced arthritis associated with fever, livedo reticularis and pANCA. Elkayam O, Yaron M, Caspi D. Ann Rheum Dis 1996; 55: 769–71.

Three women treated with long courses of oral minocycline for acne developed LR of the lower legs associated with fever, and arthritis/arthralgia associated with elevated titers of pANCA during treatment. Symptoms resolved after discontinuation of treatment but recurred following rechallenge. The specific outcome of LR following discontinuation of treatment is not clearly stated.

Livedo reticularis associated with interferon α therapy in two melanoma patients. Ruiz-Genao DP, García-F-Villalta MJ, Hernández-Núñez A, Ríos-Buceta L, Fernández-Herrera J, García-Díez A. J Eur Acad Dermatol Venereol 2005; 19: 252–4.

Two patients treated with subcutaneous interferon-α₂b three times weekly as adjuvant therapy for malignant melanoma (AJCC stages IIA and IIB, respectively) developed LR on the thighs, legs, and trunk 2 weeks after commencing treatment. LR cleared completely with no further recurrence after treatment was discontinued for other reasons.

Evidence Levels: **A** Double-blind study **B** Clinical trial ≥ 20 subjects **C** Clinical trial < 20 subjects **D** Series ≥ 5 subjects **E** Anecdotal case reports

Livedoid vasculopathy

Bethany R Hairston, Mark DP Davis

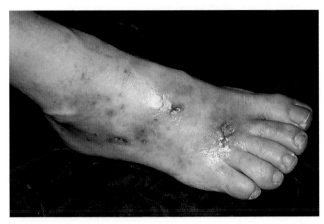

From Lebwohl MG. The Skin and Systemic Disease: A Color Atlas, 2nd edn. Churchill Livingstone 2003, with permission of Elsevier.

Livedoid vasculopathy, or livedoid vasculitis, is a painful ulcerative condition of the lower extremities with characteristic clinical and histopathologic features. The lesions of *atrophie blanche*, a term once synonymous with the disease, are typically present on the lower extremities and are characterized by smooth, porcelain-white lesions surrounded by punctate telangiectasia and hyperpigmentation. Shallow central ulceration is often present. This condition is difficult to treat and often recalcitrant to therapy.

MANAGEMENT STRATEGY

Appropriate diagnosis of livedoid vasculitis is necessary before treatment options can be considered. Histologic identification of the characteristic segmental hyalinized appearance of the dermal blood vessels is important to exclude other causes of lower extremity ulcerative disease. Increasing numbers of reports suggest that the disease has a procoagulant predisposition, with both hereditary and acquired hypercoagulable states.

Typically shallow and numerous, the ulcerations in livedoid vasculopathy are painful and slow to heal. *Wound care* is an important facet of treatment. Excellent *dressings* and topical products are available to treat chronic ulcerative diseases, and selection depends on the moisture content of the wound and the possibility of superinfection. *Topical and oral antibiotics* may be beneficial, and wounds should be cultured to determine appropriate sensitivity to medications. *Pain management* is also essential.

Because of the potential procoagulant mechanisms involved in disease etiology, medical therapy has traditionally centered on the prevention and treatment of dermal vessel thrombosis and improvement of vascular perfusion. Medical management has included *aspirin (acetylsalicylic acid)*, *niacin (nicotinic acid)*, *pentoxifylline*, *dipyridamole*, *warfarin*, *danazol*, and *ketanserin*. Systemic corticosteroids are not considered a primary therapy; however, some patients have improved with immunosuppressants used in combination therapy. *Psoralen with UVA (PUVA)* has also been used. Patients with livedoid vasculitis recalcitrant to traditional management have been treated with *minidose heparin*, *subcutaneous low molecular weight heparin injections*,

intravenous iloprost (a prostacyclin analog), *intravenous immunoglobulin (IVIG)*, and a *tissue-type plasminogen activator (tPA)*.

SPECIFIC INVESTIGATIONS

▶ Skin biopsy, including routine histology and direct immunofluorescence
▶ Wound and tissue cultures
▶ Laboratory studies: hemogram, determination of serum homocysteine, cryoglobulin, anticardiolipin antibody, factor V Leiden R506Q and prothrombin G20210A mutations, biological activity and antigen levels of protein C and S, functional and immunologic levels of antithrombin III protein, and detection of lupus anticoagulant
▶ Non-invasive venous and arterial function testing: continuous-wave Doppler, venous duplex imaging, plethysmography, and transcutaneous oximetry

Livedoid vasculopathy: further evidence for procoagulant pathogenesis. Hairston BR, Davis MD, Pittelkow MR, Ahmed I. Arch Dermatol 2006; 142: 1413–18.

This retrospective study of 45 patients with biopsy-proven livedoid vasculopathy analyzed the presence of coagulation abnormalities. The laboratory results revealed numerous heterogeneous coagulation abnormalities, including factor V Leiden mutations, protein C or S abnormalities, prothrombin G20210A gene mutations, lupus anticoagulant, anticardiolipin antibodies, and elevated homocysteine, thereby providing further evidence of procoagulant mechanisms for this disease.

Livedoid vasculopathy: what is it and how the patient should be evaluated and treated. Callen JP. Arch Dermatol 2006; 142: 1481–2.

This editorial reviews nomenclature changes with this disease.

A well presented, illustrative approach to diagnosis and review of treatments, including a 'therapeutic ladder.'

Livedoid vasculopathy: the role of hyperhomocysteinemia and its simple therapeutic consequences. Meiss F, Marsch WC, Fischer M. Eur J Dermatol 2006; 16: 159–62.

Hypercoagulability due to hyperhomocysteinemia was recognized as a potentially contributing factor to livedoid vasculopathy in a 49-year-old woman.

Livedo (livedoid) vasculitis and the factor V Leiden mutation: additional evidence for abnormal coagulation. Calamia KT, Balabanova M, Perniciaro C, Walsh JS. J Am Acad Dermatol 2002; 46: 133–7.

A case of livedo vasculitis with the factor V Leiden mutation is described.

Livedoid vasculopathy associated with heterozygous protein C deficiency. Boyvat A, Kundakci N, Babikir MO, Gurgey E. Br J Dermatol 2000; 143: 840–2.

Livedoid vasculitis in association with protein C deficiency is described in one patient.

Livedoid vasculitis: a manifestation of the antiphospholipid syndrome? Acland KM, Darvay A, Wakelin SH, Russell-Jones R. Br J Dermatol 1999; 140: 131–5.

Four patients with ulcerative livedoid vasculitis are described, all of whom had associated elevated anticardiolipin antibody levels but no other evidence of systemic disease.

Atrophie blanche: a disorder associated with defective release of tissue plasminogen activator. Pizzo SV, Murray JC, Gonias SL. Arch Pathol Lab Med 1986; 110: 517–19.

Plasma from eight patients with *atrophie blanche* was analyzed for release of vascular tPA before and after venous occlusion. The average plasma level of releasable tPA was only 0.03 IU/mL, compared to 0.70 IU/mL in 118 healthy controls.

FIRST-LINE THERAPIES

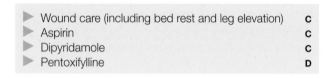

▶ Wound care (including bed rest and leg elevation)	C
▶ Aspirin	C
▶ Dipyridamole	C
▶ Pentoxifylline	D

Atrophie blanche: a clinicopathological study of 27 patients. Yang LJ, Chan HL, Chen SY, Kuan YZ, Chen MJ, Wang CN. Changgeng Yi Xue Za Zhi 1991; 14: 237–45.

Twenty-seven patients were reviewed with respect to mean age at onset, disease duration, natural course, and clinical morphology. Thirteen patients responded to local wound care, bed rest, and low-dose aspirin plus dipyridamole as treatment for the first attack or recurrent episodes.

Antiplatelet therapy in atrophie blanche and livedo vasculitis. Drucker CR, Duncan WC. J Am Acad Dermatol 1982; 7: 359–63.

Seven patients with abnormal platelet function in vitro had clinical improvement after treatment with dipyridamole and aspirin.

Pentoxifylline (Trental) therapy for the vasculitis of atrophie blanche. Sauer GC. Arch Dermatol 1986; 122: 380–1.

Six patients with livedoid vasculopathy treated with pentoxifylline had improved or healed ulcerations in 2–3 months. They remained free of ulcers as long as pentoxifylline was continued, but ulcers recurred when the drug was stopped.

Livedo vasculitis: therapy with pentoxifylline. Sams WM Jr. Arch Dermatol 1988; 124: 684–7.

Eight patients with disease unresponsive to a variety of medications were treated with pentoxifylline. Three experienced complete healing, four were much improved, and only one was unchanged after treatment.

SECOND-LINE THERAPIES

▶ Danazol	D
▶ Warfarin	D
▶ Hyperbaric oxygen	D

Low-dose danazol in the treatment of livedoid vasculitis. Hsiao GH, Chiu HC. Dermatology 1997; 194: 251–5.

Six of seven patients treated with low-dose danazol (200 mg/day orally) had rapid cessation of new lesion formation, prompt reduction in pain, and healing of active ulceration.

Ulcerations caused by livedoid vasculopathy associated with a prothrombotic state: response to warfarin. Davis MD, Wysokinski WE. J Am Acad Dermatol 2008; 58: 512–15.

Warfarin therapy healed ulcerations in a 50-year-old woman who had a lifelong history of painful ulcerations; the patient was a heterozygous carrier of factor V Leiden and prothrombin gene mutations.

A case of livedoid vasculopathy associated with factor V Leiden mutation: successful treatment with oral warfarin. Kavala M, Kocaturk E, Zindanci I, Turkoglu Z, Altintas S. J Dermatol Treat 2008; 19: 121–3.

A 19-year-old man with a 4-year history of recurrent leg ulcerations had rapid improvement with oral warfarin therapy after laboratory diagnosis of protein C and factor V Leiden mutations.

Warfarin therapy for livedoid vasculopathy associated with cryofibrinogenemia and hyperhomocysteinemia. Browning CE, Callen JP. Arch Dermatol 2006; 142: 75–8.

A 50-year-old man with abnormal cryofibrinogen and homocysteine levels had a dramatic response to oral warfarin therapy after being refractory to treatment with multiple other medications.

Livedoid vasculopathy: long-term follow-up results following hyperbaric oxygen therapy. Juan WH, Chan YS, Lee JC, Yang LC, Hong HS, Yang CH. Br J Dermatol 2006; 154: 251–5.

Eight patients completed a prospective study evaluating the efficacy of hyperbaric oxygen on healing the ulcers of livedoid vasculopathy. Leg ulcers in all eight healed completely at a mean of 3.4 weeks; however, six patients had relapses of ulceration but responded to additional hyperbaric oxygen therapy.

THIRD-LINE THERAPIES

▶ Low molecular weight heparin	D
▶ Fluindione (vitamin K antagonist)	D
▶ Intravenous immunoglobulin (IVIG)	C
▶ tPA	C
▶ Iloprost	E
▶ Sulfapyridine	D
▶ Ketanserin	E
▶ PUVA	C

Treatment of livedoid vasculopathy with low-molecular-weight heparin: report of 2 cases. Hairston BR, Davis MD, Gibson LE, Drage LA. Arch Dermatol 2003; 139: 987–90.

Two patients with livedoid vasculitis recalcitrant to conventional first- and second-line therapies had a beneficial response to subcutaneous injections of low molecular weight heparin.

Difficult management of livedoid vasculopathy. Frances C, Barete S. Arch Dermatol 2004; 140: 1011.

Fourteen of 16 patients treated with either low molecular weight heparin or a vitamin K antagonist (fluindione) had more effective results than with antiplatelet drugs. One patient responded partially to aspirin and dipyridamole; the remaining patient responded to no treatments.

402

The authors recommend that the benefit–risk ratio, cost, and quality of life be considered when prescribing either low molecular weight heparin or vitamin K antagonists.

Pulsed intravenous immunoglobulin therapy in livedoid vasculitis: an open trial evaluating 9 consecutive patients. Kreuter A, Gambichler T, Breuckmann F, Bechara FB, Rotterdam S, Stucker M, et al. J Am Acad Dermatol 2004; 51: 574–9.

The efficacy and safety of IVIG were investigated in nine patients with livedoid vasculitis; seven of them had not responded to other treatment modalities. A vast improvement in erythema, healing of ulceration, and pain was noted in all patients.

Livedoid vasculopathy associated with plasminogen activator inhibitor-1 promoter homozygosity (4G/4G) treated successfully with tissue plasminogen activator. Deng A, Gocke CD, Hess J, Heyman M, Paltiel M, Gaspari A. Arch Dermatol 2006; 142; 1466–9.

Plasminogen activator inhibitor-1, an important inhibitor of the fibrinolytic system, was elevated in a 33-year-old woman with livedoid vasculopathy. Treatment with heparin sodium and tPA dramatically improved her skin lesions, resulting in complete healing of her lower extremity ulcerations.

Tissue plasminogen activator for treatment of livedoid vasculitis. Klein KL, Pittelkow MR. Mayo Clin Proc 1992; 67: 923–33.

In a prospective study, six patients who had non-healing ulcers caused by livedoid vasculitis and in whom numerous conventional therapies had failed were treated with low-dose tPA. In five of the six a dramatic improvement with almost complete healing of the ulcers occurred during hospitalization. Several were maintained with warfarin therapy after their inpatient treatment.

Livedoid vasculopathy with combined thrombophilia: efficacy of iloprost. Magy N, Algros MP, Racadot E, Gil H, Kantelip B, Dupond JL. Rev Med Interne 2002; 23: 554–7. (In French.)

A patient with lupus anticoagulant and factor V Leiden gene mutation had a dramatic and effective response to intravenous iloprost after unsuccessful anticoagulant therapy.

Clinical studies of livedoid vasculitis (segmental hyalinizing vasculitis). Winkelmann RK, Schroeter AL, Kierland RR, Ryan TM. Mayo Clin Proc 1974; 49: 746–50.

Clinical, laboratory, and histologic studies of 37 patients with livedoid vasculitis are presented. Treatment options included niacin (nicotinic acid), which was effective because of the inhibiting effect of nicotinate on the contraction of vascular smooth muscle of the skin. Nine of 12 patients had sustained remission of their livedoid vasculopathy. Rest and wet-dressing therapy produced short remissions. Six of 11 patients responded to sulfapyridine, and three of eight responded to guanethidine. Corticosteroids, sympathectomy, and other forms of chemotherapy were not successful.

Chronic leg ulceration with livedoid vasculitis, and response to oral ketanserin. Rustin MH, Bunker CB, Dowd PM. Br J Dermatol 1989; 120: 101–5.

A patient with a 6-year history of recalcitrant painful ulcerations due to livedoid vasculitis healed rapidly after treatment with oral ketanserin.

Livedoid vasculitis responding to PUVA therapy. Lee JH, Choi HJ, Kim SM, Hann SK, Park YK. Int J Dermatol 2001; 40: 153–7.

Eight patients treated with systemic PUVA had rapid cessation of new lesion formation, notable symptom relief, and complete healing of primary lesions without unacceptable adverse effects.

Lyme borreliosis

Gopi Patel, Fran Wallach

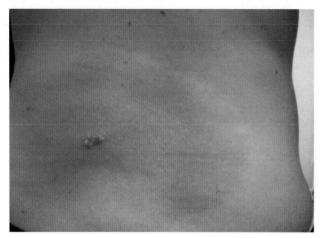

Courtesy of Jeffrey P Gumprecht, MD, New York NY.

Lyme disease is a multisystem illness caused by spirochetes of the genus *Borrelia*. In the United States the causative agent is *B. burgdorferi*. In Europe, Lyme borreliosis is caused primarily by *B. afzelii*, followed by *B. garnii*. Clinical manifestations of Lyme disease depend on the stage of illness and may be limited to the skin or involve the nervous system, joints, or heart. The disease was first described in 1977 after geographic clustering of purported juvenile rheumatoid arthritis in Lyme, Connecticut. Epidemiology suggested a tickborne illness. Today Lyme disease is the most common vector-borne disease in the United States. It is endemic in the Northeast, the mid-Atlantic, and parts of Wisconsin and Minnesota. The most common vector for Lyme disease is the *Ixodes scapularis* tick. *Ixodes pacificus* has been linked to transmission of *B. burgdorferi* in the Pacific Northwest.

Mice and deer are the major reservoirs of *B. burgdorferi*. *Ixodes* ticks feed once in each of the three stages of their 2-year lifecycle. After hatching in the spring, larvae feed in summer, acquiring *B. burgdorferi* from their preferred host, the white-footed mouse. The following spring the larvae molt into nymphs, which again feed off the white-footed mouse. The nymphs mature into adult ticks, which feed and mate in autumn and winter, usually on the white-tailed deer. *B. burgdorferi* is passed back and forth between ticks and their hosts. Humans can become accidental hosts during the spring and summer, when nymphs are actively feeding.

MANAGEMENT STRATEGY

Routine antimicrobial prophylaxis or serologic testing after a tick bite is *not* recommended. Some experts recommend prophylaxis for patients bitten by *I. scapularis* ticks that have been attached over 36 hours if exposure occurred in an endemic area. This recommendation is based on evidence that a single 200 mg dose of doxycycline prevented 87% of Lyme infections if administered within 72 hours of tick removal. An accurate and detailed exposure history, however, is often unavailable. Those with a known tick exposure should be monitored for up to 30 days for the occurrence of skin lesions or fever. Cutaneous lesions or symptoms developing within 1 month after tick removal should prompt evaluation for early Lyme disease.

The best method of preventing Lyme disease is to avoid tick-infested areas. If exposure is unavoidable, then one should *wear light-colored clothing* and *long pants tucked into socks* to prevent ticks from finding exposed skin. *Daily inspection* of the entire body, including the scalp, is recommended, as attached ticks removed within 24–36 hours are unlikely to transmit *B. burgdorferi*. *DEET-containing insect repellents* provide added protection. *Ixodes* ticks are small: larvae are less than 1 mm in size and adult females are 2–3 mm. Attached ticks should be removed with tweezers by pulling on the mouth apparatus close to the skin, taking care not to leave parts of the embedded tick behind.

Lyme disease generally occurs in stages, with different signs and symptoms at each stage. Therapeutic recommendations vary depending on the stage of disease and the presence of extracutaneous manifestations.

Early localized Lyme disease

The most common clinical manifestation of early Lyme disease is erythema migrans (EM), also known as erythema chronicum migrans. This characteristic skin lesion usually begins as an erythematous papule and develops into an expanding, erythematous, annular lesion with central clearing at the site of the tick bite. The lesion can be minimally tender. In most patients with Lyme disease EM appears 3–30 days after spirochete inoculation. The lesion may be accompanied by nonspecific symptoms, including fever, regional lymphadenopathy, arthralgias, fatigue, and headaches. About 75–80% of patients in the United States who present with EM have only a single primary lesion. Others can have secondary lesions that arise through hematogenous dissemination from the primary site. Untreated lesions usually fade within 3–4 weeks. Administration of *doxycycline* 100 mg twice daily, *amoxicillin* 500 mg three times daily, or *cefuroxime axetil* 500 mg twice daily for 14–21 days is recommended for early localized or early disseminated Lyme disease associated with EM. Doxycycline has the advantage of treating human granulocytic anaplasmosis, which can be co-transmitted with *B. burgdorferi* by *Ixodes scapularis*. Doxycycline is relatively contraindicated during pregnancy or lactation, and for children less than 8 years old.

A rare skin manifestation of early Lyme infection described predominantly in Europe is borrelial lymphocytoma (BL). This solitary bluish-red swelling occurs at the site of a tick bite, typically preceding or concomitantly with EM. Commonly involved sites are the earlobes in children and near or on the nipple in adults. BL may develop within weeks to months after a tick bite, and if untreated can persist for months to years. Treatment regimens used for EM can also be used for BL.

Early disseminated Lyme disease

In untreated infection early dissemination of the spirochete occurs via blood or lymphatics over several weeks. Secondary annular skin lesions resembling primary EM can occur and are generally smaller. Other common symptoms include fever, lethargy, myalgias, headache, and mild neck stiffness. Patients may present with atrioventricular conduction disturbances, iritis or uveitis, aseptic meningitis (lymphocytic pleocytosis in CSF), cranial nerve palsies (notably facial nerve palsies), or peripheral radiculopathy. In adults, intravenous *ceftriaxone* 2 g daily for

14–28 days is recommended for early Lyme disease presenting with neurologic or advanced cardiac conduction abnormalities. Intravenous *penicillin G* or *cefotaxime* are acceptable alternatives. Temporary pacing may be required for patients with high-degree AV block (PR≥0.30 s). Insertion of a permanent pacer is not necessary as conduction defects resolve spontaneously. Isolated facial nerve palsy and first-degree AV block can be treated with oral doxycycline (class B recommendation).

Late Lyme disease

Late Lyme disease can occur months to years after a previously untreated or inadequately treated initial infection. Lyme arthritis is the most common manifestation of late Lyme disease, although decreasing in incidence owing to improved recognition of early disease. Lyme arthritis is oligoarticular and presents as recurrent swelling of large joints, primarily the knees. Persistent swelling is atypical. Positive serologic testing is required to confirm the diagnosis, and positive PCR results from synovial fluid strengthen the diagnosis.

Late neuroborreliosis is rare and can manifest as peripheral neuropathy, encephalomyelitis, or a subacute encephalopathy. The latter is most commonly described in Europe and can be characterized by memory disturbances, mood alterations, and somnolence.

A rare dermatologic finding associated with late Lyme disease is acrodermatitis chronica atrophicans (ACA). This skin manifestation develops late after initial infection and patients present with violaceous discoloration and swelling of involved skin, usually the extremities. Over time the skin becomes atrophic. Involvement of peripheral nerves is not uncommon, causing sensory neuropathy in addition to cutaneous abnormalities. ACA is rarely seen in the United States, but is not infrequent in Europe, where it is associated with *B. afzelii* infection.

Lyme arthritis without neurologic symptoms can be treated with a 28-day oral regimen of either doxycycline 100 mg twice daily or amoxicillin 500 mg three times daily. Adults with evidence of concurrent neurologic involvement should receive intravenous ceftriaxone. Recurrent or persistent joint swelling after an oral regimen can be re-treated with another 28-day course of oral antibiotics or with a 2–4 week parenteral regimen.

Persistent arthritic complaints appear to be immunologically mediated and are most common in individuals with the HLA-DR4 haplotype. Prolonged or multiple repeated courses of antibiotics are unhelpful and may be harmful. Symptomatic treatment with non-steroidal agents, intra-articular corticosteroids, disease modifying antirheumatic drugs, or in severe non-remitting cases arthroscopic synovectomy may provide relief.

Adults with late neurologic disease should be treated with a parenteral regimen for 2–4 weeks. Repeated or prolonged therapy is not recommended.

SPECIFIC INVESTIGATIONS

▶ Serologic testing for borrelial infection

Prospective study of serologic tests for Lyme disease. Steere A, McHugh G, Damle N, Sikand V. Clin Infect Dis 2008; 47: 188–95.

Early Lyme disease is a clinical diagnosis, with 80% of patients in endemic areas presenting with erythema migrans. Only one-third of patients presenting with EM and early Lyme disease have positive serology, but sensitivity increases during the convalescent phase. Two-step testing with ELISA and Western immunoblotting remains the gold standard for diagnosing later stages of Lyme disease. In this study by Steere et al., over 90% of patients with disseminated disease and 100% of patients with late disease had a positive two-step test result. The authors were also able to demonstrate increased sensitivity using a single-step IgG C6 peptide ELISA. This test warrants further investigation in a broader patient population.

Early Lyme disease. Wormser GP. N Engl J Med 2006. 354; 2794–801.

The clinical assessment, treatment, and prevention of Lyme disease, human granulocytic anaplasmosis, and babesiosis: clinical practice guidelines by the Infectious Diseases Society of America. Wormser GP, Dattwyler RJ, Shapiro ED, et al. Clin Infect Dis 2006; 43: 1089–134.

A critical appraisal of 'chronic Lyme disease.' Feder Jr HM, Johnson BJB, O'Connell S, Shapiro ED, Steere AC, Wormser GP; Ad Hoc International Disease Group. N Engl J Med 2007; 357: 1422–30.

Practice parameter: Treatment of nervous system Lyme disease (an evidence-based review). Report of the Quality Standards Subcommittee of the American Academy of Neurology. Halperin JJ, Shapiro ED, Logigian E, Belman AL, Dotevall L, Wormser GP, et al. Neurology 2007; 69: 1–12.

FIRST-LINE THERAPIES

Early localized disease (erythema migrans, borrelial lymphocytoma)

▶ Doxycycline 100 mg twice daily for 10–21 days (contraindicated in pregnancy, children <8 years)   A
▶ Amoxicillin 500 mg three times daily for 14–21 days   A
▶ Cefuroxime axetil 500 mg twice daily for 14–21 days   A

Early disseminated disease (neurologic involvement or advanced cardiac conduction abnormalities)

▶ Ceftriaxone 2 g IV daily for 14–28 days   B
▶ Penicillin G 18–24 million units daily (divided and dosed every 4 hours) for 14–28 day   B

Late neuroborreliosis or Lyme arthritis with neurologic involvement

▶ Ceftriaxone 2 g IV daily for 14–28 days   B
▶ Cefotaxime 2 g IV 150–200 mg/kg/day (in three to four divided doses)   B
▶ Penicillin G 18–24 million units daily (divided and dosed every 4 hours) for 14–28 days   B

Lyme arthritis without neurologic involvement

▶ Doxycycline 100 mg twice daily for 28 days   B
▶ Amoxicillin 500 mg three times daily for 28 days   B
▶ If an oral regimen fails, it is reasonable to use parenteral therapy with ceftriaxone or penicillin G for 14–28 days   B

Prophylaxis with single-dose doxycycline for the prevention of Lyme disease after an *Ixodes scapularis* tick bite. Nadelman RB, Nowakowski J, Fish D, Falco RC, Freeman K, McKenna D, et al.; Tick Bite Study Group. N Engl J Med 2001; 345: 79–84.

In this investigation, 482 patients were randomized to receive 200 mg doxycycline or placebo within 72 hours of removal of an *I. scapularis* tick. One of 235 subjects (0.4%) who received doxycycline developed erythema migrans, compared to eight of 247 (3.2%) who received placebo. No asymptomatic seroconversions occurred and no subject developed extracutaneous Lyme disease. Prophylaxis was effective at reducing the development of Lyme disease. More gastrointestinal symptoms occurred with doxycycline.

Amoxicillin plus probenecid versus doxycycline for treatment of erythema migrans borreliosis. Dattwyler RJ, Volkman DJ, Conaty SM, Platkin SP, Luft BJ. Lancet 1990; 336: 1404–6.

Seventy-two adults with early Lyme disease were randomized to either amoxicillin 500 mg three times daily or doxycycline 100 mg twice daily for 3 weeks. Both groups had 100% cure rates of their erythema migrans and were asymptomatic after a 6-month follow-up period.

Comparison of cefuroxime axetil and doxycycline in the treatment of early Lyme disease. Nadelman RB, Luger SW, Frank E, Wisniewski M, Collins JJ, Wormser GP. Ann Intern Med 1992; 117: 273–80.

A randomized, multicenter, investigator-blinded trial treated 123 patients with erythema migrans for 20 days with either cefuroxime axetil 500 mg twice daily (n=63) or doxycycline 100 mg twice daily (n=60). Cure or improvement was achieved in 51 of 55 (93%) evaluable patients treated with cefuroxime axetil, and in 45 of 51 (88%) patients treated with doxycycline. At 1 year post treatment the percentage of patients who achieved a satisfactory outcome was comparable between the two groups. Cefuroxime was associated with more diarrhea than was doxycycline and is more expensive than doxycycline or amoxicillin.

Duration of antibiotic therapy for early Lyme disease. Wormser GP, Ramanathan R, Nowakowski J, McKenna D, Holmgren D, Visintainer P, et al. Ann Intern Med 2003; 138: 697–704.

In this study, 180 patients with erythema migrans were randomized to receive 10 days of oral doxycycline, with or without a single intravenous dose of ceftriaxone, or 20 days of oral doxycycline. The complete response rate at 30 months was similar in all groups: 83.9% in the 20-day doxycycline group, 90.3% in the 10-day doxycycline group, and 86.5% in the doxycycline/ceftriaxone group. Diarrhea occurred more frequently in the ceftriaxone group.

Two controlled trials of antibiotic treatment in patients with persistent symptoms and a history of Lyme disease. Klempner MS, Hu LT, Evans J, Schmid CH, Johnson GM, Trevino RP, et al. N Engl J Med 2001; 345: 85–92.

Patients with persistent symptoms after previously treated Lyme disease were randomized to receive either intravenous ceftriaxone 2 g daily for 30 days followed by oral doxycycline 200 mg daily for 60 days, or matching placebos. This study was halted after planned interim analysis of the first 107 subjects indicated that it would be unlikely to reveal a significant difference in outcomes between the groups.

SECOND-LINE THERAPIES

Treatment of the early manifestations of Lyme disease. Steere AC, Hutchinson GJ, Rahn DW, Sigal LH, Craft JE, DeSanna ET, et al. Ann Intern Med 1983; 99: 22–6.

During 1980 and 1981, the authors compared antibiotic regimens in 108 adult patients with early Lyme disease. Erythema migrans and associated symptoms improved faster in patients treated with penicillin or tetracycline than in those given erythromycin. None of 39 patients given tetracycline developed major late complications (meningoencephalitis, myocarditis, or recurrent arthritis), compared to three of 40 given penicillin and four of 29 given erythromycin. Based on this and similar studies, erythromycin is considered less efficacious than first-line therapies.

Azithromycin compared with amoxicillin in the treatment of erythema migrans. A double-blind, randomized, controlled trial. Luft BJ, Dattwyler RJ, Johnson RC, Luger SW, Bosler EM, Rahn DW, et al. Ann Intern Med 1996; 124: 785–91.

In this report, 246 adults with erythema migrans were randomized to either amoxicillin 500 mg three times daily for 20 days or azithromycin 500 mg once daily for 7 days. Those treated with amoxicillin were more likely to achieve complete resolution of disease at day 20 (88% for amoxicillin compared with 76% for azithromycin). More azithromycin recipients (16%) than amoxicillin recipients (4%) had relapses.

Lymphangioma circumscriptum

Patrick OM Emanuel

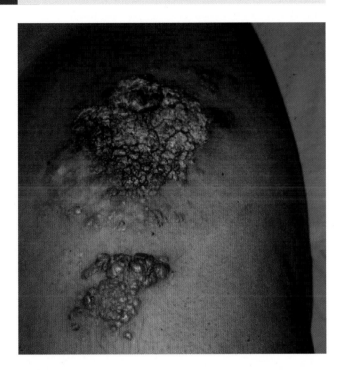

Lymphangioma circumscriptum is an uncommon subcutaneous variant of lymphangioma in which subcutaneous lymphatic cisterns communicate through dilated channels with superficial clusters of vesicles. It presents on the skin surface as grapelike groups of thin-walled translucent lymph-filled vesicles, often compared to frog spawn.

More commonly congenital, they are typically noted at birth or appear during childhood. There is a morphologically identical acquired variant related to lymphatic obstruction as a consequence of surgery, radiation, or malignancy.

MANAGEMENT STRATEGIES

Although observation is an appropriate option for many cases, cosmetic concern is the typical indication for treatment. Other indications may include persistent leakage of lymphatic fluid or blood, and recurrent infection. The risk of developing angiosarcoma and squamous cell carcinoma is trivial and certainly should not be used to rationalize full surgical excision.

Treatment is challenging and often thwarted by local recurrences owing to the persistence of deep lymphatic cisterns which may navigate deep into the subcuticular adipose tissue, skeletal muscle, and nerves. Every treatment option has associated recurrence rates/complication profiles. Consequently, there is disagreement in the literature as to which treatment option is the most effective. Although *complete surgical excision* has the lowest recurrence rates, it has the highest rate of complications; more extensive lesions may be deemed inoperable.

Sclerotherapy using a variety of sclerosants has been advocated as a less invasive and effective treatment modality which is either a first-line alternative or an adjunct to surgery.

Other authorities suggest that after definitive diagnosis and radiologic mapping, surgical excision and postoperative histologic assessment of excision margins provides the most effect treatment option.

Resurfacing of the lesions can be attempted and achieved even if proper surgical excision is not possible and/or sclerotherapy fails, but recurrence rates are usually higher than with other therapies. The high-energy, short-pulse CO_2 laser has been found to yield functionally and cosmetically acceptable results. This seals communicating channels to the deeper cisterns by vaporizing the superficial lymphatics, and is said to have fewer complications than more aggressive treatment alternatives. Other laser methods, particularly the pulsed dye laser, have also been shown to be effective in selected superficial cases.

SPECIFIC INVESTIGATIONS

> ▶ Biopsy
> ▶ Imaging studies
> ▶ MRI
> ▶ Lymphangiography
> ▶ Ultrasound

In the majority of cases the clinical diagnosis is straightforward. In some, the differential diagnosis may be broad: genital lesions are often associated with verrucous changes, which give them a warty appearance and are often confused with viral warts or squamous cell carcinoma; discoloration of the vesicles can lead to confusion with hemangiomas and even malignant melanoma; herpetic infection and dermatitis herpetiformis are less frequent differential diagnoses. Biopsy is diagnostic for clinically unusual cases and exhibits numerous thick-walled, dilated lymphatic channels encroaching on this epidermis (which may become hyperkeratotic), expanding the papillary dermis and extending deep into the dermis and subcutis. Immunostaining with VEGFR3 and D2–40 decorates the vessels and confirms their lymphatic origin.

MRI can define the entire anatomy of a lesion and, when used preoperatively, can help prevent unnecessarily extensive or incomplete surgical resection. CT, ultrasound, and lymphoscintigraphy have also been useful in determining the extent of a lesion.

Secondary lesions may be investigated for an underlying cause if the cause is not clinically obvious. Lymphangiomas may be associated with rare disorders such as Proteus, Cobb and Klippel–Trenaunay syndromes, and so appropriate investigations and consultations should be sought if these conditions are suspected.

FIRST-LINE THERAPIES

▷ Conservative/observation	A
▷ Antibiotics	D
▷ Sclerotherapy	A
▷ OK-432	A
▷ Hyperosmolar saline	D
▷ Sodium tetradecyl sulfate	E
▷ Surgery	A

Intralesional sclerotherapy with group A *Streptococcus pyogenes* of human origin (OK-432) has emerged as an effective sclerosing agent.

OK-432 therapy in 64 patients with lymphangioma. Ogita S, Tsuto T, Nakamura K, Deguchi E, Iwai N. J Pediatr Surg 1994; 29: 784–5.

A case of unresectable lymphangioma circumscriptum of the vulva successfully treated with OK-432 in childhood. Ahn SJ, Chang SE, Choi JH, Moon KC, Koh JK, Kim DY. J Am Acad Dermatol 2006; 55: S106–7.

Treatment of lymphangioma in children: our experience of 128 cases. Okazaki T, Iwatani S, Yanai T, Kobayashi H, Kato Y, Marusasa T, et al. J Pediatr Surg 2007; 42: 386–9.

Intracystic injection of OK-432: a new sclerosing therapy for cystic hygroma in children. Ogita S, Tsuto T, Tokiwa K, Takahashi T. Br J Surg 1987; 74: 690–1.

The main advantage of OK-432 over other sclerosing agents is the absence of perilesional fibrosis. OK-432 is an effective agent for cases of a single or limited numbers of cysts. In larger lesions the technique is useful as a pretreatment adjunct to surgical excision.

Lymphangioma circumscriptum: treatment with hypertonic saline sclerotherapy. Bikowski JB, Dumont AM. J Am Acad Dermatol 2005; 53: 442–4.

Hypertonic saline has been reported to be effective for the management of LC to the shoulder, although wider use of this agent in comparison with other treatments for LC has not been reported.

Percutaneous sclerotherapy of lymphangioma. Molitch HI, Unger EC, Witte CL, van Sonnenberg E. Radiology 1995; 194: 343–7.

Five patients with unresectable lymphangiomas of the pelvis (n=2), neck (n=1), abdomen (n=1), or leg (n=1) were treated at two medical centers with sclerotherapy, using doxycycline as the sclerosant.

Treatment of unusual vascular lesions: usefulness of sclerotherapy in lymphangioma circumscriptum and acquired digital arteriovenous malformation. Park CO, Lee MJ, Chung KY. Dermatol Surg 2005; 31: 1451–3.

Two cases of lymphangioma circumscriptum were treated with a sclerosant, sodium tetradecyl sulfate, and were almost cleared with several treatments of sclerotherapy.

Surgery

Treatment of lymphangioma in children: our experience of 128 cases. Okazaki T, Iwatani S, Yanai T, Kobayashi H, Kato Y, Marusasa T, et al. J Pediatr Surg 2007; 42: 386–9.

Primary surgical excision was significantly more successful than sclerotherapy, but the results are often unsatisfactory because of complications, including damage to surrounding structures, particularly nerves and blood vessels, scarring, and recurrence owing to incomplete excision. Ultrasound and magnetic resonance imaging demonstrates deep cisterns, thereby ensuring deeper excision of these structures and less risk of recurrence.

Surgical management of 'lymphangioma circumscriptum'. Browse NL, Whimster I, Stewart G, Helm CW, Wood JJ. Br J Surg 1986; 73: 585–9.

Confirmation of the completeness of excision can be obtained using frozen section analysis of the lateral and deep margins.

Lymphangioma circumscriptum of the vulva mimicking genital wart: a case report and review of literature. Sah SP, Yadav R, Rani S. J Obstet Gynaecol Res 2001; 27: 293–6.

A case report of vulval LC, clinically diagnosed as a genital wart. Following biopsy, the patient required extensive vulval surgery and there was no recurrence after 16 months.

Surgical management of penoscrotal lymphangioma circumscriptum. Latifoglu O, Yavuzer R, Demir Y, Ayhan S, Yenidünya S, Atabay K. Plast Reconstruct Surg 1999; 103: 175–8.

An extensive lymphangioma circumscriptum of the penis and scrotum that was treated by wide excision in single-stage surgery. At the 14th postoperative month the patient was free of recurrence.

Lymphangioma circumscriptum: pitfalls and problems in definitive management. Bond J, Basheer MH, Gordon D. Dermatol Surg 2008; 34: 271–5.

Two cases of surgical excision with no recurrence at 1 and 2 years. Imaging of deep communicating structures and histologic assessment of excision margins provide the greatest chance of non-recurrence.

SECOND-LINE THERAPIES

▶ Carbon dioxide laser	D
▶ Pulsed dye laser	D
▶ Radiotherapy	E
▶ Cryotherapy	D
▶ Argon laser	D
▶ Suction-assisted lipectomy	D

Carbon dioxide laser vaporization of lymphangioma circumscriptum. Bailin PL, Kantor GR, Wheeland RG. J Am Acad Dermatol 1986; 14: 257–62.

Carbon dioxide laser in a vaporization mode successfully ablated superficial cutaneous lesions in seven patients with lymphangioma circumscriptum.

Lymphangioma circumscriptum: review and evaluation of carbon dioxide laser vaporization. Eliezri YD, Sklar JA. J Dermatol Surg Oncol 1988; 14: 357–64.

Three patients were treated with carbon dioxide laser vaporization, with good to excellent cosmetic results and complete resolution of their symptoms.

CO_2 laser therapy of vulval lymphangiectasia and lymphangioma circumscriptum. Huilgol SC, Neill S, Barlow RJ. Dermatol Surg 2002; 28: 575–7.

Focal recurrence and an area of localized persistence were noted in both patients with lymphangioma circumscriptum treated with CO_2 laser therapy.

CO_2 laser therapy of vulval lymphangiectasia and lymphangioma circumscriptum. Haas AF, Narurkar VA. Dermatol Surg 1998; 24: 893–5.

A difficult case of lymphangioma circumscriptum was treated successfully with a high-energy, short-pulse CO_2 laser following two failed surgical excisions.

Evidence Levels: **A** Double-blind study   **B** Clinical trial ≥ 20 subjects   **C** Clinical trial < 20 subjects   **D** Series ≥ 5 subjects   **E** Anecdotal case reports

CO₂ laser ablation of lymphangioma circumscriptum of the scrotum. Treharne LJ, Murison MS. Lymphat Res Biol 2006; 4: 101–3.

Widespread disease of the scrotum had excellent symptomatic relief following treatment with the CO_2 laser.

Treatment of lymphangioma circumscriptum with the intense pulsed light system. Thissen CA, Sommer A. Int J Dermatol 2007; 46: 16–18.

An intense pulsed light source led to good cosmetic results.

Treatment of lymphangioma circumscriptum with combined radiofrequency current and 900 nm diode laser. Lapidoth M, Ackerman L, Amitai DB, Raveh E, Kalish E, David M. Dermatol Surg 2006; 32: 790–4.

Treatment was rated as 'excellent' in four patients and 'good' in two. Swelling, erythema, and pain were present in all patients, and ulcers and scarring in two.

Lymphangioma circumscriptum treated with pulsed dye laser. Lai CH, Hanson SG, Mallory SB. Pediatr Dermatol 2001; 18: 509–10.

A child with a symptomatic lymphangioma circumscriptum was treated with pulsed dye laser, with good results.

Radiotherapy in congenital vulvar lymphangioma circumscriptum. Yildiz F, Atahan IL, Ozhar E, Karcaaltincaba M, Cengiz M, Ozyigit G, et al. Int J Gynecol Cancer. 2007 [Epub ahead of print]

A patient was treated successfully with a course of external radiotherapy following failed attempts with sclerosing agents and surgery.

Radiotherapy is a useful treatment for lymphangioma circumscriptum: a report of two patients. Denton AS, Baker-Hines R, Spittle MF. Clin Oncol (Roy Coll Radiol) 1996; 8: 400–1.

Localized radiotherapy has been successfully used.

Lymphedema

Geover Fernández, Giuseppe Micali, Robert A Schwartz

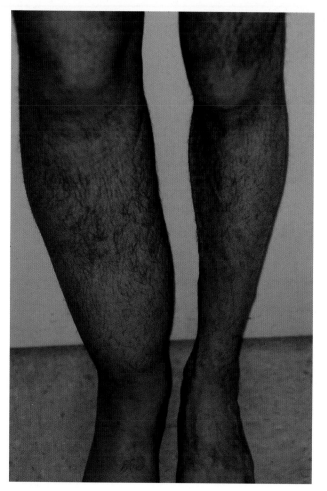

Lymphedema is a chronic, sometimes debilitating condition characterized clinically by its brawny, non-pitting edema. It is due to the accumulation of protein-rich lymph in interstitial spaces as a result of ineffective lymphatic drainage. Lymphedema is classified into primary and secondary forms. Primary lymphedema is caused by a developmental malformation of the lymphatic system. Primary congenital lymphedema (Milroy disease) is an uncommon autosomal dominant disorder due, in some families, to missense mutations that interfere with vascular endothelial growth factor receptor-3 signaling, resulting in abnormal lymphatic vascular function. Primary lymphedema may be further classified by age of onset into congenital lymphedema, lymphedema praecox, and lymphedema tarda. Secondary lymphedema is usually due to blockage or destruction of otherwise normal lymph channels. In the United States the most common causes are compression by tumor, surgical manipulation, or radiation damage. Worldwide, the most common cause is filariasis. Acquired lymphedema may predispose to an aggressive type of angiosarcoma, best documented post

mastectomy and known as the Stewart–Treves syndrome. Chronic lymphedema may result in verrucous and proliferative changes resembling elephant skin (elephantiasis).

MANAGEMENT STRATEGIES

Lymphedema must be distinguished from edema of cardiac, hepatic, and renal origin. Lymphoscintigraphy (isotope lymphography) is a first-line imaging modality to evaluate and diagnose disorders of the lymphatic vasculature. The treatment options are basically the same. A *medical, conservative approach* is the standard of treatment for lymphedema. The main management strategy is to *reduce stagnation of protein-rich lymph in the extravascular tissue* and to *improve the outflow of lymphatic circulation*.

Complete decongestive therapy represents a superb treatment plan. It is a four-component therapeutic modality composed of *multilayer compression bandage, manual lymphatic drainage, skin care*, and *exercise*. Patients should be encouraged to use compression bandages or garments continuously during the day, as well as leg elevation. *Pneumatic compression pumps* were widely used to control lymphedema, but owing to their poor outcome as a monotherapy their current use has been limited. Medications, such as *diuretics*, have shown limited or no effect on lymphedema. *Meticulous skin care and hygiene* may prevent secondary bacterial and fungal infections. At the earliest sign of infection, *topical and systemic antibiotics* should be administered to prevent sepsis. This is especially important because recurrent infections may lead to further lymphatic injury.

Surgical approaches are reserved for cases recalcitrant to conservative management. *Microsurgical lymphaticovenous implantation* combined with decongestive therapy has yielded excellent results. *Excisional surgical therapy* has been performed to reduce limb size and to improve mobility in chronic advanced cases of lymphedema.

SPECIFIC INVESTIGATIONS

▶ Lymphoscintigraphy
▶ MRI
▶ CT

Advances in imaging of lymph flow disorders. Witte CL, Witte MH, Unger EC, Williams WH, Bernas MJ, McNeill GC, et al. Radiographics 2000; 6: 1697–719.

An excellent review article illustrating multiple clinical cases in which lymphoscintigraphy, MRI, and CT were useful in the evaluation and diagnosis of patients with primary or secondary lymphedema.

The advantages and limitations of each imaging modality are reviewed.

Imaging of the lymphatic system: new horizons. Barrett T, Choyke PL, Kobayashi H. Contrast Media Mol Imag 2006; 1: 230–45.

In this article useful information on the most recent developments in soft tissue imaging, including radionuclide-based imaging positron emission tomography (PET), dynamic contrast-enhanced MRI (DCE-MRI) and color Doppler ultrasound (CDUS), and their applications are highlighted. Although none of these techniques is able to detect lymphatic flow, they may be useful to rule out secondary lymphedema in the oncology setting by providing a functional assessment of node status.

FIRST-LINE THERAPIES

▶ Decongestive lymphatic therapy   **B**

Efficacy of complete decongestive therapy and manual lymphatic drainage on treatment-related lymphedema in breast cancer. Koul R, Dufan T, Russell C, Guenther W, Nugent Z, Sun X, et al. Int J Radiat Oncol Biol Phys 2007; 67: 841–6.

This study documented a significant reduction in lymphedema volume in 250 patients with breast cancer-related lymphedema treated with combined decongestive therapy and manual lymphatic drainage with exercises.

Can manual treatment of lymphedema promote metastasis? Godette K, Mondry TE, Johnstone PA. J Soc Integr Oncol 2006; 4: 8–12.

There are several contraindications to performing complete decongestive therapy (CDT). These include hypertension, paralysis, diabetes mellitus, bronchial asthma, acute infections, and congestive heart failure. Malignant disease is also widely considered a contraindication to CDT. However, this opinion is not unequivocally supported by current cancer research.

SECOND-LINE THERAPIES

▶ Pneumatic compression therapy   **B**

Decongestive lymphatic therapy for patients with breast carcinoma-associated lymphedema. A randomized, prospective study of a role for adjunctive intermittent pneumatic compression. Szuba A, Achalu R, Rockson SG. Cancer 2002; 95: 2260–7.

A prospective randomized study of 23 patients comparing decongestive lymphatic therapy alone versus decongestive lymphatic therapy plus intermittent pneumatic compression. Intermittent pneumatic compression proved effective as an adjunct to decongestive therapy.

THIRD-LINE THERAPIES

▶ Surgery   **B**
▶ Endermologie   **B**
▶ Sorafenib   **E**

Follow-up study of upper limb lymphedema patients treated by microsurgical lymphaticovenous implantation (MLVI) combined with compression therapy. Yamamoto Y, Horiuchi K, Sasaki S, Sekido M, Furukawa H, Oyama A, et al. Microsurgery 2003; 23: 21–6.

A follow-up study of 18 patients treated by microsurgical lymphaticovenous implantation combined with compression therapy showed favorable results in 78% of patients. Average follow-up was 2 years.

Lymphatic microsurgery for the treatment of lymphedema. Campisi C, Davini D, Bellini C, Taddei G, Villa G, Fulcheri E, et al. Microsurgery 2006; 26: 65–9.

Of the 447 patients followed, 380 (85%) have been able to discontinue the use of conservative measures, with an average follow-up of more than 7 years and average reduction in excess volume of 69%. There was an 87% reduction in incidence of cellulitis after microsurgery.

Pediatric lymphedema and correlated syndromes: role of microsurgery. Campisi C, Da Rin E, Bellini C, Bonioli E, Boccardo F. Microsurgery 2008; 28: 138–42.

Microsurgical methods may provide successful and long-lasting results, with both derivative lymphaticovenous anastomoses and reconstructive lymphaticovenous–lymphatic anastomoses. Better long-term results are obtained in earlier stages, before tissue fibrosis and sclerosis ensue.

Endermologie (with and without compression bandaging)– a new treatment option for secondary arm lymphedema. Moseley AL, Esplin M, Piller NB, Douglass Jl. Lymphology 2007; 40: 129–37.

Two studies of 24 and 10 women treated respectively by LPG Endermologie combined with compression bandaging showed reductions in limb volume (134 and 185 mL), limb fluid (182 and 216 mL), truncal fluid (342 and 290 mL), as well as amelioration of fibrotic induration in some lymphatic territories, with significant improvements in subjects' reporting of heaviness, tightness, tissue hardness, and limb size.

Dramatic reduction of chronic lymphoedema of the lower limb with sorafenib therapy. Moncrieff M, Shannon K, Hong A, Hersey P, Thompson J. Melanoma Res 2008; 18: 161–2.

This paper describes a 34-year-old woman with metastatic melanoma after lymph node dissection followed by radiotherapy who had an extraordinary reduction in her chronic lymphedema while on the broad-spectrum RAF-kinase inhibitor sorafenib.

Lymphocytoma cutis

Fiona J Child, Sean J Whittaker

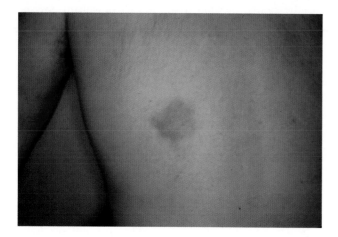

Lymphocytoma cutis (cutaneous lymphoid hyperplasia, cutaneous B-cell pseudolymphoma, Spiegler–Fendt sarcoid) is an entity encompassing a spectrum of benign B-cell lymphoproliferative diseases that share clinical and histopathologic features. Various stimuli can induce lymphocytoma cutis, but in most cases the cause is not known. It is more common in females, with a female-to-male ratio of 3:1. Most cases are characterized by localized erythematous, plum-colored nodules and plaques that may be difficult to distinguish from cutaneous B-cell lymphoma. Less frequently the generalized form may present with multiple miliary papules that measure a few millimeters in diameter. Lymphocytoma cutis secondary to *Borrelia* infection is most frequently seen at sites where skin temperature is low, such as the earlobes, nipples, nose, and scrotum.

MANAGEMENT STRATEGY

A skin biopsy for histopathology and immunohistochemistry is required to confirm the diagnosis, but the distinction between lymphocytoma cutis and cutaneous B-cell lymphoma may be difficult on both clinical and histopathologic evaluation. There are no agreed histologic criteria; however, features that suggest lymphocytoma cutis include well-formed, non-expanded, reactive germinal centers, the majority of the infiltrate consisting of small round lymphocytes with a B-:T-cell ratio of <3:1 and polytypic expression of κ and λ light chains. A further feature is the presence of numerous tingible-body macrophages within the lymphoid follicles. Molecular analysis of the immunoglobulin heavy chain gene has shown that a significant proportion harbor B-cell clones, which suggests that many cases previously thought to be lymphocytoma cutis represent indolent low-grade primary cutaneous B-cell lymphomas (PCBCL). Therefore, in cases with a detectable B-cell clone a careful evaluation to exclude systemic disease (a thorough clinical examination, thoracoabdominopelvic CT scan, and bone marrow biopsy) is required, with adequate long-term follow-up.

A history of possible stimuli known to cause lymphocytoma cutis should be sought; these include *Borrelia burgdorferi* infection, trauma, vaccinations, allergy hyposensitization injections, ingestion of drugs, arthropod bites, acupuncture, gold pierced earrings, tattoos, treatment with leeches (*Hirudo medicinalis*), and post herpes zoster scars, but the majority of cases are of unknown etiology.

The course of the disease varies but tends to be chronic and indolent, and some lesions may resolve spontaneously without treatment. There is no therapy of proven value for lymphocytoma cutis, with only anecdotal case reports and small series reported and no clinical trials in the literature.

If a cause can be identified, the causative agent should be removed. If infection with *Borrelia burgdorferi* is suspected, treatment with appropriate *antibiotics (amoxycillin* 500–1000 mg three times per day, or *doxycycline* 100 mg two to three times per day for at least 3 weeks) should be initiated.

Localized disease can be treated by simple *excision* and may respond to *intralesional injection of corticosteroids, local irradiation*, or *intralesional interferon-α*. More widespread (generalized) disease is traditionally treated with *oral antimalarials*, most commonly *hydroxychloroquine* (maximum dose 6.5 mg/kg/day); however, lesions may fail to respond to treatment or may recur following cessation of therapy. Other treatment modalities include *subcutaneous interferon-α and oral thalidomide*. Effective responses to destructive therapies, including *cryotherapy* and the *argon laser*, have been reported. A subtype of generalized lymphocytoma cutis may be exacerbated by light, and therefore *sun avoidance* and the use of *sun block* is important.

SPECIFIC INVESTIGATIONS

> ▶ Serology for *Borrelia burgdorferi* (antibodies identified in 50% of patients with borrelial lymphocytoma)
> ▶ Skin biopsy for histology, immunophenotype, and immunoglobulin gene analysis
> ▶ Patch testing (if a possible contact allergen is suspected)

The spirochetal etiology of lymphadenosis benigna cutis solitaria. Hovmark A, Asbrink E, Olsson I. Acta Dermatol Venereol (Stockh) 1986; 66: 479–84.

Of 10 patients investigated, four reported a previous tick bite. Positive *Borrelia* serology was found in six of nine patients, and spirochetes were cultivated from one of two skin biopsies.

Lymphadenosis benigna cutis resulting from *Borrelia* infection (*Borrelia* lymphocytoma). Albrecht S, Hofstadter MD, Artsob H, Chaban RT. J Am Acad Dermatol 1991; 24: 621–5.

A child who developed lymphocytoma cutis on her ear following a tick bite 6 months previously had positive *Borrelia* serology and a *Borrelia*-like organism was identified in skin biopsy sections. The lesion regressed during a 2-month course of penicillin V.

Cutaneous lymphoid hyperplasia and cutaneous marginal zone lymphoma: Comparison of morphologic and immunophenotypic features. Baldassano MF, Bailey EM, Ferry JA, Harris NL, Duncan LM. Am J Surg Pathol 1999; 23: 88–96.

The histologic and immunophenotypic features of 14 cases of lymphocytoma cutis and 16 cases of cutaneous marginal zone lymphoma were compared.

Differential diagnosis of cutaneous infiltrates of B lymphocytes with follicular growth pattern. Leinweber B, Colli C, Chott A, Kerl H, Cerroni L. Am J Dermatopathol 2004; 26: 4–13.

The histopathologic, immunophenotypic, and molecular features of *Borrelia burgdorfori*-associated lymphocytoma cutis, primary cutaneous follicle center cell lymphoma, and primary cutaneous marginal zone lymphoma were compared. Features that favored lymphocytoma cutis were the presence of tingible-body macrophages, strong proliferation rate of follicular cells, BCL-2-negative follicular cells, and the absence of monoclonality.

***Borrelia burgdorfori*-associated lymphocytoma cutis: clinicopathologic, immunophenotypic, and molecular study of 106 cases.** Colli C, Leinweber B, Müllegger R, Chott A, Kerl H, Cerroni L. J Cutan Pathol 2004; 31: 232–40.

One hundred and six cases of *Borrelia burgdorfori*-associated lymphocytoma cutis, in a region endemic for borrelia infection, were studied retrospectively. The most common sites affected were the earlobe, genital area, and nipple (these locations may be due to the predilection of *Borrelia burgdorfori* spirochetes for cooler body sites). In some cases the histopathologic, immunophenotypic, and molecular features were misleading, and it was concluded that integration of all data is necessary to obtain the correct diagnosis.

Clonal rearrangements of immunoglobulin genes and progression to B cell lymphoma in cutaneous lymphoid hyperplasia. Wood GS, Ngan BY, Tung R, Hoffman TE, Abel EA, Hoppe RT, et al. Am J Pathol 1989; 135: 13–19.

In this study, five of 14 cases of cutaneous lymphoid hyperplasia exhibited a clonal immunoglobulin rearrangement by Southern blot analysis. One of these evolved into a diffuse large B-cell lymphoma during a 2-year follow-up period, suggesting that monoclonal populations may exist in some cases of cutaneous lymphoid hyperplasia, and these may represent a subgroup more likely to evolve into lymphoma.

Immunophenotypic and genotypic analysis in cutaneous lymphoid hyperplasias. Hammer E, Sangueza O, Suwanjindar P, White CR, Braziel R. J Am Acad Dermatol 1993; 28: 426–33.

Of 11 patients with histologic and immunophenotypic features of lymphocytoma cutis, clonal rearrangements were detected in two, both of whom subsequently developed B-cell lymphoma.

Polymerase chain reaction analysis of immunoglobulin gene rearrangement analysis in cutaneous lymphoid hyperplasias. Bouloc A, Delfau-Larue M-H, Lenormand B, Meunier F, Wechsler J, Thomine E, et al. Arch Dermatol 1999; 135: 168–72.

Twenty-four patients with a diagnosis of lymphocytoma cutis according to clinical, histopathologic, and immunophenotypic criteria underwent PCR analysis of the immunoglobulin heavy chain gene using DNA from lesional skin. In one patient a B-cell clone was detected. In the other 23 a polyclonal result was obtained.

Cutaneous B-cell lymphomas are known to have a relatively high false-negative rate using PCR owing to somatic hypermutation, which affects the variable region of the immunoglobulin heavy chain gene and may prevent primer binding. The number of false-negative results may be reduced by using multiple primer sets for different parts of the variable region. This paper only used one set of primers, and therefore the detection of only one B-cell clone may be a significant underestimate.

Lymphomatoid contact reaction to gold earrings. Fleming C, Burden D, Fallowfield M, Lever R. Contact Derm 1997; 37: 298–9.

A rare entity characterized by nodules at sites of piercing with gold jewelry and the histologic features of lymphocytoma cutis. Patch tests to gold sodium thiosulfate are positive.

FIRST-LINE THERAPIES

Localized

▶ Excision	E
▶ Topical corticosteroids	E
▶ Intralesional corticosteroids	E
▶ Oral antibiotics (if positive *Borrelia* serology)	E

Generalized

▶ Antimalarials	E
▶ Sun avoidance/sunblock (light exacerbated)	E

Treatment of cutaneous pseudolymphoma with hydroxychloroquine. Stoll DM. J Am Acad Dermatol 1983; 8: 696–9.

A case report of a 40-year-old woman with generalized lymphocytoma cutis that cleared with 400 mg hydroxychloroquine daily.

A study of the photosensitivity factor in cutaneous lymphocytoma. Frain-Bell W, Magnus IA. Br J Dermatol 1971; 84: 25–31.

Patients with lymphocytoma and associated light sensitivity are reported and previous cases reviewed.

SECOND-LINE THERAPIES

Localized

▶ Superficial radiotherapy	E
▶ Intralesional interferon-α	E
▶ Argon laser	E
▶ Cryotherapy	D
▶ Topical 0.1% tacrolimus ointment	E

Generalized

▶ Subcutaneous interferon-α_{2b}	E
▶ Thalidomide	E

Cutaneous lymphoid hyperplasia: results of radiation therapy. Olson LE, Wilson JF, Cox JD. Radiology 1985; 155: 507–9.

Four cases of lymphocytoma cutis were treated with radiation therapy. Over a follow-up period of 8 months to 7 years there were no recurrences.

Local orthovolt radiotherapy in primary cutaneous B-cell lymphoma. Pimpinelli N, Vallecchi C. Skin Cancer 1999; 14: 219–24.

Data from 115 patients with PCBCL produced a 98.2% complete remission rate and a median disease-free period of 55 months; recurrences were mostly limited to the skin. In view of the difficulties in distinguishing between PCBCL and lymphocytoma cutis, many groups have used superficial radiotherapy in cases of lymphocytoma cutis, although evidence remains anecdotal.

In our experience these cases are relatively radio-resistant compared to PCBCL.

Role of the argon laser in treatment of lymphocytoma cutis. Wheeland RG, Kantor GR, Bailin PL, Bergfeld WF. J Am Acad Dermatol 1986; 14: 267–72.

The argon laser improved cosmetic appearance and alleviated symptoms of lymphocytoma cutis but failed to provide complete histological clearing in a young man who had failed to respond adequately to initial therapy with hydroxychloroquine.

Lymphocytoma cutis: a series of five patients successfully treated with cryosurgery. Kuflik AS, Schwartz RA. J Am Acad Dermatol 1992; 26: 449–52.

Five patients with lymphocytoma cutis underwent therapy with liquid nitrogen to individual lesions using a single cycle of 15–20 seconds per lesion, with complete clinical resolution of all lesions treated within 3–6 weeks.

Spiegler–Fendt type lymphocytoma cutis: a case report of two patients successfully treated with interferon alpha-2b. Hervonen K, Lehtinen T, Vaalasti A. Acta Dermatol Venereol (Stockh) 1999; 79: 241–2.

Two men, who had generalized lymphocytoma cutis and had failed to respond to other therapies, were treated with subcutaneous interferon-α_{2b} 2.5 MU three times per week, with complete resolution of all lesions by 3 months. However, lesions recurred in both men between 6 and 23 months after the completion of treatment.

Treatment of cutaneous lymphoid hyperplasia with thalidomide: report of two cases. Benchikhi H, Bodemer C, Fraitag S, Wechsler J, Delfau-Larue M-H, Gounod N, et al. J Am Acad Dermatol 1999; 40: 1005–7.

Two cases of lymphocytoma cutis involving the nose that showed complete regression following treatment with thalidomide for 3 months at a dose of 100 mg once daily for 2 months, and 50 mg once daily for the third month. There was no recurrence at respectively 36 and 31 months' follow-up.

Lymphocytoma cutis treated with topical tacrolimus. El-Dars LD, Statham BN, Blackford S, Williams N. Clin Exp Dermatol 2005; 30: 305–7.

Two cases of lymphocytoma cutis affecting the face were treated with topical tacrolimus 0.1% bd. In both cases the lesions completely resolved after 8 months' application.

Lymphogranuloma venereum

Patrice Morel

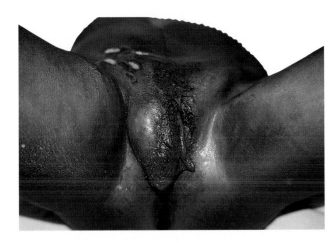

Lymphogranuloma venereum (LGV) is a sexually transmitted disease caused by serovars L1, L2, and L3 of *Chlamydia trachomatis*. LGV is endemic in some areas of Africa, Asia, South America, and the Caribbean. LGV typically presents with one or more genital ulcers, followed by the development of unilateral painful inguinal lymphadenopathy (buboes). Outbreaks of LGV among men having sex with men (MSM) with proctitis have recently been observed outside the traditionally epidemic countries.

MANAGEMENT STRATEGY

Antibiotic treatment of LGV is necessary (a) to prevent the spread of the infection, which may lead to painful inflammation and infection of the inguinal and/or femoral lymph nodes (buboes), rectal and perirectal complications with proctitis followed by abscesses, fistulas, strictures, and genital elephantiasis; (b) to prevent transmission to sexual partners; and (c) to prevent the co-transmission of HIV.

Because LGV is caused by *C. trachomatis*, treatment with either *doxycycline* or *erythromycin* for 21 days is the recommended regimen. Antibiotic treatment cures the ongoing infection and prevents further tissue damage. Patients should be followed clinically until signs and symptoms have resolved. Buboes may require *aspiration* through intact skin to relieve inguinal pain and to prevent the formation of ulcers. The late complications of LGV may necessitate surgical repair after antibiotic treatment is complete.

Patients with HIV infection should be treated with the same regimens. Anecdotal evidence suggests that LGV infection in HIV-positive patients may require prolonged therapy, and that resolution may be delayed.

Sexual partners of patients who have LGV should be examined, tested for urethral or cervical chlamydial infection, and treated if they had sexual contact with the patient during the 30 days preceding the onset of symptoms in the patient.

SPECIFIC INVESTIGATIONS

▶ Chlamydial serology
▶ Culture
▶ Molecular biological diagnostic test

Genital ulcer disease: accuracy of clinical diagnosis and strategies to improve control in Durban, South Africa. O'Farrel N, Hoosen AA, Coetzee KD, Van Den Ende J. Genitourin Med 1994; 70: 7–11.

There is a relatively poor degree of clinical suspicion for lymphogranuloma venereum in countries endemic for chancroid, donovanosis, and lymphogranuloma venereum. In Durban, the accuracy of a clinical diagnosis of lymphogranuloma venereum was 66% in men and 40% in women.

Update on lymphogranuloma venereum in the United Kingdom. Jebbari H, Alexander S, Ward H, Evans B, Solomou M, Thornton A, et al. Sex Transm Infect 2007; 83: 324–6.

An update on the UK experience of LGV between late 2004 and spring 2007: 492 cases of LGV were diagnosed. All were male, 99% of whom had sex with men. Co-infection was considerable: HIV (74 %), hepatitis C (14 %), syphilis (5 %).

Diagnostic and clinical implications of anorectal lymphogranuloma venereum in men who have sex with men: a retrospective case–control study. Van der Bij AK, Spaargaren J, Morré SA, Fennema HS, Mindel A, Coutinho RA, et al. Clin Infect Dis 2006; 42: 186–94.

The authors conducted a retrospective case–control study to identify risk factors for and clinical and diagnostic signs of anorectal LGV infection in men who have sex with men. LGV testing is recommended for these men with anorectal *Chlamydia trachomatis*. Successful treatment of LGV (serovars L1–L3) proctitis requires a 3-week course of doxycycline, whereas in the case of *C. trachomatis* proctitis caused by serovars D–K, a 1-week course is given. If routine LGV serovar typing is unavailable, the authors propose administration of the LGV regimen for men who have sex with men with anorectal *Chlamydia* and either proctitis detected by proctoscopic examination, >10 white blood cells/high-power field detected on an anorectal serovar specimen, or HIV seropositivity.

Lymphogranuloma venereum. Herring A, Richens J. Sex Transm Infect 2006; 82: iv 23–5.

The laboratory diagnosis of LGV is dependent on the detection of *C. trachomatis*-specific DNA followed by genotyping to identify serovars L1, L2, or L3. The first step is the detection of *C. trachomatis* using a nucleic acid amplification test (NAAT). Any NAAT positive for *C. trachomatis* from men who have sex with men should be sent to a reference laboratory for confirmation. Several molecular diagnostic methods specific for LGV detection have been reported (e.g., standard PCR, real-time PCR.). Culture is the most specific, but few laboratories have culture facilities. Serology (complement fixation, microimmunofluorescence IgG) may be useful if direct detection has been unsuccessful. A high titer in a patient with symptoms is highly suggestive of LGV.

A real-time quadriplex PCR assay for the diagnosis of rectal lymphogranuloma venereum and non lymphogranoloma venereum *Chlamydia trachomatis* infections. Chen C-Y, Chi KH, Alexander S, Ison CA, Ballard RC. Sex Transm Infect 2008; 84: 273–6.

A real-time quadriplex PCR assay has been developed that is capable of detecting LGV, non-LGV, or mixed infections simultaneously in rectal specimens.

FIRST-LINE THERAPIES

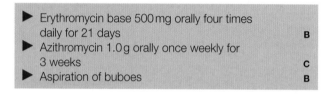

► Doxycycline 100 mg orally twice daily for 21 days **B**

Sexually Transmitted Diseases Treatment Guidelines 2006. Centers for Disease Control and Prevention. MMWR Recomm Rep 2006; 55 (RR-11): 1–94.

Several tetracycline formulations, including doxycycline, and minocycline appeared to be effective. Because of its convenient dosing (100 mg orally twice daily for 21 days) and minimal toxicity, doxycycline remains the recommended treatment for LGV.

SECOND-LINE THERAPIES

► Erythromycin base 500 mg orally four times daily for 21 days **B**
► Azithromycin 1.0 g orally once weekly for 3 weeks **C**
► Aspiration of buboes **B**

Treatment of lymphogranuloma venereum. McLean CA, Stoner BP, Workowski KA. Clin Infect Dis 2007; 44: S 147–52.

Azithromycin (1.0 g orally once weekly for 3 weeks) is likely to be effective against LGV chlamydial infections. The high tissue concentration and long half-life of azithromycin are attractive properties. However, minimal clinical data are available on the effectiveness of azithromycin in the treatment of LGV.

Lymphogranuloma venereum. Becker LE. Int J Dermatol 1976; 15: 26–33.

Buboes should not be surgically incised and drained, or allowed to rupture spontaneously. If the bubo becomes fluctuant and rupture seems likely, it should be aspirated with a large syringe using an 18 or 19-gauge needle. The bubo should be entered through normal skin, preferably superiorly, and not directly through the involved skin to reduce the possibility of sinus tract formation.

Incision and drainage versus aspiration of fluctuant buboes in the emergency department during an epidemic of chancroid. Ernst AA, Marvez-Valls E, Martin DH. Sex Transm Dis 1995; 22: 217–20.

These authors consider that incision and drainage is an effective method for treating fluctuant buboes and may be preferable to traditional needle aspiration, considering the frequency of required re-aspirations.

We do not agree completely with the conclusion of this study, as it includes patients with chancroid and LGV. We think that incision and drainage may delay recovery, facilitate a bacterial superinfection, and increase the risk of developing chronic lymphocutaneous fistulae.

THIRD-LINE THERAPIES

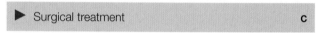

► Surgical treatment **C**

Problematic ulcerative lesions in sexually transmitted diseases: surgical management. Parkash S, Radhakrishna K. Sex Transm Dis 1986; 13: 127–33.

Anatomic changes resulting from chronic infection are not amenable to antibiotic therapy and may require surgical repair, although the patient should always receive a course of antibiotics first.

SPECIAL CONSIDERATIONS

Pregnancy

Pregnant and lactating women should be treated with erythromycin. Azithromycin might prove useful for treatment of LGV in pregnancy, but no published data are available regarding its safety and efficacy (MMWR-2006). Infection with LGV in infants born to infected women has not been addressed in the literature.

Evidence Levels: **A** Double-blind study **B** Clinical trial ≥ 20 subjects **C** Clinical trial < 20 subjects **D** Series ≥ 5 subjects **E** Anecdotal case reports

Lymphomatoid papulosis

Jacqueline M Junkins-Hopkins, Alain H Rook, Carmela C Vittorio

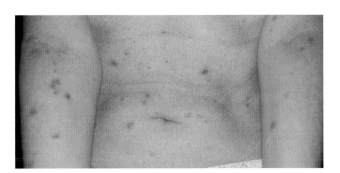

Lymphomatoid papulosis (LyP) is a distinct subset of CD30+ lymphoproliferative disorders in the World Health Organization/European Organization for the Research and Treatment of Cancer (WHO/EORTC) classification of cutaneous lymphomas, defined histologically by a variable infiltrate of CD30+ lymphocytes, in conjunction with the clinical presentation of recurrent, self-healing papulonodular eruption. The papules and nodules evolve into a crusted or necrotic stage, which often heal with a scar. Less common presentations include regional and oral disease. LyP affects adults and children as young as 11 months of age, and typically persists for years to decades. Approximately 10–20% of patients with LyP may present with or develop a lymphoproliferative malignancy, such as mycosis fungoides (MF – cutaneous T-cell lymphoma [CTCL]), anaplastic large cell lymphoma (ALCL), and Hodgkin's or non-Hodgkin's nodal lymphomas. There may be a slight risk of developing a non-hematologic neoplasm. The same clone has been documented in patients with LyP and MF, and patients with LyP may progress to CD30+ lymphoma, supporting the concept that LyP lies within the spectrum of CTCL. Clinical and histologic overlap may also be seen with LyP and pityriasis lichenoides et varioliformis acuta (PLEVA).

MANAGEMENT STRATEGY

Most importantly, the management of LyP begins with understanding the natural history of the disease. LyP is defined as a recurrent, self-healing (remission of every individual lesion), papulonodular eruption, with histology suggesting CTCL. Histologic features include CD30+ cells resembling the Reed–Sternberg cells of Hodgkin's disease, admixed with inflammatory cells (LyP type A), histology simulating MF (LyP type B), and cohesive sheets of CD30+ cells (LyP type C) resembling ALCL. Except for the rare papulonecrotic variant of generalized LyP, which may have associated fevers, a diagnosis of LyP should be reserved for patients without constitutional symptoms, hepatosplenomegaly, or lymphadenopathy. This symptomatology may indicate a co-existing nodal lymphoma, and patients with these findings should undergo a hematologic evaluation and CT

scanning to exclude a systemic lymphoma. Distinguishing LyP from primary cutaneous ALCL is important, although this may be difficult because of clinical and histologic overlap, including spontaneous regression. Persistent lesions >2–3 cm in diameter favor ALCL; however, some patients do not fit well into either category. Such borderline cases have similar biologic behavior to LyP and can be managed as such. Nodular scabies, herpes virus, and ruptured molluscum may simulate LyP histologically, further emphasizing the need for clinicopathologic correlation.

Treatment of LyP should be tailored to the disease burden, because most modalities do not alter the natural course of LyP, nor do they prevent the development of extracutaneous lymphomas. Treatment should be reserved for symptomatic or scarring disease. There may be some response to topical *corticosteroids*, but this does not induce remission. Other alternatives, such as *tetracycline and aciclovir*, have anecdotally been associated with clearance, but these options cannot replace those discussed below. In cosmetically bothersome cases *low-dose methotrexate* or *8-methoxypsoralen with UVA (PUVA)* are appropriate first-line treatments. Patients may respond to 5 mg/week of methotrexate, but may require 15–20 mg/week. A response may be seen within the first few weeks of treatment, including the development of fewer lesions, shortening of the lifecycle of individual lesions, and an induction of remission. PUVA is a valuable treatment, but conventional UVB is of less benefit. Large or borderline lesions can be treated with local radiotherapy or excision. Therapies that are beneficial in MF may also be used, including topical *carmustine (BCNU)*, topical *mechlorethamine (nitrogen mustard)*, and biologic agents such as *interferon-α* and *interferon-γ*, and the retinoid X receptor agonist bexarotene, at doses of 150–300 mg daily. In the authors' experience, topical bexarotene in a region of localized disease prevents recurrence of the condition. Similarly, topical imiquimod 5% cream can hasten resolution of lesions. LyP can recur for decades, requiring careful consideration of treatment side effects and continued monitoring for the development of lymphoma. Multiagent chemotherapy is not indicated, despite histologic features that may suggest ALCL. Use of the *308 nm excimer laser* and subcutaneous injection of *mistletoe abstract* may offer therapeutic benefit in patients who do not respond to conventional therapy.

SPECIFIC INVESTIGATIONS

- ▶ Biopsy and histologic review to confirm the diagnosis
- ▶ Exclusion of constitutional ('B') symptoms and clinically detectable hepatosplenomegaly or lymphadenopathy
- ▶ Consider staging procedures for LyP type C: chest, thoracic/abdominal/pelvic CT and bone marrow evaluation
- ▶ Ongoing surveillance for a lymphoproliferative neoplasm

Spectrum of primary cutaneous CD30 (Ki-1)-positive lymphoproliferative disorders. A proposal for classification and guidelines for management and treatment. Willemze R, Beljaards RC. J Am Acad Dermatol 1993; 28: 973–80.

The spectrum of CD30+ lymphoproliferative disease is reviewed, and guidelines for management are offered. Typical LyP, including type C, does not require staging procedures if there is a normal physical examination and review of systems. One might consider a staging work-up if there is histology that overlaps with CD30 lymphoma. Long-term follow-up is required for all subtypes. Typical LyP requires either no treatment or PUVA, topical mechlorethamine, topical carmustine, or low-dose methotrexate. Relapse occurs after discontinuation of treatment, with rare permanent remissions.

Lymphomatoid papulosis. Reappraisal of clinicopathologic presentation and classification into subtypes A, B, and C. El Shabrawi-Caelen L, Kerl H, Cerroni L. Arch Dermatol 2004; 140: 441–7.

A retrospective review of 85 patients with LyP documented histologic overlap between subtypes A, B, and C and between type B and MF. The authors also stress the tight overlap with LyP and CD30 lymphoma. A variety of clinicohistopathologic presentations of LyP, including those with histology showing follicular mucinosis, syringotropism, vesicle formation, MF-like band-like infiltrates, and associated keratoacanthoma, are discussed.

CD30/Ki-1-positive lymphoproliferative disorders of the skin – clinicopathologic correlation and statistical analysis of 86 cases: a multicentric study from the European Organization for Research and Treatment of Cancer Cutaneous Lymphoma Project Group. Paulli M, Berti E, Rosso R, Boveri E, Kindl S, Klersy C, et al. J Clin Oncol 1995; 13: 1343–54.

Four clinicopathologic categories of CD30+ lymphoproliferative disease are defined: LyP, anaplastic large cell lymphoma (ALCL), non-anaplastic CD30 lymphoma, and borderline LyP and ALCL (spontaneous resolution, but borderline histology). The prognosis was excellent and similar to that of LyP in this borderline group.

Primary and secondary cutaneous CD30+ lymphoproliferative disorders: a report from the Dutch Cutaneous Lymphoma Group on the long-term follow-up data of 219 patients and guidelines for diagnosis and treatment. Bekkenk MW, Geelen FAMJ, van Voorst Vader PC, Heule F, Geerts ML, van Vloten WA, et al. Blood 2000; 95: 3653–61.

Guidelines are proposed for the diagnosis and treatment of patients with CD30+ lymphoproliferative disorders based on long-term follow-up of 219 patients, 118 of whom had LyP (type A, type B, and type C; 4% had tumors) Staging of patients with type C LyP (based on physical examination, routine examination for blood morphology, blood chemistry, chest radiography, CT of the thorax, abdomen, and bone marrow biopsy) failed to reveal extracutaneous disease. Fifty-two of 118 patients received no treatment or topical corticosteroids. The remainder received a variety of standard treatments, none of which were associated with complete, sustained remission. Nineteen percent developed an associated lymphoma (only one with LyP C). Induction of remission of the secondary lymphoma had no effect on the natural course of LyP. The calculated risk for extracutaneous disease was 4% at 10 years.

The t(2; 5)-associated p80 NPM/ALK fusion protein in nodal and cutaneous CD30+ lymphoproliferative disorders. Su LD, Schnitzer B, Ross CW, Vasef M, Mori S, Shiota M, et al. J Cutan Pathol 1997; 24: 597–603.

The chromosomal translocation t(2; 5) and subsequent expression of ALCL tyrosine kinase (ALK) is often identified in nodal CD 30+ lymphoma. The authors found 24 cases of LyP to stain negative for this antibody.

CD30+ cutaneous lymphoproliferative disorders: the Stanford experience in lymphomatoid papulosis and primary cutaneous anaplastic large cell lymphoma. Liu HL, Hoppe RT, Kohler S, Harvell JD, Reddy S, Kim YH. J Am Acad Dermatol 2003; 49: 1049–58.

In 31 of 56 cases with LyP a higher than previously reported associated coexisting hematolymphoid malignancy (61% with one or more) was noted. Most had MF, which occurred before, during, or after the diagnosis of LyP. Some had two hematolymphoid malignancies. Three progressed to ALCL, with an interval ranging from 77 to 152 months. The overall 5- and 10-year survival of patients with LyP was 100% and 92%, respectively, and none died of LyP. Those with ALCL had a favorable course. LyP subtype did not predict the risk of associated malignancy. Treatment included topical corticosteroids, low-dose methotrexate, phototherapy, mechlorethamine ointment, and radiation. Two inadvertently received multiagent chemotherapy, which did not alter the course of the disease.

The higher association with malignancy may represent selection bias.

Increased risk of lymphoid and nonlymphoid malignancies in patients with lymphomatoid papulosis. Wang HH, Myers T, Lach LJ, Hsieh CC, Kadin ME. Cancer 1999; 86: 1240–5.

Six of 57 (10.5%) of patients with LyP and one of 67 (1.5%) matched controls followed for 8 years developed a non-lymphoid malignancy (lung, breast, and pancreatic carcinoma, and neuroblastoma). Two patients and no controls developed MF and ALCL. The calculated relative risk was 3.11 for non-lymphoid malignancies and 13.33 for malignant lymphomas in patients with LyP. There was no significant difference in survival between the two groups. The risk of malignancy was associated with advanced age (63 vs 43 years at entry into the study), but not LyP subtype.

Lymphomatoid papulosis in childhood: six case reports and a literature review. Bories N, Thomas L, Phan A, Balme B, Slameire D, Thurot-Guillou C, et al. Ann Dermatol Venereol 2008; 135: 657–62.

In a retrospective analysis of six children with LyP aged 2–11 years of age, it was found that the features and risk of malignancy were similar to those of adults with LyP. Clinical monitoring only was encouraged.

Children may also have primary and secondary ALCL arise in the skin; therefore it is important to monitor for the development of larger and/or more persistent lesions.

Single cell analysis of CD30+ cells in lymphomatoid papulosis demonstrates a common clonal T-cell origin. Steinhoff M, Hummel M, Anagnostopoulos I, Kaudewitz P, Seitz V, Assaf C, et al. Blood 2002; 100: 578–84.

The large CD30+ cells in LyP represent a single clone, whereas the CD30– cells are polyclonal.

Assessment for clonality will not help to differentiate borderline cases of LyP from ALCL or MF.

Dominance of nonmalignant T-cell clones and distortion of the TCR repertoire in the peripheral blood of patients with cutaneous CD30+ lymphoproliferative disorders. Humme D, Lukowsky A, Steinhoff M, Beyer M, Walden P, Sterry W, et al. J Invest Dermatol 2009; 129: 89–98.

The authors analyzed 126 lesional skin and corresponding peripheral blood samples from 31 patients with LyP and detected a dominant T-cell clone in the skin of 81% of patients with LyP, which was similar to ALCL (86%). A non-identical clonal T-cell population was also detected in the peripheral blood of eight of 21 patients (38%) with LyP.

The study failed to identify a blood or cutaneous compartment that may harbor clonal T cells to explain the relapsing nature of LyP, but it confirmed the clonal nature of LyP. One must use caution when using PCR analysis to 'confirm' a diagnosis of LyP, because, as was demonstrated in this study, classic LyP may be clonal, and ALCL may not have a dominant clone.

Lymphomatoid papulosis associated with mycosis fungoides: a study of 21 patients including analyses for clonality. Zackheim H, Jones C, LeBoit PE, Kashani-Sabet M, McCalmont TH, Zehnder J. J Am Acad Dermatol 2003; 49: 620–3.

Of 54 patients with LyP, 39% had MF. LyP preceded (67%), followed (19%), or was concurrent with (14%) a diagnosis of MF: 95% had type A LyP. Of those checked (seven patients) 100% had an identical clone in MF and LyP lesions.

CD30-positive T-cell lymphoproliferative disorder of the oral mucosa – an indolent lesion: Report of 4 cases. Agarwal M, Shenjere P, Blewitt RW, Hall G, Sloan P, Pigadas N, et al. Int J Surg Pathol 2008; 16: 286–90. Epub 2008 2 April.

The authors report four cases of CD30+ oral tumors, three of which presented on the tongue and one on the buccal mucosa. All regressed, and none was associated with an aggressive course. One presented as an ulcer. The histology of two cases showed features typical of LyP. Other similar cases are reviewed.

If one is not aware of this presentation, oral CD30 LPD may be erroneously diagnosed as T-cell lymphoma. This may or may not present in conjunction with cutaneous or genital mucosal lesions of LyP. The evaluation of patients with LyP should include examination of the oral mucosa. Isolated oral lesions with histology of LyP should be distinguished from ALCL and CD8+ aggressive epidermotropic CTCL, which may have overlapping clinical and histologic features.

Three cases of lymphomatoid papulosis with a CD56+ immunophenotype. Flann S, Orchard GE, Wain M, Russell-Jones R. J Am Acad Dermatol 2006; 55: 903–6.

These authors report three cases of LyP in which there was CD56 cytotoxic immunophenotype in addition to the CD30 staining. These patients otherwise had typical clinical and histologic features of LyP, including an indolent course.

Coexpression of CD56 and CD30 is a rare occurrence in LyP.

Lymphomatoid papulosis in a patient with Crohn's disease treated with infliximab. Outlaw W, Fleischer A, Bloomfeld R. Inflamm Bowel Dis 2009; 15: 965–6.

The authors report a 21-year-old man with a history of Crohn's disease, well controlled on azathioprine and infliximab, who developed LyP. This resolved, with no further recurrences over a 1-year follow-up, upon discontinuation of the inflixamab.

This association of LyP with TNF inhibitors has been reported previously, but is a rare occurrence; a true cause and effect has not been established. Nonetheless, this is something to consider in patients undergoing treatment with this therapy.

Large cell transformation mimicking regional lymphomatoid papulosis in a patient with mycosis fungoides

Nakahigashi K, Ishida Y, Matsumura Y, Kore-eda S, Ohmori K, Fujimoto M, et al. J Dermatol 2008; 35: 283–8.

The authors report a 57-year-old man with stage III MF who developed a regional eruption of either transformed MF or type C LyP on his chest. Spontaneous resolution supported the diagnosis of LyP.

The importance of differentiating LyP from large cell transformation of MF is stressed. In contrast to LyP, which is associated with a better prognosis in patients with MF, patients with large cell transformation have a worse prognosis.

Prognosis of lymphomatoid papulosis. Gruber R, Sepp, NT, Fritsch PO, Schmuth M. Oncologist 2006; 11: 955–7.

The authors report their results of a retrospective analysis of 21 patients with LyP, which found that two (9.5%) of their patients' LyP preceded the onset of lymphoma. They noted that if the course of the disease is analyzed, instead of calculating the absolute frequency of LyP, there is an increased risk for progression to lymphoma when LyP is followed up for extended time periods.

The authors further implied that the cumulative risk may represent a more relevant basis for therapeutic decisions. However, as therapeutic intervention has not been proven to alter the course in LyP, aggressive intervention is not suggested.

FIRST-LINE THERAPIES

▶ Therapy not required	B
▶ PUVA	B
▶ Low-dose methotrexate	B
▶ Topical corticosteroids	E

Primary and secondary cutaneous CD30+ lymphoproliferative disorders: a report from the Dutch Cutaneous Lymphoma Group on the long-term follow-up data of 219 patients and guidelines for diagnosis and treatment. Bekkenk MW, Geelen FAMJ, van Voorst Vader PC, Heule F, Geerts ML, van Vloten WA, et al. Blood 2000; 95: 3653–61.

In patients with relatively few non-scarring LyP lesions, active treatment is not necessary.

PUVA-treatment in lymphomatoid papulosis. Wantzin GL, Thompsen K. Br J Dermatol 1982; 107: 687–90.

Four patients with classic LyP and one with one to two tumors were treated with PUVA, 51–124 J/cm^2 and 481 J/cm^2, respectively. There was a reduction in the number of lesions and shortening of the lifecycle of each individual lesion to 1 week from 3–6 weeks. Remission was achieved in one patient.

Methotrexate is effective therapy for lymphomatoid papulosis and other primary cutaneous CD30+ lymphoproliferative disorders. Vonderheid EC, Sajjadian A, Kadin ME. J Am Acad Dermatol 1996; 34: 470–81.

A 20-year experience of methotrexate therapy in 45 patients with LyP, CD30+ lymphoma, and borderline cases is reviewed. Patients responded within 4 weeks (15–20 mg weekly). Maintenance doses were given at 10–14-day intervals (range 7–28 days); 29% had concomitant MF, requiring other therapies (mechlorethamine hydrochloride, carmustine, standard UV therapy, and PUVA), which offered some additional benefit, but the relative effectiveness was less than with methotrexate. LyP and CD30+ lymphoma responded similarly.

Three patients had diminished responsiveness, suggesting resistance to methotrexate. Severe exacerbations occurred upon abrupt drug discontinuation.

This is considered first-line therapy for symptomatic disease, but remission is rare, limiting long-term treatment with methotrexate.

Lymphomatoid papulosis: successful weekly pulse superpotent topical corticosteroid therapy in three pediatric patients. Paul MA, Krowchuk DP, Hitchcock MG, Jorizzo JL. Pediatr Dermatol 1996; 13: 501–6.

Three children with LyP were treated with halobetasol or clobetasol propionate twice daily for 2–3 weeks, followed by weekly pulsed application, resulting in complete resolution of nearly all cutaneous lesions. Adjuvant intralesional triamcinolone was used for three ulcerated lesions.

Although this modality is unlikely to alter the disease course, it is a reasonable treatment approach because it has a relatively low complication profile.

Medium-dose UVA1 therapy of lymphomatoid papulosis. Calzavara-Pinton P, Venturini M, Sala R. J Am Acad Dermatol 2005; 52: 530–1.

Seven patients with LyP were treated with fixed daily exposures of $60 J/cm^2$ UVA1 radiation, five times weekly, until complete (five patients) or partial (two patients) improvement. The mean cumulative UVA1 doses were $1071.4 \pm 485.6 J/cm^2$, and the number of exposures was 17.9 ± 8.1. Side effects included mild dryness. The subtype of LyP (A versus B) did not affect the results. Three patients with relapse responded to a second treatment cycle.

SECOND-LINE THERAPIES

▶ Topical mechlorethamine (nitrogen mustard)	B
▶ Topical carmustine	C
▶ Aciclovir	E
▶ Topical bexarotene	C

Long-term efficacy, curative potential, and carcinogenicity of topical mechlorethamine chemotherapy in cutaneous T cell lymphoma. Vonderheid EC, Tan ET, Kantor AF, Shrager L, Micaily B, Van Scott EJ. J Am Acad Dermatol 1989; 20: 416–28.

Seven patients with LyP and 17 with concomitant LyP and MF were treated with 10–20 mg of mechlorethamine dissolved in 40–60 mL water and applied once daily to the entire skin surface except for the genitalia, until at least 2 weeks after complete clearance of lesions. Four of the seven with LyP achieved a complete response, with one lasting for more than 8 years of follow-up. A slightly increased risk in the squamous and basal cell carcinomas, Hodgkin's disease, and colon cancer was noted.

A common side effect of mechlorethamine therapy is an allergic hypersensitivity reaction. There may be a reduced incidence of contact allergy when mechlorethamine is prepared in an ointment base.

Topical carmustine therapy for lymphomatoid papulosis. Zacheim HS, Epstein EH, Crain WR. Arch Dermatol 1985; 121: 1410–14.

Seven patients with LyP were treated with once-daily total skin applications of topical carmustine, prepared by dissolving a 100 mg vial of carmustine in 50 mL of 95% (or absolute) ethanol; 5 mL (10 mg) was added to 60 mL of water and applied

with a 2-inch paintbrush after showering. Total doses ranged from 280 to 1180 mg. Local treatment of individual lesions after the total skin course included twice-daily application of 2 or 4 mg/mL 95% ethanol. All patients had a rapid reduction in the number and size of lesions. Lesions cleared faster and did not scar with maintenance therapy, but remission was not seen. Rare persistent telangiectases were noted.

THIRD-LINE THERAPIES

▶ Oral bexarotene	C
▶ Recombinant interferon	C
▶ Radiotherapy	E
▶ Topical methotrexate	E
▶ Mistletoe abstract	E
▶ Imiquimod cream	E

Bexarotene is a new treatment option for lymphomatoid papulosis. Krathen RA, Ward S, Duvic M. Dermatology 2003; 206: 142–7.

Oral bexarotene, started at $300 mg/m^2$ daily, was associated with more rapid disappearance, less necrosis, and a reduction in new lesions. One of three patients had a complete response. Topical bexarotene used in patients with less than 10% body surface area involved had a similar benefit.

Oral bexarotene is often used in conjunction with thyroxine and oral fenofibrate and/or atorvastatin because of frequently seen hypothyroidism and hyperlipidemia.

Lymphomatoid papulosis: response to treatment with recombinant interferon alfa-2b. [Letter] Proctor SJ, Jackson GH, Lennard AL, Marks J. J Clin Oncol 1992; 10: 170.

Recombinant interferon-α_{2b} 1 mU injected intralesionally three times in 1 week completely cleared lesions less than 0.5 cm in diameter. Larger lesions required three to 10 injections. Maintenance with thrice-weekly 3 mU subcutaneous doses appeared to reduce recurrences.

Therapeutic use of interferon-alpha for lymphomatoid papulosis. Schmuth M, Topar G, Illersperger B, Kowald E, Fritsch PO, Sepp NT. Cancer 2000; 89: 1603–10.

Four of five patients receiving subcutaneous interferon-α, 3–15 million IU three times per week for 12–13-months, had a complete response at 6-week follow-up. All noted some response. Two had rapid recurrences after discontinuing short-term interferon-α (5–7 months), but one had a complete response when long-term therapy was instituted (17 months). Only one of six controls achieved spontaneous remission.

Interferon-α is one of the few therapies that has shown potential for altering the course of LyP. Its benefit is associated with long-term treatment courses, but the side effect profile for low-dose interferon-α is low, allowing a prolonged treatment course.

Topical methotrexate for lymphomatoid papulosis. Bergstrom JS, Jaworsky C. J Am Acad Dermatol 2003; 49: 937–9.

A 71-year-old man with LyP treated himself with a home concoction of this medication applied topically. A 2.5 mg tablet was moistened with tap water and rubbed on the bandage until the gauze turned orange. Application of the medication-soaked bandage to newly formed lesions daily (approximately one-third of a tablet, or 0.83 mg) resulted in regression of the lesions within 2–3 days.

This is a report of an innovative approach using a medication that has known efficacy in treating LyP, yet a limiting complication profile. The bioavailability of methotrexate in tap water is not known, and it is possible that the patient is achieving enough systemic absorption to clear his lesions. Further investigation is needed.

308-nm Excimer laser for the treatment of lymphomatoid papulosis and stage IA mycosis fungoides. Kontos AP, Kerr HA, Malick F, Fivenson DP, Lim HW, Wong HK. Photodermatol Photoimmunol Photomed 2006; 22: 168–71.

A patient with LyP which had failed response to PUVA and MTX was treated with the 308 nm excimer pulse laser, 13 treatments three times per week, with a maximum fluence of 500 mJ/cm². This resulted in 75% clearance, with minimal recurrence and postinflammatory hyperpigmentation.

This hand-held device allows delivery of higher fluences, with a diminished risk of carcinogenesis.

Persistent agmination of lymphomatoid papulosis: An equivalent of limited plaque mycosis fungoides type of cutaneous T-cell lymphoma. Heald P, Subtil A, Breneman D, Wilson LD. J Am Acad Dermatol 2007; 57: 1005–11.

Seven cases of regional LyP were treated as if they were localized mycosis fungoides, with local radiotherapy, resulting in long-standing remissions. The radiation doses ranged from 30 to 46 Gy, in fractionated doses. One patient also had topical bexarotene and localized electron beam therapy. At follow-up (2–6 years), six of the seven had no recurrences. One patient with recurrence subsequently achieved complete remission with interferon-α and PUVA.

Treatment of regional LyP as if it were MF may offer remission of LyP, but, as demonstrated, these patients may develop lymphoma. Long-term follow-up is critical.

Therapeutic use of mistletoe for CD30+ cutaneous lymphoproliferative disorder/lymphomatoid papulosis. Seifert, G, Tautz C, Seeger K, Hanze G, Laengler A. J Eur Acad Dermatol Venereol 2007; 21: 536–78.

An 8-year-old with ALCL associated with LyP was treated with injections of mistletoe abstract Abnoba *Viscum fraxini*, twice weekly, starting at 20 mg in the first week, then titrated to a dose that allowed a marked local reaction with mild fever and local swelling. The medication was injected subcutaneously into or adjacent to the lesions, resulting in fever to 38°C, and local swelling and redness 1 day after administration. The lesions regressed within 2 weeks. The therapy was continued at 2 mg subcutaneously per week.

Mistletoe has been used in Europe for cancer patients, and there have been no serious adverse or long-term effects reported.

Treatment of lymphomatoid papulosis with imiquimod 5% cream. Hughes PH. J Am Acad Dermatol 2006; 54: 546–7.

A 13-year-old boy with LyP was reported to have a complete response within 2 weeks with lesional application of imiquimod 5% cream three times per week.

Patients' responses to imiquimod are variable, and patients should be warned of possible inflammation. The usefulness of imiquimod is limited by its cost.

Malignant atrophic papulosis

Noah Scheinfeld

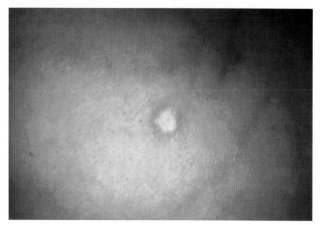

From Lebwohl MG. The Skin and Systemic Disease: A Color Atlas, 2nd edn. Churchill Livingstone 2003, with permission of Elsevier.

Malignant atrophic papulosis (MAP, Degos disease, DD) possesses purely cutaneous and systemic variants. These are divided according to their prognosis, with purely cutaneous DD being wholly benign and systemic DD usually being fatal within a few years of onset. Cutaneous DD can develop into systemic DD, but no factor has yet been defined that will predict which persons with cutaneous DD will go on to develop systemic DD.

About 300 cases of DD have been reported. It is likely that the purely cutaneous type is underdiagnosed. DD affects all ages and both sexes. A familial variant appears to exist.

Cutaneous and systemic DD have similar cutaneous eruptions. In the skin, DD occurs as erythematous, pink or red papules (2–15 mm), which evolve into scars with central, porcelain-white atrophic centers. The papules of MAP usually have a peripheral telangiectatic rim and can be domed or atrophic. The lesions may appear anywhere on the skin, except on the face. Papules can have central crusts. Urticarial, ulceropustular and/or gumma-like nodules may be observed. Purely cutaneous DD has a benign course which may wax and wane with no effect on mortality. Systemic DD has a dire prognosis, the cause of death being related to perforation of blood vessels, characteristically resulting in intestinal perforation. Systemic MAP can involve the nervous, ophthalmologic, gastrointestinal, cardiothoracic, and hepatorenal systems. Death usually occurs within 2–3 years from the onset of systemic involvement.

Pathologically, the tissue affected by DD reveals an occlusive arteriopathy involving small-caliber vessels which results in tissue infarction. The bland appearance of MAP's vasculopathy or an endovasculitis on histological examination does not equate with the serious nature of systemic DD.

No specific laboratory tests define the diagnosis of DD. Cases can be associated with antiphospholipid antibodies and antinuclear antibodies, but this is not considered pathogenic. Some reports note increased plasma fibrinogen levels, increased platelet aggregation, and a reduction in local and systemic fibrinolytic activity. The role of testing is to give assurance to patients that they do not have systemic DD. A patient with purely cutaneous DD should be given regular stool guaiac tests so they can be tested for internal bleeding.

No medical therapy has been shown to alter the course of DD. Antiplatelet drugs (e.g., *aspirin, dipyridamole*) may reduce the number of new atrophic papules and cause involution in some patients with only cutaneous involvement, although this has not been shown in a reproducible fashion. Attempts at treatment of systemic DD have mostly been unsuccessful. It has been suggested that *intravenous immunoglobulin* may have a role, but recent reports have demonstrated its lack of efficacy. Other treatments that have been tried without real benefit in all variants of DD include topical corticosteroids, phenformin and ethylestrenol, cidofovir, iodohydroxyquinoline, aspirin and dipyridamole, phenylbutazone, arsenic, sulfonamides, dextran, corticosteroids, heparin, warfarin, niacin, streptomycin, corticotropin, azathioprine, methotrexate, ciclosporin, tacrolimus, mycophenolate mofetil, pentoxifylline, clopidogrel, and infliximab.

SPECIFIC INVESTIGATIONS

> ▶ Physical examination
> ▶ Skin biopsy
> ▶ Complete blood count
> ▶ Stool guaiac
> ▶ Antinuclear antibody titer
> ▶ Protein C, protein S and factor V Lieden, antithrombin III, homocysteine levels
> ▶ Anticardiolipin antibody titer
> ▶ Antiphospholipid antibody titer
> ▶ Endoscopy of the gastrointestinal tract (i.e., stomach, esophagus, duodenum, colon, rectum)
> ▶ Laparoscopy of the intestine

FIRST-LINE THERAPIES

> ▶ Heparin   E
> ▶ Coumadin (warfarin)   E
> ▶ Aspirin   E
> ▶ Dipyridamole   E

Malignant atrophic papulosis. Degos R. Br J Dermatol 1979; 100: 21–35.

Numerous clinical manifestations have been reported that can affect the skin, mucosa, gastrointestinal tract, viscera, and CNS, and may require surgical intervention or fibrinolytic therapy. Anticoagulants have shown the most favorable responses.

Malignant atrophic papulosis: treatment with aspirin and dipyridamole. Stahl D, Thomsen K, Hou-Jensen K. Arch Dermatol 1978; 114: 1687–9.

A case report of a patient in whom treatment with aspirin 0.5 g twice daily and dipyridamole 50 mg three times daily arrested the development of both cutaneous lesions and systemic symptoms. Discontinuation of therapy resulted in no relapses 4 months post therapy.

Malignant atrophic papulosis in an infant. Torrelo A, Sevilla J, Mediero I, Candelas D, Zambrano A. Br J Dermatol 2002; 146: 916–18.

A 7-month-old girl with cutaneous lesions, vomiting, and poor weight gain was treated successfully with aspirin 12 mg/kg daily and dipyridamole 4 mg/kg daily in three divided doses.

SECOND-LINE THERAPIES

▶ Phenformin	E
▶ Ethylestrenol	E
▶ Nicotine patches	E
▶ Lansoprazole (for gastrointestinal ulceration)	E
▶ Ciclosporin	E

Effect of fibrinolytic treatment in malignant atrophic papulosis. Delaney TJ, Black MM. Br Med J 1975; 3: 415.

The further development of cutaneous disease was halted in a 42-year-old woman placed on phenformin 50 mg twice daily and ethylestrenol 2 mg four times daily. Withdrawal of therapy resulted in relapse that responded to reinstitution of therapy.

Penile ulceration in fatal malignant atrophic papulosis (Degos' disease). Thompson KF, Highet AS. Br J Dermatol 2000; 143: 1320–2.

A fatal outcome in a patient who initially presented with penile ulceration and was treated with aspirin and dipyridamole, but could not tolerate the therapy. Ciclosporin resulted in clinical improvement. Neurologic and gastrointestinal symptoms developed and lansoprazole resulted in healing of gastric ulceration. Atrial fibrillation and pleuritic pain were treated with heparin, with clinical improvement. Continued symptoms prompted trials of tacrolimus, prednisolone, azathioprine, and cyclophosphamide, without success.

A case of malignant atrophic papulosis successfully treated with nicotine patches. Kanekura T, Uchino Y, Kanzaki T. Br J Dermatol 2003; 149: 660–2.

Nicotine patches that released 5 mg every 24 h were applied daily and resulted in clearing of skin lesions. Three weeks after withdrawal of the patches the lesions recurred, and again responded to therapy. The patient had no systemic involvement.

THIRD-LINE THERAPIES

▶ Azathioprine	E
▶ Cyclophosphamide	E
▶ Tacrolimus	E
▶ Intravenous immunoglobulin	E
▶ Ultraviolet B therapy	E

Inefficacy of intravenous immunoglobulins and infliximab in Degos' disease. De Breucker S, Vandergheynst F, Decaux G. Acta Clin Belg 2008; 63: 99–102.

A 60-year-old man presented with sudden visual loss, a history of postprandial abdominal pain, malabsorption, and skin lesions typical of systemic Degos' disease. Despite anti-aggregants and prednisone the patient's status did not improve. He was given intravenous immunoglobulins followed by infliximab. Two months after the third injection of infliximab the patient developed a fatal mesenteric infarction.

The use of intravenous immunoglobulin in cutaneous and recurrent perforating intestinal Degos disease (malignant atrophic papulosis). Zhu KJ, Zhou Q, Lin AH, Lu ZM, Cheng H. Br J Dermatol 2007; 157: 206–7.

A 38-year-old Chinese woman with Degos disease, unresponsive to a variety of therapies, was treated with one course of high-dose IVIG (0.4 g /kg daily for 5 days). A week later a dramatic improvement of the lesions and her general condition was noticed. During the following 11 months of follow-up, the patient has had no new skin lesions or gastrointestinal complaints.

A fatal case of malignant atrophic papulosis (Degos' disease) in a man with factor V Leiden mutation and lupus anticoagulant. Hohwy T, Jensen MG, Tøttrup A, Steiniche T, Fogh K. Acta Dermatol Venereol 2006; 86: 245–7.

A 33-year-old man presented with a widespread skin eruption consistent with malignant atrophic papulosis. He was treated with narrowband ultraviolet B, prednisolone and, later, aspirin, pentoxifylline and warfarin without effect, and died 2.5 years after onset of the disease.

A case of systemic malignant atrophic papulosis (Köhlmeier-Degos' disease). Fernández-Pérez ER, Grabscheid E, Scheinfeld NS. J Natl Med Assoc 2005; 97: 421–5.

Despite the use of ciclosporin, prednisone, cidofovir, intravenous immunoglobulin and anticoagulant therapy, this young male patient died. The therapy had no effect on the course of his disease.

Malignant atrophic papulosis of Degos. Report of a patient who failed to respond to fibrinolytic therapy. Howsden SM, Hodge SJ, Herndon JH, Freeman RJ. Arch Dermatol 1976; 112: 1582–8.

A 21-year-old woman died of complications from MAP after therapy with phenformin, ethylestrenol, aspirin, niacin, and low molecular weight dextran.

Benign familial Degos disease worsening during immunosuppression. Powell J, Bordea C, Wojnarowska J, Farrell AM, Morris PJ. Br J Dermatol 1999; 141: 524–7.

A 61-year-old woman with Degos disease underwent a cadaveric kidney transplant. Her condition worsened with the use of prednisolone, azathioprine, and ciclosporin.

[An autopsy case of Degos' disease with ascending thoracic myelopathy]. Sugai F, Sumi H, Hara Y, Kajiyama K, Morino H, Fujimura H. Rinsho Shinkeigaku 1998; 38: 1049–53. (In Japanese.)

Aggressive therapies, including pulsed-dose methylprednisolone and cyclophosphamide, were not successful in this 44-year-old man with Degos disease complicated by thoracic transverse myelopathy; the patient ultimately died from respiratory failure.

Malignant melanoma

Orit Markowitz, Darrell S Rigel

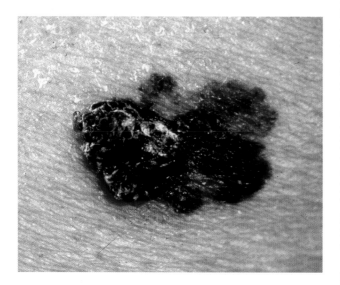

Melanoma is the leading cause of death among all cutaneous diseases in the USA. It is estimated that 62 480 new cases of invasive melanoma will be diagnosed in 2008, and that 8420 patients will die of this cancer. It has also been estimated that 54 020 cases of in situ melanoma are expected to be newly diagnosed in 2008. The principal management of primary cutaneous melanoma is surgical, and it is further estimated that long-term survival after excised primary cutaneous melanoma with a Breslow depth <1 mm is 90%.

MANAGEMENT STRATEGY

Individuals at higher risk for melanoma are fair skinned with a skin phototype I or II, a history of intermittent sunburns, and a personal or family history of multiple atypical moles or dysplastic nevi and/or melanoma, as well as inherited genetic mutations.

Helping both physicians and patients in early detection are the *ABCD signs of melanoma: Asymmetry, Border irregularity, Color variegation, and Diameter >6 mm*. These have recently been joined by 'E' for 'evolving,' demonstrating the importance of change in a lesion over time. A pigmented lesion that stands out as atypical within the context of surrounding nevi is referred to as the 'ugly duckling' sign and should also arouse suspicion of melanoma. A specificity of 0.88 and sensitivity of 0.73 has been reported if two out of three of the following characteristics are noted: irregular outline, diameter >6 mm, and color variegation. Even expert clinicians misdiagnose melanoma in up to one-third of cases, and only *biopsy and histologic examination* can provide a definitive diagnosis.

Dermoscopy, also known as skin surface microscopy or epiluminescence microscopy (ELM), increases the diagnostic sensitivity of melanoma in clinicians with some formal training. In high-risk patients, baseline photographs can be helpful in the identification of new and changing lesions. The availability of baseline images for comparison permits the detection of melanomas that are growing or changing. Three-month-interval digital dermoscopy mole monitoring has demonstrated 93% sensitivity for non-lentigo maligna in situ melanoma, and 96% sensitivity for invasive melanoma diagnosis. This non-invasive diagnostic tool helps prevent the excision of stable yet clinically concerning atypical nevi.

The ideal biopsy of a suspected primary cutaneous melanoma is complete full-thickness excision with at least a 2 mm margin of normal-appearing surrounding skin. If total excision is not practical, full-thickness incisional biopsy usually suffices. Measurement of Breslow thickness is an important determinant of patient management and prognosis. In addition, the histologic status of the sentinel lymph node (SLN) has been shown to be a significant prognostic factor. Important in the management of melanoma is *primary prevention* (risk reduction) and *secondary prevention* (early detection). Educating the public about the risks of sun exposure is a crucial part of primary prevention. Secondary prevention involves teaching high-risk patients about the ABCD signs and how to perform total body self-examinations. The NIH stresses the importance of screening programs and regular skin examinations by health professionals. The American Academy of Dermatology Task Force recommends follow-up one to four times a year for 2 years after a diagnosis of melanoma, depending on the thickness of the lesion and other risk factors, such as a family history of melanoma, and then once or twice a year thereafter.

Staging of melanoma is crucial because it not only assigns patients into well-defined risk groups, it also aids in clinical decision-making and in comparing treatment results. In 2001 the American Joint Committee on Cancer released the final version of their cancer staging system for cutaneous melanoma. Significant changes from the previous staging system include upstaging patients when ulceration is present, and describing nodal metastases in histologic terms so as to take into account information gleaned from SLN biopsies.

The primary treatment for stage IA (invasive melanoma up to 1 mm thick without ulceration, and without adverse features, including positive deep margins, extensive regression, and mitotic rate <0) is *wide local excision*. Total excision of primary melanoma with wide margins offers the best chance for cure. The National Comprehensive Cancer Network suggests that *sentinel lymph node (SLN) biopsy* be discussed with patients in those with melanomas at least 1 mm thick, or with ulceration or additional adverse features. Wide local excision with 'consideration' of an SLN biopsy is suggested for stage IA with adverse features, and 'encouragement' of SLN biopsy in stage IB (<1 mm thick but with ulceration or Clark level IV invasion) and stage II (>1 mm thick but without nodal disease) melanomas.

The SLN is detected by preoperative lymphoscintigraphy followed by intraoperative injection of a blue dye and/or – for possibly greater accuracy – a radiocolloid around the primary lesion. Once removed, the SLN is examined for melanoma, and if positive, represents a significant negative prognostic indicator. Selecting which patients should undergo SLN biopsy is a critical decision, and there is much debate as to the minimal tumor thickness requiring this procedure and the utility of the procedure in terms of survival outcome. If the SLN is histologically positive, a *selective lymphadenectomy* is recommended. The overall effect of selective lymphadenectomy following a positive SLN has yet to show survival benefit.

Elective lymphadenectomy involves removal of regional lymph nodes without preceding clinical or microscopic evidence of nodal metastases. One large study demonstrated that this procedure increases the survival rate in certain subgroups of patients with melanoma (those with ulceration and those with tumor thicknesses between 1 and 2 mm). However, it did

Evidence Levels: **A** Double-blind study   **B** Clinical trial ≥ 20 subjects   **C** Clinical trial < 20 subjects   **D** Series ≥ 5 subjects   **E** Anecdotal case reports

not show improved overall survival in all patients with melanoma. This procedure, which results in significant morbidity, remains controversial.

For those who have stage III melanoma (evidence of either microscopic or macroscopic nodal disease), in addition to wide local excision with nodal dissection, the only adjuvant therapy approved by the FDA at present is high-dose *interferon-α$_{2b}$*. (Interferon is also approved by the FDA for stage IIB and IIC disease.) Some studies have shown that interferon may increase the relapse-free interval, but there is no clear evidence that this treatment improves overall survival. Alternatively, patients with stage III disease may either be observed or entered into a clinical trial.

For patients with clinically positive lymph nodes, a diagnostic nodal biopsy (e.g., fine-needle biopsy) is recommended and, if positive, a *therapeutic lymphadenectomy* is performed.

Traditionally, patients with satellitosis or in-transit metastases on an extremity have been candidates for treatment with *isolated limb hyperthermic perfusion/infusion* with chemotherapeutic agents (the most successful of which is melphalan).

Additional treatment options for patients with stage III macrometastases or in-transit metastases include radiation therapy, local ablation therapy, intralesional BCG, topical imiquimod, and finally systemic therapy, depending on the extent of nodal involvement. Systemic therapy includes clinical trials which are preferred, as well as dacarbazine, high-dose IL-2, paclitaxel, paclitaxel/cisplatin, paclitaxel/carboplatin, and dacarbazine or temozolomide-based combination chemotherapy with cisplatin and vinblastine with or with out IL-2/IFN. Among these, only two drugs, DTIC and IL-2, have been approved by the US Food and Drug Administration (FDA) for use in these patients.

Stage IV (distant metastases) melanoma has a very poor prognosis, with patients demonstrating a <5% 5-year survival. For those in whom only a solitary metastasis can be found, *resection of the metastasis* may be feasible. Generally, at this stage, the treatment options are limited and not very effective. No randomized controlled trials have demonstrated a significant survival advantage for any of the stage IV therapies. As in advanced stage III, *chemotherapy, radiation, and immunotherapy* are some of the options available for such patients. Chemotherapy with *dacarbazine (DTIC)*, which has an approximate 20% response rate, is commonly employed. Treatment with immunotherapy (e.g., interleukin-2) has also yielded some positive results, but more double-blind controlled studies are needed. Recently, combination paclitaxel and carboplatin has shown some disease activity in a patient population that has failed DTIC and temozolomide (TMZ). Radiation may be used as primary treatment for lentigo maligna and as palliation in metastatic melanoma. Lastly, clinical trials are ongoing assessing vaccine therapies, and the first multicenter phase II/III trial demonstrated low therapeutic efficacy, which was not statistically different from that of systemic DTIC. A new and more promising approach is combining the blockage of downregulatory signals of the immune system using anti-CTLA-4 antibodies with various peptide vaccines.

SPECIFIC INVESTIGATIONS

▶ Biopsy of primary site
▶ Sentinel lymph node biopsy
▶ Laboratory and imaging studies (chest radiograph, CT, MRI, PET scans)
▶ Dermoscopy

Incisional biopsy and melanoma prognosis. Bong JL, Herd RM, Hunter JA. J Am Acad Dermatol 2002; 46: 690–4.

This article represents a large retrospective case analysis using matched controls to investigate the influence of incisional biopsy on melanoma prognosis. A total of 5727 biopsied melanoma patients were examined, 5.6% having undergone incisional biopsies. The authors conclude that melanoma prognosis is not influenced by an incisional procedure before definitive excision of the tumor. Because of the histologic limitations of this procedure, however, the authors recommend that incisional biopsies be reserved for lesions that cannot be excised primarily, or when clinical suspicion for melanoma is low.

Final version of the American Joint Committee on Cancer staging system for cutaneous melanoma. Balch CM, Buzaid AC, Soong SJ, Atkins MB, Cascinelli N, Coit DG, et al. J Clin Oncol 2001; 19: 3635–48.

This paper describes the revised staging system for cutaneous melanoma. This takes into account the presence of ulceration in the primary cutaneous melanoma as well as the histology of the SLN(s). Accurate staging is important in clinical decision-making and in comparing treatment results between different centers.

Technical details of intraoperative lymphatic mapping. Morton DL, Wen DR, Wong JH, Economou JS, Cagle LA, Storm FK, et al. Arch Surg 1992; 127: 392–9.

This was the first description of intraoperative lymphatic mapping to identify the first node in the lymphatic watershed that drains the site of the melanoma. A total of 223 patients with either stage I or stage II melanoma were evaluated.

Sentinel-node biopsy or nodal observation in melanoma. Morton DL, Thompson JF, Cochran AJ, Mozzillo N, Elashoff R, Essner R, et al.; MSLT Group. N Engl J Med 2006; 355: 1307–17.

The authors enrolled 1269 patients with intermediate-thickness (1.2–3.5 mm) primary melanomas as part of the Multicenter Selective Lymphadenectomy Trial I (MSLT-I). In evaluating the results of this trial the authors concluded that a 5-year survival rate was higher among those who underwent immediate lymphadenectomy than in those in whom lymphadenectomy was delayed following positive sentinel node biopsy. The article also suggests that sentinel node biopsy provides important prognostic information and identifies patients with nodal metastases whose survival can be prolonged by immediate selective lymphadenectomy

The Multicenter Selective Lymphadenectomy Trial II is in progress to assess the impact of this treatment on survival for thin 1 mm melanomas and for thick melanomas >4 mm.

Sentinel-node biopsy in melanoma. N Engl J Med 2007; 356: 418–19.

There are multiple commentaries on the 2006 article discussing the controversy behind the utility of SLN biopsy in terms of increased morbidity with lymphadenectomy and no increase in survival rate based on the data presented. The authors reply that early surgical intervention of the regional lymph nodes in patients with positive biopsy results improved overall survival and provided staging information for the consideration of adjuvant biologic therapy. They also concluded that sentinel node biopsy is the 'standard of care' for the staging of melanoma and hence treatment planning.

The role of sentinel lymph node biopsy for melanoma: evidence assessment. Johnson TM, Sondak VK, Bichakjian CK, Sabel MS. J Am Acad Dermatol 2006; 54: 19–27.

This is a comprehensive review of 1198 articles identified by a search for melanoma sentinel node in the National Institutes of Health National Library of Medicine. The paper discusses the evidence base behind the sentinel node hypothesis. The authors state that the available evidence overwhelmingly supports SLN status as the most powerful independent factor predicting survival, with highest sensitivity and specificity of any nodal staging test. They also discuss that SLNB results in improved regional disease control. The article claims that, based on available evidence, there is a potential subset survival benefit for subclinical detection of nodal disease followed by immediate CLND. The article reviews the MSLT-1 interim results and discusses the morbidities of SLNB. It also reviews other aspects of sentinel lymph node biopsy, including the evidence for its use in candidates for adjuvant therapy. The authors conclude that current evidence supports the use of SLNB in the management of melanoma.

National Comprehensive Cancer Network. Clinical practice guidelines in oncology. V.2,2008. Online. Houghton AN, Colt DG. Available: http://www.nccn.org/professionals/physician_gls/PDF/melanoma.pdf

The extent of initial work-up is controversial. Most agree that chest radiography and blood work are not necessary for stage IA disease. For stage IB and stage IIA melanomas, a baseline chest radiograph is optional because it is insensitive and nonspecific. Other imaging studies, such as CT, MRI, and/or PET scans, should be performed as indicated by symptoms, signs and/or laboratory values, or for stages III and IV. FNA is indicated for stage III with macrometastases or in-transit metastases, and stage IV. LDH is only indicated for stage IV. These guidelines also discuss frequency of follow-up visits and appropriate follow-up tests, both of which depend on the stage of the melanoma as well as other risk factors.

Atlas of dermoscopy. Marghoob AA, Braun R, Kopf AW, eds. London: Parthenon Publishing, 2005.

This clinician-oriented atlas is an up-to-date multiauthored text dealing with virtually every aspect of dermoscopy.

FIRST-LINE THERAPIES

▶ Surgical excision	**B**
▶ Selective lymphadenectomy	**C**
▶ Follow-up	**C**

Narrow excision (1-cm margin). A safe procedure for thin cutaneous melanoma. Veronesi U, Cascinelli N. Arch Surg 1991; 126: 438–41.

The WHO trial included 612 patients with primary melanomas 2 mm thick or less, that were excised using margins of either 1 or 3 cm. There were no differences in overall survival rates between the two groups, nor were there any statistically significant differences in local recurrence. The five local recurrences that did occur, however, were from lesions that were between 1 and 2 mm thick. Because of this non-statistically significant trend, the effectiveness of 1 cm margins for melanomas 1–2 mm deep has remained somewhat controversial. Nonetheless, the authors recommend 1 cm margins of excision for melanomas less than 2 mm thick.

Long-term results of a prospective surgical trial comparing 2 cm vs. 4 cm excision margins for 740 patients with 1–4 mm melanomas. Balch CM, Soong SJ, Smith T, Ross MI, Urist MM, Karakousis CP, et al. Ann Surg Oncol 2001; 8: 101–8.

The Intergroup Melanoma Surgical Trial included 468 patients having stage I melanoma with a thickness between 1 and 4 mm. Surgical margins of either 2 or 4 cm were used. The two groups showed no significant differences in survival or local recurrences, demonstrating the safety of using 2 cm margins in melanomas up to 4 mm thick.

Excision margins in high-risk malignant melanoma. Thomas JM, Newton-Bishop J, A'Hern R, Coombes G, Timmons M, Evans J, et al. N Engl J Med 2004; 350: 757–66.

A randomized clinical trial with 900 subjects comparing 1-cm and 3-cm margins in high-risk tumors (thickness ≥2 mm). The median follow-up was 60 months. A 1-cm margin was associated with a significantly increased risk of locoregional recurrence. There were 128 deaths attributable to melanoma in the group with 1-cm margins, compared to 105 in the group with 3-cm margins, but overall survival was similar in the two groups.

Guidelines of care for primary cutaneous melanoma. Sober AJ, Chuang TY, Duvic M, Farmer ER, Grichnik JM, Halpern AC, et al. J Am Acad Dermatol 2001; 45: 579–86.

For melanoma in situ and for primary melanoma thicker than 4 mm, there are no large prospective randomized studies examining appropriate margins. This American Academy of Dermatology Task Force recommends taking margins of 0.5 cm for melanoma in situ, and at least 2 cm for melanomas thicker than 4 mm. They also suggest, in agreement with WHO guidelines, 1 cm margins for melanomas with a depth of invasion <2 mm, and 2-cm margins for melanomas ≥2 mm deep.

Long-term results of a multi-institutional randomized trial comparing prognostic factors and surgical results for intermediate thickness melanomas (1.0 to 4.0). Intergroup Melanoma Surgical Trial. Balch CM, Soong S, Ross MI, Urist MM, Karakousis CP, Temple WJ, et al. Ann Surg Oncol 2000; 7: 87–97.

Previous prospective studies showed that elective lymphadenectomy did not benefit all patients. This trial included 740 patients. The results suggest that elective lymphadenectomy may benefit certain subgroups of patients, specifically those with primary lesions 1–2 mm thick, those without ulcerated tumors, and those under 60 years of age.

Utility of follow-up tests for detecting recurrent disease in patients with malignant melanoma. Weiss M, Loprinzi CL, Creagan ET, Dalton RJ, Novotny P, O'Fallon JR. JAMA 1995; 274: 1703–5.

The frequency of follow-up after melanoma resection is controversial. However, it is known that most recurrences of primary melanoma are discovered by history and/or physical examination. In this retrospective study of 261 patients with resected local and regional nodal melanoma, chest radiography first diagnosed about 6% of those with recurrence.

Despite that, the authors claimed that routine chest radiographs, along with routine blood work, were of limited value in the postoperative follow-up of patients with resected intermediate- and high-risk melanomas.

SECOND-LINE THERAPIES

▶ Immunotherapy	B
▶ Chemotherapy	B
▶ Regional isolation perfusion	B

Autoimmunity correlates with tumor regression in patients with metastatic melanoma treated with anti-cytotoxic T-lymphocyte antigen-4. Attia P, Phan GQ, Maker AV, Robinson MR, Quezado MM, Yang JC, et al. J Clin Oncol 2005; 28: 6043–53.

A total of 56 patients with progressive stage IV melanoma were enrolled to receive varying doses of CTLA-4 in addition to vaccination with two modified HLA-A*0201-restricted peptides from gp100. It was found that administration of anti-CTLA-4 monoclonal antibody plus peptide vaccination can cause durable objective responses secondary to induction of autoimmunity in patients with metastatic melanoma.

Prognostic significance of autoimmunity during treatment of melanoma with interferon. Gogas H, Loannovich J, Dafni U, Stavropoulou-Giokas C, Frangia K, Tsoutsos D, et al. N Engl J Med 2006; 354: 709–18.

A study of 200 patients with melanoma (stage IIB, IIC, or III) reported that those with autoantibodies or clinical manifestations of autoimmunity after treatment with high-dose interferon-α_{2b} had improved survival (both relapse free and overall).

Systematic review of systemic adjuvant therapy for patients at high risk for recurrence of melanoma. Verma S, Quirt I, McCready D, Bak K, Charette M, Iscoe N. Cancer 2006; 106: 1431–42.

A systematic review of high-dose interferon-α treatment for melanoma concluded that high-dose INF-α treatment was associated with disease-free survival in high-risk primary melanomas; however, with intermediate- to high-risk melanomas the role of adjuvant therapy remains undefined.

Practical Guidelines for the management of interferon-alpha-2b side effects in patients receiving adjuvant treatment for melanoma: expert opinion. Hauschild A, Gogas H, Tarhini A, Middleton MR, Testori A, Dreno B, et al. Cancer 2008; 112: 982–94.

This article reviews the role of high-dose adjuvant interferon-α on the survival of patients with stage II and III melanoma, and concludes that it is incompletely defined. The authors consider the importance of patient discussion detailing the benefits and potential side effects of interferon therapy when evaluating treatment options.

Palliative therapy of disseminated malignant melanoma: a systematic review of 41 randomized clinical trials. Eigentler TK, Caroli UM, Radny P, Garbe C. Lancet Oncol 2003; 4: 748–59.

Dacarbazine remains the standard treatment for distant disease. None of the combination regimens has yet to demonstrate a significant survival advantage in randomized controlled studies.

Combination of paclitaxel and carboplatin as second-line therapy for patients with metastatic melanoma. Rao RD, Holtan SG, Ingle JN, Croghan GA, Kottschade LA, Creagan ET, et al. Cancer 2006; 106: 375–82.

This was a retrospective review article including 31 patients who received combination treatment after other treatment failures, most of which were post TMZ or DTIC. The authors concluded that the clinical benefit rates appear to be at least as good as for most other therapies considered standard for metastatic melanoma, and the data provide justification for further testing of this drug combination in the first-line setting.

Locoregional cutaneous metastases of malignant melanoma and their management. Wolf IH, Richtig E, Kopera D, Kerl H. Dermatol Surg 2004; 30: 244–7.

This article discussed the benefits seen especially as palliative treatment, with application of topical imiquimod 5% cream three times weekly to cutaneous metastases with a 1-cm margin. In a five-patient sample, complete clinical and histopathologic remission of locoregional cutaneous metastases of malignant melanoma occurred in two and partial remission occurred in one, with no regression in the remaining two patients.

Treatment of lentigo maligna with imiquimod before staged excision. Cotter MA, McKenna JK, Bowen GM. Dermatol Surg 2008; 34: 147–51.

Forty patients with biopsy-confirmed LM were treated five times a week for 3 months with 5% imiquimod cream before staged excision. Tazarotene 0.1% gel was added when no clinical signs of erythema developed with imiquimod alone after 1 month (10 patients). A total of 33 of 40 patients had a complete clinical response, as determined by the absence of remaining clinical lesions on physical examination. Upon histologic review, 30 of 40 patients had no evidence of LM, whereas 10 of 40 harbored residual disease. The authors conclude that imiquimod appears to be an effective adjuvant treatment for LM but does not qualify as replacement therapy for surgery.

Management of in-transit melanoma of the extremity with isolated limb perfusion. Fraker DL. Curr Treat Options Oncol 2004; 5: 173–84.

The primary use of ILP is in the treatment of satellitosis and in-transit metastasis. ILP involves very high doses of chemotherapeutic agents, usually melphalan, administered through either femoral, iliac, or axillary vessels to isolated anatomic regions. Reports have shown that the addition of tumor necrosis factor to melphalan may improve response rates, but no clear benefit has been demonstrated.

Bcl-2 antisense (oblimersen sodium) plus dacarbazine in patients with advanced melanoma: The Oblimersen Melanoma Study Group. Bedikian AY, Millward M, Pehamberger H, Conry R, Gore M, Trefzer U, et al. J Clin Oncol 2006; 24: 4738–45.

In one of the largest randomized controlled studies in advanced melanoma, 771 patients were randomly assigned to treatment with oblimersen-dacarbazine (386 patients) and dacarbazine (385). Bcl-2 protein inhibits apoptosis and confers resistance to treatment with traditional cytotoxic chemotherapy, radiotherapy, and monoclonal antibodies. Oblimersen sodium is an antisense oligonucleotide compound designed specifically to bind to human *bcl-2* mRNA, resulting in catalytic degradation of *bcl-2* mRNA and subsequent reduction in bcl-2 protein translation. It was found that the use of oblimersen with dacarbazine safely improves multiple outcomes in patients with advanced melanoma, particularly those with normal baseline LDH. As the patients in this study had severe advanced stage III and IV melanoma, the authors suggest examination of patients with less advanced disease in whom Bcl-2 expression has been confirmed.

THIRD-LINE THERAPIES

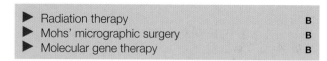

▶ Radiation therapy	**B**
▶ Mohs' micrographic surgery	**B**
▶ Molecular gene therapy	**B**

Radiotherapy for melanoma. Ang KK, Geara FB, Byers RM, Peters LJ. In: Balch CM, Houghton AN, Sober AJ, Soong S, eds. Cutaneous melanoma. Philadelphia: JB Lippincott, 1998; 389–401.

Radiation is rarely used for the primary treatment of melanoma, except in certain cases of facial lentigo maligna melanoma.

This chapter offers an excellent review of radiation treatment for melanoma, discussing studies examining radiotherapy as a palliative treatment for cutaneous, subcutaneous, osseous, and brain metastases.

A higher radiotherapy dose is associated with more durable palliation and longer survival in patients with metastatic melanoma. Kenneth R, Olivier KR, Schild SE, Morris CG, Brown PD, Markovic SN. Cancer 2007; 110: 1791–5.

In this study, 84 consecutive patients with 114 lesions that were not metastatic to the central nervous system (CNS) were evaluated for the response of the presenting symptom, the duration of response, and survival after radiotherapy (RT). The median dose delivered was 30 Gy and the median biologic effective dose (BED) was 39.0 Gy. The authors concluded that RT provided effective palliation of non-CNS metastasis from malignant melanoma and should be considered for symptomatic patients. RT doses >30 Gy and a BED >39.0 Gy were found to be associated with longer palliation, but the authors commented that their findings should be viewed with caution because the lack of data regarding performance status, as well as other unknown confounding factors, limit the applicability of a retrospective study.

Mohs micrographic surgery for the treatment of primary cutaneous melanoma. Zitelli JA, Brown C, Hanusa BH. J Am Acad Dermatol 1997; 37: 236–45.

In this large study, 535 patients with cutaneous melanoma of various thicknesses were treated with Mohs' micrographic surgery. After being divided into groups, depending on the thickness of the melanoma, the results were compared to historical controls that were treated with standard wide-margin surgical excision. The patients in this trial showed 5-year survival and metastatic rates that were equal to or better than those of historic controls.

With the lack of a randomized prospective study, this trial can only suggest the possible advantages of Mohs' surgery over standard excisional surgery in the treatment of primary cutaneous melanoma.

Mohs surgery for the treatment of melanoma in situ: A review. Dawn ME, Dawn AG, Miller SJ. Dermatol Surg 2007; 33: 395–402.

The article reviews the current literature on the benefit of Mohs' micrographic surgery to treat clinically ill-defined melanoma in situ, and concludes that there is substantial evidence to support complete margin assessment in the treatment of melanoma in situ, particularly in the head and neck region.

Mohs micrographic surgery is accurate 95.1% of the time for melanoma in situ: A prospective study of 167 cases. Bene NI, Healy C, Coldiron BM. Dermatol Surg 2008; 34: 660–4.

A total of 167 patients with melanoma in situ (MIS), including 116 with MIS in sun-exposed skin of lentigo maligna (LM) type, were treated by Mohs' surgery over a period of 12 years. The clearance rate by Mohs' technique using frozen sections was 95.1% for both melanoma in situ lentigo maligna type and non-lentigo maligna type. The cure rate was 98.2% for both MIS types for a mean follow-up of 63 months. The authors conclude that MIS can be difficult to treat, especially in sun-exposed areas, or areas such as the digits and genitals, where clear margins are harder to define. They state that their data confirm that Mohs' surgery represents a viable option for treatment of poorly defined MIS in critical locations.

Toward a molecular classification of melanoma. Fecher LA, Cummings SD, Keefe MJ, Alani RM. J Clin Oncol 2007: 1606–20.

This is an excellent review of the molecular pathways studied in melanoma and the clinical trials being conducted to target these pathways. The authors conclude that although molecular markers of potential clinical utility look promising in small-scale studies, the vast majority fail to prove clinically useful in larger-scale studies. These results appear to stem from the heterogeneous nature of melanomas and the lack of a classification scheme that would allow for tailored use of molecular markers and/or therapies. They go on to discuss that recent studies have shed new light on the molecular events associated with clinicopathologic subclasses of melanomas that have led to an evolving paradigm for classifying melanomas according to the degree of sun exposure and associated molecular defects.

Mastocytoses

Nicholas A Soter

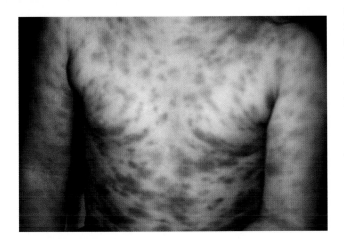

The mastocytoses are a group of disorders of mast cell proliferation that may exhibit both cutaneous and systemic features. Clinical manifestations result from mast-cell activation and from infiltration of various organs. The World Health Organization has classified mastocytosis into disease categories: cutaneous mastocytosis, indolent systemic mastocytosis, smoldering systemic mastocytosis, systemic mastocytosis with an associated clonal hematologic non-mast cell lineage, aggressive systemic mastocytosis, mast cell leukemia, mast cell sarcoma, and extracutaneous mastocytoma. The most frequent site of organ involvement in individuals with mastocytosis is the skin. Cutaneous forms include urticaria pigmentosa (shown here), mastocytoma, diffuse and erythrodermic cutaneous mastocytosis, and telangiectasia macularis eruptiva perstans. The cutaneous forms of mastocytosis may be present with or without systemic manifestations. Only the treatment of the cutaneous features will be discussed.

MANAGEMENT STRATEGY

An important aspect of therapy of the cutaneous lesions of mastocytosis is avoidance of triggering factors, which may include temperature changes, friction, physical exertion, ingestion of alcohol, the use of non-steroidal anti-inflammatory agents or opiate analgesics, and emotional stress. Of concern is the possibility of anaphylaxis after stings by *Hymenoptera* spp., which may occur even in patients receiving venom immunotherapy.

A history seeking systemic features should be undertaken, as well as a physical examination to determine the types of skin lesions and to seek lymphadenopathy and hepatosplenomegaly. The presence of specific systemic manifestations will dictate the type of specialty physician to whom a referral should be made.

Patients with systemic mastocytosis require long-term follow-up, as 10–30% may develop associated clonal hematogic non-mast cell lineage diseases, such as myelodysplastic or myeloproliferative syndromes, leukemias, or lymphomas.

A skin biopsy should be obtained in all individuals with cutaneous lesions. A complete blood count with differential analysis, a blood chemistry profile that includes liver function tests, and blood tryptase and interleukin (IL)-6 levels should be obtained in all patients with cutaneous lesions, except those with mastocytomas. If there are abnormalities of the complete blood count, a bone marrow examination should be obtained. Plasma histamine levels are not useful to screen patients. Twenty-four-hour urine levels of mast cell mediators may be obtained in patients with systemic features. Abdominal imaging studies provide a non-invasive means to assess the lymph nodes, liver, and spleen. In patients with bone pain, a ^{99}Tc bone scan is useful. Osteoporosis may be detected by bone density analysis.

In many cases cutaneous mastocytomas may involute spontaneously; it is rarely described in adults. Childhood urticaria pigmentosa regresses spontaneously in approximately 50% of cases and urticaria pigmentosa in adults in 10%. Diffuse and erythrodermic cutaneous mastocytosis usually resolves spontaneously between the ages of 15 months and 5 years. Telangiectasia macularis eruptiva perstans tends to be a chronic condition.

Most of the therapeutic reports have been in patients with urticaria pigmentosa and, to a lesser extent, in diffuse and erythrodermic cutaneous mastocytosis. The major therapeutic measure is the administration of *oral H_1 antihistamines* to alleviate pruritus and whealing. The use of antihistamines that interfere with the HERG K+ channel and cause cardiac arrhythmias should be avoided. *Oral disodium cromoglycate* has been efficacious in some individuals. The role and efficacy of topical high-potency glucocorticoid preparations with plastic-film occlusion or hydrocolloid dressings, of psoralens and ultraviolet A (PUVA) photochemotherapy, and UVA1 phototherapy have not been subjected to controlled clinical trials or remain anecdotal. There is no therapy that will eradicate the mast cells in the cutaneous lesions.

SPECIFIC INVESTIGATIONS

▶ Blood tryptase and IL-6 levels
▶ Bone density scan, 24-hour urine histamine, histamine metabolites, and prostaglandin metabolites
▶ Bone marrow examination

Diagnostic value of tryptase in anaphylaxis and mastocytosis. Schwartz LB. Immunol Allergy Clin North Am 2006; 26: 451–63.

Total and mature (β) tryptase levels are elevated in patients with systematic mastocytosis. Total tryptase levels reflect the increased burden of mast cells in patients with all forms of systemic mastocytosis. Mature tryptase levels reflect the magnitude of mast cell activation. The levels of tryptase are normal in patients with cutaneous mastocytosis.

IL-6 levels predict disease variant and extent of organ involvement in patients with mastocytosis. Brockow K, Akin C, Huber M, Metcalfe DD. Clin Immunol 2005; 115: 216–23.

In patients with systemic mastocytosis, plasma IL-6 levels were elevated and there was a significant correlation between plasma IL-6 and total tryptase levels (p<0.003). In patients with indolent systemic mastocytosis, the plasma IL-6 levels correlated with the extent of urticaria pigmentosa. Plasma levels of IL-6 in patients with cutaneous mastocytosis were not significantly different from those of healthy controls.

Elevated blood tryptase levels and IL-6 appear to be useful in differentiating patients with systemic disease from those with cutaneous disease.

Surrogate markers of disease in mastocytosis. Akin C, Metcalfe DD. Int Arch Allergy Immunol 2002; 127: 133–6.

Measurement of the histamine metabolites *N*-methylhistamine and methylimidazole acetic acid in 24-hour urine specimens is the preferred method of assessing baseline levels in patients with systemic mastocytosis, and these levels correlate with the amount of the mast cell burden. The levels of the major urinary metabolite of prostaglandin D_2 (9a, 11β-dihydroxy-15-oxo-2,3,18,19-tetranorprost-5-ene-1,20-dioxic acid) and thromboxane B_2 or its metabolites in plasma and urine are elevated in patients with systemic mastocytosis. Soluble forms of CD 25, the α chain of the interleukin-2 receptor, and CD 117, the receptor for stem cell factor, may be elevated in the circulation in systemic mastocytosis. A *c-kit* mutation may be detected in lesional tissues, such as skin and bone marrow in systemic mastocytosis.

Although these surrogate disease markers of mastocytosis are valuable tools in diagnosing the extent of disease, they should not be obtained routinely.

Histologische Charakteristika und Häufigkeit der sekundaren Osteoporose bei systemischer Mastozytose Eine retrospektive Analyse an 158 Fällen. Delling G, Ritzel H, Werner M. Pathologe 2001; 22: 132–40.

In a retrospective study of 158 untreated patients with mastocytosis, the prevalence of mastocytosis in iliac crest biopsy specimens was 1.25%, with a prevalence of 2.25% in individuals younger than 45 years. Osteopenia was present in 64% of patients with mastocytosis.

Bone marrow aspirates with biopsies in cutaneous mastocytosis should be restricted to individuals with changes in the complete blood count, organomegaly, or alterations in other organ systems. Some investigators recommend a bone marrow aspirate and biopsy in all patients with adult-onset disease.

FIRST-LINE THERAPIES

▶ H₁ antihistamines	A
▶ H₂ antihistamines	D
▶ Disodium cromoglycate	A

A double-blind, placebo-controlled, crossover trial of ketotifen versus hydroxyzine in the treatment of pediatric mastocytosis. Kettelhut BV, Berkebile C, Bradley D, Metcalfe DD. J Allergy Clin Immunol 1989; 83: 866–70.

In six children with urticaria pigmentosa and two with diffuse cutaneous mastocytosis, hydroxyzine alleviated pruritus (in seven) or the formation of bullae (in five). Ketotifen alleviated pruritus (in one) or the formation of bullae (in three).

Ketotifen is not available in the USA.

Comparison of azelastine and chlorpheniramine in the treatment of mastocytosis. Friedman BS, Santiago ML, Berkebile C, Metcalfe DD. J Allergy Clin Immunol 1993; 92: 520–6.

In a double-blind, randomized, crossover trial in 13 subjects with urticaria pigmentosa and systemic mastocytosis, the administration of both azelastine and chlorpheniramine for 4 weeks was associated with a reduction in pruritus.

Comparison of the therapeutic efficacy of cromolyn sodium with that of combined chlorpheniramine and cimetidine in systemic mastocytosis: results of a double-blind clinical trial. Frieri M, Alling DW, Metcalfe DD. Am J Med 1985; 78: 9–14.

Five of six patients had less pruritus and four of six had less urticaria while receiving chlorpheniramine and cimetidine. There was no beneficial effect in those receiving disodium cromoglycate.

Systemic mastocytosis treated with histamine H₁ and H₂ receptor antagonists. Gasior-Chrzan B, Falk ES. Dermatology 1992; 184: 149–52.

In a single patient with telangiectasia macularis eruptiva perstans and systemic mastocytosis, there was improvement in pruritus, erythema, and urticaria after the administration of cyproheptadine and cimetidine.

Cimetidine in systemic mastocytosis. Berg MJ, Bernhard H, Schentag JJ. Drug Intell Clin Pharm 1981; 15: 180–3.

An adult with systemic disease received treatment with cyproheptadine, Lomotil (diphenoxylate-atropine), and cimetidine. Prompt recurrence of gastrointestinal and dermatological symptoms occurred after stopping the cimetidine. The drug was restarted in 3 days and the symptoms subsided.

In systemic mastocytosis H₂ antagonists can play an additional role in reducing gastric hyperacidity.

Oral disodium cromoglycate in the treatment of systemic mastocytosis. Soter NA, Austen KF, Wasserman SI. N Engl J Med 1979; 301: 465–9.

In a double-blind crossover study in five patients with systemic mastocytosis and urticaria pigmentosa, in 15 of 18 trials, oral disodium cromoglycate ameliorated pruritus and whealing.

Urticaria pigmentosa treated with oral disodium cromoglycate. Lindskov R, Wantzin GL, Knudsen L, Søndergaard I. Dermatologica 1984; 169: 49–52.

In three of four patients with urticaria pigmentosa, the oral administration of disodium cromoglycate was associated with a reduction in pruritus and whealing as assessed by a diminution in dermographism.

Treatment of bullous mastocytosis with disodium cromoglycate. Welch EA, Alper JC, Bogaars H, Farrell DS. J Am Acad Dermatol 1983; 19: 349–53.

A reduction in pruritus, whealing response, and blister formation occurred in two infants with diffuse and erythrodermic cutaneous mastocytosis with bullae who were treated with oral disodium cromoglycate.

SECOND-LINE THERAPIES

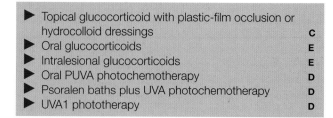

▶ Topical glucocorticoid with plastic-film occlusion or hydrocolloid dressings	C
▶ Oral glucocorticoids	E
▶ Intralesional glucocorticoids	E
▶ Oral PUVA photochemotherapy	D
▶ Psoralen baths plus UVA photochemotherapy	D
▶ UVA1 phototherapy	D

Treatment of urticaria pigmentosa with corticosteroids. Barton J, Lavker RM, Schechter NM, Lazarus GS. Arch Dermatol 1985; 121: 1516–23.

Evidence Levels: **A** Double-blind study **B** Clinical trial ≥ 20 subjects **C** Clinical trial < 20 subjects **D** Series ≥ 5 subjects **E** Anecdotal case reports

In six patients with urticaria pigmentosa, topical application of betamethasone dipropionate ointment 0.05% under occlusion for 8 hours daily for 6 weeks was associated with an absence of pruritus and Darier's sign. All patients remained clear of lesions at a mean follow-up of 11.5 months (range 9–15 months).

Urticaria pigmentosa: systemic evaluation and successful treatment with topical steroids. Guzzo C, Lavker R, Roberts LJ II, Fox K, Schechter N, Lazarus G. Arch Dermatol 1991; 127: 191–6.

In seven of nine adult patients with urticaria pigmentosa, the topical application of betamethasone dipropionate ointment 0.05% under occlusion overnight to one half of the body for 6 weeks was associated with resolution of the lesions, with a maximum response within 3–12 weeks after the cessation of treatment. Lesions began to recur between 6 and 9 months after completing therapy. Re-treatment for 6 months followed by once-weekly application of betamethasone dipropionate ointment under occlusion kept the patients clear of lesions, with the longest follow-up time being 2.5 years.

Prolonged remission of urticaria pigmentosa following topical steroid therapy under a hydrocolloid occlusion. Sidhu S, Wakelin SH, Wojnarowska F. Clin Exp Dermatol 1997; 22: 302–3.

In a single adult with urticaria pigmentosa treated with clobetasol propionate 0.05% under a hydrocolloid dressing once weekly for 6 weeks, there was a reduction in pruritus and fading of hyperpigmentation that has lasted for 6 years.

The appropriate method for using topical glucocorticoids in patients with urticaria pigmentosa needs to be determined in controlled trials.

Bullous mastocytosis treated with oral betamethasone therapy. Verma KK, Bhat R, Singh MK. Indian J Pediatr 2004; 71: 261–3.

In a 7-month-old girl with diffuse cutaneous mastocytosis with bullae and flushing, treatment with oral betamethasone 0.1 mg/kg/day caused remission within 4 weeks.

Mastocytoma: topical corticosteroid treatment. Mateo JR. J Eur Acad Dermatol Venereol 2001; 15: 492–4.

Four infants aged between 2.5 and 6 months with mastocytomas were treated with twice-daily applications of clobetasol propionate 0.05% for 6 weeks and on alternate days for 6 weeks with tapering for a total treatment of 6 months. At the end of treatment there were residual macules with atrophy and a negative Darier's sign.

Solitary mastocytoma improved by intralesional injections of steroid. Kang NG, Kim TH. J Dermatol 2002; 29: 536–8.

In a 2-month-old boy with a solitary mastocytoma treated with three intralesional injections of triamcinolone acetonide, the lesion became flat with a reduction in erythema and subjective symptoms 9 months after treatment.

Photochemotherapy (PUVA) in the treatment of urticaria pigmentosa. Vella Briffa D, Eady RAJ, James MP, Gatti S, Bleehen S. Br J Dermatol 1983; 109: 67–75.

In eight patients with urticaria pigmentosa treated with PUVA photochemotherapy twice weekly for 15–69 exposures, the amount of pruritus and whealing was reduced. The disease tended to relapse once the treatment was discontinued.

Short- and long-term effectiveness of oral and bath PUVA therapy in urticaria pigmentosa and systemic mastocytosis. Godt O, Proksch E, Streit V, Christophers E. Dermatology 1997; 195: 35–9.

In 20 patients with urticaria pigmentosa treated with PUVA photochemotherapy, improvement in pruritus was seen in eight of 15. Darier's sign was suppressed in seven and reduced in eight patients. There was follow-up for 18 years; 25% showed improvement for more than 5 years. Bath PUVA photochemotherapy with 8-methoxypsoralen was without effect. The success of PUVA photochemotherapy lasted from only a few weeks to more than 10 years.

Photochemotherapy of dominant, diffuse, cutaneous mastocytosis. Smith ML, Orton PW, Chu H, Weston WL. Pediatr Dermatol 1990; 7: 251–5.

In three infants and one child with diffuse cutaneous mastocytosis treated with oral PUVA photochemotherapy twice weekly for 3–5 months, there was reduced pruritus, reduced blister formation, and a less thick skin with persistence of dermographism.

Medium- versus high-dose ultraviolet A1 therapy for urticaria pigmentosa: a pilot study. Gobello T, Mazzanti C, Sordi D, Annessi G, Abeni D, Chinni LM, et al. J Am Acad Dermatol 2003; 49: 679–84.

In 12 patients with urticaria pigmentosa, treatment with both medium-dose (60 J/cm²) for 15 days and high-dose (130 J/cm²) for 10 days UVA1 was associated with less pruritus, with a decrease in the number of mast cells, and a change in the number of lesions over a 6-month period.

The appropriate method and schedules for the use of oral and bath PUVA photochemotherapy, UVA1 phototherapy, and even UVB phototherapy should be determined by controlled trials.

THIRD-LINE THERAPIES

▶ Interferon-α	D
▶ Leukotriene-receptor inhibitor	E
▶ Ciclosporin	E
▶ Nifedipine	E
▶ Thalidomide	E
▶ Hydrocolloid dressings	E
▶ Surgical excision	E
▶ Flashlamp-pumped pulsed dye and Nd:YAG lasers	E
▶ Electron beam radiation	E
▶ Imatinib mesylate	E
▶ Cladribine	D
▶ Omalizumab	E

Treatment of adult systemic mastocytosis with interferon [alpha]–results of a multicentre phase II trial on 20 patients. Casassus P, Caillat-Vigneron N, Martin A, Simon J, Gallais V, Beaudry P, et al. Br J Haematol 2002; 119: 1090–7.

In a prospective multicenter phase II trial of the use of daily subcutaneous injections of interferon-α$_{2b}$ in 20 adults with systemic mastocytosis, starting with 1 million units daily for 1 week, 3 million units/m² body surface daily for 2 weeks, then 5 million units/m² if tolerated for 6 months. In seven of 13 patients, attenuation of urticaria pigmentosa was noted. Relapse with reappearance of systemic symptoms occurred after withdrawal of therapy.

Leukotriene-receptor inhibition for the treatment of systemic mastocytosis. Tolar J, Tope WD, Neglia JP. N Engl J Med 2004; 350: 735–6.

In a 2-month-old boy with systemic mastocytosis and skin lesions, wheezing, and hepatomegaly, when montelukast 0.25 mg/kg twice daily was not given, wheezing and cutaneous vesicles reappeared and subsided when the drug was readministered.

The leukotriene-receptor inhibitors should be evaluated in mastocytosis in a controlled trial.

Response to cyclosporin and low-dose methylprednisolone in aggressive systemic mastocytosis. Kurosawa M, Amano H, Kanbe N, Igarashi Y, Nagata H, Yamashita T, et al. J Allergy Clin Immunol 1999; 103: S412–20.

In a single adult man with aggressive systemic mastocytosis with urticaria pigmentosa, the administration of ciclosporin 100 mg daily and methylprednisolone 4 mg daily was associated with control of pruritus and a reduction in the extent of urticaria pigmentosa.

This single anecdotal report does not allow assessment of the effect of ciclosporin.

Urticaria pigmentosa responsive to nifedipine. Fairley JA, Pentland AP, Voorhees JJ. J Am Acad Dermatol 1984; 11: 740–3.

In a single adult woman with urticaria pigmentosa, the administration of nifedipine 10 mg three times daily was associated with a reduction in urtication of the skin lesions.

Thalidomide in advanced mastocytosis. Damaj G, Bernit E, Ghez D, Claisse J-F, Schleinitz N, Harlé JR, et al. Br J Haematol 2008; 141: 249–53.

In two patients with systemic mastocytosis treated with thalidomide, the skin lesions resolved in one individual and decreased in the other, with resolution of pruritus.

Flushing due to solitary cutaneous mastocytoma can be prevented by hydrocolloid dressings. Yung A. Pediatr Dermatol 2004; 21: 262–4.

In an 8-week-old boy, a double-layer hydrocolloid dressing reduced the shearing forces and prevented flushing.

Solitary mastocytoma in an adult: treatment by excision. Ashinoff R, Soter NA, Freedberg IM. J Dermatol Surg Oncol 1993; 19: 487–8.

In a 33-year-old woman, a solitary mastocytoma was excised.

Treatment of an unusual solitary mast cell lesion with the pulsed dye laser resulting in cosmetic improvement and reduction in the degree of urticarial reaction. Rose RF, Daly BM, Sheehan-Dave, R. Dermatol Surg 2007; 31: 851–3.

In a 12-year-old girl with a solitary mast cell lesion with features of solitary mastocytoma and telangiectasia macularis eruptiva perstans treated with a 585-nm pulsed-dye laser, there was cosmetic improvement and reduction in the severity of wheals after six treatments.

The treatment of urticaria pigmentosa with the frequency-doubled Q-switch ND-YAG laser. Bedlow AJ, Gharrie S, Harland CC. J Cutan Laser Ther 2000; 2: 45–7.

In a 30-year-old woman with urticaria pigmentosa treated with a frequency-doubled Q-switched Nd:YAG laser, there was initial improvement in the clinical appearance, but the lesions recurred after 9 months.

The cosmetic treatment of uticaria pigmentosa with Nd-YAG laser at 532 nanometers. Resh B, Jones E, Glaser DA. Cosmet Dermatol 2005; 4: 78–82.

In a 19-year-old man with urticaria pigmentosa treated with a 532 nm diode-pumped Nd:YAG laser there was a reduction in the number of lesions.

The efficacy of lasers in the treatment of various forms of cutaneous skin lesions of mastocytosis remains unknown.

Treatment of telangiectasia macularis eruptiva perstans with total electron beam radiation. Monahan TP, Petropolis AA. Cutis 2003; 71: 357–9.

In a 60-year-old man with telangiectasia macularis eruptiva perstans treated with 4000 cGy in 40 fractionated treatments, both pruritus and cutaneous lesions resolved with a 1-year follow-up.

Successful treatment of progressive cutaneous mastocytosis with imatinib in a 2-year-old boy carrying a somatic KIT mutation. Hoffman KM, Moser A, Lohse P, Winkler A, Binder B, Sovinz P, et al. Blood 2008; 112: 1653–7.

In an 8-month-old boy with cutaneous mastocytosis with macules, papules, and bullae treated with imatinib for 13 months, the pruritus resolved and skin lesions improved. Within a week of discontinuing therapy the pruritus recurred and the lesions increased in size. Treatment was continued for a total of 32 months. At age 6, only non-pruritic hyperpigmented macules remain.

Cladribine therapy for systemic mastocytosis. Kluin-Nelemans HC, Oldhoff JM, van Doormaal JJ, van't Wout JW, Verhoef G, Gerrits WBJ, et al. Blood 2003; 102: 4270–6.

In each of seven patients with systemic mastocytosis and urticaria pigmentosa treated with cladribine, there was a reduction in the number of skin lesions to near disappearance and a reduction in mast cells in skin biopsy specimens.

Successful treatment of cutaneous mastocytosis and Ménière disease with anti-IgE therapy. Siebenhaar F, Kühn W, Zuberbier T, Maurer M. J Allergy Clin Immunol 2007; 120: 213–15.

In a 56-year-old woman with cutaneous mastocytosis described as red-brown macules and papules with an increase in mast cells in a skin biopsy specimen, treatment with omalizumab 150 mg every 2 weeks for 6 weeks, then maintenance monthly, controlled wheal formation and pruritus, although the skin lesions persisted.

Interferon-α, tyrosine kinase inhibitors, cytoreductive agents, and omalizumab have been used in patients with systemic mastocytosis, with improvement of the skin symptoms, or a reduction in the skin lesions, in some patients. The use of these therapeutic agents in extensive cutaneous mastocytosis without systemic disease has not been examined.

Melasma

Stephanie Ogden, Christopher EM Griffiths

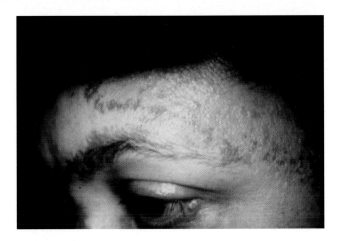

Melasma, or chloasma, a condition characterized by hyperpigmentation, occurs predominantly on the face of women of childbearing age. Several patterns of facial involvement are recognized, including central involving the forehead; cheeks, chin and upper lip; malar and mandibular. The condition may also occur on the forearms or neck with or without coexisting facial melasma. Individuals with Fitzpatrick skin type III or higher are most commonly affected. Rarely men may be affected.

Examination under Wood's or black light can be used to highlight the affected areas, thereby aiding diagnosis and monitoring of treatment. Lesional skin may demonstrate more prominent solar elastosis and increased vascularity. There are three histological subtypes of melasma: epidermal; dermal; and mixed epidermal and dermal. Epidermal melasma, which is most easily differentiated from uninvolved skin by its darkened appearance under Wood's light, is the most responsive to therapy.

The pathogenesis of melasma is not fully understood, but there is a definite relationship with high estrogen states, including pregnancy (up to 50–70% of pregnant women affected) and use of the oral contraceptive pill. There is some evidence that hormone replacement therapy can also contribute to the development of melasma. Other etiological factors include ethnicity and environmental factors, namely exposure to ultraviolet radiation (UV), and exposure to certain cosmetics containing phototoxic agents.

MANAGEMENT STRATEGY

Treatment of melasma is difficult owing to the recalcitrant and recurrent nature of the condition, although pregnancy-related melasma tends to improve spontaneously postpartum. Women taking the oral contraceptive pill may be advised to *change to an alternative low-estrogen contraceptive* or, if possible, to use an *alternative form of contraception*.

The hyperpigmentation is exacerbated by sun exposure; patients should therefore be advised regarding sun protection measures, in particular regular use of *broad-spectrum sunscreen, with good protection against UVA*. Regular sunscreen use may prevent the development of melasma in pregnant women.

Current treatment modalities include topical agents, chemical peels, and laser therapies. The response to monotherapy can be disappointing and a combination approach may yield greater success. The most frequently reported topical therapies include *2–5% hydroquinone, azelaic acid,* and *tretinoin*. More recently the use of *kojic acid, liquiritin,* and *rucinol* has been reported to improve melasma.

Overall the epidermal type of melasma responds best to topical treatments and to superficial chemical peels such as glycolic acid and Jessner's solution, which primarily remove melanin-laden keratinocytes from the epidermis.

SPECIFIC INVESTIGATIONS

> ▶ Thyroid function tests

Association of melasma with thyroid autoimmunity and other thyroidal abnormalities and their relationship to the origin of the melasma. Lufti RJ, Fridmanis M, Misiunas AL, Pafume O, Gonzalez EA, Villemur JA, et al. J Clin Endocrinol Metab 1985; 61: 28–31.

A study of 84 non-pregnant women with melasma and 24 age-matched controls found that in patients with melasma the frequency of thyroid disorders (58.3%) was four times greater than in the control group. Furthermore, 70% of women with melasma during pregnancy or while using oral contraceptives had thyroid abnormalities, compared to 39.4% with idiopathic melasma.

FIRST-LINE THERAPIES

▶ Triple combination agent (hydroquinone, tretinoin and fluocinolone)	A
▶ Hydroquinone	A
▶ Tretinoin	A
▶ Adapalene	A
▶ Sunscreen	A
▶ 'Kligman cream'	B

Treatment of melasma. Rendon M, Berneburg M, Arellano I, Picardo M. J Am Acad Dermatol 2006; 54: S272–81.

This review was performed by the Pigmentary Disorders Academy to evaluate the clinical efficacy of different treatments for melasma and provide a consensus on management. The preferred first-line therapy was topical: mainly fixed triple combinations.

Efficacy and safety of a new triple-combination agent for the treatment of facial melasma. Taylor SC, Torok H, Jones T. Cutis 2003; 72: 67–72.

Two multicentre, randomized studies compared the efficacy and safety of a formulation containing tretinoin 0.05%, hydroquinone 4.0%, and fluocinolone acetonide 0.01% with the three possible dual combinations of the three agents in 641 patients with melasma (Fitzpatrick skin types I–IV). Significantly more patients treated with the triple combination formulation experienced complete clearing of melasma, and at week 8 a 75% reduction in melasma/pigmentation was observed in more than 70% of patients treated, compared to 30% in patients treated with dual therapy.

A randomized controlled trial of the efficacy and safety of a triple fixed combination (fluocinolone acetonide 0.01%, hydroquinone 4%, tretinoin 0.05%) compared with hydroquinone 4% cream in Asian patients with moderate to severe melasma. Chan R, Park KC, Lee MH, Lee ES, Chang SE, Leow YH, et al. Br J Dermatol 2008; 159: 697–703.

Comparison of the topical triple combination as described above with hydroquinone 4% in a multicentre, randomized, investigator-blinded study of 260 Asian patients (majority skin phototype IV). A significantly higher number of patients treated with the triple combination achieved a melasma global severity score of none or mild after 8 weeks, although there were more adverse events in this group (none severe).

A new formula for depigmenting human skin. Kligman AM, Willis I. Arch Dermatol 1975; 11: 40–8.

This study demonstrated that a combination of 5.0% hydroquinone, 0.1% dexamethasone and 0.1% tretinoin ('Kligman cream') used for 3 months led to improvement in melasma, but no substantial improvement was seen when each agent was used alone.

Kligman cream is the forerunner of triple combination therapy.

Topical tretinoin (retinoic acid) improves melasma. A vehicle-controlled, clinical trial. Griffiths CEM, Finkel LJ, Ditre CM, Hamilton TA, Ellis CN, Voorhees JJ. Br J Dermatol 1993; 129: 415–21.

A study of 0.1% tretinoin once daily in 38 Caucasian women for 40 weeks found that 68% of tretinoin-treated patients were improved or much improved, compared to only 5% in the vehicle-treated group.

Adapalene in the treatment of melasma: a preliminary report. Dogra S, Kanwar AJ, Parasad D. J Dermatol 2002; 29: 539–40.

A randomized split-face study comparing adapalene 0.1% and tretinoin 0.05% for 14 weeks in 30 Indian women found no significant difference between the retinoids, with both producing a significant improvement in melasma.

The efficacy of a broad-spectrum sunscreen in the treatment of melasma. Vasquez M, Sanchez JL. Cutis 1983; 92: 95–6.

A double-blind study comparing a broad-spectrum sunscreen agent with its vehicle in 53 patients who were concomitantly using a depigmenting solution. Ninety-six percent of those who used the sunscreen showed improvement, compared to 80.7% of those who used placebo.

SECOND-LINE THERAPIES

▶ Azelaic acid	A

The treatment of melasma 20% azelaic acid versus 4% hydroquinone cream. Balina LM, Graupe K. Int J Dermatol 1991; 30: 893–5.

A double-blind randomized study of over 300 women. After the 24-week treatment period, 65% of azelaic acid-treated patients had good or excellent results. No significant treatment differences were observed with regard to overall rating, reduction in lesion size, and pigmentary intensity between azelaic acid- and hydroquinone-treated patients.

THIRD-LINE THERAPIES

▶ Liquiritin	A
▶ Rucinol	A
▶ Glycolic acid peel	A
▶ Salicylic acid peel	A
▶ Jessner's solution	A
▶ Kojic acid	B
▶ Intense pulsed light/laser(s)	B
▶ Lactic acid peel	B
▶ Dermabrasion	D
▶ N-acetyl-4-S-cysteaminylphenol	D

Topical liquiritin improves melasma. Amer M, Metwalli M. Int J Dermatol 2000; 39: 299–301.

A split-face study of twice-daily liquiritin or vehicle for 4 weeks in 20 women. Sixteen of 20 patients experienced an excellent response on the liquiritin-treated side (defined as no difference in pigmentation compared to normal surrounding skin). One patient experienced a fair response on the vehicle-treated side.

Evaluation of efficacy and safety of rucinol serum in patients with melasma: a randomized controlled trial. Khemis A, Kaiafa A, Queille-Roussel C, Duteil L, Ortonne JP. Br J Dermatol 2007; 156: 997–1004.

A double-blind, randomized study with a split-face design of rucinol serum or vehicle for 12 weeks in 28 women, which revealed a significant improvement in clinical pigmentation score in rucinol-treated compared with vehicle-treated skin.

Rucinol is a resorcinol derivative that inhibits tyrosinase and tyrosinase-related protein-1 activity in vitro.

Efficacy and safety of serial glycolic acid peels and a topical regimen in the treatment of recalcitrant melasma. Erbil H, Sezer E, Tastan B, Arca E, Kurumlu Z. J Dermatol 2007; 34: 25–30.

Twenty-eight patients were randomized to receive a cumulative total of eight glycolic acid peels every other week combined with azelaic acid 20% cream, and adapalene 0.1% gel applied at night, or the topical agents alone, over a 20-week treatment period. Both groups attained a statistically significant improvement in the Melasma Area and Severity Index (MASI) at 20 weeks, although there was greater improvement in the chemical peel group.

Tretinoin peels versus glycolic acid peels in the treatment of melasma in dark-skinned patients. Khunger N, Sarkar R, Jain RK. Dermatol Surg 2004; 30: 756–60.

A small prospective open study in 10 Indian women with melasma treated with 70% glycolic acid on one side of the face (left on for 1–3 minutes) and 1% tretinoin on the contralateral side (left on for 4 hours) on a weekly basis for 12 weeks. Equivalent lightening of melasma occurred with both agents.

Comparison of 30% salicylic acid with Jessner's solution for superficial chemical peeling in epidermal melasma. Ejaz A, Raza N, Iftikhar N, Muzzafar F. J Coll Phys Surg Pak 2008; 18: 205–8.

A double-blind randomized study of 60 Asian patients. Both peeling agents were effective in treating melasma as assessed by change in MASI scores.

434

Treatment of melasma with Jessner's solution versus glycolic acid: a comparison of clinical efficacy and evaluation of the predictive ability of Wood's light examination. Lawrence N, Cox SE, Brody HJ. J Am Acad Dermatol 1997; 36: 589–93.

Eleven women completed this study that consisted of 1–2 weeks' treatment with tretinoin 0.05%, followed by peels with 70% glycolic acid on the right side of the face and Jessner's solution on the left side on three occasions a month apart. After peeling, 0.05% tretinoin and 4% hydroquinone were used. There was no significant difference between peels, but several patients had persistent erythema.

Use of superficial peels may speed the response to topical agents.

Treatment of melasma using kojic acid in a gel containing hydroquinone and glycolic acid. Lim JTE. Dermatol Surg 1999; 25: 282–4.

A split-face study of 40 Chinese women with epidermal melasma randomized to receive 2% hydroquinone, 10% glycolic acid, and 2% kojic acid, or 2% hydroquinone and 10% glycolic acid alone for 12 weeks. Both preparations improved melasma.

A commentary on the article notes that kojic acid is considered to have high sensitizing potential.

Efficacy and safety of intense pulsed light in treatment of melasma in Chinese patients. Li Y, Chen JZS, Wei H, Wu Y, Liu M, Xu Y, et al. Dermatol Surg 2008; 34: 693–701.

Eighty-nine women with epidermal or mixed melasma were enrolled in this prospective uncontrolled study. Patients received a total of four treatments at 3-week intervals (590-/615-/640-nm filters, triple pulse for patients with mixed-type melasma). The mean MASI score decreased from 15.2 at baseline to 4.5 at the 3-month follow-up visit. Three patients developed postinflammatory hyperpigmentation.

The results in this study are far better than those of a previous smaller study. Controlled trials with longer follow-up are required to further assess the safety and efficacy of IPL in the treatment of melasma.

Erbium:YAG laser resurfacing for refractory melasma. Manaloto RM, Alster T. Dermatol Surg 1999; 25: 121–3.

All 10 women in this study had melasma resistant to topical bleaching creams and chemical peels. Resurfacing with the erbium:YAG laser calibrated to 1.0–1.5 J with a 5 mm collimated spot at 8 Hz (5.1–7.6 J/cm^2) led to an initial improvement in melasma, but was followed by significant postinflammatory hyperpigmentation. The latter improved with glycolic acid peels, topical azelaic acid, and sunscreen as tolerated.

Laser treatment is only recommended when topical treatments have failed.

Combined ultrapulse CO$_2$ laser and Q-switched alexandrite laser compared with Q-switched alexandrite laser alone for refractory melasma: split-face design. Angsuwarangsee S, Polnikorn N. Dermatol Surg 2003; 29: 59–64.

Six women were treated in this split-face study. Combination laser was better than Q-switched alexandrite laser alone. Three patients had postinflammatory hyperpigmentation.

The treatment of melasma with fractional photothermolysis: a pilot study. Rokhsar CK, Fitzpatrick RE. Dermatol Surg 2005; 31: 1645–50.

The Fraxel laser was used to treat 10 women with melasma. Four to six treatment sessions were performed at 1–2 weekly intervals. At 3 months half the patients reported their melasma to be 75–100% improved. There was one case of post-treatment hyperpigmentation.

Lactic acid chemical peels as a new therapeutic modality in melasma in comparison to Jessner's solution chemical peels. Sharquie KE, Al-Tikreety M, Al-Mashhadani. Dermatol Surg 2006; 32: 1429–36.

Chemical peeling with 92% lactic acid solution or Jessner's solution on a 3-weekly basis in a split-face study of 24 patients (four of whom were men) led to a significant improvement in MASI scores (mean 76.69% reduction). There was no significant difference between the two peels.

Dermabrasion: a curative treatment for melasma. Kunachak S, Leelaudomlipi P, Wongwaisayawan S. Aesthet Plast Surg 2001; 25: 114–17.

Of 410 patients with melasma followed up for between 1 and 9 years after treatment by mechanical dermabrasion (using a rotatory diamond fraise), 398 (97%) achieved persistent clearance of melasma. Side effects included temporary erythema (35%), hyperpigmentation (40%), pruritus, and milia. Two patients developed hypertrophic scars, and one experienced permanent hypopigmentation on the forehead.

Only recommended following failure of topical agents, associated with significant 'downtime.'

N-acetyl-4-S-cysteaminylphenol as a new type of depigmenting agent for the melanoderma of patients with melasma. Jimbow K. Arch Dermatol 1991; 127: 1528–34.

A retrospective observation of 12 patients treated with N-acetyl-4-S-cysteaminylphenol as an oil-in-water emulsion on a daily basis for 4 weeks. All patients experienced at least moderate improvement of melasma lesions.

Merkel cell carcinoma

Manjit R Kaur, Jeremy R Marsden

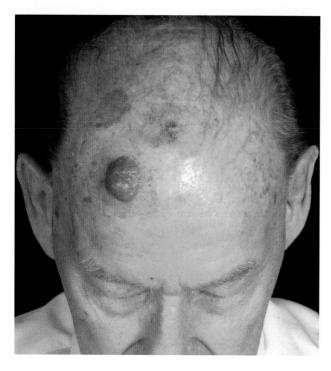

Merkel cell carcinoma (MCC) is a rare and aggressive neuroendocrine carcinoma of the skin. It is commoner in men, in white skin, and in the elderly. It presents as a rapidly enlarging red/purple papule or nodule on sun-exposed sites. Recent evidence suggests that a novel Polyomavirus may be pathogenic. There are several factors that may be contributing to the increased incidence of MCC, including increasing UV exposure, immunosuppression, an aging population, and increased detection and reporting of MCC. Although around 50 times less common than melanoma, it has a higher mortality (40–60%). The optimal management of MCC is unclear, owing to its rarity and the lack of controlled clinical trial data. Much of the existing literature is based on single center case series and retrospective reviews, which are inherently subject to bias.

MANAGEMENT STRATEGY

At present at least two different staging systems are in use for MCC, but neither accounts for the specific characteristics and prognostic factors. However, a new AJCC Staging System specifically for Merkel cell carcinoma will be published in 2009 in the seventh edition of the *AJCC Cancer Staging Manual*. The prognosis of MCC is highly dependent on the stage at presentation. Patients with primary disease have 5-year survival rates of 90%, which decreases to 60% with regional involvement, and to 10% among those presenting with distant metastatic disease, where the median survival is around 8 months. The single most consistent predictor of survival is the presence of lymph node disease (clinical or sentinel node-positive disease).

Surgical management of MCC is similar to that for melanoma. *Wide local excision* is recommended for excision of the primary, but there are no controlled trials comparing different margins. In addition, there are no consistent prognostic indicators such as Breslow thickness or tumor diameter to provide guidance. Similar to melanoma management, prophylactic nodal dissection has not been shown to provide any survival advantage.

MCC has a much higher rate of microscopic involvement of the lymph nodes (30%) than melanoma (15%). Sentinel lymph node biopsy (SLNB) permits directed adjuvant therapy of the regional lymph nodes. However, survival data are lacking, and therefore there is insufficient evidence to support its use routinely to guide treatment decisions.

Unlike melanoma, MCC is both radiosensitive and chemosensitive. There is a role for primary radiotherapy when surgery is not possible. Combined surgery plus radiotherapy may be associated with a lower locoregional recurrence rate and longer overall survival than surgery alone. However, the role of adjuvant radiotherapy is not clear, as the effect of varying surgical margins is not defined. The evidence for adjuvant chemotherapy is lacking; at present it is generally reserved for palliation of metastatic disease. Protein kinase inhibitors may be promising therapies for the future, with a phase II trial of imatinib in progress for the treatment of metastatic or inoperable MCC. Imatinib's activity includes inhibition of the expression of the proto-oncogene c-kit, which is frequently expressed in Merkel cell carcinoma.

SPECIFIC INVESTIGATIONS

> ▶ Skin biopsy with confirmatory immunohistochemical stains
> ▶ Sentinel lymph node biopsy

Merkel cell carcinoma can be distinguished from metastatic small cell carcinoma using antibodies to cytokeratin 20 and thyroid transcription factor 1. Leech SN, Kolar AJ, Barrett PD, Sinclair SA, Leonard N. J Clin Pathol 2001; 54: 727–9.

Ten of 11 MCCs stained with the antibody to CK20, but none was positive for TTF-1. All cases of small cell carcinoma stained strongly with anti-TTF-1 and none for CK-20.

This study illustrates the usefulness of immunohistochemical antibody-based stains such as CK-20 and TTF-1, which have greatly facilitated the ease and specificity of MCC diagnosis.

Sentinel lymph node biopsy for evaluation and treatment of patients with Merkel cell carcinoma: the Dana Farber experience and meta-analysis of the literature. Gupta GS, Wang LC, Penas PF, Gellenthin M, Lee SJ, Nghiem P. Arch Dermatol 2006; 142 : 685–90.

One hundred and twenty-two patients with clinically localized MCC were included (30 from Dana Farber Institute and 92 from 12 publications). Positive SLNB was seen in 32% of patients. Three-year relapse-free survival (RFS) was three times lower with a positive SLNB and was significantly improved with the use of adjuvant therapy in such patients, although detail with regard to which adjuvant therapy is superior is not apparent. The median follow-up was 12–15 months.

This is the largest and most comprehensive meta-analysis on the accuracy and usefulness of SLNB and confirms the utility of SLNB as a prognostic indicator for MCC. As the mean time to the development of distant metastatic disease is 18 months, the study was unable to assess the true impact of SLNB-guided therapeutic decisions using overall survival as an outcome measure. RFS is of uncertain value. The study is confounded by heterogeneity of treatment, lead-time bias, and small numbers.

FIRST-LINE THERAPIES

▶ Surgery **B**
▶ Surgery with adjuvant radiation **B**
▶ Radiation **D**

Adjuvant local irradiation for Merkel cell carcinoma. Lewis KG, Weinstock MA, Weaver AL, Otley CC. Arch Dermatol 2006; 142: 693–700.

This meta-analysis of 1254 cases in 132 reports is the largest collective evidence regarding the efficacy of local adjuvant radiotherapy in the management of MCC. Surgery and adjuvant radiotherapy were compared with surgery alone: there were threefold reductions in local recurrence (12% vs 39%) and twofold reductions in regional recurrence (23% vs 56%). Rates of distant metastasis and overall survival were similar. The median follow-up was 28.2 months.

The main limitation of this study was lack of uniformity of treatments in the many case series from which the data were extracted.

Adjuvant radiation therapy is associated with improved survival in Merkel cell carcinoma of the skin. Mojica P, Smith D, Ellenhorn JD. J Clin Oncol 2007; 25: 1043–7.

A retrospective analysis of 1187 MCC cases with locoregional disease from the SEER registry between 1973 and 2002. Patients receiving surgery alone (n=689) were compared to those receiving surgery plus adjuvant radiotherapy (n=477). The median overall survival for patients receiving surgery and radiotherapy was 63 months, compared to 45 months despite higher-stage disease in the radiotherapy group. Patients with larger tumours (>2 cm) had the most benefits from adjuvant radiotherapy.

This is the second retrospective study to show a survival benefit with 'any' adjuvant radiotherapy for MCC. However, the results have to be interpreted with caution because of the heterogeneity of treatments and regimens.

Radiotherapy alone for primary Merkel cell carcinoma. Arch Mortier L, Mirabel X, Fournier C, Piette F, Lartigau E. Dermatology 2003; 139: 1587–90.

Nine patients with inoperable localized tumors were treated with radiotherapy alone and none relapsed during 3 years of follow-up, compared to 17 patients treated with surgery and radiotherapy where two patients relapsed. Radiotherapy was delivered with at least 2 cm margins and the median dose was 60 Gy in five fractions, with a standardized regimen of five sessions per week. Six patients had radiotherapy to both the primary site and the regional nodal basin.

This small study makes the point that primary radiotherapy can be very effective.

SECOND-LINE THERAPIES

▶ Chemotherapy **B**

Chemotherapy for patients with locally advanced or metastatic Merkel cell carcinoma. Voog E, Biron P, Martin JP, Blay JY. Cancer 1999; 85; 2589–95.

One hundred and seven patients from 37 different centers with locally advanced or metastatic MCC on 42 different regimens were reviewed in this exhaustive literature review conducted between 1980 and 1995. Overall response rates to first-line chemotherapy were around 61%, with a median response duration of 8 months; 7.7% died from drug toxicity. Platinum-containing regimens (n=26), of which cisplatin/etoposide were the most common, had response rates of 61%. The combination of doxorubicin and cisplatin yielded a 100% response rate for seven patients with metastasis treated in five different series. 5-Fluorouracil-containing regimens also resulted in higher response rates of 92%, but were only given to 12 patients. Progression after first-line chemotherapy was associated with significantly worse survival for patients with metastases, and response rates to second and third-line chemotherapy were significantly lower.

This study indicates the efficacy of chemotherapy in MCC, but the optimal chemotherapy regimen remains to be determined.

Hyperthermic isolated limb perfusion with tumor necrosis factor alpha, interferon gamma, and melphalan for locally advanced nonmelanoma skin tumors of the extremities: a multicenter study. Olieman AF, Liénard D, Eggermont AM, Kroon BB, Lejeune FJ, Hoekstra HJ, et al. Arch Surg 1999; 134: 303–7.

Three patients with MCC were treated in a phase II study consisting of hyperthermic isolated limb perfusion with TNF-α, interferon-γ and melphalan. Limb salvage was achieved in all three patients, although only one had a complete response.

Our own experience of regional chemotherapy using isolated limb infusion indicates that it can provide very effective palliation.

THIRD-LINE THERAPIES

▶ Synchronous adjuvant chemo-radiotherapy **C**
▶ Adjuvant chemotherapy **D**

High risk Merkel cell carcinoma of the skin treated with synchronous carboplatin/etoposide and radiation: A Trans Tasman Radiation Oncology Group Study – TROG 96: 07. Poulsen M, Rischin D, Walpole E, Harvey J, Mackintosh J, Ainslie J, et al. J Clin Oncol 2003; 21: 4371–6.

A phase II non-randomized prospective study of 53 patients who had advanced localized, nodal, or recurrent disease. Radiation was delivered to the primary site and nodes at 50 Gy in 25 fractions over 5 weeks. Synchronous chemotherapy was given with carboplatin and etoposide at weeks 1, 4, 7, and 10; 87% of patients completed the chemotherapy and there were no treatment-related deaths. Grade 3/4 neutropenia was seen in 60%. Despite the high proportion of patients with nodal disease the 3-year survival rate was 76%. Locoregional and distant rates of control were also superior to those of other series.

This study indicates that synchronous chemoradiotherapy is tolerated well, but further investigation is needed to assess the true magnitude of these benefits.

Does chemotherapy improve survival in high risk stage I and II Merkel cell carcinoma of the skin? Poulsen MG, Rischin D, Porter I, Walpole E, Harvey J, Hamilton C, et al. Int J Radiat Oncol Biol Phys 2006; 64: 114–19.

Patients treated with synchronous chemoradiotherapy in the TROG study (n=42) were compared with matched historic control subjects treated with surgery and radiotherapy (n=62). No significant benefit of chemotherapy was found on overall survival, disease-specific survival, locoregional or distant metastasis. However, the study was underpowered to detect small improvements in survival.

There were several sources of bias in this study despite matching – these inherent differences in the group could have had an effect on the differences in outcome between the two arms. This study poses a very important question and requires a randomized controlled trial to answer it.

Miliaria

Christen M Mowad, Periasamy Balasubramaniam,
Warren R Heymann

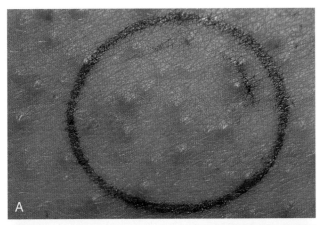

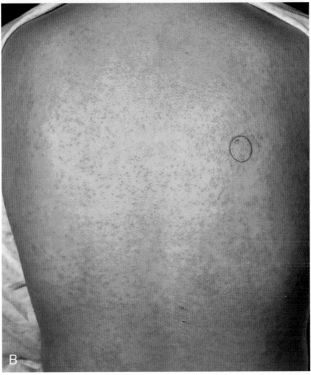

Miliaria is a benign, transient disorder caused by occlusion in the eccrine duct. It is subdivided into miliaria rubra, miliaria crystallina, and miliaria profunda, based on the level of obliteration. Miliaria rubra ('prickly heat') is the most common, presenting as numerous pruritic non-follicular papules or vesicles with surrounding erythema. The obstruction occurs within the eccrine duct in the stratum malpighii. Typically it occurs on the trunk, neck, or back, but can affect other areas and has been reported to occur under splints or braces because of the warm occlusive environment. Miliaria crystallina, the most superficial form (sudamina), occurs with occlusion of the sweat duct in the stratum corneum. It is self-limited and typically appears as clear vesicles without significant erythema. Miliaria profunda is more uncommon, the

occlusion occurring at the dermoepidermal junction or dermis. Miliaria profunda is typically seen after repeated cases of miliaria rubra in tropical settings. These patients can also have associated systemic symptoms related to overheating.

MANAGEMENT STRATEGY

Miliaria most typically occurs as a result of excessive sweating in hot, humid conditions, prolonged perspiration, or following extended febrile illness. There are other less common reports of congenital miliaria, miliaria occurring after medication administration in the intensive care setting, and in association with congenital illnesses such as pseudohypoaldosteronism. Miliaria is often exacerbated by tight clothing and high humidity. Management begins with *removal of the inciting factors,* so most of the literature has focused on identifying causative agents. There is no strong evidence for the various treatment options.

Adults often develop miliaria during travel and military service in the tropics or with heavy exercise. *Gradual exposure* helps to acclimatize to a hot and humid environment, but this may take a few months. *Loose-fitting clothing* and *cool showers* may minimize the symptoms. Mild cases may benefit from the use of light powders such as *cornstarch* or baby *talcum powder.* With the use of any topical lotion, cream, or powder, care must be taken to ensure that the product applied does not occlude the skin, further exacerbating the condition. In the case of severe itching, *antihistamines, cold packs,* and *topical corticosteroids* may be used. *Oatmeal baths* have been anecdotally reported to provide relief. However, all these measures will prove ineffective if the sweating is not reduced. All cases will respond to *air-conditioning, exposure of the involved skin,* and the use of *antipyretics,* in appropriate circumstances. Miliaria profunda has been reported to respond to oral retinoids and anhydrous lanolin.

Miliaria may be complicated by superinfection. If infection occurs, it should be treated with *systemic antibiotics* aimed at staphylococci as the likely pathogen. Clinicians should make patients aware that anhidrosis in the area of the eruption may occur and persist up to 3 weeks (or sometimes even longer) after the onset of lesions, and increased heat retention may occur if a large surface area was initially affected. Thus, patients at risk of heat exhaustion or heat stroke should take precautions to remain in air-conditioned environments during hot weather. A biopsy may be helpful in atypical cases of miliaria.

SPECIFIC INVESTIGATIONS

► None usually required

In atypical cases
► Microbiology – swab for bacteria and yeasts
► Histology

Nonneoplastic disorders of the eccrine glands. Wenzel FG, Horn TD. J Am Acad Dermatol 1998; 38: 1–7.

The histology and pathophysiology of eccrine sweat ducts are reviewed, as are normal and abnormal sweat content and formation. The erythematous macule or papule of miliaria rubra occurs with an obstruction of the sweat duct at the level of the stratum malpighii. In the case of miliaria crystallina the disruption is in the stratum corneum, and with miliaria profunda, at or beneath the dermoepidermal junction. The pathogenesis of miliaria is reviewed, describing the role of resident bacteria and PAS-positive extracellular polysaccharide substance blocking eccrine ducts.

Duct disruption, a new explanation of miliaria. Shuster S. Acta Dermatol Venereol 1997; 77: 1–3.

A hypothesis is presented that ascribes miliaria crystallina to mechanical disruption of the eccrine duct, rather than the commonly accepted pathogenesis of duct plugging. This disruption is attributed to UV irradiation causing a split between upper epidermal cells and stratum corneum.

The role of extracellular polysaccharide substance produced by *Staphylococcus epidermidis* in miliaria. Mowad CM, McGinley KJ, Foglia A, Leyden JJ. J Am Acad Dermatol 1995; 33: 729–33.

The ability of various strains of coagulase-negative staphylococci to induce miliaria under an occlusive dressing as well as microbiologic, histologic, and immunostaining features were evaluated. *Staphylococcus epidermidis* was the only strain that induced miliaria. The authors conclude that periodic acid–Schiff (PAS)-positive extracellular polysaccharide substance (EPS) produced by *S. epidermidis* plays a central role in the pathogenesis of miliaria by obstructing sweat delivery.

The pathogenesis of miliaria rubra: role of the resident microflora. Holzle E, Kligman AM. Br J Dermatol 1978; 99: 117–37.

The degree of miliaria rubra and anhidrosis induced in 55 subjects was shown to be directly correlated with the density of resident flora present on occluded areas of skin, as measured by detergent scrub and culture. A historical overview of research into the pathogenesis of miliaria rubra is included.

Miliaria crystallina in an intensive care setting. Haas N, Martens F, Henz BM. Clin Exp Dermatol 2004; 29: 32–4.

Two cases of miliaria crystallina occurring in an intensive care setting are presented. The authors hypothesize that the mechanism is secondary to transient poral closure due to the drugs used in the intensive care setting that may have stimulated sweating.

Pruritus, papules and perspiration. LaShell M, Tankersley M, Guerra A. Ann Allergy Asthma Immunol 2007; 98: 299–302.

Case report of an 18-year-old woman in Alaska who developed diffuse pruritus and water-filled pinpoint bumps on her abdomen and extremities occurring within 30 minutes of indoor exercise or hot tub exposure. This article reviews common exercise-induced eruptions, with miliaria rubra being discussed as the cause of this patient's recurring, self-limited eruption. Exercise challenge recreated the clinical picture and confirmed the diagnosis.

Neoprene splinting: dermatologic issues. Stern EB, Callinan N, Hank M, Lewis EJ, Schousboe JT, Ytterberg Sr R. Am J Occup Ther 1998; 52: 573–8.

A case of miliaria rubra developing under a neoprene splint where excess perspiration may collect under the skin in hot or cold environments. The neoprene fails to wick away perspiration from the skin, providing an ideal environment for miliaria. This needs to be differentiated from allergic contact dermatitis to neoprene.

Newborn with pseudohypoaldosteronism and miliaria rubra. Akcakus M, Koklu E, Poyrazoglu H, Kurtoglu S. Int J Dermatol 2006; 45: 1432–4.

Autosomal recessive type I pseudohypoaldosteronism as a cause of miliaria is discussed in a patient who developed miliaria rubra specifically during salt depletion crises. The rash cleared after stabilization of electrolytes and reappeared upon hyponatremia. The patient had two siblings with similar eruptions. The miliaria rubra seen in this patient was felt to be due to high concentrations of sodium chloride in the sweat directly damaging eccrine ducts.

FIRST-LINE THERAPIES

▶ Prevention	D
▶ Frequent showering	E
▶ Cornstarch powder	E
▶ Air conditioning	B
▶ Oatmeal baths	E
▶ Topical antiseptics	E
▶ Antipyretics	E

Miliaria rubra of the lower limbs in underground miners. Donoghue AM, Sinclair MJ. Occup Med (Lond) 2000; 50: 430–3.

Case series of 25 miners working in a hot and humid environment who developed miliaria. Symptoms resolved after 4 weeks of sedentary duties in the air-conditioned areas. This report also analyzed coexisting dermatological conditions in these patients.

Diseases of the eccrine sweat glands. Hurley HJ. In: Bolognia JL, Jorizzo JL, Rapini RP, eds. Dermatology. Philadelphia: Mosby, 2003; 578–9.

Cornstarch or other light powders may be used to absorb moisture and minimize the maceration that causes the early changes needed for the development of miliaria.

Goosefleshlike lesions and hypohidrosis. Dimon NS, Fullen DR, Helfrich YR. Arch Dermatol 2007; 43: 1323–8.

Numerous treatments for miliaria are described, including anhydrous lanolin, oral isotretinoin, regular bathing to remove salt and bacteria, and antibiotics.

Newborn skin: Part I. Common rashes. O'Connor NR, McLaughlin MR, Ham P. Am Fam Phys 2008; 77: 47–52.

Numerous skin conditions exist in the newborn period. These are often concerning to parents. Physicians need to identify common skin lesions in order to provide proper management and parental counseling. Miliaria is a self-limited disorder and can be treated with avoidance of overheating, removal of excessive clothing, cooling baths, and air-conditioning.

Environmental illness in athletes. Seto CK, Way D, O'Connor N. Clin Sports Med 2006; 24: 695–718.

The wide spectrum of heat-related illness is discussed in detail. Miliaria rubra occurs with exposure to high heat and humidity as a result of occluded sweat glands. Treatment involves cooling and drying, and avoidance of further sweating.

SECOND-LINE THERAPIES

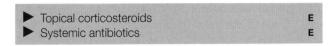

| ▶ Topical corticosteroids | E |
| ▶ Systemic antibiotics | E |

Miliaria rubra. Stearns JA. In: Dambro MR, ed. Griffith's 5-minute clinical consult. Philadelphia: Lippincott, Williams & Wilkins, 2000; 688–9.

For relief of pruritus, 0.1% betamethasone twice daily for 3 days may be applied over the affected area. In the event of superimposed infection, an antistaphylococcal agent such as dicloxacillin (flucloxacillin) 250 mg four times daily for 10 days may be used.

Prickly heat. Vicario S. In: Marx JA, ed. Rosen's emergency medicine: concepts and clinical practice, 6th edn. Vol 3. Philadelphia: Mosby, 2006; 2259.

If a case of miliaria rubra becomes pustular, oral erythromycin has been shown to be helpful. During the most acute phase of miliaria rubra, chlorhexidine lotion or cream can be used as an antibacterial agent, with salicylic acid 1% three times daily over small areas to aid in desquamation.

THIRD-LINE THERAPIES

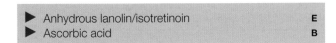

| ▶ Anhydrous lanolin/isotretinoin | E |
| ▶ Ascorbic acid | B |

Miliaria profunda. Kirk JF, Wilson BB, Chun W, Cooper PH. J Am Acad Dermatol 1996; 35: 854–6.

This case report describes a 23-year-old man with miliaria profunda successfully treated with both anhydrous lanolin and isotretinoin, after a poor response to topical corticosteroids. The impact of either as an individual treatment is therefore difficult to access. Characteristic features, pathogenesis, histopathology, and treatment are discussed.

The effects of administration of ascorbic acid in experimentally induced miliaria and hypohidrosis in volunteers. Hindson TC, Worsley DE. Br J Dermatol 1969; 81: 226–7.

Miliaria and hypohidrosis were induced in 36 subjects, half of whom were given 1 g daily of ascorbic acid and half a placebo, beginning on the day of wrapping the skin with polythene occlusion. Compared to the placebo group the ascorbic acid group developed less severe miliaria and hypohidrosis, had quicker healing of visible lesions, and notable improvement in hypohidrosis at 1 week.

Molluscum contagiosum

Patricia M Gordon, E Claire Benton

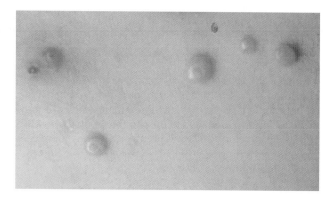

Molluscum contagiosum (MC) is a common self-limiting poxvirus infection of the skin and occasionally mucous membranes. Lesions occur in children, usually on the trunk and body folds, and in young adults, if sexually transmitted, in the genital region. They typically present as multiple 1–10 mm diameter discrete, pearly-white or flesh-coloured umbilicated papules. They may be surrounded by an eczematous reaction, which disappears on resolution of the infection. Mollusca may be very extensive and recalcitrant to treatment in all forms of cell-mediated immunosuppression, especially patients with AIDS.

MANAGEMENT STRATEGY

There is no specific antiviral therapy for molluscum contagiosum. Physical and chemical destructive methods of treatment as well as topical and systemic immunostimulatory therapies have been tried, but no single intervention has been convincingly shown to be effective. Only a few have been subjected to the rigors of placebo-controlled studies, important for a condition that has a high spontaneous resolution rate.

The choice of therapy will depend on the age and immune status of the patient as well as the number and location of the lesions. In immunocompetent patients with few lesions it is reasonable to *await spontaneous resolution*, which will usually occur within a few months. Secondarily infected MC may need *topical antiseptic or antibiotic* treatment to minimize the risk of atrophic scarring. Active intervention may be justified for cosmetic reasons, or to hasten resolution, in order to prevent autoinoculation or transmission of the virus to close contacts. Avoidance of communal bathing and restriction of the sharing of towels should also help prevent the spread of infection to others.

A commonly used and inexpensive treatment is the *manual extrusion* of individual lesions using gloved fingers or fine forceps. This has proved more effective than *cryotherapy* applied every 3–4 weeks. *Curettage and electrodesiccation* of larger lesions may result in scarring and also requires pain alleviation, especially in children, by the prior application of a eutectic mixture of local anesthetics (lidocaine and prilocaine cream). Topically applied caustic agents have been used with variable results. Good success rates are reported with topical application of 40% *silver nitrate paste*, *0.5% podophyllotoxin*,

and 10% povidone-iodine with 50% salicylic acid. A useful alternative is *5% acidified nitrite, applied nightly with 5% salicylic acid under occlusion*. Significant scarring has been documented with both potassium hydroxide and phenol, and the latter is no longer recommended. Although *cantharidin* has proved to be an effective treatment, it is not readily available in the UK and is not currently recommended by the Food and Drug Administration. The topical immune response modifier *imiquimod* has been shown to be effective and safe in several placebo-controlled studies. In patients with AIDS, both *1% imiquimod and topical cidofovir 3%*, a competitive inhibitor of DNA polymerase, have proved successful for treating MC. Recovery of immune function with *highly active antiretroviral therapy* (HAART) may also result in the resolution of MC in these patients.

SPECIFIC INVESTIGATIONS

> ▶ Methylene blue staining of a smear to look for molluscum bodies or histopathology of a curetted specimen

This is only required when the diagnosis is in any doubt.

FIRST-LINE THERAPIES

▶ Await spontaneous resolution	B
▶ Manual extrusion with gloved fingers or fine forceps	B

The natural history of molluscum contagiosum in Fijian children. Hawley TG. J Hygiene 1970; 68: 631–2.

Although the individual lesions of MC last 6–8 weeks, by autoinoculation the total duration of infection may be up to 8 months.

Scarring in molluscum contagiosum: comparison of physical expression and phenol ablation. Weller R, O'Callaghan CJ, MacSween RM, White MI. Br Med J 1999; 319: 1540.

There was no difference in overall efficacy of the two methods, but phenol resulted in significantly more scarring.

SECOND-LINE THERAPIES

▶ Topical 5% acidified nitrite co-applied with 5% salicylic acid	A
▶ Topical salicylic acid gel 12%	A
▶ Topical 10% povidone-iodine and 50% salicylic acid	B
▶ Topical 40% silver nitrate paste	B
▶ Topical 0.5% podophyllotoxin	B
▶ Cryotherapy	C

Molluscum contagiosum effectively treated with a topical acidified nitrite, nitric oxide liberating cream. Ormerod AD, White MI, Shah SAA, Benjamin N. Br J Dermatol 1999; 141: 1051–3.

A double-blind study in 30 children of sodium nitrite 5% co-applied nightly with 5% salicylic acid resulted in a cure rate of 75%, compared to 21% with salicylic acid alone.

Topical therapy with salicylic gel as a treatment for molluscum contagiosum in children. Leslie KS, Dootson G, Sterling JC. J Dermatol Treat 2005; 16: 336–40.

One hundred and fourteen children with MC were treated with 70% alcohol vehicle, phenol 10% or salicylic acid gel 12%. Salicylic acid was well tolerated and significantly better than the vehicle alone or phenol.

Molluscum contagiosum treated with iodine solution and salicylic acid plaster. Ohkuma M. Int J Dermatol 1990; 29: 443–5.

Povidone-iodine solution 10%, and 50% salicylic acid plaster applied daily to MC in 20 patients was significantly more effective than either agent used alone, with a mean duration to clearance of 26 days and with no adverse effects.

Treatment of molluscum contagiosum with silver nitrate paste. Niizeki K, Hashimoto K. Pediatr Dermatol 1999; 16: 395–7.

In 389 patients topical 40% silver nitrate paste was applied after 2% lidocaine gel; 70% cleared after one application, 97.7% after three applications. Treatment was well tolerated and no scarring was reported. It was easier to apply than a 40% aqueous solution of silver nitrate.

Podophyllotoxin in the treatment of molluscum contagiosum. Deleixhe-Mauhin F, Piérard-Franchimont C, Piérard GE. J Dermatol Treat 1991; 2: 99–101.

Twenty-four patients applied 0.5% podophyllotoxin solution daily. All cleared after less than 15 applications, without side effects apart from mild irritation.

Molluscum contagiosum in children – evidence-based treatment. White MI, Weller R, Diack P. Clin Exp Dermatol 1997; 22: 51.

This study compared the efficacy and the potential for scarring of manual extrusion, cryotherapy, and topical phenol. Manual extrusion was more effective than cryotherapy. Phenol was associated with significant scarring and is not recommended for the treatment of MC.

THIRD-LINE THERAPIES

Physical destruction	
▶ Curettage with EMLA cream	C
▶ Pulsed dye laser	C
▶ Photodynamic therapy (PDT)	D
▶ Application of duct tape	E
Topical therapy	
▶ 10% potassium hydroxide solution	A
▶ Topical 1–5% imiquimod	A
▶ Cantharidin	B
▶ Diphencyprone	C
▶ Australian lemon myrtle	C
▶ Topical cidofovir	E
▶ Tretinoin	E
▶ Adapalene	E
Systemic therapy	
▶ Candida antigen – intralesional	C
▶ Cimetidine	D
▶ Interferon-α – subcutaneous	E

Treatment of molluscum contagiosum using a lidocaine/prilocaine cream (EMLA) for analgesia. de Waard-van der Speck FB, Oranje AP, Lillieborg S, Hop WC, Stolz E. J Am Acad Dermatol 1990; 23: 685–8.

A double-blind study in 83 children showed efficacy of EMLA cream applied for less than 60 minutes in reducing the pain of curettage, though no comment was made on clearance rates.

Curettage of molluscum contagiosum in children: analgesia by topical application of a lidocaine/prilocaine cream (EMLA®). Rosdahl L, Edmar B, Gisslen H, Nordin P, Lillieborgs S. Acta Dermatol Venereol 1988; 68: 149–53.

EMLA cream provided effective local anesthesia for the curettage of MC in 55 children.

Treatment of molluscum contagiosum with the pulsed dye laser over a 28-month period. Hancox JG, Jackson J, McCagh S. Cutis 2003; 71: 414–16.

All treated lesions in 43 patients resolved, and in 15 of them no further lesions developed after two treatments.

Treatment of molluscum contagiosum with a pulsed dye laser: pilot study with 19 children. Binder B, Weger W, Komericki P, Kopera D. J Dtsch Dermatol Ges 2008; 6: 121–5.

In a non-randomized pilot study of 19 children with MC, 84.3% achieved clearance after one treatment and 100% after three treatments. Treatment was well tolerated.

Photodynamic therapy for molluscum contagiosum infection in HIV-coinfected patients: review of 6 cases. Moiin A. J Drugs Dermatol 2003; 6: 637–9.

Treatment of six patients with 5-aminolevulinic acid (ALA) and PDT resulted in a reduction in lesion count and severity.

The successful use of ALA-PDT in the treatment of recalcitrant molluscum contagiosum. Gold MH, Boring MM, Bridges TM, Bradshaw VL. J Drugs Dermatol 2004; 3: 187–90.

Case report of successful treatment with ALA-PDT of molluscum contagiosum in a patient with HIV infection.

Use of duct tape occlusion in the treatment of recurrent molluscum contagiosum. Lindau MS, Munar MY. Pediatr Dermatol 2004; 21: 609.

Case report of well-tolerated and successful home therapy of multiple MC used over 2 months.

Treatment of molluscum contagiosum with potassium hydroxide: a clinical approach in 35 children. Romiti R, Ribeiro AP, Grinblat BM, Rivitti EA, Romiti N. Pediatr Dermatol 1999; 16: 228–31.

Potassium hydroxide solution 10% was applied twice daily until lesions underwent inflammation or ulceration. Of 35 children, 32 cleared with a mean treatment period of 30 days. Hypertrophic scarring occurred in one patient, and pigmentary change was observed in nine others.

Double randomized, placebo-controlled study of the use of topical 10% potassium hydroxide solution in the treatment of molluscum contagiosum. Short KA, Fuller LC, Higgins EM. Paediatr Dermatol 2006; 23: 279–81.

A double randomized, placebo-controlled study in 24 children with MC: 70% of the active group compared with 20% of placebo group achieved complete resolution. Dosing studies are required to minimize irritancy.

Treatment of molluscum contagiosum in males with an analogue of imiquimod 1% cream: a placebo controlled, double-blind study. Syed TA, Goswami J, Ahmadpour OA, Ahmad SA. J Dermatol 1998; 25: 309–13.

One hundred male patients applied either the analogue cream or placebo to their mollusca three times daily for 5 days each week for 1 month; 82% cleared with active treatment, compared to 16% of those using placebo. The treatment was well tolerated.

Treatment of molluscum contagiosum with imiquimod 5% cream. Skinner RB. Arch Dermatol 2002; 47: 221–4.

Five patients treated for up to 8 weeks with 5% imiquimod cream showed complete resolution of multiple MC.

Comparison of the various treatment modalities available (with references).

Effectiveness of imiquimod cream 5% for treating childhood molluscum contagiosum in a double blind randomised pilot trial. Theos AU, Cummins R, Silverberg NB, Paller AS. Cutis 2004; 74: 134–8.

Complete clearance of MC occurred in 33% of 12 children, compared to 11% of the vehicle-only group.

Topical treatment of molluscum contagiosum with imiquimod 5% in Turkish children. Arican O. Pediatr Int 2006; 48: 40–5.

An open study of 12 children treated with 5% imiquimod. Three dropped out, and complete resolution was achieved in seven of the remaining nine.

Experience in treating molluscum contagiosum in children with imiquimod 5% cream. Bayerl C, Feller G, Goerdt S. Br J Dermatol 2003; 149: 25–9.

Three times weekly application for 16 weeks in 15 children gave complete remission in two and partial remission in nine; side effects included burning, redness, and itching.

Combination topical treatment of molluscum contagiosum with cantharidin and imiquimod 5% in children: a case series of 16 patients. Ross GL, Orchard GC. Aust J Dermatol 2004; 445: 100–2.

Sixteen children were treated with one application of cantharidin followed by topical imiquimod nightly for up to 5 weeks. Twelve of 16 showed over 90% clearance of MC.

Pharmokinetics and safety of imiquimod 5% cream in the treatment of molluscum contagiosum. Myhre PE, Levy ML, Eichenfield LF, Kolb VB, Fielder SL Meng TC. Paediatr Dermatol 2008; 25: 88–95.

Assessment of safety of 5% imiquimod in children treated for MC. Systemic drug levels were low after single and multiple doses of imiquimod cream.

Childhood molluscum contagiosum: experience with cantharidin therapy in 300 patients. Silverberg NB, Sidbury R, Mancini AJ. J Am Acad Dermatol 2000; 43: 503–7.

A retrospective study of topical cantharidin applied to non-facial MC for 4–6 hours was complicated by the use of other concurrent therapies. Of 300 children, over 90% cleared after a mean of 2.1 treatments; 90% experienced blistering at the treated site, but none developed bacterial infections.

Treatment of molluscum contagiosum with topical diphencyprone therapy. Kang SH, Lee D, Park JH, Cho SH, Lee SS, Park SW. Acta Dermatol Venereol 2005; 85: 529–30.

Weekly application of 0.0001% diphencyprone in 22 sensitized children over 8 weeks. There was 63.6% complete clearance over a mean treatment period of 5.1 weeks.

Essential oil of Australian lemon myrtle (*Backhousia citriodora*) in the treatment of molluscum contagiosum. Burke BE, Baillie JE, Olson RD. Biomed Pharmacother 2004; 58: 245–7.

Once-daily application of a 10% solution of *Backhousia citriodora* gave over 90% reduction in lesions in nine of 16 children, compared to none of 16 in the control group (vehicle alone).

Topical cidofovir. A novel treatment for recalcitrant molluscum contagiosum in children infected with human immunodeficiency virus 1. Toro JR, Wood LV, Patel NK, Turner ML. Arch Dermatol 2000; 136: 983–5.

Topical 3% cidofovir applied daily for 5 days per week for 8 weeks cleared previously recalcitrant lesions in two children.

Cidofovir diphosphate inhibits molluscum contagiosum virus DNA polymerase activity. J Invest Dermatol 2008; 128: 1327–9.

In vitro demonstration of inhibition of molluscum contagiosum virus DNA polymerase activity by cidofovir.

Venereal herpes-like molluscum contagiosum: treatment with tretinoin. Papa CM, Berger RS. Cutis 1976; 18: 537–40.

Twice-daily application of 0.1 or 0.05% tretinoin cleared mollusca in two patients.

Treatment of molluscum contagiosum: a brief review and discussion of a case successfully treated with adapalene. Scheinfeld N. Dermatol Online J 2007; 13: 15.

A single case report of topical adapalene therapy.

One-year experience with *Candida* antigen immunotherapy for warts and molluscum. Marron M, Salm C, Lyon V, Galbraith S. Pediatr Dermatol 2008; 25: 189–92.

One-year follow-up (by phone or clinic visit) in 25/47 patients with molluscum treated with intralesional *Candida* antigen therapy. There was complete resolution in 56%, partial clearing in 28%, and in 16% no improvement.

Treatment of molluscum contagiosum with oral cimetidine: clinical experience in 13 patients. Dohil M, Prenderville JS. Pediatr Dermatol 1996; 13: 310–12.

13 children were treated with a two-month course of oral cimetidine 40 mg/kg/day. All but three children who completed treatment experienced clearance of all lesions. These children had no new lesions but had persistence of several lesions. One child did not take the drug and did not clear. No adverse effects were observed.

Inefficiency of oral cimetidine for non-atopic children with molluscum contagiosum. Cunningham BB, Paller AS, Garzon M. Pediatr Dermatol 1998; 15: 71–2.

The response of MC to cimetidine may be better in atopic than in non-atopic children.

Interferon alpha treatment of molluscum contagiosum in immunodeficiency. Hourihane J, Hodges E, Smith J, Keefe M, Jones A, Connett G. Arch Dis Child 1999; 80: 77–9.

Molluscum contagiosum in two children with combined immunodeficiency cleared with subcutaneous interferon-α.

Interferon-alpha treatment of molluscum contagiosum in a patient with hyperimmunoglobulin E syndrome. Kilic SS, Kilicbay F. Paediatrics 2006; 117: e1253–5.

Successful treatment with 6 months of subcutaneous interferon-α of MC resistant to multiple therapies in an immunodeficient child.

Resolution of disseminated molluscum contagiosum with highly active anti-retroviral therapy (HAART) in patients with AIDS. Calista D, Boschini A, Landi G. Eur J Dermatol 1999; 9: 211–13.

Three patients with recalcitrant MC cleared 6 months after commencing HAART.

Resolution of severe molluscum contagiosum on effective anti-retroviral therapy. Horn CK, Scott GR, Benton EC. Br J Dermatol 1998; 138: 715–17.

Severe mollu scum infection in a patient with HIV disease largely disappeared after treatment of the HIV infection with ritonavir and lamivudine.

Molluscum contagiosum. Recent advances in pathogenetic mechanisms and new therapies. Smith KJ, Skelton H. Am J Clin Dermatol 2002; 3: 536–45.

A good review paper.

A prospective randomized trial comparing the efficacy and adverse effects of four recognized treatments of molluscum contagiosum in children. Hanna D, Hatami A, Powell J, Marcoux D, Maari C, Savard P, et al. Paediatric Dermatol 2006; 23: 574–9.

A prospective randomized study comparing four common treatments for MC in 124 children (curettage, cantharidin, salicylic acid plus lactic acid and imiquimod). Curettage was the most effective, with the fewest side effects. Cantharidin and salicylic acid produced irritation. Imiquimod was promising, but the optimum dosing regimen is still to be determined.

Interventions for cutaneous molluscum contagiosum. van der Wouden JC, Menke J, Gajadin S, Koning S, Tasche MJ, van Suijlekom-Smit LW, et al. Cochrane Database Syst Rev 2006,19; CD004767.

Review of all randomized controlled studies of treatment for MC. No single intervention was convincingly shown to be effective.

Morphea

Bernice R Krafchik

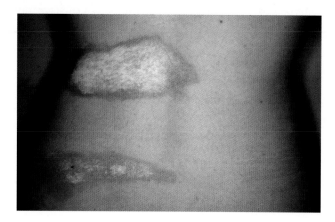

Morphea is a rare connective tissue disease affecting the skin, subcutaneous tissue, and rarely deeper tissues (muscle, fascia, and bone). Morphea is mainly classified into plaque and linear types, but there are numerous subtypes, including *en coup de sabre* and Parry–Romberg syndrome, and generalized, bullous, atrophic and pansclerotic morphea.

The disease affects children and adults, may be limited or widespread, and usually undergoes spontaneous resolution within 3–5 years; however, some cases may be active for up to 10 years, and there may be recurrences after intervals of quiescence. The fibrotic changes associated with disease activity can cause widespread local reactions with lasting effects. There can be serious cosmetic defects: skin, muscle and bone atrophy, hyperpigmentation, hypopigmentation and physical disability, including seizures in patients with *en coup de sabre* or Parry–Romberg disease. Although other internal changes such as arthralgias, arthritis, and pulmonary changes have been reported, long-lasting systemic effects are unusual. Half of cases show increased levels of autoantibodies that include positive antinuclear antibodies and rheumatoid factors, and eosinophilia is common; there is no correlation between the activity of the disease and levels of autoantibodies.

MANAGEMENT STRATEGIES

Morphea is difficult to manage and treat. The lack of a chemical marker that can monitor disease activity makes the assessment of treatment modalities almost impossible. In addition, there is a natural tendency toward regression. Once fibrosis occurs no medical intervention is helpful, and surgical strategies may be considered to correct existing defects. In recent years new therapies have emerged in an attempt to stabilize the activity and thereby lessen the long-lasting effects. Many of the treatments that were previously used, such as *penicillamine*, had so many adverse reactions that they are no longer used. Topical therapies are often attempted initially, particularly for lesions that do not have a large cosmetic impact. Nevertheless, it remains to be shown whether it is preferable to use systemic treatment immediately in areas where the cosmetic effects can be devastating, or to use a topical approach hoping that the disease process will be arrested.

Mid to super-potency topical corticosteroids are used in patients (particularly in areas that spare the face) during the initial inflammatory stages, Alternatively topical *calcipotriene* or *tacrolimus* can also be applied though controlled clinical trials are not available. There are anecdotal reports of success with all these treatments.

Psoralen plus UVA (PUVA)-bath photochemotherapy may be effective for widespread plaque and linear morphea. Patients are immersed for 20 minutes in a warm-water bath containing 1 mg/L of methoxsalen. This is followed by irradiation with UVA, 0.2–0.5 J/cm^2 for a maximum of 1.2–3.5 J/cm^2 to a mean cumulative dose of 41.1 J/ cm^2. Recently, it has been reported that low-dose UVA alone (20 J/ cm^2 for a total of 600 J/cm^2) may clear or improve severe disease. *UVA1* has also been shown to be effective, but the machine is not widely available.

Systemic therapy has gained widespread support and has been shown to effectively stop the progress of the disease. *Systemic steroids* are given both orally and by intravenous (IV) pulsing, either alone or in combination with *methotrexate*. The latter combination is now widely used as first- or second-line treatment, and has been shown to halt the progression of the disease. The pulsed or oral steroids are tapered, and the methotrexate takes effect in approximately 6 weeks. The pulsed steroid is administered intravenously as methylprednisolone (30 mg/kg for 3 days monthly) for a total period of 3 months. The dose of methotrexate is 15–25 mg/week in adults, whereas in children the dose is 0.3–0.5 mg/kg/week. It is given with folic acid daily until there is no longer any activity, continued for another year, and then tapered. If recurrence occurs, methotrexate is again introduced.

Other oral medications include oral *calcitriol*, which has been shown to be effective in localized morphea. However, unlike topical calcipotriene, oral medication may have a pronounced effect on calcium metabolism. There have been reports of the benefit of oral *ciclosporin* with PUVA and *mycophenolate mofetil*.

Physical therapy is extremely helpful in preventing and treating contractures.

Surgery, using fat implants, is now used more widely to reduce the devastating effects of Parry–Romberg disease.

SPECIFIC INVESTIGATIONS

> ▶ No diagnostic tests
> ▶ Skin biopsy (if diagnosis is in doubt)
> ▶ MRI and ultrasound of affected areas to rule out underlying involvement
> ▶ Follow-up with high-frequency ultrasound to assess disease activity

Skin imaging with high frequency ultrasound – preliminary results. Szymanska E, Nowicki A, Mlosek K, Litniewski J, Lewandowski M, Secomski W, et al. Eur J Ultrasound 2000; 12: 9–16.

It has always been difficult to assess the skin changes in patients with morphea. This study using high-frequency ultrasound demonstrated the skin changes that occurred in patients with morphea following treatment of their disease.

High-frequency ultrasound as a useful device in the preliminary differentiation of lichen sclerosus et atrophicus from morphea. Chen HC, Kadono T, Mimura Y, Saeki H, Tamaki K. J Dermatol 2004; 31: 556–9.

446

Ultrasound with high frequencies (up to 30 MHz) has the advantage of being a non-invasive and relatively inexpensive technology that is quick and easy to perform.

FIRST-LINE THERAPIES

▶ Topical corticosteroids	E
▶ Topical calcipotriene (with or without topical steroids)	C
▶ Topical imiquimod	E
▶ Topical tacrolimus	E

Treatment of scleroderma. Sapadin AN, Fleischmajer R. Arch Dermatol 2002; 138: 99–105.

In this article the authors discuss the treatment options for both systemic and localized morphea. They include the use of corticosteroids, vitamin D analogs (calcitriol, calcipotriene), UVA, and methotrexate.

Topical calcipotriol ointment in the treatment of morphea. Tay YK. J Dermatol Treat 2003; 14: 219–21.

The author presents a case of morphea unresponsive to topical corticosteroids that responded to calcipotriol ointment twice daily, with nightly occlusion to the plaque, for 9 months, and this resulted in resolution. No side effects were noted.

First case series on the use of calcipotriol-betamethasone dipropionate for morphoea. Dytoc MT, Kossintseva I, Ting PT. Br J Dermatol 2007; 157: 615–18.

Six patients were treated with the calcipotriol betamethasone preparation and their lesions were assessed ultrasonically after 1 month. Clinically and ultrasonically there was improvement, with a reduction in skin thickness. There were no side effects.

Use of imiquimod cream 5% in the treatment of localized morphea. Man J, Dytoc MT. J Cutan Med Surg 2004; 8: 166–9.

A single patient with morphea was treated with 5% imiquimod, which led to softening of the lesions. The authors suggest that interferon might interfere with the profibrotic cytokines.

First case series on the use of imiquimod for morphoea. Dytoc M, Ting PT, Man J, Sawyer D, Fiorillo L. Br J Dermatol 2005; 153: 815–20.

The authors used imiquimod 5% cream (Aldara), an inducer of interferon-γ, known to inhibit TGF-β, to treat 12 patients who were evaluated during their follow-up visits up to 6 months. The dyspigmentation, induration, and erythema improved. The histology of the skin also showed a reduction of dermal thickness.

Localized scleroderma. Laxer RM, Zulian F. Curr Opin Rheumatol 2006; 18: 606–13.

These authors verified the findings of improvement in morphea with corticosteroids and methotrexate, and phototherapy, and commented on the promise shown by the use of imiquimod.

Topical tacrolimus in the treatment of localized scleroderma. Mancuso G, Berdondini RM. Eur J Dermatol 2003; 13: 590–2.

This report involved treating two patients with the calcineurin inhibitor 0.1% twice a day, with softening of the skin.

Localized scleroderma: response to occlusive treatment with tacrolimus ointment. Mancuso G, Berdondini RM. Br J Dermatol 2005; 152: 180–2.

SECOND-LINE THERAPIES

▶ PUVA	B
▶ PUVA-bath photochemotherapy	C
▶ UVA	C
▶ UVA1	B

UVA/UVA1 phototherapy and PUVA photochemotherapy in connective tissue diseases and related disorders: a research based review. Breuckmann F, Gambichler T, Altmeyer P, Kreuter A. BMC Dermatol 2004; 4: 11.

These authors systematically review the literature on UVA/UVA1 and PUVA therapy in various skin conditions, including morphea, and conclude that significant softening of the skin occurs with all modalities used. High-dose UVA1 was of more benefit than low-dose treatment.

Different low doses of broad-band UVA in the treatment of morphea and systemic sclerosis. El-Mofty M, Mostafa W, El-Darouty M, Bosseila M, Nada H, Yousef R, et al. Photodermatol Photoimmunol Photomed 2004; 20: 148–56.

Sixty-three patients with both progressive systemic sclerosis and morphea were tested with various strengths of UVA. The results after using 5 and 10 J/cm^2 were as good as using 20 J/cm^2. This is a relatively easy treatment because many centers have UVA.

Ultraviolet A1 phototherapy. Dawe RS. Br J Dermatol 2003; 148: 626–37.

This review highlights the efficacy of both low- and high-dose UVA1 therapy in various forms of morphea. It included the report of one case where there was a marked softening of the skin in a 16-year-old with pansclerotic morphea.

Phototherapy for scleroderma: biologic rationale, results, and promise. Fisher GJ, Kang S. Curr Opin Rheumatol 2002; 14: 723–6.

These authors analyze the results of UVA1 therapy and point out that the machine and equipment required for UVA1 is very expensive, whereas UVA seemed to produce similar improvement with and without the addition of oral or bath psoralen.

Ultraviolet A sunbed used for the treatment of scleroderma. [Letter] Oikarinen A, Knuutinen A. Acta Dermatol Venereol 2001; 81: 432–3.

A letter describing the use of a UVA sunbed, its effect on softening the skin of patients with morphea, and comparing it with the expensive modality of UVA1.

Low dose broad-band UVA in morphea using a new method for evaluation. El-Mofty M, Zaher H, Bosseila M, Yousef R, Saad B. Photodermatol Photoimmunol Photomed 2000; 16: 43–9.

In this open trial of broadband UVA, 12 patients with morphea were treated with 20 J/cm^2 three times per week for 20 sessions. Softening of skin lesions and reduction in concentration of collagen on skin biopsy were reported.

THIRD-LINE THERAPIES

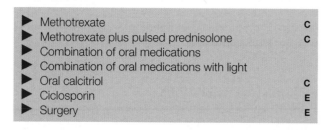

▶ Methotrexate	C
▶ Methotrexate plus pulsed prednisolone	C
▶ Combination of oral medications	
▶ Combination of oral medications with light	
▶ Oral calcitriol	C
▶ Ciclosporin	E
▶ Surgery	E

Methotrexate and corticosteroid therapy for pediatric localized scleroderma. Uziel Y, Feldman BM, Krafchik BR, Yeung RS, Laxer RM. J Pediatr 2000; 136: 91–5.

Ten patients, mean age 6.8 years, with active localized scleroderma of 4 years' mean duration, were treated with methotrexate and intravenous methylprednisolone for a 3-month period. Nine patients responded to therapy and treatment was generally well tolerated.

Good response of linear scleroderma in a child to ciclosporin. Strauss RM, Bhushan M, Goodfield MJ. Br J Dermatol 2004; 150: 790–2.

A 12-year-old child with rapidly expanding linear morphea was first treated with clobetasol twice a day. Because there was little improvement in her condition, ciclosporin 3 mg/kg daily was added to the regimen, with rapid improvement and softening of the lesion on her thigh. This took 4 months to occur. The treatment was stopped and there was no recurrence in 1 year. The authors discuss the effect of ciclosporin interfering with the cytokine IL-2, which is increased in activated lymphocytes.

Combining PUVA therapy with systemic immunosuppression to treat progressive diffuse morphoea. Rose RF, Goodfield MJ. Clin Exp Dermatol 2005; 30: 226–8.

The authors discuss the various treatments used in morphea, and comment that combination therapies may hold promise. They used a combination of ciclosporin and PUVA, and later mycophenolate mofetil and PUVA, with considerable softening of the skin.

Treatment of coup de sabre deformity with porous polyethylene implant. Copcu E. Plast Reconstruct Surg 2004; 113: 758–9.

In this article a porous polyethylene implant was used to correct an *en coup de sabre* defect, with excellent results. This highlights the future role of surgery to correct the severe cosmetic disabilities sometimes encountered in facial lesions of morphea.

Successful correction of depressed scars of the forehead secondary to trauma and morphea en coup de sabre by en bloc autologous dermal fat graft. Lapiere JC, Aasi S, Cook B, Montalvo A. Dermatol Surg 2000; 26: 793–7.

Atrophic scars of the forehead can result from various pathologic processes, including morphea *en coup de sabre* as well as trauma. A variety of surgical techniques can be used to correct these. The authors use en bloc autologous dermal fat graft harvested from the hip and inserted into a pocket created under the atrophic scar in two patients with depressed scars of the forehead. This resulted in the treated areas becoming level with the adjacent skin within 3 months. Follow-up over 12 months showed a perfectly level and stable graft, with no further resorption.

Treatment of 'en coup de sabre' deformity with porous polyethylene. Ozturk S, Acarturk TO, Yapici K, Sengezer MJ. Craniofac Surg 2006; 17: 696–701.

The authors describe the reconstruction of a facial deformity with a polyethylene implant.

This chapter is dedicated to the memory of Raul Fleischmajer, who wrote the chapter in the first edition of this book.

Methicillin-resistant *Staphylococcus aureus* (MRSA)

Dirk Elston

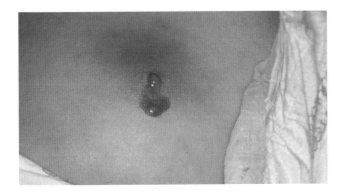

MANAGEMENT STRATEGY

Healthcare-type strains of methicillin-resistant *Staphylococcus aureus* (MRSA) are associated with sepsis and are common colonists of chronic wounds, where debridement is typically the best strategy. Community-type MRSA infections typically present as an abscess or furunculosis. The most important intervention for an abscess remains surgical drainage. Purulent material can reform rapidly, so a punch or cruciate incision is advised, as it tends to remain open longer to allow adequate drainage. A curette is used to probe the wound and ensure that all pockets of purulent material have been adequately drained. Irrigation can be helpful, but packing is discouraged as purulent material often reforms behind the packing. Evidence suggests that antibiotics are often unnecessary if an abscess is adequately drained. There are obvious reasons to avoid antibiotics when they are not needed, including the risk of Stevens–Johnson syndrome, antibiotic-associated diarrhea, and selection of resistant strains.

Patients with significant surrounding cellulitis, refractory infection, or systemic manifestations may require *antibiotic therapy*. Most CA-MRSA strains are sensitive to *trimethoprim-sulfamethoxazole*. Most strains are also sensitive to *doxycycline* and *minocycline*, but doxycycline does not penetrate well into the nares. Clindamycin resistance is emerging in many communities. For serious infections, therapy should be guided by culture and sensitivity. *Vancomycin, linezolid, dalbavancin, telavancin,* and *daptomycin* are often effective. *Rifampin* improves intracellular killing of bacteria by vancomycin. *Quinupristin-dalfopristin* and *tigecycline* may also be effective, but quinupristin-dalfopristin, like daptomycin, may not penetrate reliably into pulmonary tissue, and tigecycline has a significant incidence of nausea. *Ceftobiprole* and *oritavancin* appear promising.

Spread occurs through skin-to-skin contact and via fomites. *Decolonization* may be indicated for prevention of recurrence or prevention of serious invasive disease in close contacts.

The most effective decolonization regimens address the nares, intertriginous and anogenital sites, as well as eczematous skin. In some patients gut colonization may also be an issue.

SPECIFIC INVESTIGATIONS

▶ Culture and sensitivities
▶ Molecular studies (PCR, pulsed-field gel electrophoresis, high-performance liquid chromatography)
▶ D-zone test for inducible macrolide–lincosamide–streptogramin B resistance

Application of loop-mediated isothermal amplification technique to rapid and direct detection of methicillin-resistant *Staphylococcus aureus* (MRSA) in blood cultures. Misawa Y, Yoshida A, Saito R, Yoshida H, Okuzumi K, Ito N, et al. J Infect Chemother 2007; 13: 134–40.

A novel nucleic acid amplification technique, loop-mediated isothermal amplification, targets the spa gene and the mecA gene. The diagnostic value compared to that of duplex real-time polymerase chain reaction in this study was 92.3% vs 96.2% sensitivity, 100% specificity and positive predictive value for both, and 96.9% vs 98.4% negative predictive value.

Of the two, the LAMP method is more cost-effective.

External quality assessment of molecular typing of *Staphylococcus aureus* isolates by a network of laboratories. Deplano A, De Mendonça R, De Ryck R, Struelens MJ. J Clin Microbiol 2006; 44: 3236–44.

Some centers perform pulsed-field gel electrophoresis (PFGE) whereas others use PCR, amplified fragment length polymorphism, or spa typing. Full typability (100%) was achieved by all centers, and all but one showed 100% reproducibility in this study.

The reproducibility of results has improved dramatically since the early days of the CA-MRSA epidemic.

Rapid cost-effective subtyping of methicillin-resistant *Staphylococcus aureus* by denaturing HPLC. Jury F, Al-Mahrous M, Apostolou M, Sandiford S, Fox A, Ollier W, et al. J Med Microbiol 2006; 55: 1053–60.

Denaturing high-performance liquid chromatography allows rapid, inexpensive characterization of spaA gene amplification products and precise sizing of spa gene-repeat regions. This method, combined with heteroduplex PCR, allowed subtyping of strains in less than 5 hours.

Typing of MRSA strains is improving.

Differences in potential for selection of clindamycin-resistant mutants between inducible erm(A) and erm(C) *Staphylococcus aureus* genes. Daurel C, Huet C, Dhalluin A, Bes M, Etienne J, Leclercq R. J Clin Microbiol 2008; 46: 546–50.

The frequency of mutation to clindamycin resistance for the erm(A) isolates (mean ± standard deviation, 3.4×10^{-8} ± 2.4×10^{-8}) was only slightly higher than those for the controls. In contrast, erm(C) isolates displayed a 14-fold higher mean frequency of mutation to clindamycin resistance.

Inducible macrolide–lincosamide–streptogramin B resistance in MRSA is conferred by the erm(C) or erm(A) gene. The erythromycin–clindamycin 'D-zone' test is used to identify inducible resistance, but this study suggests that typing of the erm gene may be predictive of the risk of inducible resistance.

Detection of inducible clindamycin resistance in staphylococci by broth microdilution using erythromycin–clindamycin combination wells. Swenson JM, Brasso WB, Ferraro MJ, Hardy DJ, Knapp CC, McDougal LK, et al. J Clin Microbiol 2007; 45: 3954–7.

Broth microdilution panels correlated well with the D-zone test.

Influence of disk separation distance on accuracy of the disk approximation test for detection of inducible clindamycin resistance in *Staphylococcus* spp. O'Sullivan MV, Cai Y, Kong F, Zeng X, Gilbert GL. J Clin Microbiol 2006; 44: 4072–6.

The sensitivities of the D-tests performed at 15 mm and 22 mm were 100% and 87.7%, respectively, and specificities were 100% for both.

The use of 22-mm disk separation for the D-test results in an unacceptably high false-negative rate.

FIRST-LINE THERAPY

Treatment of MRSA abscesses	
▶ Surgical drainage alone	B
▶ Surgical drainage plus:	
▶ trimethoprim-sulfamethoxazole	B
▶ minocycline	B
▶ doxycycline	B
▶ clindamycin	B
Eradication of colonization	
Nares	
▶ Mupirocin	B
▶ Tea tree oil	B
Skin	
▶ Bleach baths	D
▶ Chlorhexidine	B
▶ Triclosan	B
▶ Tea tree oil soap	B
▶ Undecylenamidopropyltrimonium methosulphate/ phenoxyethanol	C
▶ Octenidine dihydrochloride	C

Methicillin-resistant *Staphylococcus aureus* disease in three communities. Fridkin SK, Hageman JC, Morrison M, Sanza LT, Como-Sabetti K, Jernigan JA, et al. N Engl J Med 2005; 352: 1436–44.

Initial use of an antibiotic to which the organism was resistant was paradoxically associated with fewer follow-up visits, and these patients were less likely to receive a second antibiotic.

Data from three distinct geographic areas suggest that the empiric use of an antibiotic to which the strain was resistant was not associated with a worse outcome. Drainage alone probably accounted for the good outcome of abscesses. An interesting finding was that cellulitis also responded well to β-lactam drugs. As it is difficult to isolate the actual invasive organism in cases of cellulitis, and the most common pathogen causing cellulitis is Streptococcus pyogenes, it may be that many of these patients actually had invasive streptococcal infections which would be expected to respond well to a β-lactam.

An epidemic of methicillin-resistant *Staphylococcus aureus* soft tissue infections among medically underserved patients. Young DM, Harris HW, Charlebois ED, Chambers H, Campbell A, Perdreau-Remington F, et al. Arch Surg 2004; 139: 947–51.

A study of 12 012 episodes of infection (83% *S. aureus*, 76% of these MRSA) showed that although many of the patients with MRSA received an inactive antibiotic, they had full resolution of their infections.

Methicillin-resistant *S. aureus* infections among patients in the emergency department. Moran GJ, Krishnadasan A, Gorwitz RJ, Fosheim GE, McDougal LK, Carey RB, et al. N Engl J Med 2006; 355: 666–74.

A study of patients with acute, purulent infections presenting to emergency departments found that the prevalence of MRSA was 59%; 57% of the MRSA patients who received antibiotics were given a drug with no activity against MRSA, and yet resolution was similar to that in the group given an active antibiotic.

Randomized, double-blind, placebo-controlled trial of cephalexin for treatment of uncomplicated skin abscesses in a population at risk for community-acquired methicillin-resistant *Staphylococcus aureus* infection. Rajendran PM, Young D, Maurer T, Chambers H, Perdreau-Remington F, Ro P, et al. Antimicrob Agents Chemother 2007; 51: 4044–8.

This randomized, double-blind trial of treatment in 166 patients with uncomplicated abscesses in a population at risk for CA-MRSA showed good outcomes with both placebo and cephalexin despite an 87.8% MRSA isolation rate. Clinical cure was achieved in 90.5% of the 84 placebo recipients and 84.1% of the 82 cephalexin recipients.

Management and outcome of children with skin and soft tissue abscesses caused by community-acquired methicillin-resistant *Staphylococcus aureus*. Lee MC, Rios AM, Aten MF, Mejias A, Cavuoti D, McCracken GH Jr, et al. Pediatr Infect Dis J 2004; 23: 123–7.

In this study of 69 children with CA-MRSA abscesses, drainage was performed in 96% of patients and wound packing in 65%. All were given an antibiotic, but only five (7%) were prescribed an antibiotic to which the isolate was susceptible. Initial inactive antibiotic therapy was not a significant risk factor for subsequent hospitalization (p=1.0), but an abscess >5 cm was (p=0.004). The authors concluded that drainage alone was effective management for CA-MRSA abscesses <5 cm.

Cefdinir vs. cephalexin for mild to moderate uncomplicated skin and skin structure infections in adolescents and adults. Giordano PA, Elston D, Akinlade BK, Weber K, Notario GF, Busman TA, et al. Curr Med Res Opin 2006; 22: 2419–28.

The cure rate for methicillin-susceptible staphylococcal infections was 93% (37/40) and 91% (29/32) for cefdinir and cephalexin, respectively, compared to 92% (35/38) and 90% (37/41) for MRSA infections.

These studies suggest that antibiotic therapy may not be needed in a large number of patients with MRSA abscesses if adequate drainage is performed.

Tetracyclines as an oral treatment option for patients with community onset skin and soft tissue infections caused by methicillin-resistant *Staphylococcus aureus*. Ruhe JJ, Menon A. Antimicrob Agents Chemother 2007; 51: 3298–303.

Evidence Levels: **A** Double-blind study **B** Clinical trial ≥ 20 subjects **C** Clinical trial < 20 subjects **D** Series ≥ 5 subjects **E** Anecdotal case reports

A retrospective cohort study of 282 episodes of MRSA skin infection in 276 patients showed that 95% of the MRSA strains were susceptible to tetracycline. Three-quarters of the patients presented with abscesses, followed by furuncles (13%) and a purulent focus with surrounding cellulitis (12%). Only 80% of the patients underwent incision and drainage. Most patients were treated with β-lactams; 32% were treated with doxycycline or minocycline. Treatment failure was associated with the use of a β-lactam (p=0.02).

This study is included because it suggests that the use of a β-lactam drug (or presumably no antibiotic at all) could be a risk factor for treatment failure in some patients. It should be noted that only 80% of the patients underwent incision and drainage, although all were characterized as having a purulent focus. Failure was defined as the need for a second drainage or hospital admission within 2 days.

Community-onset methicillin-resistant *Staphylococcus aureus* skin and soft-tissue infections: impact of antimicrobial therapy on outcome. Ruhe JJ, Smith N, Bradsher RW, Menon A. Clin Infect Dis 2007; 44: 777–84.

In this retrospective study of 492 patients with 531 episodes of CA-MRSA skin infection 95% of the 312 infections in patients who received an active antibiotic cleared, compared to 87% of the 219 who did not (p=0.001).

This is a second report from the same group. It is unclear how much patient overlap exists. Many patients did not receive drainage, although most infections were described as purulent.

Treatment and outcomes of infections by methicillin-resistant *Staphylococcus aureus* at an ambulatory clinic. Szumowski JD, Cohen DE, Kanaya F, Mayer KH. Antimicrob Agents Chemother 2007; 51: 423–8.

This retrospective chart review including 227 patients with MRSA skin infections found that 48.2% of isolates were resistant to clindamycin. Early in the study period most patients received a β-lactam, whereas by the end of the study 76% received trimethoprim-sulfamethoxazole. Those who received an active antibiotic had a better chance of resolution (p=0.037).

Prevalence of inducible clindamycin resistance among community- and hospital-associated *Staphylococcus aureus* isolates. Patel M, Waites KB, Moser SA, Cloud GA, Hoesley CJ. J Clin Microbiol 2006; 44: 2481–4.

The prevalence of inducible macrolide–lincosamide–streptogramin B resistance in community- and hospital-associated *S. aureus* isolates was 50% overall, but was lower in CA-MRSA (33%) than in hospital-associated MRSA (55%).

The prevalence of constitutive and inducible clindamycin resistance varies considerably in different geographic regions. In some areas clindamycin is no longer a viable option for empiric therapy.

Analysis of empiric antimicrobial strategies for cellulitis in the era of methicillin-resistant *Staphylococcus aureus*. Phillips S, MacDougall C, Holdford DA. Ann Pharmacother 2007; 41: 13–20.

A decision analysis of the costs of empiric treatment of cellulitis included initial therapy with cephalexin, clindamycin, or TMP/SMX, followed by linezolid for treatment failures. Cost estimates were based on past clinical trials and epidemiologic data. Cephalexin remained the most cost-effective initial treatment option. Clindamycin became more cost-effective when the probability of MRSA was at least 41%. TMP/SMX was cost-effective only if the probability of MRSA infection was very high.

The conclusions were based on mathematical modeling from the perspective of a third-party payer.

No decrease in clindamycin susceptibility despite increased use of clindamycin for pediatric community-associated methicillin-resistant *Staphylococcus aureus* skin infections. Szczesiul JM, Shermock KM, Murtaza UI, Siberry GK. Pediatr Infect Dis J 2007; 26: 852–4.

At an institution where 98% of CA-MRSA isolates were susceptible to clindamycin, 2 years of increasing empiric clindamycin use did not result in a reduction of susceptibility to clindamycin.

This study is somewhat reassuring, but clindamycin resistance is increasing in prevalence in most areas.

Eradication of colonization

Targeted intranasal mupirocin to prevent colonization and infection by community-associated methicillin-resistant *Staphylococcus aureus* strains in soldiers: a cluster randomized controlled trial. Ellis MW, Griffith ME, Dooley DP, McLean JC, Jorgensen JH, Patterson JE, et al. Antimicrob Agents Chemother 2007; 51: 3591–8.

A randomized, double-blind, placebo-controlled trial of intranasal mupirocin therapy in CA-MRSA-colonized soldiers found that 134 (3.9%) of the 3447 participants screened were colonized. Seven of 66 mupirocin-treated participants developed infections, compared to five of 65 placebo-treated participants. Despite eradication of nasal colonization, there was no reduction in infections and nasal eradication was ineffective in preventing new MRSA colonization in the study group.

Targeting the nares alone appears to be of little value. The skin and possibly the GI tract are important reservoirs of MRSA.

Value of whole-body washing with chlorhexidine for the eradication of methicillin-resistant *Staphylococcus aureus*: a randomized, placebo-controlled, double-blind clinical trial. Wendt C, Schinke S, Württemberger M, Oberdorfer K, Bock-Hensley O, von Baum H. Infect Control Hosp Epidemiol 2007; 28: 1036–43.

In a study of whole-body washing with chlorhexidine for 5 days together with mupirocin nasal ointment and chlorhexidine mouth rinse, groin colonization was eradicated better in the chlorhexidine group. Those with a high number of body sites positive for MRSA were less likely to be cleared.

Randomized controlled trial of chlorhexidine gluconate for washing, intranasal mupirocin, and rifampin and doxycycline versus no treatment for the eradication of methicillin-resistant *Staphylococcus aureus* colonization. Simor AE, Phillips E, McGeer A, Konvalinka A, Loeb M, Devlin HR, et al. Clin Infect Dis 2007; 44: 178–85.

A randomized study compared 2% chlorhexidine gluconate wash and 2% mupirocin ointment intranasally with chlorhexidine gluconate washes, oral rifampin, and oral doxycycline for 7 days versus no treatment. At 3 months 64 (74%) of those in the active treatment group remained clear, compared to eight (32%) of those who were not treated (p=0.0001). The difference remained significant at 8 months (p<0.0001).

This study demonstrates that sustained clearing of colonization is possible. Mupirocin resistance was associated with treatment failure (p=0.0003).

Eradication of methicillin-resistant *Staphylococcus aureus* with an antiseptic soap and nasal mupirocin among colonized patients – an open uncontrolled clinical trial. Kampf G, Kramer A. Ann Clin Microbiol Antimicrob 2004; 3: 9.

An antiseptic liquid soap containing undecylenamidopropyltrimonium methosulphate (4%) and phenoxyethanol in combination with nasal mupirocin used in 5-day cycles eradicated MRSA in 25 patients (71.4%) after a single cycle, in 91.4% after a second cycle, and in 94.2% after a third cycle.

Methicillin-resistant *Staphylococcus aureus* whole-body decolonization among hospitalized patients with variable site colonization by using mupirocin in combination with octenidine dihydrochloride. Rohr U, Mueller C, Wilhelm M, Muhr G, Gatermann S. J Hosp Infect 2003; 54: 305–9.

Intranasal mupirocin combined with an octenidine dihydrochloride bodywash for 5 days resulted in decolonization in 53.1% of patients.

Twenty-four of the 32 patients had chronic wounds. Despite this, the regimen compared favorably to other regimens.

A randomized, controlled trial of tea tree topical preparations versus a standard topical regimen for the clearance of MRSA colonization. Dryden MS, Dailly S, Crouch M. J Hosp Infect 2004; 56: 283–6.

A randomized control trial of nasal mupirocin, chlorhexidine, and silver sulfadiazine versus 10% tea tree oil cream and tea tree 5% body wash for 5 days demonstrated clearance rates of 49% and 41%, respectively.

SECOND-LINE THERAPY

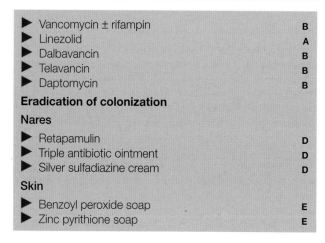

▶ Vancomycin ± rifampin	B
▶ Linezolid	A
▶ Dalbavancin	B
▶ Telavancin	B
▶ Daptomycin	B
Eradication of colonization	
Nares	
▶ Retapamulin	D
▶ Triple antibiotic ointment	D
▶ Silver sulfadiazine cream	D
Skin	
▶ Benzoyl peroxide soap	E
▶ Zinc pyrithione soap	E

A comparison of costs and hospital length of stay associated with intravenous/oral linezolid or intravenous vancomycin treatment of complicated skin and soft-tissue infections caused by suspected or confirmed methicillin-resistant *Staphylococcus aureus* in elderly US patients. McCollum M, Sorensen SV, Liu LZ. Clin Ther 2007; 29: 469–77.

A comparison of intravenous/oral linezolid vs intravenous vancomycin for complicated skin and soft-tissue infections showed that costs were lower with linezolid ($6009 vs $7329, p=0.03). Linezolid was associated with a shorter stay and a reduction in the duration of IV therapy (both p<0.001). Cure rates were comparable.

At least for hospitalized patients, linezolid therapy may be less expensive than vancomycin.

Clinical and economic outcomes of oral linezolid versus intravenous vancomycin in the treatment of MRSA-complicated, lower-extremity skin and soft-tissue infections caused by methicillin-resistant *Staphylococcus aureus*. Sharpe JN, Shively EH, Polk HC Jr. Am J Surg 2005; 189: 425–8.

An open-label study compared oral linezolid to intravenous vancomycin for complicated MRSA skin and soft-tissue infections. There were 30 patients in each treatment group. Linezolid produced a better clinical cure rate (p=0.015), a shorter duration of stay (p=0.003), and reduced outpatient costs (p<0.001). Vancomycin was associated with a higher rate of subsequent lower-extremity amputations (p=0.011).

Linezolid versus vancomycin for the treatment of infections caused by methicillin-resistant *Staphylococcus aureus* in Japan. Kohno S, Yamaguchi K, Aikawa N, Sumiyama Y, Odagiri S, Aoki N, et al. J Antimicrob Chemother 2007; 60: 1361–9.

A trial of linezolid versus vancomycin in patients with serious MRSA infections showed clinical success rates of 62.9% for the linezolid group and 50.0% for the vancomycin group at the end of therapy. The difference in microbiological eradication was even more dramatic (79.0% vs 30.0%, p<0.0001). At follow-up (1–2 weeks later), the clinical success rate was 36.7% for each group and microbiological eradication rates were 46.8% and 36.7%, respectively.

Linezolid is superior to vancomycin in the eradication of intracellular bacteria, which may account for some of the difference. The addition of rifampin to the vancomycin regimen could have evened the playing field. Linezolid side effects in this study included reversible anemia (13%) and thrombocytopenia (19%).

Linezolid versus teicoplanin in the treatment of Gram-positive infections in the critically ill: a randomized, double-blind, multicentre study. Cepeda JA, Whitehouse T, Cooper B, Hails J, Jones K, Kwaku F, et al. Antimicrob Chemother 2004; 53: 345–55.

A randomized double-blind prospective study comparing intravenous linezolid with teicoplanin showed clinical success in 71 (78.9%) linezolid-treated patients versus 67 (72.8%) patients treated with teicoplanin.

Teicoplanin resistance is emerging, and linezolid achieves better tissue penetration.

Dalbavancin and telavancin: novel lipoglycopeptides for the treatment of Gram-positive infections. Zhanel GG, Trapp S, Gin AS, DeCorby M, Lagacé-Wiens PR, Rubinstein E, et al. Expert Rev Anti Infect Ther 2008; 6: 67–81.

Dalbavancin is a glycopeptide analog of teicoplanin. Telavancin is a glycopeptide analog of vancomycin. The half-life of dalbavancin is 6–11 days, allowing for weekly administration. Telavancin has a dual mechanism of action, resulting in a low potential for the development of resistance.

In both uncomplicated and complicated skin and skin structure infections both drugs have been equivalent or superior to vancomycin. Like telavancin, fluoroquinolones have a dual mechanism of action, and yet resistance has developed.

Randomized, double-blind comparison of once-weekly dalbavancin versus twice-daily linezolid therapy for the treatment of complicated skin and skin structure infections. Jauregui LE, Babazadeh S, Seltzer E, Goldberg L, Krievins D, Frederick M, et al. Clin Infect Dis 2005; 41: 1407–15.

A phase 3 non-inferiority study compared dalbavancin (1000 mg IV on day 1500 mg IV on day 8) to linezolid (600 mg

IV or orally every 12 h for 14 days). MRSA was isolated in 51% of cultures. Dalbavancin and linezolid demonstrated similar cure rates (88.9% vs 91.2%).

Telavancin versus standard therapy for treatment of complicated skin and skin structure infections caused by gram-positive bacteria: FAST 2 study. Stryjewski ME, Chu VH, O'Riordan WD, Warren BL, Dunbar LM, Young DM, et al. Antimicrob Agents Chemother 2006; 50: 862–7.

A randomized, double-blind study of adults with complicated skin and skin structure infections evaluated telavancin 10 mg/kg intravenously every 24 h versus standard therapy (an antistaphylococcal penicillin or vancomycin 1 g q12h). Clinical cure was achieved in 96% of the patients treated with telavancin and 90% of those treated with standard therapy. Clearance rates for MRSA were 92% versus 68% (p=0.04).

A retrospective analysis of practice patterns in the treatment of methicillin-resistant *Staphylococcus aureus* skin and soft tissue infections at three Canadian tertiary care centres. Conly JM, Stiver HG, Weiss KA, Becker DL, Rosner AJ, Miller E. Can J Infect Dis 2003; 14: 315–21.

A retrospective study of hospitalized patients where MRSA treatment was initiated with intravenous vancomycin. The mean duration of hospitalization was 28.9 ± 20.8 days. Of the 70% of patients who met criteria for IV-to-oral therapy switch, only 10% received oral treatment and IV treatment continued for a mean of 13 days beyond the opportunity for a change to oral therapy.

Considerable opportunity exists for reduction in the duration of hospitalization for MRSA skin and soft tissue infections.

Daptomycin versus vancomycin for complicated skin and skin structure infections: clinical and economic outcomes. Davis SL, McKinnon PS, Hall LM, Delgado G Jr, Rose W, Wilson RF, et al. Pharmacotherapy 2007; 27: 1611–18.

This prospective, open-label study of 53 adult patients with complicated skin and skin structure infections at risk for MRSA infection compared those treated with daptomycin to a matched historical cohort of 212 patients treated with vancomycin. The study included patients with complicated cellulitis (31%), abscess (22%), and both cellulitis and abscess (37%). Microbiology differed between the groups, with *S. aureus* found in only 51% of patients in the daptomycin group compared to 79% in the vancomycin group. MRSA was found in 42% and 75%, respectively (p<0.001). Clinical improvement or resolution on days 3 and 5 were 90% versus 70%, and 98% versus 81% in the two groups (p<0.01 for both comparisons).

Although the results are confounded by differences in microbiology between the groups, those receiving daptomycin achieved more rapid resolution and had a shorter duration of inpatient therapy.

Efficacy of daptomycin in complicated skin and skin-structure infections due to methicillin-sensitive and -resistant *Staphylococcus aureus*: results from the CORE Registry. Martone WJ, Lamp KC. Curr Med Res Opin 2006; 22: 2337–43.

Data from 145 patients with MRSA infections demonstrated clinical success in 89.7%.

THIRD-LINE THERAPIES

▶ Quinupristin-dalfopristin	C
▶ Tigecycline	B
▶ Ceptobiprole	C
▶ Oritavancin	C
▶ Honey	D
▶ Confectioner's sugar	E
▶ Sugar and povidone-iodine	E
▶ Botanical extracts including gentian	D

Results of a double-blind, randomized trial of ceftobiprole treatment of complicated skin and skin structure infections caused by gram-positive bacteria. Noel GJ, Strauss RS, Amsler K, Heep M, Pypstra R, Solomkin JS. Antimicrob Agents Chemother 2008; 52: 37–44.

In a randomized, double-blind trial of ceftobiprole 50 mg every 12 h versus vancomycin 1 g every 12 h (282 receiving ceftobiprole and 277 receiving vancomycin), 91.8% of the MRSA patients treated with ceftobiprole and 90.0% of those treated with vancomycin were cured (95% confidence interval of difference, –8.4%, 12.1%). Adverse events were common and included nausea (14%) and taste disturbance (8%).

Ceftobiprole is a broad-spectrum cephalosporin active against MRSA. Although adverse effects were common, the rate was similar to that with vancomycin, and the drug had to be discontinued because of side effects in only 4% of patients.

Effect of medical honey on wounds colonised or infected with MRSA. Blaser G, Santos K, Bode U, Vetter H, Simon A. J Wound Care 2007; 16: 325–8.

In seven patients with non-healing wounds infected or colonized with MRSA who had failed other antiseptics and antibiotics, honey resulted in complete healing.

Mixture of sugar and povidone-iodine stimulates healing of MRSA-infected skin ulcers on db/db mice. Shi CM, Nakao H, Yamazaki M, Tsuboi R, Ogawa H.. Arch Dermatol Res 2007; 299: 449–56.

A trial of a topical paste composed of 70% sugar and 30% povidone-iodine accelerated healing of MRSA-infected ulcers in diabetic mice (p<0.01).

My grandmother, Anny Elston, MD, reported that as a World War I medic she used confectioner's sugar to treat infected ulcers in returning prisoners of war. All ulcers healed. The treatment is inexpensive, and resistance to the desiccating effects of sugar is unlikely.

Topical gentian violet for cutaneous infection and nasal carriage with MRSA. Okano M, Noguchi S, Tabata K, Matsumoto Y. Int J Dermatol 2000; 39: 942–4.

Topical gentian violet 0.5% was used once a day in 28 patients with skin lesions, and a 0.3% solution was applied to the nares of nine patients twice a day. Cure of skin lesions took 9.1 ± 6.0 days. Staphylococci were eliminated from nasal lesions in 15.3 ± 9.0 days.

Screening of plant extracts for antimicrobial activity against bacteria and yeasts with dermatological relevance. Weckesser S, Engel K, Simon-Haarhaus B, Wittmer A, Pelz K, Schempp CM. Phytomedicine 2007; 14: 508–16.

Usnea extract inhibited MRSA growth.

Mucoceles

Noah Scheinfeld

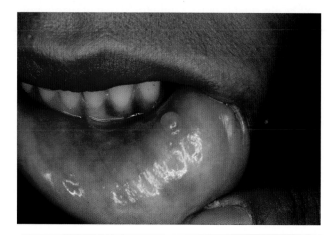

Labial mucoceles fall into two categories: mucous extravasation cysts and mucus retention cysts. The mucous extravasation cyst is a false cyst because it lacks an epithelial lining arising from the partially or totally severed salivary gland duct, resulting in the accumulation of saliva in the adjacent soft tissue. At this point the mucocele is cut off by a fibrous connective tissue pseudocapsule. Ductal epithelium lines the mucus retention cyst. The mucus retention cyst develops from partial obstruction of a duct in the presence of the salivary gland's continued secretion of mucus. The extravasation mucocele manifests most commonly and presents most often on a young person's lower lip. The retention mucocele is more apt to occur on the buccal cheek or soft palate of an older person.

MANAGEMENT STRATEGIES

Mucocele of the lip will be considered here as this is the most common type that dermatologists deal with. Mucoceles are benign lesions that may be symptomatic. As lesions may involute spontaneously, minimal inventions such as *cryotherapy* and *intralesional corticosteroids* should be tried first. Surgical approaches are reserved for cases recalcitrant to conservative treatment. *Simple incision and drainage* of lip mucoceles is not favored because the rate of recurrence is high and the procedure involves using a blade, which can be disconcerting for younger patients.

The treatment of choice for mucoceles that do not respond to minimal intervention is surgical excision. Management of complex mucoceles and mucus retention cysts may be difficult, because surgical removal may cause trauma to other adjacent minor salivary glands, prompting the formation of new mucoceles.

SPECIFIC INVESTIGATIONS

▶ Biopsy
▶ Doppler ultrasonography
▶ Color Doppler imaging

Case of superficial mucocele of the lower lip. Oka M, Nishioka E, Miyachi R, Terashima M, Nishigori C. J Dermatol 2007; 34: 754–6.

A biopsy of the mucocele can show neutrophils and erythrocytes present in the mucous epithelium with a dermal infiltrate comprising neutrophils, mononuclear lymphocytic cells, and eosinophils.

Calibre persistent labial artery: clinical features and non-invasive radiological diagnosis. Kocyigit P, Kocyigit D, Akay BN, Ustuner E, Kisnisci R. Clin Exp Dermatol 2006; 31: 528–30.

Doppler ultrasonography, which is a non-invasive and simple diagnostic tool, can help distinguish caliber-persistent labial artery (a primary arterial branch that penetrates into the submucosal tissue without division or reduction in diameter) which presents as an asymptomatic papule on the lower lip, from other entities including a varix, hemangioma, venous lake, mucocele, or fibroma.

Ultrasonography: a noninvasive tool to diagnose a caliber-persistent labial artery, an enlarged artery of the lip. Vazquez L, Lombardi T, Guinand-Mkinsi H, Samson J. J Ultrasound Med 2005; 24: 1295–301.

In three cases of caliber-persistent labial artery investigators localized and determined the extension of the intralabial artery with ultrasonography, including pulsed and color Doppler analysis, and compared the sonograms to the clinical and histopathologic findings.

FIRST-LINE THERAPIES

▶ Expectant observation	**E**
▶ Cryotherapy	**C**
▶ Intralesional corticosteroids	**D**

Expectant observation

A review of common pediatric lip lesions: herpes simplex/recurrent herpes labialis, impetigo, mucoceles, and hemangiomas. Bentley JM, Barankin B, Guenther LC. Clin Pediatr (Phila) 2003; 42: 475–82.

After a diagnosis is made treatment is often not needed, as smaller and more superficial mucoceles are likely to rupture and heal spontaneously. The patient's future as it relates to mucoceles is good whether or not surgery is involved.

Watchful waiting may be the best approach for superficial mucoceles as they may involute spontaneously.

Cryotherapy

A simple cryosurgical method for treatment of oral mucous cysts. Toida M, Ishimaru JI, Hobo N. Int J Oral Maxillofac Surg 1993; 22: 353–5.

Twelve females and six males with mucous cysts on the lower lip and the tip of the tongue were treated by direct application of liquid nitrogen with a cotton swab. Each lesion was exposed to four or five cycles composed of freezings of 10–30 seconds and thawings of double the freezing times. No anesthesia was required. All lesions had disappeared completely 2–4 weeks after one or two treatment courses of cryosurgery. In all cases, neither scarring nor recurrence was noted during the 6 months to 5 years of follow-up.

Cryotherapy furnishes a simple non-blood means for treating mucoceles that can be effective without having to use a blade.

Cryosurgical treatment of mucocele in children. Twetman S, Isaksson S. Am J Dent 1990; 3: 175–6.

Cryosurgery of superficial mucoceles located in the lower lip of eight children did not require administration of local anesthetic. Surgeons performed cryosurgery easily and small children tolerated it well, without complications or recurrence at 1 year.

Children may be more amenable to cryotherapy than to needle-based treatments.

Steroid injection

Histopathology of mucoceles infiltrated with steroids. Merida FMT. Med Cutan Ibero Lat Am 1976; 4: 15–18.

Eight cases of lip mucocele with intralesional infiltration of triamcinolone acetonide (Kenacort). In three cases there was complete regression of the lesion after a variable period between the first and the fourth infiltration. In five cases the results were negative. The patients who reacted positively to treatment were followed for a year afterwards.

Yet again we find that injection of low concentration corticosteroids can kick-start the dissipation of aberrant collections of cells without needing to use blade-based surgical interventions.

SECOND-LINE THERAPIES

▶ Punch biopsy	E

Two simple treatments for lower lip mucocoeles. Gill D. Australas J Dermatol 1996; 37: 220.

Punch biopsy is a useful technique for treating mucocele and has the added benefit of providing a histologically certain diagnosis.

THIRD-LINE THERAPIES

▶ CO$_2$ laser	B
▶ Surgical excision	B
▶ Marsupialization	D
▶ Micro-marsupialization	D

Treatment of mucocele of the lower lip with carbon dioxide laser. Huang IY, Chen CM, Kao YH, Worthington P. J Oral Maxillofac Surg 2007; 65: 855–8.

Eighty-two patients with biopsy-confirmed mucocele of the lower lip were treated with CO$_2$ laser vaporization, with no bleeding and minimal scar formation. There were two recurrences.

This can be an excellent and rapid treatment, but requires expensive equipment and trained operators.

Surgical excision

Clinicostatistical study of lower lip mucoceles. Yamasoba T, Tayama N, Syoji M, Fukuta M. Head Neck 1990; 12: 316–20.

Researchers reported 70 patients with lower lip mucoceles for their characteristics, clinical features, and histopathologic findings. Of 70 biopsies, 68 were mucous extravasation cysts and two were mucus retention cysts. Surgical excision was the treatment of choice, with recurrence of the lesion in only two cases.

Surgery is the a definitive – albeit not foolproof – method of treating mucoceles.

Marsupialization

Clinical and histopathologic study of salivary mucoceles. Kang SK, Kim KS. Taehan Chikkwa Uisa Hyophoe Chi 1989; 27: 1059–71.

In a series of 112 patients, surgeons treated 107 mucoceles (95%) by excision and only five by marsupialization. Eighteen of 112 cases had recurrence, and the recurrence rate in this study was 16%.

Large mucoceles sometimes may be best treated by marsupialization because of the risk of traumatizing the labial branch of the mental nerve. This involves creating a pouch (marsupialization) inside the lesion and then draining it. It is a more complex technique than simple excision but has its uses in complex cases.

Micro-marsupialization

Treatment of mucus retention phenomena in children by the micro-marsupialization technique: case reports. Delbem AC, Cunha RF, Vieira AE, Ribeiro LL: Pediatr Dent 2000; 22: 155–8.

Micro-marsupialization requires neither injections nor surgery, and was studied in 14 patients. It involves placing a topical anesthetic gel on the mucocele for 3 minutes, passing a 4/0 silk suture through the body of the mucocele, and tying a surgeon's knot. The suture material is removed 7 days later, at which time the mucocele is resolved. The advantages of this technique include simplicity and relative lack of pain. Micro-marsupialization is not indicated for fibrotic lesions, lesions of the palate, or lesions inside the buccal mucosa. Of the original 14 patients treated by the technique, 12 had full regression 1 week after treatment. Recurrence occurred in two cases.

This may be an excellent technique to use for complex cases in children, but is probably best performed by pediatric dentists.

Mucous membrane pemphigoid

Gudula Kirtschig, Fenella Wojnarowska

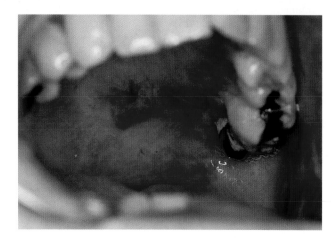

Mucous membrane pemphigoid (MMP), also known as cicatricial pemphigoid, is a rare autoimmune subepidermal bullous disease characterized by erosions and blisters of one or more mucous membranes and less commonly the skin; scarring may involve the conjunctiva, esophagus, skin, and genitals. Bullous pemphigoid affecting chiefly the skin is addressed in a separate chapter.

MANAGEMENT STRATEGY

MMP is a chronic disease and rarely remits spontaneously. The individual sites involved determine the effect on the patient's health and well-being. The best treatment for MMP is unclear, as there are only two small randomized controlled trials in ocular MMP. A multidisciplinary approach is essential. There are no known underlying diseases or associated drug triggers.

In all patients *superpotent topical corticosteroids* should be applied to affected sites. In patients with disease localized to the oral or genital mucosa, if the response to *superpotent topical corticosteroids* is inadequate, *anti-inflammatory antibiotics such as dapsone (50–200 mg/day) or tetracyclines (see below)*, alone or with medium doses of *systemic corticosteroids* (e.g., *prednisolone 0.5 mg/kg/day*) may be added.

Interventions for mucous membrane pemphigoid and epidermolysis bullosa acquisita. Kirtschig G, Murrell D, Wojnarowska F, Khumalo N. Cochrane Database Syst Rev 2003; CD004056.

The first international consensus on mucous membrane pemphigoid: definition, diagnostic criteria, pathogenic factors, medical treatment, and prognostic indicators. Chan LS, Ahmed AR, Anhalt GJ, Bernauer W, Cooper KD, Elder MJ, et al. Arch Dermatol 2002; 138: 370–9.

SPECIFIC INVESTIGATIONS

> **For diagnosis**
> ▶ Direct immunofluorescence
> ▶ Indirect immunofluorescence on salt split skin
>
> **For treatment**
> ▶ Glucose 6 phosphate dehydrogenase (G6PD)
> ▶ Thiopurine methyltransferase (TPMT)
> ▶ CBC, LFTs, renal function

FIRST-LINE THERAPIES

> ▶ Topical corticosteroids   C
> ▶ Dapsone   C
> ▶ Anti-inflammatory antibiotics   D
> ▶ Systemic corticosteroids   C
> ▶ Cyclophosphamide   C

Mild disease involving the oral mucosa, genitals, or skin

Therapeutic management of mucous membrane pemphigoid. Report of 11 cases. Carrozzo M, Carbone M, Broccoletti R, Garzino-Demo P, Gandolfo S. Minerva Stomatologica 1997; 46: 553–9.

Four of eight patients with oral MMP benefited from topical clobetasol propionate.

Treatment of severe erosive gingival lesions by topical application of clobetasol propionate in custom trays. Gonzalez-Moles MA, Ruiz-Avila I, Rodriguez-Archilla A, Morales-Garcia P, Mesa-Aguado F, Bascones-Martinez A, et al. Oral Surg Oral Med Oral Pathol Oral Radiol Endodont 2003; 95: 688–92.

Twenty-two patients with oral MMP benefited from topical steroid application using a gingival tray.

Treatment-resistant or severe disease

Upper aerodigestive tract manifestations of cicatricial pemphigoid. Hanson RD, Olsen KD, Rogers RS. Ann Otol Rhinol Laryngol 1988; 97: 493–9.

Dapsone 125–150 mg/day was beneficial in most of 142 patients and preferred to systemic corticosteroids, azathioprine, or cyclophosphamide.

Cicatricial pemphigoid: a re-evaluation of therapy. Nayar M, Wojnarowska F. J Dermatol Treat 1993; 4: 89–93.

Seven of 14 patients had some benefit from 50–150 mg/day dapsone.

Treatment of cicatricial (benign mucous membrane) pemphigoid with dapsone. Rogers RS III, Seehafer JR, Perry HO. J Am Acad Dermatol 1982; 6: 215–23.

Nineteen of 24 patients with oral and ocular MMP achieved complete or partial control of inflammation after 2–12 weeks' treatment with 75–200 mg dapsone per day.

Dapsone therapy of cicatricial pemphigoid. Rogers RS III, Mehregan DA. Semin Dermatol 1988; 7: 201–5.

Seventy-seven patients with oral, ocular or generalized MMP benefited from either 150 mg dapsone per day or 1500–3000 mg sulfapyridine per day for at least 12 weeks.

Sulphamethoxypyridazine for dermatitis herpetiformis, linear IgA disease and cicatricial pemphigoid. McFadden JP, Leonard JN, Powles AV, Rutman AJ, Fry L. Br J Dermatol 1989; 121: 759–62.

Sulfamethoxypyridazine 500–1500 mg was partially effective in 10 of 15 patients with oral and generalized MMP.

Treatment with dapsone 50–200 mg/day, and sulphonamides, 500–1500 mg sulfapyridine or sulfamethoxypyridazine, can be helpful, particularly if IgA deposits are present.

Antiepiligrin cicatricial pemphigoid of the larynx successfully treated with a combination of tetracycline and niacinamide. Sakamoto K, Mori K, Hashimoto T, Yancey KB, Nakashima T. Arch Otolaryngol Head Neck Surg 2002; 128: 1420–3.

Successful therapy with tetracycline and nicotinamide in cicatricial pemphigoid. Kreyden OP, Borradori L, Trueb RM, Burg G, Nestle FO. Hautarzt 2001; 52: 247–50.

Single case reports of effective treatment with tetracycline and nicotinamide (500–3000 mg/day).

Cicatricial pemphigoid: a re-evaluation of therapy. Nayar M, Wojnarowska F. J Dermatol Treat 1993; 4: 89–93.

Minocycline 100 mg was beneficial for oral lesions in two of 10 patients with generalized MMP.

Combination therapy with nicotinamide and tetracyclines for cicatricial pemphigoid: further support for its efficacy. Reiche L, Wojnarowska F, Mallon E. Clin Exp Dermatol 1998; 23: 254–7.

Minocycline 50–100 mg/day combined with 2.5–3 g nicotinamide per day was beneficial in five of eight patients.

Treatment with anti-inflammatory antibiotics can be helpful;, nicotinamide may confer additional benefit. The antibiotics used are tetracycline 500–2000 mg/day, doxycycline 100–300 mg/day, or minocycline 100–200 mg/day.

Cicatricial pemphigoid and erythema multiforme. Mondino BJ. Ophthalmology 1990; 97: 939–52.

In 11 patients with ocular MMP treated with prednisone 60–80 mg/day, disease progression was seen in none with stage 1 disease, in 14% with stage 2 disease, and in 53% with stage 3 disease.

Mucous membrane pemphigoid. Treatment experience at two institutions. Lamey PJ, Rees TD, Binnie WH, Rankin KV. Oral SurgOral Med Oral Pathol 1992; 74: 50–3.

Fourteen patients with oral MMP were treated with a combination of systemic and topical steroids: eight became asymptomatic, five improved, and one was unchanged.

Cicatricial pemphigoid: a re-evaluation of therapy. Nayar M, Wojnarowska F. J Dermatol Treat 1993; 4: 89–93.

Five of 15 patients with generalized MMP benefited from prednisolone 40–60 mg/day, but it was ineffective in oral disease.

Treatment with systemic corticosteroids does seem to be helpful at doses of prednisolone 0.5–2 mg/kg/day. Most studies were performed using a combination of systemic steroids and a steroid-sparing drug; a small randomized trial supported combination treatment in ocular MMP (see below).

Ocular MMP

Cicatricial pemphigoid. Foster CS. Trans Am Ophthalmol Soc 1986; 84: 527–663.

A randomized study of 24 patients with bilateral stage III ocular MMP. In all 12 patients receiving cyclophosphamide (2 mg/kg/day) plus prednisone (1 mg/kg/day) and in five of 12 receiving prednisone (1 mg/kg/day) the inflammation subsided. In a randomized study of 40 patients with stage III ocular MMP, 14 of 20 patients receiving dapsone (2 mg/kg/day) and all 20 patients receiving cyclophosphamide (2 mg/kg/day) responded within 6 months; most also received prednisone.

Dapsone combined with systemic corticosteroids seems to be a reasonable first-line treatment in moderate MMP. In treatment-resistant or rapidly progressive ocular disease cyclophosphamide (orally or intravenously) combined with prednisone is first-line treatment.

SECOND-LINE THERAPIES

▶ Topical mitomycin C	C
▶ Azathioprine	D
▶ Mycophenolate mofetil	C
▶ Methotrexate	D
▶ Ciclosporin	D

Intraoperative mitomycin C in the treatment of cicatricial obliterations of conjunctival fornices. Secchi AG, Tognon MS. Am J Ophthalmol 1996; 122: 728–30.

Intraoperative topical mitomycin was useful in four of four patients.

Subconjunctival mitomycin C for the treatment of ocular cicatricial pemphigoid. Donnenfeld ED, Perry HD, Wallerstein A, Caronia RM, Kanellopoulos AJ, Sforza PD, et al. Ophthalmology 1999; 106: 72–9.

No disease progression occurred in eight of nine eyes treated with subconjunctival mitomycin C.

Ocular cicatricial pemphigoid review. Foster CS, Sainz De La Maza M. Curr Opin Allergy Clin Immunol 2004; 4: 435–9.

No long-term reduction in inflammation was found.
Mitomycin may reduce scarring in the short term.

Cicatricial pemphigoid and erythema multiforme. Mondino BJ. Ophthalmology 1990; 97: 939–52.

Ten patients were treated with azathioprine 1.5 mg/kg/day; half had disease progression, worse than with cyclophosphamide, prednisone, or combined regimens.

Immunosuppressive therapy for ocular mucous membrane pemphigoid strategies and outcomes. Saw VP, Dart JK, Rauz S, Ramsay A, Bunce C, Xing W, et al. Ophthalmology 2008; 115: 253–61.

Azathioprine or mycophenolate mofetil were beneficial in about two-thirds of patients.

Cicatricial pemphigoid: treatment with mycophenolate mofetil. Ingen-Housz-Oro S, Prost-Squarcioni C, Pascal F, Doan S, Brette MD, Bachelez H, et al. Ann Dermatol Venereol 2005; 132: 13–16.

Mycophenolate mofetil helped to control the disease in 10 of 14 patients; most also received cyclophosphamide or dapsone.

Mycophenolate mofetil therapy for inflammatory eye disease. Thorne JE, Jabs DA, Qazi FA, Nguyen QD, Kempen JH, Dunn JP. Ophthalmology 2005; 112: 1472–7.

Nine patients with inflammatory eye disease were treated; in some the dose of prednisone was reduced from 40 to 10 mg/day after 3.5 months of treatment.

Methotrexate therapy for ocular cicatricial pemphigoid. McCluskey P, Chang JH, Singh R, Wakefield D. Ophthalmology 2004; 111: 796–801.

In 12 of 17 patients with mainly ocular MMP oral methotrexate (and topical treatment) prevented progression of scarring.

Cyclosporine therapy of life-threatening cicatricial pemphigoid affecting the respiratory tract. Williams DY, Oziemski M, Varigos G. Int J Dermatol 1995; 34: 639–41.

Ciclosporin helpful.

Ocular autoimmune pemphigoid and cyclosporine. Alonso A, Bignone ML, Brunzini M, Brunzini R. Allergol Immunopathol (Madr) 2006; 34: 113–15.

Treatment-resistant ocular pemphigoid in 82 patients was treated with ciclosporin 100 mg/day, with an attendant reduction in the dose of steroids.

There is evidence of the effectiveness of immunosuppressive agents. The most commonly used drugs are azathioprine, 1–3 mg/kg/day, and mycophenolate mofetil, 0.5–1 g twice daily. Less commonly used are methotrexate, 5–25 mg/week, and ciclosporin, 2–4 mg/kg/day.

THIRD-LINE THERAPIES

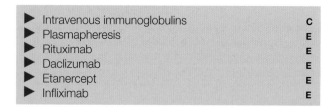

▶ Intravenous immunoglobulins	C
▶ Plasmapheresis	E
▶ Rituximab	E
▶ Daclizumab	E
▶ Etanercept	E
▶ Infliximab	E

High-dose intravenous immunoglobulins: an approach to treat severe immune-mediated and autoimmune diseases of the skin. Ruetter A, Luger T. J Am Acad Dermatol 2001; 44: 1010–24.

Consensus statement on the use of intravenous immunoglobulin therapy in the treatment of autoimmune mucocutaneous blistering diseases. Ahmed AR, Dahl MV. Arch Dermatol 2003; 139: 1051–9.

Good reviews on uses and regimes.

A nonrandomized comparison of the clinical outcome of ocular involvement in patients with mucous membrane (cicatricial) pemphigoid between conventional immunosuppressive and intravenous immunoglobulin therapies. Letko E, Miserocchi E, Daoud YJ, Christen W, Foster CS, Ahmed AR. Clin Immunol 2004; 111: 303–10.

None of eight patients with ocular MMP had progressed from stage 2 ocular disease after a 24-month treatment, compared to half of those treated with conventional immunosuppression.

Intravenous immunoglobulins and mucous membrane pemphigoid. Mignogna MD, Leuci S, Piscopo R, Bonovolontà G. Ophthalmology 2008; 115: 752.

IVIG treatment was beneficial in six patients with generalized MMP also affecting the eyes.

Intravenous immunoglobulin at doses 0.5–2 g/kg/day (over 3–5 days) initially once a month combined with other systemic treatments is justified in treatment-resistant or rapidly progressive MMP.

A case of antiepiligrin cicatricial pemphigoid successfully treated by plasmapheresis. Hashimoto Y, Suga Y, Yoshiike T, Hashimoto T, Takamori K. Dermatology 2000; 2: 58–60.

A single case of ocular MMP benefiting from plasmapheresis combined with immunosuppression.

There is inadequate evidence to recommend plasmapheresis.

Successful adjuvant treatment of recalcitrant mucous membrane pemphigoid with anti-CD20 antibody rituximab. Taverna JA, Lerner A, Bhawan J, Demierre MF. J Drugs Dermatol 2007; 6: 731–2.

A single case responded.

Rituximab in autoimmune bullous diseases: mixed responses and adverse effects. Schmidt E, Seitz CS, Benoit S, Bröcker EB, Goebeler M. Br J Dermatol 2007; 156: 352–6.

A single case was helped in some sites, but ocular disease progressed.

Treatment of ocular inflammatory disorders with daclizumab. Papaliodis GN, Chu D, Foster CS. Ophthalmology 2003; 110: 786–9.

One patient with scarring ocular MMP had a reduction in inflammation.

Successful biologic treatment of ocular mucous membrane pemphigoid with anti-TNF-alpha. John H, Whallett A, Quinlan M. Eye 2007; 21: 1434–5.

Treatment of ocular cicatricial pemphigoid with the tumour necrosis factor alpha antagonist etanercept. Prey S, Robert PY, Drouet M, Sparsa A, Roux C, Bonnetblanc JM, et al. Acta Dermatol Venereol 2007; 87: 74–5.

Successful treatment of mucous membrane pemphigoid with etanercept in 3 patients. Canizares MJ, Smith DI, Conners MS, Maverick KJ, Heffernan MP. Arch Dermatol 2006; 142: 1457–61.

Treatment of recalcitrant cicatricial pemphigoid with the tumor necrosis factor alpha antagonist etanercept. Sacher C, Rubbert A, König C, Scharffetter-Kochanek K, Krieg T, Hunzelmann N. J Am Acad Dermatol 2002; 46: 113–15.

Five patients were successfully treated with etanercept, including three with ocular disease; one patient maintained remission after cessation of the drug, and another relapsed.

Successful treatment of mucous membrane pemphigoid with infliximab. Heffernan MP, Bentley DD. Arch Dermatol 2006; 142: 1268–70.

Mucous membrane pemphigoid in a series of 7 children and a review of the literature with particular reference to prognostic features and treatment. Veysey EC, McHenry P, Powell J, Crone M, Harper JI, Allen J, et al. Eur J Pediatr Dermatol 2007; 17: 218–26.

Two cases with MMP benefited from infliximab; disease was ocular and oral in both and esophageal in one.

The biologics, particularly the anti-TNF antagonists etanercept and infliximab, seem promising, but the evidence is still anecdotal.

Mycetoma: eumycetoma and actinomycetoma

Mahreen Ameen, Wanda Sonia Robles

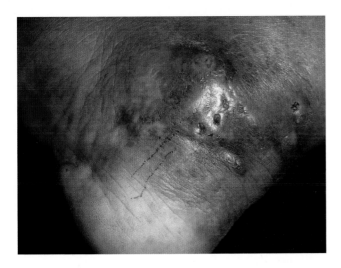

Mycetomas (Madura foot) are endemic in the tropics and subtropics. They are chronic, granulomatous, subcutaneous infections caused by either *Actinomycetes* bacteria or eumycetes fungi, giving rising to actinomycetomas and eumycetomas, respectively. The infectious agents are saprophytes existing in soil or plants, and infection usually results from traumatic inoculation into the skin. Consequently, the disease most commonly affects agriculturalists and those who are barefoot. The disease is characterized by abscesses, draining sinuses, and discharging grains, and progresses slowly with a risk of bone and visceral involvement. The discharging grains represent aggregates of fungal hyphae or bacterial filaments. Actinomycetomas are produced by agents of the genera *Nocardia, Actinomadura, Streptomyces,* and *Nocardiopsis*. *Nocardia* is the commonest agent, particularly in the Americas, but *Streptomyces somaliensis* is more common in Sudan and the Middle East. Eumycetomas are caused by a large number of fungi: *Madurella mycetomatis* is of particular significance, as it is the most prevalent causative agent in regions of India and Africa.

MANAGEMENT STRATEGY

Treatment of mycetomas is generally difficult, and management varies from a very conservative approach to chemotherapy and surgery. Effective chemotherapy is available for actinomycetomas, but eumycetomas are more refractory to drug therapy.

Eumycetomas may sometimes be managed conservatively as they are usually indolent and seldom life-threatening. Treatment is then symptomatic, with relief of pain and applications of dressings to affected areas, particularly the sinuses. Any secondary bacterial infection requires treatment. More active management consists of long courses of antifungals, for 18–24 months or even longer, together with aggressive surgical excision and debulking. Antifungal therapy is initiated before surgery and continued afterwards to reduce the risk of recurrence. Small lesions have a more favorable prognosis, as they are more easily excised completely. Advanced disease with bony involvement characteristically shows a poor response to therapy and often requires surgical amputation. Of all the antifungal drugs, the azoles have been most commonly used. Fluconazole has been found to be ineffective, but *ketoconazole* and *itraconazole* have both demonstrated efficacy, particularly at high doses (200–400 mg daily for ketoconazole and 300–400 mg daily for itraconazole). Itraconazole is preferred as it is better tolerated for longer periods and is thought to demonstrate greater efficacy than ketoconazole, although there are no published studies comparing their efficacy. There are reports of the high tolerability and efficacy of the newer broad-spectrum triazoles such as *voriconazole* and *posaconazole* against *Madurella* species and *Scedosporium apiospermum* infection. However, their high costs are prohibitive for use in most endemic regions. Griseofulvin appears to be ineffective. *Amphotericin* has shown variable responses in the few cases in which it has been used. High-dose *terbinafine* (500 mg twice daily) has demonstrated limited efficacy.

Actinomycetomas are usually amenable to antibiotic therapy, but cure rates vary widely from 60% to 90%. Combined therapy is preferred in order to prevent the development of drug resistance, as well as to eradicate any residual infection. The duration of drug therapy depends on clinical response. Cure is defined by a lack of clinical activity, absence of grains, and negative cultures. Treatment with *sulfonamides* and *sulfonamide combinations* such as *trimethoprim-sulfamethoxazole (co-trimoxazole)* are usually first line. *Aminoglycosides, tetracyclines, rifampicin, ciprofloxacin* and *amoxicillin-clavulanate* have also been successfully used. Parenteral *amikacin* and oral co-trimoxazole combination therapy is especially advocated for cases at risk of bone or visceral involvement. Actinomycetomas seldom require surgical management.

SPECIFIC INVESTIGATIONS

▶ Direct microscopy
▶ Culture
▶ Histopathology

It is imperative to differentiate between eumycetomas, which respond poorly to chemotherapy, and actinomycetomas, which generally respond well. Furthermore, species identification is important, as it has treatment and prognostic implications, some species having demonstrated a better response to some chemotherapy regimens than others.

The clinical diagnosis can be confirmed by the demonstration and identification of grains, which can be obtained by direct extraction, fine needle aspiration, or deep tissue biopsy. Direct microscopy of a crushed grain in 10% potassium hydroxide solution gives an indication of its size and shape, which provides an initial clue to the causative agent, whether bacterial or fungal. Histopathology of a deep surgical biopsy demonstrates a granulomatous, inflammatory reaction with abscesses containing grains. Culture of grains using Sabouraud or blood agar media permits species identification. However, fungal culture can be particularly difficult, as morphological differentiation of fungi may be poor or delayed. Molecular tests have therefore been developed for species identification of several black-grained eumycetomas, including species-specific polymerase chain reaction (PCR) analysis. Serological tests such as enzyme-linked immunosorbent assay (ELISA) are employed by some centers to support diagnosis as well as to assess therapy response. Radiology and ultrasound enable assessment of disease extent and bony involvement. Helical computed tomography (CT) can provide detailed assessments of soft tissue and visceral involvement.

FIRST-LINE THERAPIES

▶ Sulfonamides	B
▶ Aminoglycosides	B
▶ Itraconazole	C

The following review articles outline the diagnosis and management of mycetomas.

New aspects of some endemic mycoses. Poncio Mendes R, Negroni R, Bonifaz A, Pappagianis D. Med Mycol 2000; 38: 237–41.

This review article advocates the use of azole drugs for eumycetomas, and prefers itraconazole to ketoconazole because of its higher tolerability. Sulfonamides are suggested as first-line therapy for *Nocardia* actinomycetomas, and sulfonamides in combination with amikacin for *Actinomadura madurae*. Ciprofloxacin is suggested as a useful drug for the treatment of actinomycetomas with bony lesions.

Management of mycetoma in West Africa. Develoux M, Dieng MT, Kane A, Ndiaye B. Bull Soc Pathol Exot 2003; 96: 376–82.

A good review article highlighting the need for thorough pre-treatment assessment. This involves assessing the extent of the lesion for any bone involvement, and identifying etiologic agents. Recommended treatment for eumycetomas is with ketoconazole or itraconazole combined with surgery. For actinomycetomas, antibiotic therapy should be chosen depending on the etiologic agent.

Mycetoma: a thorn in the flesh. Fahal AH. Trans Roy Soc Trop Med Hyg 2004; 98: 3–11.

A review article based on the experiences of the Mycetoma Research Centre in Sudan. This article highlights the clinical similarities between eumycetoma and actinomycetoma infections, although actinomycetoma has a more rapid course. Combined antibiotic treatment for actinomycetomas and aggressive surgery in combination with antifungals for eumycetomas is recommended.

Mycetoma caused by *Madurella mycetomatis*: a neglected infectious burden. Ahmed AO, van Leeuwen W, Fahal A, van de Sande W, Verbrugh H, van Belkum A. Lancet Infect Dis 2004; 4: 566–74.

A good review article on developments in the clinical, epidemiologic, and diagnostic management of *Madurella mycetomatis* eumycetoma.

Mycetoma. Welsh O, Vera-Cabrera L, Salinas-Carmona MC. Dermatol Clin 2007; 25: 195–202.

A recent and comprehensive review article covering the etiopathogenesis, diagnosis, and treatment options for mycetomas. The authors describe their long experience in Mexico of using parenteral amikacin therapy (15 mg/kg per day for 3 weeks) in combination with oral trimethoprim/sulfamethoxazole (8/40 mg/kg per day for 5 weeks) for the treatment

of severe or refractory actinomycetomas. Up to four 5-weekly cycles can be given, and treatment is administered continuously to minimize the development of secondary resistance to amikacin. The authors recommend that audiometry and creatinine clearance be performed during the last 2 weeks of each cycle.

Actinomycetomas in Senegal. Study of 90 cases. Dieng MT, Niang SO, Diop B, Ndiaye B. Bull Soc Pathol Exot Filiales 2005; 98: 18–20. (In French.)

Ninety patients with actinomycetomas (*A. pelletieri*, n=60; *A. madurae*, n=25; *S. somaliensis*, n=5) in Senegal were treated with sulfamethoxazole monotherapy. Despite bone involvement in 55% of cases, cure was achieved after 1 year of treatment in 83% of patients; 50% of these cases were localized to the foot. Despite treatment, two patients died of visceral involvement.

Mycetoma in children: Experience with 15 cases. Bonifaz A, Ibarra G, Saul A, Paredes-Solis V, Carrasco-Gerard E, Fierro-Arias L. Pediatr Infect Dis J 2007; 26: 50–2.

Mycetomas are very rare in children, but their clinical presentation and course are similar to those in adults. There were 13 cases of *Nocardia* actinomycetoma and two of *M. mycetomatis* eumycetoma. Sulfonamide combinations were advocated as first-line therapy for actinomycetomas and co-amoxiclav as second-line therapy. Itraconazole and ketoconazole were used in the management of eumycetomas.

This is the largest series describing the treatment of children with mycetomas.

A modified two-step treatment for actinomycetoma. Ramam M, Bhat R, Garg T, Sharma VK, Ray R, Singh MK, et al. Ind J Dermatol Venereol Leprol 2007; 73: 235–9.

The authors emphasize that although parenteral therapy regimens demonstrate high efficacy, they are costly in terms of inpatient stays. They describe a reduced parenteral regimen (intravenous gentamicin 80 mg twice daily together with oral trimethoprim/sulfamethoxazole [co-trimoxazole] 320/1600 mg twice daily for one month), followed by a longer phase of oral medication (doxycycline 100 mg twice daily, together with co-trimoxazole at the same dose). All 21 patients demonstrated a significant clinical response at the end of the parenteral phase of treatment. The oral phase needed to be continued for 3.5–16 months (mean 9.1 months) until cure, and in the majority of patients this included a treatment period of 5–6 months after complete healing of the lesions to prevent any relapse.

Improvement of eumycetoma with itraconazole. Smith EL, Kutbi S. J Am Acad Dermatol 1997; 34: 279–80.

This study from Saudi Arabia treated 25 patients with a follow-up period of 12 years. The authors recommend a combination itraconazole drug regimen together with surgical excision or debulking. Drainage of sinuses with removal of grains that can cause inflammation reduces pain and swelling.

Clinical and mycologic findings and therapeutic outcome of 27 mycetoma patients from São Paolo, Brazil. Castro LG, Piquero-Casals J. Int J Dermatol 2008; 47: 160–3.

This article describes the treatment of 13 cases of eumycetoma (with itraconazole) and 14 cases of actinomycetoma (with co-trimoxazole). Combination drug therapy was used in more than half of the cases. There was higher efficacy in three patients with actinomycetoma treated with co-trimoxazole combined with amikacin. However, two of these patients

Evidence Levels: **A** Double-blind study **B** Clinical trial ≥ 20 subjects **C** Clinical trial < 20 subjects **D** Series ≥ 5 subjects **E** Anecdotal case reports

developed hearing loss after treatment. The authors emphasize the problems of diagnostic testing, even in secondary and tertiary health centers, and were only able to identify the etiological agent in fewer than half of their cases.

SECOND-LINE THERAPIES

▶ Amoxicillin-clavulanate	B
▶ Terbinafine	B
▶ Ketoconazole	C
▶ Posaconazole	D
▶ Voriconazole	E
▶ Imipenem	D
▶ Oxazolidinones	E

Treatment of actinomycetoma due to *Nocardia* spp. with amoxicillin-clavulanate. Bonifaz A, Flores P, Saul A, Carrasco-Gerard E, Ponce RM. Br J Dermatol 2007; 156: 308–11.

This study advocates co-amoxiclav as rescue therapy in patients with *Nocardia* spp. refractory to other therapy regimens. Twenty-one patients who had previously failed on other regimens were treated with oral amoxicillin/clavulinic acid [co-amoxiclav] 875/125 mg twice daily. There was clinical and microbiological cure in 15 (71%) patients after a mean treatment period of 10 months. Patients with bone and visceral involvement required longer treatment periods.

Clinical efficacy and safety of oral terbinafine in fungal mycetoma. N'Diaye B, Dieng MT, Perez A, Stockmeyer M, Bakshi R. Int J Dermatol 2006; 45: 154–7.

High-dose terbinafine, 500 mg twice daily, was given as monotherapy to 23 patients with eumycetomas in Senegal. After 24–48 weeks of treatment mycological cure was seen in 25% patients, and a further 55% demonstrated clinical improvement. Treatment was well tolerated.

Ketoconazole in the treatment of eumycetoma due to *Madurella mycetomii*. Mahgoub ES, Gumaa SA. Trans Roy Soc Trop Med Hyg 1984; 78: 376–9.

This trial consisted of 13 patients treated in the Sudan and Saudi Arabia. Ketoconazole was given at doses of 200–400 mg daily for 3–36 months (median 13 months). Treatment was well tolerated. Five patients were cured, and a further four improved. Response appeared to be dose dependent. The authors recommend a 400 mg daily dose of ketoconazole, and a minimum treatment period of 12 months where there is bony involvement irrespective of clinical improvement.

Given the availability of newer antifungals, there are few recent trials evaluating the use of ketoconazole for eumycetomas. However, it is a less expensive drug than itraconazole and is therefore more commonly used in endemic regions.

Posaconazole treatment of refractory eumycetoma and chromoblastomycosis. Negroni R, Tobon A, Bustamante B, Shikanai-Yasuda MA, Patino H, Restrepo A. Rev Inst Med Trop São Paolo 2005; 47: 339–46.

In this study from Argentina, posaconazole (800 mg daily in divided doses) was given to six patients with eumycetoma (*M. grisea*, n=3; *M. mycetomatis*, n=2; *S. apiospermum*, n=1) resistant to standard therapy. Complete clinical response was reported in five of the six patients. Four patients were cured

and a further patient improved. Treatment was well tolerated, even after long-term administration of more than 2 years.

***Madurella mycetomatis* mycetoma treated successfully with oral voriconazole.** Lacroix C, De Kerviller E, Morel P, Derouin F, Feuilhade de Chavin M. Br J Dermatol 2005; 152: 1067–8.

Voriconazole has been reported to be effective in the management of disseminated fungal infections with *Scedosporium* and *Fusarium* spp. This is the first report of successful treatment of a eumycetoma with oral voriconazole. The case was acquired in Mali and treated in France with voriconazole monotherapy for 16 months at a dose of 300 mg twice daily. There was no evidence of any bony involvement, the treatment was well tolerated, and the patient remained disease-free 4 years after the end of treatment.

Successful treatment of black-grain mycetoma with voriconazole. Loulergue P, Hot A, Dannaoui E, Dallot A, Poirée S, Dupont B, et al. Am J Trop Med Hyg 2006; 75: 1106–7.

A further case of *Madurella mycetomatis* eumycetoma without bone involvement, which was acquired in Senegal and treated in France. Although antifungal susceptibility testing showed high susceptibility to voriconazole, itraconazole, and terbinafine, oral voriconazole was chosen to treat the patient because of its known long-term tolerance. The patient was treated for more than 1 year at a dose of 200 mg twice daily, with an excellent clinical response. However, there are no long-term follow-up data on this case.

***Scedosporium apiospermum* mycetoma with bone involvement successfully treated with voriconazole.** Porte L, Khatibi S, Hajj LE, Cassaing S, Berry A, Massip P, et al. Trans Roy Soc Trop Med Hyg 2006; 100: 891–4.

Scedosporium apiospermum mycetoma usually requires limb amputation. This case with bone involvement was acquired in the Ivory Coast and treated in France. The patient had previously failed to respond to itraconazole, fluconazole, and co-trimoxazole, and had refused amputation. Voriconazole 400 mg daily was given for 18 months, with good clinical effect. Magnetic resonance imaging demonstrated impressive regression of bony lesions. However, treatment was discontinued because of hepatic impairment.

This report suggests voriconazole as a promising treatment option for S. apiospermum *mycetomas.*

Actinomycetoma and *Nocardia* sp. Report of five cases treated with imipenem or imipenem plus amikacin. Fuentes A, Arenas R, Reyes M, Fernández RF, Zacarías R. Gac Med Mex 2006; 142: 247–252. (In Spanish.)

These were severe cases with visceral involvement (n=2), and all were refractory to previous therapies. They were treated with intravenous imipenem monotherapy (n=2) at a dose of 500 mg three times daily, or in combination with intravenous amikacin (n=3) at a dose of 500 mg twice daily (15 mg/kg) given in cycles of 3 weeks at 6-month intervals. Oral co-trimoxazole was also given and continued between cycles. After one to two cycles of treatment two patients demonstrated complete clinical and bacteriological cure, and there was marked clinical improvement in the rest.

Clinical experience with linezolid for the treatment of *Nocardia* infection. Moylett EH, Pacheco SE, Brown-Elliott BA, Perry TR, Buescher ES, Birmingham MC. Clin Infect Dis 2003; 36: 313–18.

Oral linezolid belongs to the new broad-spectrum oxazo-lidinones. This report describes its successful use in *Nocardia* infection. There was only a single case of cutaneous infection with *N. brasilienesis*. Linezolid produced clinical cure after only 2 months of treatment at a dose of 600 mg twice daily.

THIRD-LINE THERAPIES

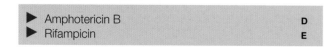

▶ Amphotericin B	**D**
▶ Rifampicin	**E**

Scedosporium infection in immunocompromised patients: successful use of liposomal amphotericin B and itraconazole. Barbaric D, Shaw PJ. Med Pediatr Oncol 2001; 37: 122–5.

A report of five cases of *Scedosporium* infection in immunosuppressed patients, three of whom died despite treatment with various combinations of amphotericin B and itraconazole. Two patients were successfully treated with liposomal amphotericin B and itraconazole.

Treatment of actinomycetoma with combination of rifampicin and co-trimoxazole. Joshi R. Ind J Dermatol Venereol Leprol 2008; 74: 166–8.

This case report from India describes the success of treatment with rifampin 600 mg daily in combination with high-dose trimethoprim/sulfamethoxazole [co-trimoxazole] 320/1600 mg twice daily. This was given to a patient with refractory infection of the foot. After 4 months of chemotherapy all the lesions had healed, and treatment was continued for a further 6 months. The patient remained disease free at follow-up 6 months later. The author recommends its use as it is an oral regimen and a relatively inexpensive treatment option.

Evidence Levels: **A** Double-blind study **B** Clinical trial ≥ 20 subjects **C** Clinical trial < 20 subjects **D** Series ≥ 5 subjects **E** Anecdotal case reports

Mycobacterial (atypical) skin infections

Vallari Majmudar, John Berth-Jones

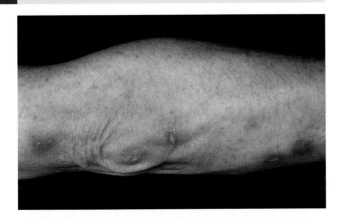

FISH TANK (SWIMMING POOL) GRANULOMA

Fish tank granuloma is an infection of the skin caused by *Mycobacterium marinum*. It is characterized by asymptomatic plaques and nodules, commonly on the upper extremities, which may spread in a sporotrichoid fashion. It occurs after minor trauma in people who come in contact with the organism. The most common sources of infection are tropical fish aquariums and swimming pools. The infection is commonly limited to the skin, but tenosynovitis, osteomyelitis, and arthritis have been reported with deeper infections. Rarely, disseminated infection may occur, especially in the immunocompromised. The average incubation period is 2–6 weeks.

MANAGEMENT STRATEGY

No controlled trials have been conducted, probably owing to the paucity of cases. Most cases seem to respond to the various *antimicrobial* regimens that are advocated as first-line therapies. The mean duration of treatment in various reports ranges between 6 weeks and 5 months. No statistical difference in efficacy between these treatments has been demonstrated. Lesions can often be effectively treated by *simple excision*, but occasionally this seems to result in a prolonged period of infection. *Heat treatment* of the infected area may have an adjunctive role according to some authors.

Although spontaneous resolution has been reported in up to 3 years, the aim of treatment is rapid recovery from infection and the prevention of progression to deeper structures.

The second-line treatments described below have been so designated as there is relatively little published information about them. The third-line treatments are probably best regarded as adjuncts to the others.

SPECIFIC INVESTIGATIONS

- ▶ Histology
- ▶ Culture
- ▶ Polymerase chain reaction (PCR) to detect mycobacterial DNA

Histology shows non-caseating granulomas, but a complete absence of epithelioid cells and multinucleate giant cells is not unusual in acute lesions. Ziehl–Nielsen staining is positive for acid-fast bacilli in 30% of biopsies. Culture of the biopsy specimen at 28–32°C yields pigmented colonies of *M. marinum*. In culture-negative cases PCR systems can provide rapid and sensitive detection of mycobacterial DNA in formalin-fixed, paraffin-embedded specimens. In vitro sensitivity studies have not been uniformly predictive of clinical response to the antibiotics. Although they do not have a routine role in directing initial treatment, they may be useful in resistant cases.

Polymerase chain reaction based detection of Mycobacterium tuberculosis in tissues showing granulomatous inflammation without demonstrable acid-fast bacilli. Pa-fan Hsiao, Chin-Yuan Tzen, Hsiu-Chin Chen, Hsin-Yi Su. Int J Dermatol 2003; 42: 281–6.

A total of 38 specimens were analysed with two different primers targeting the gene encoding for 16S ribosomal RNA and IS6110. Eighteen of these were diagnosed as *Mycobacterium tuberculosis* and four as atypical mycobacteria.

FIRST-LINE THERAPIES

▶ Minocycline 100–200 mg once daily for 6–12 weeks	D
▶ Doxycycline 100 mg twice daily for 3–4 months	D
▶ Clarithromycin 500 mg once or twice daily for 3–4 months	D
▶ Rifampin 600 mg and ethambutol 1.2 g daily for 3–6 months	D
▶ Co-trimoxazole 2–3 tablets twice daily for 6 weeks	D
▶ Clarithromycin 250 mg twice daily and ethambutol 800 mg once daily for 2–6 months	D

Sixty-three cases of Mycobacterium marinum infection. Clinical features, treatment and antibiotic susceptibility of causative isolates. Aubry A, Chosidow O, Caumes E, Robert J, Cambau E. Arch Intern Med 2002; 162: 1746–52.

One of the largest series in the literature. A national survey over 3 years identified 63 cases of *Mycobacterium marinum*. All patients were treated with antibiotics and 48% underwent surgery. Clarithromycin, doxycycline, and rifampicin were the most commonly prescribed antibiotics. Antibiotic monotherapy was given in 23 patients (14 had minocycline, five had doxycycline, four had clarithromycin). Of these, 20 had treatment success (16 had tetracyclines and four received clarithromycin) at an average of 3.5 months. Forty patients had drug combinations, commonly clarithromycin and rifampicin or tetracyclines, tetracyclines and rifampicin or ethambutol. Tetracyclines were prescribed more for skin infections but rifampicin for deeper infections. Clarithromycin was prescribed equally. The average duration of treatment for deeper structure infections was 7.5 months.

Atypical mycobacterial cutaneous infections in Hong Kong: 10 year retrospective study. Ho MH, Ho CK, Chong LY. Hong Kong Med J 2006; 12: 21–6.

Seventeen cases of *Mycobacterium marinum* were identified over a 10-year period. Thirteen responded to treatment with oral tetracycline alone (nine minocycline and four doxycycline). Two patients had antituberculous drugs initially but were subsequently switched to minocycline. One patient had a combination of isoniazid, rifampicin, ethambutol, and minocycline. The average duration of treatment was 20 weeks. The authors recommend minocycline 100 mg twice daily as the treatment of choice.

Treatment of *Mycobacterium marinum* cutaneous infections. Rallis E, Koumantaki-Mathioudaki E. Expert Opin Pharmacother 2007; 8: 2965–78.

Review article. The authors conclude that in limited superficial cutaneous infections, minocycline 100 mg twice daily, doxycycline 100 mg twice daily, clarithromycin 500 mg twice daily or co-trimoxazole 800 mg twice daily as monotherapy are effective treatment options. Ciprofloxacin 500 mg twice daily is an alternative. The literature search has found that these treatments have also been used in combination with other antibiotics, antituberculous drugs, surgery or hyperthermic treatment. In immunocompromised individuals or in cases of severe cutaneous infection a combination of rifampicin 600 mg/day and ethambutol 15–25 mg/kg/day is recommended. The average duration of treatment is 3 months and should be continued for 3–4 weeks after clinical resolution of lesions.

Mycobacterium marinum infection: A case report and review of the literature. Johnson R, Xia Y, Cho S, Burroughs R, Krivda S. Cutis 2007; 79: 33–6.

A case report of a 67-year-old man treated successfully with clarithromycin and ethambutol for 2 months. The authors conclude that determining antibiotic sensitivity is unhelpful because the organism behaves differently in vivo and in vitro. Surgical debridement is saved for refractory cases. Wearing of gloves and immediately cleansing of wounds may help prevent the disease.

Mycobacterium marinum with different responses to second-generation tetracyclines. Cummins D, Delacerda D, Tausk F. Int J Dermatol 2005; 44: 518–20.

A case report of a 23-year-old man who responded to minocycline 100 mg twice daily for 1 month but not to doxycycline 100 mg twice daily, despite being sensitive to both antibiotics. This case highlighted that in vivo and in vitro sensitivities may differ. Recent in vitro studies have shown promise with newer fluoroquinolones such as gatifloxacin, moxifloxacin, and sparfloxacin, and they remain potential future therapies.

SECOND-LINE THERAPIES

▶ Ciprofloxacin 500 mg with clarithromycin 250 mg twice daily for 4 months	E
▶ Rifabutin 600 mg with clarithromycin 500 mg twice daily and ciprofloxacin 500 mg twice daily	E

Antibiotic treatment of fish tank granuloma. Laing RB. J Hand Surg [Br] 1997; 22: 135–7.

A series of three cases is described. The author concluded that, in the light of the low toxicity profile, the combination of ciprofloxacin 500–1000 mg daily and clarithromycin 250–500 mg twice daily offers a useful alternative to existing treatments, particularly in patients who require protracted therapy. The duration of treatment varied from 8 to 12 weeks, depending on the clinical response. The authors suggest that rifabutin 600 mg may also prove valuable in cases that fail to respond to conventional antibiotic treatment.

THIRD-LINE THERAPIES

▶ Simple excision	E
▶ Curettage and electrodesiccation	E
▶ Incision and drainage	E
▶ Heat therapy by gloves, hot water or heated armlet	E
▶ Photodynamic therapy	E
▶ Cryotherapy	E

Treatment of *Mycobacterium marinum* cutaneous infections. Rallis E, Koumantaki-Mathioudaki E. Expert Opin Pharmacother 2007; 8: 2965–78.

Review article. Surgical treatment may not be necessary or may even be contraindicated in some patients, and should be reserved for cases with isolated superficial lesions that are non-responsive to systemic therapy. Cryotherapy, electrodessication, PDT and local hyperthermic therapy have also been reported with some success.

Efficacy of oral minocycline and hyperthermic treatment in a case of atypical mycobacterial skin infection by *Mycobacterium marinum*. Hisamichi K, Hiruma M, Yamazaki M, Matsushita A, Ogawa H. J Dermatol 2002; 29: 810–11.

Minocycline 200 mg daily and local hyperthermic treatment (a disposable chemical pocket warmer) was used every evening for 5–6 hours over 2.5 months. Although there have been four cases in Japan where patients have been treated with hyperthermic treatment alone, the authors advocate it to be used in conjunction with minocycline.

MYCOBACTERIUM ULCERANS

Mycobacterium ulcerans (Buruli ulcer) is the third most common mycobacterial infection after leprosy and tuberculosis in immunocompetent hosts. It occurs most commonly in wetlands of tropical and subtropical countries (Africa and Australia). Children under 15 years of age are most commonly affected. It is introduced into the skin by minor injury. After inoculation into the skin, *M. ulcerans* proliferates and produces a toxin, mycolactone, which enters the cells and causes necrosis of the dermis, panniculus, and deep fascia. Initially firm, painless nodules, papules, or plaques are seen. As the necrosis spreads, there is overlying ulceration over 1–2 months. The ulcers have a characteristic undermined edge and necrotic base. Although indolent in the majority, the ulcers can grow rapidly to more than 15 cm, with resultant extensive scarring and deformity. Up to 13% of patients may develop systemic involvement.

MANAGEMENT STRATEGY

BCG vaccination has a mild but significant protective effect. There are anecdotal reports of spontaneous resolution of cutaneous *M. ulcerans* infection, but recommended treatment is still primarily surgical. Newer reports suggest that there may be a role for adjunctive antimycobacterial agents with surgery.

SPECIFIC INVESTIGATIONS

▶ Histology
▶ Culture of tissue for mycobacteria
▶ Polymerase chain reaction (PCR)

Evidence Levels: **A** Double-blind study **B** Clinical trial ≥ 20 subjects **C** Clinical trial < 20 subjects **D** Series ≥ 5 subjects **E** Anecdotal case reports

Smears from the necrotic base of ulcers often reveal clumps of acid-fast bacilli on Ziehl–Nielsen staining. Appropriately selected biopsy specimens that include the necrotic base and the undermined edge of lesions with subcutaneous tissue are nearly always diagnostic. Histology reveals necrosis of the deep dermis and panniculitis. Inflammatory cells are few, presumably owing to the immunosuppressive activity of the toxin. With healing, there is a granulomatous response and the ulcerated area is eventually replaced by a depressed scar. *M. ulcerans* can be cultured from exudates or tissue fragments, but visible growth often requires 6–8 weeks' incubation at 33°C. Polymerase chain reaction methods may be used for quicker diagnosis.

THERAPY

▶ Oral rifampin daily at 10 mg/kg and streptomycin intramuscularly at 15 mg/kg daily for 4–12 weeks	C
▶ Wide surgical excision	C
▶ Wide surgical excision and adjunctive rifampin 10 mg/kg daily and ciprofloxacin (250–500 mg twice daily) for 3–6 months	C
▶ Local heat (40°C)	C
▶ Hyperbaric oxygenation	E

Efficacy of the combination rifampin-streptomycin in preventing growth of *Mycobacterium ulcerans* in early lesions of Buruli ulcer in humans. Etuaful S, Carbonnelle B, Grosset J, Lucas S, Horsfield C, Phillips R, et al. Antimicrob Agents Chemother 2005; 49: 3182–6.

A study of the efficacy of antibiotics in converting early lesions (nodules and plaques) from culture positive to culture negative. Lesions were excised after treatment with oral rifampin at 10 mg/kg of body weight and intramuscular streptomycin at 15 mg/kg of body weight daily for 0 (i.e., no antibiotics given), 2, 4, 8, or 12 weeks and examined by culture, PCR, and histopathology for *M. ulcerans*. Twenty-one lesions were included. Those excised without antibiotic treatment or after 2 weeks treatment were culture positive. All lesions treated for 4, 8, or 12 weeks were culture negative. No lesions became enlarged during antibiotic treatment, and most became smaller, with the greatest response of 52% reduction seen after 4 weeks.

Outcomes for *Mycobacterium ulcerans* infection with combined surgery and antibiotic therapy: findings from a south-eastern Australian case series. O'Brien DP, Hughes AJ, Cheng AC, Henry MJ, Callan P, McDonald A, et al. Med J Aust 2007; 186: 58–61.

Forty patients with *M. ulcerans* were identified in this study from Australia. The organism was confirmed by histology, culture, or PCR. There were 59 treatment episodes: 29 involved surgery alone, 26 surgery plus antibiotics, and four involved antibiotics alone. All four receiving only antibiotics failed to respond. From 55 episodes of surgery, the overall success rate was 76% (81% with antibiotics and 72% with surgery alone). Comparing surgery with antibiotics (rifampicin, clarithromycin, ciprofloxacin, ethambutol, amikacin, and azithromycin) and those treated with surgery alone, antibiotics were significantly associated with higher treatment success rates if the margins of excision were positive or the patient required major surgery (flaps and grafts). All eight patients treated with a combination of rifampicin (150–300 mg twice daily) and ciprofloxacin (250–500 mg twice daily) had successful outcomes. They were treated for 90 days, except for one with osteomyelitis who was treated successfully for 180 days. The authors suggest treatment with surgical excision and adjunctive antibiotic therapy, especially rifampicin and ciprofloxacin.

Successful treatment of *Mycobacterium ulcerans* osteomyelitis with minor surgical debridement and prolonged rifampicin and ciprofloxacin therapy: a case report. O'Brien DP, Athan E, Hughes A, Johnson PD. J Med Case Rep 2008; 2: 123.

An 87-year-old woman developed *M. ulcerans* ulcers on her lower legs and heels over a 9-month period. They were treated with surgical excision and adjunctive antibiotics (5 days of amikacin 900 mg daily, rifampicin 450 mg daily, ethambutol 800 mg daily, and clarithromycin 250 mg twice daily). Despite this, she developed four further lesions affecting both legs and the right buttock, with osteomyelitis affecting her first metatarsal. The ulcers were surgically excised with debridement of the area of osteomyelitis. Both clarithromycin and amikacin were discontinued because of side effects, but she continued on rifampicin 300 mg daily as monotherapy. She was subsequently commenced on ciprofloxacin 250 mg twice daily because of disease progression. After 6 months of combination therapy with rifampicin and ciprofloxacin there was no evidence of persistent disease. She remained disease free at 36 months follow-up. In healthy adults the authors recommend rifampicin at a dose of 10 mg/kg daily and ciprofloxacin 500–750 mg twice daily alongside surgical excision and debridement.

Mycobacterium ulcerans infection. van der Werf TS, van der Graaf WT, Tappero JW, Asiedu K. Lancet 1999; 354: 1013–18.

Excision of small and extensive pre-ulcerative lesions by either direct closure or skin grafting. In patients with extensive contractures caused by ulceration and fibrosis involving joints, physiotherapy and plastic surgery input may be required. The authors state that treatment with antimycobacterial agents has been disappointing. Despite *M. ulcerans* being sensitive to antimycobacterial agents (including aminoglycosides, ethambutol, rifampicin, and clarithromycin) in vitro, success in vivo has been poor. Studies have shown no significant effect with clofazimine, rifampicin, or co-trimoxazole. The authors suggest a need for well-designed clinical trials of antimicrobial agents for treatment of *M. ulcerans*.

Heat treatment of *Mycobacterium ulcerans* infections without surgical excision. Meyers WM, Shelly WM, Connor DH. Am J Trop Med Hyg 1974; 23: 924–9.

Eight patients from Zaire with *M. ulcerans* infection were treated by the local application of heat to maintain a temperature of approximately 40°C in the ulcerated area. All lesions healed without surgical intervention and without local recurrences during follow-up periods of up to 22 months. The authors postulated that the mechanism was primarily by direct inhibition of multiplication of *M. ulcerans*.

Treatment of *Mycobacterium ulcerans* infection by hyperbaric oxygenation. Krieg RE, Wolcott JH, Confer A. Aviat Space Environ Med 1975; 46: 1241–5.

A study on *M. ulcerans*-infected mice comparing hyperbaric oxygenation treatment with 40 controls (infected, not treated). Three groups were treated daily with 100% oxygen by three different protocols and the results compared weekly.

The hyperbaric oxygen therapy was more effective in the group treated with 2.5 atmospheres pressure for 1.25 hours twice a day. After 25 weeks two feet had been auto-amputated and there were only 12 deaths among the treated mice, compared to 18 feet amputated and 24 deaths in the control group. The authors concluded that hyperbaric oxygenation has a beneficial effect in mice and, if used in conjunction with other therapeutic procedures in humans, may be an effective therapeutic adjunct in treating *M. ulcerans* infections.

MYCOBACTERIUM KANSASII

This organism most commonly causes pulmonary disease; skin lesions are rare. The route of entry is usually through a minor injury. Most reported cases have occurred in immunocompromised subjects. The gross morphology of such lesions varies greatly and can be verrucous, nodular, pustular, ulcerated, or sporotrichoid. Cutaneous lesions may progress slowly or run an acute course.

MANAGEMENT STRATEGY

As cutaneous infection with *M. kansasii* is rare (occurring in 2.5–4.5% of *M. kansasii* infections), no firm treatment guidelines have been recommended. Although conventional combination chemotherapy with *antituberculous drugs* is effective, the choice of treatment should be determined by in vitro sensitivity.

SPECIFIC INVESTIGATIONS

> ▶ Histology
> ▶ Culture of tissue for mycobacteria

Lesions caused by *M. kansasii* may yield a variety of histopathologic features. They may be granulomatous in the chronic form, or show necrosis with an intense inflammatory infiltrate composed of polymorphonuclear cells in the more acute form. The organisms grow best on Lowenstein–Jensen culture medium at 37°C.

FIRST-LINE THERAPIES

> ▶ Combination of antituberculous drugs for
> 6–9 months **D**
> ▶ Antituberculous drugs with intramuscular
> kanamycin 500 mg three times a week for
> 3 months **E**
> ▶ Minocycline 100–200 mg daily for 16 weeks **E**
> ▶ Erythromycin 2 g daily for 6 months **E**

Mycobacterium kansasii infection with multiple cutaneous lesions. Hanke C, Temofeew R, Slama S. J Am Acad Dermatol 1987; 16: 1122–8.

A case report of a patient with *M. kansasii* diagnosed by histology and culture of the tissue is described. Following in vitro sensitivity testing she responded to combination therapy with rifampicin 300 mg twice daily and ethambutol 400 mg twice daily for 6 months. The literature is reviewed and the authors suggest long-term therapy with a combination of antimycobacterial drugs, including aminosalicylic acid, ethambutol,

isoniazid, rifampicin, streptomycin, and viomycin. One case responded completely to treatment with minocycline 50 mg four times daily for 6 weeks, followed by 100 mg daily for a further 10 weeks.

Cutaneous Mycobacteria kansasii infection presenting as cellulitis. Rosen T. Cutis 1983; 31: 87–9.

This report describes a renal transplant patient who developed a cellulitis-like lesion on the leg and periarticular soft tissue swelling due to *M. kansasii*. Rifampin 600 mg a day and isoniazid 300 mg a day were initiated. Owing to liver function abnormalities, isoniazid was substituted by ethambutol 400 mg twice a day. Kanamycin 500 mg IM three times a week was subsequently added. Three months of therapy with rifampin, ethambutol, and kanamycin resulted in clearing of skin and periarticular lesions.

Cutaneous Mycobacterium kansasii infection: case report and review. Breathnach A, Levell N, Munro C, Natarajan S, Pedler S. Clin Infect Dis 1995; 20: 812–17.

The authors review all 28 described cases of *Mycobacterium kansasii* in the literature. They conclude that monotherapy with erythromycin, minocycline, and doxycycline may be sufficient in immunocompetent patients, but immunodeficient patients may require triple therapy with antimycobacterials, and the dose of immunosuppressant should be reduced if possible.

Cutaneous Mycobacterium kansasii infection – treatment with erythromycin. Groves R, Newton J, Hay R. Clin Exp Dermatol 1991; 16: 300–2.

The authors describe a patient who was successfully treated with erythromycin 2 g daily for 6 months.

Cutaneous Mycobacterium kansasii infection associated with a papulonecrotic tuberculid reaction. Callahan EF, Licata AL, Madison JF. J Am Acad Dermatol 1997; 36: 497–8.

Treatment with isoniazid 300 mg/day, rifampin 600 mg/day, ethambutol 1200 mg daily for 9 months resulted in complete clearing of all cutaneous lesions.

MYCOBACTERIUM FORTUITUM COMPLEX (INJECTION ABSCESS)

Mycobacterium fortuitum, *Mycobacterium chelonae* and *Mycobacterium abscessus* are generally grouped together to form the *Mycobacterium fortuitum* complex. Cutaneous lesions due to *Mycobacterium fortuitum* complex usually occur after surgery, percutaneous catheter insertion, or accidental inoculation. Dark red nodules develop, with abscess formation and clear fluid drainage. Disseminated disease occurs most commonly in immunosuppressed hosts.

MANAGEMENT STRATEGY

Organisms of the *Mycobacterium fortuitum* complex should be individually identified and in vitro sensitivity tests performed prior to the initiation of chemotherapy. Susceptibility testing is recommended because of subspecies variability, and even variability within subgroups. *M. fortuitum* and *M. chelonae* are resistant to most antituberculous drugs except kanamycin and amikacin. *M. fortuitum* is more susceptible to amikacin, cefoxitin, ciprofloxacin, and imipenem; *M. abscessus* is usually sensitive to amikacin, cefoxitin, and clarithromycin; tobramycin and clarithromycin are more effective than amikacin in the treatment of *M. chelonae*. The wide variability in antibiotic sensitivity means that each case must be considered individually. For persistent non-healing cutaneous lesions, wide excisional surgery with delayed closure or skin grafting can be undertaken. The duration of therapy can vary from 6 weeks to 7 months and is dictated by clinical and microbiological response.

SPECIFIC INVESTIGATIONS

> ▶ Histology
> ▶ Culture of infected tissue
> ▶ Polymerase chain reaction (PCR) for species identification

Histology reveals polymorphonuclear microabscess and granuloma formation with foreign body-type giant cells. Acid-fast bacilli may be demonstrated in the microabscesses. Diagnosis is usually confirmed by culture. PCR systems can also be used for diagnosis and species identification in selected cases.

Atypical cutaneous mycobacteriosis diagnosed by polymerase chain reaction. Collina G, Morandi L, Lanzoni A, Reggiani M. Br J Dermatol 2002; 147: 781–4.

This paper reports two cases where *M. chelonae* and *M. fortuitum* were identified by polymerase chain reaction from tissue samples.

THERAPY

▶ Amikacin 300–400 mg IV twice daily plus doxycycline 100 mg three times daily	D
▶ Sulfamethoxazole 50 mg/kg/day for 3–6 months	D
▶ Clarithromycin 500 mg twice daily	D
▶ Surgical excision/debridement	D
▶ Minocycline 100–200 mg/day	E
▶ Levofloxacin 300 mg/daily	E
▶ Ciprofloxacin 750 mg twice daily	E
▶ Imipenem 500 mg to 1 g IV 6 hourly	E

Clinical usefulness of amikacin and doxycycline in the treatment of infection due to *M. fortuitum* and *M. chelonae*. Dalovisio JR, Pankey GA, Wallace RJ, Jones DB. Rev Infect Dis 1981; 3: 1068–74.

A series of 10 cases. The authors suggest that amikacin 300–400 mg twice daily and doxycycline 100 mg three times daily are the drugs of choice in this condition. Conventional antituberculous drugs have no place in the treatment of these infections. The authors further recommended that antimicrobial therapy should be prolonged (up to 7 months) and combined with surgical debridement.

The clinical presentation, diagnosis, and therapy of cutaneous and pulmonary infection due to the rapidly growing mycobacteria, *M. fortuitum* and *M. chelonae*. Wallace RJ. Clin Chest Med 1989; 10: 419–29.

Sulfonamide activity against *Mycobacterium fortuitum* and *Mycobacterium chelon*. Wallace RJ, Jones DB, Wiss K. Rev Infect Dis 1981; 3: 898–904.

Forty-eight clinical strains of *M. fortuitum* and 15 of *M. chelonae* were evaluated for susceptibility to sulfonamides, including trimethoprim-sulfamethoxazole (TMP-SMZ). Six patients with disease due to rapidly growing mycobacteria were treated with sulfonamides, and all showed a good response to therapy. Sulfonamides may be the treatment of choice for infections due to *Mycobacterium fortuitum*, and offer potential for the therapy of disease due to *Mycobacterium chelonae*.

Resistant cutaneous infection caused by *Mycobacterium chelonei*. Fenske NA, Millns JL. Arch Dermatol 1981; 117: 151–3.

A case report and review of the literature. The authors describe a case of *M. chelonae* which was resistant to most antituberculous drugs. Minocycline 100 mg twice a day resulted in healing of ulcerations in 8 weeks. Discontinuation of therapy 6 months later was followed by marked recrudescence, with ulceration in 1 week. Reinstitution of minocycline resulted in substantial remission but not eradication of the infection.

Development of resistance to clarithromycin after treatment of cutaneous *Mycobacterium chelonae* infection. Driscoll MS, Tyring SK. J Am Acad Dermatol 1997; 36: 495–6.

A case report and review of the literature. Initially the patient was prescribed minocycline 100 mg twice daily and advised to apply heat to the affected leg. There was no response and the treatment was changed to clarithromycin 500 mg twice daily. After 7 weeks the lesions had regressed and the treatment was discontinued. Two months later the nodules had recurred and erythromycin 400 mg three times daily was commenced. There was no response after 3 months. Subsequently, ciprofloxacin and azithromycin were tried without any response. The authors recommended that treatment should be combined with clarithromycin and a second agent chosen on the basis of antibiotic testing.

Clinical trial of clarithromycin for cutaneous (disseminated) infection due to *Mycobacterium chelonae*. Wallace RJ, Tanner D, Brennan PJ. Ann Intern Med 1993; 119: 482–6.

Fourteen patients (10 with disseminated disease) were treated with at least 3 months of therapy using clarithromycin 500 mg twice daily. All patients had an excellent response. The mean duration of therapy was 6.8 months (range 4.5–9 months).

Successful treatment of a widespread cutaneous *Mycobacterium fortuitum* infection with levofloxacin. Nakagawa K, Tsuruta D, Ishii M. Int J Dermatol 2006; 45: 1098–9.

A case report of an immunocompromised patient with *M. fortuitum* treated successfully with levofloxacin 300 mg daily.

Skin and soft tissue infections due to rapidly growing mycobacteria. Uslan D, Kowalski T, Wengenack N, Virk A, Wilson J. Arch Dermatol 2006; 142: 1287–92.

Sixty-three patients over 17 years with *M. fortuitum, chelonae* and *abscessus* were identified. The most frequently prescribed antimicrobial agents were macrolides, fluoroquinolones, aminoglycosides, cephalosporins, and tetracyclines. Most were given as combination therapy. Surgery was performed in nine patients. This should be reserved for isolated lesions.

Mycosis fungoides

Jeremy R Marsden, Sajjad F Rajpar

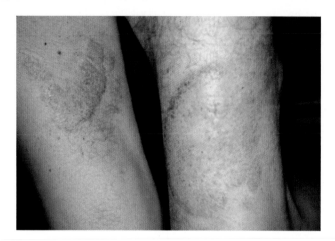

Cutaneous T-cell lymphomas (CTCL) are a rare group of disorders characterized by malignant clonal proliferation of T lymphocytes. Mycosis fungoides (MF) is the most common CTCL, accounting for 65% of cases, with an estimated annual incidence of 0.5 per 100 000 population. The prevalence of MF is much higher owing to its relatively good prognosis. MF usually presents in the sixth decade and is more common in males and individuals with black skin. Poikiloderma atrophicans vasculare and parapsoriasis en plaque are generally considered to be early MF, and so are grouped with this disorder for the purposes of management. Prognosis, mortality, and choice of treatment are related to disease stage, which can be classified as follows:

- Stage 1: Patches and plaques involving less (1A) or more (1B) than 10% of the skin
- Stage 2: As stage 1, with non-malignant lymphadenopathy (2A) or cutaneous tumors (2B)
- Stage 3: Erythroderma
- Stage 4: Malignant infiltration of lymph nodes (4A) or viscera (4B).

A revised staging system for MF, incorporating advances in molecular biology and diagnostic methodologies, has recently been proposed by the International Society for Cutaneous Lymphomas and the European Organisation of Research and Treatment of Cancer. This system may allow better stratification of patients for clinical trials, and the identification of additional prognostic variables in the future.

MANAGEMENT STRATEGY

Management starts with accurate diagnosis. Confirmation by skin biopsies is essential; frequently these need to be multiple to avoid sampling error, and may need to be repeated if equivocal in the face of continuing clinical suspicion. The key finding is epidermal invasion by abnormal lymphoid cells with a convoluted 'cerebriform' nucleus.

With the possible exception of very early disease, there is no evidence that MF is curable. Progression is often very slow or even absent; consequently, the aim of treatment is safe, effective control of symptoms. Patients with skin lymphoma should ideally be managed by a team including a dermatologist, a histopathologist familiar with skin lymphoma, and a radiation oncologist. This approach minimizes the risk of management error.

Studies claiming to cure patients with very early MF are flawed by having inadequate controls and diagnostic criteria that would not be considered adequate today. Although the possibility of cure in very early stage 1A MF cannot be excluded, this has not been proved. Nonetheless, it is reasonable to consider curative *local radiotherapy* for localized or limited disease, as this can be given with little morbidity.

The objectives of treatment are therefore to control symptoms, to slow progression, or both. Many patients will require treatment changes to induce or maintain a response, and many need treatment combinations. In stage 1 MF this can be achieved with *emollients*, but may require *potent topical corticosteroids* or *photochemotherapy (PUVA)*, with a good chance of complete response (complete response). As disease stage advances, so treatment becomes less likely to produce a complete response, but can still provide very effective control. Thus, in stage 2 MF many patients will respond to combinations of topical treatment as before with *PUVA*, or to *PUVA plus retinoids* or *PUVA plus interferon-α_{2a}*. Local radiotherapy is very effective at controlling persistent plaques or tumors, and *total skin electron beam (TSEB)* therapy is a good option when skin involvement is widespread and refractory to other approaches.

Topical chemotherapy (nitrogen mustard and BCNU) is used in the management of stage 1 and 2 MF in the USA, but not as widely in the UK. There are concerns about the safety of topical chemotherapy because of its long-term carcinogenicity in a disease that usually progresses slowly, as well as potential risks from environmental exposure to others. Whether or not these anxieties are justified, there are no published approved guidelines for the safe use of topical chemotherapy in MF, and until these are available its use in the UK is likely to remain limited.

The above treatments are of little value for stage 3 MF, which can present de novo or develop from progression of earlier stages. The principal symptom is severe and persistent itch, and this is remarkably unresponsive to treatment. The rash frequently improves with *low-dose methotrexate*, although response is often slow. The diagnosis of Sézary syndrome should be confirmed by demonstrating >5% Sézary cells per 100 circulating lymphocytes and a T-cell clone in blood in the presence of erythroderma. Sézary syndrome patients may be stage III–IVB. *Extracorporeal photopheresis (ECP)* has been used for over 20 years for Sézary syndrome; despite this, no randomized controlled trial has been performed, and reports of its efficacy are inconsistent with case series often including patients in whom a circulating clone has not been confirmed. Although some improvement often does occur, its effect on survival is unclear. Durable complete responses have been reported, however, and extracorporeal photopheresis clearly warrants further investigation.

Chemotherapy with *deoxycoformycin* is associated with significant improvement in over 50% of patients, though this rarely lasts for more than 12–18 months. Other high-dose single-agent regimens such as *fludarabine* are less effective. *Combination chemotherapy*, e.g., with CHOP, offers no therapeutic advantage and is associated with a very significant risk of neutropenic sepsis, and opportunistic infections such as *Pneumocystis* can occur even months after completion of treatment.

In stage 4 MF survival is limited; responses to combination chemotherapy are rarely complete, and as above are associated with significant risk, but may offer the best chance of improvement. Prompt relapse following treatment is common. The best

Evidence Levels: **A** Double-blind study **B** Clinical trial ≥ 20 subjects **C** Clinical trial < 20 subjects **D** Series ≥ 5 subjects **E** Anecdotal case reports

tried approach is *CHOP* at two-thirds of the normal dosage, and there are other lymphoma regimens that may offer a similar compromise between safety and efficacy. *Local radiotherapy* is useful for bulky nodal disease and symptomatic skin lesions. This group may be suitable for phase 1 trials of new chemotherapeutic agents, and for new approaches such as *allogeneic stem cell transplantation.* Effective palliation requires consideration of common symptoms such as nausea, constipation, pain, anorexia, and depression.

SPECIFIC INVESTIGATIONS

> ▶ Histology of skin and lymph nodes (if palpable) with immunophenotyping and T-cell receptor (TCR) gene analysis
> ▶ Hematology, differential white cell count and film (for Sézary cell count determination)
> ▶ T-cell receptor gene analysis on peripheral blood
> ▶ HTLV-1 serology

Revisions to the staging and classification of mycosis fungoides and Sézary syndrome: a proposal of the International Society for Cutaneous Lymphomas (ISCL) and the cutaneous lymphoma task force of the European Organization of Research and Treatment of Cancer (EORTC). Olsen E, Vonderheid E, Pimpinelli N, Willemze R, Kim Y, Knobler R, et al. Blood 2007; 110: 1713–22.

EORTC consensus recommendations for the treatment of mycosis fungoides/Sézary syndrome. Trautinger F, Knobler R, Willemze R, Peris K, Stadler R, Laroche L, et al. Eur J Cancer 2006; 42: 1014–30.

Guidelines for the management of primary cutaneous T-cell lymphomas. Whittaker SJ, Marsden JR, Spittle M, Russell Jones R. Br J Dermatol 2003; 149: 1095–107.

All patients should have skin biopsies with immunophenotyping and T-cell receptor (TCR) gene analysis using polymerase chain reaction on both the skin and peripheral blood: this is rarely abnormal in blood in stage 1A MF, but clonal T-cell expansion is found in 60% of cases of 1B disease and with increasing frequency as disease progresses. All patients should have a full blood count, differential, and film with Sézary cell count, together with CD4 and CD8 counts, indices of liver and renal function, and LDH. HTLV-1 is associated with CTCL-like skin lesions, and serology should be performed to exclude this as a cause. If lymph nodes are clinically abnormal they should be biopsied and examined for histology, immunophenotype, and TCR gene analysis, as the skin. Although evidence suggests that MF is a systemic disease even when skin involvement is limited, these staging investigations rarely detect further disease in clinical stage 1A MF, and infrequently in clinical stage 1B. Patients with clinical stage 2A disease and above require a CT scan of the thorax, abdomen, and pelvis. A bone marrow biopsy should be performed if blood involvement by Sézary cells is demonstrated, or if unexplained hematologic abnormalities exist. Tests should only be repeated on the basis of clinical evidence of progression, particularly as the radiation dose from a CT scan is significant.

FIRST-LINE THERAPIES

Stage 1 MF
▶ Emollients	E
▶ Topical corticosteroids	B

▶ PUVA or UVB	B
▶ Topical chemotherapy	B

Stage 2 MF

As above, plus:
▶ Local radiotherapy	B
▶ Interferon-α_{2a}	B

It is common to combine treatments; for instance, a patient receiving PUVA for stage 1B MF may respond well but develop a tumor on the non-exposed scalp requiring local radiotherapy. However, care should be used with drug combinations for which there are few or no published safety data.

Clinical stage 1A (limited patch and plaque) mycosis fungoides. A long term outcome analysis. Kim YH, Jensen RA, Watanabe GL. Arch Dermatol 1996; 132: 1309–13.

In a study of 122 patients with stage 1A MF and mean follow-up of 9.8 years, only 11 progressed and three died from their disease; 73 received topical mechlorethamine with 68% complete response, and 34 TSEB with 97% complete response. Despite these differences in treatment outcome, survival was similar in the two groups. Actuarial survival was no different from that of a matched normal population.

A randomized trial comparing combination electron-beam radiation and chemotherapy with topical therapy in the initial treatment of mycosis fungoides. Kaye FJ, Bunn PA, Steinberg SM, Stocker JL, Ihde DC, Fischmann AB, et al. N Engl J Med 1989; 321: 1784–90.

It is clear from this randomized trial of 103 patients that early aggressive treatment with TSEB and combination chemotherapy produces greater response rates than conservative treatment but, crucially, this does not translate into longer disease-free or overall survival.

Topical steroids for mycosis fungoides – experience in 79 patients. Zackheim HS, Kashani-Sabet M, Smita A. Arch Dermatol 1998; 134: 949–54.

In this prospective uncontrolled study, 63% of 51 stage 1A patients and 25% of 28 stage 1B patients achieved a complete response. A partial response (PR) occurred in 31% of stage 1A and 57% of stage 2A patients. Post-treatment biopsies in seven of 39 patients with a clinical complete response appeared to confirm pathological complete response. Median follow-up was 9 months, and during this period nearly half of the stage 1A complete responders progressed. Comparison with data for topical mechlorethamine suggests a lower rate of complete response with corticosteroids. There were no major adverse effects.

There is no evidence that topical corticosteroids cure MF. Consequently, there are no data showing that complete response is a necessary or even desirable endpoint; if the control of itch is the main treatment objective, then whether or not appearance improves may be of only secondary relevance. Further, many of the complete responses were transient. However, treatment is safe, and experience suggests that topical steroids offer a good compromise between efficacy and safety for the treatment of patches and plaques. A trial comparing corticosteroids with emollient placebo would be helpful.

PUVA treatment of erythrodermic and plaque type mycosis fungoides; a ten year follow up study. Abel EA, Sendagorta E, Hoppe RT, Hu CH. Arch Dermatol 1987; 123: 897–901.

The results following PUVA are presented for 29 patients, 19 of whom were pretreated with topical chemotherapy or TSEB. Fifteen were stage 1 or 2A, 10 were stage 3, and 4 were stage 4A. Seventeen patients, including seven with erythroderma, cleared in about 5 months, but the stage 3 patients tolerated only small doses of UVA. Most had relapsed by 22 months despite maintenance treatment, but the majority cleared again with PUVA. Two patients developed disseminated herpes simplex.

Ultraviolet-B phototherapy for early stage cutaneous T-cell lymphoma. Ramsay DL, Lish KM, Yalowitz CB, Soter NA. Arch Dermatol 1992; 128: 931–3.

This retrospective uncontrolled study involved 26 patients with stage 1A MF and eight with stage 1B MF. UVB treatment was given three times weekly, starting at 50–60% MED. Twenty-five patients achieved remission at a median of 5 months (range 1–33); 18 had maintenance treatment with median remission duration of 22 months. Five patients relapsed, two while on treatment. UVB was well tolerated. Patients with infiltrated plaques did not respond.

Both PUVA and UVB are effective in MF, though trials comparing the two have not taken place. There is more experience with PUVA, which is consequently the most commonly administered phototherapy for MF. UVB is usually used for patch or thin plaque stage disease. Most patients with stage 1 MF treated with PUVA will clear; it is less effective in thick plaques and ineffective for tumors, but can rather surprisingly work well in stage 3 MF. In general, the earlier the stage, the longer the remission. As maintenance treatment has not been shown to prolong remission and may increase the risk of actinic cancers, phototherapy often does not need to be continued for more than 12–16 weeks. Treatment can be repeated and still be effective, but as with many of the treatments used for MF it is unknown whether this prolongs survival.

Topical mechlorethamine therapy for early stage mycosis fungoides. Ramsay DL, Halperin PS, Zeleniuch-Jacquotte A. J Am Acad Dermatol 1988; 19: 684–91.

In a prospective study, 67 of 117 patients achieved complete response using topical mechlorethamine daily until remission, then with a reducing frequency for a further 2 years. Patients with patches cleared in a median 6.5 months, those with plaques in 41 months, and of those with tumors only four of 10 cleared in a median of 39 months. Of patients with patches, 44% relapsed in a median of 66 months; 61% with plaques relapsed in 44 months, and 100% of those with tumors within 8 months.

Long-term efficacy, curative potential, and carcinogenicity of topical mechlorethamine chemotherapy in cutaneous T cell lymphoma. Vonderheid EC, Tan ET, Kantor AF, Shrager L, Micaily B, Van-Scott EJ. J Am Acad Dermatol 1989; 20: 416–28.

This retrospective review of 331 patients identified 25 complete responses lasting more than 8 years in 116 patients with stage 1A/B MF. Of 37 patients with stage 3 MF, 22 also had a complete response. However, there is uncertainty of pathological diagnosis in some patients who had a durable complete response. Complete responses lasting more than 8 years were also described in nine patients with stage 2/3, where we know cure is very unlikely. There were significant increases in the risk of squamous cell carcinoma (SCC), basal cell carcinoma (BCC), Hodgkin's disease, and colon cancer, and maintenance treatment was continued for at least 3 years.

Topical mechlormethamine (nitrogen mustard), 10 mg in 60 mL water, or as ointment, is effective in stage 1 and 2 MF. As with phototherapy, earlier-stage disease responds more quickly and for longer. Topical carmustine (BCNU) is also effective, causes less contact allergic dermatitis, and appears to work more quickly; each treatment is limited to 3–4 weeks because of the risk of myelosuppression, which may be cumulative. Claims that topical chemotherapy can cure MF are unconfirmed, and maintenance treatment is best avoided because of the potential for secondary malignancies.

Interferon alfa 2a in the treatment of cutaneous T cell lymphoma. Olsen EA, Rosen ST, Vollmer RT, Variakojis D, Roenigk HH Jr, Diab N, et al. J Am Acad Dermatol 1989; 20: 395–407.

Twenty-two patients with all stages of CTCL were treated with either 3 MU or 36 MU interferon-α_{2a} daily for 10 weeks, then maintenance for 9.5 months. Three of eight responded to the lower dose, and 11 of 14 to the higher dose, but 86% of this group needed dose reductions. Remissions lasted 4–27.5 months. In the lower dose group, dose escalation increased responses. Mean time to complete response was 5.4 months.

Phase II trial of intermittent high-dose recombinant interferon alfa-2a in mycosis fungoides and the Sézary syndrome. Kohn EC, Steis RG, Sausville EA, Veach SR, Stocker JL, Phelps R, et al. J Clin Oncol 1990; 8: 155–60.

Twenty-four patients with advanced, pretreated MF were given very high-dose pulsed interferon – 10 MU/m^2 then 50 MU/m^2 for days 2–5 of cycle 1, then doubling the dose every 3-week cycle. Seven patients had a response but only one was complete. Dose increments did not increase responses.

Interferon alpha-2a in cutaneous T cell lymphoma. Vegna ML, Papa G, Defazio D, Pisani F, Coppola G, De Pita O, et al. Eur J Haematol 1990; 45: 32–5.

In 23 patients with CTCL, lower doses of interferon-α_{2a} produced at least 80% response rates in stage 1–2 MF, but only 57% in stage 4A.

There are no adequately powered randomized controlled trials of interferon in the treatment of MF. However, a large number of open studies have demonstrated the drug to be clearly effective, often as much as chemotherapy. Patients with stage 1 or 2 disease respond best, and many require only 3 MU of interferon-α_{2a} three times weekly; there is little evidence that larger doses are more effective, and they are more toxic. Treatment needs to be continued for a minimum of 6 months to establish a response, and thereafter for 12–18 months or longer to maintain it. Flu-like symptoms and leukopenia are common adverse effects. The former often improve in the first few weeks of treatment; the latter normally recovers promptly on drug withdrawal. Interferon can usually be reintroduced at a lower dose with careful monitoring. Liver function also needs to be checked during treatment.

Interferon alfa-2a combined with phototherapy in the treatment of cutaneous T-cell lymphoma. Kuzel TM, Gilyon K, Springer E, Variakojis D, Kaul K, Bunn PA Jr, et al. J Natl Cancer Inst 1990; 82: 203–7.

Fifteen patients with CTCL, nine with stage 1 and four with stage 2, were treated with relatively high doses of interferon-α_{2a} 6–30 MU and PUVA, each three times weekly. There were 12 complete and two partial responses, with a median duration of nearly 2 years.

Photochemotherapy alone or combined with interferon alpha-2a in the treatment of cutaneous T cell lymphoma.

Roenigk HH Jr, Kuzel TM, Skoutelis AP, Springer E, Yu G, Caro W, et al. J Invest Dermatol 1990; 95: 198s–205s.

Eighty-two patients with MF or parapsoriasis were treated with PUVA; 51 cleared, and 31 of these relapsed during follow-up. In addition, 15 patients with more advanced disease were also treated with 6–30 MU interferon-α_{2a} and 12 cleared. Median duration of response was 23 months.

These and other uncontrolled studies show that interferon plus PUVA is effective. However, it is unclear whether this combination is superior to PUVA alone, and a randomized trial is needed.

Stage 3 MF

▶ Interferon-α_{2a} **B**
▶ Low-dose methotrexate   **B**
▶ Extracorporeal photopheresis (ECP)   **B**
▶ PUVA   **C**

Low dose methotrexate to treat erythrodermic cutaneous T cell lymphoma: Results in twenty-nine patients. Zackheim HS, Kashani-Sabet M, Hwang ST. J Am Acad Dermatol 1996; 34: 626–31.

In this retrospective study 29 patients with erythrodermic CTCL were treated with methotrexate 5–12.5 mg weekly for 2–129 months; 70% had at least 10% Sézary cells, but in only two of 11 patients was bone marrow histology abnormal; 41% of patients achieved a complete response and 17% a partial response. The median duration of response was 31 months. Response was unrelated to Sézary cell count or the presence of lymphadenopathy. Toxicity was moderate, including lung fibrosis in two patients and myelosuppression in three. Median survival was 8.4 years.

These are interesting data, but the definition of erythrodermic CTCL lacks precision in the study. For instance, only 13 had skin biopsies diagnostic of CTCL; the rest were suggestive or consistent with the diagnosis. None had a T-cell clone identified, and only two of 11 had bone marrow involvement. Median survival was surprisingly long. Nonetheless, this does seem to be a potentially useful treatment and should be investigated further.

Extracorporeal photopheresis in Sézary syndrome: no significant effect in the survival of 44 patients with a peripheral blood T-cell clone. Fraser-Andrews E, Seed P, Whittaker S, Russell-Jones R. Arch Dermatol 1998; 34: 1001–5.

A retrospective analysis of outcome in 44 patients with Sézary syndrome defined by erythroderma, >10% Sézary cells, a T-cell clone, and skin histology showing CTCL. Twenty-nine patients had ECP, and their survival was no different from that of 15 patients who did not receive ECP.

UK consensus statement on the use of extracorporeal photophoresis for the treatment of cutaneous T-cell lymphoma and chronic graft versus host disease. Scarisbrick J, Taylor P, Holtick U, Makar Y, Douglas K, Berlin G, et al. Br J Dermatol 2008; 158: 659–78.

An extensive review of the literature comprising 30 small uncontrolled studies of the use of ECP in MF. Response rates ranging from 43% to 100% are reported, with a mean composite rate of 63%. This paper also provides advice on patient selection, treatment and monitoring schedules, and assessment criteria.

ECP is safe and well tolerated, and should be considered for patients with stage III or IVA MF with evidence of blood involvement, either by the presence of a T-cell clone by TCR gene rearrangement analysis,

a circulating Sézary cell count of more than 10% of total lymphocyte count, or peripheral CD4:CD8 of >10. Treatment is delivered every 2–4 weeks, with responses typically seen at 3–6 months. Median time to relapse is 18 months; whether ECP prolongs survival is uncertain. Bexarotene or interferon-α_{2a} has been combined with ECP in cases where response is poor.

Stage 4 MF

As for stages 2 and 3, plus:
▶ Combination chemotherapy   **B**
▶ Radiotherapy to lymph nodes   **E**

Systemic therapy of cutaneous T-cell lymphomas. Bunn PA, Hoffman SJ, Norris D, Golitz LE, Aeling JL. Ann Intern Med 1994; 121: 592–602.

Data exist for a large number of cytotoxic agents in MF; responses are obtained in about 65%, and are complete in 30%. No single drug stands out as preferable; methotrexate is well studied and seems effective even in low dose without folinic acid rescue. Alternatives include purine analogs, vincristine, etoposide, bleomycin, and cisplatin. Response rates are higher (80%, 40% complete response) with combination chemotherapy, but it is unlikely that this translates into a greater clinical benefit. CHOP is widely used, but is frequently associated with neutropenic sepsis; this is a particular risk in patients with ulcerated tumors, and in erythrodermic MF when normal T-cell numbers may be profoundly reduced. To minimize this risk the dose should be reduced by one-third, and suitable prophylaxis provided against opportunistic infection.

MF is often chemoresponsive, especially in patients who are not heavily pretreated – the problem is maintaining the response, which is frequently short-lived.

SECOND-LINE THERAPIES

Stage 1 MF

▶ Retinoids plus PUVA   **B**
▶ Interferon-α_{2a} **B**
▶ Total skin electron beam radiotherapy (TSEB)   **B**
▶ Oral bexarotene   **B**

Retinoids plus PUVA (RePUVA) and PUVA in mycosis fungoides, plaque stage. Thomsen K, Hammar H, Molin L, Volden G. Acta Dermatol Venereol 1989; 69: 536–8.

This small study shows that the response rate is not increased by combining PUVA with etretinate, probably because response rates to PUVA alone are so high. The total PUVA dose was reduced.

Retinoids – isotretinoin is the most studied – are effective in MF, but are often not well tolerated and seem most useful when combined with other treatments such as PUVA, so that the cumulative dose can be reduced. They may also have a place in helping to maintain remission, though any direct cancer-protective effect in MF is unproven.

Electron beam treatment for cutaneous T-cell lymphoma. Jones GW, Hoppe RT, Glatstein E. Hematol Oncol Clin North Am 1995; 9: 1057–76.

This systematic review involving nearly 1000 patients shows that complete responses of 96% can be achieved in stage 1–2A

MF, 36% in stage 2B, and 60% in stage 3. Interestingly, up to 50% with stage 1A MF have still not relapsed up to 20 years following TSEB.

TSEB is an effective treatment for refractory cutaneous disease, with better responses in early stages. A restriction to one lifetime course is no longer necessary, as patients may tolerate two or three courses. The data on 'cure' following TSEB have the same limitations as those following topical chemotherapy, and require a higher level of proof.

Phase 2 and 3 clinical trial of oral bexarotene (Targretin capsules) for the treatment of refractory or persistent early-stage cutaneous T-cell lymphoma. Duvic M, Martin AG, Kim Y, Olsen E, Wood GS, Crowley CA, et al. Arch Dermatol 2001; 137: 581–93.

This study investigated 58 patients with stage 1A/2A CTCL which had proved resistant to PUVA, UVB, total skin electron beam irradiation, or topical chemotherapy. Oral bexarotene at a dose of 300 mg/m^2 produced 50% or greater improvement in 54% of patients. Both response rates and side effects were dose related.

An EORTC phase III trial comparing PUVA vs PUVA plus bexarotene in stage 1B-2A MF is currently under way.

Stage 2 MF	
As for stage 1, plus:	
▶ Low-dose methotrexate	B
▶ Oral bexarotene	B
Stage 3 MF	
As for stage 2, plus:	
▶ Total skin electron beam radiotherapy (TSEB)	B
▶ Chlorambucil plus prednisolone	E
▶ Radiotherapy to lymph nodes	E
▶ Oral bexarotene	B

Experience with total skin electron beam therapy in combination with extracorporeal photopheresis in the management of patients with erythrodermic (T4) mycosis fungoides. Wilson LD, Jones GW, Kim D, Rosenthal D, Christensen IR, Edelson RL, et al. J Am Acad Dermatol 2000; 43: 54–60.

A retrospective, non-randomized series of 44 patients with erythrodermic MF treated with TSEB alone (n=23) or in combination with ECP (n=21). Following TSEB a complete response was seen in 32 of the 44; 2-year overall survival was 63% in 17 patients, and 88% for 15 patients also receiving ECP.

From these data TSEB does seem to be effective in stage 3 MF, although others disagree. This series includes patients from 1974 who do not meet current diagnostic criteria; whether ECP adds benefit is unclear, as the study was not randomized.

Bexarotene is effective and safe for treatment of refractory advanced-stage cutaneous T-cell lymphoma: multinational phase II-III trial results. Bexarotene Worldwide Study Group. J Clin Oncol 2001; 19: 2456–71.

This trial included 94 patients with stage 1B–4B CTCL. There was a 45–55% overall response rate, with a mean response duration of 9.8 months.

In the UK bexarotene is licenced for advanced-stage CTCL that is refractory to at least one systemic treatment. Bexarotene is a novel retinoid that interacts specifically with the RXR receptor and promotes apoptosis of malignant T cells. Median time to response is 16 weeks and median time to relapse is 43 weeks. The response is dose related, and a daily dose of 300 mg/m^2 optimizes the risk–benefit ratio. Side effects

include hypertriglyceridemia (75%) and central hypothyroidism (20%). Both are easily managed with statins, fibrates (excluding gemfibrozil, which can raise bexarotene levels, resulting in even higher triglycerides) and thyroxine. Side effects are reversible on ceasing therapy.

Efficacy for all stages of CTCL, including refractory disease and Sézary syndrome, has been demonstrated. The favorable side-effect profile and the ease of oral administration facilitate outpatient use. Bexarotene is thus gaining an increasingly important role in CTCL management, although its relatively high cost (approximately £1700 per month) may present a barrier to use for some.

Management of cutaneous lymphoma. Russell-Jones R, Spittle MF. Baillière's Clin Haematol 1996; 9: 756–7.

There are few published data to support the use of chlorambucil and prednisolone in CTCL, but experience clearly indicates their value in other low-grade non-Hodgkin's lymphomas. Treatment is cyclical to minimize the risk of myelosuppression.

Stage 4 MF	
▶ Purine analogs	B
▶ Oral bexarotene	B
▶ Denileukin diftitox (DAB-IL2)	B

Experimental therapies in the treatment of cutaneous T cell lymphoma. Foss FM, Kuzel TM. Hematol Oncol Clin North Am 1995; 9: 1127–37.

Deoxycoformycin, fludarabine, and 2-chlorodeoxyadenosine are all effective in CTCL, and were used in the hope that T cell-specific cytotoxicity would improve the therapeutic index; however, toxicity is significant and responses often short-lived. There is, however, quite good evidence to support the use of deoxycoformycin in stage 3 MF.

Pivotal phase III trial of two dose levels of denileukin diftitox for the treatment of cutaneous T-cell lymphoma. Olsen E, Duvic M, Frankel A, Kim Y, Martin A, Vonderheid E, et al. J Clin Oncol 2001; 19: 376–88.

This new biologic targets diphtheria toxin to the IL-2 receptor. This phase III study involved 71 patients with stage 1B–4A CTCL that was CD25 positive. There was a 10% complete response and 20% partial response. The median duration of response was 6.9 months.

DAB-IL2 is licenced in the USA for CTCL. Acute side effects are common and include vascular leak, flu-like syndrome, and acute hypersensitivity. Efficacy has been shown for multiply relapsed and refractory advanced-stage MF, for which DAB-IL2 may have a role. Some early evidence is available to suggest that co-treatment with bexarotene may upregulate IL2 expression and so provide a synergistic effect with DAB-IL2.

THIRD-LINE THERAPIES

Stage 1A-2A MF	
▶ Topical bexarotene gel	B
Stage 2B and stage 3 MF	
▶ Single-agent chemotherapy	B
▶ Reduced-dose combination chemotherapy	B
Stage 4 MF	
▶ Reduced-dose combination chemotherapy	B
▶ Bone marrow transplantation	D

472

Phase 1 and 2 trial of bexarotene gel for skin-directed treatment of patients with cutaneous T-cell lymphoma. Breneman D, Duvic M, Kuzel T, Yocum R, Truglia J, Stevens VJ. Arch Dermatol 2002; 138: 325–32.

Sixty-seven patients with stage IA–IIA CTCL used this topical retinoid in incremental doses. There was a 21% complete response and 42% partial response. The median time to relapse was 23 months.

Topical 1% bexarotene gel has been approved by the FDA for refractory or persistent stage 1A–2A MF. The product is not licenced in Europe. Treatment is initially applied on alternate days, increasing gradually to a maximum of four times daily. Local irritation can occur, particularly with increased frequency of application.

Haematopoietic stem cell transplantation for patients with pirmary cutaneous T-cell lymphoma. Duarte R, Schmitz N, Servitje O, Sureda A. Bone Marrow Transplant 2008; 41: 597–604.

Autologous bone marrow transplantation produces a complete response in the majority of treated patients, though relapse with in a matter of months is common. On the other hand, allogeneic stem cell transplant is associated with a graft-versus-lymphoma effect, which seems to improve time to relapse; almost two-thirds of treated patients reported in the literature have reached a median survival of 3 years. Optimal conditioning regimens and timing of transplant remain unknown, though this approach does seem deserving of further investigation.

Mycosis fungoides and Sézary syndrome. Hwang S, Janik J, Jeffe E, et al. Lancet 2008; 371: 945–57.

Increasing knowledge of the molecular biology of MF has led to novel and more targeted therapeutic approaches. This includes monoclonal antibodies, such as zanolimumab (anti-CD4), which has shown efficacy in both early- and late-stage MF, and alemtuzumab (anti-CD52), as well as vaccines and histone deacetylase inhibitors.

Myiasis

Claudia I Vidal, Robert G Phelps

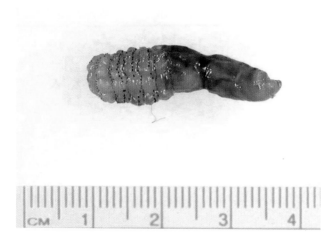

Myiasis is the infestation of human and animal tissue by the larval or pupal stages of two-winged true flies (*Diptera*), also known as maggots. Myiasis is widespread in the tropics and subtropics of Africa and the Americas, but much less prevalent in most other areas of the world. The infestation can involve numerous species, and clinical presentations include nodules, ulcers, creeping eruption, and contamination of a wound (wound myiasis). The goal of therapy is complete removal of larvae and the prevention of future infestation.

MANAGEMENT STRATEGY

At the beginning of the 20th century myiasis was a major public health and economic problem, often affecting livestock. Simple improvements in hygiene and wound care have largely eliminated this. Nevertheless, reports of human infection continue today, including nosocomial outbreaks. The mechanism of transmission of fly larvae to human hosts differs among the many species of flies; however, cutaneous invasion occurs in all species as a result of the larvae burrowing into the skin. Ultimately, the management goal is to prevent exposure to larvae.

As many cases of myiasis are acquired during travel to endemic areas, travelers should be made aware of the risk, especially in Central and South America and parts of Africa. Individuals traveling to rural areas should be covered at all times with *long-sleeved garments and hats*. At night, *sleeping under a mosquito net* is appropriate, and *insect repellents* may also be useful, as the mechanical vectors for certain larvae are blood-sucking arthropods such as mosquitoes. Certain flies deposit their eggs on fabric such as clothing. Thus, *clothing should be dried and then hot-ironed* to kill any eggs. Other flies deposit their eggs in soil, where larvae hatch and may penetrate the skin of barefooted persons. *Appropriate footwear* should be worn at all times.

To prevent wound myiasis, *simple antisepsis* is usually adequate. Wounds should be adequately cleaned and irrigated at appropriate intervals and have proper dressings. Patients with any type of wound should never sleep outside, and in an indoor or hospital environment windows should remain closed.

Once infestation has occurred, therapy consists of *removal of all larvae* with minimal trauma to the organisms. Occlusion deprives the larva of oxygen and induces it to move in search of air, allowing it to be removed manually. Alternatively, infiltration of the area with lidocaine and *surgical removal* usually suffice when few organisms are present. Care must be taken to extract the larvae whole, otherwise a considerable foreign body reaction may ensue. If there is secondary pyogenic infection, this should be treated with appropriate antibiotics.

SPECIFIC INVESTIGATIONS

▶ Detailed travel history	E
▶ Morphologic identification of the parasite	E

Scanning electron microscopy studies of sensilla and other structures of adult *Dermatobia hominis* (L. Jr., 1781) (Diptera: Cuterebridae). De Fernandes FF, Chiarini-Garcia H, Linardi PM. J Med Entomol 2004; 41: 552–60.

Molecular identification of two species of myiasis-causing Cuterebra by multiplex PCR and RFLP. Noel S, Tessier N, Angers B, Wood DM, Lapointe FJ. Med Vet Entomol 2004; 18: 161–6

The fly larvae should be extracted whole and specific identification attempted. Each larva, however, may molt and have several instars, each with a slightly different morphology. This can complicate identification. The adult fly should be identified as well, if possible. It is advisable to consult an entomologist in more difficult cases. Scanning electron microscopy and molecular studies by multiplex polymerase chain reaction (PCR) may be helpful in identifying some species.

Case report: myiasis – the botfly boil. Pallai L, Hodge J, Fishman SJ, Millikan LE, Phelps RG. Am J Med Sci 1992; 303: 245–8.

Most of the reported cases of myiasis in the continental US have been of the *Dermatobia hominis* type. Endemic foci include Belize, Costa Rica, and Brazil.

FIRST-LINE THERAPIES

Surgical therapy	
▶ Local anesthesia with or without surgical incision	E
▶ Squeezing the skin surrounding the furuncle with fingers or wooden spatulas	E
Non-surgical therapy	
▶ Vaseline therapy	E
▶ Bacon therapy	E
▶ Pork fat therapy	E
▶ Hair gel	E
▶ Occlusion with *chimo* (paste-like form of smokeless tobacco)	E
▶ Small wad of cotton soaked in the sap of the *Thevetia ahouai* (Apocynaceae) tree	E

Surgical therapy

Cutaneous myiasis. Krajewski A, Allen B, Hoss D, Patel C, Chandawarkar RY. J Plast Reconstruct Aesthet Surg 2009; (in press).

Evidence Levels: **A** Double-blind study **B** Clinical trial ≥ 20 subjects **C** Clinical trial < 20 subjects **D** Series ≥ 5 subjects **E** Anecdotal case reports

The favored treatment modality is direct and complete surgical extraction of larvae from the lesion because of the risks of secondary infection associated with retained larvae.

Myiasis in a pregnant woman and an effective, sterile method of surgical extraction. Richards KA, Brieva J. Dermatol Surg 2000; 20: 955–7.

The authors describe a method of larva removal in furuncles that consists of three parts: (1) anesthetizing the larva by injection of 1% lidocaine hydrochloride around the pore to prevent it from anchoring its spines; (2) covering the pore with sterile polymyxin B; and (3) placement of a cruciform incision next to the pore to extract the undamaged larva.

Myiasis. Millikan LE. Clin Dermatol 1999; 17: 191–5.

The author describes the preferred approach: surgically excise the organism with lidocaine anesthesia and close the wound primarily. This gives the optimal cosmetic result.

The larva of D. hominis *is anchored in subcutaneous tissue, making manual removal difficult. In a surgical approach, care should be taken to avoid lacerating the larvae because retained larval parts may precipitate a foreign body reaction.*

Cutaneous myiasis – a review and report of three cases due to *Dermatobia hominis.* Lane RP, Lowell CR, Griffiths WA, Sonnex TS. Clin Exp Dermatol 1987; 12: 40–5.

Probing the pore to determine its angle can help the surgeon anticipate the location of the larva and guide the proper placement of the cruciate incision.

A cruciate incision directly over the pore can lead to damage to the larva and incomplete removal.

Removal of *Dermatobia hominis* **larvae.** Nunzi E, Rongioletti F, Rebora A. Arch Dermatol 1986; 122: 140.

Infiltration with up to 2 mL of lidocaine hydrochloride underneath the furuncular nodule can cause sufficient pressure to push the larva out of the skin, possibly avoiding surgical incision.

Botfly stories. Johnstone B. Available at: http://www.vexman.com/stories.htm.

Digital manipulation to remove the larvae can be quite dramatic, with sudden expulsion of the larva from the skin to a distance of up to 5 or 6 feet. This method is successful only with a living larva; *if the larva dies in the tissue, it cannot be squeezed out.*

Non-surgical therapy

Cutaneous myiasis. McGraw TA, Turiansky GW. J Am Acad Dermatol 2008; 58: 907–26; quiz 927–9.

Alternatives to bacon therapy. Biggar RJ. JAMA 1994; 271: 901–2.

The authors use Vaseline over the wound to smother the larvae, which then emerge spontaneously.

Traditional methods encourage the larva to exit on its own, taking advantage of its need for oxygen, by using various occlusive dressings to suffocate it.

Bacon therapy and furuncular myiasis. Brewer TF, Wilson ME, Gonzalez E, Flesenstein D. JAMA 1993; 270: 2087–8.

Multiple strips of raw bacon were placed over the nodule with the fat occluding the central punctum. Within 3 minutes the larvae migrated sufficiently into the bacon fat to be grasped with toothed tweezers and gently removed. This treatment is both inexpensive and atraumatic. The covering should not be restrictive (e.g., nail polish) because this may asphyxiate the larvae without causing them to migrate out of the skin.

Dermal myiasis: the porcine lipid cure. Sauder DN, Hall RP, Wurster CF. Arch Dermatol 1981; 117: 681–2.

Pork fat was placed on the lesions and then covered with an occlusive tape. The emerging larvae were teased out with forceps.

SECOND-LINE THERAPIES

▶ Systemic ivermectin	E
▶ Topical ivermectin	E
▶ Chloroform/ether	E
▶ Ethanol spray	E
▶ Oil of betel leaf	E
▶ Mineral turpentine	E

Use of ivermectin in the treatment of orbital myiasis caused by *Cochliomyia hominivorax.* De Tarso P, Pierre-Filho P, Minguuini N, Pierre LM, Pierre AM. Scand J Infect Dis 2004; 36: 503–5.

Ivermectin is a broad-spectrum antiparasitic agent that stimulates and increases the receptor affinity of γ-aminobutyric acid (GABA). A single dose of ivermectin (200 µg/kg) was used for infestation with *Hypoderma lineatum*, and led to spontaneous migration of the maggots. A case of orbital myiasis caused by *C. hominivorax* was successfully treated similarly with oral ivermectin.

Larvicidal effects of mineral turpentine, low aromatic white spirits, aqueous extracts of *Cassia alata*, **and aqueous extracts, ethanolic extracts and essential oil of betel leaf (***Piper betle***) on** *Chrysomya megacephala.* Kumarasinghe SP, Karunaweera ND, Ihalamulla RL, Arambewela LS. Int J Dermatol 2002; 41: 877–80.

Myiasis: successful treatment with topical ivermectin. Victoria J, Trujillo R, Barreto M. Int J Dermatol 1999; 38: 142–4.

Four patients presented with traumatic myiasis caused by *C. hominivorax*, each infested with 50–100 larvae. A single topical treatment with 1% ivermectin in a propylene glycol solution was directly applied to the affected area. The topical solution was left for 2 hours, followed by gentle washing with normal saline or sterile water. Within 1 hour almost all the larvae stopped moving, and within 24 hours all had died.

Flies and myiasis. Elgart ML. Dermatol Clin 1990; 8: 237–44.

The application of chloroform, chloroform in light vegetable oil, or ether, with removal of the larvae under local anesthesia, is advocated for wound myiasis.

Myxoid cyst

David de Berker

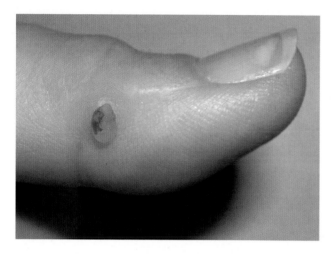

Myxoid cysts are also known as digital mucus cysts or pseudo-cysts and represent a ganglion of the distal interphalangeal joint. They arise in different forms in soft tissues, typically above or distal to the distal interphalangeal joint. The most common presentation is as a translucent nodule on the dorsum of the digit.

MANAGEMENT STRATEGY

Myxoid cysts contain gelatinous material that has escaped from the distal interphalangeal joint. Treatment can involve removal of the material combined with measures to prevent further escape from the joint. *Simple drainage* through an incision can achieve the first, but normally there is recurrence, with further synovial fluid in the myxoid cyst within a few weeks. Measures to prevent the further accumulation of fluid are directed at reducing joint pathology or blocking the pathway of escape of fluid. The first category includes the use of *injected triamcinolone*, which might reduce synovial inflammation and the pressure of fluid within the joint, and *surgery* for osteophytes. Osteophytes appear to weaken the joint capsule and possibly contribute to joint pathology and synovial fluid production. Their removal is associated with resolution of the myxoid cyst.

Blockage of the path of fluid escape is achieved by a range of traumatic and scarring procedures. The challenge is to produce an effective scar over the joint without excess morbidity or a long-term nail dystrophy.

A practical compromise of morbidity, complexity of treatment, and efficacy is to employ *cryosurgery* in the first instance. This is best used with a distal block using plain lidocaine or bupivacaine. The cyst is then incised and drained. Two 20-s freezes with liquid nitrogen are given, with a complete thaw in between. Over the next 2 weeks the wound is dressed. This results in success in about 50% of cases involving fingers. Those that fail can be re-treated in the same way or proceed to surgery. Morbidity is least when there is *precise surgery* to the path of fluid escape. This can be identified by methylene blue injection into the joint and then raising a flap in a distal to proximal path, containing the cyst in the roof of the flap.

The pathway is dyed and can be tied with absorbable ligature. The flap is sutured back in place and success is reported as 94% in the fingers. In some instances patient preference or medical considerations may mean that surgery is the first-line therapy.

SPECIFIC INVESTIGATIONS

> ▶ Transillumination
> ▶ Pricking and expression of gelatinous material (see photograph)
> ▶ MRI

Transillumination is a useful clinical aid. Where there is diagnostic doubt, simple incision can be helpful to demonstrate gelatinous material. Alternatively, high-resolution ultrasound or MRI can be employed. The first can only help define whether the structure is cystic or not. The latter provides better anatomical definition, and in over 80% of cases allows location of the pedicle communicating between the cyst and joint. Plain X-ray may reveal osteophytes of osteoarthritis, but this will not usually alter treatment.

MR imaging of digital mucoid cysts. Drapé JL, Idy Peretti I, Goettmann S. Radiology 1996; 200: 531–6.

FIRST-LINE THERAPIES

> ▶ Cryosurgery   **B**
> ▶ Repeated puncture   **D**
> ▶ Laser therapy   **C**
> ▶ Sclerosant   **C**

Myxoid cysts of the finger: treatment by liquid nitrogen spray cryosurgery. Dawber RPR, Sonnex T, Leonard J, Ralphs I. Clin Exp Dermatol 1983; 8: 153–7.

Fourteen patients were treated with two 30-s freezes and no evacuation of the cyst. Follow-up was between 14 and 40 months, with an 86% cure rate. One patient had a significant nail dystrophy as a long-term complication.

Removal of the overlying cyst or evacuation of the contents might reduce the dose of cryosurgery needed.

Specific indications for cryosurgery of the nail unit. Kuflik EG. J Dermatol Surg Oncol 1992; 18: 702–6.

Forty-nine patients were treated with a range of single cryosurgical doses, from 20 to 30 s using open spray and 30 to 40 s using the cryoprobe. This was combined with curettage in 23 and simple de-roofing in the remainder. There was resolution in 63% over the follow-up period of 1–60 months.

A simple technique for managing digital mucous cysts. Epstein E. Arch Dermatol 1979; 115: 1315–16.

Repeated puncture of myxoid cysts in 40 patients led to resolution in 72% after two to five treatments, but no follow-up period is given.

Treatment of digital myxoid cysts with carbon dioxide laser vaporization. Huerter CJ, Wheeland RG, Bailin PL, Ratz JL. J Dermatol Surg Oncol 1987; 13: 723–7.

Carbon dioxide laser cured 10 patients with follow-up of 35 months.

Evidence Levels: **A** Double-blind study   **B** Clinical trial ≥ 20 subjects   **C** Clinical trial < 20 subjects   **D** Series ≥ 5 subjects   **E** Anecdotal case reports

Treatment of mucoid cysts of fingers and toes by injection of sclerosant. Audebert C. Dermatol Clin 1989; 7: 179–81.

The sclerosant sodium tetradecyl sulphate (3%) was injected into the myxoid cyst in 15 patients. 'A few drops' were used at each injection. Four needed a second injection and one a third. The result was resolution in all cases, although the period of follow-up was not reported.

There is a chance of producing painful necrosis of the nail fold, but this is seldom extensive. The theoretical complication of sclerosant entering the joint does not appear to occur.

SECOND-LINE THERAPIES

▶ Surgery   **B**

Marginal osteophyte excision in treatment of mucous cysts. Eaton RG, Dobranski AI, Littler JW. J Bone Joint Surg 1973; 55A: 570–4.

Forty-four patients with surgery entailing tracing of the communication between cyst and joint, excision of the cyst, and in some instances surgery to the osteophytes, provided success in 43 of 44 patients, with follow-up of between 6 months and 10 years.

There is a theoretical possibility of operating on the osteophytes alone, leaving the cyst in place and allowing it to involute once the precipitating pathology has been removed.

Etiology and treatment of the so called mucous cyst of the finger. Kleinert HE, Kutz JE, Fishman JH, McCraw LH. J Bone Joint Surg 1972; 54: 1455–8.

Similar surgery, but with less emphasis on osteophyte debridement, resulted in success for all of 36 patients followed for between 12 and 18 months postoperatively.

Surgical treatment of myxoid cysts guided by methylene blue joint injection. de Berker D, Lawrence C. Br J Dermatol 1998; 139: 72.

Tracing the communication between joint and cyst with methylene blue and then ligating it with absorbable sutures resulted in cure in 29 of 31 patients followed for 8–15 months. In this procedure excision of the lesion was not required.

Ganglion of the distal interphalangeal joint (myxoid cyst): therapy by identification and repair of the leak of joint fluid. de Berker D, Lawrence C. Arch Dermatol 2001; 137: 607–10.

A study of 54 patients used methylene blue dye injected into the distal interphalangeal joint to identify the communication between the joint and the cyst. A skin flap was designed around the cyst. The communication was sutured and the flap replaced with no tissue excision. In 89% of patients the communication was identified. At 8 months, 48 patients remained cured with no visible scarring. Myxoid cysts of the toes had a higher relapse rate than those of the fingers.

THIRD-LINE THERAPIES

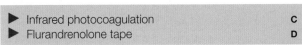
▶ Infrared photocoagulation   **C**
▶ Flurandrenolone tape   **D**

The most likely course of action after failure of surgery is either to repeat the surgery or to modify the surgical approach to include osteophyte surgery if these were not treated in the first instance. If a CO_2 laser is available this might also be chosen, given the good results reported in the small published series. Alternatively, sclerosant could be used, although again, multiple treatments could be anticipated.

Myxoid cysts treated by infra-red photocoagulation. Kemmett D, Colver GB. Clin Exp Dermatol 1994; 19: 118–20.

Infrared photocoagulation employs broad-spectrum radiation from a specialized source, delivering a metered destructive dose. In a series of 14 patients, 12 had resolution after one treatment and re-treatment cured a further one patient. There was some notching of the nail fold in three.

Treatment of myxoid cyst with flurandrenolone tape. Ronchese F. R I Med J 1970; 57: 154–5.

After the failure of electrodesiccation, five patients were treated with corticosteroid tape for 2–3 months and success was reported in all during a follow-up of 2–3 years.

Necrobiosis lipoidica

Abdul Hafejee, Ian Coulson

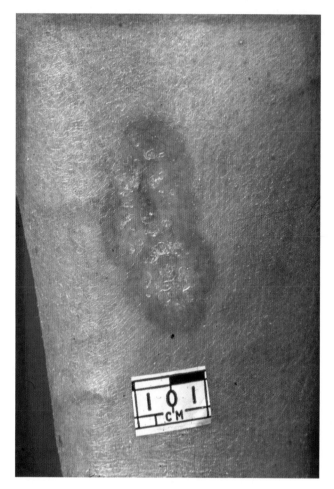

Necrobiosis lipoidica (NL) is a complication seen in 1 in 300 diabetics but may be unassociated with glucose intolerance. Both granulomatous and angiopathic mechanisms have been proposed in its etiology. NL initially appears as an atrophic plaque found over pretibial sites. Ulceration may occur after trauma, with ensuing pain. NL may rarely be complicated by squamous cell carcinoma.

MANAGEMENT STRATEGY

Smoking cessation and *avoiding trauma to the affected shins* are key factors to avoid transformation from an unsightly plaque into a painful, recalcitrant ulcer. The progression of new lesions may be halted by intralesional or occluded *potent topical corticosteroids* applied to the margins of the lesions. Once atrophy has developed there is little that will reverse this, although *topical retinoids* may be tried. Telangiectasia is often marked and has been treated with *pulsed dye laser*. Extensive lesions may justify trials of *nicotinamide* or *prednisolone*. *Antiplatelet therapy* in the form of *aspirin, dipyridamole, or ticlopidine* has its enthusiasts, though responses are inconclusive. Topical *psoralen and UVA (PUVA)* has received recent interest and may arrest progression and improve the appearance. A *variety of systemic anti-inflammatory and immu-*

nosuppressive agents have received recent attention, including *mycophenolate mofetil, fumaric acid esters, ciclosporin, antimalarials, thalidomide,* and *pentoxiphylline. Infliximab and etanercept* have also been proposed.

The chronically ulcerated lesion is a challenge; *antibiotics* deal with secondary infection, appropriate dressings may be required, and growth factors such as *becaplermin* and *granulocyte–macrophage colony-stimulating factor (GM-CSF)* may accelerate healing. As diabetics may have coexisting large vessel atherosclerosis that may contribute to ulceration, non-invasive arterial studies or angiography need to be considered if clinically indicated. Venous hypertension may also contribute to the localization and ulceration of necrobiosis. Excision and grafting may transform the patient's quality of life and improve cosmesis.

Work with the diabetologist to *optimize diabetic control.*

SPECIFIC INVESTIGATIONS

> ▶ Two-hour postprandial glucose
> ▶ Skin biopsy
> ▶ Consider angiography or venous circulation studies
> ▶ Consider a biopsy to exclude sarcoidosis, which may mimic necrobiosis lipoidica (NL), or if clinical features suggest, the rare development of squamous cell carcinoma

Squamous cell carcinoma arising in an area of long-standing necrobiosis lipoidica. Lim C, Tschuchnigg M, Lim J. J Cutan Pathol 2006; 33: 581–3.

Case report of squamous cell carcinoma arising de novo in an area of NL.

Carcinoma cuniculatum arising in necrobiosis lipoidica. Porneuf M, Monpoint S, Barnéon G, Alirezai M, Guillot B, Guilhou JJ. Ann Dermatol Venereol 1991; 118: 461–4.

Although rare, squamous cell carcinomas may complicate any condition in which papillary dermal scarring is appreciable.

Unilateral necrobiosis lipoidica of the ischemic limb – a case report. Naschitz JE, Fields M, Isseroff H, Wolffson V, Yeshurun D. Angiology 2003; 54: 239–42.

A possible ischemic pathogenesis of NL emerges from a case of unilateral large vessel arteriosclerotic ischemia with ipsilateral NL.

The author has experience of a severely ulcerated area of NL that only started to heal after the disobliteration of severe femoropopliteal atheroma.

FIRST-LINE THERAPIES

> ▶ Stop smoking and optimize diabetic control   **C**
> ▶ Intralesional or topical corticosteroids under occlusion   **D**

Necrobiosis lipoidica diabeticorum: association with background retinopathy, smoking, and proteinuria. A case controlled study. Kelly WF, Nicholas J, Adams J, Mahmood R. Diabet Med 1993; 10: 725–8.

Stop smoking and control diabetes mellitus with vigilance. Fifteen diabetics with NL were each matched with five control subjects with diabetes mellitus. Background retinopathy, proteinuria, and smoking were all more common with NL. No differences were noted between those with NL and controls in the prevalence of vascular disease and neuropathy. Glycosylated hemoglobin concentrations were higher in patients with NL.

Granuloma annulare and necrobiosis lipoidica treated by jet injector. Sparrow G, Abell E. Br J Dermatol 1975; 93: 85–9.

Three of five cases of NL underwent complete resolution and one had partial improvement with 5 mL triamcinolone injection to the edges of lesions. No serious complications of this type of treatment were observed.

Treatment of psoriasis and other dermatoses with a single application of a corticosteroid left under a hydrocolloid occlusive dressing for a week. Juhlin L. Acta Dermatol Venereol 1989; 69: 355–7.

A 0.1% betamethasone alcoholic lotion under a hydrocolloid dressing was an effective, well-tolerated treatment, and three applications only were required.

SECOND-LINE THERAPIES

▶ Systemic corticosteroids	D
▶ Aspirin and dipyridamole	C
▶ Ticlopidine	D
▶ Nicotinamide	D
▶ Clofazimine	D
▶ Topical PUVA	D
▶ Topical tacrolimus	E

Necrobiosis lipoidica: treatment with systemic corticosteroids. Petzelbauer P, Wolff K, Tappeiner G. Br J Dermatol 1992; 126: 542–5.

Oral methylprednisolone was given to six patients with non-ulcerating NL for 5 weeks; in all there was cessation of disease activity during the 7-month follow-up period. Initial dosage was 1 mg/kg daily for 1 week, then 40 mg daily for 4 weeks, followed by tapering and termination in 2 weeks. All, including the diabetics, tolerated the treatment well. There was no improvement in atrophy. Benefit was maintained at the end of the 7-month follow-up period.

Careful monitoring of blood glucose is mandatory in all diabetic patients with NL treated with systemic corticosteroids.

Ulcerating necrobiosis lipoidica effectively treated with pentoxifylline. Noz KC, Korstanje MJ, Vermeer BJ. Clin Exp Dermatol 1993; 18: 78–9.

Ulcerated NL healed completely within 8 weeks of administration of 400 mg pentoxifylline twice daily.

Healing of necrobiotic ulcers with antiplatelet therapy. Correlation with plasma thromboxane levels. Heng MC, Song MK, Heng MK. Int J Dermatol 1989; 28: 195–7.

NL in diabetics has been considered to be a cutaneous manifestation of diabetic microangiopathy. Seven diabetic patients with necrobiotic ulcers of recent onset that healed after administration of 80 mg/day of acetylsalicylic acid and 75 mg three times daily of dipyridamole had elevated thromboxane levels. Healing was associated with

depression of the elevated thromboxane levels in all seven patients.

Treatment of necrobiosis lipoidica with low-dose acetylsalicylic acid. A randomized double-blind trial. Beck HI, Bjerring P, Rasmussen I, Zachariae H, Stenbjerg S. Acta Dermatol Venereol 1985; 65: 230–4.

No response was seen with the use of 40 mg acetylsalicylic acid daily for 24 weeks, despite documented platelet aggregation inhibition.

A randomized double blind comparison of an aspirin dipyridamole combination versus a placebo in the treatment of necrobiosis lipoidica. Statham B, Finlay AY, Marks R. Acta Dermatol Venereol 1981; 61: 270–1.

Fourteen patients with a clinical and histologic diagnosis of NL were treated in a double-blind control study with either an aspirin–dipyridamole combination or a matching placebo for an 8-week period. None of the patients in the aspirin–dipyridamole group showed a significant improvement.

Necrobiosis lipoidica treated with ticlopidine. Rhodes EL. Acta Dermatol Venereol 1986; 66: 458.

When 33 patients were given an unstated dose of this antiplatelet agent, NL cleared in nine and improved in 17. The author warns that cases of agranulocytosis have been reported with ticlopidine.

High dose nicotinamide in the treatment of necrobiosis lipoidica. Handfield-Jones S, Jones S, Peachey R. Br J Dermatol 1988; 118: 693–6.

An open study of high-dose nicotinamide in the treatment of 15 patients with NL. Of 13 patients who remained on treatment for more than 1 month, eight improved. A reduction in pain, soreness, and erythema, and the healing of ulcers if present, was noted. There were no significant side effects, particularly with respect to diabetic control. Lesions tended to relapse if treatment was stopped.

Clofazimine – therapeutic alternative in necrobiosis lipoidica and granuloma annulare. Mensing H. Int J Dermatol 1989; 28: 195–7.

Ten patients with NL were treated with clofazimine 200 mg orally daily. Six of 10 patients responded; three of the responders achieved complete remission of the dermatosis. All the patients treated had reddening of the skin, but this was reversible after the end of therapy, as were the other side effects (i.e., diarrhea and dryness of the skin).

Topical PUVA treatment for necrobiosis lipoidica. McKenna DB, Cooper EJ, Tidman MJ. Br J Dermatol 2000; 143: 71.

Four of eight patients with NL responded favorably to topical PUVA using a 0.15% methoxsalen emulsion, with weekly treatments, starting with 0.5 J/cm^2 with 20% incremental increases until erythema developed at the edge of the lesions. The mean number of treatments administered was 39.

Successful treatment of chronic ulcerated necrobiosis lipoidica with 0.1% topical tacrolimus ointment. Clayton T, Harrison P. Br J Dermatol 2005; 152: 581–2.

A case report of ulcerated NL that healed successfully with 0.1% tacrolimus ointment applied twice daily for 1 month.

THIRD-LINE THERAPIES

▶ Topical retinoids	E
▶ Ciclosporin	E
▶ Heparin	E
▶ Chloroquine	E
▶ Mycophenolate mofetil	E
▶ Infliximab	E
▶ Etanercept	E
▶ Fumaric acid esters	D
▶ Promogran for ulceration	E
▶ GM-CSF for ulceration	D
▶ Becaplermin for ulceration	E
▶ Pentoxifylline	E
▶ Photodynamic therapy	E
▶ Pulsed dye laser for telangiectasia	E
▶ Surgery for ulceration	E
▶ Thalidomide	E

Necrobiosis lipoidica treated with topical tretinoin. Heymann WR. Cutis 1996; 58: 53–4.

A case is presented in which atrophy was diminished by the application of topical tretinoin.

Persistent ulcerated necrobiosis lipoidica responding to treatment with cyclosporin. Darvay A, Acland KM, Russell-Jones R. Br J Dermatol 1999; 141: 725–7.

In two patients with severe ulcerated NL the ulceration healed completely after 4 months of ciclosporin therapy, and both patients have remained free of ulceration since. Effective doses were between 3 and 5 mg/kg daily. Three other reports of the effective use of ciclosporin therapy in ulcerated NL now exist.

Minidose heparin therapy for vasculitis of atrophie blanche. Jetton RL, Lazarus GS. J Am Acad Dermatol 1983; 8: 23–6.

The authors speculate that subcutaneous heparin 5000 IU twice daily may help NL because it helped the vasculitis associated with atrophie blanche. A subsequent letter informs that perilesional low-dose heparin has been successfully used in NL by Russian dermatologists.

Necrobiosis lipoidica diabeticorum treated with chloroquine. Nguyen K, Washenik K, Shupack J. J Am Acad Dermatol 2002; 46: S34–6.

A single report of the first case of successful treatment of NL with oral chloroquine.

Successful treatment of ulcerated necrobiosis lipoidica with mycophenolate mofetil. Reinhard G, Lohmann F, Uerlich M, Bauer R, Bieber T. Acta Dermatol Venereol 2000; 80: 312–13.

A 61-year-old woman with NL for over 30 years was started on mycophenolate mofetil 0.5 g twice daily and the lesions regressed within 4 weeks. The dose was reduced to 0.5 g over the next 4 months and then stopped. Within 14 days of stopping mycophenolate mofetil the ulceration recurred.

Infliximab: a promising new treatment option for ulcerated necrobiosis lipoidica. Kolde G, Muche JM, Schulze P, Fischer P, Lichey J. Dermatology 2003; 206: 180–1.

A 33-year-old man with insulin-dependent diabetes mellitus and ulcerated NL was treated with infliximab monotherapy 5 mg/kg infusions each month. By the second infusion the ulceration had healed, but subsequent infusions were

stopped because of the development of miliary tuberculosis. The NL did not recur on stopping infliximab.

Treatment of necrobiosis lipoidica with the tumor necrosis factor antagonist etanercept. Zeichner J, Stern D, Lebwohl M. J Am Acad Dermatol 2006; 54: S120–1.

A 35-year-old woman who received 25 mg subcutaneous intralesional etanercept once weekly cleared after 8 months of treatment.

Clearance of necrobiosis lipoidica with fumaric acid esters. Gambichler T, Kreuter A, Freitag M, Pawlak FM, Brockmeyer NH, Altmeyer P. Dermatology 2003; 207: 422–4.

A 50-year-old woman with a 15-year history of recalcitrant NL was treated with Fumaderm Initial (30 mg dimethylfumarate), starting at one tablet daily increased at weekly intervals up to three tablets daily. After the third week, Fumaderm (120 mg dimethylfumarate) was started at one tablet daily and increased to a maximum dose of two tablets daily. After 6 months of treatment the NL had resolved apart from skin atrophy. Remission was maintained over a 6-month follow-up period.

Fumaric acid esters in necrobiosis lipoidica: results of a prospective noncontrolled study. Kreuter A, Knierim C, Stücker M, Pawlak F, Rotterdam S, Altmeyer P, et al. Br J Dermatol 2005; 153: 802–7.

Eighteen patients with NL were given the standard Fumaderm regimen as used in psoriasis for at least 6 months. Three discontinued therapy, but the rest gained significant clinical, ultrasonographic, and histological improvement.

The management of hard-to-heal necrobiosis with Promogran. Omugha N, Jones AM. Br J Nurs 2003; 15: S14–20.

A single case study with non-healing ulcerated NL of 3 years' duration. Treatment with a new protease-modulating matrix (freeze-dried matrix composed of collagen and oxidized regenerated cellulose) resulted in complete healing of the ulcer after 8 weeks, where other dressing regimens had failed to effect healing over a period of 2.5 years.

Healing of chronic leg ulcers in diabetic necrobiosis lipoidica with local granulocyte–macrophage colony-stimulating factor treatment. Remes K, Ronnemaa T. J Diabetes Complications 1999; 13: 115–18.

Topical recombinant human GM-CSF healed two patients with ulcerated NL within 10 weeks. A reduction in the size of the ulcers was already evident after the first topical applications. The ulcers have remained healed for more than 3 years.

Becaplermin and necrobiosis lipoidicum diabeticorum: results of a case control pilot study. Stephens E, Robinson JA, Gottlieb PA. J Diabetes Complications 2001; 15: 55–6.

Five patients with type 1 diabetes mellitus and NL were treated with topical becaplermin gel (recombinant platelet-derived growth factor). The index patient had ulcerated NL, and this healed. Three of the five patients with non-ulcerated NL reported a subjective improvement in sensation and lightening of color of the lesions. However, serial photographs and measurements over the 5-month treatment period showed no significant change in the size of the treated areas.

480

Necrobiosis lipoidica diabeticorum: response to pentoxiphylline. Brasaria S, Braga-Brasaria M. J Endocrinol Invest 2003; 26: 1037–40.

A case report of a 20-year-old diabetic with ulcerating NL almost completely healing after 6 months of pentoxyphylline 400 mg three times daily.

Successful treatment of necrobiosis lipoidica diabeticorum with photodynamic therapy. Heidenheim M, Jemec G. Arch Dermatol 2006; 142: 1548–50.

A case report of a 60-year-old woman who received six treatments with methylaminolevulinate photodynamic therapy, spaced at 1-week intervals. Both clinical and histological clearance was reported.

Necrobiosis lipoidica diabeticorum treated with the pulsed dye laser. Moreno-Arias GA, Camps-Fresneda A. J Cosmet Laser Ther 2001; 3: 143–6.

A single report of the successful eradication of unsightly telangiectasia, a prominent feature of mature NL.

The surgical treatment of necrobiosis lipoidica diabeticorum. Dubin BJ, Kaplan EN. Plast Reconstruct Surg 1977; 60: 421–8.

Seven cases treated by excision of the lesions down to the deep fascia, ligation of the associated perforating blood vessels, and the use of split-skin grafts to cover the defects. There were no recurrences.

Thalidomide for the treatment of refractory necrobiosis lipoidica. Kukreja T, Peterson J. Arch Dermatol 2006; 142: 20–2.

A 51-year-old woman was treated successfully with a dose of thalidomide 150 mg daily, tapering to 50 mg twice weekly. A response was seen after 4 months and maintained after 2 years.

Necrolytic migratory erythema

Clara-Dina Cokonis, Sarah Asch, Analisa Vincent Halpern

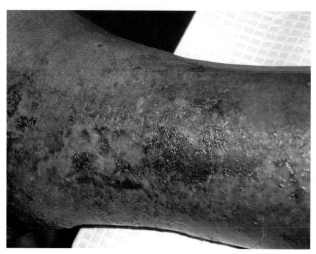

Courtesy of Dr Anna Krishtul

Necrolytic migratory erythema (NME) is classically considered a paraneoplastic cutaneous reaction pattern associated with a pancreatic islet-cell neoplasm, diabetes mellitus, weight loss, venous thromboembolism, normocytic anemia, and hyperglucagonemia as part of the glucagonoma syndrome. NME consists of an irregular annular eruption, generally in the intertriginous and acral areas, with an erythematous psoriasiform crusted edge. Lesions tend to migrate over time; bullae and hyperpigmentation may be noted. It is often mistaken for intertrigo, psoriasis, or seborrhoeic dermatitis. Parakeratosis and upper-level keratinocyte vacuolization are characteristic on histopathologic examination of early lesions. In the absence of glucagonoma, NME has also been reported with glucagon infusion-dependent states as well as hepatic disease, gluten-sensitive enteropathy, pancreatic insufficiency, and other malabsorption or malnutritional states. Excessive stimulation of basal metabolic pathways in the glucagonoma syndrome leads to a hypermetabolic state in which the patient becomes nutritionally deficient. It is thought that zinc, amino acid, and essential fatty acid deficiencies contribute to the cutaneous disease. Necrolytic acral erythema (NAE), associated with hepatitis C, is thought by some to be an acral variant of NME and may be part of the spectrum of NME.

MANAGEMENT STRATEGY

Treatment of the underlying disease is the preferred therapy for NME. In the setting of glucagonoma, *surgical excision* of the tumor is the treatment of choice, although curative resection is possible in only a minority due to frequent metastasis. Chemotherapy, primarily with *dacarbazine* and *streptozocin*, is a frequent, albeit only moderately successful, adjunctive therapy. *Octreotide and lantreotide*, long-acting somatostatin analogs, alone or in combination with *interferon-α*, are useful in the treatment of metastases or inoperable tumors, and

have shown some success in clearing NME regardless of tumor response. Some patients with NME secondary to glucagonoma have had improvement of skin lesions after intravenous infusions of *amino acids* and *fatty acids*.

The occurrence of NME in the absence of glucagonoma should make one suspect the possibility of nutritional deficiencies encountered in hepatic disease, celiac disease, Crohn's disease, enteropathies, and chronic pancreatitis. If found, any deficiency in *amino acids, essential fatty acids,* or *zinc* should be corrected.

SPECIFIC INVESTIGATIONS

▶ Serum glucagon and chromagranin A
▶ Serum zinc, amino acids (tryptophan), total protein, albumin, essential fatty acid, riboflavin, niacin, pyridoxine (vitamin B_6), cyanocobalamin (vitamin B_{12}), biotin, folic acid, panthothenic acid, methylmalonic acid, and propionic acid levels
▶ Hemoglobin/hematocrit
▶ Serum fasting glucose
▶ Serum liver function tests and hepatitis B and C profile
▶ Abdominal CT scan, endoscopic ultrasound, celiac angiography, and somatostatin receptor scintigraphy
▶ Multiple endocrine neoplasia type 1 (MEN 1) gene
▶ Skin biopsy (H&E)

Endocrine tumours of the pancreas. Oberg K, Eriksson B. Best Pract Res Clin Gastroenterol 2005; 19: 753–81.

An updated review including discussion of biochemical profiles, imaging, and medical treatment of neuroendocrine tumors.

Medical management of pancreatic neuroendocrine tumors. Delaunoit T, Neczyporenko F, Rubin J, Erlichman C, Hobday TJ. Am J Gastroenterol 2008; 103: 475–83.

A trials-based review of current medical therapies for neuroendocrine tumors, including surgical/invasive options, somatostatins and analogs, somatostatin-based radiotherapy, interferon and other immunotherapies.

Necrolytic migratory erythema: clinicopathologic study of 13 cases. Pujol RM, Wang CY, el-Azhary RA, Su WP, Gibson LE, Schroeter AL. Int J Dermatol 2004; 43: 12–18.

A series highlighting the variability of presentation and histologic diagnosis of NME, emphasizing the need for high clinical suspicion.

Necrolytic migratory erythema without glucagonoma in patients with liver disease. Marinkovich MP, Botella R, Datloff J, Sangueza OP. J Am Acad Dermatol 1995; 32: 604–9.

In the absence of glucagonoma, hepatocellular dysfunction and hypoalbuminemia appear to be the most common factors associated with NME. NME may be a cutaneous marker for various liver diseases associated with malnutrition and low-protein states.

Endocrine pancreatic tumors with glucagon hypersecretion: a retrospective study of 23 cases during 20 years. Kindmark H, Sundin A, Granberg D, Dunder K, Skogseid B, Janson ET, et al. Med Oncol 2007; 24: 330–7.

Glucagonoma is highly associated with NME. In this retrospective series, over half of patients with glucagon hypersecretion also had NME.

Evidence Levels: **A** Double-blind study **B** Clinical trial ≥ 20 subjects **C** Clinical trial < 20 subjects **D** Series ≥ 5 subjects **E** Anecdotal case reports

FIRST-LINE THERAPIES

▶ Tumor resection **B**
▶ Somatostatins **B**

Diagnosis and surgical treatment of pancreatic endocrine tumors in 36 patients: a single-center report. Liu H, Zhang SZ, Wu YL, Fang HQ, Li JT, Sheng HW, et al. Chin Med J (Engl) 2007; 120: 1487–90.

A retrospective analysis of 36 cases of pancreatic endocrine tumors. Surgical removal of the primary tumor and resectable hepatic metastases was curative in 50% of malignant cases.

Treatment with the radiolabeled somatostatin analog [177 Lu-DOTA 0,Tyr3]octreotate: toxicity, efficacy, and survival. Kwekkeboom DJ, de Herder WW, Kam BL, van Eijck CH, van Essen M, Kooij PP, et al. J Clin Oncol 2008; 26: 2124–30.

Five hundred and four patients with gastropancreatic neuroendocrine tumors were treated with a radiolabeled somatostatin analog with promising results for tumor-free survival, progression-free survival, and overall survival.

SECOND-LINE THERAPIES

▶ Nutritional supplementation with amino acids, zinc, or essential fatty acids **D**

Glucagonoma syndrome: survival 21 years with concurrent liver metastases. Dourakis SP, Alexopoulou A, Georgousi KK, Delladetsima JK, Tolis G, Archimandritis AJ. Am J Med Sci 2007; 334: 225–7.

A report of unresectable glucagonoma treated symptomatically; the rash cleared with zinc supplementation.

Peripheral amino acid and fatty acid infusion for the treatment of necrolytic migratory erythema in the glucagonoma syndrome. Alexander KE, Robinson M, Staniec M, Gluhy RG. Clin Endocrinol 2002; 57: 827–31.

Long-term intermittent peripheral intravenous administration of amino acids and fatty acids led to significant improvement in NME symptoms.

Necrolytic migratory erythema without glucagonoma in a patient with short bowel syndrome. Nakashima H, Komine M, Sasaki K, Mitsui H, Fujimoto M, Ihn HK, et al. J Dermatol 2006; 33: 557–62.

Peripheral amino acid infusions successfully treated an NME-like eruption associated with short bowel syndrome.

THIRD-LINE THERAPIES

▶ Gluten-free diet **E**
▶ Pancreatic enzyme replacement **E**
▶ Dacarbazine **D**
▶ Liver transplantation **E**
▶ Opioid abstinence **E**

Necrolytic migratory erythema: a report of three cases. Thorisdottir K, Camisa C, Tomecki KJ, Bergfeld WF. J Am Acad Dermatol 1994; 30: 324–9.

NME associated with nutritional deficiencies in a patient with inadequate pancreatic enzymes resolved with vitamin and mineral supplementation and remained clear with pancreatic enzyme supplementation. Non-compliance with avoidance of dietary gluten in a patient with NME secondary to gluten-sensitive enteropathy led to cutaneous flares, which resolved with reinstitution of adherence to the diet.

Successful treatment of glucagonoma-related necrolytic migratory erythema with dacarbazine. van der Loos TLJM, Lambrecht MC, Lambers JCCA. J Am Acad Dermatol 1987; 16: 468–72.

Intravenous dacarbazine led to prolonged remission of NME in a patient with surgically incurable glucagonoma.

Metastatic glucagonoma: treatment with liver transplantation. Radny P, Eigentler TK, Soennichsen K, Overkamp D, Raab HR, Viebahn R, et al. J Am Acad Dermatol 2006; 54: 344–7.

A case report of multiple modality treatment of metastatic glucagonoma culminating in a liver transplant, with no recurrence of disease on long-term follow-up.

Necrolytic migratory erythema in an opiate-dependent patient. Muller FM, Arseculeratne G, Evans A, Fleming C. Clin Exp Dermatol 2008; 33: 40–2.

An NME-like eruption in an opiate-dependent patient cleared after withdrawal of opiates, and recurred on subsequent rechallenge with opiates.

Nephrogenic systemic fibrosis

Eleanor A Knopp, Shawn E Cowper

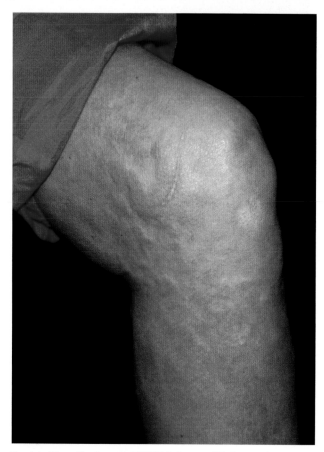

Reprinted from The Lancet, 356(9234) Cowper SE, Robin HS, Steinberg SM, Su LD, Gupta S, Le Boit PE. Scleromyxoedema-like cutaneous diseases in renal dialysis patients. 1000–1, 2000 with permission from Elsevier.

Nephrogenic systemic fibrosis (NSF) affects patients with renal impairment, most of whom have been exposed to MRI contrast. Onset is marked by cutaneous erythema, edema, hyperpigmentation, and woody induration. The clinical course commonly results in joint contractures and sometimes fibrosis of internal organs.

MANAGEMENT STRATEGY

Prevention is paramount. Patients with renal dysfunction (acute kidney injury or chronic kidney disease (estimated GFR of <30 mL/min/1.73 m²)) should avoid exposure to gadolinium-containing contrast agents (GCCA). If unavoidable, optimal dosing and follow-up should involve the managing radiologist and nephrologist. Although not proven to prevent NSF, immediate hemodialysis following exposure to GCCA is recommended.

Nephrogenic systemic fibrosis: recommendations for gadolinium-based contrast use in patients with kidney disease. Perazella MA, Reilly RF. Semin Dial 2008; 21: 171–3.

US FDA. Information on Gadolinium-Containing Contrast Agents. FDA CDER Website: *http://www.fda.gov/cder/drug/infopage/gcca/default.htm*, Accessed 07/15/2008.

SPECIFIC INVESTIGATIONS

- ▶ Deep skin biopsy (incisional or substantial deep punch) followed by histological and CD34 immunohistological evaluation
- ▶ Renal function parameters (e.g., BUN and creatinine)
- ▶ Electrophoresis to exclude a scleromyxedema-associated paraprotein
- ▶ Serological autoantibody testing (e.g., ANA, Scl-70) to exclude systemic sclerosis
- ▶ Hypercoagulability evaluation

There are no serologic tests for NSF. Diagnosis is based on clinical and histopathological correlation in a patient with renal disease. Gadolinium identification is not required to establish a diagnosis.

FIRST-LINE THERAPIES

▶ Re-establishment of renal function	E
▶ Physical therapy	E
▶ Pain management	E

Treatment of nephrogenic systemic fibrosis: limited options but hope for the future. Linfert DR, Schell JO, Fine DM. Semin Dial 2008; 21: 155–9.

Transplantation, particularly if performed soon after onset of NSF, is often the best therapeutic avenue. Significant clinical improvement may not be observed for months or years following resumption of renal function, and in some cases may not occur at all. Rigorous physical therapy is mandatory to maintain joint function.

SECOND-LINE THERAPIES

▶ Extracorporeal photopheresis (ECP)	E
▶ Imatinib mesylate	E

Nephrogenic systemic fibrosis: early recognition and treatment. Knopp EA, Cowper SE. Semin Dial 2008; 21: 123–8.

ECP has been associated with symptomatic improvements in at least nine patients in the setting of ongoing renal failure.

Extracorporeal photopheresis improves nephrogenic fibrosing dermopathy/nephrogenic systemic fibrosis: three case reports and review of literature. Mathur K, et al. J Clin Apher 2008; 236: 144–50.

An additional three patients demonstrate improvement with ECP.

Imatinib mesylate treatment of nephrogenic systemic fibrosis. Kay J, High WA. Arthritis Rheum. 2008; 58: 2543–8.

THIRD-LINE THERAPIES

► Pentoxifylline	E
► Sodium thiosulfate	E
► UVA1	E
► Photodynamic therapy with methyl aminolevulinate	E
► Plasmapheresis	E
► IVIg	E
► Corticosteroids (topical, intralesional, and systemic)	E
► Methotrexate (systemic)	E
► Azathioprine	E
► Calcipotriene	E

Gadolinium – a specific trigger for the development of nephrogenic fibrosing dermopathy and nephrogenic systemic fibrosis? Grobner T. Nephrol Dial Transplant 2006; 21: 1104–8.

Pentoxifylline was associated with improvement in two patients.

Nephrogenic systemic fibrosis: early recognition and treatment. Knopp EA, Cowper SE. Semin Dial 2008; 21: 123–8.

Most of these therapies lack reproducibility or complete information upon which to evaluate efficacy.

Notalgia paresthetica

Joanna Wallengren

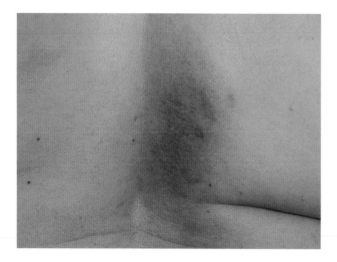

Notalgia paresthetica is a unilateral sensory neuropathy characterized by pruritus or burning pain at the medial inferior tip of the scapula, often accompanied by pigmentation or mild lichenification. Occasionally the distribution may be bilateral, and a few hereditary cases have been described.

MANAGEMENT STRATEGY

Treatment aims to reduce the itch by altering peripheral or central nerve transmission. Topical corticosteroids are generally ineffective unless secondary inflammation is present.

Topical *capsaicin* 0.025% three times daily for 5 weeks depletes sensory nerve transmitters in the skin. Local anesthesia with *EMLA (2.5% lidocaine and 2.5% prilocaine)* under hydrocolloid occlusion twice daily blocks peripheral nerve transmission. Upon discontinuation of both these treatments there is a considerable risk of relapse. The treatments may than be repeated for a few days or weeks until pruritus subsides.

Daily electrical stimulation using *TENS or CFS* for 2–5 weeks has been tried with good results, the pruritus relapsing gradually.

Deep intramuscular *acupuncture* to the paravertebral muscles in the T2–T6 dermatome once a week until the pruritus subsides, as well as spinal physiotherapy, has been reported in a few cases. Also, single treatments with *anesthetic block* or *botulinum toxin* have been described in anecdotal case reports. The reduction of itch due to these treatments may last for months or years.

Oral therapy may be preferred in patients in whom repeated topical treatments may be difficult to perform. Anticonvulsants such as *oxcarbazepin* (300 mg × 2 daily) and *gabapentin* (600 mg daily at night) alter central nerve transmission. Relapse is to be expected as soon as therapy is discontinued.

SPECIFIC INVESTIGATIONS

> ▶ Skin biopsy
> ▶ MRI of the thoracic spine

Notalgia paresthetica. Case reports and histologic appraisal. Weber PJ, Poulos EG. J Am Acad Dermatol 1988; 18: 25–30.

Skin biopsies from 14 patients revealed necrotic keratinocytes. Melanin and melanophages in the upper and mid dermis were found in biopsies of patients with brown lesions.

Symptoms of notalgia paresthetica may be explained by increased dermal innervation. Springall DR, Karanth SS, Kirkham N, Darley CR, Polak JM. J Invest Dermatol 1991; 97: 555–61.

An increased number of epidermal and dermal sensory nerve fibers was found in skin biopsies from five patients with notalgia paresthetica.

Localized pruritus–notalgia paresthetica. Massey EW, Pleet AB. Arch Dermatol 1979; 115: 982–3.

Two patients are described, their symptoms being explained as neuropathy of the thoracic nerves at the level of T2–T6. These nerves penetrate the spinal muscle at a right-angle, which predisposes them to injury from mild insults, resulting in notalgia paresthetica.

Notalgia paresthetica associated with nerve root impingement. Eisenberg E, Barmeir E, Bergman R. J Am Acad Dermatol 1997; 37: 998–1000.

An impingement of the nerve root as a possible cause of notalgia paresthetica was confirmed by MRI in one patient.

Notalgia paresthetica is a clinical diagnosis and none of the abovementioned investigations are required in the clinical situation.

FIRST-LINE THERAPIES

> ▶ Capsaicin   A
> ▶ EMLA (2.5% lidocaine and 2.5% prilocaine)   E

Successful treatment of notalgia paresthetica with topical capsaicin: vehicle-controlled, double-blind, crossover study. Wallengren J, Klinker M. J Am Acad Dermatol 1995; 32: 287–9.

This double-blind crossover comparison between capsaicin 0.025% and vehicle cream was performed in 20 patients for 10 weeks, the 4-week treatments being followed by 2 weeks of washout. The group treated with capsaicin first had a reduction of VAS from 61% to 35% during the first period, whereas in the other group VAS was reduced from 52% to 27%. Most patients relapsed within a month.

Notalgia paraesthetica – report of three cases and their treatment. Layton AM, Cotterill JA. Clin Exp Dermatol 1991; 16: 197–8.

All three patients improved upon treatment with EMLA; two relapsed, but pruritus was reduced.

SECOND-LINE THERAPIES

> ▶ Oxcarbazepin   E
> ▶ Gabapentin   E
> ▶ TENS   D
> ▶ CFS   D

Evidence Levels: **A** Double-blind study   **B** Clinical trial ≥ 20 subjects   **C** Clinical trial < 20 subjects   **D** Series ≥ 5 subjects   **E** Anecdotal case reports

Anticonvulsants

Open pilot study on oxcarbazepine for the treatment of notalgia paresthetica. Savk E, Bolukbasi O, Akyol A, Karaman G. J Am Acad Dermatol 2001; 45: 630–2.

Four patients were treated with oxcarbazepin for 6 months: two improved, VAS being reduced from 80% to 50% and from 90% to 40%, respectively.

Gabapentin treatment for notalgia paresthetica, a common isolated peripheral sensory neuropathy. Loosemore MP, Bordeaux JS, Bernhard JD. J Eur Acad Dermatol Venereol 2007; 21: 1440–1.

A case report on one patient who improved but relapsed upon discontinuation of treatment.

Electrical nerve stimulation

Transcutaneous electrical nerve stimulation offers partial relief in notalgia paresthetica patients with a relevant spinal pathology. Savk E, Savk O, Sendur F. J Dermatol 2007; 34: 315–19.

Nine of 15 patients treated with TENS for 2 weeks improved substantially, mean VAS being reduced from 100% to 45%.

Cutaneous field stimulation (CFS) in treatment of severe localized itch. Wallengren J, Sundler F. Arch Dermatol 2001; 137: 1323–5.

Seventeen patients with different disorders of neuropathic pruritus completed the study. Four of five patients with notalgia paresthetica improved after daily use of CFS for 5 weeks, VAS being reduced from 65% to 40%. Itch gradually relapsed after the discontinuation of CFS.

THIRD-LINE THERAPIES

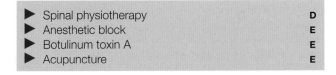

▶ Spinal physiotherapy	D
▶ Anesthetic block	E
▶ Botulinum toxin A	E
▶ Acupuncture	E

Notalgia paresthetica: clinical, physiopathological and therapeutic aspects. A study of 12 cases. Raison-Peyron N, Meunier L, Acevedo M, Meynadier J. J Eur Acad Dermatol Venereol 1999; 12: 215–21.

Pruritus was reduced in five of nine patients treated by spinal physiotherapy using ultrasound, or manipulation. According to the authors, the improvement was sustained for 1–9 years.

Successful treatment of notalgia paresthetica with a paravertebral local anesthetic block. Goulden V, Toomey PJ, Highet AS. J Eur Acad Dermatol 1998; 8: 114–16.

Paravertebral block at dermatome T3–T6 in one patient resulted in clearing of pruritus within a few days, lasting for 1 year of follow-up.

Successful treatment of notalgia paresthetica with botulinum toxin type A. Weinfeld PK. Arch Dermatol 2007; 143: 980–2.

Two patients were treated locally with botulinum toxin, reduction of itch lasting for 18 months after the treatment. One patient with notalgia paresthetica treated locally with Botox (100 U) on one occasion reported a reduction of itch from 80% to 25% 6 weeks after the treatment. At follow-up after 18 months pruritus had relapsed to 60% (Bartosik J, Wallengren J, unpublished).

Neurogenic pruritus: an unrecognised problem? A retrospective case series of treatment by acupuncture. Stellon A. Acupunct Med 2002; 20: 186–90.

Sixteen patients with different disorders of neuropathic pruritus completed the study. Four patients with notalgia paresthetica improved, mean VAS being reduced from 73% to 0%. One patient relapsed within a year. One patient was treated with local acupuncture once weekly. She improved after a few weeks, but at the follow-up after 18 months pruritus was back to 62% (Carlsson, Wallengren J, unpublished).

Neurofibromatosis, type 1

Clara-Dina Cokonis, Rhonda E Schnur

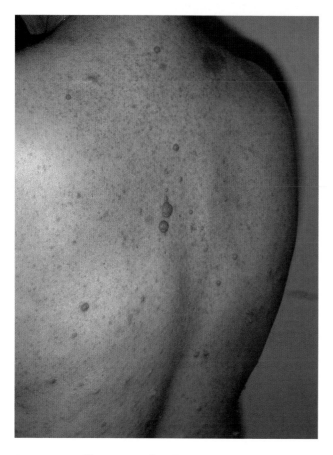

Type 1 neurofibromatosis (NF1) is an autosomal dominant neurocutaneous disorder with highly variable expression. NF1 is caused by changes in the neurofibromin gene on chromosome 17. The neurofibromin protein is a GTPase-activating protein that negatively regulates Ras protein signal transduction, limiting cell growth and malignant transformation. Neurofibromas may be benign subcutaneous lesions or deeper, larger, plexiform tumors that follow nerves and/or extend into deeper bony and visceral structures; malignant peripheral nerve sheath tumors (MPNSTs) may develop in deeper lesions.

MANAGEMENT STRATEGY

The diagnosis of NF1 is established by well-defined clinical criteria. The sensitivity of mutation analysis varies depending on the techniques used, but is improving. The nature of the mutation may affect prognosis; large deletions or null mutations are detected in a higher percentage of patients with MPNSTs.

There is currently no proven medical therapy to prevent or treat neurofibromas, but significant efforts are underway to develop targeted treatment approaches that exploit the molecular biology of NF1. *Statins* are actively being explored as potential aids in the treatment of MPNSTs, NF1-associated learning disability, and tibial fragility. *Ketotifen* has been used in the past for pain, tenderness, and pruritus of neurofibromas, but there are no recent large studies using this drug. Otherwise, standard treatment is limited to *surgery*. Benign neurofibromas, cosmetic concerns and discomfort are indications for removal. Most neurofibromas are small and can be removed by simple excision using a scalpel or punch biopsy. Although there is little morbidity, surgery is not practical for large tumors.

A wire loop connected to a *monopolar diathermy* machine in the cutting mode has been used to treat hundreds of small lesions. Hemostasis is readily obtained, healing is by secondary intention, and cosmetic outcome is good. CO_2 *laser vaporization* has been used for small tumors with healing by secondary intention, or for larger tumors in conjunction with primary closure. Hundreds of tumors can be removed in one outpatient session under local anesthesia. Unfortunately, surgery is not curative and lesions may continue to progress, requiring repeated procedures.

Treatment of plexiform neurofibromas is particularly challenging because these tumors are often highly vascular and invasive. Symptomatic lesions are evaluated by MRI or PET scans because of the risk for evolution into MPNSTs. Unexplained pain or rapid growth within a plexiform neurofibroma, and areas displaying necrosis or an unusual appearance on imaging studies, merit biopsy to exclude malignant transformation. cDNA gene expression profiling may be used in the future to help distinguish benign from premalignant and malignant lesions.

Radiofrequency therapy may be useful for treating diffuse facial plexiform neurofibromas. Non-surgical treatments for plexiform neurofibromas and MPNSTs are also under active investigation. A new generation of therapeutic agents includes angiogenesis inhibitors and anti-inflammatory agents that inhibit cell growth and induce apoptosis. Drugs that target Ras signal transduction or limit Ras post-translational processing, such as farnesyl transferase inhibitors, look promising. Rapamycin and sorafenib are currently being studied in clinical trials. Statins are being explored in the treatment of MPNSTs as well as NF1-related bone dysplasia and cognitive difficulties, because of their known inhibitory activity of p21Ras/mitogen activated protein kinase (MAPK) activity. Referral of a patient with aggressive MPNSTs to an oncologist for possible radiation and chemotherapy may be warranted. Information about ongoing clinical trials can be found at www.ctf.org/research/nf1 and www.ClinicalTrials.gov.

SPECIFIC INVESTIGATIONS

- ▶ Complete cutaneous and ocular examinations (slit-lamp and funduscopy) of the patient and first-degree relatives
- ▶ Regular blood pressure checks to screen for renal artery stenosis or pheochromocytoma
- ▶ MRI of brain, optic nerves, and spinal cord if the patient is symptomatic or has focal neurologic signs
- ▶ MRI or PET scan of deep or changing plexiform neurofibromas
- ▶ Biopsy of changing or suspicious lesions
- ▶ Radiographs if osseous involvement is suspected
- ▶ Evaluation and management of learning disability and attention deficits, as needed
- ▶ DNA analysis of proband and at-risk family members

Guidelines for the diagnosis and management of individuals with neurofibromatosis 1. Ferner RE, Huson SM, Thomas N, Moss C, Willshaw H, Evans DG, et al. J Med Genet 2007; 44: 81–8.

This is a comprehensive review of the diagnosis and management of NF1.

Neurofibromin signaling and synapses. Hsueh YP. J Biomed Sci 2007; 14: 461–6.

This is a review of the signaling pathways of neurofibromin.

Nature and mRNA effect of 282 different NF1 point mutations: focus on splicing alterations. Pros E, Gómez C, Martín T, Fábregas P, Serra E, Lázaro C. Hum Mutat 2008; Mutation in Brief #1021 m 29: E173-E193, Online.

The authors correlate various point mutations in the NF1 DNA with effects on mRNA transcription, noting that most mutations lead to frameshifts or impact splicing.

Further evidence of the increased risk for malignant peripheral nerve sheath tumour from a Scottish cohort of patients with neurofibromatosis type 1. McCaughan JA, Holloway SM, Davidson R, Lam WWK. J Med Genet 2007; 44: 463–6.

The authors estimated a lifetime risk of 5.9–10.3% in NF1 patients for developing MPNSTs, and reviewed other risk factors for these frequently aggressive tumors.

TORC1 is essential for NF1-associated malignancies. Johannessen CM, Johnson BW, Williams SM, Chan AW, Reczek EE, Lynch RC, et al. Curr Biol 2008; 18: 56–62.

The authors show that the mTOR inhibitor rapamycin potently suppresses the growth of aggressive NF1-associated malignancies in an NF1 murine model via suppression of the mTOR target cyclin D1. They conclude that cyclin D1 may be an informative biomarker for MPNSTs and prove that TORC1/mTOR is essential for tumorigenesis.

Neurofibromatosis 1. JM Friedman. Updated January 7, 2007. In: GeneReviews at GeneTests: Medical Genetics Information Resource (database online). Copyright, University of Washington, Seattle 1997–2008. Available at http://www.genetests.org. Accessed [August 23, 2008].

This is one of the most comprehensive reviews of NF1 which is frequently updated.

FIRST-LINE THERAPIES

▶ Surgical excision	C
▶ CO_2 laser	C
▶ Diathermy	D

The role of surgery in children with neurofibromatosis. Neville HL, Seymour-Dempsey K, Slopis J, Gill BS, Moore BD, Lally KP, et al. J Pediatr Surg 2001; 36: 25–9.

This is a large study of 249 pediatric patients with NF1 and NF2: 50 (48 with NF1) had surgery; 14 of the 50 had malignancies, and eight underwent multiple resections. Both surgical and postoperative management are reviewed.

Carbon dioxide laser for removal of multiple cutaneous neurofibromas. Moreno JC, Mathoret C, Lantieri L, Zeller J, Revuz J, Wolkenstein P. Br J Dermatol 2001; 144: 1096–8.

CO_2 laser under general anesthesia was used to treat hundreds of cutaneous neurofibromas in 13 patients with NF1 with minimal morbidity. Flat, smooth, depigmented scars resulted. Most patients who had previous surgical excisions considered the CO_2 laser scars to be as acceptable as those obtained with surgery.

An operation for the treatment of cutaneous neurofibromatosis. Roberts AHN, Crockett DJ. Br J Plast Surg 1985; 38: 292–3.

Rapid removal of multiple cutaneous neurofibromas was performed using a wire loop held in diathermy forceps connected to a monopolar diathermy machine. Five patients with an average of 243 lesions were treated. They were hospitalized for 2–7 days and healed completely within 3 weeks.

Malignant peripheral nerve sheath tumor: molecular pathogenesis and current management considerations. Grobmyer SR, Reith JD, Shahlaee A, Bush CH, Hochwald SN. J Surg Oncol 2008; 97: 340–9.

This is an excellent review article about the diagnosis, genetics, and standard management of MPNSTs via surgery, radiation, and chemotherapy.

Molecular, genetic, and cellular pathogenesis of neurofibromas and surgical implications. Gottfried ON, Viskochil DH, Fults DW, Couldwell WT. Neurosurgery 2006; 58: 1–16.

This reviews all current therapeutic and theoretic approaches to treatment of neurofibromas and MPNSTs.

SECOND-LINE THERAPIES

▶ Ketotifen	B

A controlled multiphase trial of ketotifen to minimize neurofibroma-associated pain and itching. Riccardi VM. Arch Dermatol 1993; 129: 577–81.

Ketotifen 2–4 mg daily reduced itching, pain, and tenderness associated with neurofibromas in 52 patients, with sustained long-term efficacy and minimal side effects.

THIRD-LINE THERAPIES

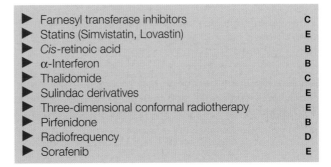

▶ Farnesyl transferase inhibitors	C
▶ Statins (Simvistatin, Lovastin)	E
▶ Cis-retinoic acid	B
▶ α-Interferon	B
▶ Thalidomide	C
▶ Sulindac derivatives	E
▶ Three-dimensional conformal radiotherapy	E
▶ Pirfenidone	B
▶ Radiofrequency	D
▶ Sorafenib	E

Molecular targets for emerging anti-tumor therapies for neurofibromatosis type 1. Dilworth JT, Kraniak JM, Wojtkowiak JW, Gibbs RA, Borch RF, Tainsky MA, et al. Biochem Pharmacol 2006; 72: 1485–92.

This is an excellent review of potential targets for medical therapy of NF1 based on the molecular biology of the protein.

Radiofrequency in the treatment of craniofacial plexiform neurofibromatosis: a pilot study. Baujat B, Krastinova-Lolov D, Blumen M, Baglin AC, Coquille F, Chabolle F. Plast Reconstr Surg 2006; 117: 1261–8.

This five-patient pilot study demonstrated partial diminution or stabilization of plexiform neurofibromas.

Hyperactive Ras as a therapeutic target in neurofibromatosis type 1. Weiss B, Bollag G, Shannon K. Am J Med Genet 1999; 89: 14–22.

Potential NF1 therapies are proposed based on the normal function of neurofibromin as a negative regulator of Ras signal transduction. Agents include farnesyl transferase inhibitors (affect post-translational RAS processing) and MEK-mitogen-activated protein kinase inhibitors (affect the downstream effector pathway). Cell differentiation inducers (e.g., retinoids), inhibitors of growth factors, and angiogenesis inhibitors (e.g., thalidomide) may also be useful.

Protein farnesyl transferase inhibitors. Ayral-Kaloustian S, Salaski EJ. Curr Med Chem 2002; 9: 1003–32.

A review of farnesyl transferase inhibitors. In addition to targeting Ras, they may also inhibit angiogenesis and induce apoptosis.

Phase I trial and pharmacokinetic study of the farnesyl-transferase inhibitor tipifarnib in children with refractory solid tumors or neurofibromatosis type I and plexiform neurofibromas. Widemann BC, Salzer WL, Arceci RJ, Blaney SM, Fox E, End D, et al. J Clin Oncol 2006; 24: 507–16.

This phase I study included 17 children with NF1 and was designed to establish a safety profile and dosing schedule for tipifarnib.

Induction of apoptosis in neurofibromatosis type 1 malignant peripheral nerve sheath tumor cell lines by a combination of novel farnesyl transferase inhibitors and lovastatin. Wojtkowiak JW, Fouad F, LaLonde DT, Kleinman MD, Gibbs RA, Reiners JJ Jr, et al. J Pharmacol Exp Ther 2008; 326: 1–11.

This study demonstrates a potential benefit in treating MPNSTs with farnesyl transferase inhibitors and lovastatin.

Sorafenib inhibits growth and mitogen-activated protein kinase signaling in malignant peripheral nerve sheath cells. Ambrosini G, Cheema HS, Seelman S, Teed A, Sambol EB, Singer S, et al. Mol Cancer Ther 2008; 7: 890–6.

The finding that nanomolar concentrations of sorafenib inhibit growth of MPNSTs in vitro warrants further study of this drug in vivo.

Isolated plexiform neurofibroma: treatment with three-dimensional conformal radiotherapy. Robertson TC, Buck DA, Schmidt-Ullrich R, Powers CN, Reiter ER. Laryngoscope 2004; 114: 1139–42.

This is a case report in which a plexiform neurofibroma of the tongue was treated with three-dimensional conformal radiotherapy, with only mild xerostomia as a side effect.

Phase I study of thalidomide for the treatment of plexiform neurofibroma in neurofibromatosis 1. Gupta A, Cohen BH, Ruggieri P, Packer RJ, Phillips PC. Neurology 2003; 60: 130–2.

Twelve patients with severe plexiform neurofibromas were treated for 1 year with thalidomide (1–4 mg/kg daily).

Although only four patients showed a small reduction in tumor size, seven had symptomatic improvement (e.g., reduced pain and paresthesia) with minimal side effects.

Plexiform neurofibromas in NF1: Toward biologic-based therapy. Packer RJ, Gutmann DH, Rubenstein A, Viskochil D, Zimmerman RA, Vezina G, et al. Neurology 2002; 58: 1461–70.

This article reviews a randomized, non-comparative phase II trial of 57 children and adults with progressive plexiform neurofibromas, using either *cis*-retinoic acid or interferon-α: 86% of retinoic acid-treated patients and 96% of interferon-treated patients were stable or improved at 18 months of follow-up.

Phase II trial of pirfenidone in adults with neurofibromatosis type 1. Babovic-Vuksanovic D, Ballman K, Michels V, McGrann P, Lindor N, King B, et al. Neurology 2006; 67: 1860–2.

In this trial, pirfenidone, an antifibrotic agent, was used to treat 24 patients with plexiform or paraspinal neurofibromas. Four tumors decreased in size, three increased, and 17 remained stable.

Sulindac derivatives inhibit cell growth and induce apoptosis in primary cells from malignant peripheral nerve sheath tumors of NF1 patients. Frahm S, Kurtz A, Kluwe L, Farassati F, Friedrich RE, Mautner VF. Cancer Cell Int 2004; 17: 4.

Results in two primary cell lines from patients with NF1 suggest that this class of anti-inflammatory compound may be of therapeutic benefit for MPNSTs.

Modelling neurofibromatosis type 1 tibial dysplasia and its treatment with lovastatin. Kolanczyk M, Kuehnisch J, Kossler N, Osswald M, Stumpp S, Thurisch B, et al. BMC Med 2008; 6: 21.

High-dose systemic lovastatin restored deficient *Runx2* gene expression and accelerated new bone formation in a murine model of NF1-related tibial dysplasia, improving cortical bone repair.

Effect of simvastatin on cognitive functioning in children with neurofibromatosis type 1: a randomized controlled trial. Krab LC, de Goede-Bolder A, Aarsen FK, Pluijm SM, Bouman MJ, van der Geest JN, et al. JAMA 2008; 300: 287–94.

Based on previous work showing that statin-mediated inhibition of 3-hydroxy-3-methylglutaryl coenzyme A reductase restored cognitive deficits in an NF1 mouse model, 62 children with NF1 were given simvastatin or placebo in a randomized, double-blind, placebo-controlled trial. Over 12 weeks there was no significant cognitive improvement.

Induction of apoptosis in neurofibromatosis type 1 malignant peripheral nerve sheath tumor cell lines by a combination of novel farnesyl transferase inhibitors and lovastatin. Wojtkowiak JW, Fouad F, LaLonde DT, Kleinman MD, Gibbs RA, Reiners JJ, et al. J Pharmacol Exp Ther 2008; 326: 1–11.

Combination treatment with farnesyl transferase inhibitors and lovastatin reduced cell proliferation and induced an apoptotic response in two NF1 malignant peripheral nerve sheath tumor (MPNST) cell lines.

Nevoid basal cell carcinoma syndrome

Saurabh Singh, Gary L Peck

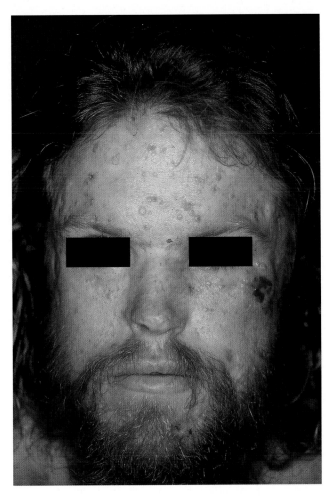

Nevoid basal cell carcinoma syndrome (NBCCS), also known as Gorlin–Goltz syndrome, is characterized by a variety of neoplasms and skeletal anomalies, the universal finding being multiple basal cell carcinomas (BCCs). In addition, more than 50% of patients exhibit palmar and plantar pits, odontogenic keratocysts, rib abnormalities, and ectopic calcification of the falx cerebri. Other neoplasms include medulloblastomas and ovarian fibromas. The chromosomal defect in this autosomal dominant disease is mapped to chromosome 9q22.3-q31, resulting in a mutation of the patched gene (PTCH), which functions as a tumor suppressor gene. The PTCH protein operates in the hedgehog signal transduction pathway and inhibits the activity of smoothened protein. Dysregulation of this transmembrane protein favors subsequent tumor formation.

MANAGEMENT STRATEGY

Affected individuals usually present with multiple primary BCCs that pose a therapeutic challenge. The goal of therapy is to achieve adequate cancer control while minimizing cosmetic disfigurement. Therapy should also include *emotional support* and *genetic counseling*. The treatment of BCCs in NBCCS is similar to that of sporadic BCCs and includes *surgical excision*, *Mohs' micrographic surgery (MMS)*, *electrodesiccation and curettage*, *cryosurgery*, *topical chemotherapy*, *topical immunomodulation*, *photodynamic therapy (PDT)*, *the use of lasers*, and *chemoprevention*. Although BCCs can occur in sunlight-protected areas in NBCCS, measures to protect against sun exposure are essential. In the past 8 years, most of the medical literature regarding the non-surgical treatment of BCC has focused on PDT, the use of lasers, topical immunomodulation with imiquimod cream, and various combinations of therapies.

SPECIFIC INVESTIGATIONS

▶ Radiologic studies
▶ Biopsy of lesions
▶ Genetic studies

Radiologic images in dermatology: nevoid basal cell carcinoma syndrome. Mirowski GW, Liu AA, Parks ET, Caldemeyer KS. J Am Acad Dermatol 2000; 43: 1092–3.

Radiologic studies detect the various skeletal and soft tissue anomalies associated with NBCCS, including odontogenic keratocysts, lamellar calcification of the falx cerebri, macrocephaly, cleft lip and/or palate, rib and vertebral anomalies, and short fourth metacarpals (Albright's sign).

Nevoid basal cell carcinoma syndrome: radiographic manifestations including cystlike lesions of the phalanges. Dunnick NR, Head GL, Peck GL, Yoder FW. Radiology 1978; 127: 331–4.

Radiographic findings of 25 NBCCS patients were analyzed: cyst-like lucencies of the phalanges were present in 46% of cases, and mandibular cysts were seen in 42% of patients. Exuberant intracranial calcifications, brachymetacarpalia, and rib and spine anomalies were also noted.

A novel polymorphism in the PTC gene allows easy identification of allelic loss in basal cell nevus syndrome lesions. Zedan W, Robinson PA, High AS. Diagn Mol Pathol 2001; 10: 41–5.

A C/T polymorphism of the PTC gene has been identified, and a PTC allelic loss has been demonstrated in NBCCS-associated BCCs and keratocysts as well as in sporadic BCCs.

Nevoid basal cell carcinoma syndrome. Gorlin RJ. Dermatol Clin 1995; 13: 113–23.

UV-specific p53 and PTCH mutations in sporadic basal cell carcinoma of sun exposed skin. Ratner D, Peacocke M, Zhang H, Ping XL, Tsou HC. J Am Acad Dermatol 2001; 44: 293–7.

FIRST-LINE THERAPIES

▶ Surgical management   **B**
▶ Mohs' micrographic surgery   **B**
▶ Protection against radiation exposure   **C**

Assessment and surgical treatment of basal cell skin cancer. Goldberg DP. Clin Plast Surg 1997; 24: 673–86.

Surgical excision, with a 2–5 mm margin of normal skin depending on tumor size, has a cure rate as high as 95–99% for primary tumors. Low-risk sporadic BCCs located on the neck, trunk, and extremities are associated with recurrence rates of 1–10%, whereas BCCs on the ear, nasolabial groove, scalp, or forehead exhibit higher recurrence rates. BCCs associated with NBCCS have a predilection to involve the embryonic cleft areas of the face, including the eyelids, periorbital, and midfacial regions. MMS, rather than simple surgical excision, is recommended for deeply invasive tumors, recurrent tumors, tumors with poorly defined margins or infiltrating histologic growth patterns, and tumors involving cartilage or bone. Extensive surgery for multiple lesions may require general anesthesia. If a skin graft is required for closure, it should be remembered that BCCs can occur within the graft in patients with NBCCS and complicate future surgery.

Guidelines for the management of BCC. Telfer NR, Colver GB, Bowers PW. Br J Dermatol 1999; 141: 415–23.

MMS has an overall 5-year cure rate of 99%, and is the treatment of choice for high-risk BCCs, such as those located on the eyelids, nose, lips, and ears, and those malignancies exhibiting infiltrative, morpheic, and micronodular growth patterns. The advantage of MMS is the maximal preservation of normal skin in cosmetically important areas such as the face, high-functioning areas such as the hands and feet, and in aggressive tumors in immunosuppressed patients.

The nevoid basal cell carcinoma syndrome: sensitivity to the ultraviolet and X-ray irradiation. Frentz G, Munch-Petersen B, Wulf HC, Niebuhr E, da Cunha Bang F. J Am Acad Dermatol 1987; 17: 637–43.

Radiation therapy should be avoided in patients with NBCCS, as these patients develop BCC as a consequence of radiotherapy within 6 months to 3 years, in contrast to the usual 20–30-year lag period for radiation-induced tumors seen in patients with sporadic BCC.

SECOND-LINE THERAPIES

▶ Electrodesiccation and curettage	B

Combined curettage and excision: a treatment method for primary basal cell carcinoma. Johnson TM, Tromovitch TA, Swanson NA. J Am Acad Dermatol 1991; 24: 613–17.

This therapy is appropriate for smaller primary BCCs located in low-risk recurrence areas such as the neck, trunk, and extremities. When used to treat non-aggressive primary lesions, the 5-year cure rate approaches 97%. Electrodesiccation and curettage should not be performed on recurrent tumors because scar tissue from the initial procedure interferes with the textural contrast needed for successful treatment with this technique. This procedure should also be avoided when tumors are large, exhibit a histologic infiltrative subtype, invade fat or other soft tissues, involve adnexal structures, or are located in high-risk areas of the midface and periorbital region.

With the multiplicity and high recurrence rate of tumors in NBCCS, electrodesiccation and curettage is certainly a therapeutic option, but should be employed after careful consideration of recurrence risk, location, and tumor size.

THIRD-LINE THERAPIES

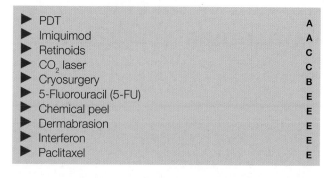

▶ PDT	A
▶ Imiquimod	A
▶ Retinoids	C
▶ CO$_2$ laser	C
▶ Cryosurgery	B
▶ 5-Fluorouracil (5-FU)	E
▶ Chemical peel	E
▶ Dermabrasion	E
▶ Interferon	E
▶ Paclitaxel	E

Photodynamic therapy using topical methyl aminolevulinate vs surgery for nodular basal cell carcinoma: results of a multicenter randomized prospective trial. Rhodes LE, de Rie M, Enström Y, Groves R, Morken T, Goulden V. Arch Dermatol 2004; 140: 17–23.

Topical methyl aminolevulinate in conjunction with a noncoherent red light (570–670 nm) at 75 J/cm^2 for the treatment of nodular BCC achieved a complete response of 91%, with a tumor-free rate of 83% at 12 months. Benefits of PDT include the ability to treat large and/or multiple tumors, better cosmesis than with surgery, and typically non-scarring results. Side effects include photosensitivity, which can last for several months, as well as localized treatment site pain, burning/stinging, and erythema.

Photodynamic therapy of multiple nonmelanoma skin cancers with verteporfin and red light-emitting diodes: two-year results evaluating tumor response and cosmetic outcomes. Lui H, Hobbs L, Tope WD, Lee PK, Elmets C, Provost N. Arch Dermatol 2004; 140: 26–32.

A complete clinical response of 98% at 6 months and 95% at 24 months was achieved when using intravenous verteporfin and a red light-emitting diode (688 nm) at a light dose of 180 J/cm^2, permitting activation of the drug within deep portions of the tumor.

Δ-Aminolevulinic acid and blue light photodynamic therapy for treatment of multiple basal cell carcinomas in two patients with nevoid basal cell carcinoma syndrome. Itkin A, Gilchrest B. Dermatol Surg 2004; 30: 1054–61.

Two patients underwent two courses of photodynamic therapy with 20% δ-aminolevulinic acid solution and 417-nm blue light source. A complete clinical response was observed in eight of nine (89%) superficial BCCs and five of 16 (31%) nodular BCCs located on the face, and in 18 of 27 (67%) superficial BCCs located on the lower extremities. The remaining 21 lesions demonstrated partial clinical resolution. No new BCCs in areas that were treated were observed during the 8-month follow-up period, and the two patients noted considerable cosmetic improvement after PDT. The most significant side effect from treatment was moderate to severe stinging during blue-light illumination.

Treatment of diffuse basal cell carcinomas and basaloid follicular hamartomas in nevoid basal cell carcinoma syndrome by wide-area 5-aminolevulinic acid photodynamic therapy. Oseroff AR, Shieh S, Frawley NP, Cheney R, Blumenson LE, Pivnick EK. Arch Dermatol 2005; 141: 60–7.

5-Aminolevulinic acid 20% was applied for 24 hours under occlusion to three children with BCCs and basaloid follicular hamartomas involving 12–25% of their body surface areas, followed by dye laser and lamp illumination. The responses varied from 85% to 98% overall clearance, with excellent cosmetic outcomes, and they were durable up to 6 years.

Broad area photodynamic therapy for treatment of multiple basal cell carcinomas in a patient with nevoid basal cell carcinoma syndrome. Chapas AM, Gilchrest BA. J Drugs Dermatol 2006; 5: 3–5.

Every 2–3 months a 73-year-old man with NBCCS underwent PDT with a 1-hour incubation of δ-aminolevulinic acid 20% topical solution applied to the entire face, followed by illumination with a blue light source. The effects of treatment included clearing of the BCCs, reduced pore size, improved cosmetic appearance of old facial scars, reduced severity of photodamage, and a significant reduction in the rate of new tumor development, precluding the need for surgical intervention.

Guidelines on the use of photodynamic therapy for nonmelanoma skin cancer: an international consensus. Braathen LR, Szeimies R, Basset-Seguin N, Bissonnette R, Foley P, Pariser D. J Am Acad Dermatol 2007; 56: 125–43.

Recommendations for the use of photodynamic therapy in the treatment of non-melanoma skin cancers are made, based on the quality of evidence for efficacy, safety/tolerability, cosmetic outcome, and patient satisfaction/preference in the medical literature. PDT is considered to be a first-line treatment for actinic keratoses, Bowen's disease, and superficial BCCs. Methyl aminolevulinate-PDT is recommended for treatment of nodular BCCs <2 mm in depth. PDT may be considered as a method for preventing BCCs in immunosuppressed patients and other high-risk individuals.

PDT, which has been employed for a range of malignancies, involves the intravenous, intralesional, or topical use of a photosensitizing agent. Upon exposure to visible light, the photosensitizing agent is activated, producing oxygen species that preferentially accumulate for longer periods in malignant cells, which are then selectively destroyed by a phototoxic reaction. The light source for PDT is often derived from a laser of appropriate wavelength as dictated by the photosensitizer used. Many studies have found that PDT is most appropriate for superficial BCCs and for those with multiple BCCs in low-risk areas when surgical options are impractical.

Imiquimod 5% cream for the treatment of superficial basal cell carcinomas: results from two phase III, randomized, vehicle-controlled studies. Geisse J, Caro I, Lindholm J, Golitz L, Stampone P, Owens M. J Am Acad Dermatol 2004; 50: 722–33.

Imiquimod is an immunomodulatory drug that is a Toll-like receptor 7 agonist which stimulates monocytes/macrophages and dendritic cells to produce interferon-α and other cytokines to stimulate cell-mediated immunity. This topical medication was initially approved for the treatment of genital and perianal warts, and subsequently for the treatment of superficial BCCs. Two identical, randomized, vehicle-controlled 6-week studies using imiquimod to treat superficial BCCs demonstrated histologic clearance rates of 79% and 82%. A 6-week, five-times-weekly regimen is recommended.

Hundreds of basal cell carcinomas in a Gorlin-Goltz syndrome patient cured with imiquimod 5% cream. Ferreres JR, Macaya A, Jucglá A, Muniesa C, Prats C, Peyrí J. J Eur Acad Dermatol Venereol 2006; 20: 877–8.

A 54-year-old man with NBCCS was lost to follow-up for 20 years and presented with hundreds of BCCs measuring <3 cm in diameter on the scalp, face, trunk, arms, and legs, in addition to 12 larger lesions. Seven of the larger lesions were surgically excised, and the remaining BCCs were subjected to 6 weeks of 5% imiquimod cream applied once daily. Over 300 superficial BCCs were completely treated. Nine lesions on the scalp and lower extremities did not respond adequately and were surgically excised. There have been no signs of recurrence after 36 months.

The use of imiquimod 5% cream for the treatment of superficial basal cell carcinomas in a basal cell nevus syndrome patient. Kagy MK, Amonette R. Dermatol Surg 2000; 26: 577–9.

These authors achieved complete regression of multiple, superficial, non-facial BCCs in a patient with NBCCS using imiquimod 5% cream, but the therapy was poorly tolerated. Side effects include localized itching and burning in most patients, pain in some cases, and rarely flu-like symptoms.

Treatment of Darier's disease, lamellar ichthyosis, pityriasis rubra pilaris, cystic acne, and basal cell carcinoma with oral 13-cis-retinoic acid. Peck GL, Yoder FW, Olsen TG, Pandya MD, Butkus D. Dermatologica 1978; 157: 11–12.

Two patients with NBCCS were treated with 13-*cis*-retinoic acid (isotretinoin) for 3 months, and a marked inflammatory response was observed in most tumors, particularly BCCs of the head and neck. Approximately 10% of the tumors demonstrated complete regression, both clinically and histologically. The malignancies that responded were 3–4 mm in diameter and located on the head and neck.

Treatment and prevention of basal cell carcinoma with oral isotretinoin. Peck GL, DiGiovanna JJ, Sarnoff DS, Gross EG, Butkus D, Olsen TG, et al. J Am Acad Dermatol 1988; 19: 176–85.

Of 270 tumors due to NBCCS, arsenic exposure, or sunlight exposure in 12 patients treated with a mean dose of oral isotretinoin 3.1 mg/kg/day for 8 months, 8% underwent complete clinical and histologic regression. Lower doses given to three patients for 3–8 years were effective for chemoprevention of new BCCs. When treatment was discontinued, multiple new BCCs appeared in the NBCCS patient but not the patient with the history of arsenic exposure, suggesting that the need to maintain chemopreventive therapy may depend on the etiology of the skin cancer.

Prevention of skin cancer in xeroderma pigmentosum with the use of oral isotretinoin. Kraemer K, DiGiovanna JJ, Moshell A, Peck GL. N Engl J Med 1988; 318: 1633–7.

Chemoprophylactic effects of isotretinoin were observed in five patients with xeroderma pigmentosa who completed a 2-year trial at a dose of 2 mg/kg/day. Treatment with isotretinoin resulted in a 63% average reduction of NMSCs compared to the number of tumors formed in the 2 years prior to isotretinoin administration. One year after the medication was stopped, tumor frequency increased a mean of 8.5-fold compared to the treatment period.

Common side effects of systemic retinoids include mucocutaneous toxicity, hypertriglyceridemia, and teratogenicity. During this study skeletal toxicity was also noted. Lower doses of isotretinoin were used after the 1-year post-treatment period and were found to be efficacious for chemoprevention.

Long-term therapy with low-dose isotretinoin for prevention of basal cell carcinoma: a multicenter clinical trial. Tangrea JA, Edwards BK, Taylor PR, Hartman AM, Peck GL, Salasche SJ, et al.; Isotretinoin-Basal Cell Carcinoma Study Group. J Natl Cancer Inst 1992; 84: 328–32.

Oral isotretinoin used as monotherapy at a low dose of 10 mg daily given for 3 years to patients with a history of sporadic BCCs was ineffective in preventing new tumors. Higher doses were not tested.

Systemic and topical retinoids in the management of skin cancer in organ transplant recipients. De Graaf YGL, Euvrard S, Bouwes Bavinck JN. Dermatol Surg 2004; 30: 656–61.

A summary of the medical literature for retinoid chemoprevention of NMSCs in organ transplant patients is presented, with the conclusion that systemic retinoids are effective in preventing NMSC development in this particular patient population. Specifically, the use of the drug acitretin is supported, as experience with isotretinoin in transplant patients is limited. Topical retinoids can be used for treatment of actinic keratoses and verrucae in organ transplant patients, but are less effective than systemic retinoids.

Skin cancer chemoprevention with systemic retinoids: an adjunct in the management of selected high-risk patients. Campbell RM, DiGiovanna JJ. Dermatol Ther 2006; 19: 306–14.

Patients with XP, NBCCS, and recipients of organ or bone transplantation are all at high risk for skin cancer and can benefit from retinoid chemoprophylaxis. Sun protection and regular follow-up with a dermatologist are integral to the early diagnosis and management of skin malignancies. Retinoid use can lead to many adverse events: short-term side effects are predominately mucocutaneous or lipid related, whereas long-term use can produce calcification of tendons and ligaments, or osteoporosis.

Chemoprevention of nonmelanoma skin cancer with systemic retinoids: practical dosing and management of adverse effects. Otley CC, Stasko T, Tope WD, Lebwohl M. Dermatol Surg 2006; 32: 562–8.

A practical guide to the administration of oral retinoids for chemoprevention of NMSCs is outlined, in addition to guidelines for prevention and management of adverse effects. Proposed dose escalation schedules for acitretin and isotretinoin are presented.

Systemic retinoids in chemoprevention of non-melanoma skin cancer. Lens M, Medenica L. Exp Opin Pharmacother 2008; 9: 1363–74.

The primary indication for retinoid chemoprophylaxis is the deterrence of NMSC development in high-risk patients who continue to actively develop new skin malignancies. The use of systemic retinoids for chemoprevention of NMSCs is reviewed, including mechanism of action, efficacy, and side effects. General and specific recommendations for patients who would benefit from retinoid chemoprevention of NMSCs are listed, one of which includes patients with NBCCS.

Beneficial effect of low-dose systemic retinoid in combination with topical tretinoin for the treatment and prophylaxis of premalignant and malignant skin lesions in renal transplant recipients. Rook AH, Jaworsky C, Nguyen T, Grossman RA, Wolfe JT, Witmer WK, et al. Transplantation 1995; 59: 714–19.

Topical tretinoin (0.025–0.05%) was effective in preventing skin cancer when used in combination with oral etretinate (10 mg daily) in renal transplant patients with multiple actinic keratoses and a history of multiple squamous cell carcinomas per year.

Etretinate is no longer available, but its use in skin cancer chemoprevention preceded that of acitretin.

Gorlin syndrome: the role of the carbon dioxide laser in patient management. Grobbelaar AO, Horlock N, Gault DT. Ann Plast Surg 1997; 39: 366–73.

Grobbelaar et al. report using a CO_2 laser to treat multiple tumors rapidly and successfully, resulting in complete destruction without recurrence at 26-month follow-up. CO_2 laser is a promising modality for treating multiple BCCs, with the advantages of a 2–3-week healing time, minimal postoperative pain, and acceptable cosmetic results. Side effects include postoperative erythema lasting up to 3 months, as well as hypo- and hyperpigmentation.

Microscopically controlled surgical excision combined with ultrapulse CO_2 vaporization in the management of a patient with the nevoid basal cell carcinoma syndrome. Krunic AL, Viehman E, Madani S, Clark RE. J Dermatol 1998; 25: 10–12.

Krunic et al. used an ultrapulse CO_2 laser in combination with MMS to treat large plaque tumors and reported no recurrence of the treated areas at 15-month follow-up.

Full-face carbon dioxide laser resurfacing in the management of a patient with the nevoid basal cell carcinoma syndrome. Doctoroff A, Oberlender SA, Purcell SM. Dermatol Surg 2003; 29: 1236–40.

A CO_2 laser was used to treat a 32-year-old woman with numerous BCCs on the face that were not amenable to other surgical modalities. Two months after the procedure she presented with two BCCs on her face, which were treated with MMS. At 10-month follow-up she presented with four BCCs on the face, three of which were removed by MMS. Imiquimod successfully treated one of the tumors, which was located on her nose.

Recent research presents CO_2 lasers as an effective therapy for patients with multiple BCCs in whom complete surgical excision and other treatment modalities are impractical. This therapy is most effective when used in combination with other treatment modalities.

Cryosurgery for cutaneous malignancy: an update. Kuflik EG. Dermatol Surg 1997; 23: 1081–7.

Cryosurgery is best suited to superficial non-infiltrating tumors with well-defined borders. It is not effective for morpheaform or infiltrating histologic subtypes, recurrent lesions, or deeply penetrating or very aggressive tumors. Advantages of this procedure include its effectiveness in treating large superficial tumors, tumors that are fixed to cartilage, and lesions located within a burn scar. This therapy also provides an alternative for high-risk surgical patients, such as the elderly and those with coagulopathy or with a pacemaker. Cryosurgery should be avoided in people of color and those with cryoglobulinemia. Reported cure rates are as high, at 98.4%, with a 5-year cure rate of 99% for primary tumors.

Cryosurgery and topical fluorouracil: a treatment method for widespread basal cell epithelioma in basal cell nevus syndrome. Tsuji T, Otake N, Nishimura M. J Dermatol 1993; 20: 507–13.

Evidence Levels: **A** Double-blind study **B** Clinical trial ≥ 20 subjects **C** Clinical trial < 20 subjects **D** Series ≥ 5 subjects **E** Anecdotal case reports

Combined therapy with cryosurgery and topical 5% 5-FU was more effective in producing complete clinical and histologic clearance of BCCs in a patient with NBCCS than either modality used alone.

Long-term management of basal cell nevus syndrome with topical tretinoin and 5-fluorouracil. Strange PR, Lang PG. J Am Acad Dermatol 1992; 27: 842–5.

The topical retinoid tretinoin has been shown to exhibit a chemopreventive benefit in skin cancer. Strange and Lang report successful treatment of a child with NBCCS for 10 years using 0.1% tretinoin and 5% 5-FU creams. They state that hundreds of superficial BCCs initially present disappeared with the combination therapy, leaving fewer than 20 at any given time, with no growth of these remaining tumors. They concluded that the regimen was both therapeutic and tumor suppressive, and had an excellent safety profile as developmental or laboratory abnormalities were not found.

Topical 5% 5-FU has been used to treat sporadic superficial BCCs as well as BCCs associated with NBCCS. Studies to date yield conflicting results of the effectiveness of 5-FU in the treatment of NBCCS. As previously mentioned, 5-FU is more effective in promoting complete tumor clearance in NBCCS when combined with another treatment modality, such as cryosurgery or tretinoin.

Nevoid basal cell carcinoma syndrome successfully treated with trichloroacetic acid and phenol peeling. Kaminaka C, Yamamoto Y, Furukawa F. J Dermatol 2007; 34: 841–3.

A 76-year-old woman with NBCCS presented with multiple superficial BCCs on the face, leg, and back. A 60% TCA and phenol peel was applied to the back until the lesions demonstrated frosting three times over the course of a month. Mild erythema and erosion occurred during treatment. Two years later, no new or recurrent lesions were observed.

Widespread basal cell carcinoma of the scalp treated by dermabrasion. Melandri D, Carruthers A. J Am Acad Dermatol 1992; 26: 270–1.

A patient with multiple confluent BCCs on the scalp developed recurrent BCC despite numerous surgical and MMS procedures. The entire scalp underwent dermabrasion, with complete healing within 6–7 days, and only one recurrent BCC formed within 6 years.

Intralesional interferon therapy for basal cell carcinoma. Cornell RC, Greenway HT, Tucker SB, Edwards L, Ashworth S, Vance JC, et al. J Am Acad Dermatol 1990; 23: 694–700.

Different treatment modalities for the management of a patient with the nevoid basal cell carcinoma syndrome. Kopera D, Cerroni L, Fink-Puches R, Kerl H. J Am Acad Dermatol 1996; 34: 937–9.

Failure of interferon alfa and isotretinoin combination therapy in the nevoid basal cell carcinoma syndrome. Sollitto R, DiGiovanna J. Arch Dermatol 1996; 132: 94–5.

In the study by Cornell et al., a patient with BCCs not associated with NBCCS received three intralesional injections per week of interferon-α_{2b} at a dose of 1.5 million IU for 3 weeks, resulting in complete regression of 81% of the lesions at 1 year with an excellent cosmetic outcome. Kopera et al. administered the same dosing and time schedule of intralesional interferon-α_{2b} to a patient with NBCCS and noted only a reduction in size and flattening of the lesions, and subsequently treated the patient with CO_2 laser. Therefore, Kopera et al. concluded that interferon-α_{2b} is inadequate in the eradication of BCCs in patients with NBCCS. Sollitto et al. combined isotretinoin 2 mg/kg daily and intralesional interferon-α, and found clearance in only one of three lesions at the end of 7 weeks in a patient with NBCCS.

To date, intralesional interferon to treat BCC has been used largely for investigational purposes. Its use is limited by its high cost and side-effect profile of flu-like symptoms. More studies are required to determine the effectiveness and clinical usefulness of intralesional interferon in NBCCS. In a number of studies, however, intralesional interferon has been shown to cause regression in noduloulcerative and superficial lesions.

Successful treatment of an intractable case of hereditary basal cell carcinoma syndrome with paclitaxel. El Sobky RA, Kallab AM, Dainer PM, Jillella AP, Lesher JL Jr. Arch Dermatol 2001; 137: 827–8.

A 54-year-man with NBCCS was treated with 19 cycles of the chemotherapeutic agent paclitaxel. The treatment was well tolerated and without toxicity. At 16-month follow-up most of his pre-existing lesions had healed without scarring. The BCCs that were still present were clinically regressing and no new ones were noted.

Nevus sebaceus

Stuart R Lessin, Clifford S Perlis

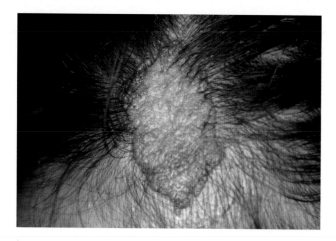

Nevus sebaceus, first described by Jadassohn in 1895, is a term for a congenital hamartoma of the epidermis and adnexal structures typically involving the scalp and face. It presents at birth or appears in early childhood as a pink, orange or yellow waxy plaque with a granular pitted surface that is often hairless. The size and configuration can be variable. During puberty the lesion thickens and becomes verrucous as glands enlarge within the dermis. Development of cutaneous and adnexal neoplasms has been reported in 10–20% of lesions after puberty and in adulthood. These neoplasms are most commonly benign. Surgical treatment addresses cosmetic issues, as well as prophylaxis or treatment of secondary neoplasms.

MANAGEMENT STRATEGY

For most lesions, clinical examination is sufficient to establish the diagnosis. A skin biopsy can confirm the clinical impression when indicated. Most neoplastic growths that arise in a nevus sebaceus do not develop until after the age of 16 years; the overwhelming majority are benign. These include syringocystadenoma papilliferum, trichoblastoma, tricholemmoma, sebaceoma, nevocellular nevus, and seborrheic keratosis. The most common malignancy that develops within a nevus sebaceous is a basal cell carcinoma, but the absolute incidence is very rare. Isolated case reports describe rare patients who have developed sebaceous carcinoma, squamous cell carcinoma, tricholemmal carcinoma, or microcystic adnexal carcinoma within a nevus sebaceus. The management strategies outlined in this chapter refer to lesions unaccompanied by extracutaneous features of the linear nevus sebaceous syndrome.

In 2000, a case series established that trichoblastoma was the most common neoplasm arising in nevus sebaceus. With this evidence of minimal risk of malignant neoplastic transformation, prophylactic surgery is not justified. Conservative management with clinical observation and biopsy of any lesions suspicious for malignancy appears to be most prudent.

Tumors arising in nevus sebaceus: A study of 596 cases. Cribier B, Scrivener Y, Grosshans E. J Am Acad Dermatol 2000; 42: 263–8.

A retrospective case series of 596 cases demonstrating a 1.7% occurrence of benign tumors in childhood. Most tumors arising in nevus sebaceus occurred in adults over 40; in these cases, 2.1% of the neoplasms were basal cell carcinomas. The authors conclude that prophylactic surgery in children is of uncertain benefit.

Should nevus sebaceus of Jadassohn in children be excised? A study of 757 cases, and literature review. Santibanez-Gallerani A, Marshall D, Duarte AM, Melnick SJ, Thaller S. J Craniofac Surg 2003; 14: 658–60.

A retrospective case series of 757 children aged 16 years or younger. No cases of basal cell cancer were found. The authors questioned the need for prophylactic excision in children.

Trichoblastoma is the most common neoplasm developed in nevus sebaceus of Jadassohn: a clinicopathologic study of a series of 155 cases. Jaqueti G, Requena L, Sánchez Yus E. Am J Dermatopathol 2000; 22: 108–18.

A retrospective case series of 155 patients failed to reveal any cases of basal cell carcinoma. Trichoblastoma was the most common (7.7%) basaloid tumor. It appears that histologic misinterpretation of trichoblastomas as basal cell carcinoma has been responsible for the erroneous reporting of an increased risk of basal cell carcinoma development within nevus sebaceus. The authors concluded that early prophylactic surgery seems inappropriate.

SPECIFIC INTERVENTIONS

▶ Skin biopsy

A skin biopsy may be performed to confirm a clinical diagnosis. Clinical changes suggestive of neoplastic transformation should be investigated by skin biopsy.

FIRST-LINE THERAPIES

▶ Observation	D
▶ Surgical excision	E

Based on recent case series and histological analyses demonstrating that the incidence of basal carcinoma is rare, particularly in children, clinical observation should be considered as the first option for any intervention. Prophylactic surgical excision is not warranted based on current data. Elective surgical excision may be considered if lesions become symptomatic, or for cosmetic reasons. In instances of biopsy-confirmed neoplastic transformation, management should be dictated by the histology of the specific tumor.

Should naevus sebaceus be excised prophylactically? A clinical audit. Barkham MC, White N, Brundler MA, Richard B, Moss C. J Plast Reconstruct Aesthet Surg 2007; 60: 1269–70.

A retrospective case series of 63 cases, 37 seen by plastic surgeons and 26 by dermatologists. Plastic surgeons excised 28 of 37 cases and dermatologists excised four of 26 cases. No malignant changes were seen in the 32 excisions; only one apocrine adenoma was found. The authors concluded that prophylactic surgery is not warranted.

Evidence Levels: **A** Double-blind study **B** Clinical trial ≥ 20 subjects **C** Clinical trial < 20 subjects **D** Series ≥ 5 subjects **E** Anecdotal case reports

SECOND-LINE THERAPIES

▶ Curettage and cautery	E
▶ Cryotherapy	E
▶ Laser resurfacing	E
▶ Photodynamic therapy	E

A variety of destructive methods have been described for the treatment of nevus sebaceus and provide an alternative to surgical excision; however, they may not be as effective at removing deeper structures.

Photodynamic therapy for nevus sebaceus with topical delta-aminolevulinic acid. Dierickx CC, Goldenhersh M, Dwyer P, Stratigos A, Mihm M, Anderson RR. Arch Dermatol 1999; 135: 637–40.

A case report of the use of photodynamic therapy with topical δ-aminolevulinic acid for elective treatment of a large nevus sebaceus of the face in a patient with cosmetic concerns who did not wish to undergo surgical excision. An excellent cosmetic result was obtained, though post-treatment skin biopsy revealed residual sebaceous tissue in the reticular dermis, underlying the normal-appearing epidermis and widened and fibrotic dermis.

Linear nevus sebaceus of Jadassohn treated with the carbon dioxide laser. Ashinoff R. Pediatr Dermatol 1993;10: 189–91.

A case report of the use of a carbon dioxide laser to electively treat a nevus sebaceus of the nose in a 10-year-old boy. Carbon dioxide laser vaporization provided partial and superficial destruction, with a good palliative appearance-enhancing result. The treatment did not eliminate the need for continued clinical surveillance.

Onchocerciasis

Michele E Murdoch

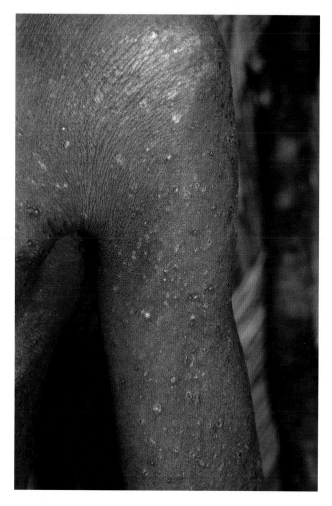

Onchocerciasis is a major tropical parasitic infection caused by the filarial worm *Onchocerca volvulus* and is transmitted by blood-sucking *Simulium* spp. blackflies, which breed near fast-flowing rivers. The disease is endemic in 30 countries in sub-Saharan Africa; small foci also exist in the Yemen and Central and Southern America (Mexico, Guatemala, Ecuador, Colombia, Venezuela, and Brazil). Recent global estimates suggest that 37 million people carry *O. volvulus*, most of whom live in Africa. A total of 90 million people are considered at risk of infection because of where they live. The first manifestation of infection is usually intense pruritus, and subsequently a wide variety of acute and chronic skin and eye changes develop.

MANAGEMENT STRATEGY

The socioeconomic consequences of onchocerciasis are most marked in hyperendemic areas in sub-Saharan Africa. Globally, approximately 270 000 people are blind and 500 000 have significant visual loss as a direct consequence of onchocerciasis. A multi-country study in Africa revealed that 42% of the adult population in endemic villages suffered from pruritus, and 28% of the population had onchocercal skin lesions.

The global control of onchocerciasis hinges on strategies to reduce the level of disease in endemic areas until it is no longer a significant public health problem. Three Regional Programs have been established to coordinate control. The Onchocerciasis Control Program (OCP, 1974–2002) successfully used *aerial larviciding* of rivers in West Africa to control the vector blackfly, and more recently it has distributed *ivermectin* to control any recrudescence. The Onchocerciasis Elimination Program in the Americas (OEPA), which has been running since 1991, aims to eliminate clinical manifestations of onchocerciasis and interrupt transmission of disease altogether using 6-monthly mass ivermectin therapy. The largest program, the African Program for Onchocerciasis Control (APOC), commenced in 1995 and has now been extended to run until 2015. It consists of large-scale annual distribution of ivermectin in 19 non-OCP countries. Ivermectin is a safe, effective microfilaricide (i.e., it kills the immature larval stages of filarial worms), but as it does not kill the adult worms; when given annually, treatment has to be repeated throughout the lifespan of the adult worm (10–14 years). A few months after dosing with ivermectin, the numbers of microfilariae in the skin gradually increase back towards pre-treatment levels, so a single dose of ivermectin per year may not completely interrupt transmission.

Recently, *Wolbachia* spp. symbiotic endobacteria have been identified as essential for the filarial worms' fertility, and offer novel targets for mass treatment. Additional treatment with *doxycycline* to sterilize the worms may thus enhance ivermectin-induced suppression of microfilaridermia and is a promising basis for blocking transmission (Onchocerciasis. Hoerauf A, Büttner DW, Adjei O, Pearlman E. Br Med J 2003; 326: 207–10).

Onchocerciasis and lymphatic filariasis commonly coexist, and current integrated control programs use repeated *annual mass treatment of endemic communities with ivermectin and albendazole.*

SPECIFIC INVESTIGATIONS

- ▶ Skin snips
- ▶ Other parasitological forms of diagnosis
- – Detection of intraocular microfilariae using a slit lamp
- – Demonstration of adult worms by collagenase digestion of excised nodules
- ▶ Full blood count (for eosinophilia)
- ▶ Mazzotti test
- ▶ Future investigative tools
- – Diethylcarbamazine (DEC) patch test
- – Serodiagnosis
- – Polymerase chain reaction (PCR)
- – Antigen detection dipstick assay on urine

FIRST-LINE THERAPIES

▶ Ivermectin	A
▶ Ivermectin combined with doxycycline	A

The effects of ivermectin on onchocercal skin disease and severe itching: results of a multicentre trial. Brieger WR, Awedoba AK, Eneanya CI, Hagan M, Ogbuagu KF, Okello DO, et al. Trop Med Int Health 1998; 3: 951–61.

Evidence Levels: A Double-blind study   B Clinical trial ≥ 20 subjects   C Clinical trial < 20 subjects   D Series ≥ 5 subjects   E Anecdotal case reports

The effects of ivermectin were assessed in 3-monthly, 6-monthly, and annual doses in 4072 villagers in forest zones of Ghana, Nigeria, and Uganda who underwent interviews and clinical examinations at baseline and at five follow-up visits. Reactive skin lesions were categorized as acute papular onchodermatitis, chronic papular onchodermatitis, and lichenified onchodermatitis. From 6 months onwards there was a 40–50% reduction in the prevalence of severe itching after ivermectin treatment compared to the placebo group. Also, a greater reduction in prevalence and severity of reactive skin lesions over time was seen in those receiving ivermectin. The differences between the various ivermectin treatment regimens were not significant.

A trial of a three-dose regimen of ivermectin for the treatment of patients with onchocerciasis in the UK. Churchill DR, Godfrey-Faussett P, Birley HDL, Malin A, Davidson RN, Bryceson ADM. Trans Roy Soc Trop Med Hyg 1994; 88: 242.

As ivermectin is also thought to suppress embryogenesis in adult worms, the efficacy of three doses of ivermectin given at monthly intervals was studied to determine whether such a regimen could lead to a greater suppression of microfilaridermia. Thirty-three patients (of whom 27 were European) with onchocerciasis were treated with a single dose of 150–200 µg/kg ivermectin and observed in hospital for 72 hours. Second and third doses were given as outpatient treatment respectively 1 and 2 months later. Patients were followed up at 3-, 6-, and 12-monthly intervals after the last dose of ivermectin. The patients with positive skin snips prior to treatment were compared with patients given a single dose of ivermectin in a previous study (Godfrey-Faussett P., et al., 1991, see below). Relapses occurred slightly less frequently after three doses.

In contrast to studies in West Africa, where reactions to ivermectin are rare, 17 patients (52%) had reactions. The authors therefore recommend that the first dose of ivermectin for lightly infected expatriates be given in hospital.

The treatment of expatriates lightly infected with onchocerciasis is therefore a single dose of 150–200 µg/kg ivermectin with observation in hospital for 72 hours, followed by two subsequent doses at monthly intervals. If there is a recurrence of itching, a typical rash, or eosinophilia, the individual may require further doses of ivermectin at 6–12-monthly intervals.

Ivermectin in the treatment of onchocerciasis in Britain. Godfrey-Faussett P, Dow C, Black ME, Bryceson ADM. Trop Med Parasitol 1991; 42: 82–4.

Thirty-one patients with early, light infection were treated with a single dose of 150–200 µg/kg ivermectin. Those who relapsed were re-treated after an interval of not less than 5 months. Approximately two-thirds relapsed within 1 year. A similar pattern was seen after the second dose. A single dose of ivermectin, repeated every 3–6 months as necessary, was considered to be the treatment of choice for patients in non-endemic areas lightly infected with *O. volvulus*. One-third of such patients may be cured with each treatment.

Effects of standard and high doses of ivermectin on adult worms of *Onchocerca volvulus*: a randomised controlled trial. Gardon J, Boussinesq M, Kamgno J, Gardon-Wendel N, Demanga-Ngangue, Duke BOL. Lancet 2002; 360: 203–10.

Ivermectin 150 µg/kg given at intervals of 0.5–3.0 months is known to cause slight but significant increased mortality of adult worms. In this randomized study of 657 Cameroonian patients with onchocerciasis, 3-monthly treatment with ivermectin killed more female adult worms than did annual treatment. There was no difference between standard (150 µg/kg) and high-dose schedules (800 µg/kg).

The feasibility of large-scale 3-monthly ivermectin treatment in endemic areas and its likely greater effect in reducing transmission have still to be determined.

An investigation of persistent microfilaridermias despite multiple treatments with ivermectin, in two onchocerciasis-endemic foci in Ghana. Awadzi K, Boakye DA, Edwards G, Opoku NO, Attah SK, Osei-Atweneboana MY, et al. Ann Trop Med Parasitol 2004; 98: 231–49.

Some individuals in endemic areas have persistent microfilaridermia despite nine treatments with ivermectin. In this open, case–control study of 21 'suboptimal' responders, seven amicrofilaridermic responders, and 14 ivermectin-naive subjects, the results revealed that the persistent microfilaridermias are mainly due to non-responsiveness of the adult female worms, raising the possibility that the worms have developed resistance to ivermectin.

Adverse systemic reactions to treatment of onchocerciasis with ivermectin at normal and high doses given annually or three-monthly. Kamgno J, Gardon J, Gardon-Wendel N, Demanga-Ngangue, Duke BO, Boussinesq M. Trans Roy Soc Trop Med Hyg 2004; 98: 496–504.

In Cameroon, after the first dose, ivermectin 150 µg/kg given at 3-monthly intervals was associated with a reduced risk of reactions (especially edematous swellings, pruritus, and back pain) compared with standard annual treatment doses of 150 µg/kg. High doses of ivermectin (800 µg/kg) at annual and 3-monthly intervals caused subjective ocular symptoms.

Endosymbiotic bacteria in worms as targets for a novel chemotherapy in filariasis. Hoerauf A, Volkmann L, Hamelmann C, Adjei O, Autenrieth IB, Fleischer B, et al. Lancet 2000; 355: 1242–3.

The activity of doxycycline against endosymbiotic *Wolbachia* spp. bacteria and the fertility of adult female worms were assessed by examination of excised subcutaneous onchocercal nodules in 22 Ghanaian individuals treated with doxycycline 100 mg daily for 6 weeks and 14 untreated controls. Immunohistology with an antibody to bacterial heat shock protein-60 was used to assess the presence or absence of *Wolbachia* spp., and the morphology of female worms was examined. In addition, PCR reactions using, first, endobacterial primers, and second, nematode primers, were performed. None of the treated worms had usual bacterial loads, and there was total suppression of normal embryonic worm development during early oocyte/morula stages, whereas nodules from untreated controls showed normal embryogenesis.

Depletion of *Wolbachia* endobacteria in *Onchocerca volvulus* by doxycycline and microfilaridermia after ivermectin treatment. Hoerauf A, Mand S, Adjei O, Fleischer B, Büttner DW. Lancet 2001; 357: 1415–16.

The Ghanian participants in this study were not randomized because this was not acceptable to the village elders. Instead, the first 55 patients were allocated to ivermectin and doxycycline, and the next 33 to ivermectin alone. Doxycycline 100 mg daily was given from the start of the study for 6 weeks. Subgroup A (31 doxycycline-treated and 24 controls) was given ivermectin 2.5 months after the start of the study and subgroup B (24 doxycycline-treated and nine controls)

6 months after the onset of the study. The results suggested a complete block in worm embryogenesis for at least 18 months after treatment with ivermectin and doxycycline.

The principle of targeting *Wolbachia* spp. with ivermectin in combination treatment offers the potential of interrupting transmission. Shorter anti-*Wolbachia* spp. regimens (either with other antibiotics or in combinations) are needed for mass treatment of endemic areas.

***Wolbachia* endobacteria depletion by doxycycline as antifilarial therapy has macrofilaricidal activity in onchocerciasis: a randomized placebo-controlled study.** Hoerauf A, Specht S, Büttner M, Pfarr K, Mand S, Fimmers R, et al. Med Microbiol Immunol 2008; 197: 295–311.

In a randomized, placebo-controlled trial in Ghana, 67 onchocerciasis patients received 200 mg/day doxycycline for 4 or 6 weeks, followed by ivermectin after 6 months. After 6, 20, and 27 months, efficacy was evaluated by onchocercoma histology, PCR, and microfilariae determination. Administration of doxycycline resulted in endobacteria depletion and female worm sterilization. The 6-week treatment was macrofilaricidal, with >60% of the female worms found dead.

A combination of doxycycline (100 mg daily for 6 weeks) plus ivermectin is now advisable for individuals leaving an onchocerciasis-endemic area for a long time.

No depletion of *Wolbachia* from *Onchocerca volvulus* after a short course of rifampin and/or azithromycin. Richards FO Jr, Amann J, Arana B, Punkosdy G, Klein R, Blanco C, et al. Am J Trop Med Hyg 2007; 77: 878–82.

In this open-label trial in Guatemala, 73 patients with 134 palpable onchocercal nodules were randomized into four treatment groups: rifampin, azithromycin, a combination of the two drugs, and controls (multivitamins). After 5 days of antibiotic treatment, all participants received a single dose of ivermectin on day 6. Nine months after treatment, the nodules were removed and the worms were examined. Skin snips to determine microfilariae were obtained at baseline and after 9 months. There were no significant differences between any of the treatment groups in the condition of the worms in the nodules, the presence of *Wolbachia* surface protein, or the number of microfilariae in skin.

Short courses with these antibiotics will not clear Wolbachia *from* O. volvulus.

Effects of 6-week azithromycin treatment on the *Wolbachia* endobacteria of *Onchocerca volvulus*. Hoerauf A, Marfo-Debrekyei Y, Büttner M, Debrah AY, Konadu P, Mand S, et al. Parasitol Res 2008; 103: 279–86.

The authors concluded that azithromycin administered alone for 6 weeks at 250 mg/day or 1200 mg once a week was not suitable for treatment of onchocerciasis. However, they suggested that daily azithromycin should be studied in combination with other drugs and with other doses.

SECOND-LINE THERAPIES

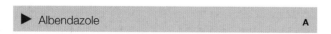

▶ Albendazole   **A**

Albendazole in the treatment of onchocerciasis: double-blind clinical trial in Venezuela. Cline BL, Hernandez JL, Mather FJ, Bartholomew R, De Maza SN, Rodulfo S, et al. Am J Trop Med Hyg 1992; 47: 512–20.

Forty-nine individuals with onchocerciasis (26 treated and 23 controls) were treated with a 10-day course of albendazole (400 mg daily) or placebo. Patients in the albendazole-treated group with baseline microfilarial densities over 5 mf/mg skin showed a significant reduction in microfilarial densities at 12 months. Albendazole was well tolerated and is believed to interfere with embryogenesis in adult *O. volvulus* worms.

The co-administration of ivermectin and albendazole – safety, pharmacokinetics and efficacy against *Onchocerca volvulus*. Awadzi K, Edwards G, Duke BO, Opoku NO, Attah SK, Addy ET, et al. Ann Trop Med Parasitol 2003; 97: 165–78.

In a randomized double-blind, placebo-controlled trial in 44 male patients with onchocerciasis in Ghana, the co-administration of ivermectin (200 μg/kg) with albendazole (400 mg) did not offer any advantage over ivermectin alone.

The safety, tolerability and pharmacokinetics of levamisole alone, levamisole plus ivermectin, and levamisole plus albendazole, and their efficacy against *Onchocerca volvulus*. Awadzi K, Edwards G, Opoku NO, Ardrey AE, Favager S, Addy ET, et al. Ann Trop Med Parasitol 2004; 98: 595–614.

Levamisole (2.5 mg/kg) given alone or with albendazole (400 mg) had little effect on *O. volvulus*. Co-administration of ivermectin (200 μg/kg) with levamisole was no more effective than ivermectin alone.

OTHER THERAPIES

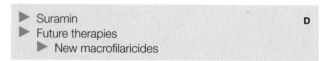

▶ Suramin   **D**
▶ Future therapies
  ▶ New macrofilaricides

Thirty-month follow-up of sub-optimal responders to multiple treatments with ivermectin, in two onchocerciasis-endemic foci in Ghana. Awadzi K, Attah SK, Addy ET, Opoku NO, Quartey BT, Lazdins-Helds JK, et al. Ann Trop Med Parasitol 2004; 98: 359–70.

A macrofilaricide is a drug that can kill adult parasite worms and hence a single course of treatment is potentially curative. Suramin is both a macrofilaricide and a microfilaricide, but unfortunately a course of suramin requires weekly intravenous infusions and may have serious adverse effects, including nephrotoxicity. After the use of ivermectin became widely established the only indications for suramin were the curative treatment of selected individuals in areas without transmission and that of individuals leaving an endemic area; and severe hyper-reactive onchodermatitis unresponsive to repeated treatments with ivermectin.

In this paper Awadzi et al. propose the use of suramin under hospital supervision in selected individuals with onchocerciasis who are resistant to multiple doses of ivermectin. The treatment regimen proposed was a total adult dose of 5.0 g (72.5–84.7 mg/kg) over 6 weeks.

The antiparasitic moxidectin: safety, tolerability, and pharmacokinetics in humans. Cotreau MM, Warren S, Ryan JL, Fleckenstein L, Vanapalli SR, Brown KR, et al. J Clin Pharmacol 2003; 43: 1108–15.

As there is now a considerable risk of the development of ivermectin resistance there is an urgent need to find a safe macrofilaricide suitable for large-scale field use. Molecules chemically related to known antiparasitic drugs are currently being evaluated. Moxidectin is already in use in veterinary medicine, and studies in animal models suggest that it is a potential macrofilaricidal agent. This preliminary study in healthy human male volunteers revealed that moxidectin is safe and well tolerated at doses of between 3 and 36 mg.

A new drug for river blindness? Kuesel A, Lazdins J. TDRnews 2007; 79: 15–19.

Moxidectin is currently being evaluated in a TDR-sponsored phase II clinical trial of 192 people in Ghana, led by Dr Kwablah Awadzi. Wyeth, the owner of moxidectin, is providing the drug and operational support. The trial has been designed to show whether moxidectin can inhibit the production of microfilariae more effectively than ivermectin, either by killing the adult worms or by sterilizing them.

Oral lichen planus

Drore Eisen

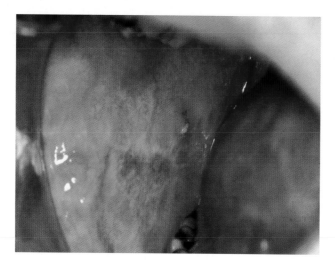

Oral lichen planus (OLP) is a common chronic inflammatory disorder which rarely undergoes complete remission even with treatment.

MANAGEMENT STRATEGY

All treatment should be aimed at eliminating erythematous and ulcerative lesions, alleviating symptoms, and potentially reducing the risk of malignant transformation. Given the uncertainty of the premalignant nature of OLP, it is important to monitor all patients carefully and long term.

Although the etiology of OLP is unknown, the possibility of a hypersensitivity reaction to a dental restoration (oral lichenoid reaction) should be considered when lesions are confined to mucosa in close proximity to amalgam restorations. In such cases, identifying allergies to dental materials by patch testing, and then removing the fillings with positive reactions, or empirically removing the filling, often results in resolution of the lesions. Another uncommon cause of oral lichenoid reactions are drugs. A thorough medication history, with emphasis on non-steroidal anti-inflammatory drugs and angiotensin-converting enzyme inhibitors, is warranted, as drug-induced reactions are reversible when the implicated drug is withdrawn.

Eliminating or minimizing exacerbating factors, including sharp or rough dental restorations, fractured teeth, and poorly fitting dental appliances, should be attempted before medical therapy is initiated. The institution of an optimal oral hygiene program that eliminates dental plaque and calculus also significantly improves gingival OLP.

All of the agents used for the treatment of oral lichen planus are for off-label indications and lack adequate efficacy studies; thus, such factors as optimal dose, duration of treatment, safety, and their true efficacy remain unknown.

The most useful agents for the treatment of OLP are *potent topical corticosteroids* such as fluocinonide or clobetasol. Patients should continue therapy on all symptomatic lesions. Asymptomatic reticular lesions do not require therapy. For OLP affecting the gingiva, custom dental trays that fit over the teeth can be filled with topical corticosteroids and worn for prolonged periods. For intractable erosive lesions, *intralesional triamcinolone acetonide* (10–20 mg/mL) can be highly effective and repeated every 2–4 weeks.

Unresponsive OLP may benefit from *topical immunomodulators* such as tacrolimus, picrolimus, and ciclosporin. These may be used as alternatives to, or in conjunction with, topical corticosteroids. Burning and stinging are the most frequent adverse effects, and relapses after cessation of therapy are to be expected. Given the potential association of these immunosuppressants with an increased risk of cancer, their long-term use for this chronic, potentially premalignant disease may be limited.

For patients with severe oral disease or with extraoral manifestations, the addition of *systemic immunosuppressives* is indicated. The author has found that methotrexate (12.5–20 mg/week), azathioprine (100–150 mg/day), mycophenolate mofetil (1–2 g/day), acitretin (25–50 mg/day), and hydroxychloroquine (400 mg/day) are the most useful systemic agents. Ciclosporin, thalidomide, and TNF-α inhibitors may be used for refractory cases, but data are limited.

Systemic corticosteroids (30–80 mg of prednisone) should be reserved for acute flares and not used as maintenance therapy. Secondary candidiasis frequently complicates all therapy and should be treated with topical or systemic antifungal agents. All treatments for OLP are palliative and not curative, and patients should expect a chronic course with intermittent acute exacerbations.

SPECIFIC INVESTIGATIONS

> ► Biopsy for confirmation; direct immunofluorescence when needed to rule out other vesiculoerosive diseases
> ► Monitoring for malignant transformation
> ► Hepatitis serologies when risk factors are present
> ► Consider lichenoid reactions

The sensitivity and specificity of direct immunofluoresence testing in disorders of mucous membranes. Helander SD, Rogers RS III. J Am Acad Dermatol 1994; 30: 65–75.

OLP gingival lesions are often non-diagnostic, and a biopsy for immunofluorescence shows characteristic shaggy fibrinogen deposition at the basement membrane zone.

Oral lichen planus: controversies surrounding malignant transformation. Gonzalez-Moles MA, Scully C, Gil-Montoya JA. Oral Dis 2008; 14: 229–43.

Although the malignant potential of OLP is still subject to controversy, the frequency of malignant change ranges from 0.4% to 3.3%, over periods of observation from 0.5 to over 20 years.

The clinical features, malignant potential, and systemic associations of oral lichen planus: a study of 723 patients. Eisen DR. J Am Acad Dermatol 2002; 46: 207–14.

The association between hepatitis infection and OLP may depend on geographic factors.

Based on the findings in this large series, routine hepatitis screening in western European and American patients is not warranted.

Oral lichen planus and allergy to dental amalgam restorations. Laeijendecker R, Dekker SK, Burger PM, Mulder PG, Van Joost T, Neumann MH. Arch Dermatol 2004; 140: 1434–8.

When patch test reactions to mercury compounds were positive, partial or complete replacement of amalgam fillings led to a significant improvement in nearly all patients.

FIRST-LINE THERAPIES

▷ Topical corticosteroids	**B**
▷ Intralesional corticosteroids	**B**

Systemic and topical corticosteroid treatment of oral lichen planus: a comparative study with long-term follow-up. Carbone M, Goss E, Carrozzo M, Castellano S, Conrotto D, Broccoletti R, et al. J Oral Pathol Med 2003; 32: 323–9.

Patients who were treated with topical clobetasol, or prednisone and then clobetasol, responded similarly, suggesting that systemic steroids should be reserved for acute exacerbations and not as an initial treatment.

Topical corticosteroids are the mainstay treatment for OLP. High-potency preparations appear to be more effective than mid-potency ones. Once the disease becomes inactive, therapy may be temporarily discontinued.

Short-term clinical evaluation of intralesional triamcinolone acetonide injection for ulcerative oral lichen planus. Xia J, Li C, Hong Y, Yang L, Huang Y, Cheng B. J Oral Pathol Med 2006; 35: 327–31.

Eighty-five percent of the 45 patients treated with intralesional triamcinolone achieved complete resolution of the treated ulcerations.

SECOND-LINE THERAPIES

Topical immunosuppressants	
▶ Tacrolimus	**A**
▶ Pimecrolimus	**A**
▶ Ciclosporin	**A**
Systemic immunosuppressants	
▶ Methotrexate	**E**
▶ Mycophenolate mofetil	**E**
▶ Azathioprine	**E**
▶ Hydroxychloroquine sulfate	**C**

Tacrolimus and pimecrolimus

A comparative treatment study of topical tacrolimus and clobetasol in oral lichen planus. Radfar L, Wild RC, Suresh L. Oral Surg Oral Med Oral Pathol Oral Radiol Endod 2008; 105: 187–93.

In this 6-week study comprising 30 patients, tacrolimus was shown to be as useful as clobetasol.

Long-term efficacy and safety of topical tacrolimus in the management of ulcerative/erosive oral lichen planus. Hodgson TA, Sahni N, Kaliakatsou F, Buchanan JA, Porter SR. Eur J Dermatol 2003; 13: 466–70.

Of 50 patients who used tacrolimus for 2–39 months, 14% had complete resolution of ulcers or erosions, 80% had partial resolution, and 6% reported no clinical benefit.

Randomized trial of pimecrolimus cream versus triamcinolone acetonide paste in the treatment of oral lichen planus. Gorouhi, F, Solhpour A, Beitollahi JM, Afshar S, Davari P, Hashemi P, et al. J Am Acad Dermatol 2007; 57: 806–13.

Pimecrolimus was as effective as 0.1% triamcinolone in 20 patients in this 2-month study.

Treatment of oral erosive lichen planus with 1% pimecrolimus cream: a double-blind, randomized, prospective trial with measurement of pimecrolimus levels in the blood. Passeron T, Lacour JP, Fontas E. Ortonne JP. Arch Dermatol 2007; 43: 472–6.

Although highly effective when used twice daily for 4 weeks, blood concentrations of pimecrolimus in this 14-patient study were consistently elevated, suggesting systemic absorption. Relapses occurred in all patients shortly after discontinuing therapy.

These studies all document the efficacy of topical applications of tacrolimus and pimecrolimus for symptomatic OLP. These drugs are not always effective: they do not result in long-term improvement, as relapses are expected when they are discontinued. Given the potential for systemic absorption and the warning that their use may be associated with an increased risk of cancer, their safety for long-term use in the oral cavity is still unknown.

Ciclosporin

Ciclosporin vs. clobetasol in the topical management of atrophic and erosive oral lichen planus: a double-blind, randomized controlled trial. Conrotto D, Carbone M, Carrozzo M, Arduino P, Broccoletti R, Pentenero M, et al. Br J Dermatol 2006; 154: 139–45.

In a 2-month study involving 40 patients, 65% of those applying ciclosporin improved, versus 95% of those who used clobetasol. Two months after discontinuing treatment, only one-third of the clobetasol group remained clear, versus three-quarters of the ciclosporin group.

Studies demonstrating the benefits of ciclosporin have been inconsistent. The high cost of swishing topical ciclosporin (500 mg/5 mL three times daily) limits its routine use, but swishing a small quantity reduces the cost, and even finger rub application using low doses (50 mg/day) in an adhesive base preparation has been shown to be beneficial.

Systemic immunosuppressants

Oral lichen planus: a case series with emphasis on therapy. Torti DC, Jorizzo JL, McCarty MA. Arch Dermatol 2007; 143: 511–15.

About 50% of OLP patients treated with low doses of methotrexate (2.5–12.5 mg/week) responded to therapy.

Successful treatment of oral erosive lichen planus with mycophenolate mofetil. Dalmau J, Puig L, Roe E, Peramiquel L, Campos M, Alomar A. J Eur Acad Dermatol Venereol 2007; 21: 259–60.

Hydroxychloroquine sulfate (Plaquenil) improves oral lichen planus: an open trial. Eisen D. J Am Acad Dermatol 1993; 28: 609–12.

Nine of 10 patients had an excellent response to hydroxychloroquine 200–400 mg daily for 6 months. Erosions required 3–6 months of treatment before they resolved.

A prospective study of findings and management in 214 patients with oral lichen planus. Silverman S Jr, Gorsky M, Lozada-Nur F, Giannotti K. Oral Surg Oral Med Oral Pathol Oral Radiol Endod 1991; 72: 665–70.

Azathioprine (50–150 mg/day) is effective but may require 3–6 months of therapy before maximal benefit is achieved.

Systemic agents appear to offer significantly better results than topical agents alone. None produces a long-term remission when discontinued, but significant clinical benefits are often achieved and maintained with long-term administration. Topical therapy should be maintained while systemic treatment continues.

THIRD-LINE THERAPIES

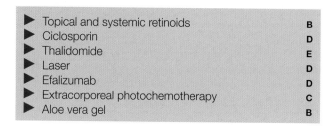

▶ Topical and systemic retinoids	B
▶ Ciclosporin	D
▶ Thalidomide	E
▶ Laser	D
▶ Efalizumab	D
▶ Extracorporeal photochemotherapy	C
▶ Aloe vera gel	B

Topical tretinoin therapy and oral lichen planus. Sloberg K, Hersle K, Mobacken H, Thilander H. Arch Dermatol 1979; 115: 716–18.

More than 70% of the 23 patients treated with 0.1% tretinoin improved.

Oral lichen planus: a preliminary clinical study on treatment with tazarotene. Petruzzi M, De Benedittis M, Grassi R, Cassano N, Vena G, Serpico R. Oral Dis 2002, 8: 291–5.

As a monotherapy, topical retinoids have limited value in OLP, but in combination with topical corticosteroids, especially for reticular lesions, modest benefits may be achieved.

Treatment of oral erosive lichen planus with systemic isotretinoin. Camisa C, Allen CM. Oral Surg Oral Med Oral Pathol 1986; 62: 393–6.

Treatment of lichen planus with acitretin: a double-blind, placebo-controlled study in 65 patients. Laurberg G, Geiger JM, Hjorth N, Holm P, Hou-Jensen K, Jacobsen KU, et al. J Am Acad Dermatol 1991; 24: 434–7.

Systemic use of isotretinoin (10–60 mg/day) produces only modest benefits for OLP, and not in all cases. In a 2-month study in 65 patients, some with OLP, acitretin (30 mg/day) resulted in remis- sion or marked improvement in most cases. The majority of patients experienced adverse effects.

Severe lichen planus clears with very low-dose cyclosporine. Levell NJ, Munro CS, Marks JM. Br J Dermatol 1992; 127: 66–7.

Systemic ciclosporin should be reserved for refractory cases and used for a limited period only.

Effective treatment of oral erosive lichen planus with thalidomide. Camisa C, Popovsky JL. Arch Dermatol 2000; 136: 1442–3.

A single report of oral erosive LP resolving with thalidomide (50–100 mg daily).

Treatment of oral lichen planus with the 308-nm UVB excimer laser – early preliminary results in eight patients. Kollner K, Wimmershoff M, Landthaler M, Hohenleutner U. Lasers Surg Med 2003; 33: 158–60.

Six of eight patients showed clinical improvement.

A single-center, open-label, prospective pilot study of subcutaneous efalizumab for oral erosive lichen planus. Heffernan MP, Smith DI, Bentley D Tabacchi M, Graves JE. J Drugs Dermatol 2007; 6: 310–14.

Four patients treated for 12 weeks with 0.7 mg/kg showed improvement, but two had serious adverse effects.

Efalizumab is no longer available because reports of progressive multifocal leukoencephalopathy in patients with long-term use of the drug.

Treatment of refractory erosive oral lichen planus with extracorporeal photochemotherapy: 12 cases. Guyot AD, Fahri D, Ingen-Housz-Oro S, Bussel A, Parquet N, Rabian C, et al. Br J Dermatol 2007; 156: 553–6.

Nine of 12 patients had complete healing of erosions which relapsed when the treatments became less frequent or stopped.

The efficacy of aloe vera gel in the treatment of oral lichen planus: a randomized controlled trial. Choonhakarn C, Busaracome P, Sripanidkulchai B, Sarakarn P. Br J Dermatol 2008; 158: 573–7.

Twenty-two of 27 patients treated with aloe vera gel had improvement after 8 weeks.

Evidence Levels: **A** Double-blind study **B** Clinical trial ≥ 20 subjects **C** Clinical trial < 20 subjects **D** Series ≥ 5 subjects **E** Anecdotal case reports

Orf

Jane C Sterling

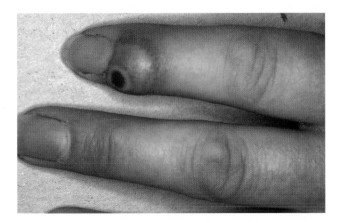

Orf is an infection by a parapoxvirus which causes inflammation and necrosis of the skin at the site of viral entry. It is predominantly an occupational disease in farmers, because the virus is carried by sheep and occasionally goats.

MANAGEMENT STRATEGY

Orf is a self-limiting infection and *treatment is usually not necessary*. The immune response to the virus usually results in resolution of the disease within 2–7 weeks without any specific treatment. There is no available treatment that is specifically antiviral for the orf virus, and no human vaccine has been produced. Treatment is usually only indicated if there is secondary bacterial infection or immunosuppression. Erythema multiforme can be triggered by orf infection: the treatment of this is as for any other case of erythema multiforme. Treatment of erythema multiforme is covered in a separate chapter.

Various treatments have been reported anecdotally. *Idoxuridine, surgery,* and *cryotherapy* have been suggested to reduce the time to healing. For immunosuppressed individuals, infection with orf may result in a more persistent infection or giant orf. In such cases interventional treatment is warranted. Surgery may be performed to remove the bulk of the infected tissue. Idoxuridine, *cidofovir,* and cryotherapy have also been reported to improve time to healing or to clear persistent infection. *Interferon,* and more recently *topical imiquimod* cream, have shown some potential benefit.

SPECIFIC INVESTIGATIONS

▶ Electron microscopy of scrapings from lesion
▶ Biopsy
▶ PCR

Diagnosis is usually clinical, but can be confirmed by the above investigations if required.

The structure of the orf virus. Nagington J, Newton A, Horne RW. Virology 1964; 23: 461–72.

An ultrastructural description of the orf virus.

Orf. Report of 19 human cases with clinical and pathological observations. Leavell UW, McNamara MJ, Muelling R, Talbert WM, Rucker RC, Dalton AJ. JAMA 1968; 204: 657–64.

Detailed description of the clinical and histological features of 19 cases of orf infection. Defines six stages of infection. Over half the lesions healed within 5 weeks.

Polymerase chain reaction for laboratory diagnosis of orf virus infections. Torfason EG, Gunadottir S. J Clin Virol 2002; 24: 79–84.

Method for molecular diagnosis of orf used as a research tool.

FIRST-LINE THERAPIES

▶ No specific treatment usually necessary

For most patients, treatment of this virus infection is unnecessary because natural clearance will occur.

Orf. Report of 19 human cases with clinical and pathological observations. Leavell UW, McNamara MJ, Muelling R, Talbert WM, Rucker RC, Dalton AJ. JAMA 1968; 204: 657–64.

Lymphangitis and lymphadenopathy occurred in three of 19 cases.

Awareness of the risk of secondary bacterial infection is important. This would merit therapy with a systemic antibiotic.

SECOND-LINE THERAPIES

▶ Surgery	D
▶ Cryotherapy	E
▶ Idoxuridine	E
▶ Cidofovir	E
▶ Interferon	E
▶ Imiquimod	D

Orf nodule: treatment with cryosurgery. Candiani JO, Soto RG, Lozano OW. J Am Acad Dermatol 1993; 29: 256–7.

A healthy female with orf received a single treatment with liquid nitrogen (two freeze–thaw cycles) and the lesion healed in 2 weeks.

A case of ecthyma contagiosum (human orf) treated with idoxuridine. Hunskaar S. Dermatologica 1984; 168: 207.

The orf lesion of a healthy female was treated with 40% idoxuridine in dimethylsulfoxide three times daily for 6 days. The lesion healed in under 4 weeks.

Parapoxvirus orf in kidney transplantation. Peeters P, Sennasael J. Nephrol Dial Transplant 1998; 13: 531.

A large lesion on the thumb recurred after excisional surgery. After 40% idoxuridine topically, further surgery, and repeated cryotherapy, the lesion resolved.

'Giant' orf of finger in a patient with a lymphoma. Savage J, Black MM. Proc Roy Soc Med 1972; 65: 766–8.

A patient who had received chemotherapy developed an enlarging orf lesion on one finger. The finger was amputated.

Giant orf in a patient with chronic lymphocytic leukaemia. Hunskaar S. Br J Dermatol 1986; 114: 631–4.

A large palmar orf lesion was excised and small local recurrences were treated with 40% idoxuridine.

A case of human orf in an immunocompromised patient treated successfully with cidofovir cream. Geerinck K, Lukito G, Snoeck R, DeVos R, DeClercq E, Varenterghe Y, et al. J Med Virol 2001; 64: 543–9.

An immunosuppressed renal transplant patient developed a persistent giant orf lesion. Treatment with 1% cidofovir cream daily for five cycles of 5 days of treatment alternating with 5 rest days plus debridement as necessary led to full resolution of the lesion.

Recurrent orf in an immunocompromised host. Tan ST, Blake GB, Chambers S. Br J Plast Surg 1991; 44: 465–7.

A tumor-like orf lesion in an immunosuppressed patient was unresponsive to surgery and idoxuridine. Temporary improvement occurred after 2 weeks of daily intralesional interferon, 1 million IU per injection, with clearance following repeat surgery with subcutaneous interferon (1 million IU daily).

Rapid improvement of human orf (ecthyma contagiosum) with topical imiquimod cream; report of four complicated cases. Erbagci Z, Erbagci I, Almila Tuncel A. J Dermatol Treat 2005; 16: 353–6.

Treatment with imiquimod 5% applied twice daily for up to 10 days to orf lesions complicated by erythema multiforme, angioedema or as giant orf; therapy possibly hastened clearance of the orf lesion and the secondary effects.

Palmoplantar keratoderma

Ravi Ratnavel

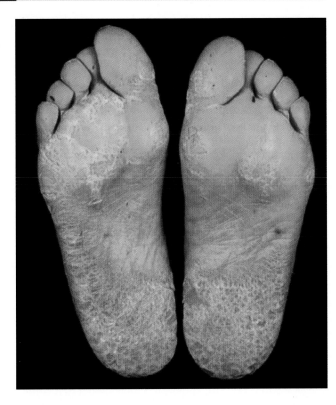

Palmoplantar keratodermas (PPKs) consist of a heterogeneous group of disorders characterized by thickening of the palms and soles. The condition may be subdivided into hereditary keratodermas, acquired forms, and syndromes with PPK as an associated feature of a specific dermatosis.

MANAGEMENT STRATEGY

PPK may be localized to the hands and feet, or develop as part of a more generalized skin disorder. It is important when making a diagnosis to establish its morphology and the presence of any associated ectodermal disease at sites other than the palms and soles. Biopsy may be necessary to distinguish between some hereditary forms of PPK. PPK can be associated with infections (dermatophytes, human papillomavirus, HIV, syphilis, and scabies), drugs (arsenic exposure), and internal malignancy, or may be a cutaneous manifestation of systemic disease (myxedema, diabetes mellitus, or cutaneous T-cell lymphoma). Hyperkeratosis of the palms and soles can also be a feature of eczema, psoriasis, and cutaneous T-cell lymphoma.

The treatment of PPK is difficult. Most therapeutic options produce only short-term improvement and are frequently compounded by unwanted adverse effects. Treatment options range from simple measures such as *salt-water soaks* with paring and *topical keratolytics*, to *systemic retinoids* and *reconstructive surgery* with total excision of the hyperkeratotic skin followed by grafting.

In patients with limited disease, *topical keratolytics* containing salicylic acid, lactic acid, or urea in a suitable base may be tried. Examples include 5–10% salicylic acid, 10–40% propylene glycol, or 10% lactic acid in aqueous cream or a combination therapy using 10% urea and 5% lactic acid in aqueous cream to be applied twice daily. These formulations can be made up on an individual basis, or the closest proprietary product prescribed. The efficacy of these agents may be increased by occlusion at night. *Topical retinoids* such as tretinoin (0.01% gel and 0.1% cream) may also be tried; treatment is often limited by skin irritation. *Potent topical corticosteroids*, such as clobetasol propionate 0.05%, with or without keratolytics, are occasionally of value in inflammatory PPK. *5-Fluorouracil 5%* has produced dramatic results in spiny keratoderma, but its use in other keratodermas has not been evaluated.

The efficacy of the *oral retinoids* in keratoderma is well established. Good responses have been seen in mal de Meleda, Papillon–Lefèvre syndrome, and erythrokeratoderma variabilis. In some types of PPK, particularly epidermolytic forms, hyperesthesia may limit the usefulness or practicality of treatment with retinoids. The potential risk of bone toxicity should also be assessed in patients on long-term therapy, although the risks are small. Periodic radiologic bone monitoring and, when possible, prescription of intermittent therapy are recommended. The optimal dosage of acitretin is between 25 and 35 mg daily in adults or 0.7 mg/kg daily in children, which may be adjusted after 4 weeks of therapy.

Psoralen plus UVA (PUVA) therapy or *re-PUVA* (a synergistic combination of oral retinoids and PUVA) may be effective in PPK secondary to psoriasis or eczema. In oculocutaneous tyrosinemia (an autosomal recessive condition characterized by focal palmoplantar keratosis, corneal ulceration, and mental retardation), *dietary restriction of phenylalanine and tyrosine* has led to resolution of PPK. *Oral administration of $1\alpha,25$-dihydroxyvitamin D_3* and *topical calcipotriol* ointment has been reported to be effective. Regular podiatry, careful selection of footwear, and treatment of secondary fungal infections is an integral part of management of all PPK. Regular intermittent use of terbinafine cream and other topical antifungals can reduce skin maceration and improve comfort. *Surgical or laser dermabrasion* is an option for some patients, with potential amelioration of symptoms and improved penetration of topical agents.

For severe refractory PPK *excision and skin grafting* may be considered. Excision should remove the hyperkeratotic skin, including dermis, epidermis, and subcutis, to prevent any risk of recurrence.

SPECIFIC INVESTIGATIONS

▶ Scrapings for mycology
▶ Thyroid function tests

An epidemiologic investigation of dermatologic fungus infections in the northernmost county of Sweden (Norbotten) 1977–81. Gamborg Nielson P. Mykosen 1984; 27: 203–10.

In a 5-year survey of dermatophyte infections in Norbotten the frequency of dermatophytosis among patients with hereditary PPK was shown to be 35%, corresponding to a prevalence of 36.7%. The predominant feature of dermatophytosis in patients with hereditary PPK was scaling and fissuring. Treatment improved the clinical signs after 2–3 months.

Hereditary palmoplantar keratoderma and dermatophytosis in the northernmost county of Sweden (Norbotten). Gamborg Nielson P. Acta Dermatol Venereol Suppl (Stockh) 1994; 188: 1–60.

In relatives of the original propositi, dermatophytosis was found in 65% of men, 22% of women, and 21% of children, resulting in a total frequency of 36.2%. Statistically, it was proved that *Trichophyton mentagrophytes* occurred more often in patients with hereditary PPK. Vesicular eruptions along the hyperkeratotic border occurred significantly more often in patients with dermatophytosis and were considered pathognomonic of secondary dermatophytosis.

Palmoplantar keratoderma in association with myxoedema. Hodak E, David M, Feuerman EJ. Acta Dermatol Venereol 1986; 66: 354–5.

A patient with myxedema and intractable PPK showed improvement after treatment with thyroid replacement therapy. The possibility of a causal relationship between hypothyroidism and PPK was questioned.

Severe palmar keratoderma with myxoedema. Tan OT, Sarkany I. Clin Exp Dermatol 1977; 2: 287–8.

A patient with myxedema and PPK showed rapid improvement in PPK after thyroxine treatment.

FIRST-LINE THERAPIES

▶ Topical keratolytics	**B**
▶ Topical retinoids	**B**

Alleviation of the plantar discomfort caused by pachyonychia congenita with topical applications of aluminum chloride and salicylic acid ointments. Takayama M, Okuyama R, Sasaki Y, Ohura T, Tagami H, Aiba S. Dermatology 2005; 211: 302.

Aluminium chloride solution is used to reduce plantar sweating, which may exacerbate blistering and hyperkeratosis in this condition.

Vitamin A acid in the treatment of palmoplantar keratoderma. Gunther SH. Arch Dermatol 1972; 106: 854–7.

Nine patients with PPK were treated with retinoic acid 0.1% in petroleum jelly and all improved within 4 months. Permanent remission ensued in two patients. Recurrence was observed in the majority of cases 8 weeks after the withdrawal of treatment. This was avoided by the topical application of vitamin A acid once or twice weekly.

Topical treatment of keratosis palmaris et plantaris with tretinoin. Touraine R, Revuz J. Acta Dermatol Venereol Suppl (Stockh) 1975; (suppl 74): 152–3.

Six patients were treated for 2 months with either tretinoin 0.1% lotion or 0.05% cream. Improvement was seen in most patients. Better results were achieved with the use of occlusive dressings, mechanical paring prior to topical application, and when a higher concentration of topical tretinoin was used (0.3%).

SECOND-LINE THERAPIES

▶ Systemic retinoids	**A**

The treatment of keratosis palmaris et plantaris with isotretinoin. A multicenter study. Bergfeld WF, Derbes VJ, Elias PM, Frost P, Greer KE, Shupack JL. J Am Acad Dermatol 1982; 6: 727–31.

Five of six patients with PPK were safely and effectively treated with isotretinoin, with dramatic clearing of the keratoderma within the first 4 weeks of therapy. The mean dose was 1.95 mg/kg daily, and mean duration of therapy was 113 days.

Acitretin in the treatment of severe disorders of keratinisation. Results of an open study. Blanchet-Bardon C, Nazzaro VV, Rognin C, Geiger JM, Puissant A, et al. J Am Acad Dermatol 1991; 24: 983–6.

An open, non-comparative study to evaluate the clinical response to acitretin of patients with non-psoriatic disorders of keratinization, and to establish the optimal dosage for efficacy and tolerance. Thirty-three patients with ichthyoses, PPK, or Darier's disease were treated for 4 months. Most showed a marked improvement. The optimal acitretin dosage providing the best efficacy with minimal side effects varied from patient to patient. The mean daily dose (± SD) was 27 ± 11 mg in adults and 0.7 ± 0.2 mg/kg in children.

A controlled study of comparative efficacy of oral retinoids and topical betamethasone/salicylic acid for chronic hyperkeratotic palmoplantar dermatitis. Capella GL, Fracchiolla C, Frigerio E, Altomare G. J Dermatol Treat 2004; 15: 88–93.

A single-blind, matched-sample investigation was carried out in 42 patients with chronic hyperkeratotic palmoplantar dermatitis, who were administered acitretin 25–50 mg daily for 1 month controlled versus a conventional topical treatment (betamethasone/salicylic acid ointment). Acitretin was significantly better than the conventional treatment after 30 days (two-sided p<0.0001). The authors suggested that acitretin should be considered a first choice treatment.

Acitretin in the treatment of mal de Meleda. Van de Kerkhof PC, Dooren-Greebe RJ, Steijlen PM. Br J Dermatol 1992; 127: 191–2.

Two patients with mal de Meleda treated with acitretin experienced a marked reduction of PPK. The optimal dosage was found to be between 10 and 30 mg daily. Higher dosages resulted in hyperesthesia. Discontinuation of acitretin resulted in relapse within days.

Keratoderma climactericum (Haxthausen's disease): clinical and laboratory findings and etretinate treatment in 10 patients. Deschamps P, Leroy D, Pedailles S, Mandard JC. Dermatologica 1986; 172: 258–62.

Etretinate 0.7–0.8 mg/kg daily brought about partial or total remission of hyperkeratosis in 10 cases of keratoderma climactericum.

Mutilating palmoplantar keratoderma successfully treated with etretinate. Wereide K. Acta Dermatol Venereol 1984; 64: 556–9.

Three patients with mutilating keratodermas were successfully treated with oral etretinate. All had constriction of one or more digits, with impending pseudoamputation. Treatment resulted in disappearance of the pseudoainhum and normalization of the digital blood circulation.

It is assumed that acitretin would provide a similar outcome.

Evidence Levels: **A** Double-blind study **B** Clinical trial ≥ 20 subjects **C** Clinical trial < 20 subjects **D** Series ≥ 5 subjects **E** Anecdotal case reports

THIRD-LINE THERAPIES

▶ Reconstructive surgery with total excision of hyperkeratotic skin followed by grafting	C
▶ Topical calcipotriol	E
▶ Oral vitamin D_3 analogs	E
▶ Topical corticosteroids with or without keratolytics	E
▶ PUVA or re-PUVA	D
▶ Dermabrasion	E
▶ CO_2 laser	B
▶ 5-Fluorouracil	E
▶ Tyrosine-restricted diet in oculocutaneous keratoderma	E

Plastic surgery in the management of palmoplantar keratoderma (palmoplantar neoplasty). Farina R. Aesthet Plast Surg 1987; 11: 249–53.

Five cases of PPK were treated successfully by grafting skin taken from the calves and thighs.

Palmoplantar keratoderma and skin grafting: postsurgical long-term follow-up of two cases with Olmsted syndrome. Bédard MS, Powell J, Laberge L, Allard-Dansereau C, Bortoluzzi P, Marcoux D. Pediatr Dermatol 2008; 25: 223–9.

A 6- and 10-year follow-up of successful surgical correction of mutilating keratoderma.

Surgical correction of pseudo-ainhum in Vohwinkel syndrome. Pisoh T, Bhatia A, Oberlin C. J Hand Surg [Br] 1995; 20: 338–41.

Successful surgical correction of constricting rings in a patient with Vohwinkel syndrome.

Surgical correction of hyperkeratosis in the Papillon–Lefevre syndrome. Peled IJ, Weinrauch L, Cohen HA, Wexler MK. J Dermatol Surg Oncol 1981; 7: 142–3.

A patient with Papillon–Lefèvre syndrome underwent successful surgical correction of hyperkeratosis of the palms.

Topical calcipotriol in the treatment of epidermolytic palmoplantar keratoderma of Vorner. Lucker GP, Van de Kerkhof PC, Steijlen PM. Br J Dermatol 1994; 130: 543–5.

A patient with hereditary epidermolytic PPK of Vorner was successfully treated with topical calcipotriol.

Efficacy, tolerability, and safety of calcipotriol ointment in disorders of keratinisation. Results of a randomized, double blind vehicle-controlled, right/left comparative study. Kragballe K, Steijlen PM, Ibsen HH, van de Kerkhof PC, Esmann J, Sorensen LH, et al. Arch Dermatol 1995; 131: 556–60.

Twenty patients with PPK showed no therapeutic benefit with topical calcipotriol.

Improvement of palmoplantar keratoderma of nonhereditary type (eczema tyloticum) after oral administration of 1 alpha 25-dihydroxyvitamin D3. Katayama H, Yamane Y. Arch Dermatol 1989; 125: 1713.

A patient with acquired PPK was successfully treated with oral $1\alpha,25$-dihydroxyvitamin D, 0.5 µg daily for 3 months, with no side effects.

Oral psoralen photochemotherapy (PUVA) of hyperkeratotic dermatitis of the palms. Mobacken H, Rosen K, Swanbeck G. Br J Dermatol 1983; 109: 205–8.

PUVA was found to be effective in five patients with chronic hyperkeratotic dermatitis of the palms.

Dermabrasion of the hyperkeratotic foot. Daoud MS, Randle HW, Yarborough JM. Dermatol Surg 1995; 21: 243–4.

A patient with acquired PPK treated with dermabrasion and then 2% crude coal tar and 5% salicylic acid in petrolatum showed no evidence of recurrence after 6 months. The indications for dermabrasion include dry, fissured hyperkeratotic heels, psoriatic keratoderma before PUVA therapy, punctate keratoderma, and generalized keratoderma.

Methods and effectiveness of surgical treatment of limited hyperkeratosis with CO_2 laser. Babaev OG, Bashilov VP, Zakharov AK. Khirurgiia (Mosk) 1993; 4: 74–9.

Five hundred and two patients with limited hyperkeratosis were treated, with a favorable clinical effect. Recurrences were noted in only 4% of cases.

Dietary management of oculocutaneous tyrosinemia in an 11 year old child. Ney D, Bay C, Scheider JA, Kelts D, Nyhan WL. Am J Dis Child 1983; 137: 995–1000.

An 11-year-old girl with oculocutaneous tyrosinemia with plantar keratosis and keratitis demonstrated resolution of her keratitis and improvement of her plantar keratosis with dietary restriction of phenylalanine and tyrosine to less than 100 mg/kg.

Palmoplantar pustulosis

Sonja Molin, Thomas Ruzicka

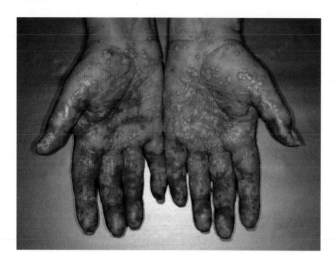

Palmoplantar pustulosis (PPP) is a chronic relapsing pustular eruption that affects the palms and soles. Because its clinical and genetic characteristics differ from those of psoriasis vulgaris, PPP should probably be considered as a distinct entity.

MANAGEMENT STRATEGY

PPP is a common disease that is often refractory to treatment and shows a high recurrence rate. Unlike psoriasis, it lacks an association with a candidate gene within the PSORS1 locus. Female predominance and a high prevalence in smokers are characteristic. *Cessation of smoking* is essential for the treatment of PPP. Consideration of the association with comorbidities such as diabetes mellitus, thyroid disease, *Helicobacter pylori* infection, celiac disease or osteoarthropathy is necessary. A *gluten-free diet* is recommended if gluten intolerance is proven. For initial therapy, as well as in patients with milder symptoms of PPP, potent *topical corticosteroids under occlusion* are the treatment of choice. *Psoralen and ultraviolet A light (PUVA)* therapy is commonly found to be effective. In more severe or recalcitrant disease systemic medication should be considered. The efficacy of *systemic retinoids* such as acitretin (starting dose 0.5 mg/kg daily) is proven, but practical use is limited by their teratogenic potential. There is evidence that the combination of PUVA and systemic retinoids is superior to the individual treatments. Modest efficacy of *tetracycline* (250 mg twice daily for 1 month) is reported. Low-dose *ciclosporin* (1 mg/kg daily) and *methotrexate* (10–25 mg once weekly) with appropriate monitoring can result in improvement of PPP. *Fumaric acid esters* (available in Germany) have been reported to be effective.

A multitude of other agents have been reported to be beneficial for the treatment of PPP. The use of *low-voltage X-ray (Grenz ray) therapy* and the retinoic acid metabolism blocking agent *liarozole* showed at least modest efficacy.

Reports on *tumor necrosis factor (TNF)-α antagonist* therapy in PPP show controversial results. They may even cause the activation or aggravation of the disease. Non-TNF-α-inhibiting biologic agents such as alefacept might be promising new therapeutic options, especially in recalcitrant cases. Larger controlled clinical trials are needed to substantiate the evidence.

SPECIFIC INVESTIGATIONS

> ▶ Screen for:
>   - ▶ *Helicobacter pylori* infection
>   - ▶ Diabetes mellitus
>   - ▶ Osteoarthropathy
>   - ▶ Gluten intolerance
>   - ▶ Thyroid diseases
> ▶ Exclude:
>   - ▶ SAPHO (synovitis, acne, pustulosis, hyperostosis and osteitis)

Palmoplantar pustulosis associated with gastric *Helicobacter pylori* infection. Sáez-Rodríguez M, Noda-Cabrera A, García-Bustínduy M, Guimerá-Martín-Neda F, Dorta-Alom S, Escoda-García M, et al. Clin Exp Dermatol 2002; 27: 720.

PPP cleared in a patient with gastric *Helicobacter pylori* infection after eradication treatment with amoxicillin and clarithromycin in combination with omeprazole. There was no relapse during a 4-year follow-up period.

Women with palmoplantar pustulosis have disturbed calcium homeostasis and a high prevalence of diabetes mellitus and psychiatric disorders: a case–control study. Hagforsen E, Michaëlsson K, Lundgren E, Olofsson H, Petersson A, Lagumdzija A, et al. Acta Dermatol Venereol 2005; 85: 225–32.

Disturbed calcium homeostasis was found significantly frequently in 60 PPP patients compared to a control group. Association with diabetes mellitus, psychiatric disorders, and gluten intolerance was found to be common.

Osteoarticular manifestations of pustulosis palmaris et plantaris and of psoriasis: two distinct entities. Mejjad O, Daragon A, Louvel JP, Da Silva LF, Thomine E, Lauret P, et al. Ann Rheum Dis 1996; 55: 177–80.

A comparison of 23 patients with PPP and 23 with psoriatic arthritis (PsoA). Clinical findings showed involvement of the anterior chest wall (e.g., the sternoclavicular joints) in 19 out of 23 patients with PPP compared to 10 of 23 with PsoA. Radiological signs of arthropathy were demonstrated in 11 PPP patients and four PsoA patients.

Skeletal involvement in pustulosis palmo-plantaris with special reference to the sterno-costo-clavicular joints. Hradil E, Gentz CF, Matilainen T, Möller H, Sanzén L, Uden A. Acta Dermatol Venereol 1988; 68: 65–73.

Increased isotope uptake in the sternocostoclavicular area was found in 16 out of 73 patients with PPP who underwent skeletal scintigraphy.

Palmoplantar pustulosis and gluten sensitivity: a study of serum antibodies against gliadin and tissue transglutaminase, the duodenal mucosa and effects of gluten-free diet. Michaelsson G, Kristjánsson G, Pihl Lundin I, Hagforsen E. Br J Dermatol 2007; 156: 659–66.

Evidence Levels: **A** Double-blind study **B** Clinical trial ≥ 20 subjects **C** Clinical trial < 20 subjects **D** Series ≥ 5 subjects **E** Anecdotal case reports

Laboratory investigation of 113 women with PPP showed IgA antibodies against gliadin in 16% and antibodies against tissue transglutaminase in 10% of cases. Celiac disease was found in 6% of patients. Gluten-free diet resulted in almost total clearance of skin symptoms and a reduction in antibody level.

Thyroid disease in pustulosis palmoplantaris. Agner T, Sindrup JH, Høier-Madsen M, Hegedüs L. Br J Dermatol 1989; 121: 487–91.

Thyroid disease was detected in 53% of 32 patients with PPP compared to 16% in the matched control group.

SAPHO syndrome: a long-term follow-up study of 120 cases. Hayem G, Bouchaud-Chabot A, Benali K, Roux S, Palazzo E, Silbermann-Hoffman O, et al. Semin Arthritis Rheum 1999; 29: 159–71.

A significant association of PPP with axial osteitis in 120 reported cases with SAPHO syndrome.

FIRST-LINE THERAPIES

▶ Oral retinoids	A
▶ Tetracycline	A
▶ PUVA	B
▶ Topical corticosteroids	C

Interventions for chronic palmoplantar pustulosis. Marsland AM, Chalmers RJ, Hollis S, Leonardi-Bee J, Griffiths CE. Cochrane Database Syst Rev 2006; CD001433.

An extensive review of the literature concerning PPP treatment shows evidence of the effectiveness of PUVA and systemic retinoids, either alone or in combination, the effectiveness of topical corticosteroids under occlusion, and probable benefit of low-dose ciclosporin, tetracycline antibiotics, and Grenz ray therapy.

A detailed survey of evidence-based PPP treatment options, including the classic publications about, for example, PUVA and systemic retinoids.

Pustulosis palmaris et plantaris. Thomsen K, Osterbye P. Br J Dermatol 1973; 89: 293–6.

A marked improvement in 42 of 59 courses compared to placebo (20 improved) in 40 PPP patients treated with tetracycline 250 mg twice daily for three 4-week periods.

A hydrocolloid occlusive dressing plus triamcinolone acetonide cream is superior to clobetasol cream in palmoplantar pustulosis. Kragballe K, Larsen FG. Acta Dermatol Venereol 1991; 71: 540–2.

Complete clearance of PPP with medium-strength topical corticosteroid under hydrocolloid occlusion in 13 out of 19 patients in a left–right comparison with a highly potent topical corticosteroid (complete remission in only three out of 19 patients).

SECOND-LINE THERAPIES

▶ Ciclosporin	A
▶ Methotrexate	B
▶ Fumaric acid esters	C

Double-blind placebo-controlled study of long-term low-dose cyclosporin in the treatment of palmoplantar pustulosis. Erkko P, Granlund H, Remitz A, Rosen K, Mobacken H, Lindelöf B, et al. Br J Dermatol 1998; 139: 997–1004.

Fifty-eight PPP patients were treated with ciclosporin in a daily dose of 1–4 mg/kg for 12 months. Low-dose treatment showed improvement in 13 of 27 patients, compared to six of 31 in the placebo group. The benefit of long-term use is only assumed.

Pustulosis palmaris et plantaris treated with methotrexate. Thomsen K. Acta Dermatol Venereol 1971; 51: 397–400.

A satisfactory response was seen in eight of 25 patients receiving weekly oral doses of 25 mg methotrexate for 2 months.

Efficacy of fumaric acid ester monotherapy in psoriasis pustulosa palmoplantaris. Ständer H, Stadelmann A, Luger T, Traupe H. Br J Dermatol 2003; 149: 220–2.

A marked reduction of PPP Area and Severity Index (PPPASI) was seen in 13 patients with PPP treated with fumaric acid esters for a period of 24 weeks.

THIRD-LINE THERAPIES

▶ Grenz ray	B
▶ Alefacept	C
▶ Liarozole	C

The effect of grenz ray therapy on pustulosis palmoplantaris. A double-blind bilateral trial. Lindelöf B, Beitner H. Acta Dermatol Venereol 1990; 70: 529–31.

A moderate response to low-voltage X-ray (Grenz ray) therapy was seen in 15 patients treated with 4 Gy on six occasions at intervals of 1 week.

Open label trial of alefacept in palmoplantar pustular psoriasis. Carr D, Tusa MG, Carroll CL, Pearce DJ, Camacho F, Kaur M, et al. J Dermatol Treat 2008; 19: 97–100.

A reduction of PPP Severity Index (PPPSI) was seen in 13 of 14 patients completing this study with 16 weeks of alefacept treatment up to a maximum dose of 30 mg/week. The mean improvement in PPPSI and PGA (Physicians' Global Assessment) was statistically significant.

Oral liarozole in the treatment of palmoplantar pustular psoriasis: a randomized, double-blind, placebo-controlled study. Bhushan M, Burden AD, McElhone K, James R, Vanhoutte FP, Griffiths CE. Br J Dermatol 2001; 145: 546–53.

There was a noticeable improvement of PPP symptoms in four of seven patients treated with liarozole (75 mg twice daily), a retinoic acid metabolism-blocking agent, compared to one of eight patients receiving placebo.

Liarozole has designated orphan drug status for use in congenital ichthyosis.

Manifestation of palmoplantar pustulosis during or after infliximab therapy for plaque-type psoriasis: report on five cases. Mössner R, Thaci D, Mohr J, Pätzold S, Bertsch HP, Krüger U, et al. Arch Dermatol Res 2008; 300: 101–5.

Five patients treated with infliximab for chronic plaque-type psoriasis developed PPP either during therapy or after its discontinuation.

The benefits of TNF-α antagonist use in PPP are variable; the efficacy as well as aggravation and initiation of PPP are reported.

Panniculitis

Robert A Allen, Richard L Spielvogel

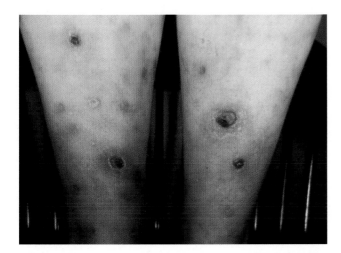

Panniculitis is a collective term for a group of inflammatory diseases that involve the subcutaneous fatty tissue. Most types present with any combination of tender subcutaneous papules, nodules, or plaques. The panniculitides are subdivided into groups based on the location of the predominant inflammation seen on a skin biopsy, either in intralobular septae or within the fat lobule itself. Erythema nodosum is the most common form of panniculitis. Whereas the inflammation in erythema nodosum involves mainly the septal tissue between fat lobules, almost all other forms of panniculitis primarily involve the fat lobule. The differential diagnosis of lobular panniculitis is variable and may be associated with systemic disease. Subtypes include infectious panniculitis, lupus profundus, Weber–Christian disease (WCD), nodular vasculitis (erythema induratum), pancreatic panniculitis, α_1-antitrypsin (A1AT) deficiency panniculitis, cytophagic histiocytic panniculitis (CHP)/forms of subcutaneous T-cell lymphoma, and the childhood or physical forms of panniculitis.

MANAGEMENT STRATEGY

A skin biopsy is helpful to determine whether the inflammation is primarily septal or lobular. The type of biopsy should be a large punch or an incisional specimen. A large amount of subcutaneous tissue is helpful for examination. This should be performed if the history and physical signs do not support a diagnosis of erythema nodosum or a subcutaneous infection. If infection is in the differential diagnosis, a small piece of the biopsy should be sent for Gram staining and culture for bacteria, mycobacteria, and fungi. If a mycobacterial infection is in the differential diagnosis, the specimen should be grown at 24, 30, 37, and 42°C. Treatment for proven infectious causes should be based on antibiotic sensitivity testing if possible.

Lupus panniculitis may herald the onset of systemic disease. Lupus profundus (panniculitis) occurs in 2–5% of cases of systemic lupus erythematosus (SLE) and tends to have a chronic course that does not involve internal organs. It is often painful, with skin lesions showing overlapping characteristics of discoid lupus erythematosus. In contrast

to erythema nodosum, its distribution is usually on the trunk and proximal extremities. Laboratory studies should include antinuclear antibody (ANA), dsDNA, ssDNA, SSA, SSB, chemistry profile, and a complete blood count (CBC). A biopsy for direct immunofluorescence should be ordered to confirm the diagnosis in cases with indeterminate histopathology. The first-line treatments are the *antimalarials,* and sunscreen use. Some cases may need *systemic corticosteroids.*

The diagnosis of WCD is one of exclusion. It is the idiopathic form of chronic lobular panniculitis without vasculitis. Patients are usually intermittently febrile. Several studies have documented other causes of panniculitis when cases of WCD are re-inspected for infection, pancreatic disease, or erythema nodosum. The work-up should include an erythrocyte sedimentation rate, liver function studies, amylase, and A1AT levels. Treatment commonly requires trials of several agents before a suitable response is obtained. *Corticosteroids, dapsone, tetracycline,* and *ciclosporin* are all reported to help in some cases. *More aggressive immunosuppression* may be required.

Some cases of nodular vasculitis are not associated with tuberculosis infections. If cultures for mycobacteria are negative, or if a rapid diagnosis is required, the tissue may be sent for polymerase chain reaction (PCR) of mycobacterial DNA. Treatment usually consists of *potassium iodide, colchicine, corticosteroids,* or *antimalarials.* Systemic vasculitis such as polyarteritis nodosa can also occur in the panniculus. However, it tends to spare veins in the biopsy specimens and has systemic involvement.

Pancreatic panniculitis can occur with any form of pancreatic tissue necrosis, including pancreatitis, pancreatic duct stricture, and pancreatic carcinoma. It is important to note that abdominal symptoms may be absent. Serum amylase and lipase levels should be measured because they are frequently elevated. A CBC with differential should be ordered to look for eosinophilia, which occurs in 60% of patients. Imaging with MRI is helpful to look for a pancreatic malignancy. Pancreatic panniculitis only resolves with treatment of the underlying cause of pancreatic inflammation.

A1AT panniculitis results from a deficiency of this enzyme. This leads to chronic inflammation in the subcutaneous fat because lipase, elastase, and other enzymes are not neutralized. An elastic tissue stain of the biopsy may be helpful to show the reduced elastic tissue and lobular or septal panniculitis characteristic of this entity. Gene phenotyping is available to determine an enzyme mutation. Treatment consists of *enzyme replacement, dapsone, colchicine,* or *liver transplantation* to permanently replace the missing enzyme.

Cytophagic histiocytic panniculitis features tender subcutaneous nodules along with fever, hepatosplenomegaly, pancytopenia, and liver dysfunction. It has been associated with viral infections (mainly Epstein–Barr), leukemias, and lymphomas. Histopathologic specimens classically show 'beanbag' cells, which are giant cells engulfing lymphocytes, neutrophils, and erythrocytes. Absence of immunoperoxidase staining with CD56 on the skin biopsy may portend a better clinical outcome. Treatment consists of *treating any underlying malignancy,* possibly with a *bone marrow transplant.* If malignancy is ruled out, ciclosporin is usually effective.

The physical forms of panniculitis, such as those resulting from cold exposure, foreign body, or factitious causes, usually resolve by *removal of the offending trigger* or surgical removal of the foreign body. This is similar to panniculitis caused by the use of silicone or paraffin that has been used for cosmetic purposes. Panniculitis can also occur in infants. It is manifested as sclerema neonatorum, or as subcutaneous fat necrosis of the newborn. The latter usually resolves spontaneously, but may be complicated by hypercalcemia. Sclerema neonatorum may be fatal.

SPECIFIC INVESTIGATIONS

> ► Skin biopsy for routine microscopy
> ► Skin biopsy for culture and sensitivity (routine, mycobacterial, fungal)
> ► Skin biopsy for PCR
> ► Skin biopsy for immunoperoxidase and gene rearrangement studies
> ► ANA and other rheumatologic serologic tests
> ► Serum A1AT
> ► Serum lipase and amylase
> ► Abdominal MRI
> ► CBC with differential

There are no specific investigations for panniculitis other than an adequate skin biopsy containing abundant fat. Further investigation should be based on history and physical findings.

LUPUS PANNICULITIS

FIRST-LINE THERAPIES

> ► Antimalarials   E
> ► Systemic or intralesional corticosteroids   E

Systemic lupus erythematosus presenting as panniculitis (lupus profundus). Diaz-Jouanen E, DeHoratius RJ, Alarcon-Segovia D, Messner RP. Ann Intern Med 1975; 82: 376–9.

A case study in which five of six patients improved after adding hydroxychloroquine to their systemic corticosteroid regimens.

Connective tissue panniculitis. Winkelmann RK, Padilha-Goncalves A. Arch Dermatol 1980; 116: 291–4.

Case report of a patient obtaining remission with hydroxychloroquine 200 mg twice daily and systemic corticosteroids. However, she developed SLE. A second patient on hydroxychloroquine was cleared of the condition after failing to respond to non-steroidal anti-inflammatory drugs (NSAIDs), potassium iodide, and corticosteroids.

Lupus erythematosus panniculitis (profundus). Maciejewski W, Bandmann HJ. Acta Dermatol Venereol (Stockh) 1979; 59: 109–12.

Case report of a patient diagnosed with lupus profundus by direct immunofluorescence and treated with chloroquine.

Lupus erythematosus presenting as panniculitis. Verbov JL, Borrie PF. Proc Roy Soc Med 1971; 64: 28–9.

A case report of the condition clearing in one patient with hydroxychloroquine 200 mg twice daily.

Treatment of chronic discoid lupus erythematosus with intralesional triamcinolone. Rowell NR. Br J Dermatol 1962; 74: 354–7.

One patient with lupus profundus and 27 patients with discoid lupus erythematosus were treated with intralesional

triamcinolone 10 mg/mL, and in 27 of the 28 the condition cleared or was clearing. All patients had failed to respond to antimalarials. The condition cleared in the lupus profundus patient.

SECOND-LINE THERAPIES

> ► Topical corticosteroids under occlusion   E

Lupus erythematosus profundus treated with clobetasol propionate under a hydrocolloid dressing. Yell JA, Burge SM. Br J Dermatol 1993; 128: 103.

A single case of a cure with clobetasol under hydrocolloid dressing occlusion, changed weekly. The patient responded after 1 month.

THIRD-LINE THERAPIES

> ► Gold   E
> ► Bismuth   E E
> ► Thalidomide   E E
> ► Ciclosporin A   E
> ► Dapsone   E

Lupus erythematosus profundus. Arnold HL Jr. Arch Dermatol 1956; 73: 14–26.

One patient had a partial response to intravenous gold followed by bismuth sodium thioglycollate.

Facets of lupus erythematosus: panniculitis responding to thalidomide. Wienert S, Gadola S, Hunziker T. J der Deutschen Dermatologischen Gesellschaft. 2008; 6: 214–16.

The dynamism of cutaneous lupus erythematosus: mild discoid lupus erythematosus evolving into SLE with SCLE and treatment-resistant lupus panniculitis. Wozniacka A, Salamon M, Lesiak A, McCauliffe DP, Sysa-Jedrzejowska A. Clin Rheumatol 2007; 26: 1176–9.

A 47-year-old woman with biopsy-proven lupus panniculitis responded to ciclosporin 4 mg/kg/day with methylprednisone. After 10 days there was improvement. The steroids were tapered and stopped after 3 months and the ciclosporin was gradually tapered to 2 mg/kg/day. The patient had failed antimalarials, systemic steroids, azathioprine, cyclophosphamide, methotrexate, and pulse doses of methylprednisolone.

Lupus erythematosus profundus successfully treated with dapsone: review of the literature. Ujiie H, Shimizu T, Ito M, Arita K, Shimizu H. Arch Dermatol 2006; 142: 399–401.

A 56-year-old woman with ulcerated, biopsy-proven lupus profundus responded to dapsone 75 mg/day after 6 weeks.

WEBER–CHRISTIAN DISEASE

FIRST-LINE THERAPIES

> ► Tetracycline   E
> ► Non-steroidal anti-inflammatory agents   E
> ► Systemic or intralesional corticosteroids   E

514

Panniculitis responsive to high dose tetracycline. Sturman SW. Arch Dermatol 1975; 111: 533–4.

One patient presented with fever, splenomegaly, and panniculitis that responded to tetracycline but recurred with two taperings. Finally, high-dose tetracycline (1 g four times daily) achieved remission. An infectious work-up did not find a causative organism.

Weber–Christian disease. Analysis of 15 cases and review of the literature. Panush RS, Yonker RA, Dlesk A, Longley S, Caldwell JR. Medicine (Baltimore) 1985; 64: 181–91.

Twelve of 13 patients with WCD improved with various therapies: 80% received corticosteroids, 33% NSAIDs, 40% antimalarials, and one patient methotrexate; 27% of patients received azathioprine after failing to respond to corticosteroids.

Panniculitis (Rothmann–Makai), with good response to tetracycline. Chan HL. Br J Dermatol 1975; 92: 351–4.

One patient responded well to low-dose tetracycline.

SECOND-LINE THERAPIES

▶ Heparin	E
▶ Ciclosporin	E
▶ Azathioprine	E
▶ Antimalarials	E
▶ Methotrexate	E

Ocular and adnexal changes associated with relapsing febrile non-suppurative panniculitis (Weber–Christian disease). Frayer WC, Wise RT, Tsaltas TT. Trans Am Ophthalmol Soc 1968; 66: 233–42.

A case report of a patient in remission with heparin.

Successful treatment of Weber–Christian disease by cyclosporin A. Usuki K, Kitamura K, Urabe A, Takaku F. Am J Med 1988; 85: 276–8.

One patient who had failed to respond to prednisone and had persistent fever achieved remission with intravenous ciclosporin followed by a change to oral therapy. The patient was disease free at 7 months.

Successful treatment of steroid-resistant Weber–Christian disease with biliary ductopenia using cyclosporin A. Hinata M, Someya T, Yoshizaki H, Seki K, Takeuchi K. Rheumatology 2005; 44: 821–3.

A 27-year-old man with WC disease and hepatic involvement including biliary ductopenia responded to ciclosporin A 225 mg/day. The treatment induced several years of remission.

Azathioprine-induced remission in Weber–Christian disease. Hotta T, Wakamatsu Y, Matsumura N, Nishida K, Takemura S, Yoshikawa T, et al. South Med J 1981; 74: 234–7.

A woman with subcutaneous nodules was originally diagnosed with dermatomyositis. After failing to respond to prednisolone and NSAIDs for 5 months, the diagnosis was changed to WCD. Azathioprine 150 mg daily resulted in clearing with minimal side effects (leukopenia). She flared upon tapering to 50 mg daily, but was stabilized at 100 mg daily for 2 years.

Weber–Christian disease. Analysis of 15 cases and review of the literature. Panush RS, Yonker RA, Dlesk A, Longley S, Caldwell JR. Medicine (Baltimore) 1985; 64: 181–91.

Twelve of 13 patients with WCD improved with various therapies: 80% received corticosteroids, 33% NSAIDs, 40% antimalarials, and one patient methotrexate; 27% of patients received azathioprine after failing to respond to corticosteroids.

THIRD-LINE THERAPIES

▶ Cyclophosphamide	E
▶ Thalidomide	E
▶ Skin grafting	E

Cyclophosphamide-induced remission in Weber–Christian panniculitis. Kirch W, Duhrsen U, Hoensch H, Ohnhaus E. Rheumatol Int 1985; 5: 239–40.

One patient with WCD failed to respond to hydroxychloroquine and prednisone. Cyclophosphamide led to rapid improvement.

Weber–Christian disease with nephrotic syndrome. Srivastava RN, Mayekar G, Anand R, Roy S. Am J Dis Child 1974; 127: 420–1.

A 5-year-old boy presented with nephrotic syndrome and WCD panniculitis. He improved initially with prednisone. However, cyclophosphamide 50 mg on alternate days with prednisone 30 mg daily was added after a flare. This resulted in rapid correction of the proteinuria and resolution of the panniculitis over the next 9 months.

Thalidomide in Weber–Christian disease. [Letter] Eravelly J, Waters MF. Lancet 1977; 1: 251.

A single patient was controlled with high-dose corticosteroids, but flared when tapering; she responded to thalidomide 300 mg daily. She was able to stop her corticosteroids and taper off the thalidomide after 13 weeks. She was disease free at 13 months.

A review of the concept of Weber–Christian panniculitis with a report of five cases. Macdonald A, Feiwel M. Br J Dermatol 1968; 80: 355–61.

A case report of two patients who healed with skin grafting after failing to improve with prednisone, antimalarials, and NSAIDs.

NODULAR VASCULITIS

FIRST-LINE THERAPIES

▶ NSAIDs	E
▶ Potassium iodide	D
▶ Treat underlying tuberculosis	B

Neutrophilic vascular reactions. Jorizzo JL, Solomon AR, Zanolli MD, Leshin B. J Am Acad Dermatol 1988; 19: 983–1005.

A review article in which nodular vasculitis is one of the causes of necrotizing vasculitis. NSAIDs may benefit some symptoms, such as serum sickness-like features, but do not help cutaneous lesions.

Potassium iodide in the treatment of erythema nodosum and nodular vasculitis. Horio T, Imamura S, Danno K, Ofuji S. Arch Dermatol 1981; 117: 29–31.

A case study in which 11 of 51 patients had nodular vasculitis. Seven of the 11 responded within 2 weeks to potassium iodide 300 mg three times daily.

Treatment of erythema nodosum and nodular vasculitis with potassium iodide. Schulz EJ, Whiting DA. Br J Dermatol 1976; 94: 75–8.

Sixteen of 17 patients responded to potassium iodide, usually with relief of symptoms within 2 days. The average duration of therapy was 3 weeks. The daily dose ranged from 360 to 900 mg.

Successul treatment of erythema induratum of Bazin following rapid detection of mycobacterial DNA by polymerase chain reaction. Degitz K, Messer G, Schirren H, Classen V, Meurer M. Arch Dermatol 1993; 129: 1619–20.

A single case of diagnosis and treatment of tuberculosis with isoniazid, rifampin (rifampicin), and ethambutol.

PCR has revolutionized the diagnosis of mycobacterial disease, confirming the long-held suspicion that many tuberculids may be due to residual mycobacterial antigens.

Erythema induratum of Bazin. Cho KH, Lee DY, Kim CW. Int J Dermatol 1996; 35: 802–8.

A retrospective study of 32 patients with proven erythema induratum of Bazin. All improved with triple therapy, but four relapsed and subsequently cleared.

Diagnosis and treatment of erythema induratum (Bazin). Feiwel M, Munro DD. Br Med J 1965; 1: 1109–11.

Twelve patients were diagnosed with erythema induratum secondary to tuberculosis and all responded well to two- to three-drug therapy, streptomycin, para-aminosalicylic acid 12.5 mg daily, and isoniazid 200–260 mg daily for 9 months.

SECOND-LINE THERAPIES

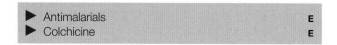

▶ Antimalarials		E
▶ Colchicine		E

Chloroquine-induced remission of nodular panniculitis present for 15 years. Shelley WB. J Am Acad Dermatol 1981; 5: 168–70.

One patient responded to chloroquine 250 mg/day within 1 month after failing to respond to various therapies for nodular panniculitis. These included corticosteroids, NSAIDs, and tetracycline.

Cutaneous necrotizing vasculitis. Lotti T, Comacchi C, Ghersetich I. Int J Dermatol 1996; 35: 457–74.

By inhibiting neutrophil chemotaxis, oral colchicine in doses of 0.6 mg twice daily, may be helpful in chronic forms of the disease.

THIRD-LINE THERAPIES

▶ Gold		E
▶ Mycophenolate mofetil		E

Nodular vasculitis (erythema induratum): treatment with auranofin. Shaffer N, Kerdel FA. J Am Acad Dermatol 1991; 25: 426–9.

One patient with nodular vasculitis responded to oral gold 3 mg twice daily and improved after 3 weeks. She had previously failed to respond to prednisone, colchicine, D-penicillamine, sulindac, and bumetanide (a loop diuretic) for suspected erythema nodosum.

Case reports: nodular vasculitis responsive to mycophenolate mofetil. Taverna JA, Radfar A, Pentland A, Poggioli G, Demierre MF. J Drugs Dermatol 2006; 5: 992–3.

A 70-year-old woman was treated with 1 g twice daily of mycophenolate mofetil. She responded slowly over the next year.

PANCREATIC PANNICULITIS

FIRST-LINE THERAPIES

▶ Treat underlying pancreatic problem	E

Resolution of panniculitis after placement of pancreatic duct stent in chronic pancreatitis. Lambiase P. Am J Gastroenterol 1996; 91: 1835–7.

One patient with pancreatitis secondary to alcohol presented with chest pain and tender skin nodules on the shins. After a skin biopsy showed panniculitis, he was diagnosed with pancreatitis without abdominal pain, but with a high amylase. A stent was placed to correct a stricture in the pancreatic duct, leading to resolution of the symptoms and skin lesions within 1 month.

Panniculitis caused by acinous pancreatic carcinoma. Heykarts B, Anseeuw M, Degreef H. Dermatology 1999; 198: 182–3.

One patient with skin nodules was found to have acinar pancreatic carcinoma upon surgical resection. She was initially unresponsive to high-dose corticosteroids and methotrexate, but the skin lesions resolved slowly after the resection. Subsequently, metastases were found in the right liver and the patient failed to respond to ledorvain and fluorouracil.

SECOND-LINE THERAPIES

▶ Octreotide	E

Liquefying panniculitis associated with acinous carcinoma of the pancreas responding to octreotide. Hudson-Peacock MJ, Regnard CFB, Farr PM. J Roy Soc Med 1994; 87: 361–2.

One patient presented with increasing numbers of painful leg nodules secondary to poorly differentiated adenocarcinoma. She failed to respond to prednisolone, but octreotide 50 μg twice daily subcutaneously halted progression of the skin nodules. However, despite the therapy, the patient died 3 weeks later.

CYTOPHAGIC HISTIOCYTIC PANNICULITIS

FIRST-LINE THERAPIES

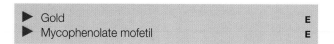

▶ Treat underlying T-cell lymphoma (chemotherapy)	E
▶ Prednisone	E
▶ Ciclosporin (if T-cell lymphoma ruled out)	E

Evidence Levels: **A** Double-blind study **B** Clinical trial ≥ 20 subjects **C** Clinical trial < 20 subjects **D** Series ≥ 5 subjects **E** Anecdotal case reports

Cytophagic histiocytic panniculitis and subcutaneous panniculitis-like T-cell lymphoma: report of 7 cases. Marzano AV, Berti E, Paulli M, Caputo R. Arch Dermatol 2000; 136: 889–96.

A report of seven cases of CHP. Five patients had subcutaneous T-cell lymphoma and died after failing to respond to various chemotherapeutic agents. One patient has done well with prednisone for 13 months, and the other living patient has done well with systemic corticosteroids, cyclophosphamide, and dapsone for 36 years.

Successful treatment of cytophagic histiocytic panniculitis with modified CHOP-E: cyclophosphamide, adriamycin, vincristine, prednisone, and etoposide. Matsue K, Itoh M, Tsukuda K, Miyazaki K, Kokubo T. Am J Clin Oncol 1994; 17: 470–4.

One patient with CHP received eight courses of modified CHOP-E every 3 weeks and has obtained a remission that has lasted 2 years.

Cytophagic histiocytic panniculitis. Case report with resolution after treatment. Alegre VA, Fortea JM, Camps C, Aliaga A. J Am Acad Dermatol 1989; 20: 875–8.

One patient with CHP for 2 months, who was investigated extensively, was treated with cyclophosphamide, vincristine, doxorubicin, and prednisone for nine cycles and achieved a cure. The authors recommend early, aggressive treatment.

Cytophagic histiocytic panniculitis – a syndrome associated with benign and malignant panniculitis: case comparison and review of the literature. Craig AJ, Cualing H, Thomas G, Lamerson C, Smith R. J Am Acad Dermatol 1998; 39: 721–36.

A case report of two patients who presented with CHP. One responded to prednisone 1 mg/kg daily plus ciclosporin 15 mg/kg daily and was well enough to be discharged home. However, 1 month later he developed fatal septicemia. An autopsy revealed no malignancy, but extensive *Aspergillus* sp. infection. Patient 2 presented with T-cell lymphoma and CHP and died during chemotherapy with cyclophosphamide, mitoxantrone, prednisone, vincristine, and X-ray therapy.

Subcutaneous pannicular T-cell lymphoma in children: response to combination therapy with ciclosporin and chemotherapy. Shani-Adir A, Lucky AW, Prendiville J, Murphy S, Passo M, Huang FS, et al. J Am Acad Dermatol 2004; 50: S18–22.

A case report of two adolescents with CHP and subcutaneous T-cell lymphoma who responded symptomatically to ciclosporin (5 and 12 mg/kg/day) with a reduction in fever and subcutaneous nodules. Complete remission was achieved in one patient with subsequent chemotherapy.

Successful treatment of severe cytophagic histiocytic panniculitis with cyclosporine A. Ostrov BE, Athreys BH, Eichenfield AH, Goldsmith DP. Semin Arthritis Rheum 1996; 25: 404–13.

A 16-year-old patient who presented with CHP initially responded to prednisone 2 mg/kg daily. A flare occurred and ciclosporin 4 mg/kg/day was instituted. A remission followed, but she was left with permanent hypothyroidism. She has remained disease free for 6 years after discontinuing the ciclosporin.

SECOND-LINE THERAPIES

▶ Bone marrow transplantation	E
▶ Potassium iodide	E
▶ Dapsone	E
▶ Cyclophosphamide	E
▶ Irradiation (total body)	E
▶ Interleukin-1 antagonist (anakinra)	E

Effective high-dose chemotherapy followed by autologous peripheral blood stem cell transplantation in a patient with the aggressive form of cytophagic histiocytic panniculitis. Koizumi K, Sawada K, Nishio M, Katagiri E, Fukae J, Fukada Y, et al. Bone Marrow Transplant 1997; 20: 171–3.

One patient with CHP secondary to an aggressive T-cell lymphoma was treated with cyclophosphamide, doxorubicin, vincristine, prednisolone, etoposide, and granulocyte–macrophage colony-stimulating factor (GM-CSF), and achieved a remission after three cycles (every 2 weeks). He was subsequently treated with an autologous bone marrow transplant and remained disease free for 1 year.

Cytophagic histiocytic panniculitis is not always fatal. White JW Jr, Winkelmann RK. J Cutan Pathol 1989; 16: 137–44.

One patient with CHP was treated with potassium iodide and achieved remission for 15 years. Another patient achieved remission with prednisone and was disease free at 28 years.

Successful treatment of a patient with subcutaneous panniculitis-like T-cell lymphoma with high-dose chemotherapy and total body irradiation. Mukai HY, Okoshi Y, Shimizu S, Katsura Y, Takei N, Hasegawa Y, et al. Eur J Haematol 2003; 70: 413–16.

One patient with CHP and subcutaneous T-cell lymphoma achieved a remission after three courses of CHOP chemotherapy, followed by high-dose chemotherapy and total body irradiation with an autologous stem cell transplant. He remained disease free at 2 years.

Interleukin 1 receptor antagonist to treat cytophagic histiocytic panniculitis with secondary hemophagocytic lymphohistiocytosis. Behrens EM, Kreiger PA, Cherian S, Cron RQ. J Rheumatol 2006; 33: 2081–4.

A 14-year-old girl with CHP who failed ciclosporin and etoposide responded to pulse methylprednisolone 1 g/day and anakinra 50 mg (2 mg/kg/day).

α_1-ANTITRYPSIN DEFICIENCY PANNICULITIS

FIRST-LINE THERAPIES

▶ Doxycycline	E
▶ Dapsone	D
▶ A1AT concentrate if emergency	E

Use of anti-collagenase properties of doxycycline in treatment of alpha 1-antitrypsin deficiency panniculitis. Humbert P, Faivre B, Gibey R, Agache P. Acta Dermatol Venereol 1991; 71: 189–94.

Three patients with recurrent A1AT panniculitis were treated with doxycycline 200 mg daily for 3 months. All achieved clearance within 8 weeks. After this period, two of the three were able to stop the medicine while the other was maintained on 100 mg daily. The authors speculate that this was due to the anticollagenase effect of the drug.

Clinical and pathologic correlations in 96 patients with panniculitis, including 15 patients with deficient levels of alpha 1-antitrypsin. Smith KC, Su WP, Pittelkow MR, Winkelmann RK. J Am Acad Dermatol 1989; 21: 1192–6.

Fifteen of 96 patients had A1AT panniculitis. Five of six of those treated with dapsone responded.

Panniculitis associated with severe alpha 1-antitrypsin deficiency. Treatment and review of the literature. Smith KC, Pittelkow MR, Su WP. Arch Dermatol 1987; 123: 1655–61.

One patient with A1AT deficiency failed to respond to prednisone, but did respond to dapsone 75 mg daily and an infusion of A1AT concentrate weekly. The patient was able to have split-thickness skin grafting after 2 weeks. Another patient had poor responses to chloroquine, azathioprine, and prednisone, but improved on the dapsone and A1AT inhibitor concentrate.

Protease-inhibitor deficiencies in a patient with Weber–Christian panniculitis. Bleumink E, Klokke HA. Arch Dermatol 1984; 120: 936–40.

One patient with tender leg nodules of A1AT panniculitis failed to respond to tetracycline, but did respond to dapsone 50 mg daily. She did have a few minor recurrences while on long-term dapsone therapy.

Treatment of alpha1-antitrypsin-deficiency panniculitis with minocycline. Ginarte M, Roson E, Peteiro C, Toribio J. Cutis 2001; 68: 27–30.

In one patient who was unable to tolerate treatment with dapsone or systemic corticosteroids the condition cleared with minocycline 100 mg twice daily. She was maintained on a dose of 100 mg once daily.

SECOND-LINE THERAPIES

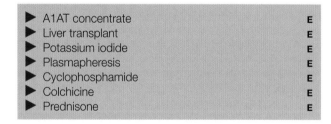

► A1AT concentrate	E
► Liver transplant	E
► Potassium iodide	E
► Plasmapheresis	E
► Cyclophosphamide	E
► Colchicine	E
► Prednisone	E

Alpha 1-antitrypsin deficiency-associated panniculitis: resolution with intravenous alpha 1-antitrypsin administration and liver transplantation. O'Riordan K, Blei A, Rao MS, Abecassis M. Transplantation 1997; 63: 480–2.

Two patients with homozygous deficiency were treated with A1AT replacement. One received a liver transplant and was cured. The other was treated with intravenous A1AT and was clear while on this medicine. She had a relapse when her free A1AT level fell below 50 µg/100 mL of serum.

Treatment of alpha-1-antitrypsin deficiency, massive edema, and panniculitis with alpha-1 protease inhibitor. Furey NL, Golden RS, Potts SR. Ann Intern Med 1996; 125: 699.

A patient with red thigh nodules was found to have A1AT deficiency panniculitis. The patient failed to respond to doxycycline

and received α_1-protease inhibitor concentrate 60 mg/kg, with great improvement within 24 hours.

Atlantic Provinces Dermatology Association Society Meeting, May 3, 1986. Miller RAW, cited by Ross JB. J Can Dermatol Assoc 1986; 13–17.

One patient with A1AT deficiency panniculitis failed to respond to prednisone and azathioprine, but responded after dapsone, potassium iodide, and plasmapheresis two to three times a week.

Cyclophosphamide therapy for Weber–Christian disease associated with alpha 1-antitrypsin deficiency. Strunk RW, Scheld WM. South Med J 1986; 79: 1425–7.

One patient with A1AT deficiency panniculitis failed to respond to prednisone 80 mg daily and heparin intravenously (given for suspected deep vein thrombosis). Cyclophosphamide was added at 150 mg/day, with a good response. The prednisone was tapered over 2 months and the cyclophosphamide was discontinued after 14 months. The patient had been disease free for 2 years after stopping the cyclophosphamide.

Necrotic panniculitis with alpha-1 antitrypsin deficiency. Viraben R, Massip P, Dicostanzo B, Mathieu C. J Am Acad Dermatol 1986; 14: 684–7.

A patient with A1AT panniculitis with necrotic plaques on the flanks and thighs failed to respond to lincomycin, prednisolone, colchicine, and cyclophosphamide. Rapid improvement followed plasma exchange infusions of 8 L once daily for 8 weeks.

Familial occurrence of alpha 1-antitrypsin deficiency and Weber–Christian disease. Breit SN, Clark P, Robinson JP, Luckhurst E, Dawkins RL, Penny R. Arch Dermatol 1983; 119: 198–202.

A report of two cases of A1AT panniculitis. Patient 1 responded to dexamethasone 5 mg intravenously every 6 hours. After 2 weeks he developed gas pain and an abdominal ileus. The dexamethasone was tapered to 6 mg four times daily and cyclophosphamide 200 mg daily was added. After 9 months the cyclophosphamide was discontinued, followed by the corticosteroids 3 months later. The patient has remained disease free for 2 years, except for small lesions at the sites of trauma. The brother of patient 1 had a similar attack and received 0.5 mg of colchicine three times daily plus dicloxacillin. The lesions resolved after 2 weeks and treatment was stopped 1 week later.

Deficiencia de alda-1-antitripsina en la panniculitis de Weber–Christian. [Abstract] Olmos L, Superby A, Lueiro M. Actas Dermato-Sifilograficas 1981; 72: 371–6.

One patient had resolution of panniculitis with prednisone. It also flared upon tapering.

Severe panniculitis caused by homozygous ZZ alpha 1-antitrypsin deficiency treated successfully with human purified enzyme (Prolastin). Chowdhury MM, Williams EJ, Morris JS, Ferguson BJ, McGregor AD, Hedges AR, et al. Br J Dermatol 2002; 147: 1258–61.

Life-threatening panniculitis and skin necrosis in one patient was cleared with Prolastin (human purified enzyme) and prednisolone. She cleared on a dose of 100 mg/kg every 6 days after being started on 60 mg/kg. She remained clear on a maintenance regimen of 6 g once weekly.

THIRD-LINE THERAPIES

▶ Ketoconazole   E

Panniculitis associated with histoplasmosis and alpha 1-antitrypsin deficiency. Pottage JC Jr, Trenholme GM, Aronson IK, Harris AA. Am J Med 1983; 75: 150–3.

A patient with nodules on the legs was found to have A1AT deficiency and histoplasmosis, which was diagnosed after exploratory thoracotomy and culture of lymph nodes. He received ketoconazole 400 mg daily for 6 months and was clear for another 9 months.

Paracoccidioidomycosis
(South American blastomycosis)

Wanda Sonia Robles, Mahreen Ameen

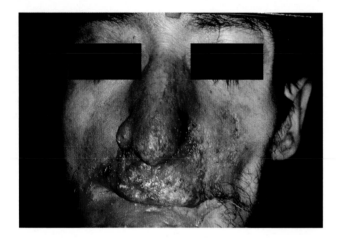

Paracoccidioidomycosis (PCM) is a chronic, progressive, granulomatous mycosis caused by the dimorphic fungus *Paracoccidioides brasiliensis*. It affects primarily the lungs and is believed to be acquired from inhalation of the fungus, which resides in soil and plants of endemic regions. PCM is restricted to Latin America, where it is the most prevalent systemic endemic mycosis. It has been reported in nearly all countries from Mexico to Argentina, with the exception of the Caribbean islands and Chile. Eighty percent of cases occur in Brazil, with the highest incidence in the state of São Paulo, followed by Venezuela, Colombia, Ecuador, and Argentina. PCM characteristically affects those working in agriculture and in rural areas. Because of the long latency period, the disease may appear many years after a person has left an endemic region. Untreated PCM has one of the highest rates of mortality of all the systemic mycoses.

There are two main clinical forms, acute or subacute, and a unifocal or multifocal chronic form. The acute form affects young people of both sexes and involves mainly the reticuloendothelial system. This form of infection is often severe and carries a worse prognosis. The chronic form most commonly affects adult men and causes pulmonary and/or mucocutaneous disease. Most cases of pulmonary infection have an indolent course. Only 2% of those infected develop the disseminated form of disease. Dissemination occurs most commonly to the mucosae of the upper airways and upper gastrointestinal tract. Cutaneous and lymph node involvement is common, and other organ systems may be involved, such as the adrenal glands (causing an addisonian syndrome), bones, and central nervous system. Oral lesions affect the gingiva, the hard palate, lips, and tongue. Nasal and pharyngeal ulcers can give rise to dysphagia and dysphonia. Ulcerative lesions can be painful, and are characterized by a punctate vascular pattern over a granulomatous base. Cutaneous lesions are highly polymorphic, consisting of verrucous and ulcerative papules, plaques and nodules. Centrofacial localization is typical and usually a result of dissemination of oral lesions. PCM is also characterized by massive and visible cervical and submandibular lymphadenopathy, which may progress to form abscesses with draining sinuses. Other lymph glands may also become enlarged. Primary mucocutaneous infection is rare, but can occur following direct inoculation of the skin or mucous membranes. It can arise from using twigs to clean the teeth, which is practiced in rural Brazil.

Disseminated infection is severe in the immunocompromised, including those co-infected with HIV. The mortality rate with HIV infection is high, ranging from 30% to 45%. However, the incidence of PCM in patients with AIDS in Latin America is low, and this has been attributed to the widespread use of trimethoprim-sulfamethoxazole as prophylaxis for *Pneumocystis carinii* pneumonia.

MANAGEMENT STRATEGY

P. brasiliensis is highly sensitive to antifungal drugs, and therefore a large therapeutic armamentarium exists to treat PCM. *Itraconazole* is the drug of choice for the treatment of mild to moderate acute and chronic clinical forms of PCM. It is given at a dose of 100–200 mg daily for a mean period of 6 months (range 3–12 months) depending on clinical response. It gives a cure rate of 90%, and recurrence rates of 0–15% have been reported after a median of 12 months, depending on comorbidities such as alcoholism, malnutrition, and AIDs. *Ketoconazole* (200–400 mg daily) is also highly effective, 90% of patients responding after 6–12 months of treatment, with only a 10% relapse rate. However, adverse effects are common, especially with long-term treatment. With the availability of newer antifungals, its use has decreased. *Sulfonamides* (sulfadiazine, sulfamethoxypyridazine, sulfadimethoxine, trimethoprim-sulfamethoxazole) are an attractive option as they are inexpensive and well tolerated. However, the duration of therapy is characteristically long, usually 2–3 years. Compliance can therefore be a problem, which might explain their lower cure rate of only 70%. In addition, they have a significant relapse rate of 35%. They are still commonly used as first agents in endemic regions because of their ready availability and low cost. *Parenteral amphotericin B* (cumulative dose of 1–2 g based on clinical response) is the drug of choice for severe or refractory infection. The cure rate is only 60%, but consideration must be given to the fact that it is usually given to the most severely ill patients. The relapse rate with amphotericin B is generally higher than with itraconazole, occurring in 20–30% of cases. Long-term maintenance therapy with an azole or sulfonamide is therefore required. In cases of central nervous system (CNS) PCM, sulfadiazine appears to be equally effective as amphotericin B. More recently, *voriconazole,* an extended-spectrum triazole, has demonstrated comparable efficacy and tolerability to itraconazole in the treatment of PCM. However, its high cost make it prohibitive for use in most endemic settings. There are few studies demonstrating the efficacy of *fluconazole* for PCM. It has been suggested that it may be useful in the management of CNS PCM given its excellent CNS penetration. Long-term follow-up after treatment of PCM is required, as relapse rates are unknown.

Evidence Levels: **A** Double-blind study **B** Clinical trial ≥ 20 subjects **C** Clinical trial < 20 subjects **D** Series ≥ 5 subjects **E** Anecdotal case reports

SPECIFIC INVESTIGATIONS

▶ Direct microscopy
▶ Culture
▶ Histology
▶ Serological tests
▶ Chest radiography
▶ Serology for HIV/AIDS infection (where relevant)

Rapid diagnosis may be achieved by direct microscopic examination of sputum or other exudates in potassium hydroxide. *P. brasiliensis* appears as large, round yeast cells with multiple budding. Culture of sputum, skin, lymph node, or bone marrow specimens on Sabouraud dextrose agar can recover the organism, but may require 20–30 days for growth. Biopsy specimens reveal granuloma formation, and Gomori methenamine silver stain reveals yeast cells. There are several serological tests that detect antibodies against the fungus, and they can provide results earlier than culture or histopathology. The most common test is immunodiffusion, which has high specificity although sensitivity varies depending on the type of antigen used. Therefore, a negative serologic response does not exclude PCM, particularly in the immunocompromised.

FIRST-LINE THERAPIES

▶ Itraconazole	B
▶ Sulfonamides	B
▶ Amphotericin B	B

The following reviews discuss the manifestations and management of PCM.

Paracoccidioidomycosis and AIDS: an overview. Goldani L, Sugar AM. Clin Infect Dis 1995; 21: 1275–81.

This is the largest published review of paracoccidioidomycosis in association with AIDS. A wide spectrum of clinical manifestations was seen in the 27 patients described, ranging from indolent infection to rapidly progressive disease. There was multiorgan involvement in 70.4% of patients (n=19), disseminated disease being the most common form of paracoccidioidomycosis. The overall mortality among patients with AIDS is high (30%). The prognosis can be improved by earlier diagnosis and aggressive therapy with amphotericin B, followed by lifelong immunosuppressive therapy with trimethoprim-sulfamethoxazole.

Paracoccidioidomycosis in patients with human immunodeficiency virus: review of 12 cases observed in an endemic region in Brazil. Paniago AM, de Freitas AC, Aguiar ES, Aguiar JI, da Cunha RV, Castro AR, et al. J Infect 2005; 51: 248–52.

This study demonstrated that the lymph nodes were the organ most commonly involved (n=10, 83.3%), followed by the lung (n=7, 58.3%). Papulonodular ulcerative skin lesions affected 50% (n=6), and oral mucosal ulcerative lesions were present in 42% (n=5). A single patient had pleural involvement with a secondary pathological rib fracture. Seven patients had multiorgan involvement. All patients were treated with trimethoprim-sulfamethoxazole, and seven patients also received amphotericin B. However, eight patients (67%) died as a result of disease progression.

Pharmacological management of paracoccidioidomycosis. Yasuda MA. Exp Opin Pharmacother 2005; 6: 385–97.

This article emphasizes the long duration of drug therapy required for both the treatment and maintenance of patients with severe infection. It explores the possibility of finding novel therapies among new classes of drugs, drug combinations, or agents capable of modulating the immune response, such as a peptide derived from the 43-kDa *P. brasiliensis* glycoprotein.

Drugs for treating paracoccidioidomycosis. Menezes VM, Soares BG, Fontes CJ. Cochrane Database Syst Rev 2006; 19: CD004967.

This was a critical evaluation of the current therapeutic armamentarium used for the treatment of paracoccidioidomycosis. On the basis of strict selection criteria, including randomized controlled trials, only a single study could be included for analysis (Shikanai-Yasuda MA et al. 2002) with a brief mention of other studies.

Treatment options for paracoccidioidomycosis and new strategies investigated. Travassos LR, Taborda CP, Colombo AL. Exp Rev Anti Infect Ther 2008; 6: 251–62.

This article highlights the significant and unresolved burden of relapses despite the use of long courses of drug therapies, which include sulfamethoxazole-trimethoprim, itraconazole, and amphotericin B. A peptide vaccine aimed at immunotherapy of paracoccidioidomycosis is being studied, and the authors suggest that it could be used as a vaccine to reduce the duration of chemotherapy and the risk of relapse.

Paracoccidioidomycosis. Ramos-E-Silva M, Saraiva Ldo E. Dermatol Clin 2008; 26: 257–69.

This review was written with dermatologists in mind, focusing on the features of mucocutaneous presentation.

Central nervous system paracoccidioidomycosis: an overview. De Almeida SM. Braz J Infect Dis 2005; 9: 126–33.

Central nervous system (CNS) involvement with paracoccidioidomycosis has been found in 13% of patients with systemic disease. This review article covers the clinical presentation, diagnostic tests, and treatments for CNS infection. Sulfas are considered the drugs of choice, sulfamethoxazole-trimethoprim (160/800 mg three times daily) being most commonly used. Amphotericin B is only used in cases of resistance or intolerance to sulfonamides. Of the azoles, itraconazole and particularly ketoconazole penetrate the blood–brain barrier poorly. Fluconazole, however, has excellent CNS penetration, making it a potentially suitable alternative to the other drug therapies.

Treatment of paracoccidioidomycosis with itraconazole. Naranjo MS, Trujillo M, Munera MI, Restrepo P, Gomez I, Restrepo A. J Med Vet Mycol 1990; 28: 67–76.

Forty-seven patients with mainly the chronic adult form of infection were treated with itraconazole 100 mg daily for a mean of 6 months (range 3–24 months). There was marked clinical improvement in 43 patients (89%) and complete resolution of disease in only one. The mycological tests (direct examination and cultures) became negative during the first month of treatment in 87% of patients, and by the end of treatment there was a decline in specific antibody titers in 72%. There was no clinical relapse in 15 patients during a 12-month follow-up period.

Randomized trial with itraconazole, ketoconazole and sulfadiazine in paracoccidioidomycosis. Shikanai-Yasuda MA, Benard G, Higaki Y, Del Negro GM, Hoo S, Vaccari EH, et al. Med Mycol 2002; 40: 411–17.

This study from Brazil included 42 patients with moderately severe paracoccidioidomycosis who were randomized to receive itraconazole 50–100 mg daily (n=14), ketoconazole 200–400 mg daily (n=14), or sulfadiazine 150 mg/kg daily (n=14) for an induction period of 4–6 months. This was followed by slow-release sulfa (sulfamethoxypyridazine) until negative serological results were obtained. The majority of patients in all arms were reported as cured after 6 months of treatment, and antibody levels reduced significantly by 10 months for all three drugs.

This study demonstrated that both sulfadiazine and the azoles were equally effective, and the cure rates for the individual drugs were similar to those in previous studies.

Paracoccidioidomycosis in children: clinical presentation, follow-up and outcome. Pereira RM, Bucaretchi F, Barison Ede M, Hessel G, Tresoldi AT. Rev Inst Med Trop São Paulo 2004; 46: 127–31.

This study from Brazil investigated 70 episodes of infection in 63 children under the age of 15 (range 2–15 years). The juvenile and disseminated form of paracoccidioidomycosis was seen in 70% of episodes, most of them presenting with a febrile lymphoproliferative syndrome. The diagnosis was confirmed by lymph node biopsy (84%), bone biopsy (9%), and skin biopsy (7%). Treatment consisted of either sulfamethoxazole-trimethoprim monotherapy (n=50), sulfamethoxazole-trimethoprim combined with amphotericin B (n=9), or ketoconazole (n=5). Follow-up revealed significant sequential improvement 1 and 6 months later. However, six patients died (9.3%) and four developed sequelae: portal hypertension in three and hypersplenism in one (6.3%). The authors attribute the deaths to the severity of disseminated infection in the context of profound immunosuppression caused by paracoccidioidomycosis as well as malnutrition. A long period of drug treatment – up to 2 years – is required to prevent any risk of relapse.

The authors suggest sulfamethoxazole-trimethoprim as first-line therapy in children because of its efficacy, low cost, and easy route of oral administration. It may also be infused intravenously for severe infection. They attributed therapy failure largely to non-compliance.

Paracoccidioidomycosis: a clinical and epidemiological study of 422 cases observed in Mato Gross do Sul. Paniago AM, Aguiar JI, Aguiar ES, da Cunha RV, Pereira GR, Londero AT, et al. Rev Soc Bras Med Trop 2003; 36: 455–9.

In terms of treatment this paper illustrates how sulfamethoxazole-trimethoprim is commonly used in endemic areas for paracoccidioidomycosis: 90.3% of patients were treated with this drug, the majority responding to treatment.

Clinical and serologic features of 47 patients with paracoccidioidomycosis treated by amphotericin B. De Campos EP, Sartori JC, Hetch ML, de Franco MF. Rev Inst Med Trop São Paulo 1984; 26: 212–17.

In this study of 47 patients with disseminated infection treated with amphotericin B (30 mg/kg, total dose 2.0–3.0 g), clinical and serological cure was obtained in 54%.

Paracoccidioidomycosis: a comparative study of the evolutionary serologic, clinical and radiologic results for patients treated with ketoconazole or amphotericin B plus sulfonamides. Marques SA, Dillon NL, Franco MF, Habermann MC, Lastoria JC, Stolf HO, et al. Mycopathologia 1985; 89: 19–23.

This was a retrospective study comparing the use of ketoconazole (400 mg daily for 30 days, followed by 200 mg daily for 18 months) in 22 patients against amphotericin B (1.5–1.75 mg/kg/day for 30–60 days) together with sulfonamide maintenance therapy for up to 18 months in 32 patients. Approximately one-third of patients in each group had the acute form of the infection, and the rest had chronic disease. Patients treated with ketoconazole demonstrated better responses, but the results were not statistically significant. There was a sharper drop in antibody titers in patients treated with ketoconazole, but there was no difference in radiological evolution between the treatments.

Failure of amphotericin B colloidal dispersion in the treatment of paracoccidioidomycosis. Dietze R, Flowler VG Jr, Steiner TS, Pecanha PM, Corey GR. Am J Trop Med Hyg 1999; 60: 837–9.

In this study four adults with the aggressive juvenile form of paracoccidioidomycosis were treated with amphotericin B colloidal dispersion. One patient was also co-infected with HIV. They all received a dose of 3 mg/kg/day for at least 28 days. Three patients, including the HIV-infected one, demonstrated a complete clinical response, but relapsed within 6 months. They were subsequently successfully treated with co-trimoxazole. The authors suggest that possible reasons for failure might have been the dose, treatment duration, the drug formulation, inadequate drug delivery to sites of infection, and impaired host immunity. The authors also describe unpublished data on five further patients with chronic paracoccidioidomycosis treated with liposomal amphotericin 4 mg/kg/day. They also responded to treatment initially, but subsequently relapsed after treatment was stopped.

These results raise concerns about the use of short courses of lipid-based formulations to treat PCM. Further and larger studies are required to investigate their efficacy.

SECOND-LINE THERAPIES

▶ Ketoconazole	B
▶ Fluconazole	B
▶ Voriconazole	B
▶ Terbinafine	E

Treatment of paracoccidioidomycosis with ketoconazole: a three-year experience. Restrepo A, Gómez I, Cano LE, Arango MD, Gutiérrez F, Sanín A, et al. Am J Med 1983; 74: 48–52.

Thirty-eight patients with active infection were treated with ketoconzole 200 mg daily for 6 months. Treatment was well tolerated. There was complete resolution of infection in 13 patients (34%), and significant improvement in the majority of the rest.

In a subsequent study, 24 of these patients were followed up for 1–2 years. Relapse was detected in only two. There are no recent studies evaluating ketoconazole for PCM, as its use has declined with the advent of newer antifungals.

A Pan-American 5-year study of fluconazole therapy for deep mycoses in the immunocompetent host. Diaz M, Negroni R, Montero-Gei F, Castro LG, Sampaio SA, Borelli D, et al.; Pan-American Study Group. Clin Infect Dis 1992; 14: S68–76.

Of 28 patients, 27 responded to treatment with fluconazole 200–400 mg daily given for at least 6 months. Treatment was well tolerated. However, relapse was noted in one patient within the first year.

This is the only reported study of fluconazole therapy for PCM. A longer period of follow-up is required in order to evaluate drug efficacy.

An open-label comparative pilot study of oral voriconazole and itraconazole for long-term treatment of paracoccidioidomycosis. Queiroz-Telles F, Goldani LZ, Schlamm HT, Goodrich JM, Espinel-Ingroff A, Shikanai-Yasuda MA. Clin Infect Dis 2007; 45: 1462–9.

This multicenter study from Brazil investigated the efficacy, safety, and tolerability of voriconazole for the long-term treatment of acute or chronic paracoccidioidomycosis, with itraconazole as the control treatment. Patients were randomized (at a 2:1 ratio) to receive oral voriconazole (n=35) or itraconazole (n=18) for 6–12 months. Voriconazole was given at an initial loading dose of 800 mg in divided doses on day 1, followed by 200 mg twice daily. The dose of itraconazole was 100 mg twice daily. There was a satisfactory response rate in 88.6% of the voriconazole group and 94.4% of the itraconazole group. The response rate among evaluable patients was 100% for both treatment groups. No relapses were observed after 8 weeks of follow-up. Both drugs were well tolerated, although liver function test values were slightly higher in patients receiving voriconazole, necessitating the withdrawal of voriconazole from two patients.

This study has demonstrated equal efficacy and tolerability of oral voriconazole and itraconazole for the long-term treatment of paracoccidioidomycosis. This study also included a case of CNS paracoccidioidomycosis which responded to treatment. Voriconazole demonstrates good CNS penetration, having been successfully used in the treatment of other mycotic CNS infections. On the basis of these results the authors suggested that intravenous voriconazole should be evaluated as an alternative to amphotericin B for the initial treatment of severe paracoccidioidomycosis, given the high relapse rate and toxicity associated with amphotericin B therapy.

Chronic paracoccidioidomycosis in a female patient in Austria. Mayr A, Kirchmair M, Rainer J, Rossi R, Kreczy A, Tintelnot K, et al. Eur J Clin Microbiol Infect Dis 2004; 23: 916–19.

Case report of a Cuban woman who was initially misdiagnosed with tuberculosis. She was successfully treated with amphotericin B (1 mg/kg/day) for 10 days, followed by voriconazole 200 mg daily for 3 months.

Paracoccidioidomycosis (South American Blastomycosis) successfully treated with terbinafine: first case report. Ollague JM, de Zurita AM, Calero G. Br J Dermatol 2000; 143: 188–91.

A case report of a 63-year-old man who presented with lesions of paracoccidioidomycosis in the perineal region. Initial treatment with trimethoprim-sulfamethoxazole failed. He was subsequently treated with terbinafine 250 mg twice daily for 6 months, which resulted in rapid resolution of all lesions without evidence of relapse for 2 years.

Terbinafine has demonstrated similar activity to itraconazole against P. brasiliensis *in vitro.*

THIRD LINE THERAPIES

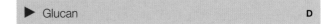

▶ Glucan   D

The use of glucan as immunostimulant in the treatment of paracoccidioidomycosis. Meira DA, Pereira PC, Marcondes-Machado J, Medes RP, Barraviera B, Pellegrino J Jr, et al. Am J Trop Med Hyg 1996; 55: 496–503.

In this clinical trial a group of 10 patients, nine of them reportedly severely infected with *P. brasiliensis*, received glucan (β1,3-polyglucose) as an immunostimulant intravenously once weekly for 1 month, followed by monthly doses of 10 mg over a period of 11 months; this was used in conjunction with antifungal drugs. The control group, which consisted of eight moderately infected patients, was treated with antifungals only (ketoconazole, co-trimoxazole, sulfonamides, amphotericin B). Patients who received glucan, despite being more seriously ill, showed a more favorable response to therapy, with only a single relapse (one of 10) compared to five of eight in the control arm.

Parapsoriasis

Alex Milligan, Rosie Davis, Graham Johnston

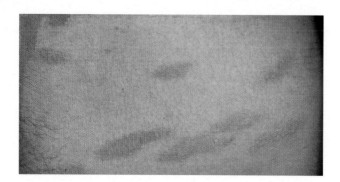

The diagnosis parapsoriasis, even as an umbrella term, continues to cause diagnostic difficulties and there is still debate as to whether the variants described in this chapter are in fact precursors of cutaneous T-cell lymphoma. This chapter covers the entities small plaque parapsoriasis (SPP: chronic superficial scaly dermatitis; persistent superficial dermatitis; digitate dermatosis; xanthoerythroderma perstans) and large plaque parapsoriasis (LPP: parakeratosis variegata; retiform parapsoriasis; atrophic parapsoriasis; poikilodermatous parapsoriasis). Confusingly, the term parapsoriasis en plaque has been used for either SPP or LPP.

Other conditions sometimes grouped under the banner of parapsoriasis are pityriasis lichenoides et varioliformis acuta (PLEVA), pityriasis lichenoides chronica, and lymphomatoid papulosis.

SMALL PLAQUE PARAPSORIASIS

SPP consists of fixed, small scaly erythematous plaques which are asymptomatic or only mildly itchy and occur mainly on the trunk. The lesions sometimes appear to run in lines parallel to the ribs (hence the name 'digitate dermatosis'). SPP runs a chronic, indolent, and benign course.

MANAGEMENT STRATEGY

The diagnosis of parapsoriasis is made on clinical grounds, with histology supporting the clinical impression, especially when early cutaneous T-cell lymphoma is in the differential diagnosis. Patches of LPP are larger than 5 cm in diameter, and often 10 cm or larger, distinguishing them from SPP, which is characterized by lesions smaller than 5 cm.

If malignancy is considered in the differential diagnosis, T-cell receptor gene rearrangement studies are more likely to demonstrate monoclonality in cutaneous T-cell lymphoma, though monoclonality is not entirely sensitive or specific for the latter. Repeat studies may be warranted if progression to cutaneous T-cell lymphoma is suspected.

Although some advocate non-aggressive therapies, such as *topical corticosteroids*, for parapsoriasis, the potential for progression to cutaneous lymphoma in patients with LPP justifies the use of *psoralen with UVA (PUVA)*. *Sunlight, broadband UVB*, and *narrowband UVB* have been used successfully as well, particularly for SPP.

SPECIFIC INVESTIGATIONS

> ► The diagnosis is principally made on clinical findings
> ► Histology is nonspecific
> ► TCR gene rearrangement studies

Assessment of TCR-beta clonality in a diverse group of cutaneous T-cell infiltrates. Plaza JA, Morrison C, Magro CM. J Cutan Pathol 2008; 35: 358–65.

Monoclonality is a reliable characteristic of CTCL, polyclonality being very infrequent. However, the authors warn that the various cutaneous lymphoid dyscrasias, including pityriasis lichenoides chronica, could manifest restricted molecular profiles in the context of an oligoclonal process or frank monoclonality.

Clonal T cell receptor gamma-chain gene rearrangement by PCR-based GeneScan analysis in the skin and blood of patients with parapsoriasis and early-stage mycosis fungoides. Klemke CD, Dippel E, Dembinski A, Pönitz N, Assaf C, Hummel M, et al. J Pathol 2002; 197: 348–54.

Although studies have shown T-cell clonality in both skin and peripheral blood, monoclonality is neither easily demonstrable nor thought to be a prerequisite for diagnosis.

FIRST-LINE THERAPIES

> ► Emollients, tar, topical corticosteroids   E
> ► PUVA   C
> ► Narrowband UVB   C
> ► UVA/UVB   E

Treatments with emollients, topical tar, and topical corticosteroid are cited in books, and appear effective in clinical practice. There have, however, been no studies or case reports to back this up, and these treatments are therefore unreferenced.

Narrowband UVB phototherapy for small plaque parapsoriasis. Aydogan K, Karadogan SK, Tunali S, Adim SB, Ozcelik T. J Eur Acad Dermatol Venereol 2006; 20: 573–7.

Forty-five patients were treated with narrowband UVB therapy three to four times weekly. There was a complete response in 33 patients with a mean cumulative dose of 14.3 J/cm² after a mean number of 29 exposures. There was a partial response in 12 of the 45. Relapses occurred in six patients within a mean of 7.5 months.

Treatment of small plaque parapsoriasis with narrow-band (311 nm) ultraviolet B: A retrospective study. Herzinger T, Degitz K, Plewig G, Rocken M. Clin Exp Dermatol 2005; 30: 379–81.

Sixteen patients had complete remission after a mean number of 32.8 exposures and a mean total dose of 35.4 J/cm². Side effects were rare and mild. Relapse occurred after an average of 29 weeks.

Narrowband (311-nm) UV-B therapy for small plaque parapsoriasis and early-stage mycosis fungoides. Hofer A, Cerroni L, Kerl H, Wolf P. Arch Dermatol 1999; 35: 1377–80.

Fourteen patients with SPP were treated with narrowband UVB, three to four times weekly for 5–10 weeks. Complete response was achieved after an average of 20 exposures.

Evidence Levels: **A** Double-blind study   **B** Clinical trial ≥ 20 subjects   **C** Clinical trial < 20 subjects   **D** Series ≥ 5 subjects   **E** Anecdotal case reports

All patients then relapsed after an average of 6 months, and topical corticosteroid therapy was effective at producing a second clearance in an unspecified number of patients.

Treatment of parapsoriasis and mycosis fungoides: the role of psoralen and long-wave ultraviolet light A (PUVA). Powell FC, Spiegel GT, Muller SA. Mayo Clin Proc 1984; 59: 538–46.

Seven patients with SPP had complete clearance with as few as 15 treatments (84 J/cm^2) of standard PUVA. Three patients experienced some recurrence at follow-up (mean of 13 months), and one of these was then successfully treated with topical corticosteroid.

UVA1 cold-light phototherapy has also been reported to be beneficial in small plaque parapsoriasis.

SECOND-LINE THERAPIES

▶ Topical nitrogen mustard   **E**

Topical carmustine (BCNU) for mycosis fungoides and related disorders: a 10-year experience. Zackheim HS, Epstein EH Jr, McNutt NS, Grekin DA, Crain WR. J Am Acad Dermatol 1983; 9: 363–74.

One patient with SPP was treated with carmustine as a subgroup of the study. A variety of treatment regimens were used and not individually specified. Complete response was achieved at follow-up, but the duration is not specified.

LARGE PLAQUE PARAPSORIASIS

Like SPP, the trunk is mainly affected but the lesions are larger, atrophic, and even poikilodermatous, with a red or yellow-orange color.

SPECIFIC INVESTIGATIONS

▶ Skin biopsy
▶ TCR gene rearrangement studies

The diagnosis is suggested clinically. Histology can vary from a mild dermatitis to epidermal atrophy, lichenoid changes at the dermoepidermal junction, and a band-like lymphocytic infiltrate in the papillary dermis.

Progression to T-cell lymphoma can occur. T-cell clonality can be demonstrated in some patients.

Large plaque parapsoriasis: clinical and genotypic correlations. Simon M, Flaig MJ, Kind P, Sander CA, Kaudewitz P. J Cutan Pathol 2000; 27: 57–60.

TCR gene rearrangement status was assessed in 12 patients. Six of the 12 showed a clonal T-cell population, one of whom developed cutaneous T-cell lymphoma after a follow-up of 8 years. The other five patients showed no such progression after follow-up of 2–21 years. The authors conclude that TCR gene rearrangement status has no prognostic significance and does not allow distinction between LPP and early mycosis fungoides.

The nosology of parapsoriasis. Lambert WC, Everett MA. J Am Acad Dermatol 1981; 5: 373–95.

Of 129 cases of LPP, 11% developed mycosis fungoides over a follow-up period ranging from 1 to 64 years.

Parapsoriasis and mycosis fungoides: the Northwestern University experience, 1970 to 1985. Lazar AP, Caro WA, Roenigk HH, Pinski KS. J Am Acad Dermatol 1989; 21: 919–23.

Of 89 patients with LPP, 30% developed mycosis fungoides. The follow-up period was not specified.

FIRST-LINE THERAPIES

▶ PUVA   **C**
▶ PUVA with 4,6,4'-trimethylangelicin (TMA)   **E**

Photochemotherapy in cutaneous T cell lymphoma and parapsoriasis en plaque. Long-term follow-up in forty-three patients. Rosenbaum MM, Roenigk HH Jr, Caro WA, Esker A. J Am Acad Dermatol 1985; 13: 613–22.

Seven patients with LPP were included as part of the above study. They were treated with oral psoralens and ultraviolet A. A complete response was achieved in all seven, though the total dosages of PUVA are not stated. Average follow-up for all 43 patients was 38.4 months (range 4–67 months), and during that time relapse was observed in five out of the seven.

Because cutaneous T-cell lymphoma is in the differential diagnosis of LPP, and PUVA is effective for both conditions, this therapy is useful in patients in whom it is difficult to distinguish between the two conditions.

Treatment of a case of mycosis fungoides and one of parapsoriasis en plaque with topical PUVA using a monofunctional furocoumarin derivative, 4,6,4'-trimethylangelicin. Morita A, Takashima A, Nagai M, Dall'Acqua F. J Dermatol 1990; 17: 545–9.

A single patient with LPP was treated with 0.1% TMA topical lotion (a monofunctional psoralen), followed 2 hours later with UVA light. Clearance was achieved after nine treatments with 24 cm^2. A control area did not have the topical TMA applied to it and clearance was not obtained even after 20 treatments.

SECOND-LINE THERAPIES

▶ Topical nitrogen mustard   **E**

Topical carmustine (BCNU) for mycosis fungoides and related disorders: a 10-year experience. Zackheim HS, Epstein EH Jr, McNutt NS, Grekin DA, Crain WR. J Am Acad Dermatol 1983; 9: 363–74.

One patient with LPP was treated with carmustine as a subgroup of the larger study. Initially a complete response was achieved, but at follow up (unknown duration) a partial response was observed. A variety of treatment regimens were used and not individually specified.

Evaluation of a one-hour exposure time to mechlorethamine in patients undergoing topical treatment. Foulc P, Evrard V, Dalac S, Guillot B, Delaunay M, Verret JL, et al. Br J Dermatol 2002; 147: 926–30.

Three patients with large plaque psoriasis were included in this study. One patient stopped treatment because of the side effects and two of the three resulted in complete remission. The mechlorethamine regimen, however, varied between the four centers included in the study and is not specified for the individual patient.

The usefulness of topical chemotherapy is limited by the development of contact dermatitis. In addition, the incidence of squamous cell carcinoma of the skin is dramatically increased in patients treated with topical nitrogen mustard and PUVA.

THIRD-LINE THERAPIES

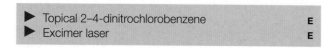

▶ Topical 2–4-dinitrochlorobenzene	E
▶ Excimer laser	E

Successful treatment of parapsoriasis en plaques with 2,4-dinitrochlorobenzene. Mandrea E. Arch Dermatol 1971; 103: 560–1.

A single patient with LPP was treated topically with twice-daily 1% 2,4-dinitrochlorobenzene in equal parts with olive oil and propylene glycol. The patient developed a painful, erythematous reaction and the treatment was stopped; 18 months later the skin remained clear.

Excimer-laser (308 nm) treatment of large plaque parapsoriasis and long-term follow-up. Gebert S, Raulin C, Ockenfels HM, Gundogan C, Greve B. Eur J Dermatol 2006; 16: 198–9.

A letter describing long-term benefit with a 308 nm laser.

Paronychia

Richard B Mallett

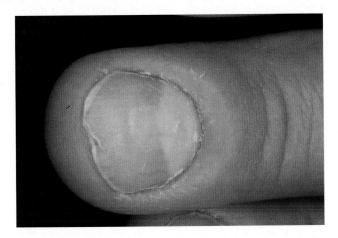

Paronychia is characterized by inflammation of the proximal and/or lateral nailfolds, the fingers being more commonly affected than the toes. Acute paronychia is a painful pyogenic infection that occurs after injury or minor trauma and is characteristically caused by *Staphylococcus aureus*, although anaerobic organisms are also found.

Chronic paronychia presents as tender erythema of the nailfolds with thickening of the tissues, loss of the cuticle, and subsequent dystrophy of the nail plate. Repetitive microtrauma and exposure to water, irritants, and allergens, resulting in a dermatitis with subsequent colonization by yeasts, and secondary bacterial infection, are causative factors in chronic paronychia, one of the commonest nail disorders. A recently recognized uncommon cause of chronic paronychia, retronychia, is characterized by disruption of the longitudinal growth of a nail due to acute injury from physical or systemic causes, with resultant embedding of the old nail in the ventral surface of the proximal nailfold as the new nail regenerates. Also, cutaneous leishmaniasis may rarely present as an unusual chronic paronychia in endemic areas.

Paronychia with pseudopyogenic granuloma may occur with systemic retinoids, antiretroviral drugs such as indinavir or lamivudine, the anti-epidermal growth factor antibody cetuximab, and epidermal growth factor tyrosine kinase inhibitors, such as gefitinib.

Tumors that may rarely present masquerading as chronic paronychia include Bowen's disease, keratoacanthomas, squamous cell carcinoma, enchondroma, and amelanotic melanoma.

MANAGEMENT STRATEGY

Acute paronychia requires urgent effective treatment to prevent damage to the nail matrix. If the infection is superficial and pointing, then *incision and drainage* without anesthesia is possible. Infection is often due to *S. aureus*, but β-hemolytic streptococci and anaerobic organisms may also be found. A swab must be taken for bacterial culture and antibiotic sensitivity, and a *broad-spectrum antibiotic* covering both aerobic and anaerobic organisms given. *Warm compresses with an astringent* (e.g., aluminum acetate lotion, if available) can help reduce edema and provide a hostile environment for bacteria. For deeper infections, antibiotic treatment should be started immediately, and if there has been no marked clinical improvement after 48 hours, *surgical treatment* undertaken. Under local anesthesia, the proximal third of the nail plate is removed and a gauze wick is laid under the proximal nailfold to allow drainage.

Chronic paronychia is most commonly a dermatitis often associated with wet work – in domestics, cooks, bartenders, fishmongers, etc. – and may be exacerbated by contact irritants or allergens. Immediate sensitivity to fresh foods can be a factor. In children, thumb sucking may initiate the condition. Eczema or psoriasis may predispose to chronic paronychia, as may poor peripheral circulation. Microtrauma, including overzealous manicuring of the cuticle, is also important. The middle and index fingers of the right hand and the middle finger of the left hand are most commonly affected, but any finger may be involved. Inflammation with bolstering of the nailfold and loss of the cuticle opens a space between the nailfold and the nail plate, which commonly becomes infected with yeast, especially *Candida* species, and a wide range of other microorganisms. Acute exacerbations due to bacterial infection may occur. Successful treatment relies on protection of the affected fingers from water, irritants, allergens, and trauma, together with anti-inflammatory treatment using moderately potent or potent *topical corticosteroids*. Swabs for yeast and bacteria should be taken, *anticandidal preparations* can be useful, and antibiotic preparations may also be needed. Treatment should be continued until the inflammation has subsided and the cuticle reformed and reattached to the nail plate (3 months or more). Applying 80% phenol with a toothpick to the groove under the proximal nailfold may encourage reattachment. Warm compresses for 10 minutes with an astringent lotion may help acute exacerbations. For frequent acute episodes, *intralesional or systemic corticosteroids plus systemic antibiotics* for a week may be useful. In cases where conservative management fails, surgery or *low-dose superficial radiotherapy* may be considered. For cases secondary to retronychia simple avulsion of the nail plate can be curative.

Drug-induced pseudopyogenic granulomatous paronychia responds to daily topical *2% mupirocin* with *clobetasol propionate* ointment.

Chronic paronychia due to cetuximab may respond to oral *doxycycline* 100 mg BD.

SPECIFIC INVESTIGATIONS

▶ Skin swabs
▶ Open patch tests

Anaerobic paronychia. Whitehead SM, Eykyn SJ, Phillips I. Br J Surg 1981; 68: 420–2.

Swabs were taken from 116 acute paronychias. Anaerobes or mixed aerobes and anaerobes were isolated in 30%. Of 81 paronychias with aerobic organisms only, *S. aureus* was isolated in 69%.

Chronic paronychia. Short review of 590 cases. Frain-Bell W. Trans St John's Hosp Dermatol Soc 1957; 38: 29–35.

On culture, *Candida albicans* was grown in 70% and bacteria, including *S. aureus*, in 10%.

An excellent overview.

Role of foods in the pathogenesis of chronic paronychia. Tosti A, Guerra L, Morelli R, Bardazzi F, Fanti PA. J Am Acad Dermatol 1992; 27: 706–10.

Nine of 20 food handlers with chronic paronychia had positive reactions to 20-minute open patch tests with suspected fresh foods, including wheat flour, egg, chicory, and tomatoes.

FIRST-LINE THERAPIES

Acute

▶ Amoxicillin with clavulinic acid   E
▶ Surgical drainage   E

Chronic

▶ Topical corticosteroid preparations   B
▶ Topical econazole lotion four times daily   B
▶ Topical clotrimazole drops   E
▶ Topical clindamycin solution   E

Due to retronychia

▶ Avulsion of nail plate   E

Drug-induced periungual granuloma

▶ Mupirocin and clobetasol propionate   E

Cetuximab-induced paronychia

▶ Doxycycline 100 mg BD   E

Paronychia: a mixed infection, microbiology and management. Brook I. J Hand Surg [Br] 1993; 18: 358–9.

Culture from 61 patients with paronychia showed a mixture of both aerobic and anaerobic bacteria in 49%. The combination of amoxicillin with clavulinic acid is suggested as first-line treatment for acute bacterial paronychia, together with appropriate surgical drainage.

Nail surgery and traumatic abnormalities. Haneke E, Baran R, Brauner GJ. In: Baran R, Dawber RP, eds. Diseases of the nails and their management, 2nd edn. Oxford: Blackwell Scientific, 1994; 408.

For acute paronychia, under local anesthesia the proximal third of the nail plate is removed and a wick laid under the proximal nailfold.

Topical steroids versus systemic antifungals in the treatment of chronic paronychia: an open, randomized double-blind and double dummy study. Tosti A, Piraccini BM, Ghetti E. J Am Acad Dermatol 2002; 47: 73–6.

An open, randomized, double-blind trial of oral itraconazole, oral terbinafine, and topical methylprednisolone aceponate. Patients were treated for 3 weeks and observed for a further 6 weeks. Of 48 nails treated with methylprednisolone aceponate, 41 (85%) were improved or cured at the end of the study, compared to only 30 of 57 (53%) with itraconazole and 29 of 64 (45%) with terbinafine.

The management of superficial candidiasis. Hay RJ. J Am Acad Dermatol 1999; 40: S35–42.

The central role of *Candida* in chronic paronychia is debatable, and other factors such as irritant or allergic dermatitis may play a role. Therefore, as well as polyenes or imidazoles, concomitant use of a topical corticosteroid is a logical approach.

Comparison of the therapeutic effect of ketaconazole tablets and econazole lotion in the treatment of chronic paronychia. Wong ESM, Hay RJ, Clayton YM, Noble WC. Clin Exp Dermatol 1984; 9: 489–96.

A randomized trial comparing oral ketaconazole 200 mg once daily versus topical econazole lotion 2 mL four times daily in 24 patients with chronic paronychia and positive cultures for *Candida* species. All patients were also advised to wear rubber gloves for wet work, to dry the hands thoroughly, and not to push back the nailfold or wear nail varnish. There was no significant difference between the two treatments, suggesting that topical econazole lotion is suitable for first-line treatment of chronic paronychia in the presence of *Candida* infection.

Diseases of the nails in infants and children: paronychia. Silverman RA. In: Callen JP, Dhal MV, Golitz LE, et al., eds. Advances in dermatology. Vol 5. Chicago: Mosby Year Book, 1990; 164–5.

Clotrimazole drops several times a day should inhibit fungal growth. Topical clindamycin solution applied to the fingers several times daily kills bacteria, has a bitter taste to discourage finger sucking, and has an alcohol–propylene glycol vehicle that dries out residual moisture. Side effects from oral absorption of these medications have not been reported.

Retronychia: report of two cases. Gahdah MJ, Kibbi AG, Ghosn S. J Am Acad Dermatol 2008: 58; 1051–3.

Two cases of paronychia due to retronychia, a term coined by Berker et al. in 1999, successfully treated with simple nail avulsion.

Paronychia associated with antiretroviral therapy. Tosti A, Piraccini BM, D'Antuono A, Marzaduri S, Bettoli V. Br J Dermatol 1999; 140: 1165–8.

Six cases of periungual pseudopyogenic granuloma induced by indinavir, lamivudine, and zidovudine responded to daily applications of clobetasol propionate and mupirocin.

Doxycycline for the treatment of paronychia induced by the epidermal growth factor receptor inhibitor cetuximab. Suh K-Y, Kindler HL, Medenica M, Lacouture M. Br J Dermatol 2006; 154: 191–2.

During treatment with cetuximab a patient developed painful paronychia, refractory to topical mupirocin and cefalexin but improved after treatment with doxycycline 100 mg twice daily.

SECOND-LINE THERAPIES

Chronic

▶ 15% sulfacetamide in 50% spirit   E
▶ Nystatin ointment   E
▶ 4% thymol in chloroform   E
▶ Intralesional or systemic corticosteroids and antibiotics   E

Management of disorders of the nails. Samman PD. Clin Exp Dermatol 1982; 7: 189–94.

Chronic paronychia can be treated with 15% sulfacetamide in 50% spirit applied frequently. Sulfacetamide is both antifungal and antibacterial.

A good overview of nail disease.

Treatment of chronic paronychia. Vickers HR. Br Med J 1979; 2: 1588.

A nystatin-containing ointment should be worked into the affected nailfold every time the patient is going to get the hands wet, for at least 6 weeks.

Paronychia and onycholysis, aetiology and therapy. Wilson JW. Arch Dermatol 1965; 92: 726–30.

Thymol has both bactericidal and antifungal properties. Apply 4% thymol in chloroform to the nailfold and allow to penetrate by capillary action. Application should be three times daily and, additionally, immediately after immersion in water.

Fungal and other infections. Hay RJ, Baran R, Haneke E. In: Baran R, Dawber RP, eds. Diseases of the nails and their management, 2nd edn. Oxford: Blackwell Scientific, 1994; 119–20.

For frequent acute exacerbations of chronic paronychia, intralesional or systemic corticosteroids plus either erythromycin 1g daily or tetracycline 1g daily for a week is recommended.

THIRD-LINE THERAPIES

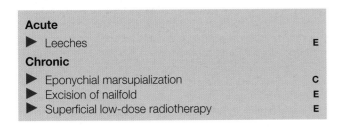

Acute	
▶ Leeches	E
Chronic	
▶ Eponychial marsupialization	C
▶ Excision of nailfold	E
▶ Superficial low-dose radiotherapy	E

Thumb paronychia treated with leeches. Graham CE. Med J Aust 1992; 156: 512.

Acute paronychia successfully treated with leeches while trekking in Tasmania.

Eponychial marsupialization and nail removal for surgical treatment of chronic paronychia. Bednar MS, Lane LB. J Hand Surg [Am] 1991; 16: 314–17.

Twenty-eight fingers with chronic paronychia were treated with marsupialization of the dorsal roof of the proximal nailfold plus complete or partial removal of the nail in those patients with associated nail abnormality. Postoperative treatment was with hydrogen peroxide soaks and oral antibiotics for 5–14 days. Twenty-seven of 28 fingers were cured.

Surgical treatment of recalcitrant chronic paronychia of the fingers. Baran R, Bureau H. J Dermatol Surg Oncol 1981; 7: 106–7.

Description of the technique of simple excision of the affected nailfold without the need for marsupialization.

How we treat paronychia. Fliegelman MT, Lafayette GO. Postgrad Med 1970; 48: 267–8.

For recalcitrant cases of chronic paronychia, triamcinolone can be injected into the affected nailfold. For the most severe cases, a course of low-dose superficial radiotherapy may be given.

Papular urticaria

Amir A Larian, Jacob Levitt

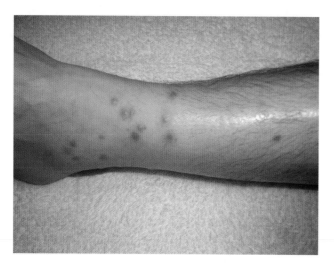

Papular urticaria (PU) is a common disease characterized by chronic or recurrent eruptions of 3–10mm pruritic papules, wheals, and/or vesicles caused by hypersensitivity to the bites of arthropods, including fleas, mosquitoes, scabies, and bedbugs. Although the antigenic stimulus cannot be identified in all cases, an eosinophilic infiltrate on histology supports that etiology. Clinically, papules tend to appear on extensor surfaces of the extremities and may have a central punctum. Acute bites can cause both reactivation of old bites at remote sites and lesions where no bite ever occurred (an id reaction). Individual lesions last between 2 and 10 days, whereas the overall eruptions can last weeks, months, and even years. Excoriations, lichenification, and secondary infections are often noted. Depending on the offending arthropod, lesions may also group around elastic bands of clothing. Eruptions are less often found on the face and neck, and typically spare the genital, perianal, and axillary regions. Cases have been reported in infants as young as 2 weeks, but are generally seen in children between the ages of 2 and 7 and in adults. There is a predilection for the spring and summer months.

MANAGEMENT STRATEGY

The exact cause of PU is often not found and thus it is a diagnosis of exclusion. Common causes are bedbugs, scabies, lice (all types), fleas, chiggers, and mosquitoes. Important differential diagnoses to consider are prurigo nodularis, allergic contact dermatitis, id reaction, atopic dermatitis, drug rash, urticaria, sarcoidosis, early varicella, pityriasis lichenoides, miliaria rubra, papulovesicular polymorphous light eruption, papular acrodermatitis of childhood (Gianotti–Crosti syndrome), linear IgA bullous dermatosis, folliculitis, delusions of parasitosis, and neurotic excoriations.

Given the lack of evidence-based treatments for PU, we have suggested a therapeutic ladder based on simultaneously addressing: 1) a presumed arthropod assault, 2) the pathophysiology of the allergic and inflammatory response, and 3) the severity of the inflammation at presentation.

The most effective treatment for PU is the *identification and removal of the offending arthropod*. This may require intense investigation by the physician and patient as to the possible sources. Because the risks are minimal and the benefit great, *empiric therapy for scabies* should be given. This can be achieved with permethrin cream 5% or malathion lotion 0.5%, done once and repeated 3–7 days later. In the case of suspected bedbugs and fleas, *fumigation of the home* is required. Fumigation of the home should also be considered in recurrent cases of PU. Clothes and bedding should be laundered before and after treatment: specifically, placed in a dryer at 60°C for 10 minutes to dehydrate and kill scabies and bedbugs. In persistent cases, the application of DEET before bed may help. If there are pets in the home, *aggressive flea control* and veterinary evaluation may be necessary. If the exposure is thought to be from the outdoors, prevention can be achieved through *protective clothing and insect repellents*.

While the cause of PU is being investigated and treated, symptomatic therapy should be implemented immediately for patient comfort. The goal of symptomatic therapy is to reduce and prevent inflammation. The degree of aggressiveness in therapy depends on the degree of inflammation at presentation. For milder cases, *topical steroids* should be prescribed, with choice of class depending on the severity of lesions. For individual refractory or severe lesions, *intralesional triamcinolone* is often helpful. When therapy with topical and intralesional steroids is ineffective, or if the inflammatory response is severe on initial presentation, proceed to systemic immunosuppression, for example a 10-day *oral prednisone* taper starting at 1 mg/kg or 1 mg/kg of intramuscular triamcinolone. Systemic corticosteroids will often permanently blunt the inflammatory reaction, provided the antigenic stimulus has been removed. When PU becomes chronic in the context of two failed courses of systemic steroids, other systemic immunosuppressants should be considered, such as *phototherapy, ciclosporin, or methotrexate*.

Pruritus control is often achieved with antihistamines. In milder cases, *non-sedating antihistamines* such as loratadine, fexofenadine, or cetirizine can help alleviate symptoms. Doses above those given on the product labeling may be necessary. With more severe itching, *diphenhydramine and hydroxyzine* are favored. In chronic or recurrent cases, T-cell-mediated lesions, in contrast to the histamine-mediated lesions of early PU, may render antihistamines ineffective. In that case, topical agents, such as *camphor/menthol, calamine lotion, crotamiton, lidocaine, and pramoxine* can help.

Secondary infection, often from scratching, is a concern, especially in children. Careful attention should be paid to any signs of infection, and appropriate *topical or oral antibiotics* should be used.

Many cases of PU persist without the offending arthropods being identified. Sometimes, hospitalizing the patient for a period of 3–7 days, while simultaneously treating for scabies on admission, results in resolution as re-exposure to arthropod antigenic stimuli ceases in the hospital environment. In refractory cases, the eruptions will continue until the patient is naturally hyposensitized over time. Hyposensitization can take years to develop, and the concept can be especially confusing to those who have no pets in the home, or for those where only one family member is affected.

SPECIFIC INVESTIGATIONS

▶ Complete blood count with differential
▶ Serum IgE

Evidence Levels: A Double-blind study **B** Clinical trial ≥ 20 subjects **C** Clinical trial < 20 subjects **D** Series ≥ 5 subjects **E** Anecdotal case reports

▶ Skin biopsy (if systemic treatment is being given)
▶ Environmental evaluation
▶ Scratch test for dermographism

Papular urticaria: A histopathologic study of 30 patients. Jordaan HF, Schneider JW. Am J Dermatopathol 1997; 19: 119–26.

Over half the cases had mild acanthosis, mild spongiosis, exocytosis of lymphocytes, mild subepidermal edema, extravasation of erythrocytes, a superficial and a deep mixed inflammatory cell infiltrate of moderate intensity with interstitial eosinophils. Four subtypes are described: lymphocytic, eosinophilic, neutrophilic, and mixed. The authors conclude that a type I hypersensitivity reaction is part of the pathogenesis of PU based on immunohistochemical evidence.

FIRST-LINE THERAPIES

▶ Elimination of arthropod	D
▶ Antihistamines	A
▶ Topical steroids	D
▶ Topical antipruritics, e.g., camphor/menthol, calamine lotion	
▶ Crotamiton, lidocaine, and pramoxine	E

Papular urticaria in children. Howard R, Frieden IJ. Pediatr Dermatol 1996; 13: 246–9.

Definitive treatment is the elimination of the arthropod source. Pets must be treated with insecticidal shampoos and be well groomed. Carpets, rugs, and cloth furniture should be thoroughly vacuumed and the vacuum bag disposed of, as eggs can fall off the pet onto these surfaces. Fumigation of fleas should include outdoor areas that the pet frequents. Veterinarians and professional exterminators should be called upon when necessary.

Zoonoses of dermatological interest. Parish LC, Scwartzman RM. Semin Dermatol 1993; 12: 57–64.

Animal fleas not only infest the pet but also live in the rugs and floors, visiting the pet for blood meals; therefore, the pet should be treated with insecticides and the house should be fumigated.

Tropical rat mite dermatitis. Theis J, Lavoipierre MM, LaPerriere R, Kroese H. Arch Dermatol 1981; 117: 341–3.

Six cases of PU caused by the tropical rat mite (*Ornithonyssus bacoti*) are presented. Rodents were present in or around the home in most cases. Patients were treated successfully with lindane, and exterminators were used to completely eliminate the source.

Flea infestation as a cause of papular urticaria. Bolam RM, Burtt ET. Br Med J 1956; 1: 1130–3.

Evidence of fleas was found in 21 of 30 cases of papular urticaria. Careful histories were taken, and home visits were done in most cases because the source was not apparent. Insecticides were advised to clear any pets of fleas, and the owners were encouraged to have a specified rug or area where the pet sleeps. This area should be cleaned regularly with insecticide dust to prevent further episodes.

Comparison of cetirizine, ebastine and loratadine in the treatment of immediate mosquito-bite allergy. Karppinen A, Kautiainen H, Petman L, Burri P, Reunala T. Allergy 2002; 57: 534–7.

A double-blind, placebo-controlled, crossover study comparing prophylactic daily cetirizine 10 mg, ebastine 10 mg, and loratadine 10 mg in 29 adults with mosquito bites. Cetirizine and ebastine significantly reduced the size of wheals and pruritus. Cetirizine was found to be most effective against pruritus but caused sedation more often than did ebastine and loratadine.

Levocetirizine for treatment of immediate and delayed mosquito bite reactions. Karppinen A, Brummer-Korvenkontio H, Petman L, Kautiainen H, Herve JP, Reunala T. Acta Dermatol Venereol 2006; 86: 329–31.

A double-blind, placebo-controlled, crossover study with levocetirizine 5 mg daily in 28 adults sensitive to mosquito bites. Patients were given the study drug for 4 days and exposed to mosquito bites on day 3. Levocetirizine reduced the size of wheals by 60% and pruritus by 62% compared to placebo.

Bullous papular urticaria. Dilaimy M. Cutis 1978; 21: 666–8.

The author reports a good response with oral antihistamines after 10–14 days in an Iraqi population of patients with bullous papular urticaria.

Papular urticaria. Pillsbury DM, Constant ER. Arch Dermatol Syphilol 1948; 57: 410–11.

Case report of a 6-year-old boy with PU who had improvement of symptoms within 20 minutes of administration of diphenhydramine. He had an 80% improvement after 1 week of treatment and showed the development of new lesions at a more rapid rate upon withdrawal of diphenhydramine.

Arthropods in dermatology. Steen CJ, Carbonaro PA, Schwartz RA. J Am Acad Dermatol 2004; 50: 819–42.

The authors advocate the identification and removal of the cause of PU while simultaneously treating symptoms with topical steroids and oral antihistamines.

A good review of arthropods and the cutaneous eruptions they can cause.

Household papular urticaria. Naimer SA, Cohen AD, Mumcuoglu KY, Vardy DA. Israel Med Assoc J 2002; 4: 911–13.

Twenty patients with PU caused by cat fleas (*Ctenocephalides felis*) are presented. Symptomatic control was achieved with calamine lotion, topical corticosteroids, and oral antihistamines. Clinical symptoms cleared within a few weeks after fumigating and spraying the areas infested by the arthropods.

Papular urticaria. Millikan LE. Semin Dermatol 1993; 12: 53–6.

Prevent PU using repellents containing DEET if repeated exposure is suspected. Use antipruritics, including menthol, camphor, and pramoxine, for pruritus.

SECOND-LINE THERAPIES

▶ Intralesional steroids, e.g., triamcinolone	E
▶ Oral steroids, e.g., prednisone or methylprednisolone	E
▶ Insect repellents, i.e., DEET	E

Insect bite-induced hypersensitivity and the SCRATCH principles: a new approach to papular urticaria. Hernandez RG, Cohen BA. Pediatrics 2006; 118: 189–96.

The authors advocate the use intralesional steroids in older children and adults to suppress pruritus if more conservative measures fail.

The role of dexamethasone in papular urticaria. El-Nasr NS. J Egypt Med Assoc 1961; 44: 340–1.

Dexamethasone 0.25 mg po bid to tid for 1–2 weeks was used with good results. Pruritus resolved within 48 hours.

Comparative activity of three repellents against bedbugs *Cimex hemipterus*. Kumar S, Prakash S, Rao KM. Indian J Med Res 1995; 102: 20–3.

Diethyl-*m*-toluamide (DEET), diethyl phenyl-acetamide (DEPA) and dimethylphthalate (DMP) were tested against bedbugs *Cimex hemipterus* on the shaven skin of rabbits. DEET was superior to the other two repellents at all concentrations tested. At 75% concentration, DEET showed 85% repellency for up to 2 hours and 52% repellency 6 hours after treatment.

Insect repellents: An overview. Brown M, Hebert AA. J Am Acad Dermatol 1997; 36: 243–9.

DEET was highly effective at repelling mosquitoes, biting fleas, gnats, chiggers, and ticks. Permethrin works as both an insecticide and a repellant against lice, ticks, fleas, mites, mosquitoes, and black flies.

THIRD-LINE THERAPIES

▶ Phototherapy	E
▶ Ciclosporin	E
▶ Hospitalization	E

Papular dermatitis in adults: subacute prurigo, American style? Sherertz EF. J Am Acad Dermatol 1991; 24: 697–702.

Twelve patients with pruritic papular eruptions were followed, and the majority were refractory to conservative symptomatic management but showed some control with oral steroids, UVB, or PUVA.

Papular urticaria and transfer of allergy following bone marrow transplantation. Smith SR, Macfarlane AW, Lewis-Jones MS. Clin Exp Dermatol 1988; 13: 260–2.

A 20-year-old man who underwent allogenic bone marrow transplantation was found to have PU as a result of transfer of allergy from the donor. The PU eruption appeared as ciclosporin was withdrawn, indicating a suppressive effect on PU from ciclosporin.

Papular urticaria; its relationship to insect allergy. Shaffer B, Jacobson C, Beerman H. Ann Allergy 1952; 10: 411–21.

The authors note cases of PU that improved when patients were hospitalized and worsened when they returned home.

Papular urticaria. Rook A, Frain-Bell W. Arch Dis Child 1953; 28: 304–10.

Multiple cases of PU are reported where the eruption cleared when patients were hospitalized. Hospitalization removes the patient from the arthropod source of PU and allows for sufficient time to rid the home of the arthropods before the patient returns home.

Parvovirus infection

Heather Salvaggio, Andrea Zaenglein

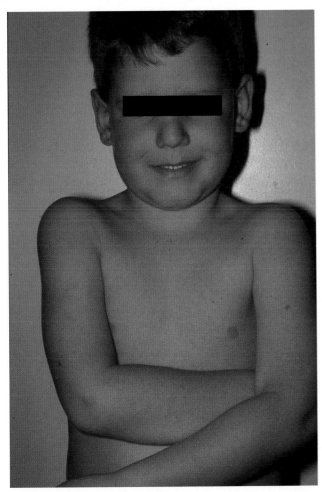

Courtesy of David R Adams MD, PhD

Infection with the human parvovirus B19 (HPB19) causes erythema infectiosum, also known as 'Fifth' disease according to the original classification of childhood exanthems. Outbreaks occur in the winter and spring, affecting school-aged children between 5 and 15 years of age. The infection is transmitted via respiratory droplets. Following a short prodrome of fever, malaise, and pharyngitis, the classic features of the exanthem appear. Bright pink macular erythema of the cheeks ('slapped cheek sign') together with circumoral pallor precedes an evanescent macular, reticulated or 'lace-like' rash over the trunk and proximal limbs. The rash may last for up to 4 weeks and may subsequently recur following sun exposure. Purpuric eruptions are also commonly reported in association with HPB19. In patients with a predisposing hematologic condition, infection with HPB19 may cause a transient aplastic crisis. Chronic and secondary infections have been encountered in immunosuppressed patients and rarely in immunocompetent patients. Primary infection during pregnancy may place the fetus at risk for hydrops fetalis.

MANAGEMENT STRATEGY

Erythema infectiosum is typically a self-resolving exanthem, so in the majority of cases *supportive care and reassurance* are all

that are required. However, the clinician should be aware of a variety of rare atypical presentations of HPB19 infection.

The rash of erythema infectiosum is immune complex-mediated, so patients are assumed to be no longer infectious by the time it appears. Once a clinical diagnosis has been made, parents can be reassured and advised on simple supportive measures such as *antipyretics, fluids,* and simple *emollients* for the rash. In the majority of immunocompetent patients the condition is self-resolving.

Infection with HPB19 is causative in several other clinical scenarios, most involving petechial eruptions. The most common is the papular–purpuric 'gloves and socks' syndrome (PPGSS). This consists of pruritic, painful edema, erythema, and petechiae of the lower legs and feet. Classically there is a sharp demarcation between the involved dorsal and the uninvolved plantar foot. This eruption may be seen together with the 'slapped cheek' sign. Oral mucosal involvement may occur, with palatal petechiae and ulcerations being most common. PPGSS is seen more often in the spring and summer and typically occurs in adolescents and young adults. Unlike in erythema infectiosum, patients with PPGSS have been reported to be viremic while the rash is present, and are thus contagious. Several cases of more generalized petechial eruptions have also been reported. These include – but are not limited to – the acropetechial syndrome, characterized by prominent perioral involvement and a petechial eruption in a bathing trunk distribution. It has been recommended by some experts that testing for parvovirus be performed in all patients with petechial rashes whose origin is undetermined.

In older patients, especially middle-aged women, the infection may cause a symmetric arthropathy similar to rheumatoid arthritis. This may accompany the rash, but frequently follows it. The arthritis is usually self-resolving, requiring only *non-steroidal anti-inflammatory drugs (NSAIDs)* for symptomatic relief. Occasionally the arthritis may lead a more chronic course.

A lupus erythematosus-like condition, which can mimic the onset of systemic lupus, has been reported. HPB19 infection can mimic various connective tissue disorders, in particular dermatomyositis and vasculitis. Infection with HPB19 has also been implicated to a play a role in the development of a multitude of other conditions, including myocarditis, hepatitis, nephritis, and neurologic disease. However, a causal relationship has not been established.

HPB19 is extremely tropic for erythroblasts. In predisposed individuals with either an underlying hemolytic state, active bleeding, or iron deficiency, HPB19 infection can cause a transient aplastic crisis. In addition to anemia, there may be moderate neutropenia and thrombocytopenia. Usually the anemia is self-limited but *transfusion* may be indicated if severe. In immunosuppressed patients, HPB19 infection may have more serious consequences. Chronic HPB19 infection can result in a chronic anemia. This can be rapidly treated with commercial *intravenous immunoglobulin infusion,* which is often curative. Potentially fatal marrow necrosis rarely occurs in very young children. Severe cases of aplastic anemia that do not respond to intravenous immunoglobulin may also be cured by *bone marrow transplantation.* Interestingly, parvovirus B19 can contaminate blood products, including bone marrow, and may have the ability to transmit infection by this means.

Hydrops fetalis is a severe anemia resulting in high-output cardiogenic heart failure and often fetal death. It occurs most commonly with primary infection, during the first trimester of pregnancy. One-third or more women of childbearing age do not have IgG antibodies to HPB19 and are susceptible to primary infection. Testing maternal serum for IgM antibodies and HPB19 DNA with PCR analysis should be carried out in pregnant women who develop symptoms of HPB19 infection or are in contact with children with a known parvovirus infection. If they have serologic evidence of primary infection, fetal ultrasonography should be performed to evaluate for signs of fetal anemia and hydrops fetalis. If present, cordocentesis to confirm the presence of anemia and *intrauterine transfusion* should be strongly considered. If the pregnancy is near or at term, delivery should be considered. Pregnant women with normal immunity and IgG antibodies to HPB19, or those with a remote history of infection, can be reassured that exposure to HPB19 during pregnancy will not have adverse outcomes on their pregnancy.

Patients with AIDS and chronic anemia secondary to HPB19 infection, who are treated with highly active antiretroviral therapy *(HAART)*, have had resolution of their anemia with documented seroconversion from IgM to IgG antiparvovirus antibodies. Other AIDS patients started on HAART experienced an immune reconstitution syndrome. With the development of renewed immunity, AIDS patients can experience overwhelming systemic involvement of the parvovirus, resulting in encephalitis, severe anemia, or other severe sequelae.

SPECIFIC INVESTIGATIONS

> ► Hematology (complete blood count)
> ► Serology

IgM antibodies to HPB19 indicate recent infection. HPB19-specfic IgG antibodies indicate past exposure and may be positive in over half the adult population.

A typical clinical appearance together with supportive serology is sufficient to establish the diagnosis in the majority of cases. In at-risk patients, or those who have symptoms of anemia, a complete blood count will establish whether there is any significant level of anemia requiring transfusion.

It is possible to detect parvovirus DNA in both the blood and lesional skin. Polymerase chain reaction techniques are considered extremely sensitive and may be useful in the following clinical scenarios: patients with an atypical presentation of HPB19 infection, where the clinical suspicion of infection is high and antibody studies are negative; and in immunocompromised patients who cannot mount an appropriate immunoglobulin response. In addition, a window exists during the first seven days after exposure when IgG and IgM are undetectable. A second period also exists where IgM has become undetectable, but the virus may still be present.

Parvovirus B19. Young NS, Brown KE. N Engl J Med 2004; 350: 586–97.

This is a comprehensive review of HPB19 infection and its manifestations.

The cutaneous manifestations of human parvovirus B19 infection. Magro CM, Dawood MR, Crowson N. Hum Pathol 2000; 31: 488–97.

This is a description of the cutaneous manifestations in a series of 14 patients who were shown to have antecedent HPB19 infection with positive serology and/or B19 genome in skin samples.

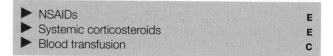

> ► Reassurance   E
> ► Antipyretics (e.g., acetaminophen [paracetamol], ibuprofen)   E

Human parvoviruses. Brown K. In: Long SS, ed. Principles and practices of pediatric infectious diseases, 3rd edn. Edinburgh: Elsevier, 2008; 1072–6.

Most children require no specific therapy. Simple supportive therapies may be used. No antiviral drug or vaccine is available. A viral vaccine is under development.

SECOND-LINE THERAPIES

> ► NSAIDs   E
> ► Systemic corticosteroids   E
> ► Blood transfusion   C

Human parvovirus infection: rheumatic manifestations, angioedema, C1 esterase inhibitor deficiency, ANA positivity and possible onset of systemic lupus erythematosus. Fawaz-Estrup F. J Rheumatol 1996; 23: 1180–5.

This is a series of nine adult patients with serological evidence of acute or recent HPB19 infection and polyarthralgia/polyarthritis. All responded to NSAIDs, although one patient also required pulsed intravenous methylprednisolone for a lupus-like illness.

In older children and adults the arthralgia/arthritis may be severe enough to warrant treatment with NSAIDs. In the majority of cases the joint symptoms settle within a few days or weeks.

Parvoviruses and bone marrow failure. Brown KE, Young NS. Stem Cells 1996; 14: 151–63.

In patients with underlying hemolytic disorders infection with HPB19 is the primary cause of a transient aplastic crisis, which may require transfusion. In immunocompromised patients, persistent infection may manifest as pure red cell aplasia and chronic anemia.

THIRD-LINE THERAPIES

> ► Immunoglobulin infusion   C
> ► Bone marrow transplantation   E
> ► Intrauterine transfusion   C
> ► HAART   E

Persistent B19 parvovirus infection in patients infected with human immunodeficiency virus type 1 (HIV-1): a treatable cause of anaemia in AIDS. Frickhofen N, Abkowitz J, Safford M, Berry JM, Antunez-de-Mayolo J, Astrow A, et al. Ann Intern Med 1990; 113: 926–33.

This is a series of seven patients who were HIV positive with persistent HPB19 infection and anemia. Six were treated with intravenous immunoglobulin and showed a rapid reduction in serum virus concentrations and subsequent resolution of their anemia. Two patients relapsed, but again responded to further immunoglobulin.

Successful bone marrow transplantation for severe aplastic anaemia in a patient with persistent human parvovirus B19

infection. Goto H, Ishida A, Fujii H, Kuroki F, Takahashi H, Ikuta K, et al. Int J Hematol 2004; 79: 384–6.

This is a single case of a previously immunocompetent 9-year-old girl with persistent HPB19 infection and aplastic anemia treated with a bone marrow transplant from an HLA-identical sibling donor.

Fetal morbidity and mortality after acute parvovirus B19 infection in pregnancy: prospective evaluation of 1018 cases. Enders M, Weidner A, Zoellner I, Searle K, Enders G. Prenat Diagn 2004; 24: 513–18.

Survival in fetuses with severe hydrops fetalis after intra-uterine transfusion was 84.6% (11/13). All fetuses with severe hydrops that were not transfused died.

Resolution of chronic parvovirus b19 induced anemia, by use of highly active antiretroviral therapy in a patient with acquired immunodeficiency syndrome. Ware AJ, Moore T. Clin Infect Dis 2001; 32: E122–3.

This is a case of an AIDS patient with transfusion-dependent anemia caused by HPB19 that resolved with HAART therapy is reported.

Pediculosis

Arpeta Gupta, Jacob O Levitt

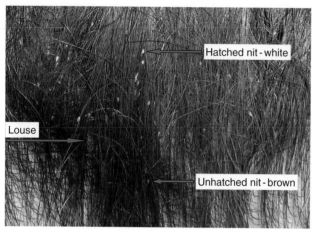

Courtesy of Jere Mammino, DO.

Lice are wingless, dorsoventrally flattened, blood-sucking insects that are obligate ectoparasites of birds and mammals. Pediculosis is an infestation by *Pediculus capitis* (head louse), *Pediculus humanus* (body louse), or *Phthirus pubis* (pubic or crab louse). The bites of lice are painless and can rarely be detected. The clinical signs and symptoms are the result of the host's reaction to the saliva and anticoagulant injected into the dermis by the louse at the time of feeding. Depending on the degree of sensitivity and previous exposure, the feeding sites produce red macules or papules hours to days after feeding. Pruritus is the most common symptom of any type of pediculosis. If left untreated, superinfection of excoriations may lead to impetiginous crusts and cervical lymphadenopathy.

PEDICULOSIS CAPITIS

MANAGEMENT STRATEGY

Infestation is most common among children 3–12 years of age and their parents. Identification of live lice is the gold standard of diagnosis; however, finding nits alone in a patient who has not been treated also warrants treatment. One study showed that about 20% of patients found to have nits alone go on to develop lice. Nits are easier to spot, especially at the nape of the neck and behind the ears. Hatched nits are white; unhatched nits are brown. Detection combing of wet hair with a fine-toothed nit comb allows for efficient recovery of lice and nits for diagnosis.

Management must take into consideration key elements of the head louse lifecycle. A nervous system develops in the egg by day 4, it takes 12 days at most to hatch, and the nymph can lay eggs as soon as 7 days after hatching. Contrary to the directions of most non-ovicidal pediculicides, one re-treatment at 7 days will not kill all viable nits. Because of this, therapies that do not kill eggs require three weekly treatments. Pediculicides that are also ovicidal require two treatments separated by 1 week. Ova less than 4 days old will not be affected by agents that act on the louse nervous system. Lice are sensitive to dehydration, but can live off the host for

up to 55 hours. Transmission is mainly by direct head-to-head contact. Indirect spread through fomites is also possible. Until definitive safety data are available, treatment of the occasional patient under the age of 2 years probably should be with mechanical methods.

Launderable items (worn clothing and used bedding, towels, scarves, and hats) should be placed in a dryer at 60°C (i.e., on high) for 10 minutes. Brushes, combs, and hair ornaments can be placed in hot water (60°C or more) for 10 minutes. Non-launderable items (i.e., certain stuffed animals) should be placed in a bag for 3 days (not 15 days, as eggs laid off a host will probably not hatch close enough to a host to obtain their first blood meal). Cloth furniture and rugs should be vacuumed. Fumigation of the home is discouraged.

Contacts of index cases, including classmates, should be screened. Empiric therapy for close household contacts, particularly if they share a bed, is justifiable. Those likely to have had head-to-head contact with the index case in the previous 4–6 weeks should be identified and screened. Children should not be excluded from school for head lice as the infestation often has been around for months prior to its detection. Hair grows 1 cm per month, and lice lay eggs close to the scalp where it is moist and warm. Nits detected 2 cm from the scalp represent a 2-month-old infestation. Therapy within a week of the detected infestation is more reasonable.

Considerations guiding therapy include safety and efficacy, which for chemical modalities depend largely on regional resistance patterns of the lice. Because of widespread resistance to *permethrin* and *lindane*, *malathion* formulated in isopropyl alcohol with *terpineol*, being both ovicidal and pediculicidal, is the most effective therapy at the time of writing. Carbaryl is a good alternative, but occasional resistance has been reported. Alternatives to agents that do not act on the louse nervous system include mechanical methods of *louse occlusion*, *cuticle disruption*, or *physical removal*. Barring *shaving the head*, these modalities are often unreliable and have the attendant problem of infestivity between treatments.

SPECIFIC INVESTIGATIONS

► Examination for nits and lice via nit combing

Louse comb versus direct visual examination for the diagnosis of head louse infestations. Mumcuoglu KY, Friger M, Ioffe-Uspensky I, Ben-Ishai F, Miller J. Pediatr Dermatol 2001; 18: 9–12.

Nit combing is four times more efficient than and twice as fast as direct visual inspection.

FIRST-LINE THERAPIES

► Malathion 0.5% lotion	**A**
► Permethrin 1% cream rinse	**A**
► Carbaryl 0.5% lotion	**B**

Therapy for head lice based on life cycle, resistance, and safety considerations. Lebwohl M, Clark L, Levitt J. Pediatrics 2007; 119: 965–74.

This paper highlights the importance of designing treatment schedules in accordance with the head louse lifecycle.

Malathion 0.5% in isopropyl alcohol 78% with terpineol 12% is a safe, resistance-breaking formulation approved by the FDA as a first-line treatment for head lice. Two treatments 1 week apart correlate with the head louse lifecycle. There is no evidence to suggest that the second application, 1 week later, is unsafe; 70–80% of cases are cured with a single treatment.

In the United States there is increasing resistance to permethrin and lindane, but not to malathion.

Effectiveness of Ovide against malathion-resistant head lice. Downs AM, Narayan S, Stafford KA, Coles GC. Arch Dermatol 2005; 141: 1318.

In this in vitro study Ovide (contains malathion, terpineol, and isopropyl alcohol) killed British head lice resistant to malathion after a 60-minute exposure. Terpineol and malathion are additive in overcoming resistance.

The authors recommend that Ovide should replace all malathion-only products to minimize the development of resistance in the United States.

A randomized, investigator-blinded, time-ranging study of the comparative efficacy of 0.5% malathion gel versus Ovide® lotion (0.5% malathion) or Nix® crème rinse (1% permethrin) used as labelled, for the treatment of head lice. Meinking TL, Vicaria M, Eyerdam DH, Villar ME, Reyna S, Suarez G. Pediatr Dermatol 2007; 24: 405–11.

Success rates were 97% for Ovide (n=30) and 45% for Nix (n=11) at day 15. At day 8, 70% of Nix versus 32% of Ovide subjects required re-treatment. Malathion had no effect on acetylcholinesterase inhibition in 94 subjects aged 2–12 years.

Efficacy of a reduced application time of Ovide lotion (0.5% malathion) compared to Nix creme rinse (1% permethrin) for the treatment of head lice. Meinking TL, Vicaria M, Eyerdam DH, Villar ME, Reyna S, Suarez G. Pediatr Dermatol 2004; 21: 670–4.

Reduced application time (20 minutes) of Ovide cured 98% (40 of 41) of subjects at day 15 versus Nix (10 minutes), which cured 55% (12 of 22); 19.5% of Ovide patients and 40.9% of Nix patients required a second treatment on day 8. Reinfestation rates were 0% for Ovide and 23% for Nix.

Permethrin 1% obtained approval with well-done studies decades ago; however, resistance has caused permethrin cure rates to decline dramatically.

Increased frequency of the T929I and L932F mutations associated with knockdown resistance in permethrin-resistant populations of the human head louse, *Pediculus capitis*, from California, Florida and Texas. Gao JR, Yoon KS, Lee SH, Takano-Lee M, Edman JD, Meinking TL, et al. Pestic Biochem Physiol 2003; 77: 115–24.

A high prevalence of *kdr* (knockdown resistance) gene mutations in head lice is reported: 45% in California, 87% in Florida, and up to 100% in parts of Texas. The *kdr* gene reduces louse voltage-gated sodium channel affinity for permethrin, rendering permethrin ineffective.

Permethrin-resistant human head lice, *Pediculus capitis*, and their treatment. Yoon KS, Gao JR, Lee SH, Clark JM, Brown L, Taplin D. Arch Dermatol 2003; 139: 994–1000.

Malathion 0.5% killed permethrin-resistant head lice with *kdr* gene mutations 10 times faster than permethrin 1% in vitro.

Pediculosis capitis: why prefer a solution to shampoo or spray? Armoni M, Bibi H, Schlesinger M, Pollak S, Metzker A. Pediatr Dermatol 1988; 5: 273–5.

At day 10, cure rates were 49/50 for carbaryl 0.5% lotion, 49/50 for malathion 0.5% solution, and 36/50 for pyrethrin 0.3%/piperonyl butoxide 3% shampoo.

Recent studies for carbaryl are lacking, and scattered reports of carbaryl resistance exist. Because of this the results of older studies may not predict efficacy today.

SECOND-LINE THERAPIES

▶ Topical crotamiton 10%	B
▶ Topical occlusion therapy	
— Dimeticone	A
— Cetaphil liquid cleanser	B
— Petroleum jelly	E
▶ Isopropyl myristate 50% in 50% ST-cyclomethicone	A
▶ Nit picking	
— Bug Busting	A
— Professional nit picking services	E

A single application of crotamiton lotion in the treatment of patients with pediculosis capitis. Karaci I, Yawalkar SJ. Int J Dermatol 1982; 21: 611–13.

Forty-seven of 49 subjects were cured with one application of crotamiton 10% lotion, and all were cured with a second application at 1 week. The trial was open-label and never independently validated.

Treatment of head louse infestation with 4% dimeticone lotion: randomised controlled equivalence trial. Burgess IF, Brown CM, Lee PN. Br Med J 2005; 330: 1423.

Cure rates of 70% after two weekly 8-hour treatments in 253 subjects were achieved.

This therapy does not appear to be ovicidal, perhaps contributing to a lower cure rate.

A simple treatment for head lice: dry-on, suffocation-based pediculicide. Pearlman DL. Pediatrics 2004; 114: e275–9.

Cetaphil cleanser is applied to the hair, dried with a hair dryer, followed by nit combing on three occasions each separated by 1 week; 133 patients were studied and 96% efficacy is claimed. The study was open-label and the results were never independently validated.

Home remedies to control head lice: assessment of home remedies to control the human head louse, *Pediculus humanus capitis* (Anoplura: Pediculidae). Takano-Lee M, Edman JD, Mullens BA, Clark JM. J Pediatr Nurs 2004; 19: 393–8.

'Home remedies' (vinegar, isopropyl alcohol, olive oil, mayonnaise, and melted butter) are neither pediculicidal nor ovicidal. Petroleum jelly was 62% pediculicidal and 94% ovicidal. The need for 8 hours of water submersion to achieve significant louse mortality makes this impractical.

Albeit not addressed in this reference, topically applied kerosene is a dangerous method that should be avoided.

North American efficacy and safety of a novel pediculicide rinse, isopropyl myristate 50% (Results). Kaul N, Palma KG, Silagy SS, Goodman JJ, Toole J. J Cutan Med Surg 2007; 11: 161–7.

In the isopropyl myristate (IPM) arm of one small, randomized trial, 18 of 30 subjects were cured at 21 days by an intention-to-treat analysis. IPM is thought to dissolve the waxy coat of the louse exoskeleton, causing fatal dehydration. As the louse eggshell is proteinaceous, this chemical is not expected to kill eggs.

Single blind, randomised, comparative study of the Bug Buster kit and over the counter pediculicide treatments against head lice in the United Kingdom. Hill N, Moor G, Cameron MM, Butlin A, Preston S, Williamson MS, Bass C. Br Med J 2005; 331: 384–7.

A cure rate of 57% (32/56) is reported for wet combing with conditioner in four sessions over 13 days.

Nit combing can be painful and time-consuming, but may be worthwhile where lice are resistant to pharmacotherapy.

THIRD-LINE THERAPIES

▶ Lindane 1%	A
▶ Oral Ivermectin	B
▶ Topical Ivermectin	B
▶ Trimethoprim/Sulfamethoxazole	B
▶ Levamisole	B
▶ Head shaving	E

Comparative in vitro pediculicidal efficacy of treatments in a resistant head lice population in the United States. Meinking TL, Serrano BA, Hard B, Entzel R, Lemard G, Rivera E, et al. Arch Dermatol 2002; 138: 220–4.

Lindane shampoo was the slowest and the least effective product, killing only 8% of lice in 1 hour. It is labelled for 4 minutes.

1% permethrin cream rinse vs 1% lindane shampoo in treating pediculosis capitis. Brandenberg K, Deinard AS, DiNapoli J, Englender SJ, Orthoefer J, Wagner D. AJDC 1986; 140: 894–6.

Lindane achieved a cure rate of 85% (214/251) at 14 days.

Current resistance patterns, toxicity, and environmental concerns make lindane an antiquated therapy for head lice.

Efficacy of ivermectin for the treatment of head lice (Pediculosus capitis). Glaziou P, Nyguyen LN, Moulia-Pelat JP. Trop Med Parasitol 1994; 45: 253–4.

A 77% (20/26) cure rate was achieved at day 14 for 26 patients aged 5–17 years after a single, open-label 200 µg/kg dose of ivermectin.

Because ivermectin is strictly pediculicidal, several doses would be required for full efficacy. The safety of this dosing schedule has not been established, especially in children.

Topical application of ivermectin for human ectoparasites. Youssef MY, Sadaka HA, Eissa MM, el-Ariny AF. Am J Trop Med Hyg 1995; 53: 652–3.

Of 25 subjects with head lice, all were cured with one application of 15–25 mL of an ivermectin 0.8% solution.

Head lice infestation: single drug versus combination therapy with one percent permethrin and trimethoprim/sulfamethoxazole. Hipolito RB, Mallorca FG, Zuniga-Macaraiq ZO, Apolinario PC, Wheeler-Sherman J. Pediatrics 2001; 107: E30.

Permethrin 1% and trimethoprim (10 mg/kg/day divided bid)/sulfamethoxazole (TMP/SMX) cured 38/40 (95%) of subjects at week 2. TMP/SMX monotherapy was 83% effective, and permethrin monotherapy was 79.5% effective.

Oral therapy of pediculosis capitis with cotrimoxazole. Shashindran CH, Gandhi IS, Krishnasamy S, Ghosh MN. Br J Dermatol 1978; 98: 699–700.

Open-label administration of trimethoprim/sulfamethoxazole (TMP/SMX) was effective given for 3 consecutive days at 160 mg/800 mg bid (n=5) or at 80 mg/400 mg bid (n=5). Monotherapy with TMP 160 mg bid (n=4) or SMX 800 mg bid (n=4) was ineffective. Repeat dosing was needed 10 days later to kill hatched nits.

In light of drug hypersensitivity and the risk of drug resistance, treatment with trimethoprim/sulfamethoxazole should be reserved for the most refractory cases.

Levamisole: a safe and economical weapon against pediculosis. Namazi MR. Int J Dermatol 2001; 40: 292–4.

Levamisole in a dose of 3.5 mg/kg administered open-label for 10 days cured 67% (18/28) of children with head lice.

PEDICULOSIS CORPORIS

MANAGEMENT STRATEGY

As body lice live in the seams of clothing, treatment revolves around *laundering of clothing and bedding* in high heat (>60°C) for at least 10 minutes. Infested mattresses should be abandoned for 3 weeks. Given that resistance patterns in head lice follow those of body lice, topical *malathion, carbaryl, or permethrin* are good first choices. Oral ivermectin is another alternative. All household contacts should be treated. Monitor for symptoms of louse-borne illness, specifically epidemic typhus (*Rickettsia prowazekii*), relapsing fever (*Borrelia recurrentis*), and trench fever (*Bartonella quintana*).

FIRST-LINE THERAPIES

▷ Laundering of clothes and bedding	E
▷ Malathion 0.5% lotion	E
▷ Carbaryl 0.5% lotion	E
▷ Permethrin 5% cream	E
▷ Oral ivermectin	E
▷ Personal hygiene	E

Human lice and their management. Burgess IF. Adv Parasitol 1995; 36: 271–342.

A comprehensive review of human lice is provided. For body lice, laundering of clothing is stressed, and the use of pediculicides on the patient is questioned. In mass eradication, fomites can be dusted with malathion or permethrin.

Given the safety of topical therapy, two treatments applied for 8–12 hours 1 week apart outweigh the risk of stray lice on the host re-establishing infestation.

538

PEDICULOSIS PUBIS

MANAGEMENT STRATEGY

Crab lice commonly affect pubic (mons and perianal), thigh, chest, and axillary hair, eyelashes, and rarely, scalp hair. Pediculicide should be applied to these areas to ensure eradication. Eyelash infestation should be treated separately (see below). Household contacts and sexual partners of the previous month should be treated. Fomites should be laundered as for head lice. Screening for other sexually transmitted diseases is advised.

FIRST-LINE THERAPIES

▶ Malathion 0.5% lotion	E
▶ Permethrin 1% crème rinse	B
▶ Permethrin 5% cream	C

Infestations. Meinking TL. Curr Probl Dermatol 1999; 11: 73–120.

A comprehensive review of pediculosis and scabies is rendered. The lifecycle of the crab louse mirrors that of the head louse, such that therapeutic strategies are analogous. Successful treatment using two applications separated by 1 week to the entire body was achieved in 27/28 (96%) patients with permethrin 1% cream rinse and 24/29 (83%) patients with lindane 1%. Meinking reports a separate study where a single total-body application of permethrin 5% cream yielded a 93% cure rate (number of patients not reported). Single application therapy is too often ineffective.

SECOND-LINE THERAPIES

▶ Lindane 1% shampoo	B
▶ Oral ivermectin	E
▶ Trimethoprim/sulfamethoxazole	E

PHTHIRIASIS PALPEBRARUM

MANAGEMENT STRATEGY

Only anecdotal reports of therapy exist. Alcoholic formulations as well as lindane are ocular irritants and should be avoided. *Physostigmine* is effective but may inhibit dark adaptation of the eye. *Petrolatum* application or mechanical removal of lice and nits seem to be the safest alternatives. Treatment of household and sexual contacts and fomites is warranted.

FIRST-LINE THERAPIES

▶ Petroleum jelly	E
▶ Mechanical lice and nit removal	E
▶ Physotigmine 0.25% or 1% ointment	E

Pediculosis ciliaris. Chin GN, Denslow GT. J Pediatr Ophtalmol Strabismus 1978; 15: 173–5.

Physotigmine 1% ointment applied to eyelid margins twice daily for 14 days is reported. Other suggestions for therapy include: 1) thick application of petroleum jelly twice daily for 8 days; 2) mechanical removal of lice and nits with forceps and cotton-tipped swabs, followed by application of yellow oxide of mercury 1–2% ointment twice daily for 1 week; 3) cryotherapy.

SECOND-LINE THERAPIES

▶ Pyrethrin ointment in vaseline (1:8)	E
▶ Cryotherapy	E
▶ Yellow oxide of mercury 1–2% ointment	E
▶ Oral trimethoprim/sulfamethoxazole	E
▶ Oral tetracycline	E

Pemphigus

Daniel Mimouni, Grant J Anhalt

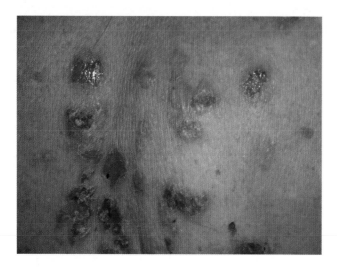

Pemphigus is an autoimmune blistering disease of the skin with an established immunological basis but unknown etiology. Its histological hallmark is the loss of cell-to-cell adhesion (acantholysis) mediated by autoantibodies to epidermal cell-surface proteins. Pemphigus has three major variants: pemphigus vulgaris, pemphigus foliaceus, and paraneoplastic pemphigus, which are differentiated by the presence/absence of intraepithelial blisters and erosions of the skin, and variable involvement of the mucous membranes. Their associated risks of morbidity and mortality vary greatly.

MANAGEMENT STRATEGY

If pemphigus vulgaris is not treated definitively and promptly, the process 'hardens,' leading to epitope spreading which makes the disease more difficult to control. Even if the initial presentation is limited, without systemic treatment it will generalize. Animal studies have clearly shown that once enough autoantibody reaches the skin, blistering will occur, and this damage cannot be prevented by anti-inflammatory agents or even pretreatment with high doses of *systemic corticosteroids*. Topical treatment of the mucous membranes or skin has no significant effect on the course of the disease, although *topical corticosteroids or intralesional injections or corticosteroids* may temporarily relieve pain and inflammation. Other factors complicate the management, and include the following:

1. Circulating autoantibodies have a degradative half-life of about 3 weeks. Lasting improvement can only occur with reduction of both existing and newly produced antibody; improvement occurs very slowly unless the antibodies are physically removed by plasmapheresis, or their catabolism is increased by administration of high doses of exogenous normal human immunoglobulins (IVIG).
2. Pemphigus is notorious in its persistence. Spontaneous remissions typically do not occur, and remissions and relapses are common. Most people require some form of treatment for life.

3. There is only a small repertoire of drugs that are effective at reducing autoantibody synthesis, and the most effective of those, cyclophosphamide, has potential toxicities that can restrict its appropriate use.
4. All forms of pemphigus are rare, and this prohibits the execution of large, controlled trials. The literature discussing therapeutic regimens is dominated by small series and case reports, which is a weak evidence base for the design of rational treatment. However, we do have excellent animal models of this disease, and understand well the pathophysiology from these studies, which are instrumental in designing our approach to treatment.

Thus, *the primary goal of treatment in all forms of pemphigus is to reduce the synthesis of autoantibodies by the immune system.* It currently consists of four basic steps.

1. *Systemic corticosteroids alone.*
2. Corticosteroids plus an antimetabolite such as azathioprine or mycophenolate mofetil.
2a. Step 2 with the additional use of IVIG or rituximab.
3. Corticosteroids plus cyclophosphamide.
4. Corticosteroids plus cyclophosphamide plus short-term plasmapheresis.

The commitment to the use of cyclophosphamide is a serious one. This drug is extremely effective, but use of this alkylating agent is accompanied by short-term leukopenia and a long-term increased risk of leukemia, lymphoma, and bladder cancer, as well as the risk of sterility in younger patients. The use of newer agents such as IVIG and rituximab is being explored as a way to avoid having to use cyclophosphamide.

Some studies have suggested other potential drugs, but they cannot yet be applied because the mechanism whereby they might effectively inhibit new antibody synthesis is unknown. This list includes tetracycline and niacin (nicotinamide), methotrexate, dapsone, and gold. A recent well-performed randomized trial showed no corticosteroid-sparing benefit of ciclosporin. It is therefore not recommended for the treatment of pemphigus vulgaris, although it may still play a role in the treatment of paraneoplastic pemphigus.

SPECIFIC INVESTIGATIONS

- ▶ Skin biopsy for routine microscopy
- ▶ Skin biopsy for direct immunofluorescence
- ▶ Serum for indirect immunofluorescence
- ▶ Enzyme-linked immunosorbent assay (ELISA)
- ▶ Malignancy screening tests in patients with paraneoplastic pemphigus

Making sense of antigens and antibodies in pemphigus. Anhalt GJ. J Am Acad Dermatol 1999; 40: 763–6.

Accuracy of indirect immunofluorescence testing in the diagnosis of paraneoplastic pemphigus. Helou J, Allbritton J, Anhalt GJ. J Am Acad Dermatol 1995; 32: 441–7.

Pemphigus vulgaris is characterized by progressively evolving fragile blisters and erosions. Oral involvement essentially 'always' occurs and is the major point to differentiate pemphigus vulgaris from pemphigus foliaceus. Histologic changes include suprabasilar acantholysis and cell surface-bound IgG. Circulating autoantibodies are specific for desmoglein 3 alone when lesions are restricted to the mouth, and for both desmoglein 3 and desmoglein 1 when cutaneous lesions are

Evidence Levels: **A** Double-blind study **B** Clinical trial ≥ 20 subjects **C** Clinical trial < 20 subjects **D** Series ≥ 5 subjects **E** Anecdotal case reports

present in addition to oral lesions. Definition of the specificity of desmoglein autoantibodies can be reliably gained by enzyme-linked immunosorbent assay (ELISA).

In pemphigus foliaceus, mucosal lesions 'never' occur. This is the major clinical feature differentiating pemphigus foliaceus from pemphigus vulgaris. The cutaneous lesions are superficial scaling erosions. Immunopathologic studies reveal subcorneal acantholysis and tissue-bound and circulating antidesmoglein 1 antibodies.

Paraneoplastic pemphigus occurs in the context of several lymphoproliferative disorders: non-Hodgkin's lymphoma, chronic lymphocytic leukemia, Castleman's disease, thymoma, and retroperitoneal sarcoma. Intractable mucositis with lichenoid erosions is the most constant clinical finding. Polymorphous cutaneous involvement with lesions that resemble erythema multiforme, pemphigus, pemphigoid, or lichenoid eruptions is observed. Histologic study shows suprabasilar acantholysis or interface/lichenoid changes. The key diagnostic finding is the presence of antibodies against desmogleins 3 and 1, and additional autoantibodies against epithelial plakin proteins, such as desmoplakin, envoplakin, and periplakin, which may be identified by immunoblotting or immunoprecipitation techniques. They may also be inferred with immunofluorescent techniques showing their reactivity with murine bladder epithelium.

FIRST-LINE THERAPIES

Pemphigus vulgaris and foliaceus	
▶ Systemic corticosteroids	B

Pemphigus: a 20 year review of 107 patients treated with corticosteroids. Rosenberg FR, Sanders S, Nelson CT. Arch Dermatol 1976; 112: 962–70.

The first-line therapy for all forms of pemphigus is *systemic corticosteroids*. Corticosteroids work relatively quickly and are relatively safe when used at appropriate doses for limited periods. In the past, regimens of rapidly accelerating doses of corticosteroids were administered, but were found to be associated with unacceptably high morbidity and mortality risks. *Initial treatment should start at 1 mg/kg daily (lean body weight)*. A good clinical response, defined as a resolution of the majority of existing lesions and absence of newly developing lesions, should be evident within 2–3 months. The dose should then be reduced to 40 mg daily and subsequently tapered over 6–9 months, ideally to a maintenance dose of 5 mg every other day. Tapering can be accomplished by reducing the prednisone by an average of 10 mg per month initially, and 5 mg per month later. There are some advantages to beginning an alternate-dose regimen at 40 mg daily, so that monthly reductions would ideally be 40/20 mg on alternate days, 40/0 mg, 30/0 mg, 20/0 mg, 15/0 mg, and 10/0 mg, and then 5/0 mg on alternate days for maintenance.

The use of a second-line therapy is certainly indicated if significant corticosteroid side effects develop or are expected to develop during the ideal prednisone taper, if the disease does not improve sufficiently to allow continuous tapering, or if the disease flares. With the introduction of better tolerated drugs such as *mycophenolate mofetil*, it is reasonable to use a second agent in all patients with moderate to severe disease from the start of therapy, in anticipation of steroid-sparing benefits.

Monthly pulse corticosteroids have been suggested as a less toxic alternative to daily oral therapy, but pemphigus is very persistent, and more consistent daily or alternate-day dosing is usually required to achieve suppression.

Patients must be monitored for corticosteroid-induced osteopenia by bone mineral density studies (DEXA scan) at the start of therapy, and annually thereafter. Patients without a history of renal calculi may be given prophylactic *supplemental calcium* 1500 mg daily and *vitamin D*, 400–800 IU daily. In patients with osteopenia or osteoporosis, additional therapies may include *hormone replacement* in women (estrogen/progesterone, or raloxifen in those with a contraindication for estrogens, such as a history of breast carcinoma) or *exogenous testosterone* in men with low serum testosterone levels, or a *bisphosphonate* such as *alendronate*, or *intranasal calcitonin*.

In pemphigus vulgaris, therapy as outlined should commence in all patients once the diagnosis is confirmed. Even in cases with limited oral lesions, the disease will progress unless treated with systemic agents, and palliative therapy with topical agents or intralesional injections just delays definitive therapy. There is clinical evidence that early intervention with definitive treatment leads to a better long-term outcome. In pemphigus foliaceus, however, not every patient requires immediate treatment. Some have a very limited and smoldering disease and can therefore benefit from some palliative treatment, such as topical corticosteroids. Paraneoplastic pemphigus is usually relentlessly progressive, justifying the immediate institution of systemic corticosteroids and a second-line treatment. If a patient has an associated benign lymphoproliferative disorder, such as thymoma, hyaline vascular Castleman's disease, or sarcoma, complete surgical removal should be attempted to prolong disease remission.

SECOND-LINE THERAPIES

▶ Mycophenolate mofetil	B
▶ Azathioprine	C
▶ High-dose IVIG	C
▶ Rituximab	D

Treatment of pemphigus vulgaris and foliaceus with mycophenolate mofetil. Mimouni D, Anhalt GJ, Cummins DL, Kouba DJ, Thorne JE, Nousari HC. Arch Dermatol 2003; 139: 739–42.

Forty-two patients were treated with mycophenolate mofetil 1.5 g twice daily, plus standard prednisone therapy. Complete clinical remission was defined as achieving no new lesions with prednisone doses <10 mg daily. This was achieved in 70% of patients with pemphigus vulgaris and 55% of those with pemphigus foliaceus. Therapy was discontinued in only two cases due to adverse effects, one secondary to febrile neutropenia and one for gastrointestinal intolerance.

For pemphigus vulgaris and foliaceus, two effective antimetabolite immunosuppressive drugs are azathioprine and mycophenolate mofetil. Mycophenolate has an excellent safety profile but is very expensive. Recent reports have associated progressive multifocal leukoencephalopathy in patients on the drug. Azathioprine appears to be equally effective and is much cheaper, but has much more frequent toxicities. These drugs are added to the systemic corticosteroids if the indications for their use are met. Once their beneficial effect is observed, the corticosteroids should be progressively tapered, while the second agent is used at full doses for up to 2–3 years to induce a durable remission. For both drugs the doses required are greater than those needed to control other cutaneous diseases, because only at high doses does one observe the required inhibition of the synthesis of autoantibodies by B cells.

Mycophenolate mofetil has approval for two dosing schedules: 1000 mg po bid in renal transplantation, and 1500 mg po bid in cardiac transplants. Both dosing regimens have been used in pemphigus, but there is insufficient evidence to recommend one over the other. Onset of action is slow, and remissions are observed in responders after 2–12 months of therapy. Complete blood count and liver enzymes should be monitored monthly, but cytopenias and hepatotoxicity are rarely observed. Some lymphopenia without neutropenia is common, but has no adverse consequences and can correlate with a good clinical effect. Some nausea and diarrhea can occur, but improve with dosage reduction. Avoidance of pregnancy is mandatory, as human fetal malformations have occurred with its use.

Azathioprine in the treatment of pemphigus vulgaris. A long term follow-up. Aberer W, Wolff-Schreiner EC, Stingl G, Wolff K. J Am Acad Dermatol 1987; 16: 527–33.

Azathioprine is given in a single daily dose of 3–4 mg/kg. At this dose there is a risk of neutropenia, thrombocytopenia, hepatotoxicity, and severe or debilitating nausea. Monitoring should consist of complete blood count and liver enzymes, initially every 2 weeks. Patients with thiopurine methyltransferase deficiency (TPMT) cannot metabolize the drug effectively and can develop severe pancytopenia during the first 2 months of therapy. Late effects include elevation of liver enzymes and drug fever. The drug also requires 6–8 weeks of therapy before its effect on the disease can be judged. It is quite effective, but even if one screens patients for TPMT deficiency before starting treatment, the incidence of side effects is greater than with mycophenolate. It is still a useful second-line agent for those who cannot afford mycophenolate. There is also concern that exposure to this drug can increase one's lifetime risk of leukemia or lymphoma, but the risk is very much less than that associated with the use of alkylating agents.

A comparison of oral methylprednisolone plus azathioprine or mycophenolate mofetil for the treatment of pemphigus. Beissert S, Werfel T, Frieling U, Böhm M, Sticherling M, Stadler R, et al. Arch Dermatol 2006; 142: 1447–54.

A prospective, multicenter, randomized, non-blinded clinical trial to compare two parallel groups of patients with pemphigus (pemphigus vulgaris and pemphigus foliaceus) treated with oral methylprednisolone plus azathioprine or oral methylprednisolone plus mycophenolate mofetil (MMF). In 13 (72%) of 18 patients with pemphigus receiving oral methylprednisolone and azathioprine, complete remission was achieved after a mean 74 days compared to 20 (95%) of 21 patients receiving oral methylprednisolone and MMF, in whom complete remission occurred after a mean 91 days. In six (33%) of 18 patients treated with azathioprine, severe adverse effects were documented, in contrast to four (19%) of 21 patients who received MMF.

Randomized controlled open-label trial of four treatment regimens for pemphigus vulgaris. Chams-Davatchi C, Esmaili N, Daneshpazhooh M, Valikhani M, Balighi K, Hallaji Z, et al. J Am Acad Dermatol 2007; 57: 622–8.

The aim of this randomized study was to compare the efficacy and safety of four treatment regimens for new-onset pemphigus vulgaris (n=121): prednisolone alone; prednisolone plus azathioprine; prednisolone plus mycophenolate mofetil; and prednisolone plus intravenous cyclophosphamide pulse therapy. Results after 1 year were better with adjuvant treatment than with corticosteroid treatment alone. The highest efficacy was noted for azathioprine, followed by cyclophosphamide (pulse therapy), and mycophenolate mofetil. Interestingly, there were no significant differences in side effects among the groups.

High-dose intravenous immune globulin for the treatment of autoimmune blistering diseases. Harman KE, Black MM. Br J Dermatol 1999; 140: 865–74.

Treatment of pemphigus with intravenous immunoglobulin. Bystryn JC, Jiao D, Natow S. J Am Acad Dermatol 2002: 358; 358–63.

Both studies used IVIG in addition to treatment with prednisone and immunosuppressive therapy. IVIG produced a rapid reduction of circulating autoantibody levels, which in some cases was accompanied by significant clinical improvement.

High-dose IVIG can be used for acute control of active pemphigus. This treatment seems to accelerate the catabolism of the autoantibody and reduce circulating levels as effectively as plasmapheresis. It is generally safe and well tolerated, but has some risk. A small number of patients can develop thrombotic complications such as deep venous thrombosis or stroke. It is enormously expensive (as much as $12,000 per treatment for a 70 kg patient), and may lose its effectiveness after repeated treatment cycles. It can be given intravenously at a dose of 2 g/kg body weight, infused in divided doses over 2–5 days monthly.

IVIG is used frequently for acute control of severe cases. It can provide disease control for several months while slower-acting drugs such as mycophenolate are used, and is safer than plasmapheresis. It can also be used effectively in combination with rituximab. The use of IVIG for extended periods to induce a remission is more controversial and requires better data.

Treatment of refractory pemphigus vulgaris with rituximab (anti-CD20 monoclonal antibody). Dupuy A, Viguier M, Bedane C, Cordoliani F, Blaise S, Aucouturier F, et al. Arch Dermatol 2004; 140: 91–6.

A single cycle of rituximab for the treatment of severe pemphigus. Joly P, Mouquet H, Roujeau JC, D'Incan M, Gilbert D, Jacquot S, et al. N Engl J Med 2007; 357: 545–53.

Twenty-one patients with pemphigus that was refractory to corticosteroids (at least two relapses despite prednisone treatment with doses higher than 20 mg/day; corticosteroid-dependent disease) or who had severe contraindications to corticosteroids were treated with four weekly infusions of rituximab, 375 mg/m^2 body-surface area. Eighteen showed complete remission at 3 months.

Two courses of rituximab (anti-CD20 monoclonal antibody) for recalcitrant pemphigus vulgaris. Faurschou A, Gniadecki R. Int J Dermatol 2008; 47: 292–4.

Two patients with recalcitrant pemphigus vulgaris were treated with two courses of four weekly infusions of rituximab, 375 mg/m^2 body-surface area with a 6-month interval. Clinical improvement was noticeable 3–6 weeks after the first infusion, and complete remission was achieved after the second course.

Treatment of pemphigus vulgaris with rituximab and intravenous immune globulin. Ahmed AR, Spigelman Z, Cavacini LA, Posner MR. N Engl J Med 2006; 355: 1772–9.

Eleven patients with severe pemphigus involving at least 30% of the body surface that was refractory to corticosteroids plus at least three or more immunosuppressive agents were treated with three weekly infusions of rituximab, 375 mg/m² body-surface area. In the fourth week, IVIG 2 g/kg was given. This course was repeated for a second cycle. This course was followed by a monthly infusion of rituximab (single infusion) and IVIG (single infusion) for 4 additional months. Of the 11 patients, nine showed complete remission lasting 22–37 months. This treatment was not associated with any significant side effects necessitating the discontinuation of treatment.

Depletion of CD20+ B cells by the use of anti-CD20 monoclonal antibody is emerging as a potentially powerful tool in many autoimmune diseases and is approved for use in rheumatoid arthritis. CD20 is not expressed on pre-B or plasma cells, so it is not profoundly immunosuppressive, and the effect only lasts 6–10 months, as the CD20+ cells are repopulated from stem cells. Currently approved dosing is 375 mg/m² weekly × 4 for lymphoma, or 1000 mg × 2, days 1 and 15 for rheumatoid arthritis (RA). The original dosing regimen for lymphoma was designed to prevent tumor lysis syndrome in patients with bulky lymphomas. The authors have used the simpler, lower-dose RA schedule in a small number of pemphigus vulgaris patients with equivalent efficacy. The toxicity of rituximab is minimal, but the addition of the drug to patients already exposed to corticosteroids and immunosuppressive drugs increases the risk of infection, including one reported fatal case of Pneumocystis carinii *pneumonia (PCP) in a patient treated with rituximab and cyclophosphamide. PCP prophylaxis should be considered with the use of this drug. The drug can cause rapid reduction of autoantibody levels in even severely affected cases, with excellent results and often dramatic recoveries. It is possible that a second course of rituximab has an important consolidation role for durable remission. The addition of IVIG to rituximab is reasonable in explosive acute cases; however, according to current studies, its added value in less acute cases is questionable. Rituximab is used most commonly in paraneoplastic pemphigus, where it has a dual role of treating the underlying lymphoproliferative disease as well as the associated autoimmune disease.*

THIRD-LINE THERAPIES

▶ Cyclophosphamide	B
▶ Cyclophosphamide plus plasmapheresis	E
▶ Chlorambucil	D

Dexamethasone–cyclophosphamide pulse therapy for pemphigus. Pasricha JS, Khaitan BK, Raman RS, Chandra M. Int J Dermatol 1995; 34: 875–82.

Alkylating agents such as cyclophosphamide have a profound effect on inhibition of autoantibody synthesis, and are the most effective agents for inducing a remission. They also have very significant potential toxicities, which restrict their use to third-line therapy.

Cyclophosphamide is the preferred agent because any neutropenia associated with its use is predictable in onset, and withdrawal of the drug results in rapid recovery of neutrophils (within 1 week to 10 days). There are four ways to administer the drug:

1. *Daily orally at 2.5 mg/kg. A single morning dose is followed by aggressive fluid consumption throughout the day to rinse metabolites from the bladder and prevent hemorrhagic cystitis. Weekly complete blood counts and urinalysis are required. With this use, a durable remission can be obtained after 18–24 months of therapy in almost all cases. This exposure probably*

increases the patient's lifetime risk of leukemia, lymphoma, or bladder cancer by as much as 5–10% over the normal population. This risk is appreciated some 20–30 years after treatment. Such treatment can also cause sterility in young patients.

2. *Monthly intravenous pulses at a dose of 750 mg/m² body surface area. Monthly intravenous administration reduces the risk of hemorrhagic cystitis, but this intermittent use is not as effective in suppressing the disease.*

3. *Monthly intravenous administration with lower dose oral daily maintenance. This can also be very effective in inducing a remission.*

4. *Single, very high-dose immunoablative therapy. This experimental treatment is effective in many autoimmune diseases. It employs a dose of intravenous cyclophosphamide of 200 mg/kg, given over 4 days, which induces profound marrow aplasia. Upon recovery patients often experience a complete remission. However, unlike the experience with disorders such as aplastic anemia, where remission may last many years, most patients with pemphigus relapse within 2 years of completing therapy, which limits its usefulness.*

Synchronization of plasmapheresis and pulse cyclophosphamide therapy in pemphigus vulgaris. Euler HH, Loffler H, Christophers E. Arch Dermatol 1987; 123: 1205–10.

Plasmapheresis is the only method by which one can rapidly reduce autoantibody levels, and is used in patients with very extensive and accelerated disease. Its use involves a total of six high-volume removals (3–3.5 L per removal, three times weekly for 2 consecutive weeks). This must be combined with the concomitant use of systemic corticosteroids and oral cyclophosphamide. If these drugs are not used, the reduction of autoantibodies removes feedback inhibition to the autoimmune B cells and causes a rebound flare of the disease. This can be blunted only by alkylating agents, owing to their preferential toxicity to rapidly proliferative B cells. This causes the induction of a durable remission, though cyclophosphamide must still be used at full doses for 18–24 months to harden that remission.

The use of chlorambucil with prednisone in the treatment of pemphigus. Shah N, Green AR, Elgart GW, Kerdel F. J Am Acad Dermatol 2000; 42: 85–8.

In patients who develop hemorrhagic cystitis from cyclophosphamide, chlorambucil can be substituted.

Chlorambucil is more difficult to use because the cytopenias induced by it are more unpredictable. When they occur, they may take months to resolve.

Ciclosporin

Ineffectiveness of cyclosporine as an adjuvant to corticosteroids in the treatment of pemphigus. Ioannides D, Chrysomallis F, Bystryn JC. Arch Dermatol 2000; 868: 505–6.

Thirty-three consecutive patients hospitalized with pemphigus vulgaris (n=29) or foliaceus (n=4) were randomized to receive either prednisolone or prednisolone plus ciclosporin 5 mg/kg daily. The groups were similar in terms of disease severity and demographics. The addition of ciclosporin produced no change in the response to treatment or the total dose of corticosteroid administered. Complications were, however, more common in those patients who received ciclosporin.

Although there are anecdotal cases reporting benefit from the use of ciclosporin, this well-performed study with an impressive number of cases is good evidence that the drug should not be used in pemphigus vulgaris and foliaceus. There is still good anecdotal evidence that ciclosporin may have a role to play in the management of paraneoplastic pemphigus, a disease with a much more complex pathophysiology.

Perforating dermatoses

Sarah Markoff, Mark G Lebwohl

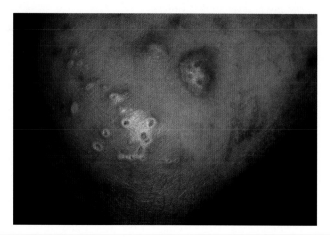

The perforating dermatoses are a varied group of conditions characterized by the transepidermal elimination of dermal material. Four primary conditions are included in the discussion of the perforating disorders:

- Reactive perforating collagenosis, which is characterized by the transepidermal elimination of collagen
- Elastosis perforans serpiginosa (EPS), characterized by transepidermal extrusion of elastic material
- Perforating folliculitis, in which epidermal perforation involves hair follicles
- Kyrle's disease, in which dermal connective tissue perforates through the epidermis.

MANAGEMENT STRATEGY

Definitive diagnosis of the perforating disorders depends on the demonstration of transepidermal elimination on skin biopsy. Differentiation between the different forms of perforating disorders can be accomplished by Masson trichrome stains for collagen (reactive perforating collagenosis), Verhoeff–van Gieson stains for elastic tissue (EPS), and step-sectioning to look for hair follicles (perforating folliculitis). Differentiation between these various disorders may be important, as EPS is associated with other diseases such as pseudoxanthoma elasticum, Down syndrome, osteogenesis imperfecta, Ehlers–Danlos syndrome, Rothmund–Thomson syndrome, Marfan syndrome, and penicillamine treatment. Reactive perforating collagenosis is commonly associated with diabetes and renal failure.

Occasionally, acquired reactive perforating collagenosis has occurred in patients treated with particular medications such as indinavir and sirolimus, and perforating folliculitis has been reported in a patient treated with tumor necrosis factor-α blockers.

Management of the perforating diseases involves determination of underlying etiologies. Most often, conditions such as diabetes mellitus and renal failure will be known to the patient who presents with perforating skin lesions. When the underlying cause is not apparent, serum chemistry for renal and liver function tests and glucose tolerance test may be helpful.

Once the diagnosis of underlying diseases is ascertained, treatment is directed at associated symptoms. Pruritus can be managed initially with *topical* or *intralesional corticosteroids, topical anesthetics and menthol*, as well as *oral antihistamines*, but the latter agents are usually not sufficiently effective. Minimizing pruritus is important because many of the perforating disorders typically exhibit a Koebner phenomenon, meaning that lesions develop in traumatized or scratched skin. Topical antipruritic agents such as menthol, phenol, or camphor, and topical anesthetics such as lidocaine and pramocaine are useful. *Topical doxepin hydrochloride* or oral antihistamines may also be of some benefit. Trimming the fingernails to minimize trauma to the skin and avoidance of scratching are key elements of treatment. *Topical tretinoin* and *topical tazarotene* have been shown to be effective for some patients. For those patients whose condition is exacerbated by sun exposure, sunscreens may be helpful. Conversely, in patients with renal disease UVB is dramatically effective for pruritus and has been reported to benefit perforating skin lesions as well. If UVB, narrowband UVB, and topical retinoids are ineffective, *oral retinoids, allopurinol* or *antibiotics* can be tried.

SPECIFIC INVESTIGATIONS

- ▶ Skin biopsy with Masson trichrome stains and Verhoeff–van Gieson stains
- ▶ Serum BUN, creatinine, ALT, AST, alkaline phosphatase, bilirubin, uric acid
- ▶ Serum glucose or glucose tolerance test
- ▶ Hepatitis C virus antibodies
- ▶ Thyroid function tests

Reactive perforating collagenosis associated with diabetes mellitus. Poliak SC, Lebwohl MG, Parris A, Prioleau PG. N Engl J Med 1982; 306: 81–4.

Reactive perforating collagenosis was found in three of 15 dialysis patients with diabetes mellitus. Typical lesions are described in six patients, all of whom had severe diabetes with retinopathy. Five of the six had chronic renal disease.

Acquired perforating dermatosis: clinicopathological features in twenty-two cases. Saray Y, Seçkin D, Bilezikçi B. J Eur Acad Dermatol Venereol 2006; 20: 679–88.

Of 22 patients with acquired perforating dermatoses, 72.7% had chronic renal failure, 50% had diabetes mellitus, 27.3% had hepatitis, 13.6% were hepatitis C virus antibody positive, and 9.1% were hypothyroid. Of the patients with diabetes mellitus, 90.9% had chronic renal failure.

FIRST-LINE THERAPIES

▷ Tretinoin 0.1%	D
▷ Tazarotene gel 0.1%	E
▷ UVB	E
▷ Narrowband UVB	D

Familial reactive perforating collagenosis: a clinical, histopathological study of 10 cases. Ramesh V, Sood N, Kubba A, Singh B, Makkar R. J Eur Acad Dermatol Venereol 2007; 21: 766–70.

Ten patients with familial reactive perforating collagenosis were studied. All responded to topical retinoic acid. The authors suggested that sunscreens may benefit patients whose lesions develop in the summer.

Familial reactive perforating collagenosis may be a distinct entity that occurs in infancy or early childhood. It is of interest that sunlight might play a role in the development of this condition, as phototherapy is used therapeutically in adults with perforating disorders.

Tazarotene is an effective therapy for elastosis perforans serpiginosa. Outland JD, Brown TS, Callen JP. Arch Dermatol 2002; 138: 169–71.

A report of two patients with EPS who responded to daily treatment with 0.1% tazarotene gel. A 22-year-old woman had been treated unsuccessfully with liquid nitrogen cryotherapy, topical tretinoin, oral isotretinoin, and CO$_2$ laser surgery. A 56-year-old woman had failed to respond to cryotherapy, corticosteroids, tretinoin, and triamcinolone acetonide. Both patients were treated with tazarotene. The skin condition of the 22-year-old greatly improved and that of the 56-year-old improved moderately.

Acquired reactive collagen disease in the adult: successful treatment with UV-B light. Vion E, Frenk E. Hautarzt 1989; 40: 448–50. (In German.)

A 77-year-old woman with reactive perforating collagenosis and severe pruritus responded to phototherapy with UVB. Both the pruritus and skin lesions improved.

UVB is a well-established modality for uremic pruritus. As many patients with perforating diseases have associated renal failure, UVB phototherapy may dramatically benefit pruritus and reduce the number of skin lesions.

Treatment of acquired perforating dermatosis with narrowband ultraviolet B. Ohe S, Danno K, Sasaki H, Isei T, Okamoto H, Horio TJ. Am Acad Dermatol 2004; 50: 892–4.

Narrowband UVB resulted in complete clearing in all five patients treated with phototherapy two to three times per week. Narrowband UVB was started at 400 mJ/cm^2 and increased up to 1500 mJ/cm^2. Clearing occurred with 10–15 treatments. Three patients recurred between 1 and 10 months after discontinuation of narrowband UVB. Two patients remained clear on narrowband UVB maintenance treatments until 7 and 8 months, respectively.

SECOND-LINE THERAPIES

▶ Allopurinol	D
▶ Isotretinoin	E
▶ PUVA	E
▶ Acitretin	E

Acquired reactive perforating collagenosis: four patients with a giant variant treated with allopurinol. Hoque SR, Ameen M, Holden CA. Br J Dermatol 2006; 154: 759–62.

All four patients failed topical and oral corticosteroids and antibiotics and were started on allopurinol 100 mg once daily despite normal serum uric acid levels. Three of the four experienced dramatic improvement at 2–4 months, with prevention of new lesions, a reduction in pruritus, and clearance of existing lesions. The fourth patient died before the follow-up examination.

Numerous anecdotal reports have documented improvement of perforating disorders with allopurinol treatment, regardless of whether uric acid levels are elevated or normal.

Reactive perforating collagenosis: a condition that may be underdiagnosed. Satchell AC, Crotty K, Lee S. Australas J Dermatol 2001; 42: 284–7.

Three patients with diabetes mellitus were treated for reactive perforating collagenosis.

A 73-year-old woman was treated with 0.5% phenol with 10% glycerine in sorbolene cream. After 1 month of treatment the itch resolved and skin lesions diminished in number and size.

A 75-year-old woman responded to treatment with narrowband UVB. The patient received phototherapy three times per week for 2 months, with resolution of lesions. When the condition recurred 6 months later, it again cleared with 3 months of narrowband UVB.

A 58-year-old woman who did not respond to corticosteroids, antihistamines, UVB, or PUVA was successfully treated with oral acitretin 25 mg daily, which resolved the itch and cleared the skin lesions.

Kyrle's disease. Effectively treated with isotretinoin. Saleh HA, Lloyd KM, Fatteh S. J Fla Med Assoc 1993; 80: 395–7. Erratum in J Fla Med Assoc 1993; 80: 467.

A 63-year-old patient with Kyrle's disease and chronic renal failure was treated with oral isotretinoin for 13 weeks. Cutaneous lesions cleared completely.

Reactive perforating collagenosis responsive to PUVA. Serrano G, Aliaga A, Lorente M. Int J Dermatol 1988; 27: 118–19.

A 21-year-old woman with a 10-year history of reactive perforating collagenosis was treated with PUVA four times per week. Improvement was noted in 2 weeks. Lesions stopped developing after completion of PUVA therapy (326 J/cm^2 total), and no new lesions were noted in over a year of post-treatment observations.

THIRD-LINE THERAPIES

▶ 0.5% phenol with 10% glycerine in sorbolene	E
▶ Surgical debridement	E
▶ Cryotherapy	E
▶ Ultrapulse laser	E
▶ Doxycycline	E
▶ Oral metronidazole	E
▶ Oral clindamycin	E
▶ Oral hydroxychloroquine	E
▶ Transcutaneous electrical nerve stimulation (TENS)	E

Successful treatment of acquired reactive perforating collagenosis with doxycycline. Brinkmeier T, Schaller J, Herbst RA, Frosch PJ. Acta Dermatol Venereol 2002; 82: 393–5.

An 87-year-old woman with acquired reactive perforating collagenosis responded to treatment with oral doxycycline 100 mg daily for 2 weeks. Within 5 days of initiation of treatment, new skin lesions ceased to form, and within 10 days of treatment most lesions had healed.

Regression of skin lesions of Kyrle's disease with metronidazole in a diabetic patient. Khalifa M, Slim I, Kaabia N, Bahri F, Trabelsi A, Letaief AO. J Infect 2007; 55: e139–40.

Metronidazole 500 mg twice daily for 1 month completely cleared lesions of Kyrle's disease. Lesions did not recur during 12 months of follow-up.

Regression of skin lesions of Kyrle's disease with clindamycin: implications for an infectious component in the etiology of the disease. Kasiakou SK, Peppas G, Kapaskelis AM, Falagas ME. J Infect 2005; 50: 412–16.

A patient with old, uninflamed hyperkeratotic lesions of Kyrle's disease and newer inflamed lesions was successfully treated with a combination of oral clindamycin and surgical removal of large lesions.

Sirolimus-induced inflammatory papules with acquired reactive perforating collagenosis. Lübbe J, Sorg O, Malé PJ, Saurat JH, Masouyé I. Dermatology 2008; 216: 239–42.

A patient with acquired reactive perforating collagenosis attributed to sirolimus following liver transplantation responded to oral hydroxychloroquine 200 mg daily even though the sirolimus was continued. Skin remained clear for 6 months, during which time the patient continued on hydroxychloroquine as well as sirolimus.

Imiquimod therapy for elastosis perforans serpiginosa. Kelly SC, Purcell SM. Arch Dermatol 2006; 142: 829–30.

A 14-year-old girl with elastosis perforans serpiginosa was treated with imiquimod cream applied every night for 6 weeks, and then three times weekly for the following 4 weeks. After 10 weeks her skin cleared completely.

A new treatment for acquired reactive perforating collagenosis. Oziemski MA, Billson VR, Crosthwaite GL, Zajac J, Varigos GA. Australas J Dermatol 1991; 32: 71–4.

A single patient with reactive perforating collagenosis was successfully treated with surgical debridement and split skin grafting of the affected areas.

Because skin lesions are often numerous, surgical removal and skin grafting may be impractical.

Elastosis performans serpiginosa: treatment with liquid nitrogen. Tuyp EJ, McLeod WA. Int J Dermatol 1990; 29: 655–6.

Liquid nitrogen was applied with a cotton-tipped applicator for approximately 10 s on six occasions over 7 months. Lesions of EPS disappeared and did not return.

Localized idiopathic elastosis perforans serpiginosa effectively treated by the coherent ultrapulse 5000C aesthetic laser. Abdullah A, Colloby PS, Foulds IS, Whitcroft I. Int J Dermatol 2000; 39: 719–20.

Portions of lesions of EPS were treated by laser, with complete clearing of treated sites but no changes in untreated sites.

Response of elastosis perforans serpiginosa to pulsed CO_2, Er:YAG, and dye lasers. Saxena M, Tope WD. Dermatol Surg 2003; 29: 677–8.

A 17-year-old male presenting with EPS on the neck was treated with CO_2 laser (UltraPulse 5000C) on the right neck and erbium:YAG laser (UltraFine; Coherent) on the left neck. Only mild improvement of EPS was achieved and subtle atrophic scarring occurred on the area treated with the CO_2 laser. The patient then received pulsed dye laser therapy on both sides of the neck, resulting only in minimal improvement of EPS.

Treatment of pruritus of reactive perforating collagenosis using transcutaneous electrical nerve stimulation. Chan LY, Tang WY, Lo KK. Eur J Dermatol 2000; 10: 59–61.

A 47-year-old woman and an 85-year-old woman, each of whom had failed to respond to treatment with topical steroids and antihistamines, received TENS therapy for 1 hour daily over the course of 3 weeks. Skin lesions cleared within 3 months of treatment in both patients.

Perioral dermatitis

Antonios Kanelleas, John Berth-Jones

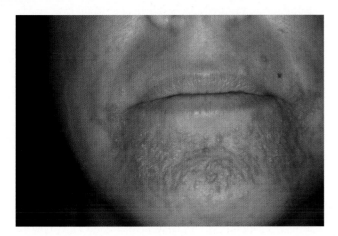

Perioral dermatitis is an eruption of inflammatory papules (and sometimes pustules) on the chin, perioral areas, and nasolabial folds, characteristically sparing the skin immediately adjacent to the vermilion border. It is usually seen in young women, but also occurs in childhood. The development of perioral dermatitis is frequently preceded by intentional or inadvertent application of potent topical corticosteroids to the facial skin. A similar eruption involving the eyelids and periorbital skin has been termed periocular dermatitis. The granulomatous subset of perioral dermatitis, which is histologically confirmed, presents with small flesh-colored or yellow-brown papules.

The suggested relationship of perioral dermatitis with infectious agents and infestations such as *Candida* spp. or *Demodex folliculorum* has not been confirmed.

Although sometimes described as a variant of rosacea, perioral dermatitis is distinguished from this disease by its distribution, by the relatively monomorphic appearance of the lesions, by the absence of flushing and telangiectasia, and by its tendency to occur in younger patients.

MANAGEMENT STRATEGY

Many cases are associated with the use of *potent topical corticosteroids*, and *withdrawal* of this medication is the most important measure in this group. Patients must be warned that the condition may initially flare after this maneuver. If the flare proves intolerable, initial use of a less potent topical corticoid can often be helpful. *Systemic tetracyclines* are also frequently employed, and a range of other modalities are used less frequently. In most cases there will be a permanent remission, but relapses may rarely occur.

SPECIFIC INVESTIGATIONS

▶ No investigation is routinely required

FIRST-LINE TREATMENT

▶ Withdrawal of topical corticoids	B
▶ Oral tetracyclines	B

Complications of topical hydrocortisone. Guin JD. J Am Acad Dermatol 1981; 4: 417–22.

Perioral dermatitis developed following the use of topical hydrocortisone.

Although usually associated with the use of potent topical corticosteroids, this case suggests that even hydrocortisone may induce perioral dermatitis.

Perioral dermatitis: aetiology and treatment with tetracycline. Macdonald A, Feiwel M. Br J Dermatol 1972; 87: 351–9.

Tetracycline 250 mg given three times daily for a week, then twice daily for 2–3 months, proved highly effective in this series of 29 cases.

Perioral dermatitis in renal transplant recipients maintained on corticosteroids and immunosuppressive therapy. Adams SJ, Davison AM, Cunliffe WJ, Giles GR. Br J Dermatol 1982; 106: 589–92.

A report of five cases where perioral dermatitis developed in patients on oral corticosteroids that could not be discontinued. A 2-month course of doxycycline was effective.

SECOND-LINE TREATMENTS

▶ Topical pimecrolimus	A
▶ Topical tetracycline	B
▶ Topical erythromycin	B
▶ Oral erythromycin	E
▶ Topical metronidazole	C
▶ Topical azelaic acid	D
▶ Oral isotretinoin	E
▶ Topical adapalene	E
▶ Photodynamic therapy	B

Pimecrolimus cream (1%) efficacy in perioral dermatitis-results of a randomized, double-blind, vehicle-controlled study in 40 patients. Oppel T, Pavicic T, Kamann S, Bräutigam M, Wollenberg A. J Eur Acad Dermatol Venereol 2007; 21: 1175–80.

Twenty patients were treated with topical pimecrolimus cream 1% twice a day for 4 weeks. The comparison group consisted of 20 patients treated with the vehicle compound. The Perioral Dermatitis Severity Index (PODSI) score was found to be significantly lower in the pimecrolimus group at the end of the treatment period, whereas no differences between the two groups were observed after a 4-week follow-up period.

There are reports linking the use of topical calcineurin inhibitors with the induction of perioral dermatitis and rosacea-like eruptions after treatment for facial inflammatory dermatoses.

Topical tetracycline in the treatment of perioral dermatitis. Wilson RG. Arch Dermatol 1979; 115: 637.

Topical tetracycline, applied twice daily, proved highly effective in this series of 30 patients. Twenty-four cleared completely after 5–28 days.

A topical erythromycin preparation and oral tetracycline for the treatment of perioral dermatitis: a placebo-controlled trial. Weber K, Thurmayr R, Meisinger A. J Dermatol Treat 1993; 4: 57–9.

A comparison of the response to topical erythromycin (33 patients), oral tetracycline (35 patients), and placebo

(31 patients). Oral tetracycline and topical erythromycin were comparable in efficacy and both were superior to placebo.

Topical therapy for perioral dermatitis. Bikowski JB. Cutis 1983; 31: 678–82.

Six cases cleared with topical erythromycin.

Identical twins with perioral dermatitis. Weston WL, Morelli JG. Pediatr Dermatol 1998; 15: 144.

Two cases responded to oral erythromycin.

Topical metronidazole in the treatment of perioral dermatitis. Veien NK, Munkvad JM, Nielsen AO, Niordson AM, Stahl D, Thormann J. J Am Acad Dermatol 1991; 24: 258–69.

A prospective, randomized, double-blind trial with 109 patients. Both groups improved, but 1% metronidazole cream applied twice daily was less effective than oxytetracycline 250 mg twice daily over 8 weeks.

Topical metronidazole gel (0.75%) for the treatment of perioral dermatitis in children. Miller SR, Shalita AR. J Am Acad Dermatol 1994; 31: 847–8.

Three children with perioral or periocular eruptions were treated with topical metronidazole gel (0.75%) twice daily. Significant improvement was observed after 2 months. Complete resolution occurred after 14 weeks.

Azelaic acid as a new treatment for perioral dermatitis: results from an open study. Jansen T. Br J Dermatol 2004; 151: 933–4.

Ten cases were treated with topical 20% azelaic acid cream applied twice daily. Complete clearing was reported in all cases after 2–6 weeks. The cream was well tolerated.

Perioral dermatitis with histopathologic features of granulomatous rosacea: successful treatment with isotretinoin. Smith KW. Cutis 1990; 46: 413–15.

Isotretinoin was used successfully in a resistant case.

Perioral dermatitis successfully treated with topical adapalene. Jansen T. J Eur Acad Dermatol Venereol 2002; 16: 175–7.

Successful treatment of one case of perioral dermatitis with topical adapalene gel once daily for 4 weeks. The patient had had no history of steroid use, and previous topical therapy with erythromycin had failed.

Photodynamic therapy for perioral dermatitis. Richey DF, Hopson B. J Drugs Dermatol 2006; 5: 12–16.

Twenty-one patients participated in this prospective split-face study. One half of the face was treated with ALA PDT once weekly for approximately 4 weeks, and the other half was treated with topical clindamycin once daily. Out of the 14 patients who completed the study, the sides treated with PDT had a mean clearance of 92.1%, compared to 80.9% for the clindamycin sides (p=0.0227). The mean patient satisfaction level for PDT was also higher.

Evidence Levels: **A** Double-blind study **B** Clinical trial ≥ 20 subjects **C** Clinical trial < 20 subjects **D** Series ≥ 5 subjects **E** Anecdotal case reports

Peutz–Jeghers syndrome

Mordechai M Tarlow, Adam S Stibich, Robert A Schwartz

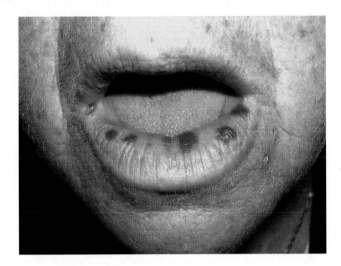

Peutz–Jeghers syndrome (PJS) is one of the more common hereditary polyposis syndromes. It is characterized by gastrointestinal polyps, periorificial pigmentation, and an increased risk of intestinal and other malignancies.

MANAGEMENT STRATEGY

The pigmented macules of PJS are typically periorificial, notably around the mouth, eyes, and anus. The hands, feet, and oral mucosa may also be transiently involved in the early years with round, oval, and irregular patches of brown to black pigment, occasionally with a bluish hue. Clinically and histologically, these are simple lentigines.

The genetic abnormality associated with this autosomal dominant disorder is a germline mutation of the STK11/LKB1 gene, located at 19p13.3, as well as a more recently identified second PJS disease locus at 19q13.4; genetic testing is not required for a diagnosis, but may aid in unclear cases as well as in genetic counseling of at-risk family members.

In patients with PJS the management strategy is to consider potential visceral complications, provide genetic counseling, and reassure that the cutaneous macules are benign in nature and that after puberty one can expect an improvement of the non-labial macules. In some cases the pigmented facial lesions are psychologically unacceptable to the patient. In these individuals there are few options, almost all of which involve the use of *laser surgery*. Treatment of systemic complications follows an evaluation for associated findings, which may include recurrent intussusceptions, gut bleeding, and a variety of visceral anomalies and intestinal and extraintestinal malignancies. Symptomatology usually begins between the ages of 10 and 30 years, but any child with recurrent unexplained abdominal pain should be evaluated for an intussusception, a medical emergency associated with PJS. Duodenal polyps may be at increased susceptibility for malignant change, but the stomach and the large and small intestines may also house cancer in this syndrome. Ovarian neoplasms, cancerous and otherwise, may be seen, especially granulosa cell tumors, sex cord tumors with annular tubules, and sex cord stromal tumors with sexual precocity. Women with PJS also appear to be at increased risk of bilateral breast cancer, whereas men may be at risk of developing testicular tumors of apparent Sertoli cell nature. Thus, the removal of cutaneous macules may hide this clinically valuable clue in a critical and compromising situation. Gastrointestinal evaluation is a key in the management of patients with PJS.

The *ruby laser (Q-switched and short pulsed)* has been used for the treatment of labial macules. The response to treatment is excellent: no sequelae or recurrences are usually noted. No anesthesia is required and no wound care is necessary. This suggests that ruby laser therapy is safe and a suitable approach for the treatment of labial macules in children with PJS.

The *CO_2, alexandrite, and argon lasers* have also been shown to be effective in the treatment of the labial macules of PJS. Cosmetic results of their use have been found to be excellent. *Intense pulsed light* has also been shown to be very effective.

Cryosurgery can be used, but does not fully eliminate the macules and may leave a hypopigmented spot. *Trichloroacetic acid* may not produce total resolution. Surgical excision, electrodesiccation, and dermabrasion commonly result in incomplete removal, scarring, or changes in normal pigmentation. Thus, these treatments give suboptimal results. In the future, chemoprevention may be an option.

SPECIFIC INVESTIGATIONS

> ▶ Histology (if diagnosis is in question)
> ▶ Gastrointestinal evaluation
> ▶ Genetic testing (in some cases)
> ▶ Psychosocial evaluation

Peutz–Jehgers syndrome. Heymann WR. J Am Acad Dermatol 2007; 57; 513–14.

A brief synopsis of the syndrome correlating molecular advances with the cutaneous, malignant, and endocrinologic features of the disorder.

Peutz–Jeghers syndrome. McGarrity TJ, Kulin HE, Zaino RJ. Am J Gastroenterol 2000; 95: 596–604.

A comprehensive review article on the intestinal as well as the extraintestinal manifestations of PJS. A management scheme for the non-cutaneous aspects is included.

Although the non-dermatologic aspects of this disease are typically in the realm of the internist and gastroenterologist, this review allows the dermatologist to offer additional patient education. It discusses all aspects, including history of the disease and genetic testing.

Peutz–Jeghers syndrome: genetic screening. Leggett BA, Young JP, Barker M. Exp Rev Anticancer Ther 2003; 3: 518–24.

A review of PJS and genetic screening.

Diagnostic and predictive genetic testing is now possible in many families owing to the identification of causative mutations in the serine/threonine kinase (STK)-11 (also known as the LKB1) gene. Such testing has now entered routine clinical practice and will allow early recognition of the condition in young, at-risk family members.

Genetic testing for polyposis: practical and ethical aspects. Jarvinen HJ. Gut 2003; 52: ii19–22.

This review delineates possible pitfalls and benefits of genetic testing as well as an appropriate approach to minimize misunderstanding and anxiety.

Peutz–Jeghers syndrome: confirmation of linkage to chromosome 19p13.3 and identification of a potential second locus, on 19q13.4. Mehenni H, Blouin JL, Radhakrishna U, Bhardwaj SS, Bhardwaj K, Dixit VB, et al. Am J Hum Genet 1997; 61: 1327–34.

This paper confirms the location of the most prevalent mutation in PJS to be the LKB1/STK11 gene at location 19p13.3, and identifies an additional locus.

This study highlights the limitation of genetic testing because PJS has not been associated with the LKB1/STK-11 gene in every case. The second gene on 19q13.4 has since been confirmed in an additional study.

Genotype–phenotype correlations in Peutz–Jeghers syndrome. Amos CI, Keitheri-Cheteri MB, Sabripour M, Wei C, McGarrity TJ, Seldin MF, et al. J Med Genet 2004; 41: 327–33.

Mutations in the STK-11 gene were found in 69% of probands with PJS. Individuals with missense mutations had a significantly delayed time to onset of first polypectomy and of other symptoms, compared to those with either truncating mutations or no detectable mutation.

This study suggests that genetic analysis may be of value beyond the diagnosis of PJS.

Harold Jeghers (1904–1990). Schwartz RA. In: Löser C, Plewig G, eds. Pantheon der Dermatologie. Berlin: Springer Verlag, 2008; 520–3.

This entity is reviewed in the context of a biography of Harold Jeghers, with original color patient photographs and a review of this syndrome.

Psychosocial impact of Peutz–Jeghers syndrome. Woo A, Sadana A, Mauger DT, Baker MJ, Berk T, McGarrity TJ. Fam Cancer 2009; 81: 59–65.

The authors have developed a questionnaire that provides specific information regarding the burden of disease and quality of life in patients affected with Peutz–Jeghers syndrome. It is useful in developing a plan of care for these patients regarding genetic counseling and surveillance strategies.

FIRST-LINE THERAPIES

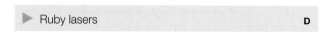

| ▶ Ruby lasers | D |

Q-switched ruby laser treatment of labial lentigos. Ashinoff R, Geronemus RG. J Am Acad Dermatol 1992; 27: 809–11.

The Q-switched ruby laser causes selective damage to pigmented cells in the skin. This laser, which has a wavelength of 694 nm and a pulse duration of 40 ns, has shown very promising results in the treatment of both amateur and professional tattoos. Fewer data are available on its ability to treat benign pigmented lesions of the skin. Three patients who had labial lentigines were treated with the Q-switched ruby laser, and dramatic clearing occurred after one or two treatments with a fluence of 10 cm^2.

Q-switched ruby laser treatment of labial lentigines in Peutz–Jeghers syndrome. DePadova-Elder SM, Milgraum SS. J Dermatol Surg Oncol 1994; 20: 830–2.

The authors report successful treatment with the Q-switched ruby laser and consider it the treatment of choice for these lesions.

Successful treatment of mucosal melanosis of the lip with normal pulsed ruby laser. Hanada K, Baba T, Sasaki C, Hashimoto I. J Dermatol 1996; 23: 263–6.

In this study, six Japanese patients with labial melanosis of PJS were successfully treated with the pulsed ruby laser. The therapy achieved rapid results without producing changes in mucosal texture or recurrence after operation.

Effective removal of certain skin pigment spots (lentigines) using the Q-switched ruby laser. Njoo MD, Westerhof W. Ned Tijdschr Geneeskd 1997; 141: 327–30. (In Dutch.)

In 15 patients Q-switched ruby laser treatment was applied to solar lentigines, labial lentigines (two), segmental lentigines (two), and lentigo simplex (one). The light energy ranged from 3 to 10 cm^2. In 11 of 15 patients, one treatment session sufficed to remove the lesion completely.

In the cases described the Q-switched ruby laser was a successful treatment for lentigines. For macules of this nature this laser is preferred to conventional forms of therapy such as cryotherapy, chemical peeling, and abrasion.

Ruby laser therapy for labial lentigines in Peutz–Jeghers syndrome. Kato S, Takeyama J, Tanita Y, Ebina K. Eur J Pediatr 1998; 157: 622–4.

Ruby laser therapy of labial lentigines in two children with PJS is described. The response to treatment was excellent and no sequelae or recurrence of the lesions were noted.

This work suggests that ruby laser therapy is safe and a suitable approach for the treatment of labial melanotic macules in children with PJS.

Q-switched ruby laser treatment of tattoos and benign pigmented lesions: a critical review. Raulin C, Schonermark MP, Greve B, Werner S. Ann Plast Surg 1998; 41: 555–65.

An excellent review on the applications of the Q-switched ruby laser, with emphasis on its particular attractiveness in removing pigmented lesions in precarious anatomic regions such as the lips and eyelids.

SECOND-LINE THERAPIES

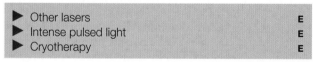

▶ Other lasers	E
▶ Intense pulsed light	E
▶ Cryotherapy	E

Treatment of labial lentigos in atopic dermatitis with the frequency-doubled Q-switched Nd:YAG laser. Akita H, Matsunaga K, Fujisawa Y, Ueda H. Arch Dermatol 2000; 136: 936–7.

Treatment of Peutz–Jeghers lentigines with the carbon dioxide laser. Benedict LM, Cohen B. J Dermatol Surg Oncol 1991; 17: 954–5.

The authors report a successful outcome in the treatment of these lentigines with the CO_2 laser.

Treatment of pigmentation of the lips and oral mucosa in Peutz–Jeghers syndrome using ruby and argon lasers. Ohshiro T, Maruyama Y, Nakajima H, Mima M. Br J Plast Surg 1980; 33: 346–9.

Three patients with punctate pigmented spots on the lips and oral mucosa accompanying PJS were successfully treated with ruby and argon lasers.

The basic principles of laser treatment, the characteristics of the different laser systems, and the skin reaction to ruby and argon lasers are discussed.

Q-switched Alexandrite laser in the treatment of pigmented macules in Laugier–Hunziker syndrome. Papadavid E, Walker NP. J Eur Acad Dermatol Venereol 2001; 15: 468–9.

Two patients with pigmented macules on their lips were treated with the Q-switched alexandrite laser.

Laugier–Hunziker syndrome presents with similar macules to those in PJS, but there are no associated gastrointestinal abnormalities. In this report one patient cleared with initial treatment, and one required repeat treatment for a relapse prior to complete clearance.

Treatment of facial lentigines in Peutz–Jeghers syndrome with intense pulsed light source. Remington BK, Remington TK. Dermatol Surg 2002; 28: 1079–81.

A case report of a series of 12 treatment sessions resulting in complete clearance; most resolved with a single course, and a few required a second.

This report offers a viable alternative to laser treatment.

Simple cryosurgical treatment of the oral melanotic macule. Yeh CJ. Clin Oral Maxillofac Surg 2000; 90: 12–13.

The author reports on the efficacy of treatment of labial melanotic macules with simple cryotherapy.

This report offers another (and less expensive) treatment option.

Chemopreventive efficacy of rapamycin on Peutz - Jeghers syndrome in a mouse model. Cancer Lett 2009; 277: 149–154.

Physical urticarias, aquagenic pruritus, and cholinergic pruritus

Clive EH Grattan, Frances Lawlor

PHYSICAL URTICARIAS

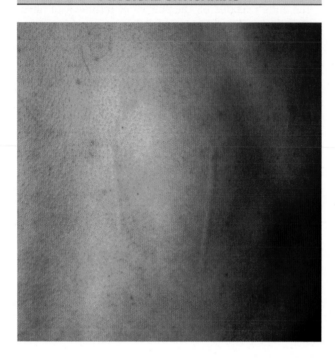

About 25% of patients with chronic urticaria have a definable and reproducible physical trigger that distinguishes them from those with ordinary urticaria and urticarial vasculitis, in which swellings are spontaneous. Physical urticarias are defined by the predominant stimulus that induces them (Table 1). More than one physical stimulus elicits urticaria in some patients, and physical urticarias can overlap with ordinary urticaria.

MANAGEMENT STRATEGY

Pharmacologic

The clinical presentation of the physical urticarias may vary considerably in severity, and so drug management should be guided more by the degree of disability and impairment in quality of life than by the specific diagnosis. For instance, cholinergic urticaria may result in occasional mild exercise-induced whealing, more extensive urticaria with angioedema, or, very rarely, anaphylaxis. The milder forms may require little more than explanation, *avoidance of situations likely to trigger an attack*, and an occasional dose of *antihistamine*, whereas a very severe attack involving anaphylaxis would require emergency treatment with *intramuscular epinephrine (adrenaline)*. Very acute presentations of physical urticaria may require short

courses of *oral corticosteroids* (e.g., prednisolone 30–40 mg daily for 5 days) in addition to regular treatment with non-sedating H_1 antihistamines, which are the cornerstone of management for all patterns. A range of other interventions can be tried if there is little or no response to antihistamines, although the evidence supporting their use is often poor.

Non-pharmacologic

The triggering physical stimulus should be avoided where possible. Aspirin and food additives have been implicated in exacerbations of some physical urticarias, but exclusion diets have little role in the management of most cases.

SPECIFIC INVESTIGATIONS

▶ Physical challenge tests
▶ Blood tests (cryoproteins, IgE)

With the exceptions of testing for cryoglobulins, in secondary cold urticaria and specific IgE in food- and exercise-induced anaphylaxis, routine laboratory investigations are unnecessary and should not be undertaken except to monitor treatment or screen for eligibility (e.g., glucose-6-phosphatase dehydrogenase in patients being considered for dapsone or sulfasalazine).

Urticaria. Dreskin SC. Immunol Allergy Clin North Am 2004; 24: 225–258.
    A good overview of the diagnosis, pathogenesis, and treatment of physical urticarias.

EAACI/GA²LEN/EDF guideline: definition, classification and diagnosis of urticaria. Zuberbier T, Bindslev-Jensen C, Canonica W, Grattan CEH, Greaves MW, Henz BM, et al. Allergy 2006; 61: 316–20.
    The section on physical urticaria testing is brief and not sufficiently detailed to be a practical guide.

Consensus meeting on the definition of physical urticarias and urticarial vasculitis. Kobza Black A, Lawlor F, Greaves MW. Clin Exp Dermatol 1996; 21: 424–6.
    Still the best available descriptive summary of physical challenge testing protocols as used in the UK. Short but proscriptive.

Cold urticaria syndromes: historical background, diagnostic classification, clinical and laboratory characteristics, pathogenesis and management. Wanderer AA. J Allergy Clin Immunol 1990; 85: 965–81.
    A well-referenced review of cold urticaria and its investigation.

Food-dependent exercise-induced anaphylaxis. Kidd JM, Cohen SH, Sosman AJ, Fink JN. J Allergy Clin Immunol 1983; 71: 407–11.
    Anaphylaxis may rarely result from exercise after a heavy food load or eating certain foods for which specific IgE can be demonstrated by skin prick or RAST testing.

Reactions to aspirin and food additives in patients with chronic urticaria, including the physical urticarias. Doeglas HMG. Br J Dermatol 1975; 93: 135–43.
    Aspirin sensitivity was demonstrated in 52% of cholinergic urticaria patients and 43% of those with delayed pressure urticaria. Exacerbations of these physical urticarias were also

Table 1 Classification of physical urticarias by the eliciting stimulus (in approximate reducing frequency of occurrence)

Symptomatic dermographism	Stroking or rubbing the skin
Cholinergic urticaria (pale, papular wheals with red flares)	Rise in core temperature and other causes of sweating (exercise, hot baths, spicy food, and stress)
Cold urticaria	Rewarming of skin after cooling (localized or systemic)
Delayed pressure urticaria	Sustained perpendicular pressure
Solar urticaria	Ultraviolet or visible solar radiation
Localized heat urticaria	Local heat contact
Adrenergic urticaria (red papular wheals with surrounding pallor)	Emotional stress
Aquagenic urticaria	Local water contact at any temperature
Exercise-induced anaphylaxis	Exercise, but not hot baths
Food and exercise-induced anaphylaxis	Exercise following a heavy food load or eating specific foods
Vibratory angioedema	Vibration

demonstrated after challenge with food additives (including tartrazine and sodium benzoate) in some patients with proven aspirin sensitivity.

FIRST-LINE THERAPIES

▶ Non-sedating ('second generation') antihistamines (Table 2)	A
▶ Classic sedating antihistamines and drugs with antihistaminic properties	A

Table 2 Examples of non- and mildly sedating antihistamines

Acrivastine	Non-sedating, three-times-daily dosing
Cetirizine	Mildly sedating, once-daily dosing
Levocetirizine	(the active enantiomer of cetirizine)
Fexofenadine	Non-sedating, once-daily dosing
Loratadine	Non-sedating, once-daily dosing
Desloratadine	(the active metabolite of loratadine)
Mizolastine	Non-sedating, once-daily dosing

Although they have not been compared against each other in a systematic way for the different patterns of physical urticaria, these drugs are probably all of similar efficacy. Cetirizine is notable for its inhibitory effects on eosinophil migration, which may be of additional benefit in delayed pressure urticaria. Mizolastine is contraindicated with drugs that inhibit cytochrome P450 oxidation, prolongation of the QT interval, and in heart failure.

Antihistamines should be used in full dose for all patterns of physical urticaria. There is a scarcity of published studies relating to second-generation H_1 antihistamines in physical urticarias. Classic sedating antihistamines may be more effective for some patients and can be given as monotherapy or in combination with second-generation antihistamines.

Therapeutic effects of cetirizine in delayed pressure urticaria: clinicopathological findings. Kontou-Fili K, Maniatakou G, Demaka P, Gonianakis M, Palaiologos G, Aroni K. J Am Acad Dermatol 1991; 24: 1090–3.

A double-blind, placebo-controlled study in 11 patients, showing a reduction in weight-induced wheal area and lesional eosinophil numbers on cetirizine 10 mg three times daily.

The use of cetirizine above the licensed dose appears to be beneficial for this indication.

A comparison of new nonsedating and classical antihistamines in the treatment of primary acquired cold urticaria. Villas-Martinez F, Contreras FJ, Lopez-Cazana JM, López Serrano MC, Martínez Alzamora F. J Invest Allergol Clin Immunol 1992; 2: 258–62.

Randomized, double-blind study showing that cetirizine, loratadine, cyproheptadine, and ketotifen were equally effective at suppression of symptoms and wheal reduction; however, more side effects were experienced with cyproheptadine.

Comparison of cinnarizine, cyproheptadine, doxepin and hydroxyzine in treatment of idiopathic cold urticaria: usefulness of doxepin. Neittaanmäki H, Myöhänen T, Fräki JE. J Am Acad Dermatol 1984; 11: 483–9.

A double-blind sequential study, with 2-week treatment periods in the first phase (n=10) and 1-week treatment periods in the second phase (n=12), in which all treatments inhibited the wheal response to local ice challenge, and doxepin offered the best subjective improvement.

The sedating and anticholinergic effects of sedating antihistamines are such that they have been largely superseded by second-generation non-sedating antihistamines for most purposes.

Effect of ketotifen treatment on cold-induced urticaria. St-Pierre JP, Kobric M, Rackham A. Ann Allergy 1985; 55: 840–3.

A placebo-controlled, double-blind, crossover study in 11 patients with primary cold urticaria, in which ketotifen increased the threshold duration for ice-induced whealing and was more effective than placebo on a four-point scale.

Classic sedating antihistamines, doxepin, and the mast-cell stabilizing antihistamine ketotifen have been extensively studied for cold urticaria in particular, but are probably no more effective than the more modern non-sedating equivalents.

SECOND-LINE THERAPIES

Symptomatic dermographism

▶ H_2 receptor antagonists	A
▶ Narrowband ultraviolet B phototherapy	C
▶ Photochemotherapy (PUVA)	C

The effect of H_1 and H_2 histamine antagonists on symptomatic dermographism. Matthews CNA, Boss JM, Warin RP, Storari F. Br J Dermatol 1979; 101: 57–61.

Ten patients were randomized to sequential 2-week periods of either cimetidine 400 mg four times daily plus chlorphenamine (chlorpheniramine) 4 mg four times daily, or active treatment alone. Chlorphenamine plus cimetidine produced a greater reduction in the wheal and flare response to a standard stroking stimulus than did chlorphenamine alone, and higher global improvement scores. Cimetidine alone appeared to worsen the subjective assessments.

In dermographic urticaria H$_2$ receptor antagonists have a small but therapeutically irrelevant additional effect compared with H$_1$ antagonists alone. Sharpe GR, Shuster S. Br J Dermatol 1993; 129: 575–9.

In this double-blind, crossover study, 19 patients were randomized to treatment with cetirizine 10 mg at night plus either ranitidine 150 mg twice daily or placebo. There was an increase in whealing threshold with additional H$_2$ blockade, but no subjective benefit.

Narrow-band ultraviolet B phototherapy is beneficial in antihistamine-resistant symptomatic dermographism: a pilot study. Borzova E, Rutherford A, Konstantinou G, Leslie K, Grattan CEH. J Am Acad Dermatol 2008; 59: 752–7.

Eight patients with antihistamine-unresponsive symptomatic dermographism showed subjective and objective improvement in itch and whealing after 6 weeks' treatment, but relapsed 6–12 weeks after stopping.

The effect of psoralen photochemotherapy (PUVA) on symptomatic dermographism. Logan RA, O'Brien TJO, Greaves MW. Clin Exp Dermatol 1989; 14: 25–8.

Five of 14 patients treated with oral PUVA experienced a useful reduction in itching after 4 weeks of treatment, but there was no difference in whealing threshold between covered and exposed skin when tested with a standardized stroking stimulus.

Cholinergic urticaria

▶ Danazol	A
▶ Anticholinergics	E

Beneficial effects of danazol on symptoms and laboratory changes in cholinergic urticaria. Wong E, Eftekhari N, Greaves MW, Milford Ward A. Br J Dermatol 1987; 116: 553–6.

Seventeen male patients were treated with danazol 200 mg three times daily in a double-blind crossover study, with sustained improvement in the number of exercise-induced wheals over 12 weeks. Levels of protease inhibitors increased over this period but declined to baseline within 1 month of stopping treatment. Anabolic steroids should only be considered for severe cholinergic urticaria not responding adequately to antihistamines, because of their potential for virilizing effects and hepatotoxicity.

Cholinergic pruritus, erythema and urticaria. A disease spectrum responding to danazol. Berth-Jones J, Graham-Brown RAC. Br J Dermatol 1989; 121: 123–7.

A male patient responded well to danazol 200 mg three times daily. The improvement in symptoms was accompanied by an increase in the serum level of the antiprotease α_1-antichymotrypsin.

This drug should be reserved for severe cases and avoided during pregnancy, as it is hepatotoxic and teratogenic.

Severe cholinergic urticaria successfully treated with scopolamine butylbromide in addition to antihistamines. Ujiie H, Shimizu T, Natsuga K, Arita K, Tomizawa K, Shimizu H. Clin Exp Dermatol 2006; 31: 978–81.

Although this case report suggests that anticholinergics may be successful for cholinergic urticaria, the general experience with this class of drugs is disappointing and unwanted effects nearly always outweigh any benefits.

Cold urticaria

▶ Cold tolerance (desensitization)	C
▶ Leukotriene receptor antagonists	E
▶ Antibiotics	E

Cold urticaria: a clinico-therapeutic study in 30 patients; with special emphasis on cold desensitization. Henquet JM, Martens BPM, van Volten WA. Eur J Dermatol 1992; 2: 75–7.

Cold desensitization in four patients with severely disabling cold urticaria resulted in symptom-free follow-up ranging from 4 to 14 years. Induction of cold tolerance took 1–2 weeks.

Patients had to take cold showers (around 15°C) for 5 minutes twice a day to maintain the tolerance, so this approach is not for the faint-hearted.

Cold urticaria: tolerance induction with cold baths. Von Mackensen YA, Sticherling M. Br J Dermatol 2007; 157: 799–846.

Nine of 23 patients desensitized with cold water immersions 15 years earlier responded to a questionnaire survey. Only one of them was able to continue the cold baths for 6 months, two for 3 months, and the others stopped almost immediately.

This report introduces a little realism concerning the likelihood of cold desensitization being an effective and well-tolerated long-term therapy for cold contact urticaria.

Improvement of cold urticaria by treatment with the leukotriene receptor antagonist montelukast. Hani N, Hartmann K, Casper C, Peters T, Schneider LA, Hunzelmann N, et al. Acta Dermatol Venereol 2000; 80: 229.

A case report of a patient with acquired cold contact urticaria responding subjectively and objectively to montelukast 10 mg daily after only 4 days.

It is not clear whether montelukast was given as monotherapy or in combination with an antihistamine.

Treatment of acquired cold urticaria with cetirizine and zafirlukast in combination. Bonadonna P, Lombardi C, Senna G, Canonica GW, Passalacqua G. J Am Acad Dermatol 2003; 49: 714–16.

Two patients with severe cold contact urticaria improved subjectively and objectively on a combination of cetirizine 10 mg once daily and zafirlukast 20 mg twice daily. Combination therapy was better than either drug alone.

Further studies are required to clarify what place (if any) leukotriene receptor antagonists have in the management of antihistamine-unresponsive cold urticaria.

Acquired cold urticaria: clinical picture and update on diagnosis and treatment. Siebenhaar F, Weller K, Mlynek A, Magerl M, Alrichter S, Vierira dos Santos R, et al. Clin Exp Dermatol 2007; 32: 241–5.

The authors write that occasional patients with acquired cold urticaria respond to high-dose antibiotics even if no underlying infection can be detected. Examples of antibiotic regimens used for this 'curative therapy' are given as phenoxymethylpenicillin 1 MU/day for 2–4 weeks, intramuscular benzylpenicillin 1 MU/day for 20 days, or doxycycline 200 mg/day for 3 weeks.

Delayed pressure urticaria

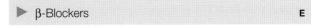

▶ Topical steroids	B
▶ Leukotriene receptor antagonists	B
▶ Sulfasalazine	E
▶ Dapsone	D

Oral corticosteroids are often used for the management of severe delayed pressure urticaria, as antihistamines are usually ineffective, but adverse effects from long-term administration are common and alternative therapies should be used whenever possible. A double-blinded study has now shown that a very potent topical steroid in a new foam formulation may be effective in the short term for patients with predominantly localized disease such as on the hands or feet.

Clobetasol propionate 0.05% in a novel foam formulation is safe and effective in the short-term treatment of patients with delayed pressure urticaria: a randomized double-blind, placebo-controlled trial. Vena G, Cassano N, D'Argento V, Milani M. Br J Dermatol 2006; 154: 353–6.

Efficacy of montelukast, in combination with loratadine, in the treatment of delayed pressure urticaria. Nettis E, Pannafino A, Cavallo E, Ferrannini A, Tursi A. J Allergy Clin Immunol 2003; 112: 212–13.

In a small randomized study objective pressure rechallenge after 15 days showed that montelukast 10 mg once daily with loratadine 10 mg once daily was more effective than either drug alone.

Desloratadine in combination with montelukast suppresses the dermographometer challenge test papule, and is effective in the treatment of delayed pressure urticaria: a randomized, double-blind, placebo-controlled study. Nettis E, Colanardi MC, Soccio AL, Ferrannini A, Vacca A. Br J Dermatol 2006; 155: 1279–82.

Although this study suggests that pressure urticaria can be controlled without steroids, clinical experience with montelukast in delayed pressure urticaria is often disappointing.

Chronic sulfasalazine therapy in the treatment of delayed pressure urticaria and angioedema. Engler RJM, Squire E, Benson P. Ann Allergy Asthma Immunol 1995; 74: 155–9.

Two patients with disabling pressure-induced wheals requiring oral corticosteroids cleared with 2–4 g daily of sulfasalazine and were able to maintain the improvement off corticosteroids.

Potential side effects include bone marrow depression and hypersensitivity reactions, so patients need careful monitoring. Sulfasalazine should only be considered in patients who are not sensitive to aspirin and other non-steroidals.

Delayed pressure urticaria. Successful treatment of 5 cases with dapsone. Gould DJ, Campbell D, Dayani A. Br J Dermatol 1991; 125: 25.

Five patients with confirmed delayed pressure urticaria cleared on dapsone 50 mg daily; four relapsed on stopping the drug.

This preliminary report has not been published as a full paper. Clinical experience with up to 150 mg dapsone/day suggests that it is useful for chronic delayed pressure urticaria when steroids might otherwise have to be used to control the disease.

Solar urticaria

▶ Induction of tolerance (phototherapy and photochemotherapy)	D

Prolonged benefit following ultraviolet A for solar urticaria. Dawe RS, Ferguson J. Br J Dermatol 1997; 137: 144–8.

Two patients with severe idiopathic solar urticaria benefited from springtime courses of ultraviolet A monotherapy.

Narrow-band UVB (TL-01) phototherapy: an effective preventative treatment for the photodermatosis. Collins P, Ferguson J. Br J Dermatol 1995; 132: 956–63.

One case of solar urticaria was treated with hardening NB-UVB in the springtime, with some benefit.

The management of idiopathic solar urticaria. Bilsland D, Ferguson J. J Dermatol Treat 1991; 1: 321–3.

The use of PUVA desensitization, with or without preceding UVA radiation, is reviewed briefly.

UVA rush hardening for the treatment of solar urticaria. Beissert S, Ständer H, Schwarz T. J Am Acad Dermatol 2000; 42: 1030–2.

Protection was achieved within 3 days of exposing three patients to multiple incremental UVA irradiations at 1-hour intervals. Rush hardening with UVA did not cause sunburn reactions, and provided protection against visible light and UVB-induced urticaria in two of the three patients.

UV-induced tolerance should be considered for patients who need more than antihistamines.

Adrenergic urticaria

▶ β-Blockers	E

Adrenergic urticaria: a new form of stress-induced hives. Shelley WA, Shelley ED. Lancet 1985; ii: 1031–2.

Two cases of a distinctive pattern of stress-induced urticaria associated with increased plasma epinephrine (adrenaline) and norepinephrine (noradrenaline) concentrations responding to propranolol. The clinical presentation and response to a β-blocker usually distinguishes adrenergic from cholinergic urticaria.

THIRD-LINE THERAPIES

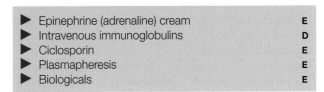

▶ Epinephrine (adrenaline) cream	E
▶ Intravenous immunoglobulins	D
▶ Ciclosporin	E
▶ Plasmapheresis	E
▶ Biologicals	E

Dyspareunia and vulvodynia: unrecognised manifestations of symptomatic dermographism. Lambiris A, Greaves MW. Lancet 1997; 349: 28.

Marked relief of pruritus and swelling was achieved by application of 2% epinephrine (adrenaline) cream to the vulval area as required, in conjunction with a systemic antihistamine.

Effect of high-dose intravenous immunoglobulin in delayed pressure urticaria. Dawn G, Urcelay M, Ah-Weng A, O'Neill SM, Douglas WS. Br J Dermatol 2003; 149: 836–40.

Three of eight patients went into remission after one or more infusions of intravenous immunoglobulin at 2 g/kg and two improved, but confirmation of pressure-induced wheals by objective testing was not done and all patients had associated ordinary chronic urticaria. It was not clear whether the benefit of treatment was mainly on the pressure urticaria component or the ordinary urticaria, which has been reported before.

Cold urticaria responding to systemic ciclosporin. Marsland AM, Beck MH. Br J Dermatol 2003; 149: 214.

One patient with acquired cold contact urticaria of over a year's duration and unresponsive to antihistamines improved within a week of starting ciclosporin at 3 mg/kg daily, and the improvement was maintained at 1.7 mg/kg daily. It was not stated what happened on stopping treatment.

There is currently no good evidence that acquired cold contact urticaria is an autoimmune disease, so the use of immunomodulating drugs should be regarded as speculative and of unproven benefit.

Cyclosporin A therapy for severe solar urticaria. Edström DW, Ros AM. Photodermatol Photoimmunol Photomed 1997; 13: 61–3.

A clinically useful reduction in sensitivity to visible or UV light occurred while taking ciclosporin at 4.5 mg/kg daily, but the symptoms recurred within 1–2 weeks of stopping treatment. The authors suggest that this treatment might be appropriate for severe disease when other treatments have failed, especially in countries where treatment is necessary only for a few months during summer.

Solar urticaria – effective treatment by plasmapheresis. Duschet P, Leyen P, Schwarz T, Höcker P, Greiter J, Gschnait F. Clin Exp Dermatol 1987; 12: 185–8.

A refractory period of at least 12 months followed a single treatment with 3L plasmapheresis.

Successful treatment of cold-induced urticaria/anaphylaxis with anti-IgE. Boyce JA. J Allergy Clin Immunol 2006; 117: 1414–18.

A single case report of complete resolution of cold urticaria after 2 months of treatment with omalizumab in a 12-year-old girl with concurrent asthma.

Successful treatment of delayed pressure urticaria with anti-TNF-α. Magerl M, Philipp S, Manasterski M, Friedrich M, Maurer M. J Allergy Clin Immunol 2007; 119: 752–4.

Single case report of a complete response of pressure urticaria symptoms within a week of starting etanercept for concurrent psoriasis.

Successful treatment of cholinergic urticaria with anti-immunoglobulin E therapy. Metz M, Bergmann P, Zuberbier T, Maurer M. Allergy 2008; 63: 247–9.

Single case report of complete resolution of cholinergic urticaria within 8 weeks of starting treatment with omalizumab.

These single case reports of apparent success with biologicals raise the possibility that they will be effective for patients with physical urticarias refractory to conventional therapies, but more evidence from controlled studies will almost certainly be necessary to persuade fund holders to pay for these expensive new drugs.

AQUAGENIC PRURITUS

Aquagenic pruritus is diagnosed when itching, prickling, burning, buzzing, or other skin discomfort, which may be intense, is provoked by contact with water. There are no visible skin changes. The sensation is associated with feelings of anger, irritability, or depression in approximately half of patients. The symptoms are provoked at any water temperature and degree of salinity. They occur within minutes rather than hours, and start either during a bath or shower or soon afterwards. The discomfort may be present for between 10 minutes and 2 hours. Any part of the body may be affected. Patients may also itch when the ambient temperature changes. Spontaneous remission is rare. The pathogenesis of the condition is not clear.

MANAGEMENT STRATEGY

Other chronic skin diseases must be ruled out by taking a full history and by clinical examination, particularly aquagenic pruritus of the elderly manifesting as xerosis, and other physical urticarias (i.e., cold urticaria, aquagenic urticaria, cholinergic urticaria, dermographism, and vibratory angioedema). Direct questioning is necessary regarding cold-induced symptoms and whealing, water-induced whealing or syncope, exercise-, heat-, or emotion-induced symptoms and whealing, and friction-induced itching and whealing. The well-recognized 'bath itch' that occurs in approximately 40% of patients with polycythemia rubra vera must be ruled out before aquagenic pruritus is diagnosed. Rarely, other hematological abnormalities have also been associated. Occasionally, antimalarial drugs have induced an aquagenic pruritus-like picture in patients with lupus erythematosus. When the diagnosis is reached, it is important to explain that aquagenic pruritus is a recognized skin condition, which, albeit very unpleasant and difficult to manage, has no immediate implications with regard to the patient's general health. It may help the sufferer to realize that he or she is not mentally unstable. Therapy is usually based on the use of *antihistamines, adding sodium bicarbonate to the water,* and *phototherapy.*

SPECIFIC INVESTIGATIONS

▶ Complete blood count (repeated yearly)
▶ Leukocyte alkaline phosphatase (repeated yearly)
▶ Water induction

FIRST-LINE THERAPIES

▶ Explanation	E
▶ Minimally sedating antihistamine	C
▶ Sodium bicarbonate added to bath water	D

Aquagenic pruritus. Greaves MW, Black AK, Eady RAJ, Coutts A. Lancet 1981; 282: 2008–11.

Aquagenic pruritus. Steinman HK, Greaves MW. J Am Acad Dermatol 1985; 13: 91–6.

Aquagenic pruritus: pharmacological findings and treatment. Greaves MW, Handfield-Jones SE. Eur J Dermatol 1992; 2: 482–4.

Antihistamines are used by these authors in the management of aquagenic pruritus. The treatment of this condition is difficult. There is no consensus regarding the first-line treatment, as the response of each patient is individual and no single treatment is effective in all cases; however, it would seem reasonable to start by advising a minimally sedating antihistamine 2 hours before the bath or shower on a regular basis. Patients may have a good response to antihistamines. Not all patients respond to antihistamine treatment, however, and of those who do, the response may consist of a diminution rather than an abolition of symptoms.

Baking soda baths for aquagenic pruritus. Bayoumi AHM, Highet AS. Lancet 1986; 11: 464.

[Idiopathic aquagenic pruritus treated with the addition of sodium bicarbonate to bath water]. Meunier L, Levy A, Costes Y, Meynadier J. Presse Med 1988; 19: 262. (In French.)

Aquagenic pruritus treatment with sodium bicarbonate and evidence for a seasonal form. Bircher AJ. J Am Acad Dermatol 1989; 21: 817.

Aquagenic pruritus may respond to the addition of sodium bicarbonate to the bath water. Advice about the amount of sodium bicarbonate to be added varies. In those who have responded, 200 g, 100 g, and 25 g have been added. The most practical approach might be to start with approximately 200 g per bath, and if there is a satisfactory response, to reduce gradually to a level that continues to suppress the itching. In a series of 25 patients, 25% improved with this treatment; however, in some cases the response may be temporary. Large quantities of sodium bicarbonate may be purchased economically at bakers' wholesalers.

SECOND-LINE THERAPIES

| ▶ | UVB | C |
| ▶ | Narrowband UVB | E |

Aquagenic pruritus. Steinman HK, Greaves MW. J Am Acad Dermatol 1985; 13: 91.

Ultraviolet phototherapy for pruritus. Rivard J, Lim HW. Dermatol Ther 2005; 18: 344–54.

Narrow band ultraviolet B in aquagenic pruritus. Xifra A, Carrascosa J. M, Ferrandiz C. Br J Dermatol 2005; 158: 1233.

Because of the necessity for hospital attendance UVB should be considered a second-line treatment for aquagenic pruritus. A response usually occurs between 2 and 4 weeks of treatment, but relapse normally occurs within months of stopping treatment, which may then be repeated.

A good response to narrowband UVB is described in two patients to whom it was administered three times per week. The improvement occurred at about 2 months of treatment and was maintained on weekly treatment in the ensuing months. In one of the patients desloratadine was added during the maintenance period. Narrowband UVB may prove to be an effective form of phototherapy.

THIRD-LINE THERAPIES

▶	Bath oil	E
▶	Emulsifying ointment in the bath water	E
▶	PUVA	E
▶	Propranolol	E
▶	Intramuscular triamcinolone	E
▶	Transdermal nitroglycerin	E
▶	Naltrexone 50 mg daily	E

The efficacy of psoralen photochemotherapy in the treatment of aquagenic pruritus. Menage HDuP, Norris PG, Hawk JLM, Greaves MW. Br J Dermatol 1993; 129: 163–5.

Photochemotherapy treatment of pruritus associated with polycythemia vera. Swerlick RA. J Am Acad Dermatol 1985; 13: 657–75.

Aquagenic pruritus responding to intermittent photochemotherapy. Holme SA, Anstey AV. Clin Exp Dermatol 2001; 26: 40–1.

Repeated PUVA treatment of aquagenic pruritus. Goodkin R, Bernhard JD. Clin Exp Dermatol 2002: 27: 164–5.

PUVA treatment has been effective in the bath itch of polycythaemia vera and has been used successfully both in a series of five patients and in individual patients, although either maintenance or repeated courses of therapy are necessary to maintain control of the condition. PUVA with oral psoralens may be regarded a third-line treatment for practical reasons.

Aquagenic pruritus responds to propranolol. Thomsen K. J Am Acad Dermatol 1990; 22: 697.

Aquagenic pruritus: effective treatment with intramuscular triamcinolone. Carson TE. Cutis 1991; 48: 382.

Sporadic patients are reported to respond to propranolol, intramuscular triamcinolone, and the addition of a bath oil or emulsifying ointment to the bath water.

Aquagenic pruritus response to the exogenous nitric oxide donor, transdermal nitroglycerin. Goihan Yahr M. Int J Dermatol 1994; 33: 752.

Transdermal nitroglycerin has been used effectively in one patient.

Efficacy and safety of naltrexone, an oral opiate receptor antagonist, in the treatment of pruritus and dermatological diseases. Metze D, Reinmann S, Beissert S, Luger T. J Am Acad Dermatol 1999; 41: 533–9.

Successful treatment of refractory aquagenic pruritus with naltrexone. Ingber S, Cohen PD. J Cutan Med Surg 2005; 9: 215–16.

Naltrexone, at a dose of 50 mg daily, controlled the condition in two patients with aquagenic pruritus to whom it was given.

CHOLINERGIC PRURITUS

Cholinergic pruritus occurs when patients itch, sting, or prickle following a rise in body temperature. The provoking stimuli are exercise (walking, running, dancing, going to the gym), including housework (ironing, vacuuming), heat (hot room, hot food, hot bath, sunny day), and emotion (excitement, stress, embarrassment) or fever. A combination of factors may cause a more pronounced itch, for example walking on a sunny day. The intensity, extent, and duration of the itching seem to be directly proportional to the strength of the eliciting stimulus. By definition, no whealing occurs on the skin during an attack. Although the prevalence of this condition is not known, it is the author's impression that many people itch when they become warm, although this itching is frequently insufficiently severe or incapacitating to present at a dermatology clinic. Cholinergic pruritus can be regarded as a variant of cholinergic urticaria. There is one case report that describes a patient presenting initially with cholinergic pruritus who progressed to cholinergic urticaria. Because there are no visible skin lesions, it is important to be aware of the condition and to differentiate it from aquagenic pruritus in those who describe itching after a bath or shower.

MANAGEMENT STRATEGY

Explaining the provoking factors and stressing that the condition is not an allergy, related to diet, or related to any underlying disease is helpful. If possible, *minimizing situations in which the itching occurs* can be helpful, and cooling the skin as quickly as possible may lessen the duration of the itching. It is not possible to tell the patient how long the condition will be present before remission takes place. Therapeutic agents typically utilized are *antihistamines,* although *danazol* has been reported to be beneficial.

SPECIFIC INVESTIGATIONS

▶ Exercise induction
▶ Warm bath induction (40–41°C)

▶ Explanation   E
▶ Minimally sedating antihistamine: cetirizine 10 mg, levocetirizine 5 mg, fexofenadine 180 mg, loratadine 10 mg, desloratadine 5 mg   E

An explanation is the most important part of treatment. The patient needs to understand the relationship between the itching and heat, and the importance of keeping cool. Treatment with minimally sedating antihistamines generally produces an improvement, although they are unlikely to suppress the condition completely. The standard dose of cetirizine, loratadine, their metabolites, or fexofenadine should be taken either regularly every morning or 2 hours before an expected stimulus, in order to assess any response. If the antihistamine proves helpful, the same dose could be repeated 9–12 hours later if necessary.

SECOND-LINE THERAPIES

▶ Danazol   C

Cholinergic pruritus, erythema, and urticaria: a disease spectrum responding to danazol. Berth-Jones J, Graham Brown RAC. Br J Dermatol 1989; 121: 235–7.

Danazol, which has been used in cholinergic urticaria, may rarely be effective in very severely affected individuals. The recommended dose is 200 mg three times daily. This dose could be continued for approximately 1 month and reduced to the minimum that controls the condition.

Pinta and yaws

Miguel Sanchez

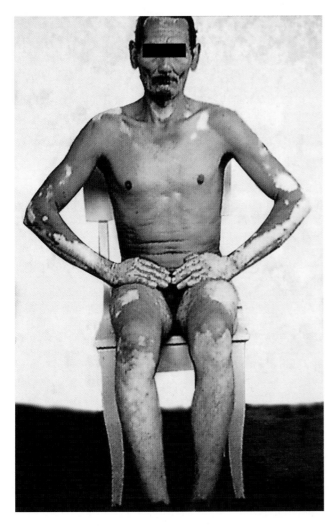

Pinta (*carate, azul, mal de pinto, empeines, lota, tina*) and yaws (*pian, frambesia, parangi, paru, buba*) are non-venereal 'endemic' spirochetal infections caused respectively by *Treponema carateum* and *Treponema pallidum* subspecies *pertenue*. Pinta was almost exclusively found in inhabitants of rural, overcrowded, poverty-stricken regions of Mexico, the Caribbean, and the northern part of South America, and has been reported most recently from scattered areas in the Brazilian rainforest. Whereas yaws was prevalent in indigent persons living in tropical, rural medically underserved areas with high humidity and rainfall within Central Africa, Southeast Asia, Central and northeast South America and some Pacific Pacific Islands, outbreaks have recently been reported from Papua New Guinea and Guyana. Most patients are children and young adults who acquire the infections by direct contact of abraded skin with another person's exudative infected lesions.

MANAGEMENT STRATEGY

Pinta and yaws are very rare, and familiarity with the types of lesion is essential to differentiate them from syphilis, psoriasis, leprosy, and leukodermas, in order to establish an appropriate treatment plan. As in syphilis, both infections have three distinct clinical stages. In pinta signs or symptoms are limited to the skin and lymph nodes, but yaws can also affect the skeletal system and mucous membranes. The *primary stage* of pinta develops after an incubation period of 15 days to months (usually 2–4 weeks). Following exposure, one to three erythematous papules erupt, usually on the face or extremities, and grow into erythematous scaly plaques that may become hypochromic or light blue in the center. Non-tender regional lymphadenopathy may appear. The *secondary stage* of pinta usually follows within 2–5 months (sometimes years later), with the appearance of erythematous papules (pintids) that enlarge to form psoriasiform plaques, which may remain for years. The plaques, which may be annular or circinate, progress through a range of colors from copper-brown to slate blue or black. Some may be hypochromic. Lymphadenopathy may be present. The *tertiary stage* is characterized by depigmented patches on the wrists, ankles, elbows, and within old lesions. These develop between 3 months and 10 years after the onset of the secondary stage. At this point patients have a combination of hyperpigmented, hypochromic, achromic, dyschromic, and polychromic patches of different sizes, imparting a mottled appearance to the skin. In 80% of cases serologic tests become reactive 2–3 months after the onset of the primary lesion, and are always reactive in late lesions.

In yaws the *primary stage* develops after an incubation period of 10 days to 3 months, with the appearance, usually on a lower extremity, of an erythematous, occasionally pruritic papulonodule ('the mother yaw') that enlarges up to 5 cm in circumference and ulcerates with exuberant granulation tissue imparting a framboesiform appearance. The *secondary stage* usually ensues over 10–16 weeks, but may be as long as 2 years after the onset of the primary stage, with an eruption of reddish, weeping, crust-covered papules ('daughter yaws') similar to, but smaller than, the primary lesion. In some patients the clinical finding are similar to those of secondary syphilis, with scaly papules and plaques, hypertrophic condyloma lata resembling lesions on body folds, or mucous patches such as lesions on mucous membranes. Nodules around the joints are common. Some patients suffer with painful osteoperiostitis of the forearm or leg and polydactylitis of the hand or foot. In approximately 10% of infected patients the disease progresses to the *tertiary stage* with infiltrated plaques and nodules that ulcerate, leaving deep ulcers with raised granulomatous edges. Skeletal changes include chronic hypertrophic osteoperiostitis which most commonly affects the tibiae (saber shins) or the superior nasal processes of the maxillae. This latter process triggers disfiguring progressive exostosis of new bone (goundou) which, in 5–20 years, results in massive destruction and perforation of the nose and the palate (rhinopharyngitis mutilans or gangosa)

The recommended treatment of pinta and yaws is a single intramuscular injection of 1.2 million units of *benzathine penicillin G* in adults, adolescents, and older children, and 0.6 million units in children under 10 years of age. Patients cease to be infectious within 24 hours. In pinta primary and secondary lesions heal in 4–12 months, but achromic lesions persist indefinitely. Penicillin-allergic patients over 8 years of age are treated with a 15-day course of *tetracycline* 250 mg four times daily or *doxycycline* 50 mg twice daily. *Erythromycin* should be reserved for penicillin-allergic children under 8 years of age (8 mg/kg four times daily) and for pregnant women (500 mg four times daily).

SPECIFIC INVESTIGATIONS

▶ Serologic tests (cardiolipin flocculation assays, treponemal-specific assays)
▶ Dark-field microscopy
▶ Direct fluorescent antibody test
▶ Histopathology

A description of the yaws infection and prevention conditions in the health district of Adzope. Konan YE, M'Bea KJ, Coulibaly A, Tetchi EO, Kpebo DO, Ake O, et al. Santé Publique 2007; 19: 111–18.

The presence of treponemes on the serous exudate of lesions examined under dark-field microscopy with negative direct fluorescent antibody test (DFA) which specifically detects *T. pallidum* suggests non-venereal treponematoid infection. No serological test is yet able to distinguish infection with any of the endemic treponematoses from each other or from venereal syphilis.

The endemic treponematoses. Antal GM, Lukehart SA, Meheus AZ. Microbes Infect 2002; 4: 83–94.

Available serologic tests cannot distinguish yaws or pinta from syphilis. Penicillin treatment often does not lead to seroreversal. Some cases of yaws and pinta may be misdiagnosed as syphilis.

Histopathological aspects of tertiary pinta. Pecher SA, Azevedo EB. Med Cutan Ibero-Latino-Americana 1987; 15: 239–42.

Treponemes are found on silver impregnation between epidermal cells in primary, secondary, and late-stage hyperpigmented lesions, but not in late hypopigmented patches.

The sequence of the acidic repeat protein (arp) gene differentiates venereal from nonvenereal *Treponema pallidum* subspecies, and the gene has evolved under strong positive selection in the subspecies that causes syphilis. Harper KN, Liu H, Ocampo PS, Steiner BM, Martin A, Levert K, et al. FEMS Immunol Med Microbiol 2008; 53: 322–32.

Only minor genetic differences have been found between the subspecies that cause venereal syphilis and yaws, after completion of the *T. pallidum* genome project. A sequence variation in the *arp* gene allows differentiation of ssp. *pallidum* from the non-venereal subspecies.

FIRST-LINE THERAPIES

▶ Penicillin   B

Treponemal infections. WHO Scientific Group. Technical Report Series No. 674. Geneva: World Health Organization, 1982.

Intramuscular benzathine penicillin is the recommended treatment for all patients with pinta or yaws. All household cases and contacts should also be treated in areas where 5% of the population is infected. In areas with 5–10% rates of infection, treatment should be administered to all children under 15 years of age; in areas with higher infection rates the entire population should be treated with penicillin.

Treatment of pinta with antibiotics. Ketchen DK. Ann NY Acad Sci 1952; 55: 1176–85.

This study on Mexican patients with pinta found that, after treatment with penicillin, skin lesions healed completely in all patients with primary lesions, in 69% with secondary lesions, and in 40% with tertiary lesions.

Nonvenereal treponematoses in tropical countries. Engelkens HJ, Vuzevski VD, Stolz E. Clin Dermatol 1999; 17: 143–52.

This review stresses that penicillin at previously recommended doses remains the treatment of choice.

Failure of penicillin treatment of yaws on Karkar Island, Papua New Guinea. Backhouse JL, Hudson BJ, Hamilton PA, Nesteroff SI. Am J Trop Med Hyg 1998; 59: 388–92.

Of 39 children, 28% developed clinical and/or serologic evidence of relapse after treatment with the recommended dose of intramuscular benzathine penicillin. All but three responded to further penicillin treatment. Resistance of yaws to penicillin has also been reported from Ecuador.

Efficacy of a targeted, oral penicillin-based yaws control program among children living in rural South America. Scolnik D, Aronson L, Lovinsky R, Toledano K, Glazier R, Eisenstadt J, et al. Clin Infect Dis 2003; 36: 1232–8.

Clinical cure of yaws lesions was achieved in 94% of 17 children with administration of oral penicillin, 50 mg/kg daily in four divided doses for 7–10 days.

Benzathine penicillin G treatment may not be possible in remote areas as the drug requires refrigeration at a temperature of 2–8°C until 7 days before use, at which time it should be stored at <30°C.

Mass treatment programs designed to eradicate endemic treponematoses expose uninfected people to adverse effects and may promote antibiotic resistance. Treatment programs that exclusively target clinically active cases can significantly reduce the prevalence of disease.

Overview of endemic treponematoses. Morand JJ, Simon F, Garnotel E, Mahe A, Clity E, Morlain B. Med Trop 2006; 66: 15–20.

The infection is highly sensitive to penicillin and resistance has not been reported. Endemic control through treatment of the entire treponemal reservoir with single-dose penicillin is highly successful.

SECOND-LINE THERAPIES

▶ Tetracycline   E
▶ Doxycycline   E
▶ Minocycline   E
▶ Erythromycin   E

Therapy for nonvenereal treponematosis. Review of the efficacy of penicillin and consideration of alternatives. Brown ST. Rev Infect Dis 1985; 7: 318–26.

This article reviews studies of treatment for pinta and yaws. Penicillin is the drug of choice. Tetracycline is also concluded to be effective, but studies were done on patients with yaws. Reports of treatment with erythromycin were few. Doxycycline and minocycline appear to be useful alternatives.

Nonvenereal treponematoses: yaws, endemic syphilis, and pinta. Koff AB, Rosen T. J Am Acad Dermatol 1993; 29: 519–35.

Tetracycline or doxycycline is the treatment of choice in older children and adults who are allergic to penicillin.

Endemic treponematosis: review and update. Farnsworth N, Rosen T. Clin Dermatol 2006; 24: 181–90.

Penicillin remains the drug of choice, but the tetracycline class of antibiotics and erythromycin also appear to be effective.

Yaws eradication: past efforts and future perspectives. Asiedu K, Amouzou B, Dhariwal A, Karam M, Lobo D, Patnaik S, et al. Bull WHO 2008; 86: 499A.

Despite once successful attempts to eradicate yaws through campaigns that involved active case finding, treatment of cases and contacts, and community mobilization, yaws is re-emerging in poor, rural, and marginalized populations of Africa, Asia, and South America.

Pitted keratolysis
(keratolysis plantare sulcatum)

Eunice Tan, John Berth-Jones

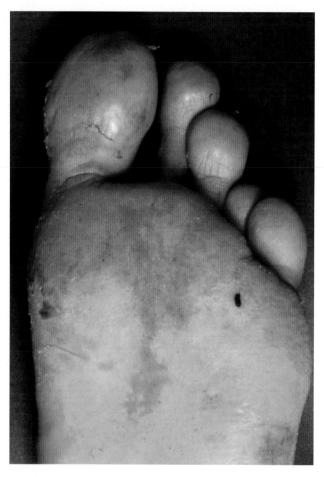

Pitted keratolysis (PK) is a superficial infection of the stratum corneum characterized by shallow punched-out circular erosions primarily on the weightbearing areas of the soles of the feet, and less commonly on the non-weightbearing areas of the feet and the palms of the hands. Hyperhidrosis, maceration, and a foul odor are common. Several species of *Corynebacterium*, *Dermatophilus*, *Actinomyces* and *Kytococcus* (formerly named *Micrococcus*) possessing enzymatic keratolytic activity have been isolated.

MANAGEMENT STRATEGY

Most patients experience little or mild irritation. Maceration, foul odor, and soreness are the main reasons for consultation. Sweat retention and immersion appear to be an important cause of PK. Industrial workers wearing rubber shoes or soldiers whose feet were continually wet have a higher prevalence of PK. Initial management strategies should include instructions on *foot hygiene* and *avoidance of occlusive footwear and friction*.

Treatment of the hyperhidrosis slowly brings the condition under control, but the usual first-line treatment includes topical *fusidic acid* with *topical aluminum chloride hexahydrate* or *formaldehyde solution soaks*.

Antibiotic resistance has been reported with *Micrococcus sedentarius* to penicillin, methicillin, ampicillin, oxacillin, and erythromycin. The topical antibiotic most commonly used by the authors is *fusidic acid*, which can be prescribed as 2% fusidic acid cream or ointment three to four times daily. Topical *1% clindamycin, 2% erythromycin, mupirocin ointment* and *tetracycline and gentamicin sulfate* cream have been reported to be effective. Although 1% clindamycin hydrochloride can be made up with 660 mg dissolved in 55 mL of 70% isopropyl alcohol and 5% propylene glycol, we suggest Dalacin T topical solution may be used instead. This can be applied twice to three times daily. Erythromycin 2% cream or ointment has been reported to be effective if used twice daily. We suggest 2% erythromycin gel, available as Eryacne, or 2% erythromycin solution, available as Stiemycin, may be used. Japanese dermatologists have had some success in treating PK with gentamicin sulfate cream, but this is unavailable in Great Britain. Mupirocin 2% ointment may be administered two to three times daily; 3% tetracycline hydrochloride ointment may be applied one to three times daily.

PK has also responded to topical antifungals such as *clotrimazole and miconazole*; 1% clotrimazole cream may be applied twice daily; 2% miconazole cream or ointment may be applied twice daily.

Systemic antibiotics are reserved for severe and resistant cases. A 7-day course of oral erythromycin at 250 mg four times daily has led to resolution of PK. The use of penicillin and sulfonamides does not seem to be effective.

Topical 20% *aluminum chloride hexadydrate* in absolute anhydrous ethyl alcohol, available as Driclor, may reduce hyperhidrosis and odor, but the pits remain. The solution is applied at night, allowed to dry, and washed off the following day. Initially it should be used daily until the condition is brought under control, when it can be used less frequently. The use of 20% aluminum chloride hexahydrate for palmoplantar hyperhidrosis has not been as successful as its use for axillary hyperhidrosis.

Topical antiseptics can be effective. Topical 4% *formaldehyde solution* applied with gauze soaks as the patient sits or stands with their feet on the gauze in a bowl for 10–15 minutes once or twice daily appears to improve the hyperhidrosis. Iontophoresis has been used in palmar and plantar hyperhidrosis and can be used in the treatment of PK where formaldehyde fails. Sympathectomy or oral anticholinergics are impractical and excessive.

Topical 2% *buffered glutaraldehyde* has been reported to have good therapeutic results but may cause sensitization. Glutaraldehyde is available in Great Britain as Cidex, used for instrument sterilization, and is hazardous to handle. Formalin ointment 40% has also had a degree of success in the treatment of PK, but is unavailable in Great Britain.

Various other agents have been tried topically but with limited success. These include 0.1% *triamcinolone acetonide* once or twice daily, *iodochlorhydroxyquin-hydrocortisone cream* (vioform-hydrocortisone) once or twice daily, *flexible collodion* as required, and *Whitfield's ointment* (6% benzoic and 3% salicylic acid ointment in a petroleum base) twice daily. Water-repellant silicone ointment has not been found to significantly reduce PK.

Evidence Levels: **A** Double-blind study   **B** Clinical trial ≥ 20 subjects   **C** Clinical trial < 20 subjects   **D** Series ≥ 5 subjects   **E** Anecdotal case reports

SPECIFIC INVESTIGATIONS

No routine investigation is required. Wood's light examination may reveal a coral red fluorescence, but this is not consistently helpful.

FIRST-LINE THERAPIES

▶ Topical fusidic acid	E
▶ Topical aluminum chloride hexahydrate	E
▶ Topical formaldehyde	E

Coexistent erythrasma, trichomycosis axillaris, and pitted keratolysis: An overlooked corynebacterial triad? Shelley WB, Shelley ED. J Am Acad Dermatol 1982; 7: 752–7.

A case report of two patients with this triad, one of whom was treated with oral erythromycin 250 mg four times daily and a solution of 20% aluminium chloride applied nightly to the soles. Three weeks later the plantar hyperhidrosis and odor were significantly reduced, but the pits remained. The other patient declined treatment for PK.

Pitted and ringed keratolysis. A review and update. Zaias N. J Am Acad Dermatol 1982; 7: 787–91.

The author has personal observations (non-controlled) that treatment of PK with topical clotrimazole, miconazole, erythromycin, tetracycline, clindamicin, glutaraldehyde, formaldehyde and oral erythromycin are curative. Penicillin has not been useful.

Road rash with a rotten odor. Schissel DJ, Aydelotte J, Keller R. Military Med 1999; 164: 65–7.

Case report of a soldier treated with topical clotrimazole cream twice a day, topical clindamycin solution twice a day, and topical ammonium chloride each evening. At his 2-week follow-up appointment, he reported resolution of the odor, tenderness, and interdigital pruritus, and at 8 weeks he had complete resolution.

SECOND-LINE THERAPIES

▶ Topical mupirocin	D
▶ Topical tetracyclines	E
▶ Topical clindamycin	E
▶ Topical erythromycin	E
▶ Topical clotrimazole	E
▶ Topical miconazole	E
▶ Oral erythromycin	E

Mupirocin ointment for symptomatic pitted keratolysis [Letter]. Vazquez-Lopez F, Perez-Oliva N. Infection 1996; 24: 55.

Four patients with symptomatic PK failing to respond to conventional treatments were treated with topical mupirocin ointment, with rapid clearance of PK.

Pitted and ringed keratolysis. A review and update. Zaias N. J Am Acad Dermatol 1982; 7: 787–91.

Topical clotrimazole, miconazole, clindamicin, erythromycin, tetracycline, and oral erythromycin are curative, as reported above.

Pitted keratolysis: A new form of treatment [Letter]. Burkhart CG. Arch Dermatol 1980; 116: 1104.

Three patients with PK were treated with topical 1% clindamycin hydrochloride solution (660 mg dissolved in 55 mL of 70% isopropyl alcohol and 5% propylene glycol). The solution was applied to the plantar surface three times daily, and within 4 weeks there was complete resolution of the clinical lesions.

Road rash with a rotten odor. Schissel DJ, Aydelotte J, Keller R. Miliatry Med 1999; 164: 65–7.

Topical clindamycin and clotrimazole, as reported above.

Pitted keratolysis: a clinicopathologic review. Stanton RL, Schwartz RA, Aly R. J Am Podiatry Assoc 1982; 72: 436–9.

Topical 2% erythromycin applied twice daily resulted in resolution of PK in both feet within 4 weeks of treatment in one case.

Painful, plaque-like, pitted keratolysis occurring in childhood. Shah AS, Kamino H, Prose NS. Pediatr Dermatol 1992: 9: 251–4.

Two children were reported with these lesions; treatment with topical 2% erythromycin solution twice a day was curative in both patients within 3 weeks of commencing treatment.

Ultrastructure of pitted keratolysis. De Almeida Jr HL, De Castro LAS, Rocha NEM, Abrantes VL. Int J Dermatol 2000; 39: 698–709.

A case report of a patient who responded to topical erythromycin with good results.

Pitted keratolysis of the palm arising after herpes zoster [Letter]. Lee H-J, Roh K-Y, Ha S-J, Kim J-W. Br J Dermatol 1999; 140: 974–5.

A case report of PK in the palm of a patient who was suffering from postherpetic neuralgia in the same area. She had been prescribed oral erythromycin 250 mg twice daily and mupirocin ointment. Four days later the lesions had resolved.

Coexistent erythrasma, trichomycosis axillaries, and pitted keratolysis: An overlooked corynebacterial triad? Shelley WB, Shelley ED. J Am Acad Dermatol 1982; 7: 752–7.

Oral erythromycin, as reported above.

Pitted kerayolysis. The role of *Micrococcus sedentarius*. Nordstrom KM, McGinley KJ, Cappiello L, Zechman JM, Leyden JJ. Arch Dermatol 1987; 123: 1320–5.

Micrococcus sedentarius isolated from PK lesions on the feet of eight patients was tested for antibiotic sensitivities and found to be resistant to penicillin, ampicillin, methicillin, and oxacillin. PK lesions were reproduced in one volunteer inoculated with *M. sedentarius* after 6 weeks of occlusion.

Isolation and characterization of micrococci from human skin, including two new species: *Micrococcus lylae* and *Micrococcus kristinae*. Kloos WE, Torrabene TG, Schleifer KH. Int J Syst Bacteriol 1974; 24: 79–101.

M. sedentarius was observed to be resistant to penicillin, methicillin, and erythromycin, which is characteristic of the genus *Micrococcus*.

THIRD-LINE THERAPIES

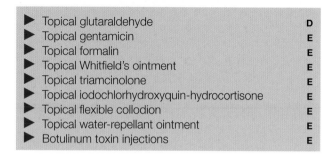

▶	Topical glutaraldehyde	D
▶	Topical gentamicin	E
▶	Topical formalin	E
▶	Topical Whitfield's ointment	E
▶	Topical triamcinolone	E
▶	Topical iodochlorhydroxyquin-hydrocortisone	E
▶	Topical flexible collodion	E
▶	Topical water-repellant ointment	E
▶	Botulinum toxin injections	E

Pitted keratolysis: forme fruste old treatments [Letter]. Gordon HH. Arch Dermatol 1981; 117: 608.

Buffered glutaraldehyde 2% used with beneficial therapeutic results on PK and hyperhidrosis (uncontrolled personal observations). The author also advises that proper instructions on foot hygiene be given and sandals worn as much as possible. He also reports sensitization to glutaraldehyde, and advises that when this occurs or when glutaraldehyde treatment has failed, then it would be advisable to use antibiotics.

Pitted keratolysis: forme fruste: A review and new therapies. Gordon HH. Cutis 1975; 15: 54–8.

Buffered glutaraldehyde 2% applied twice daily in five patients resulted in relief of signs and symptoms except in one patient addicted to wearing boots, who continued to have hyperhidrosis. Treatment with gentamicin cream resulted in improvement.

Hyperhidrosis: treatment with glutaraldehyde. Gordon HH. Cutis 1972; 9: 375–8.

Eight patients with a mixture of palmar and plantar hyperhidrosis were treated with varying strengths of 2%, 2.5%, 5%, and 10% aqueous glutaraldehyde with good results. Glutaraldehyde 10%, not alkalinized, was found to be rapidly effective but was associated with brown staining. Use of a 5% starting strength three times weekly minimized the tanning, and these patients were then placed on 2% or 2.5% strengths as required for maintenance treatment.

Contact dermatitis has been reported with the use of glutaraldehyde, but none of these patients developed this problem.

Keratolysis plantare sulcatum. Higashi N. Jpn J Clin Dermatol 1972; 26: 321–5.

Two patients with KP were treated with topical gentamicin sulfate cream and reported to have good results.

Symptomatic pitted keratolysis. Lamberg SI. Arch Dermatol 1969; 100: 10–11.

Reports of 12 military personnel with symptomatic PK treated with various topical agents. One foot was used for treatment while the other was utilized as a control without treatment or compared with another topical agent. These included steroid creams, antibiotic creams, iodochlorhydroxyquin-hydrocortisone (vioform hydrocortisone) cream, flexible collodion, Whitfield's ointment, and formalin in aquaphor (20–40%).

Formalin (40%) ointment appeared to be the most effective and was used for the remainder of both asymptomatic and symptomatic patients with PK. All cases returned to full duty with the ointment after a single outpatient visit, and on re-examination the PK had resolved.

Pitted keratolysis. Gill KA Jr, Buckels LJ. Arch Dermatol 1968; 98: 7–11.

Water-repellant silicone ointment has no effect on PK. Lesions resolved spontaneously without treatment following removal from the moist environment.

Plantar hyperhidrosis and pitted keratolysis treated with botulinum toxin injection. Tamura BM, Cucé LC, Souza RL, Levites J. Dermatol Surg 2004; 30: 1510–14.

Two patients resistant to topical and systemic treatments responded completely to one course of low-dose botulinum toxin injections to the plantar aspects of the feet.

Pityriasis lichenoides chronica

Alex Milligan, Graham Johnston

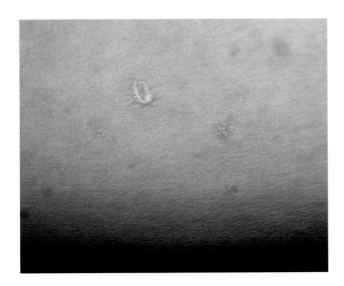

Pityriasis lichenoides chronica (PLC) typically consists of small erythematous papules, which may be purpuric. These develop a characteristic shiny mica scale attached to the center. They occur predominantly over the trunk and proximal limbs. As the name implies, PLC may persist for many years, though spontaneous resolution does occur. Patients should be warned that relapse is common and that recurrent courses of therapy may be required.

Anecdotally, PLC is said to run a more benign, self-limiting course in children, but more recently it has been shown that in children it is more likely to run an unremitting course, with greater lesional distribution, more dyspigmentation, and a poorer response to treatment. Some authors argue that there is an overlap with cutaneous lymphoma.

Pityriasis lichenoides chronica: stratification by molecular and phenotypic profile. Crowson AN, Morrison C, Li J. Hum Pathol 2007; 38: 479–90.

A prospective study of 46 patients concluded that PLC is an indolent cutaneous T-cell dyscrasia with a limited propensity for progression to mycosis fungoides.

MANAGEMENT STRATEGY

There are no controlled therapeutic trials for this condition, and case series are only small. In many therapeutic trials PLC has been grouped together with pityriasis lichenoides et varioliformis acuta (see page 568) and management strategies are therefore often similar or interchangeable.

Topical corticosteroids are only reported as effective anecdotally in textbooks rather than in studies. They are often used with *antihistamines* to reduce pruritus, but they are not reported to affect the course of the disease.

The majority of reports describe benefits with *UV therapy*, and therefore either UV alone or with *psoralen plus UVA (PUVA)*

therapy is recommended for all patients. The response appears to be unpredictable, however, and the total dose required is extremely variable.

Antibiotics do not appear to be especially helpful, though combination therapy (e.g., *tetracycline* and *topical corticosteroid*) has been suggested.

For severe or refractory cases *methotrexate, ciclosporin,* and *acitretin* have all been described as effective in small numbers of patients.

For most treatment modalities, patients who have been described as improved have usually had fewer new lesions developing, a shortened disease course, and a greater time to relapse than untreated patients.

SPECIFIC INVESTIGATIONS

▶ Consider skin biopsy

Although a skin biopsy is usually unnecessary in clinically obvious cases, it may be useful before commencing aggressive systemic therapy.

An infective etiology is often suggested, but no pathogen has yet been implicated, though an association with toxoplasmosis has been described. These reports tend to come from endemic areas, and so investigation for a triggering infection is unnecessary in cases without evidence of specific infection.

The relationship between toxoplasmosis and pityriasis lichenoides chronica. Nassef NE, Hamman MA. J Egypt Soc Parasitol 1997; 27: 93–9.

Twenty-two patients with PLC and 20 healthy controls were examined clinically and serologically for toxoplasmosis. Three (15%) of the controls had toxoplasmosis, compared to eight (36%) of the patients with PLC. Five of the latter had subsidence of skin lesions after pyrimethamine and sulfapyrimidine treatment.

Pityriasis lichenoides and acquired toxoplasmosis. Rongioletti F, Delmonte S, Rebora A. Int J Dermatol 1999; 38: 367–76.

A patient with biopsy-proven PLEVA and acute *Toxoplasma* serology is reported. His skin failed to respond to azithromycin but cleared with spiramycin followed by trimethoprim-sulfamethoxazole.

FIRST-LINE THERAPIES

▶ UVB	D
▶ Combined UVA and UVB	D
▶ PUVA	D

Comparative studies of treatments for pityriasis lichenoides. Gritiyarangsan P, Pruenglampoo S, Ruangratanarote P. J Dermatol 1987; 14: 258–61.

In this open study 30 patients with pityriasis lichenoides were recruited, although the authors did not specify how many had PLEVA and how many PLC. The first group of eight were given topical corticosteroid and half had a partial or complete response. The second group were also given oral tetracycline and the majority had a partial response. The third group of eight chronic refractory cases were given oral methoxsalen 0.6 mg/kg with UVA three times per week for an average of 2 months; five were cleared and two had a partial response.

UVB therapy of pityriasis lichenoides. Pavlotsky F, Baum S, Barzilai A, Shapiro D, Trau H. J Eur Acad Dermatol Venereol 2006; 20: 542–7.

This retrospective study of 29 patients again failed to separate PLC and PLEVA but reported a complete response in 93% of patients treated with UVB; 73% remained disease-free after 3 years.

Narrowband UVB (311 nm, TL01) phototherapy for pityriasis lichenoides. Aydogen K, Saricaoglu H, Turan H. Photodermatol Photoimmunol Photomed 2008; 24: 128–33.

TL01 phototherapy led to clearance in seven out of eight PLC patients (87.5%) with a mean cumulative dose of 18.4 J/cm² after a mean of 45.8 exposures. Relapses occurred in four patients within a mean period of 6 months.

UV-B Phototherapy for pityriasis lichenoides. Tham SN. Australas J Dermatol 1985; 26: 9–13.

Seventeen patients with PLC were treated with UVB three to five times per week with a starting dose of 80–90% of the minimal erythema dose. They received an average of 33 treatments: nine completely cleared and five had 90% clearance. Only half had relapsed at 3-year follow-up.

Phototherapy of pityriasis lichenoides. LeVine MJ. Arch Dermatol 1983; 119: 378–80.

PLC in 12 patients cleared completely after an average of 30 treatments of minimally erythemogenic doses of UVA/UVB from fluorescent sunlamps. The average UV dose required was 388 mJ/cm².

PUVA therapy of pityriasis lichenoides chronica. Han HK, Kim JK, Kook HL. Korean J Dermatol 1982; 20: 413–17.

Nine patients with PLC of relatively short duration were treated with oral methoxsalen and UVA and were cleared completely after between eight and 45 treatments.

Experience with UVB phototherapy in children. Tay Y-K, Morelli JG, Weston WL. Pediatr Dermatol 1996; 13: 406–9.

In an open study of UVB in various dermatoses in younger patients, two children with PLC were given broadband UVB three times a week for an average of 26 treatments (mean total dose 4.2 J/cm²). Both had 90% improvement in lesions and no subsequent relapse.

SECOND-LINE THERAPIES

▶ Tetracycline	D
▶ Erythromycin	E

Pityriasis lichenoides: the differences between children and adults. Wahie S, Hiscutt E, Natarajan S, Taylor A. Br J Dermatol 2007; 157: 941–5.

In this retrospective study only two of eight children cleared with erythromycin, whereas three out of four adults cleared without relapse. Phototherapy was more effective in both groups.

Pityriasis lichenoides in childhood: a retrospective review of 124 patients. Ersoy-Evans S, Greco MF, Mancini AJ, Subasi N, Paller AS. J Am Acad Dermatol 2007; 56: 205–10.

This was a retrospective study of 124 children, of whom 46 had PLC. The median age of onset was 60 months and median duration was 20 months (range 3–132 months). Two-thirds of children had at least a partial response to erythromycin.

Tetracycline for the treatment of pityriasis lichenoides. Piamphongsant T. Br J Dermatol 1974; 91: 319.

Twelve patients in Bangkok were given tetracycline 2 mg daily. All responded within 4 weeks. Seven required maintenance therapy of 1 mg daily for 6 months.

Pityriasis lichenoides in children: therapeutic response to erythromycin. Truhan AP, Hebert AA, Esterly NB. J Am Acad Dermatol 1986; 15: 66–70.

Four children aged 4–14 years with biopsy-proven PLC were given oral erythromycin 200–400 mg four times daily. Two improved within a month, and on stopping the drug after 5 and 12 months there was no recurrence. One patient improved on an increased dose and one failed to respond after 6 months of therapy.

THIRD-LINE THERAPIES

▶ Methotrexate	E
▶ Acitretin	E
▶ Acitretin plus PUVA	E
▶ Ciclosporin	E
▶ UVA1	E
▶ Topical tacrolimus	E
▶ Bromelain	E
▶ Photodynamic therapy	E

Methotrexate treatment of pityriasis lichenoides and lymphomatoid papulosis. Lynch PJ, Saied NK. Cutis 1979; 23: 635–6.

Three patients received methotrexate 25 mg/week intramuscularly or orally. All responded within weeks, but two relapsed on cessation of therapy.

Successful treatment of pityriasis lichenoides chronica with acitretin. Hay IC, Omerod AD. J Dermatol Treat 1988; 9: 53–4.

A further report of a patient with PLC who, having failed to respond to prednisolone, oxytetracycline, dapsone, methotrexate, azathioprine, UVB, and PUVA, responded to 50 mg acitretin daily.

Photochemotherapy for pityriasis lichenoides: 3 cases. Panse I, Bourrat E, Rybojad M, Morel P. Ann Dermatol Venereol 2004; 131: 201–3.

One patient with pityriasis lichenoides and two patients with PLEVA unresponsive to other therapies, including topical corticosteroids, antibiotics, and UVB, responded within weeks to acitretin plus PUVA.

Cyclosporine in dermatology. Gupta AK, Brown MD, Ellis CN, Rocher LL, Fisher GJ, Baadsgaard O, et al. J Am Acad Dermatol 1989; 21: 1245–56.

In a review of ciclosporin in a wide variety of dermatoses the authors report successful clearance within 8 weeks in a man with a 24-year history of PLC. The dose was 6 mg/kg daily, and an improvement in scaling and erythema was noticed after the first week.

Medium-dose ultraviolet A1 therapy for pityriasis lichenoides varioliformis acuta and pityriasis lichenoides chronica. Pinton PC, Capezzera R, Zane C, De Panfilis G. J Am Acad Dermatol 2002; 47: 410–14.

Evidence Levels: **A** Double-blind study **B** Clinical trial ≥ 20 subjects **C** Clinical trial < 20 subjects **D** Series ≥ 5 subjects **E** Anecdotal case reports

Eight patients (five with PLC and three with PLEVA) were treated. Three patients with PLC showed complete clinical and histological recovery. Two showed partial improvement.

Role of bromelain in the treatment of patients with pityriasis lichenoides chronica. Massimiliano R, Pietro R, Paolo S, Sara P, Michele F. J Dermatol Treat 2007; 18: 219–22.

Eight patients with PLC were treated for 3 months with oral bromelain, a crude aqueous extract of the stems and immature fruit of pineapple. The authors claim that all cleared completely and only two relapsed over 12 months.

Refractory pityriasis lichenoides chronica successfully treated with topical tacrolimus. Mallipeddi R, Evans AV. Clin Exp Dermatol 2003; 28: 456–8.

A 41-year-old woman with an 8-year history of PLC unresponsive to erythromycin, UVB, and PUVA showed almost complete clearance after 4 weeks of treatment with tacrolimus ointment. Subsequent relapses responded to further treatment.

Successful treatment of pityriasis lichenoides with topical tacrolimus. Simon D, Boudny C, Nievergelt H, Simon HU, Braathen LR. Br J Dermatol 2004; 150: 1033–5.

Two children with long-lasting refractory PLC were cleared of skin lesions after 14 and 18 weeks of treatment, respectively.

Pityriasis lichenoides chronica: good response to photodynamic therapy. Fernandez-Guarino M, Harto A, Reguero-Callerjas ME, Urrutia S, Jaen P. Br J Dermatol 2008; 158: 198–200.

A woman with 15 lesions of PLC had each occluded with methyl aminolevulinic acid for 3 hours followed by a 595 nm pulsed dye laser as a light source (one pulse for each lesion). Lesions cleared after only one treatment.

Pityriasis lichenoides et varioliformis acuta

Alex Milligan, Graham Johnston

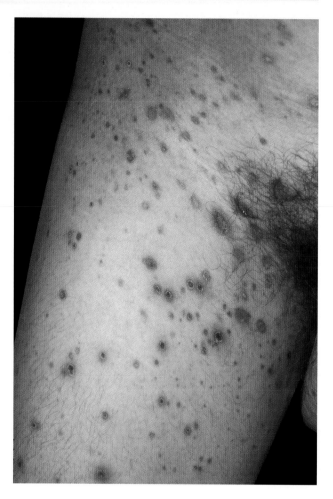

Pityriasis lichenoides et varioliformis acuta (PLEVA) is an eruption of small, erythematous papules which become vesicular and hemorrhagic. Some ulcerate and necrose, leaving pitted scars. The name refers to the morphology not the duration of the condition, because a significant proportion of cases regress with or without treatment, only to recur. Patients should be warned that relapse is common and that recurrent courses of therapy may be required. Febrile ulceronecrotic Mucha–Habermann disease is a rare and severe form of PLEVA characterized by an abrupt onset of an ulceronecrotic eruption associated with a high fever and systemic symptoms.

MANAGEMENT STRATEGY

There are only a handful of controlled trials for this condition and large series are rare. In many therapeutic trials PLEVA is often grouped together with pityriasis lichenoides chronica (see page 565) and management strategies are therefore often similar or interchangeable.

Although a 'wait and see' approach is justifiable in infants, children should be given a 6-week course of *high-dose*

erythromycin. Tetracycline should not be given because of its effects on dentition.

Second-line therapy in children, and possibly first in adults, is either *UV light* or *psoralen plus UVA (PUVA)* because the only comparative study has shown this to be more effective. *Topical corticosteroids* are only reported anecdotally in textbooks rather than in studies. They are used with *antihistamines* to reduce pruritus, but have no reported effect on disease course.

In more extensive or symptomatic disease *low-dose methotrexate* is useful, and *systemic corticosteroids* or *ciclosporin* have also been used.

Some authors have suggested that *combination therapy* (e.g., *erythromycin and PUVA* or *methotrexate and PUVA*) is effective, especially in the rare, febrile ulceronecrotic variant of Mucha–Habermann disease.

SPECIFIC INVESTIGATIONS

▶ Consider skin biopsy

A diagnostic skin biopsy is unnecessary in clinically obvious cases, but may be useful to exclude lymphomatoid papulosis or before commencing aggressive systemic therapy.

An infective etiology for PLEVA is suggested by reports of clustering of cases, resolution following tonsillectomy, and occurrence in five members of a family. Case reports exist associating PLEVA with parvovirus, adenovirus in the urine, staphylococci from throat cultures, Epstein–Barr virus, toxoplasmosis, and HIV. No organism has been cultured from lesional skin and, unless there are clinical signs of infection, routine investigation for an infective agent does not appear to be useful.

Pityriasis lichenoides: a cytotoxic T-cell-mediated skin disorder. Evidence of human parvovirus B19 DNA in nine cases. Tomasini D, Tomasini CF, Cerri A, Sangalli G, Palmedo G, Hantschke M, et al. J Cutan Pathol 2004; 31: 531–8.

This study suggests that pityriasis lichenoides is mediated by a cytotoxic T-cell effector population.

The identification of parvovirus B19 DNA in nine cases may be interpreted ambiguously.

Pityriasis lichenoides et varioliformis acuta and group-A beta hemolytic streptococcal infection. English JC III, Collins M, Bryant-Bruce C. Int J Dermatol 1995; 34: 642–4.

Biopsy-proven PLEVA in association with carriage of Gram-positive cocci cleared with ciprofloxacin in a 35-year-old woman. An identical eruption in her husband, who was found to have group A β-hemolytic streptococcus from a skin swab, cleared with erythromycin.

Pityriasis lichenoides and acquired toxoplasmosis. Rongioletti F, Delmonte S, Rebora A. Int J Dermatol 1999; 38: 367–76.

Biopsy-proven PLEVA in a patient with serology indicating acute toxoplasmosis failed to respond to azithromycin, but cleared with spiramycin followed by trimethoprim-sulfamethoxazole.

FIRST-LINE THERAPIES

▶ Oral erythromycin   **D**

Pityriasis lichenoides in childhood: a retrospective review of 124 patients. Ersoy-Evans S, Greco MF, Mancini AJ, Subasi N, Paller AS. J Am Acad Dermatol 2007; 56: 205–10.

This was a retrospective study of 124 children, 71 of whom had PLEVA. The disease was recurrent in 77%. Erythromycin was given to 79.7% of the affected children and 66.6% of these showed at least a partial response.

Pityriasis lichenoides in children: therapeutic response to erythromycin. Truhan AP, Hebert AA, Esterly NB. J Am Acad Dermatol 1986; 15: 66–70.

In this retrospective uncontrolled study, 11 children aged 2–11 years with biopsy-proven PLEVA were given oral erythromycin 200 mg three or four times daily. Nine improved within a month, and 2–6 months after stopping the drug there was only one recurrence. One patient improved on an increased dose and one failed to respond.

Mucha Habermann's disease in children: treatment with erythromycin. Shavin JS, Jones TM, Aton JK, Abele DC, Smith JG Jr. Arch Dermatol 1978; 114: 1679–80.

Three children responded rapidly to several weeks of erythromycin: 40 mg/kg in the younger patient and 1 g daily in the two adolescents. All subsequently required a second course due to relapse.

Further case reports describe response to roxithromycin and azithromycin.

SECOND-LINE THERAPIES

▶ UVB	D
▶ UVA	D
▶ PUVA	D
▶ Acitretin and PUVA	D

Pityriasis lichenoides in children: a long term follow-up of eighty-nine cases. Gelmetti C, Rigoni C, Alessi E, Ermacora E, Berti E, Caputo R. J Am Acad Dermatol 1990; 23: 473–8.

In a retrospective review of 89 cases the authors did not differentiate between the treatment of PLEVA and that of pityriasis lichenoides chronica (PLC). However, 77 of the children were treated with 4–8-week courses of UVB phototherapy, which seemed to alleviate symptoms and acute eruptions without modifying the course of the disease. The remaining 12 patients were given oral erythromycin 20–40 mg/kg daily for 1–2 weeks and the response was described as 'moderately effective.'

Comparative studies of treatment for pityriasis lichenoides. Gritiyarangsan P, Pruenglampoo S, Ruangratanarote P. J Dermatol 1987; 14: 258–61.

In this open study 30 patients with pityriasis lichenoides were recruited, although the authors did not specify how many had PLEVA and how many PLC. The first group of eight patients were given topical corticosteroid and half had a partial or complete response. The second group were given corticosteroid plus oral tetracycline and the majority had a partial response. The third group of eight patients with chronic, refractory pityriasis lichenoides were given oral methoxsalen 0.6 mg/kg with UVA three times a week for an average of 2 months; five cleared and two had a partial response.

Narrowband UVB (311 nm, TLO1) phototherapy for pityriasis lichenoides. Aydogan K, Saricaoglu H, Turan H. Photoderatol Photoimmunol Photomed 2008; 24: 128–33.

TLO1 treatment led to a complete response in 15 out of 23 PLEVA patients with a mean cumulative dose of 23 J/cm^2 after a mean of 43.4 exposures. There was a partial response in eight patients (34.8%) with a cumulative dose of 15.6 J/cm^2 after a mean of 32.3 exposures.

Erprobung von PUVA bei verscheidenen Dermatosen. Brenner W, Gschnalt F, Honigsmann H, Fritsch P. Hautzart 1978; 29: 541–4.

Five patients treated with PUVA were symptom free after 2–6 weeks of therapy.

Long-term follow-up of photochemotherapy in pityriasis lichenoides. Boelen RE, Faber WR, Lambers JCCA, Cormane RH. Acta Dermatol 1982; 62: 442–4.

Three patients required, on average, 30 PUVA exposures to clear their disease. The total energy required varied markedly. Two patients relapsed and required a further course.

Experience with UVB phototherapy in children. Tay Y-K, Morelli JG, Weston WL. Pediatr Dermatol 1996; 13: 406–9.

As part of a wider open study of UVB phototherapy, three children with PLEVA were given broadband UVB three times a week for an average of 26 treatments. All had greater than 90% improvement in lesions in this time, though two relapsed after treatment was stopped.

Psoralens and ultraviolet A therapy of pityriasis lichenoides. Powell FC, Muller SA. J Am Acad Dermatol 1984; 10: 59–64.

Two females were treated with PUVA for long-standing PLEVA. Patient 1 needed 57 treatments over 12 months (total 370.5 J/cm^2), and patient 2 required 26 treatments over 3 months (total 189 J/cm^2), at which time 80% of lesions had cleared. Patient 2 relapsed after treatment was stopped.

Photochemotherapy for pityriasis lichenoides. Panse I, Bourrat E, Rybojad M, Morel P. Ann Dermatol Venereol 2004; 131: 201–3.

Two patients, aged 6 and 18 years, presented with a 1-month and 3-month history of PLEVA, respectively. They had received different treatments without significant effect: topical corticosteroids, antibiotic, UVB therapy, and dapsone. A combination of acitretin and PUVA was described as dramatically effective within a few weeks.

THIRD-LINE THERAPIES

▶ Methotrexate	D
▶ Ciclosporin	E
▶ Dapsone	E
▶ Systemic corticosteroids	E

Methotrexate for the treatment of Mucha–Habermann disease. Cornelison RL, Knox JM, Everett MA. Arch Dermatol 1972; 106: 507–8.

Five patients were given oral methotrexate 7.5–20 mg weekly. The authors report rapid clearance of the disease, but swift relapse upon stopping therapy.

Mucha Habermann's disease. Rasmussen JE. Arch Dermatol 1979; 115: 676–7.

Four adolescents with severe progressive scarring disease unresponsive to erythromycin, tetracycline, and prednisolone all responded to a short course of methotrexate 2.5 mg given every 12 hours for three doses.

Zur Behandlung der Pityriasis lichenoides et varioliformis acuta mit Methotrexat. Schleicher H, Waldmann U, Knopf B. Dermatol Monatsschr 1975; 161: 148–52.

A 60-year-old woman responded to methotrexate 20 mg intravenously initially followed by 15 mg orally per week. She required a maintenance dose of 7.5 mg/week.

Febrile ulceronecrotic Mucha-Habermann's disease managed with methylprednisolone semipulse and subsequent methotrexate therapies. Ito N, Ohshima A, Hashizume H, Takigawa M, Tokura Y. J Am Acad Dermatol 2003; 49: 1142–8.

A 12-year-old boy with abdominal pain, hypoproteinemia, and anemia was successfully treated with methylprednisolone and subsequent methotrexate therapy.

Successful long-term use of cyclosporin A in HIV-induced pityriasis lichenoides chronica. Griffiths JK. J AIDS 1998; 18: 396.

A 42-year-old woman with AIDS developed biopsy-proven PLC, which then developed into life-threatening, febrile, ulceronecrotic PLEVA. Treatment with ciclosporin 200 mg daily produced a rapid response, though prolonged maintenance treatment was required. Interestingly, the severity of symptoms appeared to parallel the viral load.

Febrile ulceronecrotic Mucha-Habermann's disease and its successful therapy with DDS. Nakamura S, Nishihara K, Nakayama K, Hoshi K. J Dermatol 1986; 13: 381–4.

Oral dapsone 75 mg daily for 20 days, 50 mg daily for 8 days, and 25 mg daily for 6 days produced a dramatic response within 3 days in a 21-year-old man with the ulceronecrotic febrile variant of PLEVA.

Transition of pityriasis lichenoides et varioliformis acuta to febrile ulceronecrotic Mucha-Habermann disease is associated with elevated serum tumour necrosis factor-alpha. Tsianakas A, Hoeger PH. Br J Dermatol 2005; 152: 794–9.

The authors describe a child whose progression from PLEVA to Mucha–Habermann disease was accompanied by a rapid rise in serum tumour necrosis factor (TNF)-α. She was treated successfully with methotrexate.

The authors postulate that therapy with TNF antagonists may be indicated in these cases.

Evidence Levels: **A** Double-blind study **B** Clinical trial ≥ 20 subjects **C** Clinical trial < 20 subjects **D** Series ≥ 5 subjects **E** Anecdotal case reports

Pityriasis rosea

Anna Muncaster

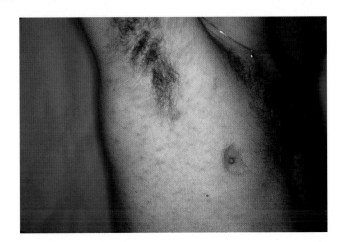

Pityriasis rosea is a common, self-limiting, papulosquamous disorder affecting the trunk and limbs, usually seen in the 10–35-year age group. It has a classical clinical appearance, is associated with little or no constitutional upset, but can have associated itching.

MANAGEMENT STRATEGY

Pityriasis rosea usually resolves spontaneously after approximately 6 weeks and, if asymptomatic, reassurance is all that is required. An infectious etiology, most likely viral, is strongly favored, and although several studies have suggested an association with human herpesviruses 6 and 7, an equal number have failed to show a causal link, therefore at present investigations are unnecessary. There have been case reports of pityriasis rosea-like eruptions after certain drugs such as captopril, ketotifen, and more recently adalimumab, but there is no evidence that pityriasis rosea is drug induced.

For patients who do require treatment, usually because of itch or embarrassment over the appearance, *topical corticosteroids* may be helpful in suppressing the inflammatory component of the disease, although evidence for this is purely anecdotal. *Emollients* and oral *antihistamines* have also been mentioned in the literature as being of some benefit. *Ultraviolet light has* been mentioned several times in the literature over the last 30 years as being helpful, and studies have shown that UVB light treatment with consecutive daily erythemogenic doses can reduce itch and disease severity. The risk of postinflammatory hyperpigmentation may be increased by phototherapy. For patients with more extensive severe eruptions *oral prednisolone* can be tried, as there are reports of improvement with 2–3 weeks of a reducing course of prednisolone. Oral corticosteroids should be used with caution, however, as there are also reports that they exacerbate the condition. A trial in India of *oral erythromycin* 250 mg four times a day for adults or 25–40 mg/kg in divided doses for children produced complete clearance after 2 weeks in the majority of patients. The best results with all these treatments have been obtained when treatment is started within the first 2 weeks of the appearance of the eruption. There has been one case

report of vesicular pityriasis rosea responding to 10 days of oral erythromycin at a dose of 250 mg four times a day, but two further trials, one using oral erythromycin and one using azithromycin, have failed to show any benefit. There has been one case report of vesicular pityriasis rosea responding to *dapsone* therapy, and one trial and case report of clearance following oral *aciclovir*.

A recent review of treatments for pityriasis rosea found very little evidence for most of the treatments given for this condition and suggested that further studies were necessary.

Interventions for pityriasis rosea. Chuh AAT, Dofitas BL, Comisel CG, Reveiz L, Sharma V, Garner SE, et al. Cochrane Database of Systematic Reviews 2007, Issue 2. Art No.: CD005068. DOI: 10.1002/14651858. CD005068.pub2.

The authors found that good evidence for the efficacy of most treatments for pityriasis rosea was lacking, and suggest more research is needed to fully evaluate erythromycin and other treatments.

SPECIFIC INVESTIGATIONS

▶ Consider mycological examination
▶ Consider syphilis serology

FIRST-LINE THERAPIES

▶ Topical corticosteroids	E
▶ Emollients	E
▶ Oral antihistamines	E

Pityriasis rosea update: 1986. Parsons JM. J Am Acad Dermatol 1986; 15: 159–67.

The author relates his own experience of using topical corticosteroids, emollients, and oral antihistamines in the treatment of pityriasis rosea. He claims all three treatments to have been of some benefit.

A comprehensive review article.

SECOND-LINE THERAPIES

▶ UVB	B

Treatment of pityriasis rosea with UV radiation. Arndt KA, Paul BS, Stern RS, Parrish JA. Arch Dermatol 1983; 119: 381–2.

Twenty patients with symptomatic and extensive pityriasis rosea were treated with UVB phototherapy in a bilateral comparison study using the left side of their body as a control. Five consecutive daily erythemogenic exposures resulted in both clinical and subjective improvement in disease severity and pruritus in 50% of the patients.

UVB phototherapy for pityriasis rosea: A bilateral comparison study. Leenitaphong V, Jiamton S. J Am Acad Dermatol 1995; 33: 996–9.

Seventeen patients with extensive pityriasis rosea were treated unilaterally with 10 daily erythemogenic doses of UVB in a bilateral comparison study using 1 J of UVA to the other half of the body as a control. This resulted in a significant reduction in disease severity in 15 out of the 17 patients, but no difference in pruritus.

UVB phototherapy for pityriasis rosea. Valkova S, Trashlieva M, Christova P. J Eur Acad Dermatol Venereol 2004; 18: 111–12.

In a letter to the editor the authors describe a study of 101 patients (including children) who received broadband UVB, either to half the body (24 patients) using UVA on the other half as a control, or to the whole body (77 patients). They showed clearance of the disease in both groups, with those patients having more severe disease requiring significantly more treatments.

THIRD-LINE THERAPIES

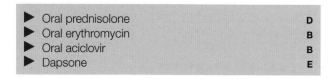

▶ Oral prednisolone	**D**
▶ Oral erythromycin	**B**
▶ Oral aciclovir	**B**
▶ Dapsone	**E**

One year review of pityriasis rosea at the National Skin Centre, Singapore. Tay YK, Goh CL. Ann Acad Med Singapore 1999; 28: 829–31.

In this retrospective case note study of 368 patients, 20 with extensive pruritic disease were treated with short reducing courses of prednisolone over 2–3 weeks, with improvement.

Pityriasis rosea: Exacerbation with corticosteroid treatment. Leonforte JF. Dermatologica 1981; 163: 480–1.

This was a case series of 18 patients, all of whom had received oral corticosteroids for pityriasis rosea. Five were observed while they received their corticosteroid course, and the other 13 were seen after completing their course. In those patients who did report an exacerbation this was worse the higher the dose of corticosteroid received, the longer the course of treatment, and in those who were treated earlier on in their disease.

Erythromycin in pityriasis rosea: A double-blind, placebo-controlled clinical trial. Sharma PK, Yadav TP, Gautam RK, Taneja N, Satyanarayana L. J Am Acad Dermatol 2000; 42: 241–4.

Ninety patients, including children, were randomly assigned to a treatment or a control group. Those in the treatment group received 2 weeks of oral erythromycin 250 mg four times a day for adults, or 25–40 mg/kg in four divided doses for children. Of patients in the treatment group, 73% had a complete response, compared to none of the controls.

Vesicular pityriasis rosea: response to erythromycin treatment. Miranda SB, Lupi O, Lucas E. J Eur Acad Dermatol Venereol 2004; 18: 622–5.

A case report of a 32-year-old woman with a 6-week history of biopsy-proven vesicular pityriasis rosea who achieved almost complete clearance after 10 days of oral erythromycin at a dose of 250 mg four times a day. No recurrence was observed during a 4-month follow-up period.

Use of high-dose acyclovir in pityriasis rosea. Drago F, Veccio F, Rebora A. J Am Acad Dermatol 2006; 54: 82–5.

In this placebo-controlled trial 87 consecutive patients were treated with either oral aciclovir (800 mg five times daily) or placebo for 1 week. At 14 days 78.6% of treated patients achieved complete regression, compared to only 4.4% of the placebo group.

Antivirals for pityriasis rosea. Castanedo-Cazares JP, Lepe V, Moncada B. Photodermatol Photoimmunol Photomed 2004; 20: 110.

In a letter to the editor the authors relate the successful treatment of a case of pityriasis rosea with a short course of oral aciclovir. Dosage and length of treatment were not stated.

Dapsone treatment in a case of vesicular pityriasis rosea. Anderson CR. Lancet 1971; 2: 493.

A case report of a 55-year-old man with histologically proven pityriasis rosea, resistant to oral prednisolone, responding to dapsone 100 mg twice daily for 1 month.

Pityriasis rubra pilaris

Anne-Marie Tobin, Brian Kirby

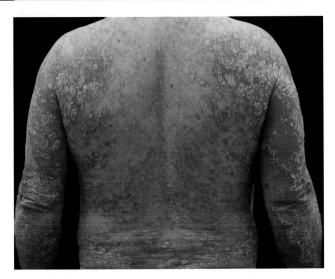

Pityriasis rubra pilaris (PRP) is a rare papulosquamous eruption which has a heterogeneous presentation and is divided into six types. The adult classic type (type I) is characterized by the development of circumscribed follicular keratoses, palmoplantar keratoderma, and erythroderma with characteristic islands of sparing in the skin. Onset is abrupt, and the rash develops in a craniocaudal direction within 2–3 months, almost always resulting in a generalized erythroderma. It can occur from the first to the eighth decade, and may occur in the setting of viral infections, notably human immunodeficiency virus (HIV), internal and external malignancies, and rheumatological conditions. The pattern of malignancy is inconsistent, and no specific associations have been reported.

MANAGEMENT STRATEGY

Eighty percent of cases resolve spontaneously within 3 years. The treatment of PRP can be difficult, and because of its relative rarity there are no randomized controlled trials reported. The retrospective case series reported suggest a variable response to most therapies, reflecting the heterogeneous characteristics of this condition.

PRP has been described in the setting of malignancy, HIV, and seronegative arthritis; at presentation, patients should have a routine physical examination, routine laboratory investigations, and a chest radiograph. Further investigations are only necessary if abnormalities are detected on history, physical examination, and laboratory tests or chest radiograph.

Patients should be given bland emollients to treat the condition; other topical treatments are ineffective, although topical corticosteroids may reduce pruritus.

Retinoids are probably the most effective treatment for PRP: some series report up to 90% response. *Etretinate* (0.75–1.0 mg/ kg daily), *isotretinoin* (1.0–1.5 mg/kg daily), and *acitretin* (0.5–1.0 mg/kg daily) have all been reported as effective. *Methotrexate* (7.5–30 mg weekly) is also effective: one case series reported clearance in 17 of 42 patients and in another series clearance

in six of eight patients. The response to methotrexate takes approximately 6–8 weeks and adequate control 3–4 months. The combination of actitretin and methotrexate may be effective in patients who do not respond to conventional doses of either drug as monotherapy. Hepatotoxicity induced by this combination has been reported in patients with psoriasis so liver function should be monitored closely.

Azathioprine has only been reported in two case series for PRP, but the response to treatment was excellent, with clearance achieved at doses of 150–200 mg daily. Some patients, however, fail to respond to similar doses (B. Kirby, personal communication).

The response to *ciclosporin* appears to be quite variable. There are reports of the use of biologic agents such as *infliximab, etanercept and efalizumab* to treat PRP, either as monotherapy or in combination with acitretin. HIV-associated PRP may be cleared with *antiretroviral therapy*.

SPECIFIC INVESTIGATIONS

> ▶ Chest radiograph
> ▶ Routine hematology
> ▶ Routine biochemistry

FIRST-LINE THERAPIES

> ▶ Retinoids   **D**
> ▶ Methotrexate   **D**

Isotretinoin treatment of pityriasis rubra pilaris. Dicken CH. J Am Acad Dermatol 1987; 16: 297–301.

Isotretinoin was reported as effective in treating PRP in 60–95% of patients after 3–6 months of treatment. The combined number of patients treated in these studies was 50. The dosing schedules varied between 0.48 and 3.19 mg/kg daily, but the usual effective dose seems to be 1.0–1.5 mg/kg daily.

There are few reports in the literature on the use of acitretin in PRP, though this drug is often used for this condition. In case reports where its success was documented it was used in combination with photo(chemo)therapy at a dose of 0.5 mg/kg daily.

Pityriasis rubra pilaris: a review of diagnosis and treatment. Cohen PR, Prystowsky JH. J Am Acad Dermatol 1989; 20: 801–7.

Etretinate was reported as being effective in the majority of patients with PRP in a number of series. The usual dose is 0.75–1.0 mg/kg daily, with dose tapering according to the response. The usual duration of therapy was 4 months; most studies report a favorable influence on disease course and prognosis.

Pityriasis rubra pilaris response to 13 *cis*-retinoic acid (isotretinoin). Goldsmith LA, Weinrich AE, Shupack J. J Am Acad Dermatol 1982; 6: 710–15.

Treatment of classic pityriasis rubra pilaris. Dicken CH. J Am Acad Dermatol 1994; 31: 997–9.

Of 15 patients treated with isotretinoin, 10 had complete clearance and two had partial clearing. Of six patients treated with etretinate, four had clearing. All eight patients treated with methotrexate had a favorable response.

Pityriasis rubra pilaris. Griffiths WAD. Clin Exp Dermatol 1980; 5: 105–12.

Methotrexate (7.5–25 mg weekly) was effective in some patients with PRP but, as with retinoids, the response is variable: only 17 of 42 patients in one series showed benefit. This retrospective report was based on patients who had received various doses of methotrexate and different dosing schedules.

Adult pityriasis rubra pilaris: a 10 year case series. Clayton BD, Jorizzo JL, Hitchcock MG, Fleischer AB Jr, Williford PM, Feldman SR, et al. J Am Acad Dermatol 1997; 36: 959–64.

In a case series of 22 patients, 11 received a combination of methotrexate and oral retinoid. Five of these had combination therapy because retinoid monotherapy failed to elicit a significant improvement.

This combination may cause hepatotoxicity, with two case reports of severe hepatitis in patients with psoriasis. Nonetheless, this combination has been used safely in a large number of patients with psoriasis.

SECOND-LINE THERAPIES

▶ Azathioprine	E
▶ Antiretroviral therapy	D
▶ Ciclosporin	E

Treatment of pityriasis rubra pilaris with azathioprine. Hunter GA, Forbes IJ. Br J Dermatol 1972; 87: 42–5.

Azathioprine was reported as effective in seven of eight patients and in four patients by Hunter and Forbes. The doses used were 50 mg three times daily, and in one case 100 mg daily.

HIV-associated pityriasis rubra pilaris response to triple antiretroviral therapy. Gonzalez-Lopez A, Velasco E, Pozo T, Del Villar A. Br J Dermatol 1999; 140: 931–4.

PRP associated with HIV infection may respond to antiretroviral therapy.

There are case reports of HIV-associated PRP responding to zidovudine. HIV-associated PRP also responds to triple antiretroviral therapy (zidovudine 20 mg 12 hourly, lamivudine 150 mg 12 hourly, and saquinavir 600 mg 8 hourly) and the response corresponds to the fall in viral load.

Three cases of pityriasis rubra pilaris successfully treated with cyclosporine A. Usuki K, Sekiyama M, Shimada T. Dermatology 2000; 200: 324–7.

Ciclosporin at 5 mg/kg daily as monotherapy was successful in patients with classic type I PRP. The response was sustained while therapy continued at a dose greater than 1.2 mg/kg daily.

Juvenile pityriasis rubra pilaris: successful treatment with ciclosporin. Wetzig T, Sticherling M. Br J Dermatol 2003; 149: 202–3.

A single case report of effective therapy of classic juvenile PRP with ciclosporin.

THIRD-LINE THERAPIES

▶ Calcipotriol	E
▶ Tazarotene	E
▶ Pimecrolimus	E
▶ Acitretin and narrowband UVB (TL-01)	E
▶ Acitretin and UVA1	E
▶ Extracorporeal photochemotherapy	E
▶ Infliximab	E
▶ Etanercept monotherapy and with acitretin	E
▶ Efalizumab	E
▶ Intravenous immunoglobulin	E

Topical treatment of pityriasis rubra pilaris with calcipotriol. Van de Kerkhof PC, Steijen PM. Br J Dermatol 1994; 130: 675–8.

Calcipotriol was reported to be effective in a small series of three patients. In this study two patients responded and one suffered irritation.

Response of juvenile circumscribed pityriasis rubra pilaris to topical tazarotene treatment. Karimian-Teherani D, Parissa M, Tanew A. Paediatr Dermatol 2008; 25: 125–6.

A single case report of sustained remission following use of tazarotene in a 12-year-old.

Treatment of pityriasis rubra pilaris with pimecrolimus cream 1%. Gregoriou S, Argyriou G, Christofidou E, Vranou A, Rigopoulos D. J Drugs Dermatol 2007; 6: 340–2.

Pimecrolimus cream 1% applied to PRP limited to the face and scalp resulted in complete clearance after 2 weeks.

Pityriasis rubra pilaris treated with acitretin and narrow band ultraviolet B (Re-TL-01). Kirby B, Watson R. Br J Dermatol 2000; 142: 376–7.

Narrowband UVB phototherapy (TL-01) has been reported as effective when combined with retinoid (Re-TL-01) in a single case of juvenile PRP. This patient had not responded to broadband ultraviolet B and it is speculated that TL-01 may have different biological effects than either broadband UVB or photochemotherapy.

One further case of PRP treated with TL-01 has been reported: this patient developed blisters in lesional skin. It is also worth noting that there are documented cases of photoaggravated and photosensitive PRP.

Combined ultraviolet A1 radiation and acitretin therapy as a treatment option for pityriasis rubra pilaris. Herbst RA, Vogelbruch M, Ehnis A, Kiehl P, Kapp A, Weiss J. Br J Dermatol 2000; 142: 574–5.

This is a single successful case report of long-wave UVA (UVA1) in combination with acitretin for the treatment of classic PRP.

Extracorporeal photochemotherapy for the treatment of erythrodermic pityriasis rubra pilaris. Hofer A, Mullegger R, Kerl H, Wolf P. Arch Dermatol 1999; 135: 475–6.

This is a single case report of the successful treatment of PRP with extracorporeal photochemotherapy.

Extracorporeal photochemotherapy for the treatment of exanthemic pityriasis rubra pilaris. Haenssle HA, Bertsch HP, Wolf C, Zutt M. Clin Exp Dermatol 2004; 29: 244–6.

Again, this is a single case report of the effective use of extracorporeal photochemotherapy in recalcitrant type II chronic adult PRP.

Successful treatment of type I adult-onset pityriasis rubra pilaris with infliximab. Manohoran S, White S, Gumparthy K. Australas J Dermatol 2006; 47: 124–9.

Evidence Levels: **A** Double-blind study **B** Clinical trial ≥ 20 subjects **C** Clinical trial < 20 subjects **D** Series ≥ 5 subjects **E** Anecdotal case reports

A single case refractory to systemic and topical treatments, treated with infliximab 5 mg/kg for six infusions, with good remission.

Pityriasis rubra pilaris successfully treated with infliximab. Ruiz-Genao DP, Lopez-Estebaranz JL, Naz-Villalba E, Gamo-Villegas R, Clazado-Villarreal L, Pinedo-Moraleda F. Acta Dermatol Venerol 2007; 87: 552–3.

Type III juvenile pityriasis rubra pilaris: a successful treatment with infliximab. Ruzzetti M, Saraceno R, Carboni I, Papoutsaki M, Chimenti S. J Eur Acad Dermatol 2008; 22: 117–18.

Again, these are two single case reports of the successful use of infliximab 5 mg/kg.

There are also two reports of infliximab failing to induce a response, one as monotherapy and one in combination with acitretin.

Successful use of etanercept in type I pityriasis rubra pilaris. Seckin D, Tula E, Ergun T. Br J Dermatol 2008; 158: 642–4.

This is a case report of etanercept used at a dose of 50 mg twice weekly subcutaneously with good effect.

Clinical improvement of pityriasis rubra pilaris with combination etanercept and acitretin therapy. Davis KF, Murase JE, Rosenberg FR, Sorenson EP, Meshkinpour A. Arch Dermatol 2007; 143: 1597–9.

These are both single case reports of the use of etanercept in combination with acitretin with good effect in PRP.

Clinical improvement of pityriasis rubra pilaris with efalizumab in a paediatric patient. Gomez M, Ruelas ME, Welsh O, Arcaute HD, Ocampo-Candiani J. J Drugs Dermatol 2007; 6: 337–9.

This case report documents the success of efalizumab 1 mg/kg weekly following the failure of multiple treatments, including etanercept, in a 10-year-old boy.

Type II adult-onset pityriasis rubra pilaris successfully treated with intravenous immunoglobulin. Kerr AC, Ferguson J. Br J Dermatol 2007; 156: 1055–6.

This is a report of a single patient treated with IVIG successfully at a dose of 2 g/kg administered over 3 days and repeated at 4-week intervals. The patient had failed multiple therapies, including anti-TNF-α, and at the time of publication had good control for up to 80 doses of IVIG.

Polyarteritis nodosa

Jeffrey P Callen

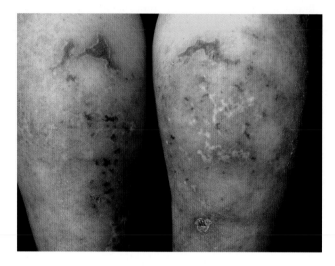

Polyarteritis nodosa (PAN) is a necrotizing vasculitis that involves small or medium-sized arterioles. Classic PAN is characterized by fever, weight loss, cutaneous ulcers, livedo reticularis, myalgias and weakness, arthralgias or arthritis, neuropathy, abdominal pain, ischemic bowel, testicular pain, hypertension, and renal failure. Microscopic polyarteritis (MPA) involves the same-sized vessels as well as smaller vessels, and is manifest clinically as a glomerulonephritis and a pulmonary capillaritis with alveolar hemorrhage. Patients with MPA may develop small vessel vasculitis (palpable purpura), livedo reticularis with or without nodules, and/or ulcerations of the skin. Cutaneous PAN (cPAN), sometimes termed benign cutaneous polyarteritis, is characterized by livedo reticularis, nodules and ulceration, usually of the leg; it has been postulated to be a localized necrotizing arteritis that does not affect internal organs, and runs a chronic but benign course. Many reports, however, have linked cPAN to inflammatory bowel disease, or hepatitis B or C infection. Occasional reports have linked cPAN to antiphospholipid antibodies, cryoproteins, or antineutrophil cytoplasmic antibodies. Some cases have occurred in patients treated with propylthiouracil and minocycline (cPAN appears to be more prevalent in children). Although it is generally benign, there have been reports of associated neuropathy, as well as visceral involvement.

MANAGEMENT STRATEGY

cPAN causes pain and discomfort and may ulcerate, thereby causing disability. These manifestations warrant therapy. Therapy may include local measures, such as *gradient pressure stockings*, or *systemic therapies*, including *systemic corticosteroids, methotrexate, azathioprine, pentoxifylline*, and *intravenous immunoglobulin (IVIG)*. As there are few cases of this disease, most of the reports are anecdotes or small case series. There is no uniformly accepted approach to these patients.

SPECIFIC INVESTIGATIONS

- ▶ Skin biopsy
- ▶ Serology for hepatitis B and C, antineutrophil cytoplasmic antibody, antiphospholipid antibodies, and cryoproteins
- ▶ Assessment for systemic involvement
- ▶ Assessment for inflammatory bowel disease
- ▶ Assessment for drugs that have been linked to cPAN

Cutaneous periarteritis nodosa: a clinicopathological study of 79 cases. Daoud MS, Hutton KP, Gibson LE. Br J Dermatol 1997; 136: 706–13.

This retrospective analysis of 79 patients evaluated the clinical and histological features of cPAN and attempted to identify any clinical, pathological, and immunological differences that may distinguish those cases likely to have a prolonged course. During the course of their illness 39 patients had ulcers. Women were affected more than men. Painful nodules on the lower extremities, with edema and swelling, were the most common clinical finding; 22% of patients had some evidence of neuropathy. Most of the laboratory findings were nonspecific. There was no evidence for hepatitis B infection in the 37 patients tested, and hepatitis C infection was present in only one of the 20 patients tested. Five patients had inflammatory bowel disease (four had Crohn's disease and one had ulcerative colitis). Ten patients had rheumatoid arthritis. Most patients (60%) had no associated medical condition. The disease course was prolonged but benign, and systemic PAN did not develop in any patient. The ulcerative form of disease was more prolonged and frequently associated with neuropathy. Therapy was varied, and the patients with non-ulcerative disease responded better than those with ulcers. Observations suggested that agents such as corticosteroids, azathioprine, pentoxifylline, and hydroxychloroquine were effective in individual patients.

This study highlights the associations that might occur in up to 40% of patients, the fact that neuropathy is relatively common, and that the course and response to treatment are dependent on the presence of ulceration.

Cutaneous polyarteritis nodosa. Díaz-Pérez JL, De Lagrán ZM, Díaz-Ramón JL, Winkelmann RK. Semin Cutan Med Surg 2007; 26: 77–86.

This review updates the Mayo Clinic experience with this disorder and suggests that therapy with non-steroidal anti-inflammatory agents or short courses of oral corticosteroids is usually effective.

Cutaneous polyarteritis nodosa associated with Crohn's disease. Report and review of the literature. Gudbjornsson B, Hallgren R. J Rheumatol 1990; 17: 386–90.

A single patient with cPAN developed gastrointestinal symptoms and was found to have Crohn's disease. Resected bowel did not reveal a vasculitis. Prior to the recognition of the bowel disease, her disease was controlled with corticosteroids and cyclophosphamide. Eventually, oral sulfasalazine was effective in controlling the bowel disease and the cPAN.

cPAN has been reported in conjunction with inflammatory bowel disease on numerous occasions. A careful focused history is the preferred method of evaluation. Radiologic or endoscopic studies are not generally necessary.

Cutaneous polyarteritis nodosa in a patient with ulcerative colitis. Volk DM, Owen LG. J Pediatr Gastroenterol Nutr 1986; 5: 970–2.

A child with cPAN and ulcerative colitis is reported.

Hepatitis C virus infection in cutaneous polyarteritis nodosa: a retrospective study of 16 cases. Soufir N, Descamps V, Crickx B, Thibault V, Cosnes A, Bécherel PA, et al. Arch Dermatol 1999; 135: 1001–2.

These authors studied 16 patients with cPAN and found antibodies to hepatitis C in five. One patient was coinfected with HIV, and one had evidence of a prior hepatitis B infection.

Hepatitis C serology should be performed in patients with cPAN. Livedo reticularis with cryoglobulinemia can be seen with hepatitis C infection.

Perinuclear antineutrophilic cytoplasmic antibody-positive cutaneous polyarteritis nodosa associated with minocycline therapy for acne vulgaris. Schaffer JV, Davidson DM, McNiff JM, Bolognia JL. J Am Acad Dermatol 2001; 44: 198–206.

This is the first case linking cPAN to minocycline therapy.

Vasculitic conditions mimicking cPAN have been reported with isotretinoin and amphetamines.

FIRST-LINE THERAPIES

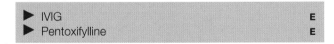

▶ Local measures – support stockings, local wound care	E
▶ Systemic corticosteroids	E
▶ Immunosuppressants – azathioprine, methotrexate	D

Low-dose weekly methotrexate for unusual neutrophilic vascular reactions: cutaneous polyarteritis nodosa and Behçet's disease. Jorizzo JL, White WL, Wise CM, Zanolli MD, Sherertz EF. J Am Acad Dermatol 1991; 24: 973–8.

These authors reported three patients with cPAN who responded dramatically to low-dose weekly methotrexate therapy.

SECOND-LINE THERAPIES

▶ IVIG	E
▶ Pentoxifylline	E

Intravenous immunoglobulin therapy in a child with cutaneous polyarteritis nodosa. Uziel Y, Silverman ED. Clin Exp Rheumatol 1998; 16: 187–9.

In this report a 9-year-old boy who developed cPAN was treated with high-dose IVIG, with an immediate favorable response.

Successful treatment of cutaneous PAN with pentoxifylline. Calderon MJ, Landa N, Aguirre A, Diaz-Perez JL. Br J Dermatol 1993; 12: 706–8.

A patient who failed to respond to aspirin and penicillin was treated with pentoxifylline. Withdrawal of the pentoxifylline resulted in a relapse that again responded to therapy.

THIRD-LINE THERAPIES

▶ Tamoxifen	E
▶ Infliximab	E
▶ Tonsillectomy	D

Estrogen-sensitive cutaneous polyarteritis nodosa: response to tamoxifen. Cvancara JL, Meffert JJ, Elston DM. J Am Acad Dermatol 1998; 39: 643–6.

Tamoxifen, an antiestrogenic agent, at a dose of 10–20 mg daily, led to control of disease in a patient that seemed to worsen with conjugated estrogen therapy. Relapse occurred within 5 days of interruption of the therapy and rapidly responded with reinitiation of the tamoxifen.

Successful response to infliximab in a patient with undifferentiated spondyloarthropathy coexisting with polyarteritis nodosa-like cutaneous vasculitis. Garcia-Porrua C, Gonzalez-Gay MA. Clin Exp Rheumatol 2003; 21: S138.

This is a report of an observation in a single patient.

Successful treatment of childhood cutaneous polyarteritis nodosa with infliximab. Vega Gutierrez J, Rodriguez Prieto MA, Garcia Ruiz JM. J Eur Acad Dermatol Venereol 2007; 21: 570–1.

This is a single case report documenting efficacy of infliximab.

Cutaneous polyarteritis nodosa: therapy and clinical course in four cases. Misago N, Mochizuki Y, Sekiyama-Kodera H, Shirotani M, Suzuki K, Inokuchi A, et al. J Dermatol 2001; 28: 719–27.

In this report of four patients, two treated with tonsillectomy had resolution of their disease. The authors proposed that chronic streptococcal disease might be responsible for cPAN.

Polymorphic light eruption

Warwick L Morison

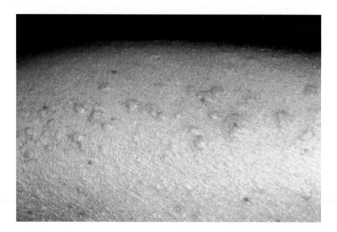

Polymorphic light eruption is the most common photodermatosis and develops hours to a day or more following specific exposure to sunlight. The morphology varies, with papular or papulovesicular forms being most common. Plaques, insect-bite type, and erythema multiforme variants are much less common. In most patients the tendency to develop polymorphic light eruption diminishes with repeated exposures to sunlight, a phenomenon called hardening.

MANAGEMENT STRATEGY

The treatment of polymorphic light eruption consists of two phases: treatment of established disease after the rash has appeared; and the prevention of the rash in patients known to have the disease. Application of a *mid-potency* or *high-potency corticosteroid cream* or *ointment*, two or three times daily, is usually sufficient to reduce symptoms and clear the rash in most patients with established disease. A few patients with extensive disease and marked symptoms require *oral prednisone* in a dose of 60–80 mg for a few days, followed by rapid reduction of the dose over a week.

Preventive management is the best choice for patients diagnosed with the disease. The majority of patients with polymorphic light eruption have high-threshold disease, so they require prolonged exposure to sunlight or artificial sources of ultraviolet (UV) radiation to trigger the reaction. Most of these individuals do not seek medical advice but learn to limit their exposure to levels below their threshold or, in some cases, to prevent the disease by use of sunscreens. Patients seeking medical advice usually have low-threshold disease, often triggered by 15–30-minute exposures to sunlight, leading to marked limitation of outdoor activities.

The initial approach to the prevention of polymorphic light eruption is *avoidance of exposure to sunlight* using a combination of reduced time spent outdoors, restriction of exposure to early morning and late afternoon hours, wearing of protective clothing, and application of *broadband sunscreens* that protect against both UVA and UVB wavelengths. This strategy is most

likely to be effective in patients with high-threshold disease and those triggered by UVB radiation.

The most effective approach for patients with low-threshold disease is desensitization using a course of *PUVA (psoralen/UVA), narrow-band (311-nm) UVB phototherapy or broadband UVB phototherapy* in spring, followed by regular exposures to sunlight during summer to maintain tolerance. This approach is successful in preventing polymorphic light eruption in up to 90% of patients, but requires planning as treatment lasts for about a month. Patients who develop polymorphic light eruption while on treatment should continue therapy and may require topical or oral corticosteroids to control the rash.

Hydroxychloroquine, β-carotene, and *nicotinamide* are reported to provide moderate and safe protection in polymorphic light eruption and may be considered in patients unable to undertake, or who are unresponsive to, desensitization therapy. Hydroxychloroquine is sometimes a useful preventive measure during a brief winter vacation in a warm climate. It should be started 3 days before the vacation in a dose of 400 mg daily, and continued throughout the vacation.

SPECIFIC INVESTIGATIONS

▶ Skin biopsy
▶ Phototesting
▶ Lupus serologies

Histopathologic findings in papulovesicular light eruption. Hood AF, Elpern DJ, Morison WL. J Cutan Pathol 1986; 13: 13–21.

The histologic pattern of this subgroup is characteristic but not pathognomonic; there is little histologic similarity to lupus erythematosus.

Polymorphous light eruption. Holzle E, Plewig G, von Kries R, Lehmann P. J Invest Dermatol 1987; 88: 32–8s.

The histologic patterns in less common subtypes are reviewed. Phototesting reproduced lesions in about 60% of patients, and the action spectrum was confined to UVA in 75%, UVB in 10%, and 15% for both wavebands.

An optimal method for experimental provocation of polymorphic light eruption. van de Pas CB, Hawk JLM, Young A, Walker SL. Arch Dermatol 2004; 140: 286–92.

Solar-simulated radiation was effective in inducing the rash in almost 70% of patients and there was no difference in success rate between previously affected and previously unaffected skin.

Because 100% of patients have developed polymorphic light eruption from exposure to sunlight or an indoor source of UV radiation such as a suntan parlor, the most reliable method of reproducing the eruption is to request the patient to deliberately expose their skin to the source of light that produced their rash, and to return for inspection and biopsy.

The prevalence of antinuclear antibodies in patients with apparent polymorphic light eruption. Murphy GM, Hawk JLM. Br J Dermatol 1991; 125: 448–51.

Of 142 patients with a history consistent with polymorphic light eruption, 6% had a positive Ro antibody test or subsequently developed lupus erythematosus. A lupus panel of tests is essential in patients being considered for active desensitization treatment.

Evidence Levels: **A** Double-blind study **B** Clinical trial ≥ 20 subjects **C** Clinical trial < 20 subjects **D** Series ≥ 5 subjects **E** Anecdotal case reports

FIRST-LINE THERAPIES

▶ Restriction of sun exposure	E
▶ Sunscreens	B
▶ Protective clothing	E

New broad-spectrum sunscreen for polymorphic light eruption. Proby M, Baker CS, Morton O, Hawk JLM. Lancet 1993; 341: 1347–8.

Application of a broad-spectrum sunscreen containing octyl methoxycinnamate, avobenzone and microfined titanium dioxide (SPF 30 for UVA and UVB) applied prior to sun exposure and repeated hourly and after swimming, provided complete protection in 27% of patients and partial protection in another 60%. The sunscreen was cosmetically acceptable and there were no adverse reactions.

Textiles and sun protection. Robson J, Diffey BL. Photodermatol Photoimmunol Photomed 1990; 7: 32–4.

Transmission of UV radiation through clothing varies greatly, providing an 'SPF' in this study from 2 for a polyester blouse to 1571 for cotton denim jeans. The tightness of the weave is the main variable determining transmission of light. Transmission of UV radiation for all fabrics is increased when a fabric is wet.

Clothing and hats are now available specifically designed to provide protection from sunlight while maintaining a high level of comfort.

SECOND-LINE THERAPIES

▶ PUVA therapy	C
▶ Narrowband (311-nm) phototherapy	C
▶ Broadband UVB phototherapy	C

UVB phototherapy and photochemotherapy (PUVA) in the treatment of polymorphic light eruption and solar urticaria. Addo HA, Sharma SC. Br J Dermatol 1987; 116: 539–47.

Patients were treated with a regular schedule of oral PUVA or high-dose (erythemogenic) broadband UVB phototherapy three times weekly for 5 weeks during the spring, and were then instructed to maximize their exposure to sunlight during summer. Ninety percent of PUVA-treated patients and about 70% of UVB-treated patients were free of symptoms of polymorphic light eruption during the summer. Development of the eruption during the active treatment was common, usually mild, and did not interfere with treatment.

A comparison of narrowband (TL-01) and photochemotherapy (PUVA) in the management of polymorphic light eruption. Bilsland D, George SA, Gibbs NK, Aitchison T, Johnson BE, Ferguson J. Br J Dermatol 1993; 129: 708–12.

A regular schedule of oral PUVA therapy or narrowband (311-nm) phototherapy was given to patients three times a week for 5 weeks in the spring, resulting in about 85% of patients in each treatment group being adequately protected from developing polymorphic light eruption during the summer. The necessity for regular sun exposure every week during the summer may not have been emphasized.

THIRD-LINE THERAPIES

▶ Prednisolone	A
▶ Hydroxychloroquine	A
▶ β-Carotene	C
▶ Nicotinamide	B
▶ Azathioprine	E
▶ Ciclosporin	E
▶ Flavonoid antioxidant	A
▶ *Polypodium leukotomas*	B

Efficacy of short-course oral prednisolone in polymorphic light eruption: a randomized controlled trial. Patel DC, Bellaney GJ, Seed PT, McGregor JM, Hawk JLM. Br J Dermatol 2000; 143: 828–31.

A 7-day course of 25 mg prednisolone daily was superior to placebo when started at the onset of the rash. This low dose of steroid is suitable for managing patients who are on brief vacations in a sunny climate.

Prednisone would be a suitable alternative.

Hydroxychloroquine in polymorphic light eruption: a controlled trial with drug and visual sensitivity monitoring. Murphy GM, Hawk JLM, Magnus IA. Br J Dermatol 1987; 116: 379–86.

Hydroxychloroquine in a dose of 400 mg daily for 1 month, and 200 mg daily for 2 months, was superior to placebo in preventing development of the rash; however, almost all patients did have a rash and irritation during the trial. The degree of protection was judged to be moderate and was related to serum level of the drug; the dose of 400 mg daily provided better protection. No visual toxicity was observed.

Comparison of PUVA and beta-carotene in the treatment of polymorphous light eruption. Parrish JA, Le Vine MJ, Morison WL, Gonzalez E, Fitzpatrick TB. Br J Dermatol 1979; 100: 187–91.

β-Carotene (3.0 mg/kg) in a twice-daily divided dose given for the entire summer provided full protection for 30% of patients and partial protection for another 20%. There were no adverse effects.

Treatment of polymorphous light eruption with nicotinamide: a pilot study. Neumann R, Rappold E, Pohl-Markl H. Br J Dermatol 1986; 115: 77–80.

Nicotinamide given in a dose of 1 g orally three times daily starting 2 days before sun exposure provided complete protection in 60% of patients. The dose was reduced to 2 g daily after 1 week, and about half of these patients developed polymorphic light eruption. A few patients had mild fatigue.

Successful treatment of severe polymorphous light eruption with azathioprine. Norris PG, Hawk JLM. Arch Dermatol 1989; 125: 1377–9.

Two patients with year-round photosensitivity triggered by as little as 1–2 minutes of sun exposure and unresponsive to all standard treatments were treated with 0.8–2.5 mg/kg of azathioprine daily for 3 months, with complete remission of symptoms and normal sun tolerance.

The erythemal responses to UVB radiation were reduced in both patients and to UVA radiation in one, which is an unusual finding in typical cases of polymorphic light eruption.

Prophylactic short-term use of cyclosporin in refractory polymorphic light eruption. Lasa O, Trebol I, Gardeazabal J, Diaz-Perez JL. J Eur Acad Dermatol Venereol 2004; 18: 747–8.

Ciclosporin in a dose of 3–4 mg/kg/day over 2 or 4 weeks was effective in preventing the development of an eruption in three patients during a short vacation in a sunny climate. The patients had not responded to other preventive measures. No adverse effects were observed, and this appears to have promise as a prophylactic treatment in patients resistant to other therapies.

Polymorphous light eruption (PLE) and a new potent antioxidant and UVA-protective formulation as prophylaxis. Hadshiew IM, Treder-Conrad C, Bülow RV, Klette E, Mann T, Stäb F, et al. Photodermatol Photoimmunol Photomed 2004; 20: 200–4.

A flavonoid antioxidant plus a broad-spectrum sunscreen was more effective in preventing PLE than sunscreen alone or placebo.

Photoprotective activity of oral polypodium leucotomos extract in 25 patients with idiopathic photodermatoses. Caccialanza M, Percivalle S, Piccinno R, Brambilla R. Photodermatol Photoimmunol Photomed 2007; 23: 46–7.

Daily oral administration of *Polypodium leucotomos* extract provided improvement in over 40% of patients in terms of tolerance to sun exposure without developing PLE.

Pompholyx

Anne E Burdick, Ivan D Camacho

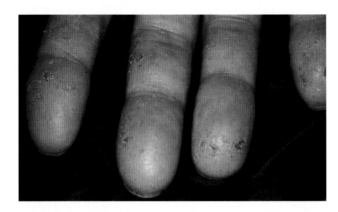

Pompholyx, also known as dyshidrosis or dyshidrotic eczema, is a recurrent, pruritic vesicular eruption of the palms, soles, and lateral aspects of the fingers. It is of unknown etiology and is considered a reaction pattern to various endogenous and exogenous factors, including atopy, hyperhidrosis, dermatophytosis, contact allergic dermatitis to nickel, chromium, balsams and cobalt, irritant dermatitis, and possibly emotional stress and seasonal changes. Pompholyx has also been reported to be induced by intravenous immunoglobulin therapy, during the immune reconstitution inflammatory syndrome, and by mycophenolate mofetil.

MANAGEMENT STRATEGY

Although pompholyx may resolve spontaneously, treatment is aimed at controlling pruritus and the formation of vesicobullae. Evaluation is required to exclude dermatophytosis, irritant or allergic contact dermatitis, impetigo, pustular psoriasis, herpes simplex, pemphigus vulgaris, and bullous pemphigoid.

Topical corticosteroids are the mainstay of treatment. For mild localized disease, *mid- to-high-potency corticosteroid* creams or ointments are recommended. *Antipruritic topicals containing pramoxine* are useful for control of symptoms, as are *oral antihistamines*. *Emollients* are also beneficial. A course of *oral antibiotics* (*cephalosporins or erythromycin*) is recommended for secondary impetiginization. Vesicles and bullae can be treated with *10% aluminum acetate* (*Burow's solution*) compresses in a 1:40 dilution. Large bullae can be mechanically drained in a sterile manner, leaving the roof intact.

Topical tacrolimus or *pimecrolimus* are useful in refractory cases once or twice daily, alone or in combination with a corticosteroid. For severe disease, *systemic corticosteroids* are indicated: daily *prednisone* 0.5–1.0 mg/kg/day tapered over 2 weeks, or intramuscular *triamcinolone acetonide* (40–60 mg). Hand and foot *UVA or UVA1*, alone or with oral or *topical psoralen* is also effective.

Severe refractory pompholyx may respond to *immunosuppressive agents* such as *azathioprine, methotrexate, ciclosporin, mycophenolate mofetil* or *etanercept*.

Intradermal botulinum toxin A and *tap water iontophoresis* may be helpful as adjuvant therapy. *Nickel chelators* such as *disulfiram* may be used in nickel-sensitive patients who demonstrate a positive provocation test. The furanochrome *khellin* may be used in combination with sun exposure in recalcitrant cases.

SPECIFIC INVESTIGATIONS

▶ Potassium hydroxide preparation
▶ Bacterial culture
▶ Patch testing

Severe dyshidrosis in two patients with HIV infection shortly after starting highly active antiretroviral (HAART) treatment. Colebunders R, Zolfo M, Lynen L. Dermatol Online J 2005; 11: 31.

Onset of pompholyx occurred 5 and 17 days after HAART treatment.

Vesicular eczema after intravenous immunoglobulin therapy for treatment of Stevens–Johnson syndrome. Young PK, Ruggeri SY, Galbraith S, Drolet BA. Arch Dermatol 2006; 142: 247–8.

The patient developed pompholyx 10 days after initiation of IVIG therapy.

Pompholyx induced by intravenous immunoglobulin (IVIG) therapy. Llombart M, García-Abujeta JL, Sánchez-Pérez RM, Hernando de Larramendi C. J Invest Allergol Clin Immunol 2007; 17: 277–8.

A patient with a history of hand eczema developed pompholyx 5 days after the standard dose of IVIG.

Mycophenolate mofetil-induced dyshidrotic eczema. Semhoun-Ducloux S, Ducloux D, Miguet JP. Ann Intern Med 2007; 132: 417.

A liver transplant recipient developed biopsy-proven dyshidrotic eczema after 3 days of 2 g/day mycophenolate mofetil, with recurrence on reinstitution of a lower dose.

A 3-year causative study of pompholyx in 120 patients. Guillet MH, Wierzbicka E, Guillet S, Dagregorio G, Guillet G. Arch Dermatol 2007; 143: 1504–8.

A prospective survey of 120 patients reported allergic contact pompholyx in 67.5% of cases (31.7% to cosmetic and hygiene products and 16.7% to metals), 15% idiopathic, 10% secondary to dermatophytes, and 6.7% due to ingestion of drugs, food, or nickel.

Role of contact allergens in pompholyx. Jain V, Passi S, Gupta S. J Dermatol 2004; 31: 188–93.

Patch testing with the Indian Standard Patch Test Battery was performed on 50 subjects and 40% reacted to one or more allergens. Nickel sulfate was the most common allergen, followed by potassium dichromate, phenylenediamine, nitrofurazone, fragrance mix, and cobalt.

Relation between vesicular eruptions on the hands and tinea pedis, atopic dermatitis and nickel allergy. Bryld L, Agner T, Menne T. Acta Dermatol Venereol 2003; 83: 186–8.

A statistically significant risk for vesicular eruptions with tinea pedis was reported in three of 16 patients (19%).

FIRST-LINE THERAPIES

▶ Topical corticosteroids	A
▶ Topical calcineurin inhibitors	C
▶ Oral antibiotics	D
▶ Oral antihistamines	E
▶ Oral corticosteroids	D
▶ Topical antipruritics	D
▶ Emollients	D

Dyshidrosis: epidemiology, clinical characteristics, and therapy. Lofgren SM, Warshaw EM. Dermatitis 2006; 17: 165–81.

A comprehensive review.

Therapeutic options for chronic hand dermatitis. Warshaw EM. Dermatol Ther 2004; 17: 240–50.

Useful table on lifestyle management for patients.

Topical tacrolimus (FK 506) and mometasone furoate in treatment of dyshidrotic palmar eczema: a randomized, observer-blinded trial. Schnopp C, Remling R, Mohrenschlager M, Weigl L, Ring J, Abeck D. J Am Acad Dermatol 2002; 46: 73–7.

Topical tacrolimus 0.1% ointment was as effective as 0.1% mometasone furoate ointment after 4 weeks of twice-daily application, reducing the Dyshidrotic Area and Severity Index (DASI) to approximately 50% in 16 patients.

An open-label pilot study to evaluate the safety and efficacy of topically applied tacrolimus ointment for the treatment of hand and/or foot eczema. Thelmo MC, Lang W, Brooke E, Osborne BE, McCarty MA, Jorizzo JL, et al. J Dermatol Treat 2003; 14: 136–40.

Tacrolimus ointment 0.1% three times daily for 8 weeks in 25 patients with hand and foot dermatitis showed significant improvement in erythema, scaling, induration, fissuring, and pruritus from baseline, with recurrence of most symptoms after 2 weeks of discontinuation. There was no effect on vesiculation.

Pimecrolimus cream 1%: a potential new treatment for chronic hand dermatitis. Belsito DV, Fowler JF Jr, Marks JG Jr, Pariser DM, Hanifin J, Duarte IA, et al. Cutis 2004; 73: 31–8.

Pimecrolimus 1% cream twice daily with overnight occlusion for 3 weeks in 294 patients with mild to moderate chronic hand dermatitis showed a statistical trend toward improvement.

SECOND-LINE THERAPIES

▶ Psoralen and UVA (PUVA)	C
▶ UVA	C
▶ UVA1	A
▶ Topical PUVA	C
▶ Intradermal botulinum A toxin	C

Comparison of localized high-dose UVA1 irradiation versus topical cream psoralen-UVA for treatment of chronic vesicular dyshidrotic eczema. Petering H, Breuer C, Herbst R, Kapp A, Werfel T. J Am Acad Dermatol 2004; 50: 68–72.

Twenty-seven patients treated with UVA1 irradiation to one hand and cream psoralen-UVA (PUVA) to the other showed similar improvement with both treatments.

A double-blind placebo-controlled trial of UVA-1 in the treatment of dyshidrotic eczema. Polderman M, Govaert J, le Cessie S, Pavel S. Clin Exp Dermatol 2003; 28: 584–7.

Twenty-eight patients who received UVA1 irradiation five times a week for 3 weeks had significant improvement of DASI and Visual Analogue Scores (VAS).

Treatment of recalcitrant dermatosis of the palms and soles with PUVA-bath versus PUVA-cream therapy. Grundmann-Kollmann M, Behrens S, Ru P, Kerscher M. Photodermatol Photoimmunol Photomed 1999; 15: 87–9.

PUVA-cream therapy was as effective as PUVA-bath therapy in 12 patients.

Regression of relapsing dyshidrotic eczema after treatment of concomitant hyperhidrosis with botulinum toxin-A. Kontochristopoulos G, Gregoriou S, Agiasofitou E, Nikolakis G, Rigopoulos D, Katsambas A. [Letter] Dermatol Surg 2007; 33: 1289–90.

Two patients treated with 100 units of botulinum toxin A (BTX-A) to each hand showed significant improvement of their dyshidrosis 1 week later, with no relapse after 8 weeks.

Adjuvant botulinum toxin A in dyshidrotic hand eczema: a controlled prospective pilot study with left-right comparison. Wollina U, Karamfilov T. J Eur Acad Dermatol Venereol 2002; 16: 40–2.

Eight patients received daily topical corticosteroids and 100 units of BTX-A on the more severely affected hand. After 8 weeks, the mean DASI score had decreased from 28 to 17 with topical therapy alone and from 36 to 3 with adjuvant BTX-A. No relapses were seen in the BTX-A group.

THIRD-LINE THERAPIES

▶ Ciclosporin	B
▶ Methotrexate	D
▶ Azathioprine	C
▶ Mycophenolate mofetil	D
▶ Etanercept	D
▶ Iontophoresis	B
▶ Retinoids	D
▶ Khellin	D

Long-term follow-up of eczema patients treated with cyclosporine. Granlund H, Erkko P, Reitamo S. Acta Dermatol Venereol 1998; 78: 40–3.

Twenty-seven patients with chronic hand eczema treated with ciclosporin 3 mg/kg/day for 6 weeks had reduced disease activity of 54% and sustained improvement for 1 year.

Comparison of cyclosporine and topical betamethasone-17,21-dipropionate in the treatment of severe chronic hand eczema. Granlund H, Erkko P, Eriksson E, Reitamo S. Acta Dermatol Venereol 1996; 76: 371–6.

Ciclosporin A 3 mg/kg daily for 6 weeks was as effective as topical 0.05% betamethasone dipropionate (BDP) in 41 patients. Disease activity scores decreased to 57% of baseline. Relapses occurred to the same extent in both groups.

Evidence Levels: **A** Double-blind study **B** Clinical trial ≥ 20 subjects **C** Clinical trial < 20 subjects **D** Series ≥ 5 subjects **E** Anecdotal case reports

Low-dose oral methotrexate treatment for recalcitrant palmoplantar pompholyx. Egan CA, Rallis TM, Meadows KP, Krueger GG. J Am Acad Dermatol 1999; 40: 612–14.

In five patients with severe pompholyx 12.5–22.5 mg of methotrexate weekly resulted in a reduced dose or discontinuation of prednisone. Superpotent corticosteroids were continued topically.

Azathioprine in dermatological practice. An overview with special emphasis of its use in non-bullous inflammatory dermatoses. Scerri L. Adv Exp Med Biol 1999; 455: 343–8.

Six patients with severe pompholyx received azathioprine monotherapy 100–150 mg daily initially and then 50–100 mg daily for maintenance after resolution of lesions; three had excellent, one had good, and two had fair responses.

Dyshidrotic eczema treated with mycophenolate mofetil. Pickenacker A, Luger TA, Schwarz T. Arch Dermatol 1998; 134: 378–9.

One patient with recurrent dyshidrotic eczema refractory to topical and systemic corticosteroids and UVA1 had complete resolution after 4 weeks of 1.5 g twice daily and 12 months of 1 g daily.

Successful treatment of dyshidrotic hand eczema using tap water iontophoresis with pulsed direct current. Odia S, Vocks E, Rakoski J, Ring J. Acta Dermatol Venereol 1996; 76: 472–4.

Twenty patients treated with topical tar and zinc oxide paste to both palms and iontophoresis to one palm showed significantly less itching and vesicle formation on the iontophoresis-treated side.

Recalcitrant hand pompholyx: variable response to etanercept. Ogden S, Clayton TH, Goodfield MJ. Clin Exp Dermatol 2006; 31: 145–6.

One patient responded significantly to etanercept 25 mg twice weekly for 6 weeks. The remission lasted 4 months. A subsequent flare was unresponsive to etanercept 50 mg twice weekly.

Successful treatment of chronic hand eczema with oral 9-*cis*-retinoic acid. Bollag W, Ott F. Dermatology 1999; 199: 308–12.

Thirty-eight patients with refractory hand eczema were treated with 20 mg or 40 mg of oral 9-*cis*-retinoic acid: 55% showed a very good response and 34% a good response. Remission lasted between 1 month and more than a year.

Topical khellin and natural sunlight in the outpatient treatment of recalcitrant palmoplantar pompholyx: report of an open pilot study. Capella GL. Dermatology 2005; 211: 381–3.

Four patients treated with daily khellin 3% gel and sunlight exposure showed improvement in the DASI score from 9.5 to 2.5.

Porokeratoses

Agustin Martin-Clavijo, Antonios Kanelleas,
Christina Vlachou, John Berth-Jones

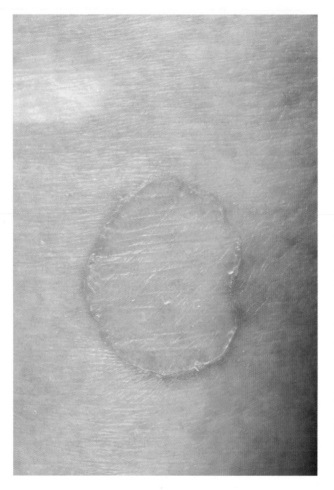

The porokeratoses are a group of disorders of keratinization characterized by lesions with a peripheral keratotic ridge, manifesting histologically as a cornoid lamella. Terminology and classification are debated, but five main forms are recognized: 1) the disseminated form, of which disseminated superficial actinic porokeratosis (DSAP) is predominant; 2) porokeratosis of Mibelli (PM); 3) giant porokeratosis; 4) palmoplantar porokeratosis (porokeratosis palmaris, plantaris et disseminata – PPPD); 5) linear porokeratosis (LP). An autosomal dominant mode of inheritance has been reported in the disseminated form. Overexpression of the p53 tumour suppression protein has been identified in the cornoid lamella. Porokeratotic lesions are progressive and carry malignant potential, especially large long-standing lesions and the linear variants. In addition, the lesions can cause pruritus and represent a cosmetic problem for some patients.

MANAGEMENT STRATEGY

The family history should be reviewed and patients' immune function assessed, particularly with the disseminated forms. Discontinuation of immunosuppression has led to resolution of lesions in some patients.

Treatment of porokeratoses may be indicated, not only for cosmetic benefit and symptomatic relief, but also to reduce the risk of malignancy. Optimal therapy is dependent on the type and extent of porokeratosis, and the level of concern over malignant progression. Management should include avoidance of irradiation (UV or X-rays) and observation for signs of malignant transformation (squamous cell carcinoma, basal cell carcinoma, Bowen's disease).

The lesions are usually asymptomatic. When present, pruritus associated with disseminated lesions is often responsive to *topical corticosteroids*. The palmoplantar variant may cause functional disability due to pain and discomfort.

Localized disease responds to 'surgical' methods such as *cryotherapy, CO$_2$ laser*, or *excision*, but these can result in significant scarring, especially when the lesions are numerous.

Topical 5-fluorouracil, imiquimod, and vitamin D analogs can be helpful, but only partial responses are likely in DSAP. Inflammatory reactions are likely when using 5-fluorouracil or imiquimod and indicate a greater likelihood of response. With some caution, these modalities can be used under occlusion, treating one area at a time. In the authors' experience results are inconsistent, even with occlusion.

Systemic retinoids have been effective in localized and systemic disease, but there have been reports of exacerbation of pre-existing lesions. Recurrence is common on discontinuation of therapy, and a long-term maintenance dose may be required. This modality might also reduce the risk of malignant transformation.

There is one report of genital DSAP responding partially to *topical diclofenac*, but a subsequent case series demonstrated very limited benefit. There are also reports of the effectiveness of *topical retinoids, dermabrasion, pulsed dye laser, Nd:YAG laser, corticosteroids*, and *topical photodynamic therapy*.

SPECIFIC INVESTIGATIONS

- ▶ Skin biopsy
- ▶ Dermoscopy
- ▶ Assessment of immune function

Porokeratosis of Mibelli. Overview and review of the literature. Schamroth JM, Zlotogorski A, Gilead L. Acta Dermatol Venereol 1997; 77: 207–13.

The pathological hallmark of porokeratosis is the cornoid lamella, which is typically found at the border of the lesion. The cornoid lamella forms a column of parakeratosis extending through the orthokeratotic stratum corneum. The granular layer beneath the cornoid lamella is usually absent, or markedly reduced in thickness. Dyskeratotic and vacuolated cells are often seen in the spinous layer beneath the cornoid lamella. An inflammatory infiltrate is seen in the dermis.

A good review article.

Gene expression profiling of porokeratosis demonstrates similarities with psoriasis. Hivnor C, Williams N, Singh F, VanVoorhees A, Dzubow L, Baldwin D, et al. J Cutan Pathol 2004; 31: 657–64.

The gene expression profile of a cornoid lamella was similar to those found in psoriasis.

This study supports the hypothesis that porokeratosis is a disorder of hyperproliferative keratinocytes exhibiting similarity to psoriasis at a molecular level. Consequently, some therapeutic maneuvers valuable in psoriasis may be beneficial in porokeratotic lesions.

584

Dermoscopy for the diagnosis of porokeratosis. Delfino M, Argenziano G, Nino M. J Eur Acad Dermatol Venereol 2004; 18: 194–5.

Dermoscopic examination of DSAP showed a characteristic central scar-like area with a single or double 'white track' structure at the margin. The histopathologic correlate of the linear structure was shown to be the cornoid lamella.

FIRST-LINE THERAPIES

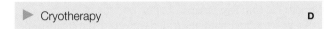

▶ Cryotherapy   **D**

Porokeratosis of Mibelli: successful treatment with cryosurgery. Dereli T, Ozyurt S, Osturk G. J Dermatol 2004; 31: 223–7.

Eight patients with 20 lesions received treatment with 30-second cycles of cryospray followed by sharp dissection of the lesion border. Most lesions resolved after one treatment; two required one further treatment.

Cryosurgery of porokeratosis plantaris discreta. Limmer BL. Arch Dermatol 1979; 115: 582–3.

Twenty-one lesions of porokeratosis in 11 patients were treated with cryotherapy, resulting in a cure rate of 90.5%. The lesions were pared prior to treatment. There was no evidence of recurrence over an average follow-up period of 22 months.

SECOND-LINE THERAPIES

▶ 5-Fluorouracil   **D**
▶ Imiquimod   **E**
▶ Vitamin D$_3$ analogs   **E**

Disseminated superficial porokeratosis: rapid therapeutic response to 5-fluorouracil. Shelley WB, Shelley ED. Cutis 1983; 32: 139–40.

Resolution of porokeratosis was observed after 3 weeks of daily application of 5% 5-fluorouracil cream. There was no recurrence at 5-month follow-up.

Fluorouracil ointment treatment of porokeratosis of Mibelli. Gonçalves JC. Arch Dermatol 1973; 108: 131–2.

Six patients with facial lesions were treated with 5% fluorouracil ointment three times daily. The treatment was maintained for 8–10 days after a strong inflammatory response occurred. There was no recurrence at 9-month follow-up.

Porokeratosis of Mibelli: successful treatment with 5% imiquimod cream. Agarwal S, Berth-Jones J. Br J Dermatol 2002; 146: 338–9.

A 3-cm lesion of PM on the leg was initially treated with topical imiquimod 5% cream five times a week for 3 months, with no improvement. Subsequent treatment with imiquimod 5% cream five times a week under occlusion with an adhesive polythene dressing was successful. There was no recurrence at 1 year.

Porokeratosis of Mibelli: successful treatment with topical 5% imiquimod cream. Harrison S, Sinclair R. Australas J Dermatol 2003; 44: 281–3.

Clinical and histological clearance of a large PM on the shin was achieved with 6 weeks of three times a week application of 5% imiquimod cream without occlusion. A marked inflammatory response was observed. There was no recurrence at 24 months.

Disseminated superficial actinic porokeratosis: treatment with topical tacalcitol. Bohm M, Luger TA, Bonsmann G. J Am Acad Dermatol 1999; 40: 479–80.

DSAP responded to 5 months of topical daily treatment with 0.0004% tacalcitol and remained clear on alternate-day maintenance therapy.

Disseminated superficial actinic porokeratosis responding to calcipotriol. Harrison PV, Stollery N. Clin Exp Dermatol 1994; 19: 95.

Three patients were treated with topical calcipotriol daily for 6–8 weeks. An overall improvement of 50–75% was noted and maintained for up to 6 months in two patients.

THIRD-LINE THERAPIES

▶ Systemic retinoids	**D**
▶ Topical retinoids	**E**
▶ CO$_2$ laser	**D**
▶ Nd:YAG laser	**E**
▶ Pulsed dye laser	**E**
▶ Fractional photothermolysis	**E**
▶ Photodynamic therapy	**E**
▶ Dermabrasion	**E**
▶ Fluorhydroxy pulse peel	**E**
▶ Corticosteroids	**E**
▶ Diclofenac 3% gel	**E**

Generalized linear porokeratosis treated with etretinate. Goldman GD, Milstone LM. Arch Dermatol 1995; 131: 496–7.

A patient treated with etretinate 50–75 mg daily showed significant improvement within 4 weeks.

Disseminated porokeratosis Mibelli treated with RO 10–9359. Bundino S, Zina AM. Dermatologica 1980; 160: 328–36.

Two patients with DSAP were treated with 50–75 mg daily of etretinate, with significant clinical improvement after 5 weeks; 25 mg daily was sufficient to maintain the results. Recurrence was observed 3–4 weeks after cessation of treatment.

Etretinate in the treatment of disseminated porokeratosis of Mibelli. Hacham-Zadeh S, Holubar K. Int J Dermatol 1985; 24: 258–60.

A 30-year-old man received 50–75 mg of etretinate daily, with significant clinical improvement after 2 weeks.

Etretinate improves localized porokeratosis of Mibelli. Campbell JP, Voorhees JJ. Int J Dermatol 1985; 24: 261–3.

A patient received etretinate 0.6–1 mg/kg daily for psoriasis, resulting in resolution of a single plaque of porokeratosis on her thigh. No recurrence was seen at 17 months' follow-up.

Treatment of disseminated superficial actinic porokeratosis with a new aromatic retinoid (Ro 10–9359). Kariniemi A, Stubb S, Lassus A. Br J Dermatol 1980; 102: 213–14.

Treatment with 50–100 mg daily of etretinate led to significant clinical improvement and resolution of pruritus within 40 days. A dose of 25 mg on alternate days was required to maintain the results. After 6 months of treatment the patient developed follicular hyperkeratosis with tiny keratin horns on the skin of both forearms.

Porokeratosis plantaris, palmaris, et disseminata. Report of a case and treatment with isotretinoin. McCallister RE, Estes SA, Yarbrough CL. J Am Acad Dermatol 1985; 13: 598–603.

A patient with familial PPPD received treatment with 1 mg/kg daily of isotretinoin. Significant clinical improvement was noted after 3 months of treatment. Two months after discontinuation of treatment a gradual recurrence was observed.

Porokeratosis plantaris, palmaris et disseminata. Marschalko M, Somlai B. Arch Dermatol 1986; 122: 890–1.

A case of familial PPPD was successfully treated with 25–50 mg daily of etretinate. Marked improvement was noted after 3 weeks of treatment.

Topical tretinoin in Indian male with zosteriform porokeratosis. Agrawal SK, Gandhi V, Madan V, Bhattacharya SN. Int J Dermatol 2003; 42: 919–20.

Once-daily application of topical tretinoin 0.1% gel led to resolution of lesions within 4 months.

Treatment of porokeratosis of Mibelli with CO_2 laser vaporization versus surgical excision with split-thickness skin graft. Rabbin PE, Baldwin HE. J Dermatol Surg Oncol 1993; 19: 199–202.

CO_2 vaporization resulted in better cosmetic and functional improvement than split skin grafting in one patient.

Reticulate porokeratosis – successful treatment with CO_2-laser vaporization. Merkle T, Hohenleutner U, Braun-Falco O, Landthaler M. Clin Exp Dermatol 1992; 17: 178–81.

CO_2 laser vaporization of mainly flexural lesions resulted in regression of lesions with slight atrophic scarring and lessening of pruritus. No further treatment was required in a 12-month follow-up period.

Treatment of lichen amyloidosis (LA) and disseminated superficial porokeratosis (DSP) with frequency-doubled Q-switched Nd:YAG laser. Liu HT. Dermatol Surg 2000; 26: 958–62.

A patient's face and arms were treated four times, 1 month apart, resulting in marked improvement, but not complete clearance of the lesions.

Successful treatment of porokeratosis with 585 nm pulsed dye laser irradiation. Alster TS, Nanni CA. Cutis 1999; 63: 265–6.

This is a case of LP that responded to a series of 585 nm pulsed dye laser treatments.

Fractional photothermolysis: a novel treatment for disseminated superficial actinic porokeratosis. Chrastil B, Glaich AS, Goldberg LH, Friedman PM. Arch Dermatol 2007; 143: 1450–2.

Two patients received three to six courses of fractioned photothermolysis (erbium-doped fiber laser). Both patients reported 50% improvement.

Successful treatment of disseminated superficial actinic porokeratosis with methyl aminolevulinate-photodynamic therapy. Cavicchini S, Tourlaki A. J Dermatol Treat 2006; 17: 190–1.

This case demonstrated a striking improvement in response to two treatments, 1 week apart, using methyl aminolevulinate cream 160 mg/g applied with occlusion for 3 hours before illumination with a red light (Aktilite) 37 J/cm².

Topical photodynamic therapy in disseminated superficial actinic porokeratosis. Nayeemuddin FA, Wong M, Yell J, Rhodes LE. Clin Exp Dermatol 2002; 27: 703–6.

A report on three patients treated with 20% ALA cream under occlusion for 5 hours prior to illumination with 100 J/cm² of broadband red light (Waldmann 1200). Resolution of two lesions of DSAP was observed in one case, but the response could not be reproduced in this or two other cases.

Successful treatment of porokeratosis of Mibelli with diamond fraise dermabrasion. Spencer JM, Katz BE. Arch Dermatol 1992; 128: 1187–8.

No recurrence observed at 15-month follow-up, but the lesion healed with slight hyperpigmentation and mild hypertrophy in a 79-year-old Filipino woman.

Linear porokeratosis: successful treatment with diamond fraise dermabrasion. Cohen PR, Held JL, Katz BE. J Am Acad Dermatol 1990; 23: 975–7.

An excellent cosmetic result. No recurrence or scarring observed after 8 months.

The use of fluor-hydroxy pulse peel in actinic porokeratosis. Teixeira SP, de Nascimento MM, Bagatin E, Hassun KM, Talarico S, Michalany N. Dermatol Surg 2005; 31: 1145–8.

This is a case of DSAP treated with a combination of a 70% glycolic peel and a 5% 5-fluorouracil solution every 2 weeks for 4 months. The result was improvement in the appearance and texture of the treated areas and reduced dyskeratosis and epidermal atypia.

Dexamethasone pulse treatment in disseminated porokeratosis of Mibelli. Verma KK, Singh OP. J Dermatol Sci 1994; 7: 71–2.

A familial case of progressive porokeratosis received pulses of 100 mg dexamethasone in 5% dextrose intravenously on 3 consecutive days in a month. No new lesions appeared after the first pulse, and clinical improvement was noted after four pulses. There was an 80% improvement after 18 pulses. The patient was then lost to follow-up.

Genital porokeratosis: treatment with diclofenac topical gel. Kluger N, Dereure O, Guilhou JJ, Guillot B. J Dermatol Treat 2007; 18: 188–90.

A partial response was observed in a case of genital porokeratosis after applying 3% diclofenac gel twice daily for 3 months.

Treatment of disseminated superficial actinic porokeratosis with topical diclofenac gel: a case series. Vlachou C, Kanelleas A, Martin-Clavijo A, Berth-Jones J. J Eur Acad Dermatol Venereol 2008; 22: 1343–5.

Eight patients with DSAP were treated with 3% diclofenac gel (Solaraze gel) twice daily for at least 6 months. At 6 months a partial improvement was seen in two cases, but no improvement in the others.

Evidence Levels: **A** Double-blind study **B** Clinical trial ≥ 20 subjects **C** Clinical trial < 20 subjects **D** Series ≥ 5 subjects **E** Anecdotal case reports

Porphyria cutanea tarda

Maureen B Poh-Fitzpatrick

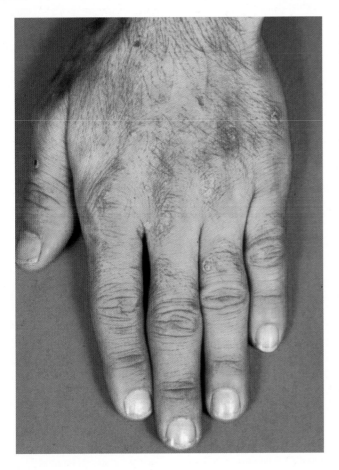

The term porphyria cutanea tarda (PCT) encompasses several related inherited or acquired disorders in which insufficient hepatic uroporphyrinogen decarboxylase enzyme activity causes overproduction of polycarboxylated porphyrins. These porphyrins mediate cutaneous photosensitivity manifested as fragility, bullae, hypertrichosis, dyspigmentation, sclerodermoid features, and scarring. Multiple factors may contribute to disease expression: mutant uroporphyrinogen decarboxylase genes, hemochromatosis genes or other predisposing genetic determinants; exposure to ethanol, estrogen, iron, hepatitis and human immunodeficiency viruses; hepatotoxic aromatic hydrocarbons and, rarely, hepatic tumors. Symptomatic PCT untreated over many years has been associated with hepatocellular carcinoma in older men with advanced liver pathology due to chronic ethanol abuse and/or viral hepatitis. Hepatic siderosis due to these disorders or to hemochromatosis is carcinogenic, as is porphyrin crystallization in hepatocytes.

MANAGEMENT STRATEGY

Because optimal management consists of induction of remission using strategies inappropriate for other porphyrias or pseudoporphyrias, a precise diagnosis is essential. Associated disorders that may influence management, such as viral infections, hemochromatosis, or other causes of excess iron storage, lupus erythematosus, diabetes mellitus, and anemias, should also be identified.

Eliminating exacerbating factors and pursuing ferrodepletion by *serial phlebotomy, deferoxamine (desferrioxamine) chelation,* or *erythropoietin bone marrow stimulation* can induce biochemical and clinical remission. Skin should be protected from sunlight exposure and mechanical trauma until full clinical remission is achieved. Porphyrin excretion can be increased using *chloroquine* or *hydroxychloroquine, enteric sorbents,* or *metabolic alkalinization.* *Interferon-α* or *antiretroviral drugs* may benefit PCT associated with hepatitis C or AIDS, respectively. Children can be treated by phlebotomy protocols adjusted for pediatric parameters. Rare reports of chloroquine or hydroxychloroquine treatment of children suggest that cautious low-dose schedules may be safe and effective. *Vitamins E and C, plasmapheresis or plasma exchange, high-flux hemodialysis,* and *cimetidine* have been reported as beneficial alternative or adjunctive therapies. Hepatoerythropoietic porphyria, caused by coinheritance of two uroporphyrinogen decarboxylase gene mutations, resists induction of remission, and so requires lifelong vigilant skin photoprotection. *Photothermolysis* using selected wavelengths may reduce persistent hypertrichosis.

SPECIFIC INVESTIGATIONS

> ▶ Porphyrin concentrations and types in erythrocytes, serum or urine, feces
> ▶ Hematological and iron profiles, serum ferritin, hemochromatosis gene analysis
> ▶ Liver function profile; serum α-fetoprotein level, liver imaging, and liver biopsy if clinically indicated
> ▶ Hepatitis A, B, and C viral serology
> ▶ HIV serology if risk factors are present
> ▶ Fasting blood glucose
> ▶ Serum antinuclear antibody

Porphyria cutanea tarda: clinical features and laboratory findings in forty patients. Grossman ME, Bickers DR, Poh-Fitzpatrick MB, DeLeo VA, Harber LC. Am J Med 1979; 67: 277–86.

Abnormalities of liver function, glucose tolerance, antinuclear antibody titers, other laboratory parameters, clinical manifestations, skin and liver histopathology, and experience with phlebotomy are surveyed in a large population.

Porphyria cutanea tarda, hepatitis C, and HFE gene mutations in North America. Bonkovsky HL, Poh-Fitzpatrick MB, Pimstone N, Obando J, Di Bisceglie A, Tattrie C, et al. Hepatology 1998; 27: 1661–9.

Of 70 American patients with PCT 53% had evidence of hepatitis C infection, and 43% of 26 patients had HFE gene mutations associated with hereditary hemochromatosis.

Iron overload in porphyria cutanea tarda. Sampietro M, Fiorelli G, Fargion S. Haematologica 1999; 84: 248–53.

Most patients with PCT have some degree of iron overload, and ferrodepletion leads to remission.

Excess liver iron triggers symptomatic PCT. Increased stored iron accompanies chronic alcoholism, hepatitis C, hemochromatosis, and end-stage renal disease. Iron-dependent partial oxidation of uroporphyrinogen to uroporphomethene, a competitive inhibitor of uroporphyrinogen decarboxylase, appears to be the mechanism by which its enzymatic activity is reduced in PCT (Phillips et al. Proc Natl Acad

Sci USA 2007; 104: 5079–84). Iron-enhanced complete oxidation of uroporphyrinogen substrate accumulated due to inhibited enzyme activity yields photoactive uroporphyrin.

Hepatocellular carcinoma risk in patients with porphyria cutanea tarda. Gisbert JP, Garcia-Buey L, Alonso A, Rubio S, Hernandez A, Pajares JM, et al. Eur J Gastroenterol Hepatol 2004; 16: 689–92.

These authors recommend that patients presenting with PCT should undergo serological viral hepatitis testing and liver biopsy, and those with concomitant hepatitis C infection or advanced fibrosis/cirrhosis should be monitored with semiannual ultrasonography and serum α-fetoprotein testing.

The decision for liver biopsy should be weighed carefully. Patients without risk factors for hepatic siderosis or other pathology (i.e., women with estrogen use as the only identifiable PCT-inducing factor) may not need this invasive procedure.

An unhappy triad: hemochromatosis, porphyria cutanea tarda, and hepatocellular carcinoma – a case report. Mogi M, Pascher A, Presser SJ, Schwalbe M, Neuhaus P, Nuessler N. World J Gastroenterol 2007; 13: 1998–2001.

Hepatic siderosis is a risk factor for liver cancer.
Porphyrin crystals in hepatocytes may also be carcinogenic.

FIRST-LINE THERAPIES

▶ Serial phlebotomies	**B**
▶ Chloroquine, hydroxychloroquine	**B**

The effect of phlebotomy therapy in porphyria cutanea tarda. Ippen H. Semin Hematol 1977; 14: 253–9.

Repeated venesection led to reduction of porphyrins and serum iron, improvement of photocutaneous lesions, and normalization of liver function tests in the majority of 351 patients.

Phlebotomy schedules should be adjusted to the tolerance of individual patients, typically ranging from 200 to 500 mL of whole blood at twice-weekly to fortnightly or monthly intervals. Keeping hemoglobin over 10–11 g/dL minimizes symptoms of iatrogenic anemia.

Childhood-onset familial porphyria cutanea tarda: effects of therapeutic phlebotomy. Poh-Fitzpatrick MB, Honig PJ, Kim HC, Sassa S. J Am Acad Dermatol 1992; 27: 896–900.

Phlebotomy guidelines for children are described.

Plasma ferritin levels as a guide to the treatment of porphyria cutanea tarda by venesection. Ratnaike S, Blake D, Campbell D, Cowen P, Varigos G. Australas J Dermatol 1988; 29: 3–8.

Phlebotomy can be terminated when iron stores, as reflected by plasma ferritin concentration, have fallen to low normal levels.

Reduction of porphyrins in plasma or serum or urine and clinical improvement typically begin during therapy and continue for weeks to months after venesection stops; patients should avoid sunlight and trauma after treatment until photosensitivity remits completely. Clinical improvement precedes full biochemical normalization.

Treatment of porphyria cutanea tarda with chloroquine. Korda V, Semrádová M. Br J Dermatol 1974; 90: 95–100.

Twenty-one adults received oral chloroquine 125 mg twice a week until cutaneous blistering and fragility ceased and urinary uroporphyrins fell below three times the normal limit. Mean duration of treatment was 8.5 months (range 4–11 months) in 19 patients. Serum transaminases and urinary uroporphyrins rose during initial weeks of therapy, and then progressively diminished.

Chloroquine risks include irreversible retinopathy after large cumulative doses (>100–300 g), but retinal toxicity is infrequent at dose rates less than 4 mg/kg daily (<6.5 mg/kg daily for hydroxychloroquine). Ophthalmologic examinations at baseline and 6-monthly intervals are recommended. The risk of hemolysis can be minimized by pretreatment testing for glucose-6-phosphate dehydrogenase deficiency and interval monitoring of hematological profiles during therapy.

Childhood-onset porphyria cutanea tarda: successful therapy with low-dose hydroxychloroquine (Plaquenil). Bruce AJ, Ahmed I. J Am Acad Dermatol 1998; 38: 810–14.

A 4-year-old child given hydroxychloroquine 3 mg/kg twice weekly for 14 months, plus vitamin E 200 U/day, achieved remission without adverse side effects.

Choice of therapy in porphyria cutanea tarda. Adjarov D, Naydenova E, Ivanov E, Ivanova A. Clin Exp Dermatol 1996; 21: 461–2.

The effectiveness of phlebotomy (500 mL weekly for 4 weeks, then monthly) versus oral chloroquine 250 mg twice weekly alone versus combined phlebotomy/chloroquine therapies was retrospectively analyzed in unequal groups totaling 115 patients. Remissions occurred more quickly and reliably with phlebotomy than with chloroquine. Combined therapy shortened the mean total treatment course by approximately 1.5 months only when initial urinary uroporphyrin levels exceeded 3000 nmol/24 h.

Others found that remissions occurred more quickly with chloroquine versus venesection (10.2 months in 24 patients, 12.5 months in 15 patients, respectively), whereas combination therapy was most rapid (3.5 months in 20 patients) (Seubert et al. Z Hautkr 1990; 65: 223–5).

Hemochromatosis (HFE) gene mutations and response to chloroquine in porphyria cutanea tarda. Stolzel U, Kostler E, Schuppan D, Richter M, Wollina U, Doss MO, et al. Arch Dermatol 2003; 139: 379–80.

Chloroquine was effective in heterozygotes with one of the major HFE mutations (C282Y, H63D), or compound heterozygotes, but C282Y homozygotes failed to improve, and serum iron decreased only in patients with PCT and wild-type HFE. Phlebotomy is the recommended therapy for patients with PCT and HFE gene mutations.

SECOND-LINE THERAPIES

▶ Deferoxamine (desferrioxamine)	**B**
▶ Erythropoietin	**D**

Liver iron overload and desferrioxamine treatment of porphyria cutanea tarda. Rocchi E, Cassanelli M, Borghi A, Paolillo F, Pradelli M, Pellizzardi S, et al. Dermatologica 1991; 182: 27–31.

Ferrodepletion by desferrioxamine 1.5 g subcutaneous pump infusions 5 days/week (18 patients) or 200 mg/kg infused intravenously once weekly (five patients), or by serial phle-

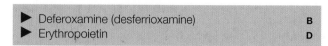

botomies (22 patients) led to clinical remission after nearly 6 months with all treatments. Normalization of serum ferritin and uroporphyrins occurred at approximately 11 months with chelation, and approximately 13 months with venesection; liver function improved with both modalities.

Chelation is expensive and cumbersome, and thus best reserved for cases in which first-line therapies are inadequate or inappropriate.

Haemodialysis-related porphyria cutanea tarda and treatment by recombinant human erythropoietin. Yaqoob M, Smyth J, Ahmad R, McClelland P, Fahal I, Kumar KA, et al. Nephron 1992; 60: 418–31.

A patient receiving erythropoietin 50 U/kg thrice weekly over several months, without adjunctive phlebotomy, exhibited lowered serum ferritin and porphyrin levels and resolution of bullous dermatosis.

Erythropoiesis may be sufficiently stimulated in patients with pre-existing anemias to support serial phlebotomies at judicious volumes and intervals, thereby accelerating ferrodepletion. Doses up to 150 U/kg three times weekly may be needed to gain this level of response.

Successful treatment of haemodialysis-related porphyria cutanea tarda with deferoxamine. Pitche P, Corrin E, Wolkenstein P, Revuz J, Bagot M. Ann Dermatol Venereol 2003; 130: 37–9.

Intravenous deferoxamine 40 mg/kg weekly for 6 weeks led to normalization of clinical and biological signs of PCT in the setting of end-stage renal disease and chronic hemodialysis in one patient that persisted for 12 months.

This rapid and persistent improvement remains to be confirmed in larger trials.

THIRD-LINE THERAPIES

▶ Antiretroviral therapy	E
▶ Interferon-α	E
▶ Vitamins E and C	D
▶ Plasmapheresis, plasma exchange	D
▶ High-flux hemodialysis	D
▶ Enteric sorbents (cholestyramine, activated charcoal)	D
▶ Metabolic alkalinization by oral sodium bicarbonate	D
▶ Cimetidine	E
▶ Photothermolysis	E

Highly active antiretroviral therapy leading to resolution of porphyria cutanea tarda in a patient with AIDS and hepatitis C. Rich JD, Mylonakis E, Nossa R, Chapnick RM. Dig Dis Sci 1999; 44: 1034–7.

The association between PCT and HIV infection is less well established than the association of PCT with the hepatitis C virus. It is possible that the hepatitis C virus may trigger PCT in patients with HIV infection.

Dramatic resolution of skin lesions associated with porphyria cutanea tarda – interferon-alpha therapy in a case of chronic hepatitis C. Shiekh MY, Wright RA, Burruss JB. Dig Dis Sci 1998; 43: 529–33.

Anecdotal reports of PCT improvement during interferon treatment of concurrent hepatitis C infection must be balanced against those of PCT appearing 1–4 months after initiation of hepatitis C treatment with interferon/ribavirin protocols (Thevenot, et al. J Hepatol 2005; 42: 607–8). Ribavirin-induced hemolysis may increase liver iron, thereby triggering PCT. Measures to reduce liver iron (i.e., phlebotomy) prior to initiation of interferon, especially when combined with ribavirin, are recommended in patients with viral hepatitis and coincident symptomatic PCT or indices of excess tissue iron stores.

High-dose vitamin E lowers urine porphyrin levels in patients affected by porphyria cutanea tarda. Pinelli A, Trivulzio S, Tomasoni L, Bertolini B, Pinelli G. Pharmacol Res 2002; 45: 355–9.

Oral vitamin E (1 g daily) reduced urinary uroporphyrin levels and attenuated skin lesions during a 4-week trial.

Removal of plasma porphyrins with high-flux hemodialysis in porphyria cutanea tarda associated with end stage renal disease. Carson RW, Dunnigan EJ, DuBose TD Jr, Goeger DE, Anderson KE. J Am Soc Nephrol 1992; 2: 1445–50.

High-flux hemodialysis may remove porphyrins more effectively than conventional hemodialysis.

Treatment of hemodialysis related porphyria cutanea tarda with plasma exchange. Disler P, Day R, Burman N, Blekkenhorst G, Eales L. Am J Med 1982; 72: 989–93.

This may aid patients with PCT and chronic renal failure for whom other treatments are unavailable.

The adsorption of porphyrins and porphyria precursors by sorbents: a potential therapy for the porphyrias. Tishler PV, Gordon RJ, O'Connor JA. Meth Find Exp Clin Pharmacol 1982; 4: 125–31.

Metabolic alkalinization therapy in porphyria cutanea tarda. Perry HO, Mullanax MG, Weigand SE. Arch Dermatol 1970; 102: 359–67.

Cimetidine in the treatment of porphyria cutanea tarda. Horie Y, Tanaka K, Okano J, Ohgi N, Kawasaki H, Yamamoto S, et al. Intern Med 1996; 35: 717–19.

In this report cimetidine reduced porphyrin levels within 2 weeks. This benign treatment may be of value in patients unwilling or unable to try standard therapeutic approaches.

Management of porphyria cutanea tarda in the setting of chronic renal failure – case report and review. Shieh S, Cohen JL, Lim HW. J Am Acad Dermatol 2000; 42: 645–52.

This survey of therapies applicable in the context of renal failure includes additional references for several third-line agents listed above.

Successful and safe treatment of hypertrichosis by high-intensity pulses of noncoherent light in a patient with hepatoerythropoietic porphyria. Garcia-Bravo M, Lopez-Gomez S, Segurado-Rodriguez MA, Morán-Jiménez MJ, Méndez M, Enriquez de Salamanca R, et al. Arch Dermatol Res 2004: 296: 139–40.

Hypertrichosis was almost completely removed after seven sessions without development of skin lesions.

Port wine stains

Brandie J Metz, Lawrence F Eichenfield

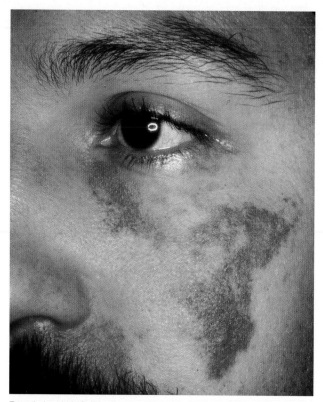

From Lebwohl MG. The Skin and Systemic Disease: A Color Atlas, 2nd edn. Churchill Livingstone 2003, with permission of Elsevier.

Port wine stains (PWS) are congenital benign capillary malformations of the superficial cutaneous vasculature. They usually present early in life as light pink to red patches that may darken and develop surface irregularities with time. The head and neck are sites of predilection, but any part of the integument can be affected. PWS are not only cosmetically distressing, but may be associated with serious physical, social, and psychological sequelae.

MANAGEMENT STRATEGY

Many therapeutic modalities have been used to treat PWS, including surgical excision and grafting, dermabrasion, cryotherapy, radiation therapy, electrotherapy, and tattooing. All have been associated with unfavorable outcomes. Various *lasers* have been used, including CO_2, Nd:YAG, and copper vapor laser, but results have been unsatisfactory. At one stage the argon laser was considered the best therapeutic method for PWS. However, hypertrophic scarring as a major complication of argon laser has limited its use.

Flashlamp-pumped pulsed dye laser is considered by most authorities as the treatment of choice for PWS. Wavelengths of 585–595 nm and pulse durations of 450–3000 μs allow for a deep, safe, and specific action that is confined to the targeted vasculature. Lightening and/or reduction in size of the stain is directly related to the number of treatments. Initial treatments usually give the highest percentage of improvement.

Measures to overcome the pain and anxiety associated with laser use include topical anesthetics such as a eutectic mixture of lidocaine and prilocaine, liposomal 4% lidocaine, S-Caine Peel, local lidocaine infiltration, nerve block, and general anesthesia. New generations of flashlamp-pumped pulsed dye lasers with cooling devices markedly reduce the pain of laser procedures.

PWS can either occur as isolated findings or be associated with eye or central nervous system (CNS) structural abnormalities. They may also be associated with limb overgrowth (Klippel–Trenaunay syndrome), or with other vascular malformations (e.g., capillary–venous, capillary–venous–lymphatic, capillary–arteriovenous).

SPECIFIC INVESTIGATIONS

- ▶ Ophthalmologic examination
- ▶ CT or MRI

Facial port wine stain and Sturge–Weber syndrome. Enjolras O, Riche MC, Merland JJ. Pediatrics 1985; 76: 48–51.

Sturge–Weber syndrome (SWS) was present in 28.5% of patients with PWS covering the V1 trigeminal sensory area alone or in association with V2 and V3, and 9.5% had glaucoma. None of the patients with PWS located in the V2 and/or the V3 areas had ocular or pial vascular abnormalities.

Location of port wine stains and the likelihood of ophthalmic and/or central nervous system complications. Tallman B, Tan OT, Morelli JG, Piepenbrink J, Stafford TJ, Trainor S, et al. Pediatrics 1991; 87: 323–7.

Among patients with trigeminal PWS, 8% had evidence of eye and/or CNS involvement. PWS of the eyelids, bilateral distribution, and unilateral PWS involving all three branches of the trigeminal nerve were associated with a significantly higher likelihood of having eye and/or CNS complications.

Patients with such presentations should be screened for glaucoma, and the risk of CNS involvement should be discussed with the family and appropriate testing considered.

Sturge–Weber syndrome: age of onset of seizures and glaucoma and the prognosis for affected children. Sujansky E, Conradi S. J Child Neurol 1995; 10: 49–58.

In this study of 171 patients with SWS, seizures were present in 80% and were almost always associated with PWS in V1 alone or V1 and V2 trigeminal dermatomes. Glaucoma was present in 48% of patients; 92% of the patients with glaucoma had PWS in V1 and V2 areas, whereas 8% had only V1 involvement. Glaucoma was diagnosed during the first year of life in 61% and by 5 years of age in 72%.

Sturge–Weber syndrome and dermatomal facial port wine stains: Incidence, association with glaucoma, and pulsed tunable dye laser treatment effectiveness. Hennedige AA, Quaba AA, Al-Nikib K. Plast Reconstruct Surg 2008; 121: 1173–80.

In this study of 874 patients Sturge–Weber syndrome occurred in 3% of all patients with facial port wine stains and 10% of those whose port wine stains were in a dermatomal distribution. Although both SWS and glaucoma occurred in patients with only V1 involvement, the risk increased substantially with V1+V2 and V1+V2+V3 involvement. No patients with only V3 involvement had eye or CNS findings.

Evidence Levels: **A** Double-blind study **B** Clinical trial ≥ 20 subjects **C** Clinical trial < 20 subjects **D** Series ≥ 5 subjects **E** Anecdotal case reports

Children at risk of SWS should have ophthalmologic examination in the neonatal period and require ophthalmologic follow-up because glaucoma may develop subsequent to initial presentation.

Sturge–Weber syndrome. The current neuroradiologic data. Boukobza M, Enjolras O, Cambra M, Merland J. J Radiol 2000; 81: 765–71.

A neonatal neuroimaging work-up using CT or MRI may not demonstrate the pial anomaly and may be delayed or repeated after 6–12 months in an at-risk infant with V1 PWS.

FIRST-LINE THERAPIES

▶ Pulsed dye laser   **B**

Anatomic differences of port wine stains in response to treatment with pulsed dye laser. Renfro L, Geronemus RG. Arch Dermatol 1993; 129: 182–8.

Centrofacial lesions and lesions involving dermatome V2 responded less favorably than lesions located elsewhere on the head and neck.

Port wine stains. An assessment of 5 years of treatment. Orten SS, Waner M, Flock S, Roberson PK, Kincannon J. Arch Otolaryngol Head Neck Surg 1996; 122: 1174–9.

Fewer treatments were required for nevus flammeus (NF), forehead and temple, lateral aspect of the face, neck, chest, and shoulder lesions. Lesions involving facial dermatomes, medial and central aspect of the face, midline of the face (excluding NF), and the extremities required more treatments. Recurrence rate following completion of treatment was 3.1%, 20.8%, and 50% at 1, 2, and more than 3 years, respectively.

Facial port wine stains in childhood: prediction of the rate of improvement as a function of the age of the patient, size and location of the port wine stain and the number of treatments with the pulsed dye (585 nm) laser. Nguyen CM, Yohn JJ, Huff C, Weston WL, Morelli JG. Br J Dermatol 1998; 138: 821–5.

Major determinants of treatment response in order of decreasing importance are PWS location, size, and patient age. The most successful responses are seen in young patients (under 1 year of age) with small PWS ($<20\,cm^2$) located over bony areas of the face, such as the central forehead. The greatest percentage of size reduction occurred after the first five treatments. There was less reduction in size with subsequent treatments.

Efficacy of early treatment of facial port wine stains in newborns: A review of 49 cases. Chapas AM, Eickhorst K, Geronemus RG. Lasers Surg Med 2007; 39: 563–8.

Patients who received treatment with the cryogen spray-cooled 595-nm pulsed dye laser before 6 months of age achieved a mean 88.6% clearance after 1 year, after an average of nine treatments. Higher clearance rates were observed for smaller lesions and V1 dermatome lesions.

Treatment of children with port wine stains using the flash lamp pulsed tunable dye laser. Tan OT, Sherwood K, Gilchrest BA. N Engl J Med 1989; 320: 416–21.

Children less than 7 years of age required fewer sessions than older children.

Treatment of port wine stains (capillary malformations) with the flash lamp pumped pulsed dye laser. Goldman MP, Fitzpatrick RE, Ruiz-Esparza J. J Pediatr 1993; 122: 71–7.

Clinical improvement correlated with number of treatments. Initial treatment in children with PWS results in approximately 40% improvement, and each subsequent treatment up to six adds a further increment of 10% improvement. Treatments should be continued as long as there is incremental improvement.

Effect of the timing of treatment of port wine stains with the flash lamp pumped pulsed dye laser. Van der Horst CM, Koster PH, de Borgie CA, Bossuyt PM, Van Gemert MJ. N Engl J Med 1998; 338: 1028–33.

No difference in laser treatment outcome was noticed among different age groups. There were four age groups: 0–5 years, 6–11 years, 12–17 years, and 18–31 years.

Few patients under the age of 12 months were included in this study, making it difficult to compare with others.

High-fluence modified pulsed dye laser photocoagulation with dynamic cooling of port wine stains in infancy. Geronemus RG, Quintana AT, Lou WW, Kauvar AN. Arch Dermatol 2000; 136: 942–3.

Early intervention during infancy using a modified pulsed dye laser with a longer wavelength (595 nm), broader pulse width (1.5 ms), dynamic cooling spray, and high-energy fluences can result in lightening or clearing of PWS with minimal risk of adverse effects.

Redarkening of port-wine stains 10 years after pulsed-dye-laser treatment. Huikeshoven M, Koster PH, deBorgie CA, Beek JF, van Gemert MJ, van der Horst CM. N Engl J Med 2007; 356: 1235–40.

In this study of patients from a previously published prospective study, the median duration of follow-up was 9.5 years. Port wine stains were, on average, darker than when measured after the last of the five initial treatments, although still lighter than when measured before treatment.

Patients should be counseled that due to progressive ectasia of PWS vessels 'recurrence,' or re-darkening of the stain, is a possibility.

Pain relief measures and cooling devices

Effects of percutaneous local anaesthetics on pain reduction during pulse dye laser treatment of port wine stains. McCafferty DF, Woolfson AD, Handley J, Allen G. Br J Anaesth 1997; 78: 286–9.

Both EMLA and 4% tetracaine gel were statistically superior to placebo in reducing pain caused by the laser treatment.

The S-Caine peel: a novel topical anesthetic for cutaneous laser surgery. Bryan HA, Alster TS. Dermatol Surg 2002; 28: 999–1003.

Patients who received S-Caine Peel experienced a significant reduction in pain vs placebo when treated with 595 nm pulsed dye laser. Application for 20 and 30 minutes was as effective as application for 60 minutes.

Effect of the topical anesthetic EMLA on the efficacy of pulsed dye laser treatment of port wine stains. Ashinoff R, Geronemus RG. J Dermatol Surg Oncol 1990; 16: 1008–11.

The use of topical anesthetic creams or sedating agents has been shown not to interfere with laser therapy.

Cryogen spray cooling and higher fluence pulsed dye laser treatment improve port wine stain clearance while minimizing epidermal damage. Chang CJ, Nelson JS. Dermatol Surg 1999; 25: 767–72.

A retrospective study of 196 patients with head and neck PWS, indicating the statistically significant advantage of using a cryogen spray-cooling device with pulsed dye laser by permitting higher light dosages and a subsequent higher clearance rate without increasing the rate of complications.

General anesthesia for pediatric dermatologic procedures: risks and complications. Cunningham BB, Gigler V, Wang K, Eichenfield LF, Friedlander SF, Garden JM, et al. Arch Dermatol 2005; 141: 573–6.

A review of 881 cases performed on 269 pediatric patients, 88% of which were pulsed dye laser treatment of vascular lesions, including PWS. There were no life-threatening events and the mortality rate was zero.

The use of general anesthesia for dermatologic procedures performed in a children's hospital setting is safe with a low rate of complications.

SECOND-LINE THERAPIES

▶ Intense pulsed light source		**B**
▶ Neodymium:yttrium–aluminum–garnet (Nd:YAG) laser		**B**

Treatment of port wine stain with a non-coherent pulsed light source: a retrospective study. Raulin C, Schroeter CA, Weiss RA, Keiner M, Werner S. Arch Dermatol 1999; 125: 679–83.

Between 70% and 100% clearing of PWS in 28 of 40 patients treated by intense pulsed light source after an average of four treatments for pink PWS (100% clearance), 1.5 for red PWS (100% clearance), and 4.2 for purple PWS (70–99% clearance).

Intense pulsed light source for the treatment of dye laser resistant port-wine stains. Bjerring P, Christiansen K, Troilius A. J Cosmet Laser Ther 2003; 5: 7–13.

A greater than 50% reduction was achieved after four treatments with intense pulsed light source in 46.7% of 15 patients with PWS previously treated by pulsed dye laser. None of the lesions located in V2 responded.

There are several case reports of successful treatment of resistant PWS with intense pulsed light source. However, controlled studies are needed to confirm this observation.

Long-pulsed neodymium:yttrium–aluminum–garnet laser treatment for port wine stains. Yang MU, Yaroslavsky AN, Farinelli WA, Flotte TJ, Rius-Diaz F, Tsao S, et al. J Am Acad Dermatol 2005; 52: 480–90.

Treatment achieved similar 50–75% clearing with both the pulsed dye laser and the Nd:YAG laser at minimum purpura dose (MPD). The pulsed dye laser performed significantly better than the Nd:YAG at fluences lower than 1 MPD, and scarring occurred in the only patient who was treated with the Nd:YAG laser at a fluence greater than 1 MPD.

Nd:YAG may be an alternative treatment option, although there is a narrow margin at which this laser is both safe and effective.

A direct comparison of pulsed dye, alexandrite, KTP and Nd: YAG lasers and IPL in patients with previously treated capillary malformations. McGill DJ, MacLaren W, Mackay IR. Lasers Surg Med 2008; 40: 390–98.

Patients with PWS previously treated with PDL were treated using the alexandrite, KTP, and Nd:YAG lasers and intense pulsed light (IPL), with additional PDL patches as a control. Fifty-five percent of patients achieved some lightening with the alexandrite laser, although a high percentage also developed hyperpigmentation or scarring. Thirty-three percent achieved some lightening with IPL, 11% each for KTP and Nd:YAG, and 28% with further PDL pulses.

THIRD-LINE THERAPIES

▶ Potassium titanyl phosphate (KTP) laser		**B**

Potassium titanyl phosphate laser treatment of resistant port-wine stains. Chowdhury MU, Harris S, Lanigan SW. Br J Dermatol 2001; 144: 814–17.

A greater than 50% reduction was seen in 17% of 30 patients with PWS previously treated by pulsed dye laser; 20% of patients experienced side effects, including scarring or hyperpigmentation.

Treatment of PWS with KTP laser is advocated by some, although studies have shown it to have limited utility and an increased incidence of scarring.

Evidence Levels: **A** Double-blind study **B** Clinical trial ≥ 20 subjects **C** Clinical trial < 20 subjects **D** Series ≥ 5 subjects **E** Anecdotal case reports

Pregnancy dermatoses

Wolfgang Jurecka

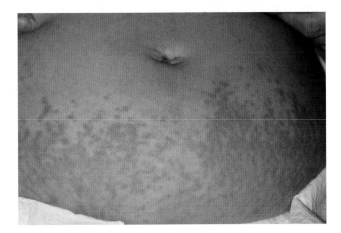

Skin changes during pregnancy may range from normal (physiologic) changes that occur with almost all pregnancies through common or pre-existing skin diseases that are not associated with, but are influenced by the pregnancy, to eruptions that appear to be specifically associated with pregnancy and the puerperium. A group of three well-defined dermatoses of pregnancy has been generally accepted. These are: pruritic urticarial papules and plaques of pregnancy (PUPPP), pemphigoid gestationis, and pruritus gravidarum (cholestasis of pregnancy). Recently, owing to their considerable clinical overlap, eczema in pregnancy, prurigo of pregnancy, and pruritic folliculitis of pregnancy were summarized as atopic eruption of pregnancy (AEP) in the group of pregnancy dermatoses. This is a misleading definition, as they are only manifestations of atopic eczema during pregnancy.

PRURITIC URTICARIAL PAPULES AND PLAQUES OF PREGNANCY

Pruritic urticarial papules and plaques of pregnancy (PUPPP) is a common, intensely pruritic dermatosis that usually begins in the third trimester of the first pregnancy, but may be delayed until a few days postpartum. It occasionally recurs, albeit less severely, in subsequent pregnancies.

MANAGEMENT STRATEGY

Most women who have PUPPP are relieved to learn that the condition is not serious, that all should be well with them and their baby, and that the rash will disappear at or within a few days after delivery. However, treatment is usually demanded to provide relief from the intense itching. The skin lesions may closely resemble the very early (urticarial) stage of pemphigoid gestationis. Direct and/or indirect immunofluorescence microscopy of perilesional skin or serum should be performed if pemphigoid gestationis is suspected. All similar eruptions that occur in non-pregnant women may also occur in pregnancy and should not be confused with those dermatoses that are pregnancy specific. Thus erythema multiforme, drug eruptions, contact dermatitis, urticaria, and insect bites should be excluded. In women with localized disease, intense (several times daily) application of *mid-strength or potent topical corticosteroids* provides symptomatic relief after a few days in almost all cases. *Ointments* containing substances such as *betamethasone, mometasone,* or *methylprednisolone* can be regarded as safe during pregnancy. New lesions usually stop appearing within 2 or 3 days, and the frequency of applications can be tapered. As the pregnancy continues many patients require therapy only once a day, or can even stop treatment before delivery. Topical antipruritic preparations are normally not useful. *Oral H_1 antihistamines,* especially the older sedating antihistamines, may offer some benefit in severely pruritic patients at bedtime. In more widespread or generalized cases and those which do not respond adequately to topical corticosteroids, a systemic corticosteroid treatment may need to be considered. *Oral methylprednisolone 20–40 mg daily* or its equivalent for 5 days, tapered over the following 2 weeks is very effective. For systemic treatment during pregnancy prednisone, prednisolone, and methylprednisolone are regarded as safer than betamethasone, dexamethasone, cortisone, and hydrocortisone, which may be associated with some risk of malformation.

One striking clinical feature of PUPPP is its onset in the third trimester in association with severe striae. It usually affects first pregnancies, in which striae are more common. There have been conflicting reports questioning whether PUPPP is associated with fetal weight and maternal weight gain, resulting in excessive abdominal distension. Some patients have therefore been delivered early, with the expectation that this will terminate the PUPPP. This has appeared to be the outcome in some cases, but the resolution of PUPPP is not necessarily related to delivery.

SPECIFIC INVESTIGATIONS

▶ Biopsy for direct immunofluorescence
▶ Serum for indirect immunofluorescence

A comparative study of toxic erythema of pregnancy and herpes gestationis. Holmes RC, Black MM, Dann J, James DC, Bhogal B. Br J Dermatol 1982; 106: 499–510.

A comparison of 30 patients with PUPPP and 24 with pemphigoid gestationis showed a broad overlap in the morphology of their skin lesions, which may lead to difficulties in the diagnosis of early (urticarial) pemphigoid gestationis. Immunofluorescence is consistently positive in pemphigoid gestationis.

A comparative histopathological study of polymorphic eruption of pregnancy and herpes gestationis. Holmes RC, Jurecka W, Black MM. Clin Exp Dermatol 1983; 8: 523–9.

There was a broad overlap in the histopathologic changes of skin lesions in patients with PUPPP and pemphigoid gestationis, allowing a clear distinction only when pemphigoid gestationis appears with typical subepidermal blisters.

An immunoelectron microscopy study of the relationship between herpes gestationis and polymorphic eruption of pregnancy. Jurecka W, Holmes RC, Black MM, McKee P, Das AK, Bhogal B. Br J Dermatol 1983; 108: 147–51.

This highly sensitive method showed that PUPPP and pemphigoid gestationis are clearly separate entities.

Polymorphic eruption of pregnancy: clinicopathology and potential trigger factors in 181 patients. Rudolph CM, Al-Fares S, Vaughan-Jones SA, Müllegger RR, Kerl H, Black MM. Br J Dermatol 2006; 154: 54–60.

Although pruritic urticarial papules and plaques are the main morphological features at disease onset, more than half of the patients later develop polymorphous features, including erythema, vesicles, and targetoid and eczematous lesions, favoring the term polymorphic eruption of pregnancy (PEP). Multiple-gestation pregnancies and excessive maternal weight gain, but not fetal weight and gender, were significantly associated with PEP.

FIRST-LINE THERAPIES

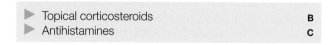

▶ Topical corticosteroids	**B**
▶ Antihistamines	**C**

Pruritic urticarial papules and plaques of pregnancy. Clinical experience in twenty-five patients. Yancey KB, Hall RP, Lawley TJ. J Am Acad Dermatol 1984; 10: 473–80.

Of 25 patients, 22 were successfully treated with frequent applications of high-potency topical corticosteroids, providing relief from the pruritus and controlling the eruption.

Pruritic urticarial papules and plaques of pregnancy (PUPPP). A clinicopathologic study. Callen JP, Hanno R. J Am Acad Dermatol 1981; 5: 401–5.

In 15 cases PUPPP cleared prior to delivery (five cases), within 1 week of delivery (nine cases), and at 6 weeks postpartum (one case). Treatment was performed with various potent topical corticosteroids and antihistamines, namely diphenhydramine, in all cases except one. Two cases required additional treatment with hydroxyzine.

Pruritic urticarial papules and plaques of pregnancy. Ahmed AR, Kaplan R. J Am Acad Dermatol 1981; 4: 679–81.

Two patients were treated with topical corticosteroids and diphenhydramine with good results.

Dermatological therapy during pregnancy and lactation. Sasseville D. In: Harahap M, Wallach R, eds. Skin changes and diseases in pregnancy. New York: Marcel Dekker, 1996; 249–319.

First-generation H_1 blockers (antihistamines) are grouped by their chemical structure into six different classes. Chlorpenamine (chlorpheniramine), diphenhydramine, tripelenamine, cyclizine and meclizine, and cyproheptadine are considered safer for use in pregnancy than other antihistamines.

Pregnancy outcome after gestational exposure to terfenadine: a multicenter prospective controlled study. Loebstein R, Lalkin A, Addis A, Costa A, Lalkin I, Bonati M, et al. J Allergy Clin Immunol 1999; 104: 953–6.

One hundred and eighteen women were exposed to terfenadine during pregnancy. Among those exposed during the first trimester (n=65), only the birthweight of the newborns was significantly lower than in a matched control group. All other parameters were comparable between the groups. On the basis of the limited sample size of this study, it appears that terfenadine is not associated with an increased incidence of malformations. However, further studies will be needed.

Pregnancy outcome after gestational exposure to loratadine or antihistamines: a prospective controlled cohort study. Diav-Citrin O, Shechtman S, Aharonovich A, Moerman L, Arnon J, Wajnberg R, et al. J Allergy Clin Immunol 2003; 111: 1239–43.

This study, which was powered to find a threefold increase, suggests that there is no major teratogenic risk for loratadine compared to astemizole, chlorpheniramine, terfenadine, hydroxyzine, promethazine, and dimetindene.

SECOND-LINE THERAPIES

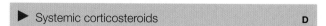

▶ Systemic corticosteroids	**D**

Pruritic urticarial papules and plaques of pregnancy. Clinical experience in twenty-five patients. Yancey KB, Hall RP, Lawley TJ. J Am Acad Dermatol 1984; 10: 473–80.

Systemic corticosteroids were efficacious in three patients with extensive disease.

Prurigo of late pregnancy. Cooper AJ, Fryer JA. Aust J Dermatol 1980; 21: 79–84.

Four of five patients were treated successfully with oral prednisone (20 mg daily, tapering by 5 mg every 2 days).

Pruritic urticarial papules and plaques of pregnancy (polymorphic eruption of pregnancy): two unusual cases. Vaughan Jones SA, Dunnill MG, Black MM. Br J Dermatol 1996; 135: 102–5.

One of two cases required a short course of systemic corticosteroids.

Although only a limited numbers of cases are reported in the literature describing treatment of severe cases of PUPPP with oral corticosteroids, nowadays it is generally accepted that this treatment is effective and safe if prednisone, prednisolone, or methylprednisolone are chosen. However, larger series and prospective studies are lacking.

Pregnancy outcome after first trimester exposure to corticosteroids: a prospective controlled study. Cur C, Diav-Citrin O, Shechtman S, Arnon J, Ornoy A. Reprod Toxicol 2004; 18: 93–101.

This study, which was powered to find a 2.5-fold increase, supports that glucocorticosteroids do not represent a major teratogenic risk in humans.

THIRD-LINE THERAPIES

▶ Early delivery	**E**

Severe polymorphic eruption of pregnancy occurring in twin pregnancies. Bunker CB, Erskine K, Rustin MHA, Gilkes JJH. Clin Exp Dermatol 1990; 15: 228–30.

Early delivery was performed to terminate the PUPPP.

Pruritic urticarial papules and plaques of pregnancy: a severe case requiring early delivery for relief of symptoms. Baltrani VP, Baltrani VS. J Am Acad Dermatol 1992; 26: 266–7.

Early delivery led to relief of symptoms.

Pruritic urticarial papules and plaques of pregnancy. Carruthers A. J Am Acad Dermatol 1993; 29: 125.

Resolution of PUPPP is unrelated to delivery, therefore early delivery should not be performed to treat PUPPP.

Treating an uncomfortable but non-serious dermatosis by such invasive methods with a potential risk for both mother and newborn is, in the author's view, not indicated and should not be performed, especially as other adequate treatments are available.

PEMPHIGOID GESTATIONIS

Pemphigoid gestationis (herpes gestationis) is a rare, intensely itchy, urticarial or polymorphic or vesiculobullous eruption. It affects approximately 1 in 60 000 pregnancies and usually appears in the second or third trimester, but it may also be associated with hydatidiform mole or choriocarcinoma. The term pemphigoid gestationis is preferable because this condition shows many clinical and immunologic similarities with bullous pemphigoid and has no relationship with herpes virus infection.

MANAGEMENT STRATEGY

Although pemphigoid gestationis is a rare disorder, correct diagnosis and optimal management are essential. It occurs only in the presence of paternal tissue (fetus, hydatidiform mole, or choriocarcinoma). Once it has manifested, its course may be significantly modulated by changes in estrogen and progesterone levels. Exacerbations may occur postpartum, with oral contraceptives, and during the menstrual cycle, and are commonly more severe in subsequent pregnancies. Circulating autoantibodies are directed against the same target antigens as in bullous pemphigoid, although more commonly against BP 180 antigen than BP 230 antigen. The autoantibodies react with the basement membrane of amnion placenta, resulting in the findings of immune activation in the placenta and evidence of placental insufficiency. Thus skin biopsies for dermatohistopathology and direct immunofluorescence, and serum for indirect immunofluorescence investigations or ELISA to confirm the diagnosis and to differentiate non-bullous pemphigoid gestationis from PUPPP are recommended. This is especially important because most patients with pemphigoid gestationis need treatment with systemic corticosteroids, at least for a while, and are therefore at risk of side effects from this treatment. Most cases resolve within a few months postpartum, with just a few urticarial eruptions during the year after delivery. However, some cases have been reported with recurrences more than 10 years postpartum. Even more important is the fetal prognosis. In the older literature an increased risk for fetal morbidity and mortality has been discussed. However, cases with a serious outcome are more likely to be reported. Furthermore, in view of the findings that the placenta is also involved in pemphigoid gestationis, a more severe impact of the disease on the fetus seems reasonable in the pre-corticosteroid era. More recent studies have recorded a much better fetal prognosis. Patients who have been treated with systemic corticosteroids were no more likely to have children that were small for dates than were those who were not treated with systemic corticosteroids. The current view is that pemphigoid gestationis is associated with premature delivery and a risk of low birthweight. Thus pregnancies of mothers with pemphigoid gestationis should be carefully followed in special units.

The goal of treatment is to suppress blister formation and to give the patients relief from the intense pruritus. Thus, in mild cases of pemphigoid gestationis, *topical potent or very potent corticosteroids* combined with *a systemic antihistamine* may be sufficient. First-generation antihistamines are favored over second-generation antihistamines. Substances such as *chlorpheniramine, diphenhydramine, tripelenamine, cyclizine, meclizine, hydroxyzine,* and *cyproheptadine* may be used (see also discussion above about the use of antihistamines in PUPPP). However, most patients require *systemic corticosteroid* treatment during the course of their disease. Initially doses of prednisolone or its equivalent in the range of 20–40 mg daily may be tried, and then adjusted depending on the response. In severe cases 1 mg/kg body weight or even higher doses of prednisolone may be necessary to prevent blister formation. If the eruption resolves well the prednisolone can be reduced fairly rapidly in steps, initially twice weekly, later once a week, to a much lower maintenance dose. Some patients then respond to doses of prednisolone of 5–10 mg daily or every second day. Frequently the eruption flares immediately postpartum, and then a temporary increase in prednisolone treatment is required (for the use of systemic corticosteroids during pregnancy see also the discussion of their use in PUPPP above).

Newborns of mothers suffering from pemphigoid gestationis may develop bullous lesions similar to those of their mother by passive transfer of the antibasement membrane zone antibody across the placenta. These lesions are transient and require no therapy. If the mother has received high doses of prednisolone for a longer time the infant should be carefully examined by a neonatologist for evidence of adrenal insufficiency.

In severe cases of pemphigoid gestationis that do not respond satisfactorily to prednisolone alone, or in cases where prolonged treatment with corticosteroids is contraindicated, *plasmapheresis* may be considered. Postpartum treatment may cause difficulties for several reasons:

- If the mother wishes to breastfeed, the drugs pass into the breast milk. Antihistamines may cause drowsiness in the baby, and corticosteroids may cause adrenal suppression. The pediatrician should therefore be informed in this situation.
- In general, pemphigoid gestationis tends to improve postpartum: however, it may take weeks, months, or even years until there is complete remission. In those cases *alternative drugs that are contraindicated during pregnancy or while the mother is breastfeeding may be used*. Owing to its close relationship to bullous pemphigoid, in this situation similar treatment to that of bullous pemphigoid may be tried (see page 107). *Azathioprine, dapsone, sulfapyridine (sulphapyridine),* and *pyridoxine* may be tried as adjunctive therapy either with oral corticosteroids or alone. Other drugs that may be used are *goserelin* and *ritodrine. High-dose intravenous immune globulin* alone or in combination with *ciclosporin* or *cyclophosphamide* has been tried with success in rare cases for its corticosteroid-sparing effect.
- Pemphigoid gestationis tends to exacerbate with menstruation. There may also be dramatic flares with oral contraceptives. Thus, patients should be recommended to *avoid oral contraceptives* as long as the disease is still active.

SPECIFIC INVESTIGATIONS

- ▶ Biopsy for histopathology and direct immunofluorescence
- ▶ Serum for indirect immunofluorescence and/ or enzyme-linked immunosorbent assay (ELISA) (immunoblot)

A comparative study of toxic erythema of pregnancy and herpes gestationis. Holmes RC, Black MM, Dann J, James DC, Bhogal B. Br J Dermatol 1982; 106: 499–510.

A comparative histopathological study of polymorphic eruption of pregnancy and herpes gestationis. Holmes RC, Jurecka W, Black MM. Clin Exp Dermatol 1983; 8: 523–9.

An immunoelectron microscopy study of the relationship between herpes gestationis and polymorphic eruption of pregnancy. Jurecka W, Holmes RC, Black MM, McKee P, Das AK, Bhogal B. Br J Dermatol 1983; 108: 147–51.

The disease most often confused with pemphigoid gestationis is PUPPP. There may be a broad clinical and histopathologic overlap between these two entities, which are immunologically distinct, with linear C3 deposits (in 100%) and linear IgG deposits (in approximately 30%) along the basement membrane zone in pemphigoid gestationis.

Clinically, pemphigoid gestationis may present either with prominent annular wheals or target lesions or with grouped vesicles, and then may be confused with either erythema multiforme or dermatitis herpetiformis. However, these two diseases should be easily distinguished from pemphigoid gestationis by histopathology and direct immunofluorescence.

Herpes gestationis autoantibodies recognize a 180kD human epidermal antigen. Morrison LH, Labib RS, Zone JJ, Diaz LA, Anhalt GJ. J Clin Invest 1988; 81: 2023–6.

Usefulness of BP 180 NC 16a enzyme-linked immunosorbent assay in the serodiagnosis of pemohigoid gestationis and in differentiating between pemphigoid gestationis and pruritic urticarial papules and plaques of preganancy. Powell AM, Sakuma-Oyama Y, Oyama N, Albert S, Bhogal B, Kaneko F, et al. Arch Dermatol 2005; 141: 705–10.

This ELISA is highly sensitive and highly specific in differentiating pemphigoid gestationis from PUPPP and a valuable tool in the serodiagnosis of pemphigoid gestationis.

ELISA is a sensitive tool for the detection of autoantibodies to bullous pemphigoid antigen 180 in patients with pemphigoid gestationis, and is useful for monitoring autoantibody serum levels.

FIRST-LINE THERAPIES

▶ Topical corticosteroids	C
▶ Systemic corticosteroids	B
▶ Antihistamines	C

Clinical features and management of 87 patients with pemphigoid gestationis. Jenkins RE, Hern S, Black MM. Clin Exp Dermatol 1999; 24: 255–9.

This review summarizes the clinical data on 142 pregnancies in 87 patients with pemphigoid gestationis. Most patients received chlorpheniramine to suppress the pruritus. Thirteen of 69 (18.8%) patients were treated with topical corticosteroids alone without systemic treatment. Fifty-six of the 69 (81.2%) required systemic corticosteroids with initial doses of prednisolone in the range of 5–110 mg daily, resulting in suppression of blistering in most cases.

Hitherto this is the largest series of patients ever published, giving a good overview of the clinical presentation, immunologic findings, and management strategies. Some patients have also been treated with azathioprine, dapsone, pyridoxine, sulfapyridine, androgenic

steroids, and goserelin. Plasmapheresis was also used, with some temporary relief.

Fetal and maternal risk factors in herpes gestationis. Lawley TJ, Stingl G, Katz SI. Arch Dermatol 1979; 114: 552–5.

Forty-one cases of immunologically proven herpes gestationis were reviewed. Systemic treatment with corticosteroids was frequently necessary to control maternal signs and symptoms of herpes gestationis. In eight patients topical application of corticosteroids alone was sufficient. Twenty-nine patients were treated systemically with corticosteroids in doses ranging from 20 to 180 mg of prednisone daily. In three of these cases azathioprine was also used postpartum. Most of the cases responded well to the treatment.

Herpes gestationis: clinical and histologic features of twenty-eight cases. Shornick JK, Bangert JL, Freemann RG, Gillian JN. J Am Acad Dermatol 1983; 8: 214–24.

Prednisone was used during 34 pregnancies, in initial doses between 20 and 80 mg daily. There was extreme variability in the need for protracted treatment. Some women were able to stop prednisone within 5 days of delivery, whereas others needed treatment for up to 18 months. The typical treatment was for 6–10 weeks postpartum.

Although topical and systemic corticosteroids alone or together are regarded as first-line treatments in pemphigoid gestationis, their use has been based only on anecdotal reports and not on controlled studies.

SECOND-LINE THERAPIES

▶ Plasmapheresis	E

Plasma exchange in herpes gestationis. Van de Wiel A, Hart HC, Flinterman J, Kerckhaert JA, Du Boeuff JA, Imhof JW. Br Med J 1980; 281: 1041–2.

Herpes gestationis: studies on the binding characteristics, activity and pathogenetic significance of the complement-fixing factor. Carruthers JA, Ewins AR. Clin Exp Immunol 1978; 31: 38–41.

In single cases it has been shown that if corticosteroid treatment proves unsuccessful or is contraindicated, then plasmapheresis should be considered as well, both during pregnancy and postpartum (see also above).

THIRD-LINE THERAPIES

▶ High-dose intravenous immunoglobulin	E
▶ Azathioprine	E
▶ Cyclophosphamide	E
▶ Ciclosporin	E
▶ Dapsone	E
▶ Sulfapyridine	E
▶ Pyridoxine	E
▶ Ritodrine	E
▶ Goserelin	E

High-dose intravenous immune globulin

High dose intravenous immune globulin for the treatment of autoimmune blistering diseases: an evaluation for its use

in 14 cases. Harman KE, Black MM. Br J Dermatol 1999; 40: 865–74.

A retrospective report on the experience of the use of high-dose intravenous immunoglobulin in several autoimmune blistering diseases. The treatment had a corticosteroid-sparing effect with a transient response, and repeated courses were required.

Immunosuppressive agents

Fetal and maternal risk factors in herpes gestationis. Lawley TJ, Stingl G, Katz SI. Arch Dermatol 1978; 114: 552–5.

In three of 41 cases, besides high doses of corticosteroids, an additional treatment with azathioprine was necessary postpartum.

A severe persistent case of pemphigoid gestationis treated with intravenous immunoglobulin and cyclosporin. Hern S, Harman K, Bhogal BS, Black MM. Clin Exp Dermatol 1998; 23: 185–8.

A patient with severe pemphigoid gestationis in whom the disease persisted for 1.5 years postpartum was treated with immunoglobulin and ciclosporin.

Chronic herpes gestationis and antiphospholipid antibody syndrome successfully treated with cyclophosphamide. Castle SP, Mather-Mondrey M, Bennion S, David-Bajar K, Huff C. J Am Acad Dermatol 1996; 34: 333–6.

Treatment with pulse-dose intravenous cyclophosphamide produced an excellent clinical response.

Immunosuppressive agents for the treatment of pemphigoid gestationis can only be used in the postpartum period while the mother is not breastfeeding.

Other therapies

Clinical features and management of 87 patients with pemphigoid gestationis. Jenkins RE, Hern S, Black MM. Clin Exp Dermatol 1999; 24: 255–9.

Dapsone, sulfapyridine, and pyridoxine were occasionally used as adjunctive therapy with oral corticosteroids.

The benefit of these drugs on the course of the disease remains questionable.

Herpes gestationis and ritodrine. Dobson RL. J Am Acad Dermatol 1988; 18: 1145–6.

Ritodrine is a β-adrenergic drug used to prevent premature labor. There has been some support for the suggestion that it may be of benefit in the treatment of pemphigoid gestationis.

Pemphigoid gestationis: response to chemical oophorectomy with goserelin. Garvey MP, Handfield-Jones SE, Black MM. Clin Exp Dermatol 1992; 17: 443–5.

Goserelin is a gonadotropin-releasing hormone (GnRH) analog and had only initial success in the treatment of continuing disease several years postpartum.

PRURITUS GRAVIDARUM

Pruritus gravidarum, also known as intrahepatic cholestasis of pregnancy, or a mild form of benign recurrent intrahepatic cholestasis, is a hepatic condition that usually occurs in late pregnancy. It first manifests with severe generalized pruritus and may be followed by the clinical appearance of jaundice. Its incidence has been estimated at 0.02–2.4% of pregnancies. It is likely that the irritation results from abnormal hepatic excretion of bile acids induced by endogenous estrogen and progesterone. The itching usually subsides rapidly after delivery.

MANAGEMENT STRATEGY

The first symptom of pruritus gravidarum is itch, followed by secondary excoriations. In mild cases the diagnosis is based on exclusion by differentiating pruritus gravidarum from other itchy conditions that may occur by chance during pregnancy. Thus scabies, eczema, urticaria, drug eruptions, or other conditions, and early cases of PUPPP and pemphigoid gestationis, must be excluded. Liver function tests may occasionally be abnormal with a raised alkaline phosphatase. Total serum bile acid levels are markedly elevated and correlate with impaired fetal prognosis. In fully developed cases numerous excoriations may be seen in conjunction with icterus. The pruritus and the cholestasis usually remit within a few days after delivery. The incidence of prematurity and low birthweight is increased in the offspring of patients with pruritus gravidarum, and the pregnancies should be followed carefully. Pruritus gravidarum may recur with subsequent pregnancies and the use of oral contraceptive pills. In mild disease attempts should be made to control pruritus by the frequent application of *cooling lotions or creams* and *topical antipruritic agents*. A *1% menthol lotion* or the addition of *6–10% polidocanol* may be helpful. In more severe cases *oral antihistamines* are the therapy of choice. First-generation antihistamines are preferable to second-generation antihistamines (for the use of oral antihistamines during pregnancy see also the discussion of their use in PUPPP above). From the author's experience *phototherapy with UVB* (290–320 nm) or *UVA* (320–400 nm) may also be of benefit in some cases. *Cholestyramine* and, as shown in numerous recent studies, the administration of *ursodeoxycholic acid* may give adequate relief of symptoms and improves fetal prognosis (prematurity)

SPECIFIC INVESTIGATIONS

▶ IgE level
▶ Liver function tests, serum bile acid

Specific pruritic disease of pregnancy. A prospective study of 3192 pregnant women. Roger D, Vaillant L, Fignon A, Pierre F, Bacq Y, Brechot JF, et al. Arch Dermatol 1994; 130: 734–9.

Causes of pruritus during pregnancy include not only the specific dermatoses of pregnancy, but also scabies and eczema. The incidence of prematurity and low birthweight is increased in newborns of patients with pruritus gravidarum.

Intrahepatic cholestasis of pregnancy: relationships between bile acid levels and fetal complication rates. Glantz A, Marschall HU, Mattsson LA. Hepatology 2004; 40: 287–8.

No increase in fetal risk was detected in patients with intrahepatic cholestasis of pregnancy and bile acid levels <40 μmol/L.

The importance of serum bile acid level analysis and treatment with ursodeoxycholic acid in intrahepatic cholestasis of pregnancy: a case series from central Europe. Ambros-Rudolph CM, Glatz M, Trauner M, Kerl H, Müllegger RR. Arch Dermatol 2007; 143: 757–62.

Elevated total serum bile acid levels are the clue to diagnosis. Close obstetric surveillance and prompt treatment with ursodeoxycholic acid is warranted and may prevent prematurity.

FIRST-LINE THERAPIES

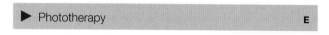

| ▶ Emollients and topical antipruritic agents | D |
| ▶ Antihistamines | D |

Skin changes and diseases in pregnancy. Lawley TJ, Yancey KB. In: Freedberg IM, Eisen AZ, Wolff K, et al., eds. Dermatology in general medicine, 6th edn. New York: McGraw-Hill, 2003; 1361–6.

Emollients and topical antipruritic agents should be tried. Antihistamines are of some benefit.

SECOND-LINE THERAPIES

| ▶ Phototherapy | E |

It is the author's experience that phototherapy with UVB (290–320 nm) or UVA (320–400 nm) is helpful in the treatment of pruritus gravidarum. No studies are available.

THIRD-LINE THERAPIES

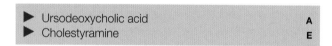

| ▶ Ursodeoxycholic acid | A |
| ▶ Cholestyramine | E |

Bile acids and progesterone metabolites in intrahepatic cholestasis of pregnancy. Reyes H, Sjovall J. Ann Med 2000; 32: 94–106.

With the administration of ursodeoxycholic acid to patients with intrahepatic cholestasis of pregnancy, pruritus and liver enzyme values are improved.

Intrahepatic cholestasis of pregnancy: changes in maternal-fetal bile acid balance and improvement by ursodeoxycholic acid. Brites D. Ann Hepatol 2002; 1: 20–8.

This review focuses on the altered bile acid profiles in maternal and fetal compartments during intrahepatic cholestasis of pregnancy and its recovery by ursodeoxycholic acid administration.

Ursodeoxycholic acid in the treatment of cholestasis of pregnancy: a randomized, double-blind study controlled with placebo. Palma J, Reyes H, Ribalta J, Hernández I, Sandoval L, Almuna R, et al. J Hepatol 1997; 27: 1022–8.

Ursodeoxycholic acid is effective and safe in patients with intrahepatic cholestasis of pregnancy, attenuating pruritus and correcting some biochemical abnormalities in the mother. Relevant aspects of fetal outcome were also improved in patients receiving ursodeoxycholic acid (1 g daily) compared to placebo.

Effect of cholestyramine and phenobarbital on pruritus and serum bile acid levels in cholestasis of pregnancy. Laatikainen M. Am J Obstet Gynecol 1978; 132: 501–6.

Doses of 4 g cholestyramine two or three times daily have produced a reduction in serum bile acid levels and a relief from pruritus in some patients.

The use of phenobarbital may be contraindicated during pregnancy.

PRESCRIBING IN PREGNANCY

The decision to treat a pregnant woman with a drug should be made by the physician and the pregnant woman together on the best benefit-to-risk ratio. Thus, the prescription should fulfill each of the following criteria:

- There should be a strict indication that requires a precise knowledge of the diagnosis and the course of the disease.
- A drug with as few active components as possible should be selected.
- The pharmacology of the active component and its safety during pregnancy should be established.
- A precise knowledge of the duration of the pregnancy (weeks of gestation) is essential.
- A drug that shows the best benefit-to-risk ratio should be selected.

Pretibial myxedema

Carrie Wood Cobb, Warren R Heymann

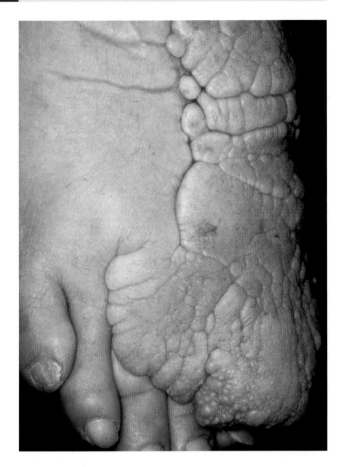

Pretibial myxedema, more accurately termed 'thyroid dermopathy,' is characterized by non-pitting edema and skin-colored to violaceous nodules or plaques. These are most commonly distributed pretibially, but can sometimes be seen over the arms, shoulders, head, and neck.

MANAGEMENT STRATEGY

Pretibial myxedema is an autoimmune phenomenon which tends to occur following treatment of patients with Graves' disease. The condition can, however, develop in hypothyroid and euthyroid patients. It is helpful to look for other clinical signs of thyroid disease, including thyroid acropachy and the presence of a goiter. Pretibial myxedema typically follows the onset of ophthalmopathy, often years after the diagnosis of hyperthyroidism. Goals of treatment include cosmesis and the prevention of long-term side effects such as elephantiasis or foot drop from neural entrapment. Resolution may occur without treatment.

Patients with significant thyroid dermopathy should be started on a trial of *high-potency topical corticosteroids*, alone or under occlusion, for at least 2 months. If symptoms persist, *intralesional corticosteroids* may be effective. A combination of the above in conjunction with *compression bandages* can be beneficial when monotherapy proves inadequate. Both *oral* and *intravenous corticosteroids* have also been shown to improve lesions in several patients. However, their use is limited by systemic side effects.

Pentoxifylline, an analog of the methylxanthine theobromine, has been shown to reduce the extent of lesions and can also be used in conjunction with topical and/or intralesional corticosteroids. Although there are conflicting data, the use of *intravenous immunoglobulin (IVIG)* in doses of 400 mg/kg daily given over 3–4 hours on 5 consecutive days for three cycles, followed by maintenance therapy, may improve lesions of pretibial myxedema. Subcutaneous or intralesional *octreotide*, a somatostatin analog, shows conflicting results. *Plasmapheresis* has been reported to be beneficial in improving severe cases.

Temporary improvement with *cytotoxic agents* has been observed. Pretibial myxedema is not a life-threatening condition, and so the use of such agents should be limited to severe, debilitating cases. *Surgical excision* has been shown to be effective in a minority of cases. The high risk of recurrence makes surgical intervention an infrequently used modality. *Complete decongestive physiotherapy* has shown some success in treating the elephantiasic form of pretibial myxedema.

Pretibial ultrasonography to measure skin thickness may be useful in assessing treatment response. Measuring serum hyaluronic acid levels to follow therapeutic response may also be of value.

SPECIFIC INVESTIGATIONS

- ▶ Thyroid function tests
- ▶ Antithyroglobulin and antithyroid peroxidase antibodies
- ▶ Anti-thyroid-stimulating hormone (TSH) receptor antibodies
- ▶ Pretibial ultrasound
- ▶ Serum hyaluronic acid

Pretibial myxedema. Fatourechi V. In: Heymann WR (ed) Thyroid disorders with cutaneous manifestations. London: Springer Verlag, 2009; 103–119.

Pretibial myxedema: pathophysiology and treatment options. Fatourechi V. Am J Clin Dermatol 2005; 6: 295–309.

Excellent reviews of therapeutic approaches for patients with all forms of thyroid dermopathy, ranging from mild disease to the severe elephantiasic variant.

Current treatment modalities for thyroid dermopathy and acropachy are at best palliative. Better and safer means of immunomodulation await discovery.

Pretibial myxedema as the initial manifestation of Graves' disease. Georgala S, Katoulis AC, Georgala C, Katoulis EC, Hatziolou E, Stavrianeas NG. J Eur Acad Dermatol Venereol 2002; 16: 380–3.

A 28-year-old Greek woman presented initially with asymptomatic pretibial myxedema, which ultimately led to a diagnosis of Graves' disease. This patient had elevated anti-TSH-receptor antibodies.

An assessment of thyroid function is warranted because most patients with pretibial myxedema have clinical or laboratory evidence of autoimmune thyroid disease.

Elephantiasic thyroid dermopathy. Tiu SC, Choi CH. Hong Kong Med J 2006; 12: 159–60.

A case of a 48-year-old man with Graves' disease who developed a severe case of elephantiasic thyroid dermopathy unresponsive to local treatments and systemic immunotherapy.

This case is a graphic example of how debilitating this variant of pretibial myxedema may be, and how recalcitrant the disorder may be to therapy.

FIRST-LINE THERAPIES

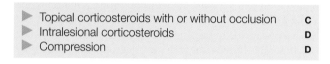

▶ Topical corticosteroids with or without occlusion	**C**
▶ Intralesional corticosteroids	**D**
▶ Compression	**D**

Therapy with occlusive dressings of pretibial myxedema with fluocinolone acetonide. Kriss JP, Pleshakov V, Rosenblum A, Sharp G. J Clin Endocrinol Metab 1967; 27: 595–604.

All 11 patients treated with topical 0.2% fluocinolone acetonide cream under occlusive dressing at bedtime improved significantly.

Dermopathy of Graves disease (pretibial myxedema): review of 150 cases. Fatourechi V, Pajouhi M, Fransway AF. Medicine 1994; 73: 1–7.

Treatment with topical 0.05–0.1% triamcinolone acetonide cream under occlusion for 2–10 weeks led to partial remission in 29 of 76 patients in this retrospective study; 1% had complete remission.

Intralesional triamcinolone therapy for pretibial myxedema. Lang PG, Sisson JC, Lynch PJ. Arch Dermatol 1975; 111: 197–202.

Seven of nine patients treated with monthly injections of 8 mL or less of intralesional triamcinolone acetonide solution (5 mg/mL, 1 mL per injection site) had complete remission of pretibial myxedema after a total of three to seven visits. The other two patients, despite withdrawing from the study prematurely for non-medical reasons, showed a partial improvement.

Pretibial myxedema: a review of the literature and case report. Frisch DR, Roth I. J Am Podiatr Med Assoc 1985; 75: 147–52.

A 29-year-old woman with pretibial myxedema was treated with rest, elevation, and topical 0.05% fluocinonide cream under occlusion. Outpatient therapy included weekly intralesional Celestone Soluspan injections followed by topical 0.05% fluocinonide cream under occlusion. Compression dressings with an Unna boot were applied weekly. After 2 months the lesions were greatly improved.

Compression stockings may also be beneficial. Unless contraindicated, compression should be used in conjunction with any therapeutic approach for this disorder.

Pathogenesis and treatment of pretibial myxedema. Kriss JP. Endocrinol Metab Clin North Am 1987; 16: 409–15.

Refractory cases of pretibial myxedema, including the elephantiasic form, may benefit from combined therapy with local corticosteroids under occlusion and an Unna boot.

SECOND-LINE THERAPIES

▶ Pentoxifylline	**E**
▶ Pentoxifylline with topical and/or intralesional steroid	**E**

Pentoxifylline inhibits the proliferation and glycosaminoglycan synthesis of cultured fibroblasts derived from patients with Graves' ophthalmopathy and pretibial myxedema. Chang CC, Chang TC, Kao SC, Kuo YF, Chien LF. Acta Endocrinol 1993; 129: 322–7.

Pentoxifylline caused an in-vitro dose-dependent decrease in fibroblast proliferation and glycosaminoglycan synthesis in fibroblast cultures taken from pretibial sites. A preliminary trial with a dose of 400 mg intravenously and 800 mg orally daily of pentoxifylline reduced the size of pretibial myxedema lesions within 1 week.

Successful combined pentoxifylline and intralesional triamcinolone acetonide treatment of severe pretibial myxedema. Engin B, Gumusel M, Ozdemir M, Cakir M. Dermatol Online J 2007; 13: 16.

A 32-year-old man achieved partial remission with clobetasol under occlusion combined with pentoxifylline 400 mg three times daily with intralesional triamcinolone (5 mg/mL).

THIRD-LINE THERAPIES

▶ Intravenous immunoglobulin	**D**
▶ Systemic corticosteroids (including pulse corticosteroid therapy)	**D**
▶ Octreotide	**E**
▶ Plasmapheresis	**D**
▶ Cytotoxic therapy	**E**
▶ Surgery	**E**
▶ Complete decongestive physiotherapy	**E**

Pretibial myxedema and high-dose intravenous immunoglobulin treatment. Antonelli A, Navarranne A, Palla R, Alberti B, Saracino A, Mestre C, et al. Thyroid 1994; 4: 399–408.

Improvement of pretibial myxedema began after a few weeks in six patients treated with 400 mg/kg daily of high-dose intravenous γ-globulin given over 3–4 hours on 5 consecutive days. The cycle was repeated three times every 21 days. Maintenance therapy of 400 mg/kg for 1 day was then administered for from seven to 15 more cycles every 21 days. Total treatment ranged from 7 to 12 months, with maximum response occurring after an average of 6 months.

Lack of response of elephantiasic pretibial myxoedema to treatment with high-dose intravenous immunoglobulins. Terheydem P, Kahaly GJ, Zillikens D, Brocker EB. Clin Exp Dermatol 2003; 28: 224–6.

IVIG did not significantly improve the lesions of a patient with elephantiasic pretibial myxedema.

Corticoid therapy for pretibial myxedema: observations on the long-acting thyroid stimulator. Benoit FL, Greenspan FS. Ann Intern Med 1967; 66: 711–20.

Oral prednisolone, begun at 60 mg then tapered, and methylprednisolone starting at 40 mg cleared the pretibial lesions of four patients and improved the lesions of two others. Of the various corticosteroid treatments studied, the best results were obtained with high-dose systemic corticosteroids for 2 weeks.

Localized myxedema, associated with increased serum hyaluronic acid, and response to steroid pulse therapy. Ohtsuka Y, Yamamoto K, Goto Y, Mizuta T, Ozaki I, Setoguchi Y, et al. Intern Med 1995; 34: 424–9.

Evidence Levels: **A** Double-blind study **B** Clinical trial ≥ 20 subjects **C** Clinical trial < 20 subjects **D** Series ≥ 5 subjects **E** Anecdotal case reports

This is a case report of a 66-year-old man with Graves' disease and localized myxedema over the legs, feet, hands, and face. The patient improved with two courses of methylprednisolone pulse therapy (1 g daily) for 3 days each, followed by an oral prednisolone taper begun at 60 mg daily and continued at 10 mg daily for 1.5 years. The patient's serum hyaluronic acid levels decreased as skin lesions improved.

Refractory pretibial myxoedema with response to intralesional insulin-like growth factor 1 antagonist (octreotide): downregulation of hyaluronic acid production by the lesional fibroblasts. Shinohara M, Hamasaki Y, Katayana I. Br J Dermatol 2000; 143: 1083–6.

Intralesional octreotide 200 μg daily improved the lesions of pretibial myxedema in a male patient with Graves' disease after 4 weeks of therapy.

Octreotide inhibits insulin-like growth factor-1-induced hyaluronic acid secretion by lesional fibroblasts, which may play a role in the pathogenesis of pretibial myxedema.

Octreotide and Graves' ophthalmopathy and pretibial myxoedema. Chang TC, Kao SC, Huang KM. Br Med J 1992; 304: 158.

Three patients with pretibial myxedema were successfully treated with 100 μg of octreotide three times daily.

The authors do not comment on the route of administration of the octreotide acetate. According to the Physicians' Desk Reference, *the drug may be administered either by subcutaneous injection or intravenously.*

Lack of effect of long-term octreotide therapy in severe thyroid-associated dermopathy. Rotman-Pikielny P, Brucker-Davis F, Turner ML, Sarlis NJ, Skarulis MC. Thyroid 2003; 13: 465–70.

Three women did not show a statistically significant benefit from octreotide 300 μg.

The conflicting results from these small studies regarding the use of octreotide for thyroid dermopathy mandates that only larger, controlled studies will verify whether it is a useful modality for this condition.

Effect of plasmapheresis and steroid treatment on thyrotropin binding inhibitory immunoglobulins in a patient with exophthalmos and a patient with pretibial myxedema. Kuzuya N, DeGroot LJ. J Endocrinol Invest 1982; 5: 373–8.

Two patients, one with elephantiasis-like lesions, were treated with 16 exchanges over 4–5 months with 1–2 L of the patient's plasma removed and replaced with 1300 mL of purified protein fraction and 700 mL 0.9% saline. Immunoglobulin G fraction was separated out, thereby reducing total thyrotropin-binding inhibitory immunoglobulin (TBII) activity per unit of serum. The pretibial myxedema was partially and temporarily improved with plasmapheresis, and abnormal antibodies were reduced.

Beneficial effects of plasmapheresis followed by immunosuppressive therapy in pretibial myxedema. Noppen M, Velkeniers B, Steenssens L, Vanhaelst L. Acta Clin Belg 1988; 43: 381–3.

A patient with pretibial myxedema unresponsive to topical corticosteroids was cured after 5 days of plasmapheresis followed by 100 mg of azathioprine twice daily for 3 months. Azathioprine was tapered to 50 mg twice daily and continued for a year, at which time no recurrence was noted.

Pretibial myxedema (elephantiasic form): treatment with cytotoxic therapy. Hanke CW, Bergfeld WF, Guirguis MN, Lewis LJ. Cleve Clin Q 1983; 50: 183–8.

Fibroblasts from pretibial myxedema sites of a 44-year-old man showed reduced DNA content in vitro with the use of cytotoxic agents. Melphalan, which reduced hyaluronic acid levels to the greatest extent, was given orally (8 mg daily) for 4 days, and repeated monthly for 6 months. This regimen provided transient improvement, but the patient's condition then worsened.

Surgical excision of pseudotumorous pretibial myxedema. Pingsmann A, Ockenfels HM, Patsalis T. Foot Ankle Int 1996; 17: 107–10.

In this case of a 56-year-old woman with Graves' disease who had undergone subtotal thyroidectomy, surgical excision of the reticular dermis was useful in the elimination of pseudotumorous pretibial myxedema recalcitrant to oral and topical corticosteroids.

Successful combined surgical and octreotide treatment of severe pretibial myxoedema reviewed after 9 years. Felton J, Derrick EK, Price ML. Br J Dermatol 2003; 148: 825–6.

A 56-year-old man with pretibial myxedema was treated with surgical shave removal followed by daily subcutaneous octreotide injections for 6 months. His lesions did not recur over a 9-year follow-up period.

Pretibial myxedema. Matsuoka LY, Wortsman J, Dietrich JG, Pearson R. Arch Dermatol 1981; 117: 250–1.

A 47-year-old woman with hypothyroidism had recurrence of pretibial myxedema in a split-thickness skin graft 3 years after placement.

Pretibial myxedema: recurrence after skin grafting. Kucer KA, Herbert A, Luscombe HA, Kauh YC. Arch Dermatol 1980; 116: 1076–7.

A patient with recurrence of pretibial myxedema in graft sites after wide excision had a good response to topical fluorinated halcinonide cream under occlusion at night, and intralesional triamcinolone acetonide every month.

Elephantiasic pretibial myxedema: a novel treatment for an uncommon disorder. Susser WS, Heermans AG, Chapman MS, Baughman RD. J Am Acad Dermatol 2002; 46: 723–6.

A 67-year-old woman with elephantiasic pretibial myxedema had a 47% reduction of leg edema after 6 weeks of intensive complete decongestive physiotherapy. This response was sustained for 2 years after treatment.

Complete decongestive physiotherapy consists of manual massage of the lower extremities to promote lymphatic drainage, followed by compressive bandages, exercise, and skin care.

Prurigo nodularis

Christopher Rowland Payne

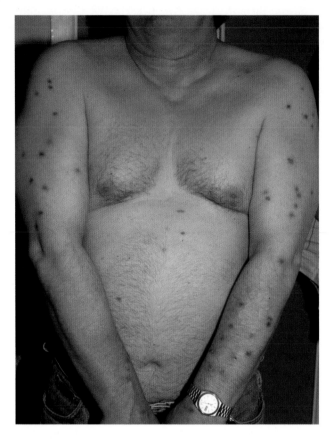

Prurigo nodularis (PN) is an excoriated eruption characterized by lichenified nodules. It favors the distal parts of the extensor aspects of the limbs and may be considered a localized form of lichen simplex chronicus.

PN affects all ages and the sex ratio is equal. Pruritus is episodic and disabling. Excoriation is always severe. The eruption is polymorphic and favors the periphery. PN has many clinical and histological similarities with eczema. Neural hyperplasia is minimal or absent.

PN usually has an identifiable cause. In half of patients it is due to a *cutaneous* disorder – usually atopic dermatitis, sometimes gravitational eczema, lichen simplex, nummular eczema, or insect bites, and occasionally subclinical dermatitis herpetiformis or subclinical bullous pemphigoid (known as pemphigoid nodularis). In one-third, the cause is *metabolic,* and in the remainder it is *psychological* – usually depression, sometimes anxiety or psychosis. The diverse metabolic disorders that cause PN induce itching by a small number of shared mechanisms, most commonly nutritional deficiency, hepatic dysfunction, and uremia, and occasionally thyroid disorder, hypercalcemia, neurological disorder (e.g., stroke), or lymphoma. Nutritional deficiency (the marker of which is reduced iron saturation) usually results from dietary deficiency, such as iron deficiency in women (in which dietary intake is not sufficient to compensate for menstrual loss), and sometimes results from malabsorption (more often postoperative than gluten-sensitive) or gastrointestinal bleeding.

In PN, remission can be expected when there is good patient compliance with symptomatic measures. However, cure is dependent on resolution of the underlying disorder.

MANAGEMENT STRATEGY

The best therapeutic results are achieved by symptomatic treatment of the cutaneous eruption while concurrently identifying and treating the underlying cause of the itch. To do this, a full medical history, complete physical examination, and a range of simple investigations are needed to determine the driver for the itching, whether metabolic, psychological or cutaneous.

Symptomatic treatment is very effective. In all patients it is essential to overcome all itching by using full doses of sedating *oral antihistamines,* such as promethazine 25–50 mg (which is best given 11 hours before rising, rather than at bedtime). Patients may be helped to restrain themselves from excoriation by cutting their nails to the quick, by wearing mittens, or by using *occlusive dressings,* such as hydrocolloid dressings. Occlusive bandaging or even plaster of Paris casts can be applied in resistant cases. The most potent *topical corticosteroids* are necessary and should be applied accurately to individual lesions in a cream form or as an impregnated tape (Cordran Tape, Haelan Tape). *Intralesional injection of corticosteroids* is also helpful (triamcinolone acetonide 40 mg/mL can be injected, 0.1 mL/nodule, and repeated at 6-weekly intervals). *Topical capsaicin* and/or *cryotherapy* may be added. When lesions are too numerous to treat topically or by injection, phototherapy with *UVB* or *PUVA* may be helpful. In severe and therapy-resistant cases oral *thalidomide* may be considered.

Treatment of the underlying cause is essential in order to achieve cure. Each specific etiology requires its own specific treatment.

When atopic dermatitis is the cause, treatments aimed at atopic dermatitis are likely to be the most successful. These would include emollients, sedative antihistamines, and potent or very potent topical corticosteroids, sometimes under occlusion.

In PN of metabolic origin, hepatic cases carry the best prognosis: when liver function tests return to normal, a successful outcome can be expected. Nutritional deficiency is common. Although this is often associated with iron deficiency anemia, iron supplements alone are not always helpful. If those deficient of iron are also deficient in other bloodborne nutrients, it may be more logical to advise eating 50 mg of dark meat daily and 50 mg of animal liver each week. Uremia, thyroid disorder, and lymphoma clearly need their own specific treatments.

In patients who scratch for psychological reasons, treatment depends on the underlying disturbance. The most frequent is depression, and this often responds to tricyclic antidepressants such as dothiepin. Not every case of PN is pruritic, but all are excoriated. Excoriation of biopic severity or excoriation without itching indicate a psychological origin.

SPECIFIC INVESTIGATIONS

- ▶ Complete blood count, ESR
- ▶ BUN, creatinine
- ▶ Liver function tests
- ▶ Iron saturation (iron/total iron-binding capacity or iron/transferrin) (Ferritin is not as good a test)

Evidence Levels: **A** Double-blind study **B** Clinical trial ≥ 20 subjects **C** Clinical trial < 20 subjects **D** Series ≥ 5 subjects **E** Anecdotal case reports

- ▶ Calcium and albumin
- ▶ Thyroid function tests
- ▶ Pemphigoid and coeliac antibodies
- ▶ Chest X-ray
- ▶ Possibly HIV serology
- ▶ Possibly serum IgE
- ▶ Possibly non-lesional biopsy for direct immunofluorescence

FIRST-LINE THERAPIES

▶ Sedative antihistamines	D
▶ Occlusion	E
▶ Topical superpotent corticosteroids	D
▶ Topical corticosteroids with occlusion	D
▶ Intralesional corticosteroids	E

Prurigo nodularis. Rowland Payne CME. In: Bernhard JD, ed. Itch – mechanisms and management of pruritus. New York: McGraw-Hill, 1994; 103–119.

Based on a series of 67 patients, the overall patient management of PN is discussed comprehensively.

Nodular prurigo: a clinicopathological study of 46 patients. Rowland Payne CME, Wilkinson JD, McKee PH, Jurecka W, Black MM. Br J Dermatol 1985; 113: 431–44.

The underlying causes of PN are reviewed in this paper.

Treatment of nodular prurigo with cyclosporin (treat the disease, not just the symptoms). Koblenzer CS. Br J Dermatol 1996; 135: 330–1.

Koblenzer emphases the importance of treating the underlying cause of the itching rather than simply trying to suppress the symptoms with ciclosporin or any other drug.

Use of occlusive membrane in prurigo nodularis. Meyers LN. Int J Dermatol 1989; 28: 275–6.

Four patients with PN responded to weekly application of an occlusive hydrocolloid pad (Duoderm). All lesions resolved, but recurred several weeks later in one patient and several months later in a second. One of these patients responded to application of an occlusive pad and an unspecified tranquilizer. The other again cleared with application of the occlusive pad.

Occlusive pads physically prevent scratching, eliminating the chief aggravating factor in PN.

SECOND-LINE THERAPIES

▶ Capsaicin	B
▶ Cryotherapy	E
▶ UVB phototherapy	E
▶ Narrowband UVB	C
▶ PUVA or bath PUVA	C

Treatment of prurigo nodularis with topical capsaicin. Stander S, Luger T, Metze D. J Am Acad Dermatol 2001; 44: 471–8.

Thirty-three patients with PN were treated with topical capsaicin (0.025–0.3%) four to six times daily for periods of between 2 weeks and 10 months. Pruritus resolved in all patients within 12 days, but returned in 16 of 33 patients within 2 months of discontinuation of capsaicin.

Cryotherapy improves prurigo nodularis. Waldinger TP, Wong RC, Taylor WB, Voorhees JJ. Arch Dermatol 1984; 120: 1598–600.

A black woman resistant to multiple therapies, including topical corticosteroids, oral hydroxyzine hydrochloride, phototherapy, and tar, was successfully treated with liquid nitrogen.

Cryotherapy to the point of blistering can lead to scarring and hypopigmentation, as it did in this patient.

Treatment of prurigo nodularis: use of cryosurgery and intralesional steroids plus lidocaine. Stoll DM, Fields JP, King LE Jr. J Dermatol Surg Oncol 1983; 9: 922–4.

Two patients were treated with liquid nitrogen applied with a cotton-tipped applicator for a freeze time of 10 seconds, followed by intralesional injection of triamcinolone acetonide (10 mg/mL) mixed with lidocaine (lignocaine) 0.75%. All lesions resolved after four to eight injections at 4–6-week intervals.

UV treatment of generalised prurigo nodularis. Hans SK, Cho MY, Park YK. J Am Acad Dermatol 1990; 29: 436–7.

Two patients were treated with UVB administered three times a week for 24–30 treatments. Itching resolved and most lesions cleared. Residual large lesions were treated with intralesional injection of corticosteroids and with topical PUVA.

Narrow-band ultraviolet B phototherapy in patients with recalcitrant nodular prurigo. Tamagawa-Mineoka R, Katoh N, Ueda E, Kishimolo S. J Dermatol 2007; 34: 691–5.

Once-weekly narrowband ultraviolet B phototherapy notably improved 10 patients with recalcitrant nodular prurigo. At 1-year follow-up only one had relapsed. The other nine continued to derive long-term benefit.

Phototherapy in nodular prurigo. Divekar PM, Palmer RA, Keefe M. Clin Ex Dermatol 2003; 28: 92–102.

Phototherapy of various types (broadband UVB, bath PUVA and oral PUVA) was administered to 14 patients with nodular prurigo. The patients were given 19 courses of treatment (nine to 34 visits). Partial improvement occurred in two-thirds, complete remission in three (but two of these had recurrence within 1 year).

Longterm results of topical trioxalen PUVA in lichen planus and nodular prurigo. Karoven J, Hannuksela M. Acta Dermatol Venereol (Stockh) 1985; 120: 53–5.

Bath and ointment trioxsalen PUVA was given to 63 patients with nodular prurigo, with good effect in 81%. In most patients the disease relapsed and further treatment was needed to maintain the result. After 1–6 years of follow-up 18% of patients were totally healed.

Local photochemotherapy in nodular prurigo. Vaatainen N, Hannuksela M, Karvonen J. Acta Dermatol Venereol 1979; 59: 544–7.

Fifteen patients with PN responded to trioxsalen baths and UVA. Moderate (seven patients) or good (eight patients) results were achieved in 3 weeks. Itching improved markedly in 4–6 days. Initial doses of 0.1–0.2 J/cm² were given daily, and doses increased by approximately 50% every third day.

THIRD-LINE THERAPIES

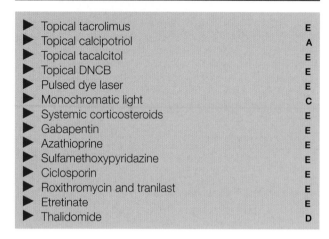

▶ Topical tacrolimus	E
▶ Topical calcipotriol	A
▶ Topical tacalcitol	E
▶ Topical DNCB	E
▶ Pulsed dye laser	E
▶ Monochromatic light	C
▶ Systemic corticosteroids	E
▶ Gabapentin	E
▶ Azathioprine	E
▶ Sulfamethoxypyridazine	E
▶ Ciclosporin	E
▶ Roxithromycin and tranilast	E
▶ Etretinate	E
▶ Thalidomide	D

Nodular prurigo responding to topical tacrolimus. Edmonds EV, Riaz SN, Francis N, Bunker CB. Br J Dermatol 2004; 150: 1216–17.

One patient responded to topical tacrolimus.

Topical vitamin D$_3$ (tacalcitol) for steroid-resistant prurigo. Katayama I, Miyazaki Y, Nishioka K. Br J Dermatol 1996; 135: 237–40.

Four cases with PN were treated using topical vitamin D$_3$ ointment (tacalcitol) with a useful clinical response.

Double-blind, right/left comparison of calcipotriol ointment and betamethasone ointment in the treatment of prurigo nodularis. Wong SS, Goh CL. Arch Dermatol 2000; 136: 807–8.

A prospective, randomized, double-blind right–left comparison of calcipotriol ointment and betamethasone valerate ointment in the treatment of PN.

Successful immunotherapy of chronic nodular prurigo with topical dinitrochlorobenzene. Yoshizawa Y, Kitamura K, Maibach HI. Br J Dermatol 1999; 14: 387–9.

Nodular prurigo successfully treated with the pulsed dye laser. Woo PN, Finch TM, Hindson C, Foulds IS. Br J Dermatol 2000; 143: 215–16.

A patient with recalcitrant nodular prurigo, resistant to topical and intralesional steroids as well as PUVA, responded well to treatment with pulsed dye laser (595 nm).

Monochromatic excimer light (308nm) in the treatment of prurigo nodularis. Saraceno R, Nistico SP, Capriotti E, de Felice C, Rhodes LE, Chimenti S. Photodermatol Photoimmunol Photomed 2008; 24: 43–5.

Partial or complete clinical and histological remission occurred in all 11 patients treated by weekly monochromatic excimer light (308 nm) for an average of eight sessions.

Gabapentin for the treatment of recalcitrant chronic prurigo nodularis. Dereli T, Karaca N, Inanir I, Ozturk G. Eur J Dermatol 2008; 18: 85–6.

Nodular prurigo responsive to azathiaprine. Lear JT, English JS, Smith AG. Br J Dermatol 1996; 134: 1151.

Two patients with nodular prurigo responded to azathiaprine 50 mg bd.

Sulfamethoxypyriadazine-responsive pemphigoid nodularis: a report of two cases. Gach JE, Wilson NJ, Wojnarowska F, Ilchyshyn A. J Am Acad Dermatol 2005; 53: S101–4.

Antipruritic effect of cyclosporine microemulsion in prurigo nodularis: Results of a case series. Siepmann D, Lugar TA, Stander S. J Dtsch Dermatol Ges 2008; 6: 941–6. Epub 28 April 2008.

Nodular prurigo responds to cyclosporin. Berth-Jones J, Smith SG, Graham-Brown RAC. Br J Dermatol 1995; 132: 795–9.

Two women with PN improved markedly while taking oral ciclosporin 3–4.5 mg/kg daily, but neither cleared completely.

As well as the usual risks of the renal complications, reversible ascending motor neuropathy has also been reported from ciclosporin given for nodular prurigo.

Uncontrollable prurigo nodularis effectively treated by roxithromycin and tranilast. Horiuchi Y, Bae S, Katayama J. J Drugs Dermatol 2006; 5: 363–5.

Three cases of uncontrollable PN were treated with a combination of 300 mg/day roxithromycin and 200 mg/day tranilast. Complete and/or marked regression of PN was observed within 4–6 months.

Prurigo nodularis (Hyde) treated with Tigason. Gip L. Dermatologica 1984; 169–260.

Etretinate and nodular prurigo. Rowland Payne CME. Br J Dermatol 1988; 118–36.

Thalidomide treatment of prurigo nodularis. Winkelmann RK, Connolly SM, Doyle JA, Padilha-Goncalves A. Acta Dermatol Venereol 1984; 64: 412–17.

Four patients with PN were treated with oral thalidomide, resulting in rapid resolution of itching and subsequent resolution of nodules. Doses of 100–300 mg daily were required. Three of the four had elevated IgE levels that decreased during treatment. In one patient the lesions recurred after discontinuation of the treatment, but responded again to further oral thalidomide. Two patients achieved long-term remission.

Fatigue, constipation, peripheral neuropathy, and even toxic pustuloderma are frequent and/or important and limiting adverse effects of this treatment. Thalidomide is hazardous to give to women of childbearing potential because of the potential for severe birth defects.

Sequential combined therapy with thalidomide and narrowband (TL01) UVB in the treatment of prurigo nodularis. Ferrandiz C, Carrasocsa JM, Just M, Bielsa I, Ribera M. Dermatology 1997; 195: 359–61.

Four patients with PN were started on thalidomide and subsequently treated with narrowband UVB for up to 37 treatments. One patient who relapsed after 5 months was controlled anew with a further course of UVB without thalidomide.

Thalidomide treatment for prurigo nodularis in human immunodeficiency virus-infected subjects: efficacy and risk of neuropathy. Maurer T, Poncelet A, Berger T. Arch Dermatol 2004; 140: 845–9.

Eight HIV-infected patients with prurigo were treated with thalidomide 100 mg daily. After the first month patients were randomized to receive 100 mg or 200 mg daily and the dose was adjusted if side effects developed. All had a more than 50% reduction in itching within an average of 3.4 months. Seven of eight had a greater than 50% reduction in skin lesions within an average of 5 months. Thalidomide peripheral neuropathy developed in three patients.

In the author's own experience, six of 10 patients with nodular prurigo improved with thalidomide. Adverse effects occurred in all 10 and led to discontinuation of treatment in six. Adverse effects from thalidomide are common, serious, and unpredictable. Thalidomide cannot be recommended as a safe treatment for PN in anything but exceptional circumstances.

Prurigo pigmentosa

Yukiko Tsuji-Abe, Hiroshi Shimizu

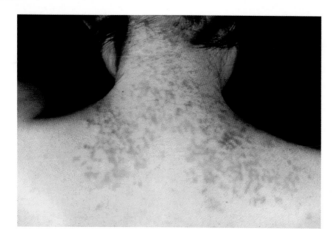

Prurigo pigmentosa has a distinct clinical appearance that starts with pruritic, urticarial papules or papulovesicles followed by a peculiar reticular pigmentation. The majority of reported patients are Japanese, with a female preponderance, but non-Japanese patients are also described.

MANAGEMENT STRATEGY

The pathogenesis of prurigo pigmentosa remains unknown. Friction from clothing can trigger the disease. In some cases, ketosis caused by diabetes mellitus, sudden weight loss, or anorexia nervosa precedes prurigo pigmentosa, and treatment of these conditions can resolve the lesions in some cases. There are several case reports of individuals who developed this condition in association with other disorders or conditions, including contact allergic reactions to certain chemical agents, *Helicobacter pylori* infection, atopic diathesis, and pregnancy. *Minocycline* (100–200 mg daily) and *dapsone* (25–100 mg daily) are usually very effective for prurigo pigmentosa. The effects are mostly observed within a few days or a week after treatment, with a reduction in both itch and papular lesions. Minocycline might be the first-line therapy, because it produces fewer adverse reactions, and the remission time has been reported as being longer than with dapsone treatment. Topical or systemic corticosteroids or antihistamines are usually ineffective.

SPECIFIC INVESTIGATIONS

▶ Fasting blood sugar and urinalysis for ketones

Prurigo pigmentosa on a patient with soft-drink ketosis. Mitsuhashi Y, Suzuki N, Kawaguchi M, Kondo S. J Dermatol 2005; 32: 767–8.

Bullous prurigo pigmentosa and diabetes. Kubota Y, Koga T, Nakayama J. Eur J Dermatol 1998; 8: 439–41.

Prurigo pigmentosa in a pregnant woman. Leone L, Colato C, Girolomoni G. Int J Gynaecol Obstet 2007; 98: 261–2.

The patient was in the 13th week of pregnancy and had been on a restricted diet for severe vomiting. Her urinary ketones were elevated. Application of emollients, intravenous fluid treatment, and return to a normal diet were associated with progressive resolution of skin lesions in 1 month.

Prurigo pigmentosa (Nagashima) associated with anorexia nervosa. Nakada T, Sueki H, Iijima M. Clin Exp Dermatol 1998; 23: 25–7.

A young woman with anorexia nervosa developed prurigo pigmentosa. After she gained weight, the lesions resolved completely.

In all these reports, prurigo pigmentosa was associated with ketosis. Disease activity sometimes correlated with the amount of urinary ketones. In some cases, lesions resolved simply as a result of treating the causative condition.

FIRST-LINE THERAPIES

▶ Minocycline	C
▶ Dapsone	C
▶ Treatment for ketosis or any other causative factors	D

Prurigo pigmentosa: a distinctive inflammatory disease of the skin. Böer A, Misago N, Wolter M, Kiryu H, Wang XD, Ackerman AB. Am J Dermatopathol 2003; 25: 117–29.

Out of 25 cases, 16 responded well to minocycline (100–200 mg daily) and seven responded well to dapsone (25 mg daily).

Bullous prurigo pigmentosa and diabetes. Kubota Y, Koga T, Nakayama J. Eur J Dermatol 1998; 8: 439–41.

A patient with diabetes mellitus developed a severe vesicular form of prurigo pigmentosa. Minocycline was very effective. In addition, the eruption subsided when the urinary glucose and ketone levels were controlled.

Prurigo pigmentosa – clinical observations of our 14 cases. Nagashima M. J Dermatol 1978; 5: 61–7.

This is the first report of prurigo pigmentosa. The author suggests that friction from clothing can trigger this condition. Dapsone was used in some cases and was highly effective.

Prurigo pigmentosa associated with diabetic keratoacidosis. Ohnishi T, Kisa H, Ogata E, Watanabe S. Acta Dermatol Venereol 2000; 80: 447–8.

Eighteen cases of prurigo pigmentosa were associated with diabetic ketoacidosis. Treatment of ketoacidosis improved the eruption in eight cases, treatment with topical corticosteroid improved the rash in one case, and progress was unknown in one case.

Minocycline and dapsone are usually very effective against prurigo pigmentosa. The effects are mostly observed within a few days or a week after treatment, with a reduction in pruritic and papular lesions. Minocycline might be the first-line therapy, because it produces fewer adverse reactions, and the remission time has been reported as being longer than with dapsone.

SECOND-LINE THERAPIES

▶ Doxycycline	**D**
▶ Roxithromycin	**E**
▶ Clarithromycin	**E**

Prurigo pigmentosa: not an uncommon disease in the Turkish population. Baykal C, Buyukbabani N, Akinturk S, Saglik E. Int J Dermatol 2006; 45: 1164–8.

Out of six cases of prurigo pigmentosa, three responded well to doxycycline 100 mg daily and another three responded well to tetracycline 500 mg daily.

The successful treatment of prurigo pigmentosa with macrolide antibiotics. Yazawa N, Ihn H, Yamane K, Etoh T, Tamaki K. Dermatology 2001; 202: 67–9

Two cases of prurigo pigmentosa responded well to 300 mg daily roxithromycin, and another two cases responded well to 400 mg daily of clarithromycin. In all cases, the effect appeared quickly and the pruritus and papules disappeared within a week.

Prurigo pigmentosa. Gürses L, Gürbüz O, Demirçay Z, Kotiloglu E. Int J Dermatol 1999; 38: 924–5.

Of two cases, one responded well to doxycycline 200 mg daily, and the other resolved spontaneously.

Prurigo pigmentosa. Gür-Toy G, Güngör E, Artüz F, Aksoy F, Alli N. Int J Dermatol 2002; 41: 288–91.

Roxithromycin 300 mg daily was effective in two cases of prurigo pigmentosa, and clarithromycin 400 mg daily was effective in another two.

Doxycycline and macrolide antibiotics are effective for prurigo pigmentosa. These therapies are recommended for use in patients who respond poorly or have contraindications to first-line medication because of adverse reactions.

THIRD-LINE THERAPIES

▶ Isotretinoin	**E**
▶ Potassium iodide	**E**
▶ Sulfamethoxazole	**E**

Vesiculous prurigo pigmentosa in a 13-year-old girl: good response to isotretinoin. Requena Caballero C, Nagore E, Sanmartín O, Botella-Estrada R, Serra C, Guillén C. J Eur Acad Dermatol Venereol 2005; 19: 474–6.

This patient was initially diagnosed as having a vesiculobullous form of Darier's disease and treatment with isotretinoin 40 mg/day was started, with a good response in 10 days. The lesion relapsed 5 months later, and treatment with minocycline 100 mg/day cleared it within 7 days.

Prurigo pigmentosa successfully treated with low-dose isotretinoin. Akoglu G, Boztepe G, Karaduman A. Dermatology 2006; 213: 331–3.

An 18-year-old woman was successfully treated with isotretinoin 20 mg daily (0.3 mg/kg/day). Pruritus and erythematous macules resolved in less than 1 month after therapy began.

Prurigo pigmentosa: 3rd non-Japanese case. Harms M, Merot Y, Polla L, Saurat JH. Dermatologica 1986; 173: 202–4.

A 23-year-old woman was first treated with dapsone 50 mg daily, but the disease recurred shortly after stopping therapy. Potassium iodide 500 mg daily was then prescribed and the lesions cleared.

Prurigo pigmentosa: a possible mechanism of action of sulfonamides. Miyachi Y, Yoshioka A, Horio T, Imamura S, Niwa Y. Dermatologia 1986; 172: 82–8.

A 31-year-old woman with a 4-year history of recurrent prurigo pigmentosa responded well to sulfamethoxazole 2.0 g daily.

Most patients with prurigo pigmentosa respond well to first- or second-line therapies or undergo spontaneous remission, but these alternatives might be useful in exceptional cases.

Pruritus

Amit Garg, Jeffrey D Bernhard

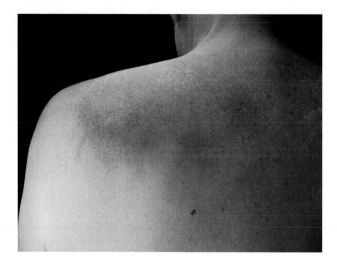

Pruritus is a cutaneous sensation (usually unpleasant) that evokes an urge to scratch, rub, pick, and in extreme cases mutilate the skin in an attempt to obtain relief. Itch/pruritus (the terms are used interchangeably) can occur in the absence of visible cutaneous disease, as a characteristic feature of a multitude of diseases of the skin, or as an unusual sign of systemic diseases. Pruritus in the absence of a detectable rash, whether localized or generalized, may pose both a diagnostic and a therapeutic dilemma to even the most seasoned dermatologist. New appreciation for the neurophysiology of itch has led to specific therapies targeting particular pathways in the nervous system.

MANAGEMENT STRATEGY

Management of pruritus is directed towards its cause, which may not always be apparent, regardless of whether dermatitis is present. Many dermatoses itch, and it is beyond the scope of this chapter to discuss them all. Xerosis and scabies deserve mention because both can have subtle findings, with the intensity of pruritus out of proportion to the rash. In xerosis, an adequate skin care regimen and emollients are indispensable. One of the more common and embarrassing errors is to miss the diagnosis of scabies, and consideration of this diagnosis may avoid delays in treatment and undue suffering in pruritic patients.

Failure to diagnose a primary skin disease does not rule out the possibility that one is present; time, repeated observation, and laboratory tests such as a skin biopsy may be required. When no rash is present, or when a rash is present but cannot be diagnosed, a full medical history and physical examination are indicated, including a precise medication review and full review of systems. The physical examination should include palpation for organomegaly and lymphadenopathy. On the complete integumentary examination one should not be misled by nonspecific secondary changes caused by rubbing, scratching, or secondary infection. Laboratory investigations are often essential to the clinical assessment of generalized pruritus, whether a rash is present or not.

The most serious error is to miss the diagnosis of an underlying systemic disease associated with pruritus. Some of the many systemic diseases that may cause pruritus include hematologic and solid malignancies, lymphoproliferative disease, HIV, thyroid disease, iron deficiency, renal disease, hepatobiliary disease, connective tissue disease, neurologic disease, and drug hypersensitivity. Periodic re-evaluation for associated systemic disease should be undertaken, as pruritus may precede the diagnosis of a systemic disease by many months (as in primary biliary cirrhosis).

In general, the implementation of good general skin hygiene measures, including bathing in tepid water, using fragrance-free moisturizing soaps, using emollients or unscented bath oils liberally after bathing, maintaining a cool moisture-rich environment with a humidifier, and wearing loose-fitting clothing is fundamental. In the management of pruritus that does not respond to simple measures, treatment should be individualized and stepwise based on etiology, severity, and regard for safety.

SPECIFIC INVESTIGATIONS

Screening
- ► Complete medical history
- ► Thorough review of systems
- ► Complete physical examination

Laboratory investigations
- ► Complete blood count with differential
- ► Blood urea nitrogen, creatinine
- ► Fasting glucose
- ► Hepatic function testing
- ► Thyroid function testing
- ► Chest radiograph (posteroanterior and lateral)
- ► Age-appropriate cancer screening

Additional testing to consider
- ► Scraping for scabies
- ► Hepatitis B and C profiles
- ► HIV testing
- ► Erythrocyte sedimentation rate
- ► Serum iron and ferritin
- ► Serum protein electrophoresis, urine protein electrophoresis
- ► Stool for ova and parasites
- ► Skin biopsy

Itch and pruritus: what are they and how should itches be classified? Bernhard JD. Dermatol Ther 2005; 18: 288–91.

Clinical classification of itch: a position paper of the International Forum for the Study of Itch. Ständer S, Weisshaar E, Mettang T, Szepietowski JC, Carstens E, Ikoma A, et al. Acta Dermatol Venereol 2007; 87: 291–4.

These two papers provide a definition of itch and discuss the terms used to signify different categories of pruritic disorder.

Neurophysiological and neurochemical basis of modern pruritus treatment. Stander S, Weisshaar E, Luger TA. Exp Dermatol 2008; 17: 161–9.

This review highlights the modern neurophysiological and neurochemical therapeutic strategies on the basis of neuronal mechanisms underlying chronic pruritus.

Evaluation of the patient with generalized pruritus. Kantor GR. In: Bernhard, JD, ed. Itch: mechanisms and management of pruritus. New York: McGraw-Hill, 1994; 337–46.

The diagnostic and therapeutic approach to idiopathic generalized pruritus. Yosipovitch G, David M. Int J Dermatol 1999; 38: 881–7.

These are two comprehensive reviews that describe the evaluation, work-up, and subsequent treatment of patients without a clear etiology for their itch. The second touches on new findings in the neural pathways and physiology of itch.

Ultraviolet phototherapy for pruritus. Rivard J, Lim HW. Dermatol Ther 2005; 18: 344–54.

Ultraviolet-based therapy is used to treat a variety of pruritic conditions. In this review, mechanisms of action for phototherapy are discussed. Treatment limitations, side effects, and common dosing protocols are reviewed.

Pruritus in chronic liver disease: mechanisms and treatment. Bergasa NV. Curr Gastroenterol Rep 2004; 6: 10–16.

This is an excellent and succinct review of cholestatic pruritus. It presents what is known about the pathophysiology of itch and cholestasis, and discusses targeted treatment strategies in cholestatic disease.

NEUROPATHIC ITCH

Neuropathic itch arises as a consequence of pathology at one or more points along the afferent (sensory) pathway of the peripheral or central nervous system. In brachioradial pruritus (BRP) and notalgia paresthetica (NP), it is believed that dorsal spinal nerve radiculopathy, usually secondary to degenerative disease of cervical and thoracic vertebral bodies, respectively, results in persistent itching, paresthesia, hypesthesia, or pain. There may be hyperpigmentation and/or excoriation of the involved area. These forms of localized pruritus may go undiagnosed for quite some time. By the time patients fail to respond to various treatments and obtain a dermatology referral, the itch has often been going on for months and may in fact have become generalized, with secondary changes that may be mistaken for a primary dermatosis.

Repeated application of *capsiacin cream*, which depletes axonal stores of substance P, may be a safe and highly effective approach to treating localized areas of neuropathic pain or itch. Although evidence for the use of gabapentin in BP and NP is anecdotal, it is increasingly being used with success for more widespread or otherwise recalcitrant neuropathic dysesthesias. Doses as high as 2400 mg or more daily, if tolerated, may be required. Pregabalin, an analog of gabapentin, has also been effective in neuropathic pain syndromes such as postherpetic neuralgia and diabetic neuropathy; there is preliminary evidence that it may be effective in types of itch.

Successful treatment of notalgia paresthetica with topical capsaicin: vehicle-controlled, double-blind, crossover study. Wallengren J, Klinker M. J Am Acad Dermatol 1995; 32: 287–9.

In this 10-week study, 20 patients with notalgia paresthetica were treated with capsaicin cream or placebo five times daily for 1 week and then three times daily for 3 weeks. Treatment was stopped for 2 weeks prior to all patients using capsaicin cream on the same schedule as before. Seventy percent of patients treated with capsaicin cream had improved symptoms, compared to only 30% on placebo. Pruritus did not intensify during the washout period in patients who received capsaicin cream in the first 4 weeks.

Solar (brachioradial) pruritus – response to capsaicin cream. Knight TE, Hayashi T. Int J Dermatol 1994; 33: 206–9.

In this open-label trial of capsaicin cream, 10 of 13 patients completing the study found significant relief (itching much improved or gone) from itch on the treated arm after 3 weeks compared to the untreated control arm.

Gabapentin treatment for notalgia paresthetica, a common isolated peripheral sensory neuropathy. Loosemore MP, Bordeaux JS, Bernhard JD. J Eur Acad Dermatol Venereol 2007; 21: 1440–1.

An 82-year-old man was treated with gabapentin 600 mg at night with resolution of symptoms. Symptoms recurred when gabapentin was stopped, and then resolved with reinitiation of the medication.

Brachioradial pruritus: report of a new case responding to gabapentin. Kanitakis J. Eur J Dermatol 2006; 16: 311–12.

A 54-year-old man with BRP noted significant (90%) improvement in pruritus with gabapentin 600 mg tid and the use of an antipruritic cream containing 8% calamine and essential fatty acids. He initially had diarrhea and sleepiness at this dose. Pruritus returned with discontinuation of gabapentin, and again resolved with its reinitiation.

Gabapentin treatment for brachioradial pruritus. Bueller HA, Bernhard JD, Dubroff LM. J Eur Acad Dermatol Venereol 1999; 13: 227–8.

Ehrchen J, Stander S. Pregabalin in the treatment of chronic pruritus. J Am Acad Dermatol 2008; 58: S36–7.

CHOLESTATIC ITCH

Cholestasis, a reduction of bile flow, results from a variety of hepatic as well as extrahepatic diseases. Although the pathophysiologic link between cholestasis and pruritus is not fully understood, it may be a consequence of increased levels of endogenous opioids. Pruritus of cholestasis is typically widespread, characteristically involves the palms and soles, and may be accompanied by jaundice. Therapeutic interventions have focused on the *removal of presumed pruritogens* from the circulation (through the use of *ursodeoxycholic acid, cholestyramine*), induction of hepatic enzymes (*rifampin*), antagonism of endogenous opioid receptors (*naltrexone, nalaxone, nalmefene*), modulation of serotonin neurotransmission (*sertraline*), activation of cannabinoid receptors (*dronabinol*), and clearing water-soluble and protein-bound pruritogens through *albumin-based dialysis* (Molecular Adsorbent Recycling System, Prometheus). *Ultraviolet B phototherapy* and *parenteral lidocaine* are further therapeutic considerations.

CHOLESTASIS

FIRST-LINE THERAPIES

▶ Rifampin	A
▶ Natrexone, nalmefene, nalaxone	A

SECOND-LINE THERAPIES

▶ Cholestyramine	A
▶ Ursodeoxycholic acid	A
▶ Sertraline	A

THIRD-LINE THERAPIES

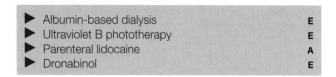

▶ Albumin-based dialysis	E
▶ Ultraviolet B phototherapy	E
▶ Parenteral lidocaine	A
▶ Dronabinol	E

Rifampin is safe for treatment of pruritus due to chronic cholestasis: a meta-analysis of prospective randomized-controlled trials. Khurana S, Singh P. Liver Int 2006; 26: 943–8.

This meta-analysis includes five prospective randomized controlled trials with 61 patients who had pruritus associated with chronic liver disease. Complete or partial resolution of symptoms occurred in 77% of patients taking rifampin 300–600 mg daily.

The efficacy and safety of bile acid binding agents, opioid antagonists, or rifampin in the treatment of cholestasis-associated pruritus. Tandon P, Rowe BH, Vandermeer B, Bain VG. Am J Gastroenterol 2007; 102: 1528–36.

In this review of 12 randomized controlled trials, both rifampin and opioid antagonists significantly reduced cholestasis-associated pruritus. There were insufficient data to assess the efficacy of cholestyramine.

Efficacy and safety of oral naltrexone treatment for pruritus of cholestasis, a crossover, double blind, placebo-controlled study. Terg R, Coronel E, Sordá J, Muñoz AE, Findor J. J Hepatol 2002; 37: 717–22.

In this double-blind randomized placebo-controlled crossover trial of 20 patients with cholestasis-associated pruritus, nine of 20 patients taking naltrexone 50 mg daily experienced a greater than 50% reduction in symptoms relative to baseline, including five whose pruritus disappeared completely. Adverse effects included a short-lived opioid withdrawal-like phenomenon.

Oral nalmefene therapy reduces scratching activity due to the pruritus of cholestasis: a controlled study. Bergasa NV, Alling DW, Talbot TL, Wells MC, Jones EA. J Am Acad Dermatol 1999; 41: 431–4.

In a randomized double-blind placebo-controlled study with pruritus associated with chronic liver disease, nalmefene therapy was associated with a 75% reduction in the mean hourly scratching activity and a reduction in the mean visual analog score of the perception of pruritus in all eight patients.

Effects of naloxone infusions in patients with the pruritus of cholestasis. A double-blind, randomized, controlled trial. Bergasa NV, Alling DW, Talbot TL, Swain MG, Yurdaydin C, Turner ML, et al. Ann Intern Med 1995; 123: 161–7.

In this double-blind placebo-controlled crossover trial in 29 patients with liver disease, naloxone infusions resulted in significantly improved visual analog scale scores and hourly scratching activity compared to placebo.

Double-blind placebo-controlled clinical trial of microporous cholestyramine in the treatment of intra- and extra-hepatic cholestasis: relationship between itching and serum bile acids. Di Padova C, Tritapepe R, Rovagnati P, Rossetti S. Methods Find Exp Clin Pharmacol 1984; 6: 773–6.

In this double-blind placebo-controlled trial in 10 patients, microporous cholestyramine 3 g three times daily over a 4-week period significantly reduced itch intensity and serum bile acids compared to placebo.

Randomised controlled trials of ursodeoxycholic-acid therapy for primary biliary cirrhosis: a meta-analysis. Goulis J, Leandro G, Burroughs AK. Lancet 1999; 354: 1053–60.

In this meta-analysis, ursodeoxycholic acid was effective in treating pruritus associated with primary biliary cirrhosis in two of 11 randomized controlled trials.

Sertraline as a first-line treatment for cholestatic pruritus. Mayo MJ, Handem I, Saldana S, Jacobe H, Getachew Y, Rush AJ. Hepatology 2007; 45: 666–74.

In this randomized double-blind placebo-controlled trial, 21 patients with pruritus associated with chronic liver disease experienced significant improvements in perceived itch and in physical evidence of scratching while taking sertraline 75–100 mg daily.

Treatment of severe refractory pruritus with fractionated plasma separation and adsorption (Prometheus). Rifai K, Hafer C, Rosenau J, Athmann C, Haller H, Peter Manns M, et al. Scand J Gastroenterol 2006; 41: 1212–17.

Seven patients with recalcitrant pruritus associated with liver disease were treated with Prometheus for three to five sessions. All six patients with bile acid elevations reported a significant improvement in pruritus, which was also associated with a parallel decrease in serum bile acids. The patient with no initial bile acid elevation did not report an improvement in pruritus. In four of six patients the improvement lasted at least 4 weeks.

Therapy of intractable pruritus with MARS. Acevedo Ribó M, Moreno Planas JM, Sanz Moreno C, Rubio González EE, Rubio González E, Boullosa Graña E, et al. Transplant Proc 2005; 37: 1480–1.

All three patients with intractable pruritus associated with primary biliary cirrhosis who underwent two to three sessions of the molecular adsorbent recirculating system had marked improvement of pruritus and reduced bilirubin levels. Improvement lasted only a few days in all cases.

Extracorporeal albumin dialysis: a procedure for prolonged relief of intractable pruritus in patients with primary biliary cirrhosis. Pares A, Cisneros L, Salmeron JM, Caballería L, Mas A, Torras A, et al. Am J Gastroenterol 2004; 99: 1105–10.

Four patients with recalcitrant pruritus associated with primary biliary cirrhosis were treated with two extracorporeal albumin dialysis sessions 1 day apart. Two patients reported resolution of itch, and the other two a reported marked reduction in pruritus. Scratching reduced in a parallel fashion to reduced pruritus. Pruritus eventually recurred over months in all four patients.

Phototherapy for primary biliary cirrhosis. Perlstein SL. Arch Dermatol 1981; 117: 608.

In this case report, two patients with pruritus treated with weekly UVB phototherapy improved.

Efficacy of lidocaine in the treatment of pruritus in patients with chronic cholestatic liver diseases. Villamil AG, Bandi JC, Galdame OA, Gerona S, Gadano AC. Am J Med 2005; 118: 1160–3.

Evidence Levels: **A** Double-blind study **B** Clinical trial ≥ 20 subjects **C** Clinical trial < 20 subjects **D** Series ≥ 5 subjects **E** Anecdotal case reports

In this double-blind trial, 18 patients were randomized (2:1) to receive parenteral lidocaine 100 mg or placebo. Patients receiving lidocaine reported significantly reduced severity of pruritus and fatigue compared to placebo.

Preliminary observation with dronabinol in patients with intractable pruritus secondary to cholestatic liver disease. Neff GW, O'Brien CB, Reddy KR, Bergasa NV, Regev A, Molina E, et al. Am J Gastroenterol 2002; 97: 2117–19.

In this report, three patients with intractable cholestatic related pruritus were started on 5 mg of dronabinol (Δ-9-THC) at bedtime, a reduction in pruritus, marked improvement in sleep, and eventual return to work. Resolution of depression occurred in two of the three.

ITCH ASSOCIATED WITH CHOLESTASIS OF PREGNANCY

CHOLESTASIS OF PREGNANCY

FIRST-LINE THERAPIES

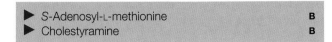

▷ Ursodeoxycholic acid	A

SECOND-LINE THERAPIES

▶ S-Adenosyl-L-methionine	B
▶ Cholestyramine	B

Intrahepatic cholestasis of pregnancy: Amelioration of pruritus by UDCA is associated with decreased progesterone disulphates in urine. Glantz A, Reilly SJ, Benthin L, Lammert F, Mattsson LA, Marschall HU. Hepatology 2008; 47: 544–51.

In this randomized controlled trial, women with intrahepatic cholestasis of pregnancy treated with ursodeoxycholic acid experienced amelioration of pruritus which was associated with increased hepatobiliary excretion of progesterone disulphates.

Intrahepatic cholestasis of pregnancy: a randomized controlled trial comparing dexamethasone and ursodeoxycholic acid. Glantz A, Marschall HU, Lammert F, Mattsson LA. Hepatology 2005; 42: 1399–405.

In this randomized double-blind placebo-controlled trial consisting of 130 women with intrahepatic cholestasis of pregnancy, 3 weeks of ursodeoxycholic acid 1 g daily resulted in significant relief from pruritus and marked reduction of serum bile acids.

Randomized prospective comparative study of ursodeoxycholic acid and S-adenosyl-L-methionine in the treatment of intrahepatic cholestasis of pregnancy. Binder T, Salaj P, Zima T, Vítek L. J Perinat Med 2006; 34: 383–91.

In this study, 78 women with intrahepatic cholestasis of pregnancy treated with ursodeoxycholic acid, S-adenosyl-L-methionine, or a combination of the two experienced a significant improvement in pruritus. Only ursodeoxycholic acid monotherapy and combination therapy led to improvement in serum concentrations of bile acids and transaminases, with the combination therapy leading to faster results.

Efficacy and safety of ursodeoxycholic acid versus cholestyramine in intrahepatic cholestasis of pregnancy. Kondrackiene J, Beuers U, Kupcinskas L. Gastroenterology 2005; 129: 894–901.

In this study, 84 women with intrahepatic cholestasis of pregnancy and pruritus were randomized to receive either ursodeoxycholic acid 8–10 mg/kg body weight daily or cholestyramine 8 g daily for 14 days. The group receiving ursodeoxycholic acid had greater improvement in pruritus, deliveries that were closer to term, greater reductions in serum alanine and aspartate aminotransferase activities, greater reductions in endogenous serum bile acid levels, and fewer adverse effects than the group receiving cholestyramine.

UREMIC ITCH

Patients with renal itch tend to have dry skin, have increased numbers of dermal mast cells, and may have a variety of unidentified circulating pruritogens, possibly including opioid peptides. Pruritus associated with chronic renal failure is usually an unremitting generalized itch which is more common among hemodialysis patients. Some dialysis patients experience itch localized to the shunt arm. The presence or intensity of pruritus does not correlate with blood urea or creatinine levels. The condition is difficult to manage and the only reliably effective treatment remains to be *kidney transplantation*. Fortunately, the incidence of uremic pruritus is decreasing as dialysis membranes with improved biocompatibility are being used. Optimizing general skin care measures with *emollients* to improve xerosis should be a fundamental part of the treatment plan. Antihistamines are generally not helpful for uremic pruritus. However, the tricyclic antihistamine *doxepin*, whose use in renal itch is not described in the literature, may be helpful because of its sedating and antidepressant properties. Whereas *UVB phototherapy* is the mainstay of treatment, *gabapentin* and *naltrexone* have also shown efficacy in trials. A number of other less conventional therapeutic interventions have reported success.

UREMIA

FIRST-LINE THERAPIES

▷ Emollients with high water content	A
▷ Narrowband UVB phototherapy	B
▷ Broadband UVB phototherapy	B
▷ Gabapentin	A
▷ Naltrexone	A

SECOND-LINE THERAPIES

▶ Acupuncture – Quchi (LI11) acupoint	A
▶ Homeopathic treatment with verum	A

THIRD-LINE THERAPIES

▶ Cholestyramine	A
▶ Activated charcoal	A
▶ Erythropoietin	A
▶ Thalidomide	B
▶ Parathyroidectomy	B

Treatment of uremic pruritus with narrowband ultraviolet B phototherapy: an open pilot study. Ada S, Seçkin D, Budakoglu I, Ozdemir FN. J Am Acad Dermatol 2005; 53: 149–51.

In this study, 20 patients with uremic pruritus were treated with narrowband ultraviolet B phototherapy for 6 weeks. Of the 10 that completed the study, eight showed 50% or more improvement in pruritus scores. Of the 10 patients that left the study before 6 weeks, six were satisfied with their response. In the 6-month follow-up period, three of seven responders who could be examined were in remission; in the remaining four, pruritus recurred within a mean of 2.5 months.

Generalized pruritus treated with narrowband UVB. Seckin D, Demircay A, Akin O. Int J Dermatol 2007; 46: 367–70.

Fifteen patients with uremic pruritus included in the analysis of this open-label trial were treated with narrowband UVB phototherapy three times weekly, with a mean number of 22 treatments having a mean cumulative UVB dose of 24 540 mJ/cm. These patients showed more than 50% improvement in visual analog and pruritus grading scores. Of the six patients who were followed up at a mean of 5.3 months, two remained in remission.

Ultraviolet phototherapy of uremic pruritus. Long-term results and possible mechanism of action. Gilchrest BA, Rowe JW, Brown RS, Steinman TI, Arndt KA. Ann Intern Med 1979; 91: 17–21

This is the classic study of 38 patients with uremic pruritus treated with UVB phototherapy. A comparison of three schedules varying from one to three treatments weekly showed that the percentage of patients responding was not influenced by frequency of UVB exposure, though patients treated more intensively improved faster. Patients receiving only half-body treatments improved as well, indicating a systemic rather than local effect. Overall, 32 of 38 patients improved after a course of six or eight UVB exposures.

Gabapentin: a promising drug for the treatment of uremic pruritus. Naini AE, Harandi AA, Khanbabapour S, Shahidi S, Seirafiyan S, Mohseni M. Saudi J Kidney Dis Transpl 2007; 18: 378–81.

In this double-blind placebo-controlled trial of 34 hemodialysis patients, those that received gabapentin 400 mg twice weekly after hemodialysis sessions for 4 weeks reported significantly improved pruritus scores compared to those who had placebo.

Gabapentin therapy for pruritus in haemodialysis patients: a randomized, placebo-controlled, double-blind trial. Gunal AI, Ozalp G, Yoldas TK, Gunal SY, Kirciman E, Celiker H. Nephrol Dial Transplant 2004; 19: 3137–9.

In this double-blind, placebo-controlled, crossover study of 25 haemodialysis patients, those who received gabapentin 300 mg thrice weekly after each haemodialysis session for 4 weeks reported a significantly improved pruritus score compared to placebo.

Naltrexone does not relieve uremic pruritus: results of a randomized placebo-controlled crossover study. Pauli-Magnus C, Mikus G, Alscher DM, Kirschner T, Nagel W, Gugeler N, et al. J Am Soc Nephrol 2000; 11: 514–19.

In this double-blind placebo-controlled crossover study, 23 patients taking naltrexone 50 mg daily showed no difference in reported pruritus and intensity of pruritus scores compared to those who took placebo.

Randomised crossover trial of naltrexone in uraemic pruritus. Peer G, Kivity S, Agami O, Fireman E, Silverberg D, Blum M, et al. Lancet 1996; 348: 1552–4.

Naltrexone 50 mg daily was given to 15 hemodialysis patients with severe resistant pruritus. All 15 responded to treatment, and the median pruritus scores were significantly reduced compared to baseline values.

Kappa-opioid system in uremic pruritus: multicenter, randomized, double-blind, placebo-controlled clinical studies. Wikström B, Gellert R, Ladefoged SD, Danda Y, Akai M, Ide K, et al. J Am Soc Nephrol 2005; 16: 3742–7.

In this multicenter, randomized, double-blind placebo-controlled study involving 144 patients with uremic pruritus, those that received post-hemodialysis intravenous nalfurafine for 2–4 weeks reported significant reductions in itch intensity, sleep disturbances, and excoriations compared to those who had placebo.

Effect of skin care with an emollient containing a high water content on mild uremic pruritus. Okada K, Matsumoto K. Ther Apher Dial 2004; 8: 419–22.

In this placebo-controlled trial involving 20 hemodialysis patients with mild pruritus, twice-weekly application of an aqueous gel containing 80 g of water for 2 weeks significantly improved reported pruritus scores and xerosis compared to the control group.

Acupuncture in haemodialysis patients at the Quchi (LI11) acupoint for refractory uraemic pruritus. Che-Yi C, Wen CY, Min-Tsung K, Chiu-Ching H. Nephrol Dial Transplant 2005; 20: 1912–15.

In this randomized controlled study involving 40 patients with refractory uremic pruritus, those who received acupuncture applied unilaterally at the Quchi (LI11) acupoint thrice weekly for 1 month reported significantly reduced pruritus scores after acupuncture and at the 3-month follow-up, compared to those who received acupuncture applied at a non-acupoint.

Effects of homeopathic treatment on pruritus of haemodialysis patients: a randomised placebo-controlled double-blind trial. Cavalcanti AM, Rocha LM, Carillo R Jr, Lima LU, Lugon JR. Homeopathy 2003; 92: 177–81.

In this double-blind placebo-controlled randomized trial of 28 hemodialysis patients, those who received verum reported significantly reduced pruritus scores throughout the trial compared with placebo. Patients reported a 49% reduction in the pruritus score at the end of the study.

Relief of pruritus and decreases in plasma histamine concentrations during erythropoietin therapy in patients with uremia. De Marchi S, Cecchin E, Villalta D, Sepiacci G, Santini G, Bartoli E. N Engl J Med 1992; 326: 969–74.

In this double-blind placebo-controlled crossover study, eight of 10 patients treated with intravenous erythropoietin experienced improvement in pruritus. The pruritus returned within 1 week after discontinuation of therapy. The improvement was not related to the change in hemoglobin level.

Cholestyramine in uraemic pruritus. Silverberg DS, Iaina A, Reisin E, Rotzak R, Eliahou HE. Br Med J 1977; 1: 752–3.

This randomized double-blind placebo-controlled study showed that cholestyramine 5 g twice daily for 4 weeks improved pruritus in four of five subjects.

Relief of idiopathic generalized pruritus in dialysis patients treated with activated oral charcoal. Pederson JA, Matter BJ, Czerwinski AW, Llach F. Ann Intern Med 1980; 93: 446–8.

Oral charcoal 6 g daily for 8 weeks improved pruritus in 10 of 11 hemodialysis patients in this double-blind placebo-controlled crossover study.

Thalidomide for the treatment of uremic pruritus: a crossover randomized double-blind trial. Silva SR, Viana PC, Lugon NV, Hoette M, Ruzany F, Lugon JR. Nephron 1994; 67: 270–3.

Twenty-nine patients in this study were assigned to receive thalidomide or placebo at bedtime for 7 days. After a washout period of 7 days, drugs were crossed over. Over half of the patients had a greater than 50% reduction in pruritus while on thalidomide.

A study on pruritus after parathyroidectomy for secondary hyperparathyroidism. Chou F, Ji-Chen H, Shun-Chen H, Shyr-Ming S. J Am Coll Surg 2000; 190: 65–70.

Thirty-seven dialysis patients with secondary hyperparathyroidism underwent parathyroidectomy. Twenty-two had pruritus prior to parathyroidectomy, and in those patients with itch, pruritus scores improved significantly. This was accompanied by improvement in the calcium-phosphorus product.

ITCH ASSOCIATED WITH MALIGNANCY

Pruritus associated with malignancy is a common occurrence among patients with lymphomas and advanced malignancy. It may be one of the most bothersome symptoms to a cancer patient, and its management is challenging. The best evidence to date in the treatment of pruritus associated with malignancy exists for *paroxetine*.

MALIGNANCY-ASSOCIATED PRURITUS

FIRST-LINE THERAPIES

▶ Paroxetine	A

SECOND-LINE THERAPIES

▶ Mirtazapine	E
▶ Butorphanol	E

Paroxetine in the treatment of severe non-dermatological pruritus: a randomized, controlled trial. Zylicz Z, Krajnik M, Sorge AA, Costantini M. J Pain Symptom Manage 2003; 26: 1105–12.

This is a prospective randomized double-blind placebo-controlled crossover study involving 26 patients, of whom 17 had solid tumors, four had hematological malignancies, and five had various non-malignant conditions associated with pruritus. Patients reported significantly reduced pruritus

intensity scores during treatment with paroxetine 20 mg daily. Nine of 24 patients completing the study experienced at least 50% reduction of intensity of pruritus. Onset of antipruritic action was observed usually after 2–3 days.

Mirtazapine for pruritus. Davis MP, Frandsen JL, Walsh D, Andresen S, Taylor S. Pain Symptom Manage 2003; 25: 288–91.

In this case series of four patients with cholestasis, lymphoma, and uremic pruritus, each patient showed improvement in pruritus with mirtazapine 15–30 mg daily.

Butorphanol for treatment of intractable pruritus. Dawn AG, Yosipovitch G. J Am Acad Dermatol 2006; 54: 527–31.

In a patient with non-Hodgkin's lymphoma and intractable pruritus, butorphanol 1 mg daily improved itch and sleep after only one dose, without improvement of daytime itch. After undergoing chemotherapy with concurrent butorphanol 3 mg daily, the patient's pruritus resolved as the cancer regressed. Butorphanol is currently unavailable in the United States.

ITCH ASSOCIATED WITH HEMATOLOGIC DISORDERS

Pruritus associated with hematologic diseases, such as polycythemia vera and myelodysplastic syndrome, is often severe and intractable to the limited therapies available. *Phototherapy* remains the primary line of therapy for these patients.

HEMATOLOGIC DISORDER-ASSOCIATED PRURITUS

FIRST-LINE THERAPIES

▶ Narrowband UVB phototherapy	D
▶ Psoralen photochemotherapy	D

SECOND-LINE THERAPIES

▶ Paroxetine	D
▶ Fluoxetine	E

THIRD-LINE THERAPIES

▶ Pregabalin	E

Narrowband (TL-01) ultraviolet B phototherapy for pruritus in polycythaemia vera. Baldo A, Sammarco E, Plaitano R, Martinelli V, Monfrecola. Br J Dermatol 2002; 147: 979–81.

In this series, 10 patients with pruritus associated with polycythemia vera were treated with narrowband ultraviolet B phototherapy thrice weekly. In eight 8 of the 10 complete remission of pruritus occurred within 2–10 weeks of treatment, with a median cumulative dose of 5371.46 mJ/cm².

Efficacy of photochemotherapy on severe pruritus in polycythemia vera. Jeanmougin M, Rain JD, Najean Y. Ann Hematol 1996; 73: 91–3.

In this series, 10 of 11 patients with polycythaemia rubra vera improved with psoralen photochemotherapy, and maintenance therapy was generally necessary.

Selective serotonin reuptake inhibitors are effective in the treatment of polycythemia vera-associated pruritus. Tefferi A, Fonseca R. Blood 2002; 99: 26–7.

In this series of patients with polycythemia vera-associated intractable pruritus, nine were treated with paroxetine 20 mg daily and one received fluoxetine 10 mg daily. All patients had a favorable initial response and eight experienced complete or near-complete resolution of pruritus. Response occurred within 48 hours in most patients.

Pregabalin in the treatment of chronic pruritus. Ehrchen J, Ständer S. J Am Acad Dermatol 2008; 58: S36–7.

Two patients with aquagenic pruritus and one with idiopathic pruritus that had severe generalized itch were all treated with pregabalin, initially at 75 mg twice daily and increased to 150 mg twice daily. The patients reported greater than 70% reduction of symptoms 5–8 weeks after starting therapy. The longest follow-up period was 6 months, at which time the effects of pregablin were stable. Weight gain, somnolence, dizziness, and peripheral edema were observed side effects.

Evidence Levels: **A** Double-blind study **B** Clinical trial ≥ 20 subjects **C** Clinical trial < 20 subjects **D** Series ≥ 5 subjects **E** Anecdotal case reports

Pruritus ani

Gabriele Weichert

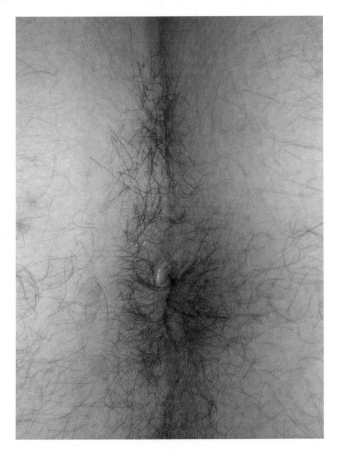

Pruritus ani represents a chronic, idiopathic intensely pruritic sensation of perianal skin. Long-standing cases are associated with significant discomfort, embarrassment, agitation, and sleep disturbance. Chronic primary pruritus ani is characterized clinically by lichenification and excoriations of the perianal area in the absence of primary skin disorders, infections, or neoplasms.

MANAGEMENT STRATEGY

When evaluating a patient with pruritus ani, any contributing primary skin disorders must be identified. These may include atopic dermatitis, psoriasis, or lichen sclerosis. Neoplasms, hemorrhoids and anal fissures should be ruled out. Infectious etiologies such as genital warts, tinea, candidiasis, infestations (i.e., pinworms, scabies), and bacterial infections (i.e., β-hemolytic *Streptococcus*) must be ruled out by clinical examination and laboratory sampling (KOH, bacterial culture swab, skin scrapings) if necessary. With this approach, most causes of acute pruritus ani can be identified and treated with directed therapy. It is the patient in whom none of the above factors are identified who suffers from chronic or idiopathic pruritus ani. History may reveal atopy or sensitive skin, leading to an increased itch sensation from all causes. A history of the management, including cleansing habits, may reveal a sensitizer causing a degree of contact dermatitis. Over-cleansing is not uncommon and may be irritating. Many of these patients

suffer from low-grade fecal incontinence. This is often evident on examination of the underclothes or of the perianal skin. A history of sleep disturbance may be revealed and can be the most frustrating aspect for many patients.

Management should include *discontinuation of any irritating topical treatments* or overzealous cleansing routines. Potential topical sensitizers should be stopped. A biopsy should be performed if the diagnosis is in doubt. *Avoidance of toilet paper* to cleanse the area after bowel movements can be helpful, as toilet paper may be abrasive. Patients are instructed to cleanse the perianal skin twice a day and after bowel movements using cotton balls or cotton squares (such as those sold in pharmacies to remove facial make-up) moistened with warm water or a liquid cleanser. Patients identified with low-grade fecal incontinence should perform this cleansing routing several times a day. Cleansing routine has been shown to be as effective as topical steroids. A short (few-weeks) course of a *low-to mid-potency topical steroid* is recommended. Caution must be taken with prolonged high-potency steroid use, as this area is prone to atrophy. Potency should be reduced as symptoms improve. Topical *zinc paste* can limit the degree of irritant dermatitis in patients with fecal incontinence. An evening *sedating antihistamine* may provide welcome sleep in the early weeks of treatment. If a patient fails to improve, anoscopy, proctosigmoidoscopy, or colonoscopy should be considered to rule out neoplastic disease. *Patch testing* should be performed in patients who continue to use potential allergens. Avoidance of caffeine and increased dietary fiber may be helpful. For second-line therapy, topical capsaicin 0.006% three times a day for 4 weeks could be used. Capsaicin will cause perianal irritation in most patients during the therapy. Finally, *intralesional steroid* injections to the perianal skin may be considered. *Intradermal methylene blue injections* are reported to damage dermal nerve endings and provide relief. *Injection with phenol in almond oil* has been reported, as has *topical PUVA therapy*.

SPECIFIC INVESTIGATIONS

▶ Bacterial swab
▶ Fungal microscopy and culture
▶ Biopsy
▶ Skin scrapings for scabies
▶ Patch testing
▶ GI investigations

Allergic contact dermatitis in patients with anogenital complaints. Bauer A, Geier J, Elsner P. J Reprod Med 2000; 45: 649–54.

A 5-year collection of patients patch tested for consideration of allergic anogenital contact dermatitis demonstrated an increased incidence of benzocaine and (chloro-)- methylisothiazolinone allergy. Of 1008 patients, a diagnosis of allergic contact dermatitis was made in 34.8%. The authors recommend using the standard tray plus dibucaine, propolis, bufexamac, and other ingredients gained from the patient's history.

Treatment of persistent pruritus ani in a combined colorectal and dermatological clinic. Dasan S, Neill SM, Donaldson DR, Scott HJ. Br J Surg 1999; 86: 1337–40.

In a series of 40 patients with pruritus ani, 34 had a recognizable dermatosis and 18 had a positive patch test result. The authors suggest early assessment by a dermatologist may be appropriate.

Abnormal transient internal sphincter relaxation in idiopathic pruritus ani: physiological evidence from ambulatory monitoring. Farouk R, Duthie GS, Pryde A, Bartolo DC. Br J Surg 1994; 81: 603–6.

Abnormal rectal sphincter tone was demonstrated in patients with pruritus ani. This may well be the contributing factor in patients who have occult fecal leakage as a component of their itch.

Pruritus ani. Causes and concerns. Daniel GL, Longo WE, Vernava AM. Dis Colon Rectum 1994; 37: 670–4.

In this series of 104 patients presenting with pruritus ani as their primary symptom, 52% had anorectal disease (including hemorrhoids, anal fissures, genital warts and fistulas) and 23% had an existing colorectal neoplasm found with investigations. In those without neoplasia, there was a direct correlation between increased caffeine intake and severity of irritation. Patients with primary pruritus ani improved with dietary restrictions (not defined), dietary fiber, steroid creams, and drying agents.

TREATMENT STRATEGIES

FIRST-LINE THERAPIES

▶ Topical corticosteroids	A
▶ Hygeine	B

1% hydrocortisone ointment is an effective treatment of pruritus ani: a pilot randomized control crossover trial. Al-Ghnaniem R, Short K, Pullen A, Fuller LC, Rennie JA, Leather AJ. Int J Colorectal Dis 2007; 22: 1463–7.

Nineteen patients were randomized to 1% hydrocortisone in paraffin twice daily or paraffin base for 2 weeks followed by cross-over treatment for 2 weeks. Blinded analysis of visual analog score (VAS) showed a 68% reduction in VAS with steroid treatment.

Idiopathic perianal pruritus: washing compared with topical corticosteroids. Oztas MO, Oztas P, Onder M. Postgrad Med J 2004; 80; 295–7.

In this study, 28 patients applied topical methylprednisolone cream twice daily for 2 weeks. In a separate group, 32 patients were instructed to cleanse the perianal area twice daily with a liquid cleanser. Effectiveness was similar at 92.3% in the first and 90.6% in the second group (p>0.05).

SECOND-LINE THERAPIES

▶ Topical capsaicin	A

Topical capsaicin – a novel and effective treatment for idiopathic intractable pruritus ani: a randomised, placebo controlled, crossover study. Lysy J, Sistiery-Ittah M, Israelit Y, Shmueli A, Strauss-Liviatan N, Mindrul V, et al. Gut 2003; 52: 1323–6.

In this double-blind placebo-controlled cross-over study, capsaicin 0.006% cream was applied three times a day for 1 month, followed by 1 month of control treatment using 1% menthol cream. Of 44 patients, 31 experienced partial relief of symptoms while using the capsaicin cream (p<0.0001). All patients experienced some degree of perianal burning with use of the capsaicin cream. The menthol cream was not effective.

THIRD-LINE THERAPIES

▶ Intralesional corticosteroids	C
▶ Intradermal methylene blue	B
▶ Subcutaneous phenol injection	B
▶ Topical PUVA	E

The use of intralesional triamcinolone hexacetonide in the treatment of idiopathic pruritus ani. Minvielle L, Hernandez VL. Dis Colon Rectum 1969; 12: 340–3.

Nineteen patients were treated weekly for 4 weeks with intralesional triamcinolone at doses of 5–20 mg/week. At the end of the treatment period, nine of 19 (73.6%) patients had excellent progress, two of 19 reported fair improvement, and three failed to improve. No perianal atrophy was noted at the end of 4 weeks.

Intradermal methylene blue injection for the treatment of intractable idiopathic pruritus ani: results of 30 cases. Mentes BB, Akin M, Leventoglu S, Gultekin FA, Oguz M. Tech Coloproctol 2004; 8: 11–14.

In this series, 30 patients were treated with a 15 mL injection of 1% methylene blue to the perianal area. One month later, 24 patients (80%) were symptom free. Four of five partial responders had complete relief with a second injection. After 12 months of follow-up, 23 patients (76.7%) continued to be symptom free.

Methylene blue has been shown by electron microscopy to cause damage to dermal nerve endings. This is the proposed mechanism of action for this modality.

Intra-dermal methylene blue, hydrocortisone and lignocaine for chronic, intractable pruritus ani. Botterill ID, Sagar PM. Colorectal Dis 2002; 4: 144–6.

Twenty-five patients were treated with perianal injection of 5 mL of 1% methylene blue, 100 mg of hydrocortisone and 15 mL of lidocaine. After one injection, 16/25 (64%) reported symptom relief. Repeat injection in non-responders led to a total response rate of 22/25 (88%). Three patients failed to respond.

A new concept of the anatomy of the anal sphincter mechanism and the physiology of defecation. XXIII. An injection technique for the treatment of idiopathic pruritus ani. Shafik A. Int Surg 1990; 75: 43–6.

In this series, 67 patients were treated with an injection of 5% phenol in almond oil: 62/67 (92.4%) experienced complete relief. Five patients relapsed after a period of remission. Repeat injection led to cure.

Treatment of genital-anal lesions in inflammatory skin diseases with PUVA cream phototherapy. Reichrath J, Reinhold U, Tilgen W. Dermatology 2002; 205: 245–8.

In an open series, four patients with pruritus vulvae improved with topical PUVA. Improvement was seen with fewer than 10 treatments in three of the four patients. All patients improved with treatment.

Pruritus vulvae and pruritus ani are felt to be similar conditions and these results could be extrapolated to pruritus ani patients. Topical PUVA would have some technical limitations, however, given the physical location of the problem!

616

Pruritus vulvae

Ginat Mirowski, Bethanee J Schlosser

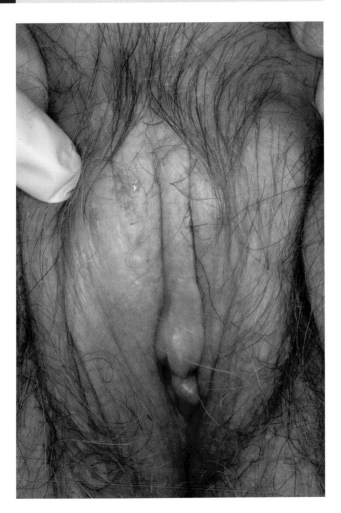

Table 1 Differential diagnosis of pruritus vulvae

Infections	*Candida albicans, Trichomonas vaginalis,* group B β-hemolytic streptococcus, *Enterobius vermicularis, Phthirius pubis, Sarcoptes scabiei,* tinea cruris, human papillomavirus, herpes simplex virus, *Chlamydia trachomatis, Gardnerella vaginalis, Neisseria gonorrhoeae,* human immunodeficiency virus
Dermatoses	Allergic contact dermatitis, irritant contact dermatitis, atopic dermatitis, psoriasis, lichen planus, seborrheic dermatitis, lichen sclerosus et atrophicus, Fox–Fordyce disease, lichen simplex chronicus, desquamative inflammatory vaginitis, fixed drug eruption, estrogen deficiency (atrophic vaginitis/vulvitis), syringomas
Systemic diseases	Diabetes mellitus, hepatic failure, renal failure, polycythemia vera, hypothyroidism, Sjögren syndrome, iron-deficiency anemia, malignant and premalignant squamous cell carcinoma, lymphoma, vulvar intraepithelial neoplasia, Bowen's disease (squamous cell carcinoma in situ), extramammary Paget's disease

Pruritus vulvae is an external sensation of itching that results in a need to scratch or rub the affected vulvar region. Over time the skin becomes lichenified, and occasionally excoriations and pigmentary changes occur. Pruritus vulvae may be primary; secondary to infections, malignancy, a wide number of dermatoses, and a number of neurologic conditions; or multifactorial. Essential pruritus vulvae is the condition in which no primary etiology can be identified.

MANAGEMENT STRATEGY

Pruritus vulvae describes a symptom, not a specific disorder of physical discomfort, that may be both psychologically distressing and socially embarrassing. An underlying etiology should be sought by obtaining a thorough history and physical examination. The differential diagnosis includes infections, dermatoses, systemic diseases, and malignant or premalignant lesions (Table 1).

Appropriate treatment should be instituted when a specific etiology is found, and an adequate course of therapy should be initiated before determining treatment failure.

If no cause is found, then symptomatic relief is a priority. The tenet of treatment is to interrupt the itch–scratch cycle, restore the skin barrier, and reduce inflammation.

The mainstay in treatment of pruritus vulvae is to *identify and remove all potential local irritants.* The patient should be instructed to discontinue all local products, including soaps, sanitary pads, OTC medications, and occlusive/synthetic clothing. They should bathe with lukewarm (not hot) water only, pat (not rub) dry, wipe from front to back, change underpants daily, and launder clothing using a double rinse cycle in the washing machine. Patients may be resistant to these measures, as they may believe that they must maintain a 'clean' vulvar region and that natural secretions and odors are offensive and 'unclean.' The patient may have developed elaborate home regimens that contribute to local irritation and contact sensitivity, and may confound or be the primary cause of persistent pruritus. Toilet (tissue) paper and commercial wipes should be avoided as their use may contribute to irritation, especially when used to rub or scratch the area. Both may contain allergens such as formaldehyde, benzalkonium chloride, and fragrances. Urine, stool, and excessive cervical or vaginal secretions may contribute to local irritation. Efforts to treat urinary incontinence and to limit contact with stool (i.e., stool bulking agents) and the use of fragrance-free products (sanitary pads or tampons) may be helpful. Cotton washcloths may be used to clean the area. Cool water or Sitz baths are recommended to clean the perineum after urination and defecation. Sitz baths provide relief and dilute irritants.

The use of *barrier petrolatum- and zinc-based ointments*, typically used to prevent diaper rash in both children and adults, helps to seal in moisture and protect the affected skin. In low-estrogen states the use of topical or systemic estrogen helps restore normal vaginal and vulvar mucosa.

Systemic or topical steroids are used to reduce inflammation. Topical preparations may contribute to an allergic or irritant contact dermatitis. Ointment-based formulations are preferred because they are less likely to contain allergens or irritants. Corticosteroid ointment, used sparingly, should be applied once or twice a day. Close clinical supervision is necessary to limit secondary changes such as striae, folliculitis, and atrophy. Systemic agents should be used to treat infections and to provide symptomatic relief of pruritus in order to limit secondary complications of local agents. Intralesional triamcinolone acetonide injection and systemic corticosteroids are effective for recalcitrant pruritus.

Although steroids reduce pruritus while reducing inflammation, they are often not sufficient to interrupt the itch–scratch cycle. Nightly sedating *antihistamines* such as hydroxyzine or doxepin are recommended. For daytime pruritus a low-dose *selective serotonin reuptake inhibitor (SSRI)* is more effective than non-sedating antihistamines.

The use of intradermal alcohol injection to treat recalcitrant cases is not advocated. This procedure requires general anesthesia, and there is a risk of cellulitis and tissue sloughing. There are no recent data on this procedure, and it is no longer recommended. For severe or refractory pruritus vulvae, CO_2 laser and the Mering procedure, used to partially denervate the area, provide relief of symptoms. Psychotherapy, acupuncture, and hypnosis are non-invasive methods that have demonstrated efficacy.

SPECIFIC INVESTIGATIONS

> ► Clinical visual and manual examination of the vulva, vagina, oral cavity, conjunctivae, total body skin, scalp and nails
> ► Clinical palpation of inguinal lymph nodes
> ► Sensory testing for light touch and Q-Tip evaluation of vulva and vaginal vestibule
> ► Normal saline wet mount of vaginal secretions (*Trichomonas vaginalis*, bacterial vaginosis, atrophic vaginitis)
> ► Whiff test (bacterial vaginosis)
> ► KOH (fungi, scabies infestation)
> ► pH paper (bacterial vaginosis, atrophic vaginitis)
> ► Tape test (*Enterobius vermicularis or pinworm*)
> ► Microbiologic cultures (bacterial, fungal, viral)
> ► Laboratory tests (fasting blood glucose, liver/renal/thyroid function, CBC with differential, iron studies including ferritin)
> ► Biopsy (H&E, immunofluorescence, special stains)
> ► Wood's lamp (erythrasma)
> ► Patch testing
> ► Coloscopy (gynecology consultation for yeast, viropathic changes or dysplasia)

The prevalence and clinical diagnosis of vaginal candidosis in non-pregnant patients with vaginal discharge and pruritus vulvae. Wright HJ, Palmer A. J Roy Coll Gen Pract 1978; 28: 719–23.

Seventeen (45%) of 38 women with pruritus vulvae were diagnosed with *C. albicans*. Yeast was not identified in the other patients, and the etiology of their symptoms was not reported.

Pruritus in diabetes mellitus: investigation of prevalence and correlation with diabetes. Neilly JB, Martin A, Simpson N, MacCuish AC. Diabetes Care 1986; 9: 273–5.

Three hundred diabetic and 100 non-diabetic outpatients were evaluated for the presence of generalized and localized pruritus. Pruritus vulvae, the most common symptom, was noted in 18.4% of diabetic women. This was significant ($p<0.05$), as only 5.6% of non-diabetic women had pruritus vulvae. Symptoms correlated with glycosylated hemoglobin.

The study suggested that diabetes mellitus should be considered in the differential diagnosis of pruritus vulvae.

Vulvar intraepithelial neoplasia with superficially invasive carcinoma of the vulva. Herod JJ, Shafi MI, Rollason TP, Jordan JA, Luesley DM. Br J Obstet Gynecol 1996; 103: 453–6.

In this retrospective study of 26 women with VIN, pruritus vulvae, the most common symptom, was present in 18 (69%).

This study suggested that VIN should be considered in patients with pruritus vulvae.

Contact sensitivity in pruritus vulvae: patch test results and clinical outcomes. Lewis FM, Shah M, Gawkrodger DJ. Am J Contact Dermatitis 1997; 8: 137–40.

Patch testing was used to evaluate 121 women with pruritus vulva. Fifty-seven (49%) had one or more relevant reactions. Common allergens identified included medications and components of medications, including preservatives, lanolins, quinolone, benzocaine, and fragrances.

Patients with a relevant allergy were significantly (p<0.001) more likely to improve than those without an allergy.

FIRST-LINE THERAPIES

> ► Avoidance of irritants   E
> ► Hygiene   E
> ► Topical corticosteroids   B
> ► Topical estrogen   E
> ► Topical pimecrolimus   B

The treatment of vulvar lichen sclerosus with a very potent topical steroid (clobetasol propionate 0.05%) cream. Dalziel KL, Millard PR, Wojnarowska F. Br J Dermatol 1991; 124: 461–4.

A series of 13 patients with lichen sclerosus were treated with clobetasol propionate 0.05% cream to determine efficacy. All 13 showed marked clinical improvement after 12 weeks of therapy.

The common problem of vulvar pruritus. Bornstein J, Pascal B, Abramovici H. Obstet Gynecol Surv 1993; 48: 111–18.

The authors of this review article recommend stopping use of all soaps, douches, and perfumed deodorants, keeping the vulvar area dry, wearing cotton underpants, and avoiding tight pants as basic principles in the treatment of pruritus vulvae.

Evidence Levels: A Double-blind study **B** Clinical trial ≥ 20 subjects **C** Clinical trial < 20 subjects **D** Series ≥ 5 subjects **E** Anecdotal case reports

Vulvovaginal dryness and itching. [Letter] Margesson LJ. Skin Ther 2001; 6: 3–4.

Author reviews the vulvar signs of estrogen deficiency and offers treatment options.

Contact dermatitis of the vulvae. Margesson LJ. Dermatol Ther 2004; 17: 20–7.

A comprehensive review of common vulvar irritants and their treatments.

Pruritus vulvae in prepubertal children. Paek SC, Merritt DF, Mallory SB. J Am Acad Dermatol 2001; 44: 795–802.

This paper reviews the causes and treatments of vulvar pruritus in prepubertal girls by retrospective evaluation of 44 records: 75% had nonspecific pruritus, and lichen sclerosus, bacterial infections, yeast infection, and pinworm infestation were seen in a minority of patients. The authors conclude that in prepubertal girls poor hygiene and irritants are major contributors to pruritus vulvae.

An approach to the treatment of anogenital pruritus. Weichert GE. Dermatol Ther 2004; 17: 129–33.

Reviews the common causes of acute and chronic anogenital pruritus with a focus on vulvar pruritus. The therapeutic approach to the management of pruritus vulvae in the absence of a clear cause is discussed.

Lichen simplex chronicus (atopic/neurodermatitis) of the anogenital region. Lynch P. Dermatol Ther 2004; 17: 8–19.

This paper suggests diagnostic tips and a differential diagnosis for vulvar LSC. The management of LSC is divided into four categories: identification of any underlying disease, repair of the barrier layer function, reduction of inflammation, and breaking of the itch–scratch cycle. Treatment options for each category are discussed.

Efficacy of topical pimecrolimus in the treatment of chronic vulvar pruritus: A prospective case series – a non-controlled, open-label study. Sarifakioglu E, Gumus II. J Dermatol Treat 2006; 17: 276–8.

This paper showed that in 15 patients with chronic vular pruritus, 1% pimecrolimus cream applied twice daily for 1 month resulted in a complete response in 10 patients and improvement in three; two patients did not return for follow-up.

SECOND-LINE THERAPIES

▶ Subcutaneous triamcinolone	B
▶ Topical antihistamine	A

Subcutaneous injection of triamcinolone acetonide in the treatment of chronic vulvar pruritus. Kelly RA, Foster DC, Woodruff JD. Am J Obstet Gynecol 1993; 169: 568–70.

A series of 45 patients with chronic pruritus vulvae were treated with subcutaneous intralesional injection of triamcinolone acetonide into the vulva. Thirty-five experienced relief of pruritus for more than 1 month (mean 5.8 months).

Efficacy of topical oxatomide in women with pruritus vulva. Origoni M, Garsia S, Sideri M, Pifarotti G, Nicora M. Drugs Exp Clin Res 1990; 16: 591–6.

A double-blind, controlled European study to determine the efficacy of topical oxatomide, an antihistamine not currently available in the United States, in treating pruritus vulvae. The drug was under experimental clinical research. All 29 patients reported improvement in both the intensity and the duration of itching. Seven patients experienced complete regression. These results were statistically significant (p<0.001) compared to placebo.

THIRD-LINE THERAPIES

▶ Intradermal alcohol injection	A
▶ Surgery	D
▶ CO$_2$ laser	D
▶ Psychotherapy	C
▶ Acupuncture	D
▶ Hypnosis	E
▶ Gonadotropin-releasing hormone	E

Treatment of pruritus vulva by multiple intradermal injections of alcohol. A double-blind study. Sutherst JR. Br J Obstet Gynecol 1979; 86: 371–3.

A double-blind controlled study reports on the efficacy of intradermal alcohol injections in the treatment of pruritus vulvae. Fourteen of 17 patients reported complete relief of pruritus only on the side treated with alcohol. Pruritus persisted on the placebo-treated side. Treatment with alcohol was significantly better than with placebo (p<0.05).

A surgical approach to intractable pruritus vulvae. Mering JH. Am J Obstet Gynecol 1952; 64: 619–27.

A series of 16 women with intractable pruritus vulvae were surgically treated with the Mering procedure (wide undermining of the skin of the vulva, vaginal mucous membranes, and anus). Fifteen patients had immediate relief of symptoms of pruritus. No recurrence was reported at 3 months' to 3 years' follow-up.

Chronic vulvovaginal pruritus treated successfully with GnRH analogue. Banerjee AK, de Chazal R. Postgrad Med J 2006; 82: e22.

A single case report of a 35-year-old woman with intractable cyclical vulvovaginal itching. Suppression of ovulation and empiric treatment with intramuscular injection of leuprorelin acetate (a GnRH analog (Depot)) for 4 weeks resulted in complete resolution of her symptoms. Autoimmune progesterone dermatitis was hypothesized as primary etiology. The patient declined a progesterone challenge test. Pruritus did not recur with resumption of normal menses.

56 cases of chronic pruritus vulvae treated with acupuncture. Huang WY, Guo ZR, Yu J, Hu XL. J Trad Chin Med 1987; 7: 1–3.

Fifty-four of 56 patients with intractable pruritus vulvae experienced symptomatic and clinical improvement with up to seven sessions of acupuncture.

Hypnosis in a case of long-standing idiopathic itch. Rucklidge JJ, Saunders D. Psychosom Med 1999; 61: 355–8.

This is a case report of a single patient with long-standing pruritus vulvae and ani. She experienced complete relief of symptoms with training in self-hypnosis.

Pseudofolliculitis barbae

Gary J Brauner

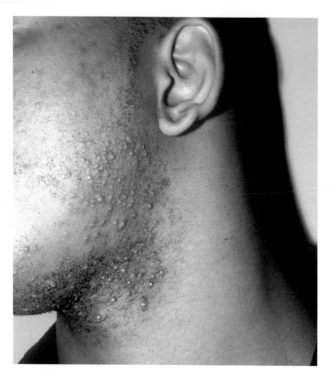

Pseudofolliculitis barbae (PFB) is a chronic inflammatory disease of hair-bearing areas induced by shaving or plucking of curved hairs, with resultant transepithelial or transfollicular penetration by the sharpened hair remnant and a foreign body reaction. It is characterized clinically by papules, papulopustules, focal or diffuse postinflammatory hyperpigmentation, growth grooves, and rarely hypertrophic or keloidal scarring.

MANAGEMENT STRATEGY

Because this process is induced by shaving its cure is simple: by not shaving or plucking at all and allowing the hairs to grow to beyond 1 cm in length, the disease will spontaneously involute. If a clean-shaven appearance is preferred or deemed necessary by occupational or social demands, management involves three elements:

- *Extraction of the foreign body* by lifting the embedded distal sharpened ends of hairs.
- *Prevention of further embedding* by proper shaving technique or permanent disruption of the follicle's ability to produce new hair.
- *Treatment of postinflammatory hyperpigmentation* or hypertrophic scarring.

Embedded hairs should be *lifted*, not plucked, just prior to shaving. A safety razor set on its 'gentlest' setting, or a preadjusted razor such as the PFB Bumpfighter, should be used, but with the *opposite hand kept off the face* to prevent skin stretching. Shaving is performed in the direction of hair growth, not against it, again to prevent too-close shaving and transfollicular penetration. A *long presoak* with a hot wet facecloth will allow hairs to swell and lift; a shaving cream that lathers and holds well will keep those hairs saturated and elevated. Shaving must be performed daily; by 2–3 days of no shaving transepidermal re-entry penetration will occur. If morning shaving is routine, the affected areas should be gently *buffed* or brushed the evening before with a toothbrush, a rough dry washcloth, or a Buf Puf to loosen hairs about to embed.

Hair clippers will cut hair closely but not so close as to allow transfollicular penetration. Because razor shaving is much closer, clippers should be used at least twice daily to avoid a permanent '5 o'clock shadow.'

Powder chemical depilatories are not practical. They are messy to use, hard to mix accurately, difficult to remove rapidly, and, because they are so irritating, can not be used more than every 3 days, which already allows PFB to recur. Lotion depilatories are much easier to apply and remove and, being less irritant, can be used every 2 days to produce a satisfactory cosmetic appearance.

Antibiotics are not necessary topically because this is a sterile foreign body reaction not a pyoderma. Irritants such as *retinoic acid* or *glycolic acid* may enhance lifting of hairs and diminish hyperpigmentation.

Several longer-wavelength long pulsed *lasers* (alexandrite, 810 nm diode, and Nd:YAG) combined with epidermal protective chilling devices can be used to produce dramatic long-lasting remission, even in Fitzpatrick types IV, V, and VI patients, and represent a breakthrough treatment for recalcitrant disease.

SPECIFIC INVESTIGATIONS

- ▶ Skin biopsy in rare instances
- ▶ K6hf gene analysis

No investigations are necessary for usual cases of PFB. Because it is induced by hair manipulation (i.e., shaving or plucking) it is not associated with other diseases. Differentiation of true bacterial folliculitis, requiring systemic antibiotics, must sometimes be considered. Rarely, yeast folliculitis may mimic PFB. Careful clinical inspection and possibly skin biopsy should be performed to rule out granulomatous disease such as sarcoidosis or dental sinusitis in the presence of apparently hypertrophic or keloidal scars. Rarely, ciclosporin therapy may induce a pseudofolliculitis-like condition. Recent French literature cites necrotic folliculitis-like lesions and pathergy as common cutaneous presentations of Behçet's syndrome; this 'pseudofolliculitis' is not the PFB of ingrowing hairs.

Scar sarcoidosis in pseudofolliculitis barbae. Norton S, Chesser R, Fitzpatrick J. Military Med 1991; 156: 369–71.

A man with hilar adenopathy had smooth firm purplish papules (lupus pernio) on his face and PFB in his beard area. Biopsies of papules of both the lupus pernio and the PFB revealed non-caseating granulomas consistent with sarcoidosis.

Evidence Levels: **A** Double-blind study **B** Clinical trial ≥ 20 subjects **C** Clinical trial < 20 subjects **D** Series ≥ 5 subjects **E** Anecdotal case reports

Disseminated cryptococcosis presenting as pseudofolliculitis in an AIDS patient. Coker L, Swain R, Morris R, McCall C. Cutis 2000; 66: 207–10.

A 42-year-old African-American man with AIDS had countless dome-shaped excoriated papules on his trunk, arms, and face, initially diagnosed as folliculitis (not pseudofolliculitis of ingrowing hairs) with biopsy-proven disseminated cutaneous cryptococcosis.

Hyperplastic pseudofolliculitis barbae associated with cyclosporin. Lear J, Bourke JF, Burns DA. Br J Dermatol 1997; 136: 132–3.

A condition resembling keloid reactions in PFB is reported as an unusual reaction to ciclosporin.

Hypertrophic pseudofolliculitis in white renal transplant recipients. Lally A, Wojnarowska F. Clin Exp Dermatol 2007; 32: 268–71.

Five cases of hyperplastic PFB in white patients with renal transplants and ciclosporin immunosuppression are reported with chin involvement in all, but two also had involvement of the nose and occiput, which is otherwise never seen. The photographs reveal folliculitis papillaris not PFB.

An unusual Ala12Thr polymorphism in the 1A alpha-helical segment of the companion layer-specific keratin K6hf: evidence for a risk factor in the etiology of the common hair disorder pseudofolliculitis barbae. Winter H, Schissel D, Parry D, Smith TA, Liovic M, Birgitte Lane E, et al. J Invest Dermatol 2004; 122: 652–7. Comment in: J Invest Dermatol 2004; 122: xi–xiii.

The authors identify a family with two curly-haired white males with PFB and one straight-haired non-PFB-afflicted female with an unusual dominantly inherited single-nucleotide polymorphism, which gives rise to a disruptive Ala12Thr substitution in the 1A α-helical segment of the companion layer-specific keratin K6hf of the hair follicle. In transfected cells this gene seems to be disruptive of filament assembly. A test group of 100 black people, 82% of whom had PFB, and 110 white people (a very high 18% of whom had PFB) showed this unusual gene in 9% of whites but only 36% of blacks (97% of whom had PFB). The authors somehow conclude that this gene represents a significant genetic risk factor for PFB.

Epiluminescence dermatoscopy enhanced patient compliance and achieved treatment success in pseudofolliculitis barbae. Chuh A, Zawar V. Australas J Dermatol 2006; 47: 60–2.

This anecdotal single case report of PFB in a straight-haired Chinese man is a unique example of inappropriate overuse of sophisticated and moderately expensive technology to illustrate ingrown hairs to a patient when they are viewable with the naked eye.

FIRST-LINE THERAPIES

▶ Beard growth	D
▶ Razor shaving technique	D
▶ Hair clippers	D
▶ Chemical depilatories	D
▶ Adjunctive hair extraction	D

Pseudofolliculitis of the beard. Strauss J, Kligman A. Arch Dermatol Syphilol 1956; 74: 533–42.

The first modern description of the pathogenesis of this disease and the rationale for allowing beard growth and spontaneous involution.

Pseudofolliculitis barbae. Medical consequences of interracial friction in the US Army. Brauner G, Flandermeyer K. Cutis 1979; 23: 61–6.

PFB is a minor disease affecting only, and almost all, black people who shave. Because of a continued requirement by the US Army for clean-shaven faces, significant interracial turmoil and animosity has been aroused. Unclear standards of care of the disease and haphazard policing of shaving habits led to a chaotic process, with effective dermatologic care almost paralyzed by the hostile parties. During the Vietnam War era randomly approached lower-ranking enlistees and draftees were much more likely to complain about their disease, even if minor, and were more likely to refuse to shave and be unkempt even without permission to grow a beard (in contravention of Army regulations). Career black enlistees are likely to underreport the severity of their disease and not seek medical help, possibly because of fear of continuous harassment and inability to be promoted by their superiors. Lotion depilatories or hair clippers, combined with routine lifting of ingrown hairs, are the most effective treatments, though complete cessation of shaving is required first.

Pseudofolliculitis barbae. 2. Treatment. Brauner G, Flandermeyer K. Int J Dermatol 1977; 16: 520–5.

The disease can be cured only by complete cessation of shaving, but it can be adequately controlled in most patients by carefully shaving the hairs neither too close nor too long, and by meticulous lifting out of penetrating hairs.

A variety of practical methods of shaving are described in detail.

Pseudofolliculitis barbae and related disorders. Halder R. Dermatol Clin 1988; 6: 407–12.

Not all regimens will work for each patient. This thorough review discusses beards, triple 'O' electric clippers, chemical depilatories, safety razors including the foil-guarded system to reduce cutting edge, electric razors including the adjustable three-headed rotary razor, manual lifting of hairs, tretinoin lotion, electrolysis, and surgical depilation.

Evaluation of a foil-guarded shaver in the management of pseudofolliculitis barbae. Alexander A. Cutis 1981; 27: 534–7, 540–2.

Pseudofolliculitis barbae and acne keloidalis nuchae. Kelly A. Dermatol Clin 2003; 21: 645–53.

Concise review with good descriptions of various and specific shaving devices.

SECOND-LINE THERAPIES

▶ Retinoic acid	E
▶ Glycolic acid	B
▶ Topical clindamycin	A

Pseudofolliculitis of the beard and topically applied tretinoin. Kligman A, Mills O. Arch Dermatol 1973; 107: 551–2.

Tretinoin solution is described as a useful adjunctive treatment.

Pseudofolliculitis – revised concepts of diagnosis and treatment. Report of three cases in women. Hall J, Goetz C, Bartholome C, Livingood C. Cutis 1979; 23: 798–800.

Three cases of pseudofolliculitis are described in black American women. Topical retinoic acid cream was useful in all three.

Pseudofolliculitis barbae. Chu T. Practitioner 1989; 233: 307–9.

In a limited open study, 1% topical clindamycin was found anecdotally effective for pseudofolliculitis and acne keloidalis.

Twice-daily applications of benzoyl peroxide 5%/clindamycin 1% gel versus vehicle in the treatment of pseudofolliculitis barbae. Cook-Bolden F, Barba A, Halder R, Taylor S. Cutis 2004; 73: 18–24.

Seventy-seven men with 16–100 combined papules and pustules on the face and neck were randomized to receive twice-daily benzoyl peroxide 5%/clindamycin 1% (BP/C) gel or vehicle for 10 weeks; 77.3% of the participants were black. All patients were required to shave at least twice a week with a disposable Bumpfighter razor, and to use a standardized shaving regimen. At weeks 2, 4, and 6, mean percentage reductions from baseline in combined papule and pustule counts were statistically significantly greater with BP/C gel than with vehicle, but for both were >50% by 10 weeks, particularly in black men. There was a significant change in non-black men, but no difference between test and controls.

Although 77% of test patients thought they were much better compared to 47% in the control vehicle group, the authors do not explain the remarkable improvement in the control group, nor why or how they assume their test product alone 'worked.'

Treatment of pseudofolliculitis barbae with topical glycolic acid: a report of two studies. Perricone N. Cutis 1993; 52: 232–5.

The studies consisted of two placebo-controlled trials in 35 adult men. The results showed that glycolic acid lotion was significantly more effective than placebo in treating PFB. There was a reduction of over 60% in lesions on the treated side, which allowed daily shaving with little irritation.

THIRD-LINE THERAPIES

▶ Laser depilation	B
▶ Surgical depilation	C

Pseudofolliculitis barbae. Quarles F, Brody H, Johnson B, Badreshia S, Vause SE, Brauner G, et al. Dermatol Ther 2007; 20: 133–6.

Anecdotal comments by each member of a large panel of experts concerning useful approaches to the treatment of PFB.

Modified superlong pulse 810 nm diode laser in the treatment of pseudofolliculitis barbae in skin types V and VI. Smith E, Winstanley D, Ross E. Dermatol Surg 2005; 31: 297–301.

Ten of 13 patients with type V or VI skin treated with superlong-pulse 810 nm diode laser at 2-week intervals three

times with a mean 29 J/cm² and 438 ms for type V and 26 J/cm² at 450 ms for type VI skin, and then followed up to only 3 months, showed clinical improvement of PFB papules which was statistically significant. The authors note that the 26 J/cm² maximum tolerable dose may not be sufficient to cause long-term reduction in hair growth. The follow-up of the study was not long enough to determine such reduction either. The authors claim that the ratio of minimal damaging fluence to minimum effective fluence in very dark skin was 1.2:1, versus the safer 1.5–2:1 for long-pulse Nd:YAG laser for PFB.

Treatment of pseudofolliculitis barbae using the Q-switched Nd: YAG laser with topical carbon suspension. Rogers C, Glaser D. Dermatol Surg 2000; 26: 737–41.

Nine patients were given two treatments 1 month apart on the neck and mandible. Evaluation only as long as 2 months after the last treatment showed a statistically significant reduction in number of papules and pustules compared to the control side.

This laser is no longer popular because of the lack of permanence of hair loss.

Pseudofolliculitis of the neck and the shoulder: a new effective treatment with alexandrite laser. Valeriant M, Terracina F, Mezzana P. Plast Reconstruct Surg 2002; 110: 1195–6.

Two Caucasian men with chronic folliculitis and pseudofolliculitis of the neck and shoulders were treated with 790 nm alexandrite laser for 30 ms with 10 mm spot size and 16–18 J/cm² for four sessions at 6-week intervals. They had a hair loss of 60–70% and 90% improvement in PFB, which persisted during 1-year follow-up.

Laser treatment of pseudofolliculitis barbae. Kauvar A. Annual Meeting American Society for Dermatologic Surgery; 2 Nov 2000. [Abstract]

Ten subjects with skin types I–IV having PFB of the beard, axilla, or bikini areas were treated with three laser treatments at 6–8-week intervals using an 810 nm diode laser for 15–30 ms at 30–38 J/cm², and were followed up 3 months after the last session. There was a hair growth delay of 3–4 weeks and more than 75% improvement of papules. Long-pulsed alexandrite laser was used in 19 patients with skin types I–IV with 3 ms bursts at 16–18 J/cm² for three laser treatments 6–8 weeks apart. All patients had more than 50% reduction in papules and pustules. There were no pigmentary changes and clinical remission was 6 months.

Treatment of pseudofolliculitis with a pulsed infrared laser. Kauvar A. Arch Dermatol 2000; 136: 1343–6.

Ten women with Fitzpatrick skin types III–V and a history of pseudofolliculitis on the face, axilla, or groin for at least 1 year had three consecutive treatments at 6–8-week intervals with an 810 nm diode laser and a chill tip at 30–38 J/cm² and 20 ms pulse duration. After their last visit all showed more than 75% improvement in the pseudofolliculitis and had a 50% reduction in hair growth. No blistering occurred.

Laser-assisted hair removal for darker skin types. Battle E, Hobbs L. Dermatol Ther 2004; 17: 177–83.

The authors carefully review the rationale for use of diode, especially long-pulsed diode, and Nd:YAG lasers for highly pigmented patients, as well as testing, dosing, and cooling precautions to improve patient safety.

Treatment of pseudofolliculitis barbae in skin types IV, V, and VI with a long-pulsed neodymium:yttrium aluminum garnet laser. Ross E, Cooke L, Timko A, Overstreet KA, Graham BS, Barnette DJ. J Am Acad Dermatol 2002; 47: 263–70.

Thirty-seven patients with pseudofolliculitis and Fitzpatrick skin types IV, V, and VI were tested with Nd:YAG laser. There was 33, 43, and 40% hair reduction on the thigh for the 50, 80, and 100 J/cm^2 fluences, respectively, after 90 days. The highest doses tolerated by the epidermis were 50, 100, and 100 J/cm^2 for types VI, V, and IV skin, respectively. After testing on the face, mean papule counts after 90 days were 6.95 and 1.0 for the control vs treatment sites, respectively.

Treatment of pseudofolliculitis barbae using the long-pulse Nd: YAG laser on skin types V and VI. Weaver S, Sagaral E. Dermatol Surg 2003; 29: 1187–91.

Twenty subjects with Fitzpatrick type V and VI skin and PFB on the neck or mandible were given two 2 × 2 cm treatments with Nd:YAG laser and 10 mm spot size at 40–50 ms and 24–40 J/cm^2 3–4 weeks apart, and were assessed by photographic papule/pustule and hair counts at 1, 2, and 3 months after the final treatment and compared to a neighboring untreated site. The 76–90% reduction in the number of papules/pustules was statistically significant. Hair reduction of 80% 1 month after testing diminished to 23% by 3 months.

Although side effects were noted as transient and without blistering, the two illustrated patients both show scarring.

Long-pulsed Nd: YAG laser-assisted hair removal in pigmented skin: a clinical and histologic evaluation. Alster T, Bryan H. Annual Meeting American Society for Dermatologic Surgery; 2 Nov 2000. [Abstract]

Twenty women with skin types IV–VI were treated by 3-monthly applications of long-pulsed Nd:YAG laser through a cooling disk at 50 ms with 40 J/cm^2 for the face, 45 J/cm^2 for the leg, and 50 J/cm^2 for the axilla. Prolonged hair loss and improvement of PFB held for 6 months after the last treatment, and were best in the axilla and worst for the face.

Surgical depilation for the treatment of pseudofolliculitis or local hirsutism of the face: experience in the first 40 patients. Hage J, Bouman F. Plast Reconstruct Surg 1991; 88: 446–51.

Forty patients, all but three of whom were Caucasian, were operated on over a 15-year period for local hirsutism in 24, pseudofolliculitis in 11, and beard growth in 12 transgender procedures. The skin of the affected areas was incised and everted in a dermal-subcutaneous plane and the hair bulbs were excised. Marked diminution of hair numbers occurred, but 15 patients required further electrolysis. Side effects were significant, with wound edge necrosis in eight, seroma or hematoma in eight, and significant subcutaneous scar formation in 15, which was later preventable by postoperative long-term (at least 3 months) pressure bandages. See also Comments in Plast Reconstruct Surg 1992; 90: 332–3.

Pseudoxanthoma elasticum

Kenneth H Neldner

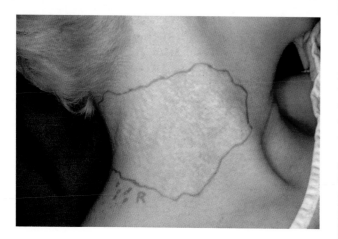

Pseudoxanthoma elasticum (PXE) is a rare autosomal recessive disorder causing abnormal calcification of the elastic fibers in the skin, retina, and cardiovascular system. The major clinical features include slightly thickened, leather-like skin lesions most commonly seen in flexural skin, retinal angioid streaks and hemorrhages, with central vision loss. Cardiovascular problems are less common, intermittent claudication in the lower extremities being the most common. Gastrointestinal bleeding is reported in about 10% of patients, which may also be due to non-PXE related factors. The prevalence of PXE in the population is approximately 1:70 000. For unknown reasons there is an approximately 2:1 predominance in females.

The chromosome carrying the PXE gene(s) was found on chromosome 16p13.1 and a specific gene(s) has been identified in the ABCC6 group of genes.

MANAGEMENT STRATEGY

Establishing the diagnosis of PXE may be difficult during the early stages of the disorder. The initial clinical signs appear most commonly during the early teenage years in flexural skin sites on the neck, axillae, antecubital fossae, and groins, as variably sized patches of slightly thickened, leathery-looking skin. The diagnosis is often missed during these early years. Larger patches gradually develop with age. Angioid streaks in the retina usually appear later, beginning in the late teens or early 20s. Frank retinal hemorrhages begin most commonly in the fifth decade, causing central vision loss. Cardiovascular changes are rarely noted in children, although rare cases have been reported.

SPECIFIC INVESTIGATIONS

- ► Complete skin examination, with special reference to all flexural skin sites and oral mucosa
- ► A 3–4 mm punch biopsy of suspicious lesions and a von Kossa stain to detect calcified elastic fibers to establish a diagnosis

- ► General physical examination and routine laboratory tests
- ► Retinal examination and photographs for evidence of angioid streaks and hemorrhages
- ► Family history for evidence of similar problems
- ► Genetic studies may be used to verify the diagnosis of PXE in questionable cases. They are expensive and not readily available, and are rarely essential to confirm the diagnosis

Pseudoxanthoma elasticum. Neldner KH. Clin Dermatol 1988; 6: 1–159.

For the interested physician, patients, or their families, this is the only book devoted solely to PXE. It is out of print from the publisher but can be obtained in paperback with full color clinical photos from the National Association for PXE, 8760 Manchester Road, St Louis, MO 64144–2724; email: NAPEstlouis@sbcglobal.net.

FIRST-LINE THERAPIES

- ► Thorough discussion of PXE with the patient and family, stressing the importance of lifelong follow-up and potential complications **B**
- ► Attention to current PXE medical literature for new therapies **E**
- ► Good nutrition; avoidance of *trans* fats; dietary calcium intake based on patient age and the current recommended dietary intake **B**
- ► Regular exercise program, with care to avoid sports with potential for head or eye injury **B**
- ► Vigorous control of hypertension and abnormal lipid profiles **C**
- ► Avoid long-term use of anticoagulants (GI bleeding) **C**
- ► Retinal referral and follow-up on regular basis with a retinal specialist familiar with PXE. If early or threatened retinal hemorrhages, check for possible treatment with bevacizumab (Avastin) **C**

Pseudoxanthoma elasticum – a connective tissue disease or a metabolic disorder at the genome/environment interface? Uitto J. J Invest Dermatol 2004; 122: ix-x.

Pseudoxanthoma elasticum is a metabolic disease. Jiang Q, Endo M, Dibra F, Wang K, Uitto J. JID advance online publication, 7 August 2008, doi: 10.1038/jid.2008.212.

Intravitreal bevacizumab for the management of choroidal neovascularization in pseudoxanthoma elasticum. Bhatnagar P, Freund KB, Spaide R, Klancnik JM Jr, Cooney MJ, Ho I, et al. Retina 2007; 24: 897–902.

Yannuzzi and his group, as well as other ophthalmologists, have had experience with injecting bevacizumab directly into the retinae of PXE patients. The results have shown some improvement, with stabilization of the neovascular process in the eyes.

A large study has not yet been carried out in PXE.

SECOND-LINE THERAPIES

- ► Consider cardiology referral for signs of mitral valve prolapse (MVP) **B**

Evidence Levels: **A** Double-blind study **B** Clinical trial ≥ 20 subjects **C** Clinical trial < 20 subjects **D** Series ≥ 5 subjects **E** Anecdotal case reports

Pseudoxanthoma elasticum and mitral valve prolapse. Lebwohl MG, Distefano D, Prioleau PG, Uram M, Yannuzzi LA, Fleischmajer R. N Engl J Med 1982; 307: 228–32.

Mitral valve prolapse (MVP) is quite common in PXE patients as well as the general population (exact frequencies are unknown). It is of no clinical significance unless accompanied by a heart murmur over the mitral valve. If this is present, the patient should take antibiotics prior to surgical and dental procedures. An echocardiogram is the best way to diagnose the presence of MVP.

THIRD-LINE THERAPIES

▶ Referral to cosmetic surgeon for removal of objectionable lesions if desired by patient for cosmetic reasons   **B**

▶ Observe pregnant women more carefully. Incidence of GI hemorrhage is questionably increased during pregnancy   **C**

▶ Encourage the patient and their family to follow the medical literature available on PXE at various computer sites. Provide information on joining one or both PXE support groups: National Association for PXE (NAPE) and PXE International. Check the internet for websites and details on updates regarding new therapies   **E**

OTHER THERAPIES

There are several important new studies under way in 2008 that could have significant long-term benefits in the management of PXE if they prove successful. A brief list is presented below.

Pseudoxanthoma elasticum: oxidative stress and antioxidant diet in a mouse model (Abcc6-/-). Li Q, Jiang Q, Uitto J. J Invest Dermatol 2008; 128: 1160–4.

Uitto and his group have developed a knockout mouse without ABCC6 genes. These mice lack calcium in normally calcified facial vibrissae. Many studies potentially related to calcium metabolism are currently under way in these knockout mice.

Vitamin K metabolites

Does the absence of ABCC6 (multidrug resistance protein 6) in patients with pseudoxanthoma elasticum prevent the liver from providing sufficient vitamin K to the periphery? Borst P, van de Wetering K, Schlingemann R. Cell Cycle 2008; 7: 1575–9.

Ninety percent of vitamin K_1 is of dietary origin, found mainly in green vegetables. It is metabolized by the liver and various good intestinal bacteria to vitamins K_2 and K_3. These are known to be essential for normal bone growth and other, currently unproven, factors in calcium metabolism. A possible role in PXE is being studied. Several medications are known to interfere with vitamin K_1 metabolism, such as warfarin.

Fetuin-A

Role of serum fetuin-A, a major inhibitor of systemic calcification, in pseudoxanthoma elasticum. Hendig D, Schulz V, Arndt M, Szliska C, Kleesiek K, Götting C. Clin Chem 2006; 52: 227–34.

Secreted by the liver, fetuin (AHSG, or fetuin-A) is a major calcification-regulating glycoprotein in the circulation; it is known to inhibit soft tissue calcification. Low levels of fetuin-A cause an increased risk for heart calcification.

Bevacizumab (Avastin)

Intravitreal bevacizumab for choroidal neovascularization associated with pseudoxanthoma elasticum. Finger RP, Charbel Issa P, Ladewig M, Holz FG, Scholl HP. Br J Opthalmol 2008; 92: 485–7.

Retinal hemorrhage with visual loss is the complication most feared by PXE patients. Age-related macular degeneration (AMD) is a very common disorder worldwide. The wet type results in retinal hemorrhage with central vision loss, similar to PXE but having a different etiologic mechanism. A great deal of research has produced treatments for AMD involving the injection of medication (Avastin) directly into the retina, with variably good results. Some PXE patients have tried this and report some improvement. Such therapy is currently untested in prolonged controlled studies and so cannot be recommended, although future studies in PXE are strongly indicated.

Psoriasis

Mark G Lebwohl, Peter van de Kerkhof

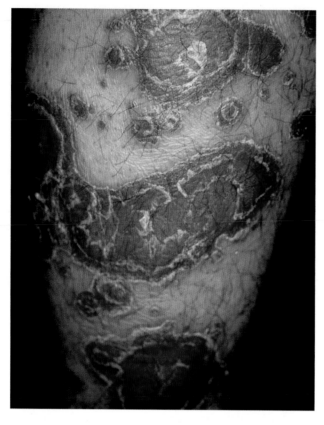

Plaque psoriasis is a common disorder in which environmental factors contribute to the development of sharply demarcated erythematous scaling plaques in genetically predisposed individuals. Because there is an overlap in treatments, guttate psoriasis, inverse psoriasis, and impetigo herpetiformis will be discussed under 'Management Strategy' below. Erythrodermic psoriasis and pustular psoriasis will be discussed at the end of the chapter. Palmoplantar pustulosis is addressed in its own chapter.

MANAGEMENT STRATEGY

The treatment of psoriasis must take many factors into account, including the extent of involvement, areas of involvement, the patient's lifestyle, and other health problems and medications. For example, patients who live far from phototherapy centers may not have the option to be treated with psoralen and UVA (PUVA), but a home phototherapy unit can be ordered for patients who can be taught to administer their own UVB therapy. In sunny climates, sun exposure can be added to the therapeutic regimen. If patients are taking medications such as lithium that are known to exacerbate psoriasis, alternatives should be sought. In patients who have had multiple skin cancers, PUVA and ciclosporin should be avoided as they increase the tendency to develop skin cancers; acitretin, which suppresses the development of skin cancers, should be considered for these individuals.

The body surface area affected in patients with psoriasis is important in the selection of therapies. In individuals with less than 5% body surface area involvement, topical therapy is usually started unless the patient has previously failed topical therapy or the psoriasis is debilitating because of the site of involvement. In patients with mild localized plaques, *mild, mid-potency or potent topical corticosteroids* can be prescribed, or other topical agents such as *calcipotriol (calcipotriene), calcitriol* or *tazarotene* can be tried. *Anthralin preparations* have fallen into disfavor because they are messy, but they still offer an effective alternative to corticosteroids. In Europe anthralin preparations are used in some day-care centers. Often patients have been using a topical medication that is inadequate as monotherapy, and in such cases combination therapy is warranted. The combination of a superpotent corticosteroid and calcipotriol or tazarotene is often effective when monotherapy with either of the agents does not work, and new formulations that combine betamethasone dipropionate with calcipotriol are available.

Some areas may be limited in extent, but require alternative treatments. For example, involvement of the palms and soles can be debilitating, and these areas are notoriously difficult to treat. Pustular psoriasis of the palms and soles, for example, only occasionally responds to topical therapy. Although the palms and soles involve only a small percentage of the body surface area, treatment with oral medications or injected medications or *phototherapy* may be warranted. The combination of *acitretin* 25 mg daily with *'bath-PUVA'* – applied by soaking the hands in a water-filled basin to which *methoxsalen* has been added, followed by UVA irradiation – has been used successfully. The *excimer* laser can also be effective for palm and sole psoriasis, as can o*ral methotrexate, acitretin* and *ciclosporin*. Although no longer available due to reports of progressive multifocal leukoencephalopathy in patients in efalizumab, double-blind placebo-controlled trials have demonstrated the efficacy of efalizumab for palm and sole psoriasis, and it is likely that other biologics also work for this difficult form of the disease.

Involvement of the scalp is common and requires gels, solutions, or foams that are not as messy as ointments and creams. *Shampoos containing tars, salicylic acid, or corticosteroids* are useful adjunctive therapies for the scalp.

The face and intertriginous sites are highly responsive to topical medications, but are particularly sensitive to the side effects of many topical agents. Topical corticosteroids cause cutaneous atrophy, telangiectasia, and striae. Therefore, only milder, safer corticosteroids should be used on the face and intertriginous sites, and alternating with non-corticosteroids may be optimal if psoriasis recurs. The topical immunomodulators *tacrolimus 0.1% ointment* and *pimecrolimus 1% cream* are effective and safe for facial and intertriginous psoriasis, but not as effective on thick plaques on the rest of the body. *Calcipotriol* (50 μg/g) can be irritating on facial or intertriginous psoriasis, but alternative vitamin D analogs such as calcitriol and tacalcitol are less irritating and therefore particularly suited for facial or flexural psoriasis. *Tazarotene* may be too irritating to use on genital skin, but it can be used on the face. The irritation of tazarotene can also be minimized by using it in a regimen with topical corticosteroids.

With 5–10% body surface involvement, topical therapy is usually prescribed, but may require the addition of *phototherapy* or *oral medications*. In those with more than 10% body surface involvement, topical therapy may be impractical for all lesions but may provide a useful adjunct to phototherapy or systemic therapy.

Evidence Levels: **A** Double-blind study **B** Clinical trial ≥ 20 subjects **C** Clinical trial < 20 subjects **D** Series ≥ 5 subjects **E** Anecdotal case reports

Phototherapy with *UVB* has been in use in the treatment of psoriasis since the 1920s and has a proven record of safety and efficacy. It is particularly useful in patients who have responded well to sun exposure. Patients who have failed UVB or have not done well with sun exposure often respond to *narrowband UVB*. *PUVA* is one of the most effective treatments for psoriasis and offers long remissions for many patients. Because of its increased risk of cutaneous malignancy, PUVA is usually reserved for those who do not achieve adequate remissions with UVB.

In patients who have not achieved satisfactory results with these treatments, *low-dose oral retinoids* can be added. *Acitretin* in doses of 10–25 mg daily dramatically improves the response to UVB and to PUVA. By keeping the dose at 25 mg or less, the side effects of acitretin can be minimized. For those who are not candidates for UVB phototherapy or PUVA, *oral methotrexate* is highly effective in combination with other treatments or as monotherapy. It is associated with hepatic fibrosis in some patients and regular monitoring of liver function tests in addition to blood counts is necessary. Current guidelines in the USA call for periodic liver biopsies in selected patients treated with methotrexate. In parts of Europe, the serum level of the aminoterminal propeptide of type III procollagen has been used as a marker for hepatic fibrosis as an alternative to routine use of liver biopsy. *Ciclosporin* is also dramatically effective as monotherapy for psoriasis, but is associated with nephrotoxicity as well as hypertension and a theoretical risk of malignancy with long-term use. Consequently, current guidelines call for limiting use of ciclosporin to 1 or 2 years.

In recent years, the ability to create new drugs that target specific parts of the immune system has led to the development of biologic agents for psoriasis. These drugs are not associated with the nephrotoxicity of ciclosporin or the hepatotoxicity and bone marrow toxicity of methotrexate. The long-term side effects of biologics are not known, however, and their cost is often prohibitive. Psoriasis experts are divided on the point at which biologics should be considered. Some consider them first-line therapy when the disease is too extensive for topical therapy. Because of their expense, biologics are used by others only after phototherapy or other systemic therapies have been tried.

At least eight biologic agents have been approved or have completed large clinical trials for psoriasis. Agents that block tumor necrosis factor-α (TNF-α), including etanercept, infliximab, adalimumab, and certolizumab, are ideal for patients with psoriatic arthritis. TNF-blocking agents have unique side effects, including the reactivation of latent tuberculosis, exacerbation of multiple sclerosis, and the development of antinuclear antibodies. Agents that block T-cell activation include efalizumab and alefacept. The latter achieves 75% improvement in the psoriasis area and severity index (PASI 75) in less than 25% of patients, but many patients who achieve remission remain clear for many months. In contrast to alefacept, doses of efalizumab, like those of infliximab, are adjusted according to body weight. The latter two drugs are therefore appropriate for patients who are obese and hence less likely to respond to fixed-dose therapies. Following the development of progressive multifocal leukoencephalopathy in at least 3 efalizumab-treated patients, this drug was withdrawn from the market in 2009.

Two drugs that block the p40 component of IL-12 and IL-23 have recently been introduced and are highly effective for psoriasis. Ustekinumab has been studied in 45 mg and 90 mg doses; dose elevation can be beneficial in overweight patients. The drug can be administered as infrequently as every 3 months. ABT-874 works by the same mechanism and is also likely to gain approval for psoriasis.

Because of the toxicities of psoriasis therapy, several concepts have evolved for controlling the disease while minimizing side effects. *Rotational therapy*, for example, involves treating psoriasis with a medication such as methotrexate for varying periods, followed by switching to PUVA, retinoids, or ciclosporin for limited periods. The different treatments used in rotation are determined by patient response. Because biologic therapies have not been associated with major organ toxicity, they are often used long term without the need for rotation.

Combination therapy involves the mixing of two or more treatments. Topical therapies are often used in combination with phototherapy and systemic therapy. Phototherapy with UVB or PUVA is often combined with oral retinoids or methotrexate, thereby minimizing the number of treatments and the toxicity of each of the therapies. Phototherapy has also been used with many of the biologic agents for psoriasis, resulting in improved response rates. Low doses of methotrexate and ciclosporin can be used in combination to minimize the nephrotoxicity of ciclosporin and the hepatotoxicity of methotrexate. The latter combination can be effective in patients who have failed monotherapy with either agent. Biologics have been used in combination with methotrexate, ciclosporin, and acitretin. Because acitretin is not immunosuppressive, it is an ideal agent for combination therapy with the new drugs that target the immune system. Many advocate combining infliximab with methotrexate, not only to achieve better results, but to reduce the development of human antichimeric antibodies which are associated with increased infusion reactions and reduced efficacy of infliximab.

Sequential therapy refers to the concept of treatment in which potent agents are used to clear the disease, and safer but less effective agents are used to maintain remission. For example, ciclosporin can be used to clear psoriasis and patients can then be switched to oral retinoids in combination with UVB for maintenance or to a biologic agent. Similarly, sequential therapy can be applied to topical medications. Calcipotriol or tazarotene can be used in combination with superpotent corticosteroids to clear psoriasis and to reduce irritation induced by calcipotriol or tazarotene monotherapy. The corticosteroid can then be tapered to a regimen where it is used only 2 days per week or eliminated altogether, while the non-corticosteroid agent can be continued.

GUTTATE PSORIASIS

Guttate psoriasis is characterized by widespread erythematous, scaling papules. The management of guttate psoriasis is very similar to that of extensive plaque psoriasis. Because streptococcal infection often precedes guttate psoriasis, underlying infection should be sought and treated. Lesions are usually too widespread for topical therapy, so most patients are started on *phototherapy with UVB*. If that is ineffective, *oral retinoids* can be added or patients can be switched to *narrowband UVB or PUVA*. This form of psoriasis frequently responds to phototherapy, so it is only occasionally necessary to resort to more aggressive second-line or third-line therapies listed below.

INVERSE PSORIASIS

Patients with inverse psoriasis develop lesions in the axillae, between the buttocks, on the medial aspects of the thighs, and in the umbilicus. These sites are easily treated with *mild topical corticosteroids*, but are more susceptible to corticosteroid side effects such as atrophy and formation of striae. Consequently, non-steroidal treatments can be attempted. *Calcipotriol* (50 μg/g) can be irritating on intertriginous sites but is nevertheless effective. *Other vitamin D analogs (calcitriol, tacalcitol)* cause less irritation. *Tazarotene* can be used on the face, but is usually too irritating to use in the axillae or groin. *Tars and anthralin* are likewise irritating in intertriginous sites. *Topical tacrolimus ointment* and *pimecrolimus cream*, albeit not approved for psoriasis, are highly effective for facial and intertriginous psoriasis, but less effective for thick plaques elsewhere on the body.

IMPETIGO HERPETIFORMIS

Impetigo herpetiformis is characterized by a generalized pustular eruption with fever and leukocytosis developing during pregnancy. Many consider this to be a variant of pustular psoriasis that occurs during pregnancy. If *bed rest, emollients, compresses,* and *mild topical corticosteroids* are ineffective, *systemic corticosteroids* have been used effectively in the past. More recently, *oral ciclosporin* has proved effective for impetigo herpetiformis. This drug, which has a pregnancy category C rating, is administered in two divided doses totaling 4–5 mg/kg daily. Concerns about cumulative toxicity, such as nephrotoxicity, are less worrisome in impetigo herpetiformis because the disorder may resolve at the end of pregnancy, limiting the amount of ciclosporin prescribed. Although there is not as much experience in the use of biologic agents for impetigo herpetiformis, the limited data available for these agents suggest that they are relatively safe during pregnancy. Most are rated as pregnancy category B, meaning that there is no evidence of fetal toxicity in animal studies; however, the risk to the fetal immune system and postnatal immune function is unknown. Therefore, these drugs should only be used during pregnancy if clearly needed. Efalizumab was rated pregnancy category C.

SPECIFIC INVESTIGATIONS

> ► Skin biopsy (if the clinical diagnosis of psoriasis is uncertain)
> ► Laboratory investigations
> > ► Serum electrolytes and calcium for patients with pustular psoriasis
> > ► ASO or bacterial cultures for patients with guttate psoriasis
> > ► Appropriate drug-related monitoring for patients on systemic therapies

Investigation is not required in the majority of cases. Skin biopsy may be helpful if the diagnosis is in question, but is usually not needed.

As discussed below, a range of investigations are required for screening and monitoring when using systemic therapies.

Routine screening for tuberculosis has been advised for patients treated with infliximab, adalimumab, and etanercept. Because methotrexate, ciclosporin, and other biologics are also immunosuppressive, skin testing for tuberculosis and, if positive, chest radiography have been suggested prior to treatment with these agents. Ciclosporin guidelines call for frequent monitoring of blood pressure and chemistry screening, with particular attention to serum creatinine and magnesium.

Methotrexate guidelines call for periodic monitoring of CBC and platelet counts, and chemistry screening with liver function tests. Assays for hepatic fibrosis such as the serum aminoterminal propeptide of type III procollagen, or liver biopsies, are advised in certain patients. Monitoring for viral hepatitis or HIV infection should be considered in populations at risk for those disorders. Serum cholesterol and triglycerides are particularly important in patients treated with oral acitretin.

From the Medical Board of the National Psoriasis Foundation: monitoring and vaccinations in patients treated with biologics for psoriasis. Lebwohl M, Bagel J, Gelfand JM, Gladman D, Gordon KB, Hsu S, et al. J Am Acad Dermatol 2008; 58: 94–105.

Apart from history, physical examination, routine chemistry screening, CBC and platelet counts, skin testing for tuberculosis is advised for patients treated with all of the biologics. Liver function tests should be monitored more frequently in patients treated with infliximab; CD4 counts should be checked every 2 weeks in patients treated with alefacept; and live vaccines should be avoided in patients on biologic therapies.

Cyclosporine Consensus Conference: with emphasis on the treatment of psoriasis. Lebwohl M, Ellis C, Gottlieb A, Koo J, Krueger G, Linden K, et al. Am Acad Dermatol 1998; 39: 464–75.

Oral ciclosporin in doses up to 5 mg/kg daily is dramatically effective for psoriasis, but is limited by the development of nephrotoxicity.

This article presents guidelines regarding dosage and monitoring, drug interactions, and complications of ciclosporin.

In patients treated with ciclosporin, blood and platelet counts as well as comprehensive serum chemistries are warranted, including blood urea nitrogen, creatinine, potassium, magnesium, uric acid, liver function tests, and lipids. Two baseline serum creatinine levels and two baseline blood pressure measurements should be obtained prior to starting ciclosporin therapy.

Methotrexate and psoriasis: 2009. National Psoriasis Foundation Consensus Conference. Kalb R, Strober B, Weinstein G, Lebwohl M. J Am Acad Dermatol 2009; 60: 824–37.

Methotrexate in psoriasis: consensus conference. Roenigk HH Jr, Auerbach R, Maibach H, Weinstein G, Lebwohl M. J Am Acad Dermatol 1998; 38: 478–85.

Methotrexate remains one of the most effective systemic agents for psoriasis. Following an initial test dose of 2.5–7.5 mg, weekly doses ranging from 15 to 30 mg can be used to clear psoriasis in most patients. The most worrisome side effects are hepatotoxicity and bone marrow suppression.

These articles review many of the publications on methotrexate and covers laboratory monitoring guidelines, including blood work and liver biopsy, dosage guidelines, drug interactions, and side effects.

Patients treated with methotrexate should have baseline blood and platelet counts as well as liver function tests and creatinine. If baseline liver function tests are elevated, serological studies for hepatitis B and hepatitis C are warranted. In Europe, assays for the aminoterminal propeptide of type III procollagen are obtained. In patients without risk factors for hepatic fibrosis (such as obesity), liver biopsies may not be required or their frequency markedly reduced. Many dermatologists in the USA and Europe still obtain periodic liver biopsies to monitor hepatic fibrosis.

Evidence Levels: **A** Double-blind study **B** Clinical trial ≥ 20 subjects **C** Clinical trial < 20 subjects **D** Series ≥ 5 subjects **E** Anecdotal case reports

FIRST-LINE THERAPIES

▶ Anthralin (dithranol)	B
▶ Coal tar	A
▶ Salicylic acid	C
▶ Topical corticosteroids	A
▶ Vitamin D analogs	A
▶ Tazarotene	A
▶ Sun exposure	B
▶ Tacrolimus ointment	A
▶ Pimecrolimus cream	A

A randomized, double-blind, vehicle-controlled study of a novel liposomal dithranol formulation in psoriasis. Saraswat A, Agarwal R, Katare OP, Kaur I, Kumar B. J Dermatol Treat 2007; 18: 40–5.

Twenty patients were enrolled in a bilateral comparison controlled trial of 0.5% dithranol entrapped in phospholipid liposomes on one side of the body compared to the vehicle (10 patients) or a conventional 1.15% dithranol, 1.15% salicylic acid, and 5.3% coal tar preparation (10 patients) applied daily, using a 30-minute short-contact regimen for 6 weeks. Both active preparations resulted in significant improvement in psoriasis, but there was less perilesional erythema and skin staining on the side treated with the liposome preparation than with the conventional cream.

Anthralin preparations have been used successfully for psoriasis for decades, but staining and irritation have limited their acceptance by both patients and physicians. Attempts to formulate non-staining, non-irritating versions of anthralin have had limited success.

Efficacy of topical 5% liquor carbonis detergens vs. its emollient base in the treatment of psoriasis. Kanzler MH, Gorsulowsky DC. Br J Dermatol 1993; 129: 310–14.

Liquor carbonis detergens 5% resulted in more improvement in psoriasis than its vehicle emollient base in a bilateral-paired comparison study.

Tars are available in gels, creams, emollient creams, and ointments, and are also available in emulsions that are added to the bath. There is a general belief that more cosmetically elegant preparations are better tolerated by patients but less effective. Crude coal tar is quite effective, but quite messy.

The role of salicylic acid in the treatment of psoriasis. Lebwohl M. Int J Dermatol 1999; 38: 16–24.

Salicylic acid is a keratolytic agent that removes scale and allows other topical medications to penetrate. There is a marked increase in penetration of topical corticosteroids when combined with 2–10% salicylic acid. Combinations of salicylic acid and tar or anthralin have also been used successfully, but salicylic acid inactivates calcipotriol. Moreover, salicylic acid blocks UVB and should therefore not be applied prior to phototherapy.

Evaluation of the efficacy and safety of clobetasol propionate spray in the treatment of plaque-type psoriasis. Jarratt MT, Clark SD, Savin RC, Swinyer LJ, Safley CF, Brodell RT, et al. Cutis 2006; 78: 348–54.

The efficacy and tolerability of clobetasol propionate foam 0.05% in the treatment of mild to moderate plaque-type psoriasis of nonscalp regions. Gottlieb AB, Ford RO, Spellman MC. J Cutan Med Surg 2003; 7: 185–92.

Clobetasol propionate shampoo 0.05%: a new option to treat patients with moderate to severe scalp psoriasis. Jarratt M, Breneman D, Gottlieb AB, Poulin Y, Liu Y, Foley V. J Drugs Dermatol 2004; 3: 367–73.

The efficacy of topical corticosteroids for psoriasis has been demonstrated in numerous double-blind, placebo-controlled trials of large numbers of patients. Topical corticosteroids are available in many vehicles, including foams, emollient foams, sprays, shampoos, solutions, lotions, creams, emollient creams, ointments, tapes, and gels.

Superpotent corticosteroids such as clobetasol can be associated with cutaneous and systemic side effects. Clinically significant adrenal suppression is seldom considered, and tests for adrenal function are virtually never performed. Practicing dermatologists are more concerned with the side effects of atrophy, telangiectasia, striae, and tachyphylaxis. For all the above reasons, superpotent corticosteroid use should be limited to 2–4 weeks, and less than 50 g/week. Superpotent corticosteroids should not be occluded and should not be used on the face or intertriginous sites. If at all possible, they should be avoided in children.

An investigator-masked comparison of the efficacy and safety of twice daily applications of calcitriol 3 μg/g ointment vs. calcipotriol 50 μg/g ointment in subjects with mild to moderate chronic plaque-type psoriasis. Zhu X, Wang B, Zhao G, Gu J, Chen Z, Briantais P, et al. J Eur Acad Dermatol Venereol 2007; 21: 466–72.

In this investigator-blinded study, 250 subjects were treated twice daily for 12 weeks with either calcitriol or calcipotriol ointments. Both agents were comparably effective, but there were more local cutaneous adverse events in patients treated with calcipotriol than those treated with calcitriol.

Because local irritation occurs in up to 20% of patients treated with calcipotriol on facial or intertriginous skin, calcitriol may be a better therapeutic option for those sites.

Once daily treatment of psoriasis with tacalcitol compared with twice daily treatment with calcipotriol. A double-blind trial. Veien NK, Bjerke JR, Rossmann-Ringdahl I, Jakobsen HB. Br J Dermatol 1997; 137: 581–6.

Tacalcitol ointment applied once daily proved to be slightly less effective than calcipotriol ointment twice daily in this 8-week, double-blind study conducted in 287 patients.

A 52-week randomized safety study of a calcipotriol/betamethasone dipropionate two-compound product (Dovobet/Daivobet/Taclonex) in the treatment of psoriasis vulgaris. Kragballe K, Austad J, Barnes L, Bibby A, de la Brassinne M, Cambazard F, et al. Br J Dermatol 2006; 154: 1155–60.

Six hundred and thirty-four patients were treated once daily for 4 weeks with a combination ointment containing calcipotriol and betamethasone dipropionate. After 4 weeks they were randomized to receive either the combination product or the combination product alternating with calcipotriol ointment at 4-week intervals; or calcipotriol ointment alone as needed for 48 weeks in this double-blind trial. The combination product was consistently more effective than calcipotriol, and patients treated throughout with combination product had the fewest side effects. Cutaneous atrophy occurred in four (1.9%) of those randomized to receive the combination ointment for 52 weeks.

Calcipotriol is a relatively unstable molecule which is inactivated upon mixing with many other topical agents, so the availability of a stable combination ointment of calcipotriol with a corticosteroid is desirable. Long-term therapy with any product containing a topical corticosteroid should be done with caution to avoid cutaneous atrophy, and especially the development of striae. To minimize local cutaneous side effects, avoid strong corticosteroids on the face and intertriginous sites. Use intermittent dosing such as weekend therapy for maintenance of therapeutic effect.

Tazarotene cream in the treatment of psoriasis: Two multicenter, double-blind, randomized, vehicle-controlled studies of the safety and efficacy of tazarotene creams 0.05% and 0.1% applied once daily for 12 weeks. Weinstein GD, Koo JY, Krueger GG, Lebwohl M, Love NJ, Menter MA, et al; Tazarotene Cream Clinical Study Group. J Am Acad Dermatol 2003; 48: 760–7.

Tazarotene creams 0.1% and 0.05% were compared to vehicle once daily for 12 weeks in this double-blind study. Tazarotene 0.1% was more effective but also more irritating than the 0.05% cream, and both were superior in efficacy to vehicle.

Tazarotene creams are slightly less effective but also less irritating than tazarotene 0.1% and 0.05% gels.

Tacrolimus ointment is effective for facial and intertriginous psoriasis. Lebwohl M, Freeman AK, Chapman MS, Feldman SR, Hartle JE, Henning A; Tacrolimus Ointment Study Group. J Am Acad Dermatol 2004; 51: 723–30.

One hundred and sixty-seven patients were treated in this double-blind, placebo-controlled trial of tacrolimus 0.1% ointment applied twice daily for 8 weeks for facial and intertriginous psoriasis. At the end of 8 weeks 65.2% of tacrolimus ointment-treated patients and 31.5% of vehicle-treated patients were clear or almost clear.

Pimecrolimus cream 1% in the treatment of intertriginous psoriasis: a double-blind, randomized study. Gribetz C, Ling M, Lebwohl M, Pariser D, Draelos Z, Gottlieb AB, et al. J Am Acad Dermatol 2004; 51: 731–8.

In this double-blind study 57 patients were treated with 1% pimecrolimus cream or placebo. At the end of week 8, 71% of pimecrolimus-treated patients were clear or almost clear, compared to 41% of vehicle-treated patients.

Topical calcineurin inhibitors are valuable alternatives for psoriasis in facial and intertriginous sites which are particularly susceptible to corticosteroid side effects and easily irritated by calcipotriol or tazarotene.

The percentage of patients achieving PASI 75 after 1 month and remission time after climatotherapy at the Dead Sea. Harari M, Novack L, Barth J, David M, Friger M, Moses SW. Int J Dermatol 2007; 46: 1087–91.

Sixty-four patients were treated with climatotherapy at the Dead Sea, which included bathing in Dead Sea water and gradually increasing sun exposure. All patients achieved PASI 50 and 75.9% achieved PASI 75. The median time to recurrence of a lesion of psoriasis was 23.1 weeks and the median duration of effect, defined as the time to 50% relapse in the PASI improvement, was 33.6 weeks.

The Dead Sea is the lowest point on earth and has the highest concentration of minerals of any body of water on the earth. The mineral haze in the atmosphere through which sunlight passes results in a unique spectrum of sunlight which accounts for the exceptional therapeutic responses. Two to four weeks of Dead Sea sun exposure and bathing are required to achieve significant benefit.

SECOND-LINE THERAPIES

▶ UVB	A
▶ Narrowband UVB	A
▶ PUVA	A
▶ Acitretin	A
▶ Adalimumab	A
▶ Alefacept	A
▶ Etanercept	A
▶ Infliximab	A
▶ Ustekinumab	A
▶ Methotrexate	A
▶ Ciclosporin	A

Components of the Goeckerman regimen. Le Vine MJ, White HA, Parrish JA. J Invest Dermatol 1979; 73: 170–3.

The efficacy of UVB phototherapy is improved by the addition of a topical tar preparation or lubricating base; 5% crude coal tar is no more effective than lubricating base when combined with a phototherapy regimen.

The original Goeckerman regimen involved inpatient application of crude coal tar, which was removed prior to daily UVB phototherapy. Most current phototherapy regimens involve outpatient treatment three times per week with topical application of mineral oil or petrolatum.

Narrowband UV-B produces superior clinical and histopathological resolution of moderate-to-severe psoriasis in patients compared with broadband UV-B. Coven TR, Burack LH, Gilleaudeau R, Keogh M, Ozawa M, Krueger JG. Arch Dermatol 1997; 133: 1514–22.

Twenty-two patients were treated in a bilateral comparison study with narrowband UVB on one side and broadband UVB on the other. The side treated with narrowband UVB cleared more quickly and more completely than the side treated with broadband UVB.

Randomized double-blind trial of the treatment of chronic plaque psoriasis: efficacy of psoralen-UV-A therapy vs. narrowband UV-B therapy. Yones SS, Palmer RA, Garibaldinos TT, Hawk JL. Arch Dermatol 2006; 142: 836–42.

In this double-blind study 93 patients were treated twice weekly with either narrowband UVB or PUVA until clearance or up to a maximum of 30 sessions. In patients with skin types 1–4, PUVA was significantly more effective than UVB, with 84% of PUVA-treated patients clearing compared to 65% of narrowband UVB-treated patients. PUVA cleared patients after a median of 17 treatments, compared to 28.5 treatments for narrowband UVB. Six months after the last treatment 68% of patients treated with PUVA remained clear, compared to 35% of patients treated with narrowband UVB.

Although PUVA is more effective than narrowband UVB, it is more difficult to administer and has an increased risk of phototoxicity and carcinogenicity.

PUVA therapy for psoriasis: comparison of oral and bathwater delivery of 8-methoxypsoralen. Lowe NJ, Weingarten D, Bourget T, Moy LS. J Am Acad Dermatol 1986; 14: 754–60.

Bath-water delivery of methoxsalen (bath-PUVA) is as effective as oral PUVA, but requires less UVA and is not associated with systemic side effects such as nausea. Phototoxicity may be increased.

Evidence Levels: A Double-blind study B Clinical trial ≥ 20 subjects C Clinical trial < 20 subjects D Series ≥ 5 subjects E Anecdotal case reports

Side effects of burning, sun sensitivity, and, especially, photocarcinogenicity are of concern. Topically applied methoxsalen has also been shown to be effective for psoriasis, but is associated with more phototoxicity.

Trioxsalen bath plus UVA effective and safe in the treatment of psoriasis. Hannuksela M, Karvonen J. Br J Dermatol 1978; 99: 703–7.

Seventy-four patients with psoriasis were treated with trioxsalen baths, resulting in good or excellent responses in 92%.

Trioxsalen may be associated with less photosensitivity than methoxsalen.

Baseline and annual eye examinations have been suggested for patients treated with PUVA, but initial concerns about the development of cataracts in these patients have not been borne out over time. Baseline serologies for lupus were once recommended prior to starting patients on PUVA, but are now only obtained in patients who have other signs or symptoms of the disease.

Efficacy and safety results from the randomized controlled comparative study of adalimumab vs. methotrexate vs. placebo in patients with psoriasis (CHAMPION). Saurat JH, Stingl G, Dubertret L, Papp K, Langley RG, Ortonne JP, et al. Br J Dermatol 2008; 158: 558–66.

Adalimumab 40 mg every other week following an 80 mg loading dose was compared to methotrexate 7.5 mg orally, increased according to clinical response up to 25 mg per week or placebo for 16 weeks. Of adalimumab-treated patients, 79.6% achieved PASI 75, compared to 35.5% of those patients treated with methotrexate and 18.9% of those treated with placebo. Methotrexate patients suffered the most adverse events leading to study discontinuation, mostly related to hepatic complications.

This was the first placebo-controlled trial of methotrexate for psoriasis. The trial design has been criticized for starting methotrexate at a low dose. Nevertheless, the clear efficacy of adalimumab and the side effects of methotrexate were demonstrated by this study.

A double-blind, placebo-controlled trial of acitretin for the treatment of psoriasis. Olsen EA, Weed WW, Meyer CJ, Cobo LM. J Am Acad Dermatol 1989; 21: 681–6.

In a double-blind study 15 patients were treated with a daily acitretin dose of 25 or 50 mg or placebo for 8 weeks. All were then treated in an open-label study with either 25 or 75 mg of acitretin daily. Improvement in psoriasis was only moderate.

Acitretin plus UVB therapy for psoriasis. Comparisons with placebo plus UVB and acitretin alone. Lowe NJ, Prystowsky JH, Bourget T, Edelstein J, Nychay S, Armstrong R. J Am Acad Dermatol 1991; 24: 591–4.

Photochemotherapy for severe psoriasis without or in combination with acitretin: a randomized, double-blind comparison study. Tanew A, Guggenbichler A, Hönigsmann H, Geiger JM, Fritsch P. J Am Acad Dermatol 1991; 25: 682–4.

This was a double-blind study of 60 patients treated with either PUVA alone or PUVA in combination with acitretin. Ninety-six percent of patients treated with acitretin and PUVA achieved marked or complete clearing, compared to 80% of patients treated with PUVA alone. The cumulative UVA dose used for the acitretin + PUVA group was 42% lower than for the patients treated with PUVA alone.

Acitretin monotherapy has limited benefit for psoriasis, partly because of its limited efficacy and partly because higher dosing

results in more mucocutaneous side effects, such as hair loss and cheilitis. In combination with other treatments such as UVB or PUVA, even low doses of acitretin result in dramatically enhanced efficacy. It is also useful in combination or monotherapy for palm and sole psoriasis.

Methotrexate versus cyclosporine in moderate-to-severe chronic plaque psoriasis. Heydendael VM, Spuls PI, Opmeer BC, de Borgie CA, Reitsma JB, Goldschmidt WF, et al. N Engl J Med 2003; 349: 658–65.

Eighty-eight patients were randomized to treatment with either methotrexate starting at 15 mg and adjusted according to clinical response or ciclosporin starting at 3 mg/kg and adjusted according to clinical response. Psoriasis improved in both groups, with a slightly greater response in the ciclosporin group. Twelve of 44 patients in the methotrexate group had to discontinue treatment because of liver function test abnormalities.

An international, randomized, double-blind, placebo-controlled phase 3 trial of intramuscular alefacept in patients with chronic plaque psoriasis. Lebwohl M, Christophers E, Langley R, Ortonne JP, Roberts J, Griffiths CE; Alefacept Clinical Study Group. Arch Dermatol 2003; 139: 719–27.

Five hundred and seven patients with psoriasis were treated with placebo, alefacept 10 mg, or alefacept 15 mg, administered weekly for 12 weeks; 33% of patients treated with 15 mg achieved 75% improvement in PASI scores at some point during the course of therapy or 12 weeks of follow-up. Of patients who achieved 75% improvement in PASI scores (PASI 75), 50% reduction in PASI (PASI 50) was maintained throughout the 12-week follow-up in 71%. Reductions in CD4 counts were noted in some patients.

Long remissions are the primary advantage of this agent, which does not achieve PASI 75 in the majority of treated patients. Improvement is slow, with maximal benefit usually occurring several weeks after the last injection. More patients improve with additional therapy, and longer remissions are achieved following two courses of treatment. Baseline total lymphocyte and CD4 counts must be obtained prior to starting patients on alefacept, and current guidelines recommend that these be repeated every 2 weeks during therapy.

Etanercept treatment for children and adolescents with plaque psoriasis. Paller AS, Siegfried EC, Langley RG, Gottlieb AB, Pariser D, Landells I, et al.; Etanercept Pediatric Psoriasis Study Group. N Engl J Med 2008; 358: 241–51.

Two hundred and eleven patients age 4–17 years participated in this double-blind trial of weekly injections of placebo or 0.8 mg/kg of etanercept. Fifty-seven percent of etanercept-treated children achieved PASI 75, compared to 11% of those treated with placebo.

In adults etanercept can be administered in doses of 50 mg twice weekly. In the US, after 3 months the dosage is lowered to 50 mg administered subcutaneously once weekly, but in other countries the twice-weekly dosing can continue. As in adults, the pediatric dose of 0.8 mg/kg is effective in children with psoriasis and psoriatic arthritis.

Adalimumab therapy for moderate to severe psoriasis: A randomized, controlled phase III trial. Menter A, Tyring SK, Gordon K, Kimball AB, Leonardi CL, Langley RG, et al. J Am Acad Dermatol 2008; 58: 106–15.

In this 1212-patient double-blind, placebo-controlled trial of adalimumab 40 mg every other week for 15 weeks, 71% of adalimumab-treated patients achieved PASI 75, compared to 7% of placebo-treated patients.

Even higher response rates were achieved in patients treated with adalimumab 40 mg subcutaneously every week. A loading dose of 80 mg of adalimumab results in much faster clinical responses.

A randomized comparison of continuous vs. intermittent infliximab maintenance regimens over 1 year in the treatment of moderate-to-severe plaque psoriasis. Menter A, Feldman SR, Weinstein GD, Papp K, Evans R, Guzzo C, et al. J Am Acad Dermatol 2007; 56: 31.e1–15.

In this double-blind study 835 patients with moderate-to-severe psoriasis were treated with either infliximab 3 mg/kg or 5 mg/kg or placebo at weeks 0, 2, and 6. PASI 75 was achieved by 75.5% of patients in the 5 mg/kg group, compared to 70.3% in the 3 mg/kg group. At week 14, infliximab-treated patients were re-randomized to continuous or intermittent maintenance regimens. Greater improvements in psoriasis occurred with continuous rather than intermittent treatment, and with the 5 mg/kg dose.

Continuous infliximab therapy may suppress the development of human antichimeric antibodies, which have been associated with more infusion reactions and reduced responsiveness to the drug.

Efficacy and safety of ustekinumab, a human interleukin-12/23 monoclonal antibody, in patients with psoriasis: 52-week results from a randomised, double-blind, placebo-controlled trial (PHOENIX 2). Papp KA, Langley RG, Lebwohl M, Krueger GG, Szapary P, Yeilding N, et al. Lancet 2008; 371: 1675–84.

In this double-blind study 1230 patients were treated with ustekinumab 45 mg or 90 mg or placebo. The drug was administered subcutaneously at weeks 0 and 4, and every 12 weeks thereafter. Of those treated with 45 mg, 66.7% achieved PASI 75 compared to 75.7% of those treated with 90 mg and 3.7% of those treated with placebo. At week 28 partial responders (i.e., those who achieved PASI 50 but not PASI 75) were re-randomized to increase dosing to every 8 weeks, or to continue every 12 weeks. Of those who increased to 90 mg of ustekinumab every 8 weeks, 68.8% achieved PASI 75 by week 52, compared to only 33.3% of those who continued dosing every 12 weeks.

Safety and efficacy of ABT-874, a fully human interleukin 12/23 monoclonal antibody, in the treatment of moderate to severe chronic plaque psoriasis: results of a randomized, placebo-controlled, phase 2 trial. Kimball AB, Gordon KB, Langley RG, Menter A, Chartash EK, Valdes J; ABT-874 Psoriasis Study Investigators. Arch Dermatol 2008; 144: 200–7.

This was a double-blind, placebo-controlled trial of ABT-874, another anti-IL-12/23 antibody. One hundred and eighty patients received five different dose regimens or placebo for psoriasis. Of those treated with a single subcutaneous injection of ABT-874 200 mg, 63% achieved PASI 75. At least 90% in all of the other treatment groups, ranging from 200 mg weekly for 4 weeks up to 200 mg weekly for 12 weeks, achieved PASI 75, except for placebo-treated patients, of whom only 3% achieved PASI 75.

Anti-IL-12/IL-23 therapies are highly effective for psoriasis, but long-term side effects are not yet known.

THIRD-LINE THERAPIES

▶ Combination therapy	A
▶ Topical 5-fluorouracil	C
▶ Topical propylthiouracil	C
▶ Intralesional 5-fluorouracil	C
▶ Sulfasalazine (sulphasalazine)	A
▶ Mycophenolate mofetil	B
▶ Hydroxyurea	B
▶ 6-Thioguanine	C
▶ Azathioprine	C
▶ FK-506	A
▶ Fumaric acid esters	B
▶ Antibiotics	C
▶ Colchicine	C
▶ Propylthiouracil	B
▶ Laser (excimer, pulsed dye)	C
▶ Cryotherapy	C
▶ Grenz rays	B
▶ Photodynamic therapy	C
▶ CTLA4Ig	A
▶ Leflunomide	A

Proceedings of the psoriasis combination and rotation therapy conference. Deer Valley, Utah, October 7–9, 1994. Menter MA, See JA, Amend WJ, Ellis CN, Krueger GG, Lebwohl M, et al. J Am Acad Dermatol 1996; 34: 315–21.

The side effects of psoriasis treatments can be minimized and efficacy enhanced by combining low doses of different therapies. Rotational therapy refers to a method in which patients cleared with one psoriasis therapy are subsequently treated with different therapies to minimize the cumulative toxicity of any given treatment. Thus, the hepatotoxicity of cumulative doses of methotrexate, the nephrotoxicity of ciclosporin, and the carcinogenicity of PUVA can be minimized.

The most commonly used combinations involve retinoids and UVB, and retinoids and PUVA. UVB and PUVA have been used in combination with one another as well as with methotrexate. Retinoids are among the safest systemic agents for psoriasis and have been combined with methotrexate and ciclosporin, though liver function tests should be watched carefully when methotrexate and acitretin are used together. The combination of methotrexate and ciclosporin is a dramatically effective therapy, as is the combination of ciclosporin and hydroxyurea. Methotrexate has also been used with hydroxyurea, but blood counts must be watched very carefully.

Although this conference predated the introduction of biologic therapies for psoriasis, all of the currently approved biologics have been administered with methotrexate, acitretin, ciclosporin, and phototherapy. Because methotrexate and ciclosporin are immunosuppressive, they should be used cautiously with biologics and for as short a period of combination as possible. An exception may be the combination of methotrexate with inflixmab, as concomitant methotrexate has been shown to reduce the development of antichimeric antibodies.

Clinical efficacy of a 308 nm excimer laser for treatment of psoriasis vulgaris. He YL, Zhang XY, Dong J, Xu JZ, Wang J. Photodermatol Photoimmunol Photomed 2007; 23: 238–41.

Evidence Levels: **A** Double-blind study **B** Clinical trial ≥ 20 subjects **C** Clinical trial < 20 subjects **D** Series ≥ 5 subjects **E** Anecdotal case reports

In this open-label study 40 patients were treated twice weekly for up to 15 treatments. PASI scores improved by approximately 90%.

The excimer laser is a useful therapy for localized plaques of psoriasis. Its main side effect is local cutaneous burning.

Targeted UVB phototherapy for psoriasis: a preliminary study. Lapidoth M, Adatto M, David M. Clin Exp Dermatol 2007; 32: 642–5.

This high-intensity targeted UVB lamp (290–320 nm; Be Clear®) resulted in significant improvement in localized plaques without treating normal surrounding skin.

Efficacy of the pulsed dye laser in the treatment of localized recalcitrant plaque psoriasis: a comparative study. Erceg A, Bovenschen HJ, van de Kerkhof PC, Seyger MM. Br J Dermatol 2006; 155: 110–14.

Pulsed dye laser was compared to the combination calcipotriol/betamethasone dipropionate ointment in an open-label, bilateral comparison study. Twelve weeks after treatment there was 62% improvement in psoriasis severity scores on the PDL-treated side, compared to 19% reduction on the combination calcipotriol/betamethasone dipropionate side.

Weekly pulse dosing schedule of fluorouracil: a new topical therapy for psoriasis. Pearlman DL, Youngberg B, Engelhard C. J Am Acad Dermatol 1986; 15: 1247–52.

Fourteen patients were treated with topical 5-fluorouracil with occlusion 2–3 days per week for a mean of 15.7 weeks. Eleven patients achieved 90% clearing of treated lesions, compared to 6% for placebo.

Because of concern about absorption, topical 5-fluorouracil should only be used on isolated plaques. Irritation is the main side effect.

Weekly psoriasis therapy using intralesional fluorouracil. Pearlman DL, Youngberg B, Engelhard C. J Am Acad Dermatol 1987; 17: 78–82.

Eleven patients were treated with intralesional injection of 1 mL of fluorouracil (50 mg/mL). Injections were repeated at 1–2-week intervals, with each patient receiving an average of two injections. Nine of 11 patients improved, with maximal clearing occurring 4 weeks after the first injection. There were no systemic side effects, but local irritation and hyperpigmentation occurred.

A controlled trial of topical propylthiouracil in the treatment of patients with psoriasis. Elias AN, Dangaran K, Barr RJ, Rohan MK, Goodman MM. J Am Acad Dermatol 1994; 31: 455–8.

Nine patients with psoriasis were treated in a double-blind study in which some lesions were treated with topical propylthiouracil and others with placebo. Study medications were applied three times daily for 4–8 weeks. There was greater clearing of lesions treated with propylthiouracil, including near complete clearing in two patients. Systemic side effects did not occur.

Sulfasalazine improves psoriasis. A double-blind analysis. Gupta AK, Ellis CN, Siegel MT, Duell EA, Griffiths CE, Hamilton TA, et al. Arch Dermatol 1990; 126: 487–93.

Fifty patients participated in this double-blind, placebo-controlled trial. Marked improvement was reported in 41% of the sulfasalazine-treated patients, and moderate improvement in another 41%. Over one-quarter of the sulfasalazine-treated patients discontinued the study because of side effects of rash or nausea.

Mycophenolate mofetil (CellCept) for psoriasis: a two-center, prospective, open-label clinical trial. Zhou Y, Rosenthal D, Dutz J, Ho V. J Cutan Med Surg 2003; 7: 193–7.

Twenty-three patients were treated in an open-label study of mycophenolate mofetil 2–3 g daily for 12 weeks. At the end of 12 weeks PASI scores improved by 47%. Only 22% of patients did not have a significant response. Five patients developed nausea and one developed transient leukopenia.

Mycophenolate mofetil is highly effective in a subset of psoriasis patients. Gastrointestinal side effects can be limited by administering the drug in four divided daily doses instead of the twice-daily dosing recommended in the package insert. An enteric-coated form is also helpful in reducing nausea.

Hydroxyurea in the management of therapy resistant psoriasis. Layton AM, Sheehan-Dare RA, Goodfield MJ, Cotterill JA. Br J Dermatol 1989; 121: 647–53.

Eighty-five patients with psoriasis were treated with long-term hydroxyurea in doses of 0.5–1.5 g daily. Remissions occurred in 61%. Reversible bone marrow suppression occurred in 35% of patients. Four patients developed cutaneous side effects.

6-Thioguanine treatment of psoriasis: experience in 81 patients. Zackheim HS, Glogau RG, Fisher DA, Maibach HI. J Am Acad Dermatol 1994; 30: 452–8.

This was a retrospective study of 81 patients treated with 6-thioguanine for psoriasis. Improvement was maintained in nearly 50% of patients for a median of 33 months. Treatment with 6-thioguanine had to be discontinued most commonly because of reversible bone marrow suppression.

Pulse dosing of thioguanine in recalcitrant psoriasis. Silvis NG, Levine N. Arch Dermatol 1999; 135: 433–7.

Bone marrow suppression can be avoided by treating patients with oral thioguanine two to three times per week with maintenance doses ranging from 120 twice weekly to 160 three times weekly. In this open study a marked improvement was noted in 10 of 14 patients.

Azathioprine in psoriasis. Greaves MW, Dawber R. Br Med J 1970; 2: 237–8.

Azathioprine can be effective monotherapy for psoriasis, but its use is limited by bone marrow toxicity.

As with 6-thioguanine and hydroxyurea, the therapeutically effective dose of azathioprine is close to doses that are toxic to the bone marrow. With all three of these drugs, frequent blood counts are essential.

Systemic tacrolimus (FK 506) is effective for the treatment of psoriasis in a double-blind, placebo-controlled study. European FK 506 Multicentre Psoriasis Study Group. Arch Dermatol 1996; 132: 419–23.

Fifty patients with psoriasis were treated for 9 weeks in this double-blind, placebo-controlled study. Starting doses were 0.05 mg/kg daily and could be increased up to 0.15 mg/kg daily. Tacrolimus-treated patients had significantly greater improvements in PASI scores than those receiving placebo. Diarrhea, paresthesias, and insomnia were the most commonly reported side effects.

Treatment of psoriasis with fumaric acid esters: results of a prospective multicentre study: German Multicentre Study. Mrowietz U, Christophers E, Altmeyer P. Br J Dermatol 1998; 138: 456–60.

Of 101 patients who started this prospective study, 70 completed 4 months of treatment. There was an 80% reduction in PASI scores. Side effects consisted of lymphocytopenia, gastrointestinal complaints, and flushing.

Although not noted in this study, nephrotoxicity has been a recognized side effect of fumaric acid therapy.

Use of rifampin with penicillin and erythromycin in the treatment of psoriasis. Preliminary report. Rosenberg EW, Noah PW, Zanolli MD, Skinner RB Jr, Bond MJ, Crutcher N. J Am Acad Dermatol 1986; 14: 761–4.

All nine patients with streptococcal-associated psoriasis responded to a 5-day course of rifampin (rifampicin) combined with 10–14 days of oral penicillin or erythromycin.

The use of oral antibiotics has been championed by Rosenberg and colleagues. Although supported by sound theories and numerous anecdotes, the use of antibiotics for psoriasis has not been supported by controlled clinical trials. Other agents that have been used include oral nystatin and oral fluconazole; even tonsillectomy has been advocated.

Therapeutic trials with oral colchicine in psoriasis. Wahba A, Cohen H. Acta Dermatol Venereol 1980; 60: 515–20.

Twenty-two patients were treated in an open trial of colchicine 0.02 mg/kg daily for 2–4 months. Of the nine patients with thin papules and plaques, eight noted marked improvement or clearing, but there was little improvement in patients with thick plaques.

Propylthiouracil in psoriasis: results of an open trial. Elias AN, Goodman MM, Liem WH, Barr RJ. J Am Acad Dermatol 1993; 29: 78–81.

Propylthiouracil at a dose of 100 mg was administered orally every 8 hours for 8 weeks to ten patients with psoriasis. Seven had marked improvement in their psoriasis and the others showed moderate improvement. Thyroid function tests were unaffected, except for a mild increase in serum thyroid-stimulating hormone after 6 weeks of therapy in a single patient.

Cryotherapy for psoriasis. Nouri K, Chartier TK, Eaglstein WH, Taylor JR. Arch Dermatol 1997; 133: 1608–9.

Target plaques of psoriasis were treated with cryotherapy, resulting in improvement. Local reactions including pain and vesiculation were the only side effects other than discoloration.

As with lasers, cryotherapy is only practical for isolated, localized plaques. Despite the Koebner phenomenon, psoriasis does not commonly occur in frozen plaques, but scarring or discoloration can occur.

Psoriasis of the scalp treated with Grenz rays or topical corticosteroid combined with Grenz rays. A comparative randomized trial. Lindelof B, Johannesson A. Br J Dermatol 1988; 119: 241–4.

Forty patients were treated with either Grenz rays or Grenz rays plus topical corticosteroids for scalp psoriasis. Grenz rays were administered at a dosage of 4 Gy at weekly intervals for six treatments; 84% of the Grenz ray-treated patients and 72% of the Grenz ray plus corticosteroid group healed. The addition of topical corticosteroids offered little benefit.

The association between X-ray therapy and squamous cell carcinomas, particularly in patients subsequently treated with PUVA, has led to less use of this valuable modality.

Administration of DAB389IL-2 to patients with recalcitrant psoriasis: a double-blind, phase II multicenter trial. Bagel J, Garland WT, Breneman D, Holick M, Littlejohn TW, Crosby D, et al. J Am Acad Dermatol 1998; 38: 938–44.

A double-blind, placebo-controlled study of DAB389IL-2 was conducted to examine the safety and efficacy of this medication in psoriasis. Patients received either placebo, or 5, 10, or 15 µg/kg intravenously for 3 consecutive days each week. At least 50% improvement was achieved in 41% of patients during the course of this regimen, compared to 25% of controls. Ten patients discontinued treatment because of adverse effects, including flu-like symptoms and, in one patient, vasospasm and coagulopathy.

Diphtheria fusion toxin has been demonstrated to be effective for psoriasis, but is limited by its side effects. Because it is already approved for the treatment of cutaneous T-cell lymphoma, efforts are under way to see if it can be made tolerable for psoriasis.

CTLA4Ig-mediated blockade of T-cell costimulation in patients with psoriasis vulgaris. Abrams JR, Lebwohl MG, Guzzo CA, Jegasothy BV, Goldfarb MT, Goffe BS, et al. J Clin Invest 1999; 103: 1243–52.

In this 26-week, open-label, dose-escalation study in which 43 patients received four intravenous infusions of this fusion protein, 46% achieved 50% or greater improvement, with significantly greater responses in patients treated with higher doses.

Efficacy and safety of leflunomide in the treatment of psoriatic arthritis and psoriasis: a multinational, double-blind, randomized, placebo-controlled clinical trial. Kaltwasser JP, Nash P, Gladman D, Rosen CF, Behrens F, Jones P, et al.; Treatment of Psoriatic Arthritis Study Group. Arthritis Rheum 2004; 50: 1939–50.

One hundred and ninety patients with psoriasis and psoriatic arthritis were treated in this double-blind, placebo-controlled trial.

Leflunomide proved to be effective for psoriatic arthritis but only modestly effective for psoriasis.

ERYTHRODERMIC PSORIASIS

Erythrodermic psoriasis is characterized by marked erythema and scaling affecting the entire cutaneous surface. All the protective functions of the skin are lost, including protection against infection, temperature control, and prevention of fluid loss. Loss of nutrients through the skin leads to anemia and electrolyte imbalance. The most common precipitating cause of erythrodermic psoriasis is the withdrawal of systemic corticosteroids; this should be avoided in patients with psoriasis. Excessive use of topical superpotent corticosteroids, phototherapy burns, and infections have also been implicated as causes of erythrodermic psoriasis.

Patients may require hospitalization with bed rest, emollients, and application of mild topical corticosteroids. Because sepsis and shock are complications of erythrodermic psoriasis, monitoring of temperature, blood pressure, urine output, and weight may be important, depending on the severity of the condition. In males and in females not of childbearing potential, oral retinoids are among the safest treatments for erythrodermic psoriasis, but are not as reliably effective as infliximab, ciclosporin, or methotrexate. Acitretin can be started in doses of 25 mg daily and can be increased to 50 mg or higher. Ciclosporin in doses of 4–5 mg/kg daily results in rapid improvement. Oral methotrexate starting at 15 mg per week and gradually increasing up to 30 mg/week is effective within a few weeks. Once erythema has cleared with topical or systemic agents, patients can occasionally be switched to phototherapy or PUVA or to other long-term therapies, including the biologics. Infliximab is rapidly effective for erythrodermic psoriasis, and is emerging as an important treatment option. Because antichimeric antibodies are more likely to develop against this agent if treatments are not maintained, long-term therapy with infliximab infusions must be considered if this treatment is chosen. Other biologics are likely to emerge as potential therapies for erythrodermic psoriasis; etanercept has been used with some success, but it is slower acting than infliximab.

When the above agents either do not work or cannot be used, many of the third-line therapies listed for psoriasis are effective. For example, there are anecdotal reports of 6-thioguanine, mycophenolate mofetil, azathioprine, and hydroxyurea working for erythrodermic psoriasis. Combination therapy such as the combination of methotrexate and ciclosporin in low doses, or the combination of methotrexate and infliximab, can also be effective. There are also anecdotal reports of carbamazepine clearing erythrodermic psoriasis.

FIRST-LINE THERAPIES

▶ Emollients	D
▶ Topical corticosteroids	D

SECOND-LINE THERAPIES

▶ Retinoids	B
▶ Ciclosporin	B
▶ Infliximab	E
▶ Etanercept	D
▶ Methotrexate	B

THIRD-LINE THERAPIES

▶ Combination therapy	D
▶ 6-Thioguanine	E
▶ Mycophenolate mofetil	E
▶ Hydroxyurea	E
▶ Azathioprine	E
▶ Carbamazepine	E

Use of short-course class 1 topical glucocorticoid under occlusion for the rapid control of erythrodermic psoriasis. Arbiser JL, Grossman K, Kaye E, Arndt KA. Arch Dermatol 1994; 130: 704–6.

Erythrodermic psoriasis will respond rapidly to oral corticosteroids or to superpotent corticosteroids with occlusion, but withdrawal of these agents often results in a more severe flare. Consequently, these treatments are avoided in patients with erythrodermic psoriasis.

Management of erythrodermic psoriasis with low-dose cyclosporine. Studio Italiano Muticentrico nella Psoriasi (SIMPSO). Dermatology 1993; 187: 30–7.

Thirty-three patients with erythrodermic psoriasis were treated with ciclosporin, starting with up to 5 mg/kg daily;

67% achieved complete remission in a median of 2–4 months, and another 27% noted substantial improvement.

Life-threatening pustular and erythrodermic psoriasis responding to infliximab. Lewis TG, Tuchinda C, Lim HW, Wong HK. J Drugs Dermatol 2006; 5: 546–8.

The authors report a rapid response of life-threatening erythrodermic psoriasis to intravenous infliximab.

There have been a number of anecdotal reports citing infliximab's successful treatment of erythrodermic psoriasis.

Treatment of erythrodermic psoriasis with etanercept. Esposito M, Mazzotta A, de Felice C, Papoutsaki M, Chimenti S. Br J Dermatol 2006; 155: 156–9.

Ten patients were treated with open-label etanercept 25 mg subcutaneously twice weekly. By week 12, 50% had achieved at least 75% improvement in psoriasis severity scores, and that number increased by week 24.

Erythrodermic psoriasis can be a life-threatening condition requiring more rapid-acting agents than etanercept. The latter biologic can be useful in more chronic and stable forms of the disease.

Treatment of pustulous and erythrodermic psoriasis with PUVA therapy and methotrexate. Lekovic B, Dostanic I, Konstantinovic K, Kneitner I. Hautarzt 1982; 33: 284–5. (In German.)

The combination of PUVA and methotrexate successfully treated five patients with erythrodermic psoriasis and two with pustular psoriasis. According to the authors, annual methotrexate doses could be reduced by 50% by adding PUVA to the regimen.

It is difficult to distinguish a PUVA burn from erythrodermic psoriasis. Nevertheless, some patients with erythrodermic psoriasis are successfully controlled with PUVA. Monotherapy with methotrexate is used more typically.

The treatment of psoriasis with etretinate and acitretin: a follow up of actual use. Magis NL, Blummel JJ, Kerkhof PC, Gerritsen RM. Eur J Dermatol 2000; 10: 517–21.

In a retrospective review of 94 patients treated with retinoids, there were no serious side effects after 10 years of follow-up. The efficacy of retinoids for pustular and erythrodermic psoriasis was stressed.

Accidental success with carbamazepine for psoriatic erythroderma. Smith KJ, Skelton HG. N Engl J Med 1996; 335: 1999–2000.

A patient with HIV infection and erythrodermic psoriasis was inadvertently treated with carbamazepine instead of etretinate. The patient's erythroderma cleared.

Carbamazepine in doses of 200–400 mg daily has been reported to clear erythrodermic psoriasis in some but not all patients. Further controlled clinical studies are warranted.

PUSTULAR PSORIASIS

Management of pustular psoriasis begins with the *removal of precipitating causes*. Lithium, antimalarials, diltiazem, propranolol, and irritating topical therapy with tar have all been implicated, but the most common cause is the withdrawal of systemic corticosteroids. As in erythrodermic psoriasis, all the protective functions of skin are compromised and patients are susceptible to infection, fluid loss, electrolyte imbalance, loss of nutrients through the skin, and loss of temperature control.

Supportive care and treatment of infection are mandatory. *Oral acitretin* results in rapid improvement. In women of childbearing potential *isotretinoin* may be preferred because the period of teratogenicity of this drug is shorter than that of acitretin. *Ciclosporin, infliximab, adalimumab,* and *methotrexate* are also highly effective for this life-threatening condition. Caution should be exercised with the use of TNF blockers, however, as there have been rare cases of pustular psoriasis caused by their use. Additionally, cases of pustular psoriasis have been precipitated by the abrupt withdrawal of efalizumab. *Hydroxyurea, 6-thioguanine, mycophenolate mofetil, azathioprine, dapsone,* and *colchicine* have also been used in isolated patients.

FIRST-LINE THERAPIES

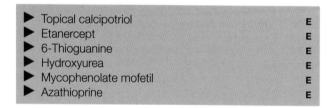

▶ Topical corticosteroids	E
▶ Retinoids	B
▶ Ciclosporin	E
▶ Infliximab	E
▶ Adalimumab	E
▶ Methotrexate	B

SECOND-LINE THERAPIES

▶ Topical calcipotriol	E
▶ Etanercept	E
▶ 6-Thioguanine	E
▶ Hydroxyurea	E
▶ Mycophenolate mofetil	E
▶ Azathioprine	E

Isotretinoin vs etretinate therapy in generalized pustular and chronic psoriasis. Moy RL, Kingston TP, Lowe NJ. Arch Dermatol 1985; 121: 1297–301.

Although isotretinoin was less effective than etretinate for plaque psoriasis, 10 of 11 patients with pustular psoriasis responded.

Many consider acitretin or isotretinoin to be the treatment of choice for patients with pustular psoriasis. Apart from the shorter period of teratogenicity of isotretinoin, it also causes less hair loss than acitretin.

Generalized pustular psoriasis (von Zumbusch) responding to cyclosporine A. Meinardi MM, Westerhof W, Bos JD. Br J Dermatol 1987; 116: 269–70.

This is one of numerous case reports documenting the dramatic response of pustular psoriasis to ciclosporin.

Ciclosporin in doses of 4–5 mg/kg daily is usually effective in the treatment of pustular psoriasis.

Infliximab in recalcitrant generalized pustular arthropatic psoriasis. Vieira Serrão V, Martins A, Lopes MJ. Eur J Dermatol 2008; 18: 71–3.

This is a case report of a patient with psoriatic arthritis and acute generalized pustular psoriasis refractory to acitretin, methotrexate, and corticosteroids which responded rapidly to treatment with infliximab, with complete clearing of lesions by week 12, along with improvement in psoriatic arthritis.

Pustular psoriasis induced by infliximab. Thurber M, Feasel A, Stroehlein J, Hymes SR. J Drugs Dermatol 2004; 3: 439–40.

Despite several reports describing the efficacy of infliximab in pustular psoriasis, there are a small number of reports of pustular psoriasis developing in patients treated with infliximab for other indications.

Several reports of psoriasis, and specifically pustular psoriasis, developing after treatment with TNF-α blockers have emerged. Nevertheless, these agents can be highly useful for the treatment of pustular psoriasis.

Long-term efficacy of adalimumab in generalized pustular psoriasis. Zangrilli A, Papoutsaki M, Talamonti M, Chimenti S. J Dermatol Treat 2008; 19: 185–7.

Adalimumab 40 mg subcutaneously once weekly resulted in rapid remission of chronic pustular psoriasis. The remission persisted throughout 72 weeks of treatment.

Etanercept at different dosages in the treatment of generalized pustular psoriasis: a case series. Esposito M, Mazzotta A, Casciello C, Chimenti S. Dermatology 2008; 216: 355–60.

Six patients with generalized pustular psoriasis who failed to respond to conventional treatments were treated with etanercept 25–50 mg twice weekly for 48 weeks, with good efficacy.

Because etanercept can be slower acting than other systemic or biologic agents, and because generalized pustular psoriasis can be life-threatening, a more rapid-acting agent should be considered for severe disease.

Generalised pustular psoriasis: response to topical calcipotriol. Berth-Jones J, Bourke J, Bailey K, Graham-Brown RA, Hutchinson PE. Br Med J 1992; 305: 868–9.

Three cases of pustular psoriasis responded to topical application of calcipotriol and the treatment was well tolerated.

It is important to monitor serum calcium when using calcipotriol in this way. Although irritation was not a problem in the reported cases, some care is required in case this develops.

Systemic corticosteroids and folic acid antagonists in the treatment of generalized pustular psoriasis. Evaluation and prognosis based on the study of 104 cases. Ryan TJ, Baker H. Br J Dermatol 1969; 81: 134–45.

Despite the short-term benefit of systemic corticosteroids for pustular psoriasis, once the dose is reduced rebound flares occur. In this study a significant proportion of patients treated with systemic corticosteroids died.

Methotrexate remains a highly effective modality for the treatment of pustular psoriasis. Doses beginning at 15 mg per week (following an initial test dose) are used.

THIRD-LINE THERAPIES

▶ Colchicine	E

Colchicine in generalized pustular psoriasis: clinical response and antibody-dependent cytotoxicity by monocytes and neutrophils. Zachariae H, Kragballe K, Herlin T. Arch Dermatol Res 1982; 274: 327–33.

Three of four patients with pustular psoriasis cleared within 2 weeks of starting oral colchicine.

Colchicine 0.6 mg twice daily can be effective for pustular psoriasis. The dose can be increased by one pill daily, but side effects of diarrhea frequently intervene.

Evidence Levels: **A** Double-blind study   **B** Clinical trial ≥ 20 subjects   **C** Clinical trial < 20 subjects   **D** Series ≥ 5 subjects   **E** Anecdotal case reports

Psychogenic excoriation

Robert E Accordino, John Koo

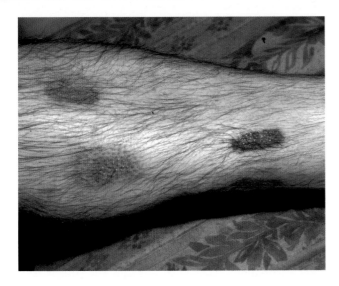

Psychogenic excoriation, also known as neurotic excoriation, is a psychodermatologic condition in which patients participate in compulsive scratching and picking of normal skin or skin with minor surface irregularities. Such behaviors may cause self-inflicted ulcers, abscesses, or scars that can ultimately become disfiguring. Psychogenic excoriation has been associated with both obsessive–compulsive disorder (in the anxiety disorder spectrum) as well as borderline personality disorder, and is thought to be related to emotional stress. Depression may also be a common underlying psychopathology. Treatment strategies may vary depending on the individual patient or clinician, because there is a lack of evidence-based practice in the medical literature regarding a systematic approach to these patients. Very few recent investigations into psychogenic excoriation have been published.

MANAGEMENT STRATEGY

Before diagnosing a patient with psychogenic excoriation, it is important to rule out other psychodermatologic disorders, such as dermatitis artefacta (often associated with damage done with objects and not just fingernails, secrecy about the etiology of lesions, and a potentially demanding and manipulative personality), or delusions of parasitosis (associated with delusional thinking, particularly the strongly held belief of microbes infesting the skin). These two conditions may respond to other forms of therapy. Since psychogenic excoriation is primarily a psychiatric disorder, psychopharmacology could be a very effective line of therapy. The condition may be associated with several psychopathologic states, including anxiety, stress, depression, and psychosis. As such, pharmacologic agents directed toward these conditions can be of benefit. Generally speaking, however, psychogenic excoriation is probably best treated with the *tricyclic antidepressant doxepin* as a first-line treatment. There is an insufficient number of

clinical trials demonstrating its efficacy in this condition, but the authors believe that it is useful due to its combined antidepressant and antihistaminic/antipruritic activity, which may be critical in breaking the itch–scratch cycle. Doxepin is usually started at 10–25 mg at bedtime, with a gradual increase in dose of 10–25 mg/week until the patient is taking up to 100 mg every evening, which is the typical effective dose, particularly if the underlying psychopathology is major depression. If the patient requires even higher dosages, a maximum of up to 300 mg daily may be used, provided there are no side effects. Doxepin can prolong the QT interval, so a screening ECG is recommended for patients over the age of 55 or any patient with a past history of cardiac dysrhythmia. Syncope, seizures, sedation, weight gain, and orthostatic hypotension are other potential side effects.

Selective serotonin reuptake inhibitors (SSRIs), antidepressants that include *fluoxetine, sertraline,* and *fluvoxamine,* have also been shown in several reports to be effective in patients with psychogenic excoriation. These drugs have better safety profiles than doxepin and are less associated with sedation and cardiac conduction abnormalities. There has even been a recent case report that *paroxetine,* another SSRI, improved a case of psychogenic excoriation. Other *tricyclic* antidepressants, such as *clomipramine* and *amitriptyline,* and various *benzodiazepines* are third-line therapies that should only be considered if the patient does not respond to the more conventional treatments outlined above or cannot tolerate the side effects. *Pimozide,* a traditional antipsychotic; *olanzapine,* an atypical antipsychotic; *aripiprazole,* a second-generation antipsychotic; and *naltrexone,* an opioid antagonist, may also have a role for some patients in treating psychogenic excoriation, especially if the underlying pathology involves psychosis.

Treating associated infection and pruritus through the prudent use of *antibiotics* and *antihistamines (oral or topical),* respectively, and using *topical corticosteroids* may provide additional symptomatic benefit for patients with psychogenic excoriation. Lastly, *psychotherapy* and *cognitive behavioral techniques,* including aversion therapy and habit reversal treatments, have been reported in certain cases to be effective for this disorder, although a lack of substantial evidence should render this an adjunctive therapy at best. There are two case reports of the efficacy of *cognitive psychotherapy with laser irradiation* of disfiguring skin lesions, as well as a recent case report on the efficacy of *hypnosis* to alleviate psychogenic excoriation.

As mentioned previously, psychogenic excoriation is primarily a psychiatric disorder, so close follow-up with a primary care physician and a psychiatrist (if the patient is willing) may help to maintain lasting remission.

SPECIFIC INVESTIGATIONS

Close follow-up with a primary care physician or psychiatrist is recommended because of the high incidence of comorbid psychiatric conditions.

Psychogenic excoriation. Clinical features, proposed diagnostic criteria, epidemiology and approaches to treatment. Arnold LM, Auchenbach MB, McElroy SL. CNS Drugs 2001; 15: 351–9.

A review article that outlines the clinical features of psychogenic excoriation, as well as comorbid psychiatric conditions, treatments demonstrated to be effective, and potential criteria for diagnosis.

Characteristics of 34 adults with psychogenic excoriation. Arnold LM, McElroy SL, Mutasim DF, Dwight MM, Lamerson CL, Morris EM. J Clin Psychiatry 1998; 59: 509–15.

Patients with psychogenic excoriations have a high prevalence of concurrent psychiatric illnesses such as mood disorders (68%), anxiety disorders (41%), somatoform disorders (21%), substance abuse (12%), and eating disorders (12%).

Neurotic excoriations and dermatitis artefacta. Koblenzer CS. Dermatol Clin 1996; 14: 447–55.

A good review article.

Dermatology and conditions related to obsessive–compulsive disorder. Stein DJ, Hollander E. J Am Acad Dermatol 1992; 26: 237–42.

Patients with psychogenic excoriations often have obsessive–compulsive symptoms and may therefore respond to specific therapies aimed at this type of disorder.

FIRST-LINE THERAPIES

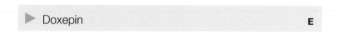

▷ Doxepin	E

Psychopharmacology for dermatologic patients. Koo J, Gambla C. Dermatol Clin 1996; 14: 509–24.

Describes in further detail the use of doxepin in psychogenic excoriations.

Improvement of chronic neurotic excoriations with oral doxepin therapy. Harris BA, Sherertz EF, Flowers FP. Int J Dermatol 1987; 26: 541–3.

Case report of two patients who responded to doxepin 30 mg and 75 mg daily.

SECOND-LINE THERAPIES

▶ Sertraline	B
▶ Paroxetine	E

Sertraline in the treatment of neurotic excoriations and related disorders. Kalivas J, Kalivas L, Gilman D, Hayden CT. Arch Dermatol 1996; 132: 589–90.

Sertraline was started at 25–50 mg daily and titrated upward to 100–200 mg daily as necessary, with improvements seen in 19 of 28 patients (68%) at an average of 4 weeks.

Paroxetine in a case of psychogenic pruritus and neurotic excoriations. Biondi M, Arcangeli T, Petrucci RM. Psychother Psychosom 2000; 69: 165–6.

This is one case report demonstrating success with the SSRI paroxetine. The medication was chosen based on the personality of the patient and was thought to work secondary to its anticompulsive activity.

THIRD-LINE THERAPIES

▶ Fluoxetine	A
▶ Fluvoxamine	C
▶ Venlafaxine	E

▶ Escitalopram	D
▶ Clomipramine	E
▶ Amitriptyline	E
▶ Benzodiazepines	E
▶ Pimozide	E
▶ Olanzapine	D
▶ Aripiprazole	E
▶ Naltrexone	E
▶ Psychotherapy	D
▶ Cognitive behavioral therapy	E
▶ Hypnosis	E

A double-blind trial of fluoxetine in pathologic skin picking. Simeon D, Stein DJ, Gross S, Islam N, Schmeidler J, Hollander E. J Clin Psychiatry 1997; 58: 341–7.

Fluoxetine was started at 20 mg daily and increased by 20 mg/week up to a maximum of 80 mg daily. Improvements in the treatment arm were statistically significant (based on an intent-to-treat analysis) at 6 weeks, with an average dose of 55 mg daily.

This trial is limited by a small sample (10 patients in the study arm and 11 in the placebo arm), a high dropout rate (40% in the fluoxetine group), and a study period of only 10 weeks, but the study did substantiate earlier case reports.

An open clinical trial of fluvoxamine treatment of psychogenic excoriation. Arnold LM, Mutasim DF, Dwight MM, Lamerson CL, Morris EM, McElroy SL. J Clin Psychopharmacol 1999; 19: 15–18.

Fluvoxamine was started at 25–50 mg daily and increased by up to 50 mg/week to a maximum of 300 mg daily for 12 weeks. Although all 14 participants demonstrated significant improvements in six of eight self-reported scales, the seven subjects who completed the study (50%) had improvements in only two of eight self-reported scales.

Use of escitalopram in psychogenic excoriation. Pukadan D, Antony J, Mohandas E, Cyriac M, Smith G, Elias A. Aust NZ J Psychiatry 2008; 42: 435–6.

Escitalopram was administered at 10 mg/day to two patients: a 63-year-old woman with a 1-month history of diffuse pruritus and excessive excoriation, as well as major depressive disorder; and a 24-year-old man with a 10-year history of repeated nail biting and features of major depressive disorder. In both patients the scratching abated within 2 weeks.

Neurotic excoriations: a review and some new perspectives. Gupta MA, Gupta AK, Haberman HF. Compr Psychiatry 1986; 27: 381–6.

A case report of successful treatment using clomipramine 50 mg every evening for 6 months.

Neurotic excoriations: a personality evaluation. Fisher BK, Pearce KI. Cutis 1974; 14: 251–4.

Successful treatment with amitriptyline 50–75 mg daily was reported.

Neurotic excoriations. Fisher BK. Can Med Assoc J 1971; 105: 937–9.

This is a case report on the success of various benzodiazepines prior to the availability of SSRIs. In general, benzodiazepines may be useful only if anxiety is the primary cause of psychogenic excoriations.

Evidence Levels: A Double-blind study B Clinical trial ≥ 20 subjects C Clinical trial < 20 subjects D Series ≥ 5 subjects E Anecdotal case reports

Clinical experience with pimozide: emphasis on its use in post-herpetic neuralgia. Duke EE. J Am Acad Dermatol 1983; 8: 845–50.

This case report primarily demonstrates the efficacy of pimozide (2 mg two or three times daily) in the treatment of post-herpetic neuralgia (eight patients) and psychogenic excoriations (two patients).

Olanzapine may be an effective adjunctive therapy in the management of acne excoriée: a case report. Gupta MA, Gupta AK. J Cutan Med Surg 2001; 5: 25–7.

This is a case report on the success of olanzapine, an atypical antipsychotic, for psychogenic excoriations.

Efficacy of olanzapine in the treatment of psychogenic excoriation. Blanch J, Grimalt F, Massana G, Navarro V. Br J Dermatol. 2004; 151: 714–16.

This article describes a series of six patients with psychogenic excoriation who improved dramatically after treatment with olanzapine 2.5–10 mg daily. The authors also report that it is often difficult to get patients to take an atypical antipsychotic medication such as olanzapine.

The treatment of psychogenic excoriation and obsessive compulsive disorder using aripiprazole and fluoxetine. Curtis AR, Richards RW. Ann Clin Psychiatry 2007; 19: 199–200.

This is a case report on the success of aripiprazole, a second-generation antipsychotic, and fluoxetine in an 18-year-old woman with psychogenic excoriations and obsessive–compulsive disorder.

Aripiprazole augmentation of venlafaxine in the treatment of psychogenic excoriation. Carter WG 3rd, Shillcutt SD. J Clin Psychiatry 2006; 67: 1311.

This case report discusses the success of aripiprazole and venlafaxine, which is a selective norepinephrine, serotonin, and dopamine reuptake inhibitor, in a 50-year-old woman with psychogenic excoriation, major depressive disorder, and generalized anxiety disorder who had been previously unresponsive to a serotonin–norepinephrine reuptake inhibitor alone.

Naltrexone for neurotic excoriations. Smith KC, Pittelkow MR. J Am Acad Dermatol 1989; 20: 860–1.

This article discusses the reported efficacy of naltrexone for psychogenic excoriations.

Psychotherapeutic strategy and neurotic excoriations. Fruensgaard K. Int J Dermatol 1991; 30: 198–203.

This article reports a positive impact of goal-directed psychotherapy in 22 patients followed over a period of approximately 5 years for psychogenic excoriations.

Treatment of facial scarring and ulceration resulting from acne excoriée with 585-nm pulsed dye laser irradiation and cognitive psychotherapy. Bowes LE, Alster TS. Dermatol Surg 2004; 30: 934–8.

Two case reports of successful treatment of acne excoriée with a pulsed dye laser to improve the appearance of scars and ulcers, as well as cognitive psychotherapy to maintain improvement.

Acne excoriée – a case report of treatment using habit reversal. Kent A, Drummond LM. Clin Exp Dermatol 1989; 14: 163–4.

This is a case report on the success of habit reversal, a cognitive behavioral technique, for psychogenic excoriations.

The behavioral treatment of neurodermatitis through habit reversal. Rosenbaum MS, Ayllon J. Behav Res Ther 1981; 19: 313–18.

This article reports a response to habit reversal therapy for neurodermatitis in three patients.

Treatment of neurodermatitis by behavior therapy: a case study. Ratcliffe R, Stein N. Behav Res Ther 1968; 6: 397–9.

This is a case report in which neurodermatitis secondary to psychogenic excoriation improved in a 22-year-old woman as a result of aversion therapy, a cognitive behavioral technique.

Using hypnosis to facilitate resolution of psychogenic excoriations in acne excoriée. Shenefelt PD. Am J Clin Hypn 2004; 46: 239–45.

In this case report, the acne excoriée in a pregnant woman was successfully alleviated through hypnotic suggestion.

Pyoderma gangrenosum

John Berth-Jones

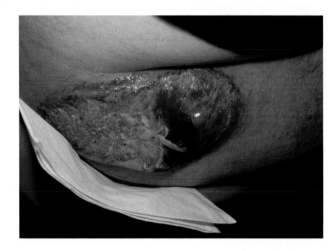

Pyoderma gangrenosum (PG) is a clinically diagnosed entity presenting as pustules which enlarge, forming ulcers with a dark, necrotic, undermined margin. Any skin site may be affected. Although PG is usually self-limiting there is a danger of disfiguring scarring.

MANAGEMENT STRATEGY

No treatment for PG is always effective. The most consistent results are reported with *systemic corticosteroids* and ciclosporin, and these effective but potentially toxic modalities can be employed when the severity of the disease justifies the risks (e.g., when there is facial involvement or rapid progression). *Infliximab* has been shown to be beneficial in a controlled trial. The evidence regarding other modalities is less conclusive. PG tends to resolve spontaneously, so some of the reports of therapeutic success may simply be the result of the disease following its natural course.

In cases where scarring is not a major concern, consideration should be given to conservative treatment with *wound dressing* only, as most lesions resolve spontaneously. When required, relatively non-toxic first-line treatments should be tried first and second-line modalities employed if there is no response. Topical tacrolimus offers an interesting novel approach to first-line therapy. A wide variety of potentially hazardous and expensive treatments are employed occasionally, and these third-line modalities should be considered only when others are ineffective.

The many recognized associations with PG include rheumatoid disease, inflammatory bowel disease, myeloproliferative disease such as acute myeloblastic leukemia, plasma cell dyscrasias, and Wegener's granulomatosis. These may warrant investigation, and may also influence the choice of treatment. Effective management of an underlying pathology such as ulcerative colitis often seems to result in improvement of the PG.

PG may demonstrate the Koebner phenomenon (pathergy); care should be taken to avoid trauma to the skin. When surgery is unavoidable in patients with a history of PG, the surgeon should be made aware of this risk. Surgical incisions should be kept as short as possible. Careful wound closure may be helpful. *Prophylactic systemic corticoids or ciclosporin* may be indicated perioperatively.

SPECIFIC INVESTIGATIONS

- ▶ Hematology
- ▶ Plasma protein electrophoresis
- ▶ Rheumatoid factor
- ▶ ANCA

In selected patients where clinically indicated
- ▶ GI work-up for inflammatory bowel disease

Pyoderma gangrenosum associated with Wegener's granulomatosis: partial response to mycophenolate mofetil. Le Hello C, Bonte I, Mora JJ, Verneuil L, Noel LH, Guillevin L. Rheumatology (Oxford) 2002; 41: 236–7.

In addition to more familiar associations, there are now many reports of PG lesions developing as a feature of Wegener's granulomatosis.

FIRST-LINE THERAPIES

▶ Topical tacrolimus	C
▶ Topical corticoids	D
▶ Dapsone	D
▶ Intralesional corticoids	D
▶ Minocycline	D
▶ Nicotine cream	E
▶ Nicotine chewing gum	E
▶ Topical pimecrolimus	E
▶ Sodium cromoglycate	D
▶ Sulfasalazine (sulphasalazine)	D

Topical tacrolimus for pyoderma gangrenosum. Reich K, Vente C, Neumann C. Br J Dermatol 1998; 139: 755–7.

Tacrolimus ointment 0.1% proved effective when used in combination with systemic ciclosporin, and also when used alone. The formula comprised 100 mg FK506 powder obtained from tablets of Prograf, mixed into 100 g of hydrophilic petrolatum (white petrolatum with 8% bleached beeswax, 3% stearyl alcohol, and 3% cholesterol).

Topical tacrolimus in the management of peristomal pyoderma gangrenosum. Lyon CC, Stapleton M, Smith AJ, Mendelsohn S, Beck MH, Griffiths CEM. J Dermatol Treat 2001; 12: 13–17.

Seven out of 11 cases of peristomal PG healed completely after 2–10 weeks of applying tacrolimus 0.3% in carmellose sodium paste (Orabase). Serum levels of tacrolimus were undetectable in all cases. In this open study the results were at least as good as those from clobetasol propionate.

Topical tacrolimus would seem to be safe enough to use as a first-line treatment, although experience remains limited.

Pyoderma gangrenosum of the scalp. Peachey RDG. Br J Dermatol 1974; 90: 106.

Evidence Levels: **A** Double-blind study **B** Clinical trial ≥ 20 subjects **C** Clinical trial < 20 subjects **D** Series ≥ 5 subjects **E** Anecdotal case reports

A case of PG involving the scalp showed slow but steady improvement on treatment with 0.1% betamethasone valerate lotion applied under polythene occlusion at night.

The efficacy of systemic corticosteroids would suggest that topical application might also be beneficial. However, there are only sparse anecdotal reports to support their efficacy. Potent compounds are generally used, e.g., betamethasone dipropionate 0.05% cream or clobetasol propionate 0.05% cream applied once daily to the lesion under an occlusive dressing of paraffin gauze or hydrocolloid.

Sulfapyridine and sulphone-type drugs in dermatology. Lorincz AL, Pearson RW. Arch Dermatol 1962; 85: 42–56.

Dapsone was successfully employed in the treatment of PG at doses of up to 400 mg daily. Low cost and the familiarity of dermatologists with this drug probably contribute to its popularity.

Dapsone has often been used in combination with other modalities, especially systemic corticosteroids. There are also many published cases in which this drug has proved ineffective. Dapsone has been successfully used in children with PG. The mechanism of action is believed to be inhibition of neutrophil migration and the myeloperoxidase system.

Triamcinolone and pyoderma gangrenosum. Gardner LW, Acker DW. Arch Dermatol 1972; 106: 599–600.

A case of multifocal PG responded to intralesional triamcinolone acetonide 10 mg/mL. Doses ranging from 40 to 200 mg were injected at any one time.

Intralesional or perilesional injection of corticosteroids appears to be very helpful in some cases. The corticosteroid is usually injected into the skin around the active margins of lesions. The risk of inducing cutaneous atrophy is small using these concentrations, and is not unacceptable in view of the scarring that will develop without treatment.

The successful use of minocycline in pyoderma gangrenosum – a report of seven cases and review of the literature. Berth-Jones J, Tan SV, Graham-Brown RAC, Pembroke AC. J Dermatol Treat 1989; 1: 23–5.

Seven cases responded to minocycline at doses of 100 mg twice daily or 200 mg twice daily. Improvement was often observed within a few days.

Successful treatment of pyoderma gangrenosum with topical 0.5% nicotine cream. Patel GK, Rhodes JR, Evans B, Holt PJ. J Dermatol Treat 2004; 15: 122–5.

Two cases responded to topical application of 0.5% nicotine in cetamacrogol cream.

Nicotine for pyoderma gangrenosum. Kanekura T, Usuki K, Kanzaki T. Lancet 1995; 345: 1058.

This is an isolated report of PG responding to nicotine chewing gum three tablets daily, each tablet containing 2 mg nicotine.

Successful treatment of severe pyoderma gangrenosum with pimecrolimus cream 1%. Bellini V, Simonetti S, Lisi P. J Eur Acad Dermatol Venereol 2008; 22: 113–15.

A patient was cleared of PG lesions within 8 weeks using pimecrolimus cream twice daily.

Pyoderma gangrenosum. A study of nineteen cases. Perry HO, Brunsting LA. Arch Dermatol 1957; 75: 380–6.

Six out of seven patients with PG associated with colitis demonstrated a good response to sulfasalazine 0.5 g every

3 hours. A good response was also seen in three of four cases of PG when colitis was not present. This drug may be particularly useful in cases of PG associated with inflammatory bowel disease, and it can also be effective in those which are not. The initial dose ranges from 0.5 to 2 g four times daily. Doses at the upper end of this range are usually reduced for maintenance therapy.

The treatment of pyoderma gangrenosum with sodium cromoglycate. De Cock KM, Thorne MG. Br J Dermatol 1980; 102: 231–3.

Two cases responded to sodium cromoglycate aqueous solution (2% W/V, Rynacrom nasal spray). In one patient, healing occurred within 3 weeks.

This is a remarkably safe treatment. Solutions of this drug have been applied to lesions of PG in concentrations ranging from 1% to 4%. Various nasal sprays and nebulizer solutions have proved suitable for direct application to PG lesions. The solution can be sprayed on to the ulcer, or applied on gauze or under occlusion with a hydrocolloid dressing. This drug may act by inhibiting neutrophil migration or cytotoxicity.

SECOND-LINE THERAPIES

| ▶ Ciclosporin | C |
| ▶ Systemic corticoids | C |

Treatment of pyoderma gangrenosum with cyclosporine: results in seven patients. Elgart G, Stover P, Larson K, Sutter C, Scheibner S, Davis B, et al. J Am Acad Dermatol 1991; 24: 83–6.

Six of seven patients, including cases associated with rheumatoid disease and cryoglobulinemia, improved on ciclosporin, four healing completely.

The response to ciclosporin seems to be fairly consistent. As the toxicity of this drug is largely related to prolonged use it can be a reasonably safe approach to gaining control of PG, which is often a brief, self-limiting illness. High doses have been used (5–10 mg/kg/day) and are probably safe for a few days in an urgent situation. However, it is likely that lower doses of 5 mg/kg/day will often be adequate.

Pyoderma gangrenosum. Clinical and laboratory findings in 15 patients with special reference to polyarthritis. Holt PJA, Davies MG, Saunders KC, Nuki G. Medicine 1980; 59: 114–33.

Twelve of these patients received, and responded to, corticosteroid treatment. Doses of up to 100 mg daily were required to induce remission.

Systemic corticosteroids (prednisone/prednisolone) have been one of the most frequently used treatments for PG, and extensive published experience indicates that they are generally considered highly effective. High doses of 40–100 mg/day may be required and the morbidity may be considerable. Lower doses of 7.5–20 mg daily are sometimes adequate for maintenance. Other systemic and topical agents are usually employed simultaneously in order to minimize the dose.

Pulse therapy

Therapeutic efficacy in the treatment of pyoderma gangrenosum. Johnson RB, Lazarus GS. Arch Dermatol 1982; 118: 76–84.

Intravenous doses of methylprednisolone 1 g daily for 5 days induced prompt responses in three cases.

THIRD-LINE THERAPIES

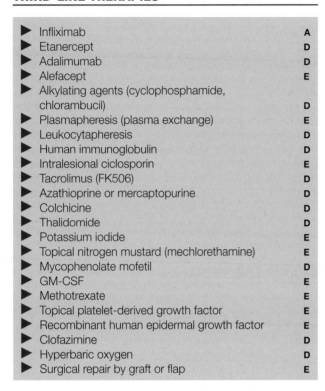

▶ Infliximab	A
▶ Etanercept	D
▶ Adalimumab	D
▶ Alefacept	E
▶ Alkylating agents (cyclophosphamide, chlorambucil)	D
▶ Plasmapheresis (plasma exchange)	E
▶ Leukocytapheresis	D
▶ Human immunoglobulin	D
▶ Intralesional ciclosporin	E
▶ Tacrolimus (FK506)	D
▶ Azathioprine or mercaptopurine	D
▶ Colchicine	D
▶ Thalidomide	D
▶ Potassium iodide	E
▶ Topical nitrogen mustard (mechlorethamine)	E
▶ Mycophenolate mofetil	D
▶ GM-CSF	E
▶ Methotrexate	E
▶ Topical platelet-derived growth factor	E
▶ Recombinant human epidermal growth factor	E
▶ Clofazimine	D
▶ Hyperbaric oxygen	D
▶ Surgical repair by graft or flap	E

Infliximab for the treatment of pyoderma gangrenosum: a randomised, double blind, placebo controlled trial. Brooklyn TN, Dunnill MG, Shetty A, Bowden JJ, Williams JD, Griffiths CE, et al. Gut 2006; 55: 505–9.

A placebo-controlled trial with 30 subjects. Two weeks after an infusion of infliximab 5 mg/kg or placebo, significantly more patients in the infliximab group had improved. In a later, open-label phase, 29 patients received infliximab with 20 demonstrating a response.

Improvement of pyoderma gangrenosum and psoriasis associated with Crohns disease with anti-tumor necrosis factor alpha monoclonal antibody. Tan MH, Gordon M, Lebwohl O, George J, Lebwohl MG. Arch Dermatol 2001; 137: 930–3.

Numerous case reports have further established the response to infliximab.

Treatment of pyoderma gangrenosum with etanercept. McGowan JW 4th, Johnson CA, Lynn A. J Drugs Dermatol 2004; 3: 441–4.

Several cases are reported responding to etanercept.

Systemic pyoderma gangrenosum responding to infliximab and adalimumab. Hubbard VG, Friedmann AC, Goldsmith P. Br J Dermatol 2005; 152: 1059–61.

An unusual case with splenic and psoas abscesses in addition to florid cutaneous pyoderma. Prompt and convincing responses were observed to infliximab and adalimumab on separate occasions.

Adalimumab therapy for recalcitrant pyoderma gangrenosum. Fonder MA, Cummins DL, Ehst BD, Anhalt GJ, Meyerle JH. J Burns Wounds 2006; 5: e8.

In this case improvement occurred on treatment with adalimumab after infliximab had failed to improve the pyoderma.

Adalimumab for treatment of pyoderma gangrenosum. Pomerantz RG, Husni ME, Mody E, Qureshi AA. Br J Dermatol 2007; 157: 1274–5.

Improvement occurred in a case that had failed to respond to etanercept.

There is also a paradoxical report of pyoderma developing in a patient receiving adalimumab for seronegative arthropathy.

An open-label pilot study of alefacept for the treatment of pyoderma gangrenosum. Foss CE, Clark AR, Inabinet R, Camacho F, Jorizzo JL. J Eur Acad Dermatol Venereol 2008; 22: 943–9.

Four patients were treated with intramuscular alefacept 15 mg weekly for 20 weeks. Remission was reported in one case and improvement in the others.

Pyoderma gangrenosum. Response to cyclophosphamide therapy. Newell LM, Malkinson FD. Arch Dermatol 1983; 119: 495–7.

A very refractory case of PG responded to cyclophosphamide 150 mg daily. Healing was evident after 14 days and almost complete after 109 days.

Intravenous cyclophosphamide pulses in the treatment of pyoderma gangrenosum associated with rheumatoid arthritis: Report of 2 cases and review of the literature. Zonana-Nacach A, Jimenez-Balderas FJ, Martinez-Osuna P, Mintz G. J Rheumatol 1994; 21: 1352–6.

Two patients improved on pulsed intravenous cyclophosphamide at doses of 500 mg/m², combined with oral corticosteroid. The first received three pulses over 5 weeks and the second seven pulses over 14 weeks. In both cases remission was subsequently maintained using oral cyclophosphamide 100 mg daily.

Chlorambucil is an effective corticosteroid-sparing agent for recalcitrant pyoderma gangrenosum. Burruss JB, Farmer ER, Callen JP. J Am Acad Dermatol 1996; 35: 720–4.

Chlorambucil was successfully used in six cases, both alone and in combination with systemic corticosteroids. The doses used ranged from 2 to 4 mg daily.

Pyoderma gangrenosum – response to topical nitrogen mustard. Tsele E, Yu RCH, Chu AC. Clin Exp Dermatol 1992; 17: 437–40.

The application of nitrogen mustard 20 mg/100 mL in aqueous solution on gauze swabs proved helpful in a single case associated with IgA paraprotein which had resisted many other treatment modalities. Patients can prepare this solution at home using tap water. Plasmapheresis was also helpful in this case. This was performed weekly for 2 years, successfully controlling the PG during this time.

Plasmapheresis is a relatively safe treatment involving removal of plasma while returning the blood cells to the circulation. Exchanges have generally been performed once to three times weekly, and prompt responses have been reported.

Leukocytapheresis treatment for pyoderma gangrenosum. Fujimoto E, Fujimoto N, Kuroda K, Tajima S. Br J Dermatol 2004; 151: 1090–2.

Efficacy of granulocyte and monocyte adsorption apheresis for three cases of refractory pyoderma gangrenosum. Seishima M, Mizutani Y, Shibuya Y, Nagasawa C, Aoki T. Ther Apher Dial 2007; 11: 177–82.

Three patients improved after weekly treatments for 10 or 11 weeks.

Granulocyte and monocyte adsorption apheresis for pyoderma gangrenosum. Kanekura T, Maruyama I, Kanzaki T. J Am Acad Dermatol 2002; 47: 320–1.

These treatments, which involve the extracorporeal removal of leukocytes, are now reported to have been effective in several cases of PG occurring both in isolation and in association with ulcerative colitis and rheumatoid disease. Treatment was performed once weekly for 4–5 weeks.

Efficacy of human intravenous immune globulin in pyoderma gangrenosum. Gupta AK, Shear NH, Sauder DN. J Am Acad Dermatol 1995; 32: 140–2.

This patient was treated for 5 days at 0.4 g/kg/day, followed by a course of 1 g/kg/day for 2 days; ciclosporin and prednisone were continued.

Successful treatment of pyoderma gangrenosum with intravenous human immunoglobulin. Dirschka T, Kastner U, Behrens S, Altmeyer P. J Am Acad Dermatol 1998; 39: 789–90.

This patient received 2-day courses of 1 g/kg daily repeated every month until complete healing was achieved after 4 months, while also receiving prednisone which was gradually reduced from 60 mg to 10 mg daily.

Intravenous immunoglobulin is effective as a sole immunomodulatory agent in pyoderma gangrenosum unresponsive to systemic corticosteroids. Suchak R, Macedo C, Glover M, Lawlor F. Clin Exp Dermatol 2007; 32: 205–7.

Infusions of 0.4 g/kg/day for 5 days were repeated at monthly intervals, with complete healing after five cycles.

Intravenous human immunoglobulin has proved effective in cases that had previously failed to respond to high doses of systemic corticosteroids and ciclosporin. However, this treatment is somewhat costly and, as IVIG is derived from pooled plasma, carries a theoretical risk of transmitting infection.

Clearing of pyoderma gangrenosum by intralesional cyclosporin A. Mrowietz U, Christophers E. Br J Dermatol 1991; 125: 498–9.

A lesion on the shoulder improved after two injections in one week of 35 mg ciclosporin into the active edges and beneath the lesion. The injection was formulated by diluting Sandimmun with normal saline in a ratio of 1:3.

Resolution of severe pyoderma gangrenosum in a patient with streaking leukocyte factor disease after treatment with tacrolimus (FK506). Abu-Elmagd K, Van Thiel DH, Jegasothy BV, Jacobs JC, Carroll P, Rodriquez-Rilo H, et al. Ann Intern Med 1993; 119: 595–8.

These authors used an initial dose of 0.15 mg/kg twice daily and reduced this gradually to the lowest effective dose.

Recalcitrant pyoderma gangrenosum treated with systemic tacrolimus. Lyon CC, Kirby B, Griffiths CE. Br J Dermatol 1999; 140: 562–4.

A refractory case of periostomal PG responded to tacrolimus 0.15 mg/kg/day.

Successful therapy of refractory pyoderma gangrenosum and periorbital phlegmona with tacrolimus (FK506) in ulcerative colitis. Baumgart DC, Wiedenmann B, Dignass AU. Inflamm Bowel Dis 2004; 10: 421–4.

Two cases of PG associated with ulcerative colitis responded to tacrolimus 0.1 mg/kg/day.

Combination oral and topical tacrolimus in therapy-resistant pyoderma gangrenosum. Jolles S, Niclasse S, Benson E. Br J Dermatol 1999; 140: 564–5.

Tacrolimus ointment 0.1% was used concomitantly with systemic administration of this drug at a dose of 0.3 mg/kg/day after higher systemic doses had proved too nephrotoxic. The addition of the topical application was followed by healing over 3 months.

Pyoderma gangrenosum treated with 6-mercaptopurine and followed by acute leukemia. Maldonado N, Torres VM, Mendez-Cashion D, Perez-Santiago E, Caceres de Costas M. J Pediatr 1968; 72: 409–14.

These authors reported a response to mercaptopurine used alone, at the relatively high dose of 2.5 mg/kg/day, although the patient, a 7-year-old boy, subsequently developed leukemia.

Crohn's disease with cutaneous involvement. Parks AG, Morson BC, Pegum JS. Proc Roy Soc Med 1965; 58: 241.

Mercaptopurine was used at the lower dose of 75 mg/day in combination with prednisone 20 mg/day.

Azathioprine has often been employed for treatment of PG, both alone and as a steroid-sparing agent. Doses have generally ranged from 100 to 150 mg daily. Less often, higher doses of up to 2.5 mg/kg/day are used. This drug seems to be useful in some cases, but results are not consistent. Mercaptopurine is the active metabolite of azathioprine.

Treatment of pyoderma gangrenosum with colchicine. Paolini O, Hebuterne X, Flory P, Charles F, Rampal P. Lancet 1995; 345: 1057–8.

Colchicine was effective and well tolerated in PG associated with Crohn's colitis. The dose used was 1 mg daily.

Colchicine in pyoderma gangrenosum. Rampal P, Benzaken S, Schneider S, Hebuterne X. Lancet 1998; 351: 1134–5.

Response was maintained using 1 mg/day for 3 years, and the drug was well tolerated.

Case report: Severe pyoderma associated with familial Mediterranean fever – Favorable response to colchicine in three patients. Lugassy G, Ronnen M. Am J Med Sci 1992; 304: 29–31.

Colchicine was effective in three cases of PG associated with familial Mediterranean fever. Treatment was commenced at 2 mg/day and reduced to 1 mg/day for maintenance.

Pyoderma gangrenosum with severe pharyngeal involvement. Buckley C, Bayoumi AHM, Sarkany I. J Roy Soc Med 1990; 83: 590–1.

An adult patient refractory to several other modalities responded to thalidomide 100 mg daily.

Pyoderma gangrenosum chez un enfant: traitement par la thalidomide. Venencie PY, Saurat J-H. Ann Pediatr 1982; 1: 67–9.

A 3-year-old child refractory to other treatments responded well to thalidomide 150 mg daily.

Pyoderma gangrenosum associated with Behçet's syndrome – response to thalidomide. Munro CS, Cox NH. Clin Exp Dermatol 1988; 13: 408–10.

A case refractory to prednisolone 100 mg daily combined with dapsone 100 mg daily responded within 48 hours to thalidomide 400 mg daily.

This drug may be of particular value in cases associated with Behçet's disease, as it is also reportedly effective in severe aphthous ulceration.

Successful treatment of pyoderma gangrenosum with potassium iodide. Akihiko A, Yohei M, Yayoi T, Hiroshi M, Kunihiko T. Acta Dermatol Venereol 2006; 86: 84–5.

Oral potassium iodide (KI) 900 mg/day was added to a regimen of prednisolone 17.5 mg, dapsone 50 mg, and minocycline 200 mg daily which had not been effective. Improvement was observed within a few days. The dose of KI was increased to 1200 mg/day after 2 weeks, and the PG had disappeared almost completely after 1 month.

KI has also been used to treat Sweet's syndrome.

Mycophenolate mofetil and cyclosporin treatment for recalcitrant pyoderma gangrenosum. Hohenleutner U, Mohr VD, Michel S, Landthaler M. Lancet 1997; 350: 1748.

This drug proved useful for a severe case of PG in combination with ciclosporin, intravenous corticosteroids, and topical application of platelet-derived wound-healing factors. The effective dose was 2 g daily.

Treatment of recalcitrant ulcers in pyoderma gangrenosum with mycophenolate mofetil and autologous keratinocyte transplantation on a hyaluronic acid matrix. Wollina U, Karamfilov T. J Eur Acad Dermatol Venereol 2000; 14: 187–90.

This patient improved when mycophenolate 2 g daily was used in combination with IV infusion of prednisolone 100 mg/day.

Mycophenolate mofetil in pyoderma gangrenosum. Lee MR, Cooper AJ. J Dermatol Treat 2004; 15: 303–7.

Mycophenolate 1–2.5 g daily was used in combination with prednisolone in three cases and as monotherapy (with 500 mg twice daily) in one.

Mycophenolate has most often been used in combination with other agents, such as ciclosporin and corticoids.

Pyoderma gangrenosum in myelodysplasia responding to granulocyte macrophage-colony stimulating factor (GM-CSF). Bulvic S, Jacobs P. Br J Dermatol 1997; 136: 637–8.

This case responded to GM-CSF in a dose of 400 mg daily injected subcutaneously.

Pyoderma gangrenosum successfully treated with perilesional granulocyte-macrophage colony stimulating factor. Shpiro D, Gilat D, Fisher-Feld L, Shemer A, Gold I, Trau H. Br J Dermatol 1998; 138: 368–9.

In this case the GM-CSF was injected perilesionally at a weekly dose of 400 mg for 4 weeks.

The use of this agent has also been reported to aggravate PG. A variety of hypersensitivity reactions, including anaphylaxis, have occasionally occurred.

Treatment of pyoderma gangrenosum with methotrexate. Teitel AD. Cutis 1996; 57: 326–8.

A case of PG failing to respond to prednisone 60 mg daily improved within 2 weeks of adding methotrexate 15 mg weekly.

Topical platelet-derived growth factor accelerates healing of myelodysplastic syndrome-associated pyoderma gangrenosum. Braun-Falco M, Stock K, Ring J, Hein R. Br J Dermatol 2002; 147: 829–31.

Complete healing occurred over 9 weeks in this case after platelet-derived growth factor (becaplermin) was added to the treatment regimen.

Recombinant human epidermal growth factor enhances wound healing of pyoderma gangrenosum in a patient with ulcerative colitis. Kim TY, Han DS, Eun CS, Chung YW. Inflamm Bowel Dis 2008; 14: 725–7.

Another case reported to improve in response to topical application of a growth factor.

Clofazimine. A new agent for treatment of pyoderma gangrenosum. Michaelsson G, Molin L, Ohman S, Gip L, Lindstrom B, Skogh M. Arch Dermatol 1976; 112: 344–9.

These authors used clofazimine with the rationale that its ability to enhance neutrophil phagocytosis would be beneficial in PG. A good response was observed in eight cases and was often apparent within a few days. The dose used was 300–400 mg daily.

This relatively safe drug has become very difficult to obtain.

Pyoderma gangrenosum treated with hyperbaric oxygen therapy. Wasserteil V, Bruce S, Sessoms SL, Guntupalli KK. Int J Dermatol 1992; 31: 594–6.

Hyperbaric oxygen has been reported as beneficial in several cases of PG. However, like all other treatments, it is not effective in all cases. This treatment may be worth trying when facilities are available.

Split skin grafts in the treatment of pyoderma gangrenosum: A report of four cases. Cliff S. Dermatol Surg 1999; 25: 299–302.

Free flap coverage of pyoderma gangrenosum leg ulcers. Classen DA, Thomson C. J Cutan Med Surg 2002; 6: 327–31.

Surgical approaches are generally best avoided in PG, at least while the disease is active, as it is likely to develop in sites of trauma.

Although the use of split skin grafts and microvascular free flaps has been reported to successfully accelerate healing, surgery is probably best reserved for use once the disease is inactive.

Pyogenic granuloma

Danielle M DeHoratius

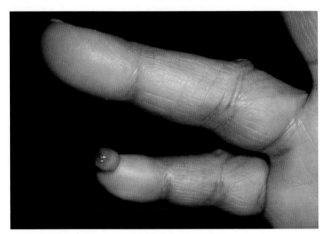

Courtesy of Manisha J. Patel, MD, Assistant Professor, Department of Dermatology. Johns Hopkins School of Medicine

Pyogenic granuloma (PG), also known as a lobular capillary hemangioma, is a common benign vascular growth. It can rapidly appear and is a solitary, erythematous papule. Pyogenic granulomas are often friable and can frequently ulcerate. They most commonly occur in children and young adults. The etiology is unclear, although reactive neovascularization is suspected because of their occurrence at sites of previous trauma. There is no gender or racial predominance. The most common locations are the head and neck region (including the oral mucosa, especially in pregnant women, *granuloma gravidarum*) and digits. Occasionally, pyogenic granulomas have been found in subcutaneous or intravascular locations. The term pyogenic granuloma, however, is a misnomer, as there is not an infectious or a granulomatous component to these lesions. Over time they can resolve on their own.

MANAGEMENT STRATEGY

Pyogenic granulomas are most commonly managed by *destruction*. This can be completed through shave excision with *electrocautery* to the base, *curettage with electrodessication*, or *cryotherapy*. Histologic confirmation is beneficial as other disorders may clinically mimic pyogenic granulomas, examples being amelanotic melanoma, Kaposi's sarcoma, and bacillary angiomatosis. There is a possibility of recurrence and/or the development of satellite lesions, but these options are less invasive and do not result in significant scarring. Complete *excision* requiring sutures may lower the recurrence rate and reduce the possibility of bleeding; however, a linear scar will be present. Hemostasis can be obtained by either electrocautery, silver nitrate, or argon laser photocoagulation, as all are shown to be effective. Because this is a benign growth, it is important to consider the cosmetic outcome of the therapeutic intervention.

Cryotherapy is also effective. With this modality, patients should be seen within 1–2 weeks to assess the response and need for additional treatments. Because the PG is not completely removed, there is a possibility of recurrence; additionally, no tissue is obtained for sampling.

Vascular *lasers* also destroy these lesions using selective photothermolysis. Usually multiple treatments are required, and there is no histologic confirmation. This modality has proved to be more successful with smaller lesions. *Sclerotherapy* also destroys these vascular lesions and has been reported to have a very high cure rate in experienced hands. Anecdotally, *imiquimod* 5% has been reported to resolve these lesions, presumably owing to its anti-angiogenic properties.

SPECIFIC INVESTIGATIONS

> ▶ Histology
> ▶ History to assess previous trauma, medication, and topical exposures

In general, clinical suspicion is very useful in diagnosing pyogenic granulomas, although histologic confirmation is important. Pyogenic granulomas should be differentiated from other vascular lesions, especially bacillary angiomatosis. Amelanotic melanoma has been reported to mimic a pyogenic granuloma. The remainder of the differential includes angiosarcoma, basal cell carcinoma, and Kaposi's sarcoma. Because many of the methods described below result in removal, this tissue can be sent to confirm the clinical diagnosis.

Some drugs have been reported to cause pyogenic granulomas. These are oral contraceptives, isotretinoin, reverse transcriptase inhibitors, epidermal growth factor inhibitors, systemic 5-fluorouracil, and topical tretinoin.

Pyogenic granuloma. Lin RL, Janniger CK. Cutis 2004; 74: 229–33.

Amelanotic melanoma presenting as a pyogenic granuloma. Elmets CA, Ceilley RI. Cutis 1980; 25: 164–8.

A 62 year-old man presented with a non-healing area on his right great toe. The lesion was initially treated as a superficial infection, but enlarged and was presumed to be a pyogenic granuloma. It was treated with shave excision and fulguration of the base; however, the tissue was not submitted for sampling. When the lesion recurred he was referred and sampling revealed an amelanotic melanoma.

FIRST-LINE THERAPIES

> ▶ Simple shave excision/curettage with electrocautery of the base   A
> ▶ Full-thickness skin excision   A
> ▶ Cryotherapy   A
> ▶ Silver nitrate cautery   D

Pyogenic granuloma in children. Pagliai KA, Cohen BA. Pediatr Dermatol 2004; 21: 10–13.

A retrospective study of 128 children with pyogenic granulomas and a follow-up phone interview of 76 patients. Of these, 72.3% underwent a shave excision with electrocautery. The second most common treatment was laser therapy (16.9%). Fifty-five percent of the children in the first group reported a subtle scar, and 33% of the CO_2 laser group and 44% of the pulsed dye laser group reported a similar scar. All patients were pleased with the cosmetic result.

Comparison of cyrotherapy and curettage for the treatment of pyogenic granuloma: a randomized trial. Ghodsi SZ, Raziel M,

Taheri A, Karami M, Mansoori P, Farnaghi F. Br J Dermatol 2006; 154: 671–5.

Eighty-nine patients were randomized for treatment with either liquid nitrogen cryotherapy or curettage followed by electrodessication. Of the 86 patients who completed the study, all had complete resolution of the lesions after one to three sessions (mean 1.42) in the cryotherapy group, and after one to two sessions (mean 1.03) in the curettage group. No scar or residual pigmentation was reported in 57% of the cryotherapy group or in 69% of the curettage group. The authors concluded that although both treatments were safe and effective, curettage should be first-line as fewer treatment sessions were necessary and cosmesis was better.

Treatment of pyogenic granuloma by shave excision and laser photocoagulation. Kirschner R, Low D. Plast Reconstruct Surg 1999; 104: 1346–9.

The shave excision technique was performed on the exophytic portion and photocoagulation of the base through a glass slide. The lasers used were an argon, argon-pumped tunable yellow dye, or KTP laser. All treatments were performed until complete hemostasis was achieved. Complete resolution was seen in 18 of the 19 patients after a single treatment. Of note, the preoperative diagnosis was erroneous in 18.8% of the cases.

Although the final diagnoses were benign in nature, this technique allows the clinical diagnosis to be confirmed and minimizes scar formation.

The efficacy of silver nitrate cauterization for pyogenic granuloma of the hand. Quitkin HM, Rosenwasser MP, Strauch RJ. J Hand Surg [Am] 2003; 28: 435–8.

Thirteen lesions were treated with simple removal and cautery of the base using silver nitrate. Postoperative care was to keep the area completely dry for 2 weeks, as the authors previously observed that recurrence was more common in moist environments. Eighty-five percent of the lesions had complete resolution with an average of 1.6 treatments. The average time to complete healing was 3.5 weeks. There was no need for expensive equipment, and this was simple and cost-effective.

Pyogenic granuloma (lobular capillary hemangioma): a clinicopathologic study of 178 cases. Patrice SJ, Wiss K, Mulliken JB. Pediatr Dermatol 1991; 8: 267–76.

A retrospective analysis of 178 patients. A majority of the 149 lesions were treated by full-thickness skin excision and linear closure, resulting in no recurrences. The remainder were treated with tangential excision and cautery (n=16) or cautery alone (n=7). The recurrence rate in this second group was 43.5%.

An excellent review.

Pyogenic granuloma – the quest for optimum treatment: Audit of treatment of 408 cases. Giblin AV, Clover AJ, Athanassopoulos A, Budny PG. Plast Reconstruct Aesthet Surg 2007; 60: 1030–5.

A retrospective study of 408 cases analyzed between 1994 and 2004 assessing the most successful form of treatment on the basis of multiple parameters. The excision and direct closure group had the fewest recurrences, although all techniques investigated showed an acceptably low recurrence rate.

Whatever technique is used, it must yield material for histologic analysis to ensure the exclusion of other diagnoses.

Cryotherapy in the treatment of pyogenic granuloma. Mirshams M, Daneshpazhooh M, Mirshekari A, Taheri A, Mansoori P, Hekmat S. J Eur Acad Dermatol Venereol 2006; 20: 788–90.

A prospective observational study of 135 patients treated with liquid nitrogen cryotherapy using a cotton-tipped applicator. Patients required anywhere from one to four treatments (mean 1.58). All patients had complete resolution, with 96.2% occurring after three treatments. Minor scars were reported in 11.8%, and 5.1% had hypopigmentation.

These authors report that cryotherapy should be considered first-line as it is an easy and inexpensive technique; however, the main limitation is that no tissue is obtained for histology.

SECOND-LINE THERAPIES

▶ Pulsed dye	B
▶ CO₂ laser	B
▶ Nd:YAG	E

Treatment of pyogenic granuloma in children with the flashlamp-pumped pulsed dye laser. Tay YK, Weston WL, Morelli JG. Pediatrics 1997; 99: 368–70.

Twenty-two children with solitary lesions were treated with a vascular-specific (585 nm), pulsed (450 ms) dye laser using a 5-nm spot size with a laser energy of 6–7 J/cm² without anesthesia. This treatment was successful in 91% and all healed without scarring. Fifteen patients required from two to six treatments at 2-week intervals, and seven required three or more. The two patients who did not respond had larger lesions (0.5–1 cm). No recurrences were reported during the follow-up period (6 months to 3 years). The limitation of this laser modality was that the depth of penetration was only 1 mm.

This can be a useful modality in children, as no anesthesia is required and there is minimal scarring. The drawback is that no tissue is obtained for histology.

The combined continuous-wave/pulsed carbon dioxide laser for treatment of pyogenic granuloma. Raulin C, Greve B, Hammes S. Arch Dermatol 2002; 138: 33–7.

One hundred patients were selected from a population-based sample and underwent treatment with the carbon dioxide (CO₂) laser. The laser was first used in the continuous mode (power 15 W) and then in the pulsed mode (pulse length 0.6–0.9 ms; energy fluence 500 mJ/pulse). Follow-up was 6 weeks and 6 months, and 98 of 100 patients had complete resolution after one treatment. In 88 patients there were no visible scars, and 10 had only slight textural changes. No erythema or pigmentary changes were observed.

Treatment of pyogenic granulomas with the Nd-YAG laser. Bourguignon R, Paquet P, Piérard-Franchimont C, Piérard GE. J Dermatol Treat 2006; 17: 247–9.

Three patients presented with large pyogenic granulomas in areas difficult to treat. Each case was histologically confirmed and previously treated using cryotherapy and electrocoagulation. The lesions were treated with an Nd:YAG laser under local anesthesia with the overlapping technique (settings used: fluence 150 J/cm², wavelength 1064 nm, triple-pulse mode combined with a pulse width of 7.5 ms, delay of 10 ms, and a 10 mm spot size). Patients reported a persistent burning sensation. One lesion responded to one treatment, but two required two sessions. No recurrence was present at 1-year follow-up. This laser beam penetrated to the mid-dermis, significantly deeper than the pulsed-dye laser.

THIRD-LINE THERAPIES

▶ Ligation	E
▶ Imiquimod 5%	E
▶ Sclerotherapy	D
▶ Intralesional corticosteroids	E

Surgical pearl: ligation of the base of a pyogenic granuloma-an atraumatic, simple, and cost-effective procedure. Holbe HC, Frosch PJ, Herbst RA. J Am Acad Dermatol 2003; 49: 509–10.

This demonstrated a pedunculated PG that was ligated using an absorbable suture tightly tied at the base. Over a few days the lesion became necrotic and fell off.

This was atraumatic and required no anesthesia, but there was also no histologic confirmation.

Successful treatment of a therapy-resistant pyogenic granuloma with topical imiquimod 5% cream. Goldenberg G, Krowchuk DP, Jorizzo JL. J Dermatol Treat 2006; 17: 121–3.

A 58-year-old man with a recurrent PG on his right third digit previously treated with shave excision and base electrocautery twice, applied imiquimod twice weekly for a total of 14 weeks. He experienced complete resolution as well as a satisfactory cosmetic outcome.

Pyogenic granuloma: a complete remission under occlusive imiquimod 5% cream. Georgiou S, Monastirli A, Pasmatzi E, Tsambaos D. Clin Exp Dermatol 2008; 33: 454–6.

The authors report an older man with a recurrent PG on his right hand formerly treated with electrocautery. He applied imiquimod 5% cream twice daily under occlusion for 3 weeks, and at 8 months' follow-up there was no recurrence.

He reported only a mild erythematous reaction in the surrounding skin.

Subungual pyogenic granuloma treated by sodium tetradecyl sulfate sclerotherapy. Moon SE. Dermatol Surg 2008; 34: 846–7.

A 33-year-old woman had a subungual mass on her right thumb slowly injected with 0.5% sodium tetradecyl sulfate solution until blanching was observed. One week after the treatment there was only a small residual lesion, and a second injection was performed. The lesion disappeared and the total volume of solution used was 0.1 mL.

This treatment can be considered for larger lesions or those in challenging locations.

Treatment of pyogenic granuloma by sodium tetradecyl sulfate sclerotherapy. Moon SE, Hwang EJ, Cho KH. Arch Dermatol 2005; 141: 644–6.

Fifteen pyogenic granulomas were injected with 0.5% sodium tetradecyl sulfate until blanching appeared. Follow-up was every 1–2 weeks, and at 6 weeks 80% showed complete resolution. In two patients a small shallow vascular area remained which responded to the CO_2 laser.

The authors felt that this treatment can be an alternative to excision because of its simplicity and lack of scarring; however, multiple treatments may be necessary to achieve resolution. There is no tissue for histologic sampling.

Recurrent intraoral pyogenic granuloma with satellitosis treated with corticosteroids. Parisi E, Glick PH, Glick M. Oral Dis 2006; 12: 70–2.

A 33-year-old woman originally presented with gingival swelling. Over the course of her treatment she had eight excisional biopsies and one cautery procedure. The lesions did not respond, and additional lesions appeared after the final surgical procedure. These were then treated using serial injections of a dilution of 0.1 mL of triamcinolone 40 mg/mL with 0.5 mL of 0.5% bupivacaine over 9 weeks. The mechanism of action was thought to be the anti-inflammatory and vasoconstrictive properties of the corticosteroids.

Radiation dermatitis

Joshua A Zeichner

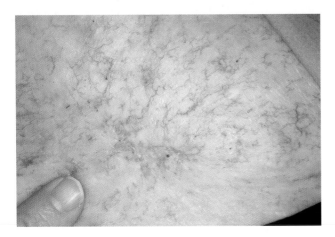

Radiation dermatitis refers to skin changes that occur after cutaneous radiation exposure, for example during interventional radiologic procedures or treatment of malignancies. The dermatitis may be categorized as either acute or chronic. Appendageal structures and basal layer cells are the most sensitive to radiation exposure, and their damage leads to the acute skin changes. These include pruritus, dry and moist desquamation, erythema, epilation, edema, and blistering. Atrophy, hyper- or hypopigmentation, telangiectasia, fibrosis, ulceration, and necrosis are later effects that depend more on dermal and vascular damage. Certain chemotherapeutic drugs such as doxorubicin and dactinomycin may induce similar skin changes at sites of previous radiation exposure, referred to as radiation recall dermatitis.

MANAGEMENT STRATEGY

Treatment of radiation dermatitis begins with prevention, and the severity of skin changes correlates with the cumulative dose of ionizing radiation the patient receives. Radiation therapy is an integral part of many cancer treatment regimens, however, and cannot always be avoided. Therefore, much of the management of radiation dermatitis consists of supportive care, pain control, and prevention of infection.

Topical therapies are the mainstay of treatment for acute radiation dermatitis. *Cornstarch and emollient creams* help dry desquamation (painless peeling of the skin). Management of moist desquamation (painful, full-thickness loss of the epidermis) is similar to that for burns, with *occlusive dressings and care to prevent infections. Topical corticosteroids* control pruritus and reduce inflammation, particularly in sun-damaged areas. Patients should also avoid friction on the skin from tight-fitting clothing. *Topical antifungal ointments* treat and may provide prophylaxis against fungal infections of the skin, especially in the intertriginous areas. Patients may gently wash the skin with water and mild soap. In addition, a topical trolamine-containing cream (Biafine) has been shown to improve wound healing and has been used in acute radiation dermatitis.

Like acute changes, chronic radiation dermatitis is treated symptomatically. Topical emollient creams and corticosteroids can be employed as needed. Skin necrosis or ulceration must be carefully monitored for signs of infection. Some recommend physical massage of the skin to improve fibrosis.

SPECIFIC INVESTIGATIONS

> ▶ History of previous radiation exposure and chemotherapeutic drugs
> ▶ Evaluation of affected skin for development of malignancy

Radio-induced malignancies of the scalp about 98 patients with 150 lesions and literature review. Maalej M, Frikha H, Kochbati L, Bouaouina N, Sellami D, Benna F, et al. Cancer Radiother 2004; 8: 81–7.

Basal cell carcinomas are the most common malignancies to develop in the skin at sites of previous radiation exposure, especially on the head and the neck.

FIRST-LINE THERAPIES

Prevention	
▶ Avoidance of excessive ionizing radiation exposure	
Acute radiation dermatitis	
▶ Emollient creams	E
▶ Topical corticosteroids	A
▶ Topical trolamine-containing emulsion	A
▶ Topical calendula	A
▶ Dexpanthenol	A
Chronic radiation dermatitis	
▶ Emollient creams	E

The prevention and management of acute skin reactions related to radiation therapy: a systematic review and practice guideline. Bolderston A, Lloyd NS, Wong RK, Holden L, Robb-Blenderman L; Supportive Care Guidelines Group of Cancer Care Ontario Program in Evidence-Based Care. Support Care Cancer 2006; 14: 802–17.

This article reviews the literature, and the authors conclude that gentle washing of the skin with water alone, or with mild soap, may help prevent acute radiation dermatitis.

There is not enough evidence to make conclusions on the efficacy of topical or oral agents. However, plain, fragrance- and lanolin-free emollient creams as well as mild corticosteroid creams may be beneficial.

Prevention and treatment of acute radiation dermatitis: a literature review. Wickline MM. Oncol Nurs Forum 2004; 31: 237–47.

This review discusses the current therapies available for prevention and treatment of acute radiation dermatitis. It is unclear whether many products on the market are effective.

Newer agents that are available include a trolamine-containing emulsion (Biafine), some herbal creams and ointments, and topical vitamin C. The benefit of aloe vera gel is still unclear. Certain skin dressings, sucralfate cream, and corticosteroids have been shown to improve radiation dermatitis.

Potent corticosteroid cream (mometasone furoate) significantly reduces acute radiation dermatitis: results from a double blind, randomized study. Bostrom A, Lindman H, Swartling C, Berne B, Bergh J. Radiother Oncol 2001; 59: 257–65.

Evidence Levels: **A** Double-blind study   **B** Clinical trial ≥ 20 subjects   **C** Clinical trial < 20 subjects   **D** Series ≥ 5 subjects   **E** Anecdotal case reports

Topical corticosteroid treatment is effective in improving skin outcome after radiation treatment.

Topical corticosteroid therapy for acute radiation dermatitis: a prospective, randomized, double-blind study. Schmuth M, Wimmer MA, Hofer S, Sztankay A, Weinlich G, Linder DM, et al. Br J Dermatol 2002; 146: 983–91.

The authors of this article found that neither topical corticosteroids nor topical dexpanthenol prevented the onset of radiation dermatitis. However, both reduced the severity of the skin changes compared to the control group, and the members of the topical corticosteroid group showed less severe skin reactions than the dexpanthenol group.

Phase III randomized trial of Calendula officinalis compared with trolamine for the prevention of acute dermatitis during irradiation for breast cancer. Pommier P, Gomez F, Sunyach MP, D'Hombres A, Carrie C, Montbarbon X. J Clin Oncol 2004; 22: 1447–53.

This randomized trial compared the use of topical calendula to topical trolamine (Biafine) at sites of irradiation in patients receiving radiation treatment for breast cancer. In this study, acute radiation dermatitis developed in a higher percentage of patients using trolamine than in those using calendula.

Trolamine-containing topical emulsion: clinical applications in dermatology. Del Rosso JQ, Bikowski J. Cutis 2008; 8: 209–14.

This agent has been shown to promote wound healing. By recruiting macrophages and increasing the ratio of IL-1 to IL-6, the emulsion expedites the formation of granulation tissue as well as synthesis of new collagen. It has been used in several settings, including postoperatively and in radiation dermatitis.

Skin treatment with Bepanthen cream versus no cream during radiotherapy – a randomized control trial. Lokkevik E, Skovlund E, Reitan JB, Hannisdal E, Tanum G. Acta Oncol 1996; 35: 1021–6.

This study demonstrated the efficacy of dexpanthenol-containing cream in treating radiation dermatitis.

SECOND-LINE THERAPIES

▶ Silver leaf dressings (under investigation)	A
▶ Dead Sea products (under investigation)	A
▶ Amifostine	B
▶ Pentoxifylline (under investigation)	A
▶ Celecoxib (under investigation)	E

Phase 2 study of silver leaf dressing for treatment of ration-induced dermatitis in patients receiving radiotherapy to the head and neck. Vavassis P, Gelinas M, Chabot Tr J, Nguyen-Tân PF. J Otolaryngol 2008; 37: 124–9.

In this study, silver leaf dressings seem to reduce the severity of skin reactions after radiation. In addition, it accelerated healing and provided improved pain control. The results of the study warrants further investigation.

Silver leaf nylon dressing to prevent radiation dermatitis in patients undergoing chemotherapy and external beam radiotherapy to the perineum. Vuong T, Franco E, Lehnert S, Lambert C, Portelance L, Nasr E, et al. Int J Radiat Oncol Biol Phys 2004; 59: 809–14.

Silver leaf nylon dressings have antimicrobial and healing properties in patients with skin burns and grafts. This study suggested that silver leaf nylon dressings are also effective in reducing radiation dermatitis, perhaps owing to their antimicrobial properties.

Assessing the effectiveness of Dead Sea products as prophylactic agents for acute radiochemotherapy-induced skin and mucosal toxicity in patients with head and neck cancers: a phase 2 study. Matceyevsky D, Hahoshen NY, Vexler A, Noam A, Khafif A, Ben-Yosef R. Israel Med Assoc J 2007; 9: 439–42.

In this phase 2 study from Israel, products made using water from the Dead Sea were shown to reduce skin and mucosal toxicity in patients receiving radiation and chemotherapy for cancers of the head and neck.

The cytoprotective effect of amifostine in acute radiation dermatitis: a retrospective analysis. Kouvaris J, Kouloulias V, Kokakis J, Matsopoulos G, Myrsini B, Vlahos L. Eur J Dermatol 2002; 12: 458–62.

Amifostine is a cytoprotective drug used to reduce toxicities from cancer chemotherapy and radiation therapy. In this retrospective analysis, the authors found a significant protective effect in the skin in patients receiving radiation therapy.

Prophylactic effect of pentoxifylline on radiotherapy complications: a clinical study. Aygenc E, Celikkanat S, Kaymakci M, Aksaray F, Ozdem C. Otolaryngol Head Neck Surg 2004; 130: 351–6.

Many late changes in radiation dermatitis are thought to be due to vascular insufficiency. In this trial, the group taking pentoxifylline had less severe fibrosis and necrosis than the placebo group. This report is the only case series of its kind in the literature.

Pentoxifylline is still under investigation for this application. Confirmatory studies have not yet been published.

Celecoxib reduces skin damage after radiation: selective reduction of chemokine and receptor mRNA expression in irradiated skin but not irradiated mammary tumor. Liang L, Hu D, Liu W, Williams JP, Okunieff P, Ding I. Am J Clin Oncol 2003; 26: S114–21.

In a mouse model, celecoxib was shown to reduce necrosis, inflammatory infiltrate, and chemokine expression in irradiated skin. This effect was selective for the skin, without affecting the irradiated tissue of the tumor in question.

Cyclooxygenase-2 (COX-2) inhibitors are currently not a standard part of treatment for radiation dermatitis, but this discovery warrants further investigation.

THIRD-LINE THERAPIES

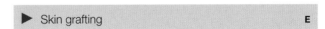

▶ Skin grafting	E

Chronic radiodermatitis injury after cardiac catheterization. Barnea Y, Amir A, Shafir R, Weiss J, Gur E. Ann Plast Surg 2002; 49: 668–72.

The authors present two patients with painful, non-healing wounds at the site of chronic radiation dermatitis. The patients underwent wound excision with skin grafting. The skin healed completely, but the pain was only partially relieved. In practice, skin grafting is extremely rare.

Raynaud's disease and phenomenon

Sameh S Zaghloul, Najat Marraiki, Mark JD Goodfield

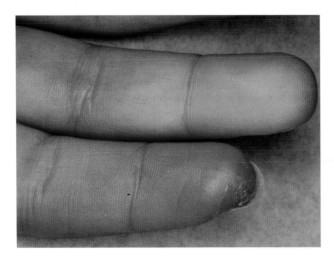

Raynaud's phenomenon (RP) is characterized by intermittent peripheral vasoconstriction leading to pallor, cyanosis, and reactive vasodilatation of the arterioles of the fingers and toes. It is caused by vasospasm in response to cold, emotion, hormones, and certain vasospastic drugs. Primary Raynaud's disease is a milder, idiopathic form, whereas secondary Raynaud's phenomenon coexists with autoimmune connective tissue disorders such as systemic lupus erythematosus and systemic sclerosis, or other conditions that reduce blood flow, such as localized structural abnormalities.

The pathogenesis of Raynaud's phenomenon is not fully understood. However, the last 20 years have witnessed significant increases in our understanding of the different mechanisms, which, either singly or in combination, may contribute. The pathogenesis and pathophysiology vary between the primary (idiopathic) and the secondary forms.

MANAGEMENT STRATEGY

Raynaud's is often mild and may not require treatment; the use of *warming devices* such as hand or toe warmers is beneficial; however, with secondary Raynaud's there is not only vasospasm but often fixed blood vessel damage, so the ischemia can be more severe. Complications can include digital ulcers and could, rarely, lead to amputation. Treatment is often non-pharmacological including avoiding cold and smoking cessation. *Calcium channel antagonists,* such as *nifedipine (10–60 mg daily),* are often considered when treatment is needed; however, the adverse effects of these drugs can include hypotension, vasodilatation, peripheral edema, and headaches. Other treatments have been studied in ran-domized, controlled trials, including classes of drugs such as *angiotensin II inhibitors, selective serotonin reuptake inhibitors, phosphodiesterase-5 inhibitors (e.g., sildenafil, 25–50 mg up to four times a day), nitrates (topical or oral),* and for more serious Raynaud's or its complications, *prostacyclin* agonists may be used. This may be particularly useful for RP associated with connective tissue disease. There are also two large studies demonstrating that endothelin receptor blockade with *bosentan (62.5 mg bd)* can reduce the number of new digital ulcers in scleroderma patients. However, it does not affect the healing period.

Avoidance of triggers such as cold (especially sudden drops in temperature) and vibration (in cases where vibration is the precipitant) should be stressed. Drugs that may exacerbate the condition include β-blockers, bleomycin, caffeine, cisplatin, ergot preparations, interferon, methylsergide, nicotine, oral contraceptives, reboxetine, tegaserod, and vinblastine.

SPECIFIC INVESTIGATIONS

- ► Nailfold capillaroscopy
- ► Screening serology – ANF estimation
- ► Anticentromere and anti-Scl-70 antibodies
- ► Rheumatoid factor
- ► Cryoglobulins
- ► Chest X-ray
- ► Pulmonary function tests
- ► Echocardiography

Careful history taking and clinical examination followed by investigation to detect potential underlying disease are essential: capillaroscopy and specific autoantibody tests are the most productive in aiding diagnosis.

Nailfold digital capillaroscopy in 447 patients with connective tissue disease and Raynaud's disease. Nagy Z, Czirjak L. J Eur Acad Dermatol Venereol 2004; 18: 62–8.

The conclusion of this article is that the scleroderma capillary pattern is often present in systemic sclerosis and dermato/polymyositis. Furthermore, patients with Raynaud's phenomenon and undifferentiated connective tissue disease may also occasionally exhibit this pattern. Therefore, capillarmicroscopy seems to be a useful tool for the early selection of those who are potential candidates for developing scleroderma spectrum disorders.

Assessment of nailfold capillaroscopy by × 30 digital epiluminescence (dermoscopy) in patients with Raynaud phenomenon. Beltran E, Toll A, Pros A, Carbonell J, Pujol RM. Br J Dermatol 2007; 156: 892–8.

The sclerodermic pattern showed a sensitivity of 76.9% and a specificity of 90.9% in SS. A typical capillaroscopic pattern of SS was observed in 73% of cases of limited SS and in 82% of cases of diffuse SS. Patients with Sjögren's syndrome and dermatopolymyositis-SS showed a nonspecific capillaroscopic pattern. All patients with primary RP presented a normal capillaroscopic pattern. A normal capillaroscopic pattern was also observed in 11 of 12 patients with pre-SS. Digital epiluminescence seems to be a useful and reliable technique in the evaluation of capillary nailfold morphological changes. This technical variation allows the identification of specific capillaroscopic patterns associated with connective tissue

Evidence Levels: **A** Double-blind study **B** Clinical trial ≥ 20 subjects **C** Clinical trial < 20 subjects **D** Series ≥ 5 subjects **E** Anecdotal case reports

diseases. It also permits us to differentiate primary RP from secondary RP. The results obtained with this technique are similar to those previously reported using standard capillary microscopy, but this is much easier.

FIRST-LINE THERAPIES

▷ Calcium channel blockers	A
▷ Glyceryl trinitrate	A
▷ Prostacyclin analogs	A

Controlled double-blind trial of the clinical effect of nifedipine in the treatment of idiopathic Raynaud's phenomenon. Gjorup T, Kelbaek H, Hartling OJ, Nielsen SL. Am Heart J 1986; 111: 742–5.

In this study, 26 patients with idiopathic Raynaud's phenomenon participated in a double-blind crossover clinical trial comparing the clinical effect of nifedipine (10–60 mg daily) with that of placebo. Nifedipine proved to be effective in the treatment of idiopathic Raynaud's phenomenon, but side effects should be expected in some 30%.

Comparison of intravenous infusions of iloprost and oral nifedipine in treatment of Raynaud's phenomenon in patients with systemic sclerosis: a double blind randomised study. Rademaker M, Cooke ED, Almond NE, Beacham JA, Smith RE, Mant TG, et al. Br Med J 1989; 298: 561–4.

This study was performed to compare the long-term effects of short-term intravenous infusions of iloprost (0.5–2 ng/kg/min) with those of oral nifedipine in patients with Raynaud's phenomenon associated with systemic sclerosis. It was concluded that both iloprost and nifedipine are beneficial in the treatment of Raynaud's phenomenon. With nifedipine, however, side effects are common. Short-term infusions of iloprost provide long-lasting relief of symptoms, and side effects occur only during the infusions and are dose dependent.

A double-blind placebo controlled crossover randomized trail of diltiazem in Raynaud's phenomenon. Rhedda A, McCans J, Willan AR, Ford PM. J Rheumatol 1985; 12: 724–7.

The results showed a significant reduction in both frequency and duration of attacks of vasospasm in the hands using diltiazem 60–240 mg/day. There was no detectable difference in response between patients with primary and those with secondary Raynaud's phenomenon.

Digital vascular response to topical glyceryl trinitrate, as measured by laser Doppler imaging, in primary Raynaud's phenomenon and systemic sclerosis. Anderson ME, Moore TL, Hollis S, Jayson MIV, King TA, Herrick AL. Rheumatology 2002; 41: 324–8.

This study investigated digital microvascular responses to topical glyceryl trinitrate (GTN) 0.4% in patients with primary Raynaud's phenomenon (PRP), limited cutaneous systemic sclerosis (LCSSc), and healthy controls using laser Doppler imaging. It was concluded that an exogenous supply of nitric oxide by topical GTN ointment causes local endothelial-independent vasodilatory responses in PRP, LCSSc patients, and control subjects.

Iloprost treatment in patients with Raynaud's phenomenon secondary to systemic sclerosis and the quality of life:

a new therapeutic protocol. Milio G, Corrado E, Genova C, Amato C, Raimondi F, Almasio PL, et al. Rheumatology 2006; 45: 999–1004.

In this randomized study 30 patients were treated with iloprost, given by intravenous infusion at progressively increasing doses (from 0.5 to 2 ng/kg/min) over a period of 6 hours each day for 10 days in 2 consecutive weeks, with repeated cycles at regular intervals of 3 months for 18 months. The results were compared with those obtained in 30 other patients who received the same drug but with different dosing regimens. The total average daily duration of the attacks, the average duration of a single attack, and the average daily frequency of the attacks were reduced significantly in all treatment groups, but the comparison between the groups demonstrated significant differences between patients treated with the new protocol and the others at later times (12 and 18 months).

Oral iloprost in Raynaud's phenomenon secondary to systemic sclerosis: a multicentre, placebo-controlled, dose-comparison study. Black CM, Halkier-Sorensen L, Belch JJ, Ullman S, Madhok R, Smit AJ, et al. Br J Rheumatol 1998; 37: 952–60.

Oral iloprost 50 μg or 100 μg twice a day was effective in reducing the duration of attacks, but not the severity or frequency. In this study of 103 patients the 50 μg dose was better tolerated.

Negative reports about beraprost (another oral prostacyclin analog) and oral iloprost also exist.

SECOND-LINE THERAPIES

▶ Selective serotonin reuptake inhibitors (fluoxetine)	B
▶ Endothelin receptor antagonist (bosentan)	B
▶ Angiotensin II -receptor type I antagonist (losartan)	B
▶ Serotonin antagonists (ketanserin)	B
▶ Phosphodiesterase inhibitors	B
▶ Oral vasodilators	B
▶ Hexopal	B

Oral vasodilators for primary Raynaud's phenomenon. Vinjar B, Stewart M. Cochrane Database Syst Rev (2): CD006687, 2008.

Two trials examined the effects of captopril; the rest were single trials of single drugs. For captopril, beraprost, dazoxiben, and ketanserin there was no evidence of an effect on the frequency, severity, or duration of attacks. Beraprost and moxisylyte gave significantly more adverse effects than placebo.

Treatment of Raynaud's phenomenon with the selective serotonin reuptake inhibitor fluoxetine. Coleiro B, Marshall SE, Denton CP, Howell K, Blann A, Welsh KI, et al. Rheumatology 2001; 40: 1038–43.

This pilot study compared fluoxetine, a selective serotonin reuptake inhibitor, (20–60 mg/day), with nifedipine as treatment for primary or secondary Raynaud's phenomenon. The results confirmed the tolerability of fluoxetine and suggest that it would be effective as a novel treatment for Raynaud's phenomenon.

Successful treatment of patients with severe secondary Raynaud's phenomenon with the endothelin receptor antagonist bosentan. Selenko-Gebauer N, Duschek N, Minimair G, Stingl G, Karlhofer F. Rheumatology 2006; 45: 45–8.

This paper concluded that treatment with bosentan (62.5 mg bd) appears to reduce the daily impact of Raynaud's disease and improve peripheral thermoregulation in patients with secondary RP, independent of digital ulcers.

Losartan therapy for Raynaud's phenomenon and scleroderma: clinical and biochemical findings in a fifteen-week, randomized, parallel group, controlled trial. Dziadzio M, Denton CP, Smith R, Howell K, Blann A, Bowers E, et al. Arthritis Rheum 1999; 42: 2646–55.

Treatment with losartan (50 mg daily) was shown to reduce the severity and frequency of Raynaud's attacks in patients with scleroderma RP.

Phosphodiesterase inhibitors in Raynaud's phenomenon. Levien TL. Ann Pharmacother 2006; 40: 1388–93.

An evaluation of the efficacy of phosphodiesterase type 5 (PDE5) inhibitors in the treatment of Raynaud's phenomenon. Available evidence suggests that sildenafil (12.5–100 mg/day) may be associated with improved microcirculation, symptomatic relief, and ulcer healing in patients with secondary Raynaud's phenomenon. Limited information suggests similar effects with tadalafil (5–20 mg alt. days) and vardenafil (10 mg bd). Improved blood flow and clinical improvements have also been observed in some patients with primary Raynaud's phenomenon treated with PDE5 inhibitors.

A double-blind randomized placebo controlled trail of Hexopal in primary Raynaud's disease. Sunderland GT, Belch JJ, Sturrock RD, Forbes CD, McKay AJ. Clin Rheumatol 1988; 7: 46–9.

Although the mechanism of action remains unclear, Hexopal (hexanicotinate inositol) (2–4 g daily) is safe and is effective in reducing the vasospasm of primary Raynaud's disease during the winter months.

THIRD-LINE THERAPIES

▶ Prostaglandin E₁ (alprostadil)	B
▶ Dipyridamole and low-dose acetylsalicylic acid	B
▶ Calcitonin gene-related peptide	C
▶ ʟ-Arginine	D
▶ H-O-U therapy	C
▶ T₃	C
▶ *Helicobacter pylori* treatment	B
▶ Sympathectomy	C
▶ Low-level laser therapy	C
▶ Acupuncture	C
▶ Evening primrose oil supplementation	C
▶ Fish oil supplementation	B
▶ Biofeedback	C
▶ Botulinum toxin	D
▶ Spinal cord stimulation	E

Efficacy evaluation of prostaglandin E1 against placebo in patients with progressive systemic sclerosis and significant Raynaud's phenomenon. Bartolone S, Trifilatti A, De Nuzzo G, Scamardi R, Larosa D, Sottilotta G, et al. Minerva Cardioangiol 1999; 47: 137–43.

Alprostadil infusions at 60 μg in 250 mL for 6 days reduced the frequency and severity of attacks in patients with secondary RP.

A double-blind controlled trail of low dose acetylsalicylic acid and dipyridamole in the treatment of Raynaud's phenomenon. Van der Meer J, Wouda AA, Kallenberg CG, Wesseling H. Vasa 1987; 18: 71–5.

This analgesic and antithrombotic combination (aspirin 50–100 mg/day, dipyridamole 200 mg bd) is safe and helpful in treating patients with RP who have severe digital ulceration.

Calcitonin gene-related peptide in treatment of severe peripheral vascular insufficiency in Raynaud's phenomenon. Bunker CB, Reavley C, O'Shaugnessy DJ, Dowd PM. Lancet 1993; 342: 80–3.

Calcitonin gene-related peptide, a potent vasodilator, given intravenously (0.6 μg/min for 3 hours/day for 5 days) resulted in an increase in blood flow, ulcer healing, and effective vascular dilation in patients with severe RP.

Oral ʟ-arginine can reverse digital necrosis in Raynaud's phenomenon. Rembold CM, Ayers CR. Mol Cell Biochem 2003; 244: 139–41.

The authors demonstrate a beneficial response to oral ʟ-arginine therapy (up to 8 g daily), which reversed digital necrosis and improved the symptoms of severe RP. This evidence suggests that a defect in nitric oxide synthesis or metabolism is associated with RP and demonstrates the potential effectiveness of ʟ-arginine therapy.

Treatment of severe Raynaud's syndrome by injection of autologous blood pretreated by heating, ozonation, and exposure to ultraviolet light (H-O-U) therapy. Cooke ED, Pockley AG, Tucker AT, Kirby JD, Bolton AE. Int Angiol 1997; 16: 250–4.

Treatment was successful in patients with severe RP. Results included reduction of attacks for at least 3 months, and, for some, no attacks at all.

Triiodothyronine treatment for Raynaud's phenomenon: a controlled trial. Dessin PH, Morrison RC, Lamparelli RD, van der Merwe CA. J Rheumatol 1990; 17: 1025–8.

In this trial T₃, 80 μg/day, increased finger skin temperature and reduced recovery times after cold exposure. Treatment is recommended for patients with severe RP and digital ulcers.

Helicobacter pylori **eradication ameliorates primary Raynaud's phenomenon.** Gasbarrini A, Massari I, Serrichio M, Tondi P, De Luca A, Franceschi F, et al. Dig Dis Sci 1998; 43: 1641–5.

Of 46 RP patients, 36 were infected with *H. pylori*. After treatment to eradicate *H. pylori*, RP disappeared in 17% of patients; 72% of the remaining patients noticed a reduction in frequency and duration of their vasospastic attacks.

The use of digital artery sympathectomy as a salvage procedure for severe ischemia of Raynaud's disease and phenomenon. McCall TE, Petersen DPM, Wong LB. J Hand Surg [Am] 1999; 24: 173–7.

In six of seven patients the use of digital artery sympathectomy was effective; the patients' digital ulcers healed and amputation was avoided.

Double-blind, randomised, placebo controlled low laser therapy study in patients with primary Reynaud's phenomenon. Hirschl M, Katzenschlager R, Ammer K, Melnizky P, Rathkolb O, Kundi M, et al. Vasa 2002; 31; 91–4.

This study examined 15 patients with primary RP and demonstrated that low-level laser therapy reduced the intensity of the attacks during laser irradiation without significantly affecting the frequency of attacks. Additionally, after laser irradiation the temperature gradient following cold exposure was reduced, but there was no effect on the number of fingers showing prolonged rewarming.

Treatment of primary Raynaud's syndrome with traditional Chinese acupuncture. Appiah R, Hiller S, Caspary L, Alexander K, Creutzig A. J Intern Med 1997; 241: 119–24.

Thirty-three patients with primary Raynaud's disease (16 controls, 17 treatment) were studied. Overall, attacks were reduced by 63%.

Evening primrose oil (Efamol) in the treatment of Raynaud's phenomenon: a double-blind study. Belch JJ, Shaw B, O'Dowd A, Saniabadi A, Leiberman P, Sturrock RD, et al. Thromb Haemost 1985; 54: 490–4.

Twenty-one patients were studied. Evening primrose oil (12 capsules daily) provided symptomatic improvement.

Fish-oil dietary supplementation in patients with Raynaud's phenomenon: a double blind controlled, prospective study. DiGiacomo RA, Kremer JM, Shah DM. Am J Med 1989; 86: 158–64.

In this trial involving 32 patients supplementation with omega-3 fatty acids (3.96 g eicosapentaenoic acid and 2.64 g docosahexaenoic acid) was shown to be of benefit in patients with primary, but not secondary, RP.

Use of biofeedback training treatment of Raynaud's disease and phenomenon. Yocum DE, Hodes R, Sundstrom WR, Cleeland CS. J Rheumatol 1985; 12: 90–3.

Biofeedback training elevates baseline temperatures. Reserved for the well-motivated patient.

Botulinum toxin in the treatment of Raynaud's phenomenon: a pilot study. Sycha T, Graninger M, Auff E, Schnider P. Eur J Clin Invest 2003; 34: 312–13.

Based on clinical evaluation in addition to laser Doppler interferometry measurements, data from this study demonstrate a beneficial effect of botulinum toxin A in two patients with primary and secondary RP. Additionally, both patients seemed to experience mild systemic effects in fingers that were not injected.

Clinical and objective data on spinal cord stimulation for the treatment of severe Raynaud's phenomenon. Neuhauser B, Perkmann R, Klingler PJ, Giacomuzzi S, Kofler A, Fraedrich G, et al. Am Surg 2001; 67: 1096–7.

Spinal cord stimulation was shown to effectively improve red blood cell velocity, capillary density, and capillary permeability in a 77-year-old woman with severe RP.

Reactive arthritis

Leslie Castelo-Soccio, Abby S Van Voorhees

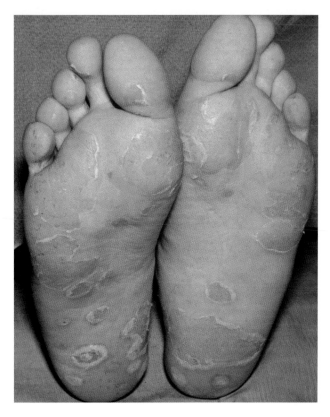

Reactive arthritis is one of the reactive forms of seronegative spondyloarthropathy. It is both a genetically determined and an immunologically mediated disease which primarily affects the skin and joints a few weeks after a gastrointestinal or urinary tract infection. It is characterized by a triad of urethritis, conjunctivitis, and oligoarthritis. The classic skin manifestations include keratoderma blenorrhagica and circinate balanitis. Reactive arthritis was formerly known as Reiter's syndrome, but was renamed when the Nazi war crime past of Hans Reiter was revisited.

MANAGEMENT STRATEGY

The mucocutaneous lesions of uncomplicated reactive arthritis are self-limited and clear within a few months. Initial therapy for limited skin disease includes *topical steroids, calcipotriene,* and *tazarotene.* In severe, extensive and chronic cutaneous presentations a number of agents have been used successfully. *UVB* and *systemic retinoids* has been shown to be effective. Likewise, *methotrexate, ciclosporin,* and *anti-TNF agents* (including etanercept and infliximab) can be effective for severe or refractory disease. There are limited data for the effectiveness of ciclosporin, presumably because the potential side effects with this medication can be avoided by using other agents. Although reactive arthritis has been reported in association with HIV disease, some data show that HIV is not an independent risk factor for reactive arthritis. Nonetheless, reactive arthritis in the context of HIV can be more refractory. Caution should be used with immunosuppressive medications

because of the potential for worsening of HIV disease. Still, there are case reports and a few small trials of methotrexate and anti-TNF agents being used successfully in severe refractory cases of reactive arthritis in HIV-positive patients.

Antibiotic therapy

The effects of short- and long-term antibiotic therapy for reactive arthritis are controversial. Although there is some evidence that antibiotics may be beneficial during the infectious phase before arthritis has developed, it is not clear whether the introduction of antibiotics after the development of arthritis modifies the course of disease. One large double-blind, placebo-controlled study suggests no effect, but another small study reports a beneficial effect of combination treatment with *doxycycline* and *rifampin* for chronic spondyloarthritis induced by *Chlamydia* infection. Therefore, the decision to use antibiotics varies with each individual case. If the inciting organism is documented by culture or PCR, antibiotics are indicated. The beneficial antibiotic, dose, and duration, as well as the effect on severity of disease, remain to be clarified. Reactive arthritis seems to occur more severely and progressively in HIV-infected patients and is often refractory to treatment. There is one case where this is not true: new-onset reactive arthritis as part of immune reconstitution syndrome is rapidly responsive to a 2-week course of doxycycline.

The symptoms of arthritis and inflammation of the peripheral ligamentous or muscular attachments (enthesis) usually dictate the focus of treatment in most patients with reactive arthritis. *Non-steroidal anti-inflammtory drugs (NSAIDs)* are the first-line therapy. *Corticosteroids injections* can provide temporary relief of the pain caused by arthritis or bursitis. Some suggest that short courses of *oral corticosteroids* may be beneficial in severe disease. *Sulfasalazine* and *methotrexate* have been shown to be effective and well tolerated in cases refractory to NSAIDs. *TNF inhibitors* have shown efficacy in treating severe refractory disease.

Transient and mild conjunctivitis does not require specific therapeutic intervention. Symptoms of eye pain or blurred vision require immediate ophthalmologic referral to determine whether these symptoms are due to conjunctivitis or a more serious eye problem, such as uveitis or iritis. Treatment often involves topical steroids, systemic corticosteroids, and other immunosuppressants such as methotrexate.

SPECIFIC INVESTIGATIONS

- ▶ Skin biopsy
- ▶ Urinalysis
- ▶ Urethral, cervical and stool cultures
- ▶ Serum antibodies to *Chlamydia*
- ▶ Erythroctye sedimenation rate and C-reactive protein
- ▶ HIV testing/status
- ▶ Rheumatoid factor and ANA – negative in reactive arthritis
- ▶ Synovial fluid analysis
- ▶ Radiographic imaging
- ▶ HLA-B27 typing
- ▶ Ophthalmologic slit lamp examination
- ▶ ECG in chronic disease to assess conduction abnormalities

Evidence Levels: **A** Double-blind study **B** Clinical trial ≥ 20 subjects **C** Clinical trial < 20 subjects **D** Series ≥ 5 subjects **E** Anecdotal case reports

Reactive Arthritis. Scand J Rheumatol 2005; 34: 251–9.

Reactive arthritis was known as Reiter's disease or Fiessinger-Leroy disease for nearly 100 years. Gram-negative microbes (*Yersinia, Salmonella, Shigella, Camplyobacter*) are the most common enteric infections associated with reactive arthritis. *Chlamydia trachomatis* is the most common cause of reactive arthritis following urethritis; 60–80% of patients with reactive arthritis are HLA-B27 positive; the presence of HLA-B27 predicts a more severe and prolonged form of the disease.

Post-infectious arthritis. Medicine 2006; 34: 413–16.

Laboratory tests such as ESR and C-reactive protein can help confirm the inflammatory nature of the disease. However, ESR and CRP will return to normal after initial inflammation. A normal value can be consistent with diagnosis. Rheumatoid factor and ANA will be negative in reactive arthritis. Radiographs of affected joints are usually normal initially. Radiography may demonstrate peripheral joint erosions or sacroiliitis in chronic cases. Synovial fluid and tissue cultures are negative.

Reiter's syndrome: The classic triad and more. Wu I, Schwartz R. J Am Acad Dermatol 2008; 59: 113–21.

An association of Reiter's syndrome and AIDS was first postulated in 1987, and many others have reported such an association since, but data on this association are mixed. Data from three cohort studies report that reactive arthritis occurs in less than 1% of patients with HIV, suggesting that HIV is not an independent association with reactive arthritis. Reactive arthritis in patients with HIV/AIDS is more recalcitrant to therapy. Caution is advised with the use of immunosuppressive drugs such as systemic corticosteroids, methotrexate, and ciclosporin. There are two reports from the 1980s where methotrexate use resulted in leukopenia and Kaposi's sarcoma in patients with AIDS. Acitretin appears safe for use in patients who are immunocompromised, and can improve skin symptoms. There are cases of familial aggregates which may relate to the association with HLA-B27. HLA-B27 positivity is associated with more frequent skin lesions.

FIRST-LINE THERAPIES

▶ Topical steroids	D
▶ Calcipotriene (calcipotriol)	E
▶ Tazarotene	E

As treatment in reactive arthritis is typically directed towards the musculoskeletal component and urethritis, there is a paucity of studies designed for the treatment of cutaneous disease. However, despite the lack of controlled studies, topical steroids are accepted in practice as first-line therapy for mild cutaneous lesions.

Successful treatment of chronic skin disease with clobetasol proprionate and a hydrocolloid dressing. Volden G. Acta Dermatol Venereol 1992; 72: 69–71.

Two patients described as having skin lesions of reactive arthritis and 19 patients with palmoplantar pustulosis responded to clobetasol proprionate lotion once a week under an occlusive patch. The mean interval to complete remission was 3 weeks for the skin lesions of reactive arthritis, and 2.2 weeks for palmoplantar pustulosis.

Reiter's disease in a homosexual HIV-positive male. Vaughan Jones SA, McGibbon DH. Clin Exp Dermatol 1994; 19: 430–3.

A case report of a 32-year-old man with AIDS whose widespread psoriasiform lesions improved after 2 weeks of topical corticosteroids and a course of flucloxacillin.

Reiter's disease in a 6-year-old girl. Arora S, Arora G. Indian J Dermatol Venereol Leprol 2005; 71: 285–6

A case report of a 6-year-old child with reactive arthritis whose primary keratoderma blenorrhagica lesions were treated with topical salicylic acid and hydrocortisone, with complete resolution in 3 weeks.

The use of topical calcipotriene/calcipotriol in conditions other than plaque-type psoriasis. Thiers BH. J Am Acad Dermatol 1997; 37: S69–71.

A 47-year-old man with relapsing reactive arthritis, with pustules and hyperkeratotic plaques on his palms and soles, as well as circinate balanitis, responded to a 14-day regimen of oral doxycycline (100 mg twice daily) and topical calcipotriene.

Treatment of keratoderma blenorrhagicum with tazarotene gel 0.1%. Lewis A, Nigro M, Rosen T. J Am Acad Dermatol 2000; 43: 400–2.

A case report of a 64-year-old man with reactive arthritis who responded to once-daily application of tazarotene gel 0.1% to his soles.

SECOND-LINE THERAPIES

▶ Systemic retinoids	C
▶ UVB/PUVA	E
▶ Antiretroviral therapy	E

There is no clear algorithm for choosing therapy for more severe cutaneous disease. Severe cutaneous disease is generally treated in the same manner as pustular psoriasis. Although there is more evidence for systemic retinoids than for methotrexate and anti-TNF agents, this probably represents the increased use of retinoids in the 1980s and 1990s for this disease. The evidence for both methotrexate and ciclosporin use in reactive arthritis is both older and more limited, but these medications should be considered in the right clinical scenario, including severe cutaneous disease. There are now increasing reports of anti-TNF agent use in this disorder. Antiretroviral medications should be added to therapy for patients with severe cutaneous manifestations and untreated HIV disease. For these patients, there is some evidence for improvement in cutaneous and joint manifestations in the setting of antiretroviral therapy alone.

Acitretin and AIDS-related Reiter's disease. Blanche P. Clin Exp Rheum 1999; 17: 105–6.

A case report of a 46-year-old patient with AIDs and Reiter's syndrome whose arthritis and skin lesions responded dramatically after 2 weeks of acitretin (25 mg daily). The acitretin was continued for 5 months; however, there was a recurrence several months after the acitretin was stopped and while the patient was maintained on antiretroviral therapy. Acitretin was resumed at the same dosage, resulting in prompt resolution of disease, and continued for 6 months. No recurrence was observed after 13 months.

Reiter's syndrome-like pattern in AIDS-associated psoriasiform dermatitis. Romani J, Puig L, Baselga E, De Moragas JM. Int J Dermatol 1996; 35: 484–8.

A retrospective review of seven HIV-positive patients with Reiter's-like psoriasiform dermatitis. Etretinate alone and RePUVA (etretinate 1 mg/kg daily, 8-methoxypsoralen 0.6 mg/kg, followed by UVA) were safe and effective in controlling skin disease. Methotrexate (15 mg weekly in three divided doses) was effective, but was complicated by hematologic toxicity in two patients. Ciclosporin (2.5 mg/kg daily) was moderately effective and was not associated with progression of AIDS.

Successful treatment of severe Reiter's syndrome associated with human immunodeficiency virus infection with etretinate. Report of 2 cases. Louthrenoo W. J Rheumatol 1993; 20: 1243–6.

A report of two cases of HIV-related reactive arthritis responding dramatically to etretinate (0.5–1.0 mg/kg daily) after 4 weeks of treatment.

Human immunodeficiency virus associated spondyloarthropathy: pathogenic insights based on imaging findings and response to highly active antiretroviral treatment. McGonagle D, Reade S, Emery P. Ann Rheum Dis 2001; 60: 696–8.

This is a case report of a 31-year-old HIV-positive man with severe HIV-associated reactive arthritis with extensive polyenthesitis and osteitis. His arthritis worsened despite treatment including indometacin, tramadol, and sulfasalazine, but improved dramatically after antiretroviral treatment (lamivudine, ritonavir, and stavudine). Improvement was accompanied by a significant rise in CD4 T-lymphocyte counts.

THIRD-LINE THERAPIES

▶ Methotrexate	C
▶ Ciclosporin	E
▶ Anti-TNF agents	E

A review of methotrexate therapy in Reiter syndrome. Lally EV, Ho G Jr. Semin Arthritis Rheum 1985; 15: 139–45.

This is a case report and review of the literature. Eighteen of 20 patients noted dramatic improvement in skin lesions within 2 weeks of receiving methotrexate. There was also significant improvement in arthritis in 15 of 20 patients, although the response was generally slower than that of skin lesions. Methotrexate was generally well tolerated, but the drug had to be discontinued in three cases due to adverse effects. The majority of patients who received methotrexate were treated for exacerbations and were discontinued successfully from the drug after clinical improvement. The usual dosage was 10–50 mg/week, administered either orally or parenterally.

Successful treatment of Reiter's syndrome in a patient with AIDS with methotrexate and corticosteroids. Berenbaum F, Duvivier C, Prier A, Kaplan G. Br J Rheum 1996; 35: 295–301.

This is a case report of a 37-year-old man with AIDS and severe Reiter's syndrome who responded to prednisone 20 mg daily and methotrexate 20 mg/week. This was combined with antiretroviral therapy, chemoprophylaxis of infection, and aggressive therapy of Kaposi's sarcoma, without exacerbation of his AIDS.

Successful treatment of severe recurrent Reiter's syndrome with cyclosporine. Kiyohara A., Ogawa H. J Am Acad Dermatol 1997; 36: 482–3.

A case report of a 48-year-old man with post-*Chlamydia* reactive arthritis unresponsive to topical steroids and etretinate treated successfully with 5 mg/kg daily ciclosporin, which was slowly tapered over 84 days. No recurrence of the disease noted at 18 months.

Infliximab in the treatment of an HIV positive patient with Reiter's syndrome. Gaylis N. J Rheumatol 2003; 30: 2.

A case report of a 41-year-old man with Reiter's syndrome who responded to infliximab added to a regimen of methotrexate and systemic corticosteroids. During therapy his arthritis resolved, as did the severe onycholysis and keratoderma blenorrhagica of the soles. The patient was able to discontinue systemic corticosteroids and was maintained on intravenous infliximab at a dose of 300 mg (3 mg/kg) every 6–7 weeks and intramuscular methotrexate at a dose of 15 mg/week for 18 months without a reduction in his CD4 cells or a rise in his viral load.

Decreased pain and synovial inflammation after etanercept therapy in patients with reactive and undifferentiated arthritis: an open-label trial. Flagg S, Meador R, Schumacher HR. Arthritis Rheum 2005; 53: 613–17.

A 6-month open trial of efficacy and safety of etanercept (25 mg subcutaneous twice weekly) in 16 patients with undifferentiated or reactive arthritis. Seven patients met the criteria for reactive arthritis and nine had a similar pattern of arthritis without evidence of infection. Ten patients completed the trial. Three tested positive for HLA-B27. All patients had been on NSAIDs and 11 had been treated with sulfasalazine and/or methotrexate. Of the 10 completers, nine were classified as responders, with less tender joints and decreased swelling of joints. The tenth had improvement in pain but no change in the number of tender or swollen joints.

Successful use of infliximab in the treatment of Reiter's syndrome: a case report and discussion. Gill H, Majithia V. Clin Rheumatol 2008; 27: 121–3.

A case report of a 28-year-old man with HIV and reactive arthritis complicated by circinate balanitis, arthritis, onycholysis and keratoderma blenorrhagica on the soles who did not respond to aggressive treatment with NSAIDs, prednisone (60–20 mg/day) and methotrexate (15 mg/week) for 3 months. He was treated with infliximab 200 mg (3 mg/kg) intravenously at 0, 2, 6, and 14 weeks, with rapid improvement of severe skin lesions and arthritis. This regimen was well tolerated. The patient was subsequently lost to follow-up.

Use of adalimumab in poststreptococcal reactive arthritis. Sanchez-Cano, D, Callejas-Rubio, JL, Ortego-Centeno N. J Clin Rheum 2007; 13: 176.

A case report describing a 21-year-old woman with oligoarthritis affecting the lower extremities after pharyngitis and 2 weeks prior to the onset of arthritis. NSAIDs, prednisone (1 mg/kg/day), hydroxychloroquine (6 mg/kg/day) and methotrexate (25 mg/week) were not effective. Adalimumab (40 mg subcutaneously every 15 days) was tried and a clinical response was achieved 8 weeks after the introduction of adalimumab, with continued use for maintenance. Steroids and methotrexate were discontinued; no side effects were observed after 1 year of treatment with adalimumab.

Evidence Levels: **A** Double-blind study **B** Clinical trial ≥ 20 subjects **C** Clinical trial < 20 subjects **D** Series ≥ 5 subjects **E** Anecdotal case reports

The use of anti-tumor necrosis factor therapy in HIV-positive individuals with rheumatic disease. Cepeda E, William F, Ishimori M, Weisman M, Reveille J. Ann Rheum Dis 2008; 67: 710–12.

Eight HIV-positive patients with rheumatic diseases (two with rheumatoid arthritis, three with psoriatic arthritis, one with reactive arthritis, one with undifferentiated spondyloarthritis, and one with ankylosing spondyloarthritis) refractory to disease-modifying antirheumatic drugs who has a CD4 count >200 mm^3, an HIV viral load of <60 000 copies/mm^3, and no active concurrent infections, were treated with anti-TNF blockers. Patients were monitored for adverse effects and clinical response for 28 months. No significant clinical adverse effects were noted. CD4 counts and HIV viral loads remained stable. Three patients on etanercept and two on infliximab had sustained improvement in their rheumatic disease.

Relapsing polychondritis

Paul H Bowman, Donald Rudikoff

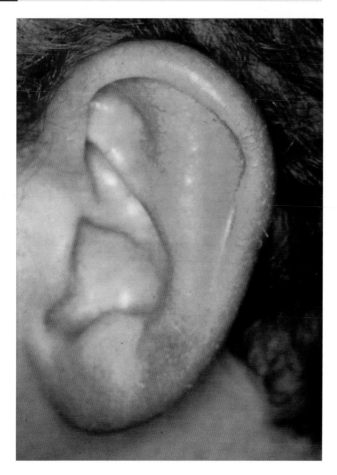

Relapsing polychondritis is a rare, multisystemic disease of unknown etiology, characterized by recurrent inflammation of cartilage and connective tissue. Patients with the MAGIC syndrome (Mouth And Genital ulcers with Inflamed Cartilage), an overlap of Behçet's disease and relapsing polychondritis, may also benefit from the treatment strategy outlined in this chapter.

MANAGEMENT STRATEGY

Treatment of relapsing polychondritis is aimed at reducing inflammation, which often progressively destroys affected structures in the ears, nose, eyes, joints, respiratory tract, and cardiovascular system. The most common cause of mortality is laryngotracheal involvement. A multidisciplinary approach is crucial to evaluate and treat the multiple organ systems that can be affected.

Systemic corticosteroids are the cornerstone of therapy, and doses of 80–100 mg daily can reliably abate acute attacks in most patients. Maintenance use (10–25 mg daily) can reduce the frequency and severity of recurrences, but does not stop disease progression in more aggressive cases. In addition, long-term side effects necessitate the use of steroid-sparing agents. *Non-steroidal*

anti-inflammatory agents (NSAIDs) such as aspirin and indometacin are safer first-line agents, but as monotherapy often do not fully control the disease. *Dapsone* should also be tried, as some patients show excellent improvement when it is used either as monotherapy or combined with steroids. When present, the response to dapsone usually occurs within 1–2 weeks, although higher doses (200 mg daily) are often required.

Azathioprine (50–150 mg daily) and *cyclophosphamide* (100–150 mg daily) have both traditionally been used as steroid-sparing agents. More recently, *ciclosporin* has shown good response in several cases at doses of 5–15 mg/kg daily, and has been effectively used at lower doses in combination with steroids. Medium-dose *methotrexate* (10–15 mg/week) has been effectively used to lower steroid requirements, and at higher doses (20–25 mg/week) has been successful as monotherapy.

A trial of *colchicine* (0.6 mg twice daily) may be worthwhile as it is a comparatively benign drug, although it has been reported to be successful in only a minority of patients. For relapsing polychondritis unresponsive to other therapies, *salazosulfapyridine* and *plasmapheresis* have each been effective when combined with first- and second-line agents. Recently anti-TNF agents and IVIG have been shown to have some efficacy in treating relapsing polychondritis. In late-stage disease with significant functional pulmonary involvement, interventions such as *tracheostomy* and/or *tracheobronchial stent placement* may improve respiratory function.

SPECIFIC INVESTIGATIONS

▶ Pulmonary evaluation
  ▶ Chest radiograph and/or computed tomography/ magnetic resonance imaging (CT/MRI)
  ▶ Dynamic expiratory CT examination
  ▶ Pulmonary function tests (especially flow/volume loops)
  ▶ Endobronchial ultrasonography
▶ Cardiovascular examination
  ▶ Electrocardiogram and/or echocardiogram (CT/ MRI may also be useful)
▶ Ophthalmologic examination
  ▶ Audiometry
▶ Complete blood count
▶ Erythrocyte sedimentation rate

Relapsing polychondritis: prevalence of expiratory CT airway abnormalities. Lee KS, Ernst A, Trentham DE, Lunn W, Feller-Kopman DJ, Boiselle PM. Radiology 2006; 240: 565–73.

Dynamic expiratory CT scans demonstrated abnormalities such as tracheomalacia and air trapping, yet only half of these patients demonstrated abnormalities on routine inspiratory CT scans.

Expiratory CT scans show clinically relevant bronchopulmonary abnormalities earlier than standard inspiratory CT scans, allowing earlier institution of aggressive therapy to prevent disease progression.

Pulmonary function in patients with relapsing polychondritis. Mohsenifar Z, Tashkin DP, Carson SA, Bellamy PE. Chest 1982; 81: 711–17.

The authors describe detailed physiologic and radiographic studies of the respiratory tract in five patients having pulmonary involvement with relapsing polychondritis.

Airway manifestations are ultimately present in over 50% of patients with relapsing polychondritis, and are the leading cause of death from this disease. Airway obstruction may be asymptomatic in the earlier stages, detected only on pulmonary function testing. Other sources stress the importance of plain radiography, CT, and MRI for early detection of tracheal narrowing and upper airways disease.

Cardiovascular involvement in relapsing polychondritis. Del Rosso A, Rosa Petrix N, Pratesi M, Bini A. Semin Arthritis Rheum 1997; 26: 840–4.

Cardiovascular complications eventually occur in half of all patients with relapsing polychondritis, and are the second most frequent cause of mortality. Aortic valve inflammation, the most common cardiac manifestation of relapsing polychondritis (10% of patients), has been reported in asymptomatic patients, and can silently progress during seemingly effective systemic corticosteroid therapy. Atrioventricular block, mitral regurgitation, and acute pericarditis have also been reported.

Surgical treatment of the cardiac manifestations of relapsing polychondritis: Overview of 33 patients identified through literature review and the Mayo Clinic records. Dib C, Moustafa SE, Mookadam M, Zehr KJ, Michet CJ Jr, Mookadam F. Mayo Clin Proc 2006; 81: 772–6.

Clinically important aortic or mitral regurgitation occurs in about 10% of relapsing polychondritis patients, aortic regurgitation being the more common and more urgent. In this retrospective series and literature review the mean time between initial onset of relapsing polychondritis and surgery was about 5 years. In contrast to previous reports of 70% 1-year mortality after valve replacement, in this analysis 50% of patients were alive 1 year after surgery.

Aortic regurgitation is a serious complication of relapsing polychondritis. Baseline chest CT, MRI, or transesophageal echocardiography should be performed upon diagnosis and repeated every 6 months. All aortic segments should be regularly evaluated because involvement of multiple thoracic and abdominal aneurysms has been reported in several patients.

Scleritis in relapsing polychondritis. Hoang-xuan T, Foster CS, Rice BA. Ophthalmology 1990; 97: 892–8.

Ocular inflammation is one of the most constant features of relapsing polychondritis, developing in up to 63% of patients. It can affect almost any part of the eye, and reduce vision. The authors stress the importance of early detection of this serious consequence of the disease.

Otolaryngological aspects of relapsing polychondritis: course and outcome. Yettser S, Inal A, Taser M, Ozkaptan Y. Rev Laryngol Otol Retinol 2001; 122: 195–200.

An analysis of the otolaryngologic manifestations of relapsing polychondritis in seven patients.

Several of the reviews referenced below (McAdam et al. 1976, Trentham et al. 1998) also discuss the importance of screening audiometry in patients with relapsing polychondritis. Up to 46% of patients suffer from impaired hearing, and inadequately treated cases can suffer permanent hearing loss.

Association of myelodysplastic syndrome and relapsing polychondritis: further evidence. Hebbar M, Brouillard M, Wattel E, Decoulx M, Hatron PY, Devulder B, et al. Leukemia 1995; 9: 731–3.

Twenty-eight percent of all patients (five of 18 cases) diagnosed with relapsing polychondritis at the authors' institution over a period of 13 years were also found to have myelodysplastic syndromes. Many other such cases have been reported elsewhere in the literature.

Anemia is a poor prognostic sign in patients with relapsing polychondritis; those with concurrent myelodysplasia often develop refractory anemia requiring transfusions. Several patients have progressed to leukemia.

McAdam et al. (1976, below) and others suggest that as the erythrocyte sedimentation rate is generally increased during periods of disease activity, it may be useful in monitoring response to therapy.

Endobronchial ultrasonography in the diagnosis and treatment of relapsing polychondritis with tracheobronchial malacia. Miyazu Y, Miyazawa T, Kurimoto N, Iwamoto Y, Ishida A, Kanoh K, et al. Chest 2003; 124: 2393–5.

In two cases of relapsing polychondritis, endobronchial ultrasonography revealed a poorly defined bronchial wall structure with two patterns of cartilaginous damage: fragmentation and edema. Successful treatment was achieved by the implantation of nitinol stents, the sizes of which were determined by endobronchial ultrasonography.

FIRST-LINE THERAPIES

▶ Systemic corticosteroids	C
▶ NSAIDs	D
▶ Dapsone	C

Relapsing polychondritis: prospective study of 23 patients and review of the literature. McAdam LP, O'Hanlan MA, Bluestone R, Pearson CM. Medicine (Baltimore) 1976; 55: 193–215.

In this classic report, 18 of 23 patients were treated with prolonged systemic corticosteroid therapy (average prednisone maintenance dose 25 mg daily), and six of 23 were well controlled using NSAIDs (aspirin, indometacin, phenylbutazone).

Although the use of systemic corticosteroids for relapsing polychondritis has not been evaluated with controlled clinical trials, multiple small series in the literature report corticosteroids as being the most uniformly reliable therapy in abating acute exacerbations and reducing the frequency and severity of recurrences. Unfortunately, they do not always halt disease progression.

Relapsing polychondritis: excellent response to naproxen and aspirin. Kremer J, Gates SA, Parhami N. J Rheumatol 1979; 6: 719–20.

A case report of a 59-year-old man with an acute flare of relapsing polychondritis which responded well to a combination of naproxen (250 mg twice daily) and salicylate (975 mg four times daily). The authors suggest that mild cases of relapsing polychondritis (and even some acute flares) usually respond to NSAIDs.

Treatment of relapsing polychondritis with dapsone. Barranco VP, Monor DB, Solomon H. Arch Dermatol 1976; 112: 1268–88.

Three patients were successfully treated with dapsone (100–200 mg daily), each showing complete resolution of an acute attack of relapsing polychondritis within 2 weeks of starting therapy.

Although not all patients respond to dapsone, those that do are usually reported as having a dramatic improvement within 1–2 weeks of initiating therapy. The effectiveness of dapsone seems to be dose dependent, with 200 mg daily being the most commonly reported effective dose.

Relapsing polychondritis – report of ten cases. Damiani JM, Levine HL. Laryngoscope 1979; 89: 929–44.

In this report of 10 cases of relapsing polychondritis seen at the Cleveland Clinic over a 20-year period, systemic steroids and dapsone were each reliable in abating episodes of disease activity and in reducing recurrences. Based on their review of the 211 case reports of relapsing polychondritis existing at the time, the authors proposed that response to steroids and/or dapsone should be a diagnostic criterion for the disease.

Although one might expect a synergistic anti-inflammatory effect from a combination regimen of steroids and dapsone, this has not been conclusively shown to be advantageous over either agent alone.

Relapsing polychondritis in HIV-infected patients: a report of two cases. Dolev JC, Maurer TA, Reddy SG, Ramirez LE, Berger T. J Am Acad Dermatol 2004; 51: 1023–5.

Two cases of relapsing polychondritis as a possible manifestation of immune reconstitution following highly active antiretroviral therapy (HAART) are presented. In one case, dapsone plus prednisone, and in the other dapsone alone, were effective treatments.

SECOND-LINE THERAPIES

▶ Azathioprine	D
▶ Ciclosporin	D
▶ Methotrexate	D
▶ Cyclophosphamide	E

Relapsing polychondritis in a Latin American man. Waller ES, Raebel MA. Am J Hosp Pharm 1979; 36; 806–10.

In this case report of a 33-year-old man with severe relapsing polychondritis, including respiratory tract chondritis requiring tracheostomy, the addition of azathioprine 150 mg daily allowed a reduction in prednisone dosage from 60 mg daily to 25 mg daily.

Cyclosporin A in the treatment of relapsing polychondritis with severe recurrent eye involvement. Priori R, Paroli MP, Luan FL, Abdulaziz M, Pivetti Pezzi P, Valesini G. Br J Rheumatol 1993; 32: 352.

A 54-year-old woman with relapsing polychondritis and severe recurrent necrotizing nodular scleritis was refractory to steroids and azathioprine but achieved complete remission with ciclosporin 5 mg/kg daily.

This and other case reports suggest that ciclosporin may be especially useful for ocular manifestations of relapsing polychondritis when they are refractory to other therapies.

Relapsing polychondritis. Trentham DE, Le CH. Ann Intern Med 1998; 129: 114–22.

In this review of the authors' experience with 36 patients with relapsing polychondritis, 23 of 31 patients were able to reduce their prednisone dose from an average of 19 mg daily to 5 mg daily by adding methotrexate (average weekly methotrexate dose 15.5 mg).

A good review article.

A case of life-threatening refractory polychondritis successfully treated with combined intensive immunosuppressive therapy with methotrexate. Yamaoka K, Saito K, Hanami K, Nakayamada S, Nawata M, Iwata S, et al. Mod Rheumatol 2007; 17: 144–7.

Relapsing polychondritis with glomerulonephritis: improvement with prednisone and cyclophosphamide. Ruhlen JL, Huston KA, Wood WG. JAMA 1981; 245: 847–8.

A 32-year-old man with relapsing polychondritis and life-threatening upper airway obstruction responded to high-dose corticosteroid therapy but subsequently developed progressive renal insufficiency despite continued treatment. The addition of oral cyclophosphamide, 150 mg daily, led to substantial improvement in renal function and sustained improvement for 21 months of follow-up, despite subsequent reduction of the prednisone dose. The authors suggest monitoring renal function in relapsing polychondritis, and suggest a regimen of prednisone and cyclophosphamide in cases with glomerulonephritis.

THIRD-LINE THERAPIES

▶ Colchicine	E
▶ Minocycline	E
▶ Pentoxifylline	E
▶ Salazosulfapyridine	E
▶ Plasmapheresis	E
▶ Tracheostomy/tracheobronchial stent placement	D
▶ Infliximab	D
▶ Adalimumab	E
▶ Etanercept	E
▶ Intravenous immunoglobulin	E

Colchicine and indomethacin for the treatment of relapsing polychondritis. Mark KA, Franks AG. J Am Acad Dermatol 2002; 46: S22–4.

One patient with steroid-dependent disease had marked improvement and reduced steroid doses after adding colchicine, 0.6 mg two to four times daily, and indometacin, 25 mg three times daily.

Antibiotic therapy for rheumatoid arthritis: scientific and anecdotal appraisals. Trentham DE, Dynesius-Trentham RA. Rheum Dis Clin North Am 1995; 21: 817–34.

Oral minocycline, as used for rheumatoid arthritis, was associated with improvement in a patient who had developed methotrexate toxicity.

Mouth and genital ulcers with inflamed cartilage (MAGIC syndrome): a case report and literature review. Imai H, Motegi M, Mizuki N, Ohtani H, Komatsuda A, Hamai K, et al. Am J Med Sci 1997; 314: 330–2.

A 39-year-old woman with relapsing polychondritis and Behçet's disease (MAGIC syndrome) had improvement in oral ulcers, erythema nodosum, and arthritis when treated with a combination of methotrexate (5 mg weekly) and pentoxifylline (300 mg daily).

[A refractory case of relapsing polychondritis]. Nosaka Y, Nishio J, Nanki T, Koike R, Kubota T, Miyasaka N. Nihon Rinsho Meneki Gakkai Kaishi 1998; 21: 80–6. [In Japanese.]

A 15-year-old girl with severe relapsing polychondritis was initially partially responsive to separate courses of oral corticosteroids and ciclosporin, but later had a complete remission when both these agents were used in combination with salazosulfapyridine.

[Auricular chondritis, malignant glomerulonephritis and pulmonary hemorrhage]. Dracon M, Noel C, Ramon P, Wallaert B, Tonnel AB, Gosselin B, et al. Nephrologie 1991; 12; 139–41. [In French.]

A 41-year-old man with auricular chondritis, subacute renal failure, and pulmonary involvement had rapid improvement with plasmapheresis and prednisone treatment.

Because antibodies to type II collagen seem to be important in the pathogenesis of relapsing polychondritis, plasmapheresis may have a role in the management of these patients.

Management of airway manifestations of relapsing polychondritis: case reports and review of the literature. Sarodia SD, Dasgupta A, Mehta AC. Chest 1999; 116: 1669–75.

Five patients with severe respiratory involvement from relapsing polychondritis (three of whom required continuous mechanical ventilation due to airway collapse) benefited from placement of self-expandable metallic tracheobronchial stents. A total of 17 stents of varying sizes were placed in these patients over a period of 3 years, with favorable overall outcome in four patients.

When severe, progressive disease leads to extensive destruction of the tracheobronchial tree despite maximal medical therapy, tracheostomy or tracheobronchial stent placement may preserve or improve respiratory function and reduce patients' reliance on mechanical ventilation.

Successful treatment of relapsing polychondritis with infliximab. Richez C, Dumoulin C, Coutoly X, Schaeverbeke T. Clin Exp Rheumatol 2004; 22: 629–31.

One patient had marked improvement in symptoms 4 days after an infusion of 4 mg/kg infliximab. Control was maintained with repeat treatments every 6–8 weeks.

Infliximab seems to be an effective therapy for relapsing polychondritis unresponsive to conventional therapy, as well as a steroid-sparing agent.

Severe septicemia in a patient with polychondritis and Sweet's syndrome after initiation of treatment with infliximab. Matzkies FG, Manger B, Schmitt-Haendle M, Nagel T, Kraetsch HG, Kalden JR, et al. Ann Rheum Dis 2003; 62: 81–2.

A 51-year-old diabetic man with relapsing polychondritis had an excellent clinical response to infliximab 3 mg/kg, but then developed a parasternal abscess 11 days later, caused by penicillin-resistant *Staphylococcus aureus*, and died from subsequent septicemia.

This report emphasizes the importance of monitoring at-risk patients closely for infection.

Sustained response to etanercept after failing infliximab, in a patient with relapsing polychondritis with tracheomalacia. Subrahmanyam P, Balakrishnan C, Dasgupta B. Scand J Rheumatol 2008; 37: 239–40.

A 54-year-old woman with relapsing polychondritis complicated by tracheomalacia experienced a dramatic improvement in her symptoms and an 18-month sustained response after etanercept was substituted for infliximab.

Prolonged response to anti-tumor necrosis factor treatment with adalimumab (Humira) in relapsing polychondritis complicated by aortitis. Seymour MW, Home DM, Williams RO, Allard SA. Rheumatology 2007; 46: 1739–41.

A 43-year-old woman with relapsing polychondritis who had undergone aortic valve replacement continued to experience aortitis despite a variety of immunosuppressive drugs and cytotoxic agents. Despite an initial good response to infliximab, after 10 months her symptoms returned. Switching her anti-TNF agent to adalimumab and continuing methotrexate and a corticosteroid resulted in improvement; she has subsequently been maintained on adalimumab and low-dose corticosteroids.

The latter two reports suggest that switching anti-TNF agents may benefit patients with recalcitrant relapsing polychondritis.

Complete remission in refractory relapsing polychondritis with intravenous immunoglobulins. Terrier B, Aouba A, Bienvenu B, Bloch-Queyrat C, Delair E, Mallet J, et al. Clin Exp Rheumatol 2007; 25: 136–8.

A young woman with relapsing episodes of nasal chondritis and severe scleritis with scleromalacia received IVIG every 3 then every 4 weeks (2 g/kg on 2 days) in association with 25 mg/day of prednisone after treatment with corticosteroids, infliximab, methotrexate, mycophenolate, and cyclophosphamide failed to control her symptoms. Dramatic improvement of symptoms was sustained for 11 months, but when IVIG treatments were spaced every 6 weeks hearing loss and episcleritis recurred. Reinstitution of a treatment frequency of every fourth week brought her symptoms under control.

Successful treatment of relapsing polychondritis with mycophenolate mofetil. Goldenberg G, Sangueza OP, Jorizzo JL. J Dermatol Treat 2006; 17: 158–9.

A 50-year-old man with bilateral ear pain was successfully treated with a prednisone taper and mycophenolate 3 g/day (increased from an initial dose of 2 g/day). At 17 months' follow-up the patient maintained his improvement on prednisone 5 mg daily and mycophenolate 3 g/day.

Rhinophyma

John Berth-Jones

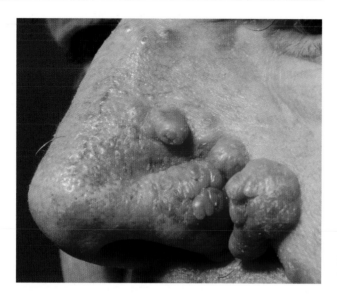

Phymas, of which rhinophyma is much the most common, are localized swellings of facial soft tissues due to a variable combination of fibrosis, sebaceous hyperplasia, and lymphedema. These occur on the nose (rhinophyma) and, less often the ears, forehead, or chin. They are seen much more frequently in males than in females. Rhinophyma may develop in patients with a long history of rosacea, when it is often regarded as a complication or 'end stage' of the disease. However, rhinophyma is also seen in patients who have no history of rosacea. Occasionally rhinophyma is complicated by the development of a malignancy.

MANAGEMENT STRATEGY

Phymas require physical ablation or removal, usually by surgery. Remodeling is most often achieved simply by paring off the excess tissue with a scalpel. Other techniques that can be useful in the hands of those with the necessary expertise include electrosurgery, excision/vaporization with argon, carbon dioxide, Nd:YAG or erbium:YAG lasers, and cryotherapy. Ionizing radiation has been used in cases with coexisting malignancy. Systemic isotretinoin can significantly reduce the bulk of rhinophyma, although it does not restore normal skin contours. It is possible, but not established, that treatment of rosacea may inhibit the development of rhinophyma.

SPECIFIC INVESTIGATIONS

> ▶ Biopsy is occasionally indicated to exclude malignancy

Rhinophyma and coexisting occult skin cancers. Lutz ME, Otley CC. Dermatol Surg 2001; 27: 201–2.

Rhinophyma can be complicated by the development of a malignancy, which can be difficult to recognize.

FIRST-LINE TREATMENTS

▶ Surgical paring	C

Triple approach to rhinophyma. Curnier A, Choudhary S. Ann Plast Surg 2002; 49: 211–14.

The authors report pleasing results in six patients treated by tangential excision for debulking, the use of scissors for sculpting, and mild dermabrasion for final contouring.

SECOND-LINE TREATMENTS

▶ Electrosurgery	C
▶ Argon laser	C
▶ Carbon dioxide laser	C
▶ Nd:YAG laser	E
▶ Erbium:YAG laser	D
▶ Cryotherapy	D
▶ Isotretinoin	C
▶ Microdebrider	E
▶ Shaw scalpel	E
▶ Radiotherapy	E
▶ Hydrosurgery	D

Electrosurgical treatment of rhinophyma. Clark DP, Hanke CW. J Am Acad Dermatol 1990; 22: 831–7.

This treatment was inexpensive and associated with few complications, and gave good or excellent cosmetic results in 13 cases.

Surgical management of rhinophyma: report of eight patients treated with electrosection. Rex J, Ribera M, Bielsa I, Paradelo C, Ferrándiz C. Dermatol Surg 2002; 28: 347–9.

Eight male patients were treated using radiofrequency electrosurgery to remove thin layers of tissue until the nose shape was recreated. All patients achieved acceptable cosmetic results.

Rhinophyma treated by argon laser. Halsbergen-Henning JP, van Gemert MJ. Lasers Surg Med 1983; 2: 211–15.

Thirteen cases were treated. This laser is believed to work by selectively coagulating capillaries causing redness of the nose and which feed the hypertrophic regions, as well as by direct coagulation shrinkage of the hypertrophic connective tissue. The result was a smooth and more natural appearance of the nose without redness. Pustulosis was also reduced.

Comparison of CO_2 laser and electrosurgery in the treatment of rhinophyma. Greenbaum SS, Krull EA, Watnick K. J Am Acad Dermatol 1988; 18: 363–8.

The results from the CO_2 laser and electrosurgery were compared in three patients by treating one side of the nose by each method. There was little to choose between them in terms of results, but electrosurgery was more cost-effective.

Spectrum of results after treatment of rhinophyma with the carbon dioxide laser. El Azhary RA, Roenigk RK, Wang TD. Mayo Clin Proc 1991; 66: 899–905.

A review of 30 patients treated with the carbon dioxide laser and followed up for 1–4 years. Milder cases were treated with laser vaporization, more severe cases with CO_2 laser excision and then vaporization. Dilated pores developed in many patients. Leukoderma, unilateral alar lift, and mild hypertrophic scarring developed in single cases.

Excision of rhinophyma with Nd:YAG laser: a new technique. Wenig BL, Weingarten RT. Laryngoscope 1993; 103: 101–6.

Treatment of rhinophyma with Er:YAG laser. Orenstein A, Haik J, Tamir J, Winkler E, Frand J, Zilinsky I, et al. Lasers Surg Med 2001; 29: 230–5.

Use of a dual-mode erbium:YAG laser for the surgical correction of rhinophyma. Fincher EF, Gladstone HB. Arch Facial Plast Surg 2004; 6: 267–71.

In each of these reports six cases of rhinophyma were treated, with satisfactory outcomes. The Er:YAG laser provides both controlled ablation of tissue and hemostasis.

Rhinophyma treated by liquid nitrogen spray cryosurgery. Sonnex TS, Dawber RPR. Clin Exp Dermatol 1986; 11: 284–8.

Five cases were treated using two freeze–thaw cycles, each freeze lasting 30 seconds after the ice field was established, with a 4-minute intervening thaw. A pethidine and diazepam premedication was used. In three cases small residual prominent areas responded to further treatment after 2 months. The final result was satisfactory in each case, with no scarring.

Isotretinoin in the treatment of rosacea and rhinophyma. Irvine C, Kumar P, Marks R. In: Marks R, Plewig G, eds. Acne and related disorders. London: Martin Dunitz, 1989; 311–15.

A study in which nine men with rhinophyma were treated with isotretinoin 1 mg/kg daily for up to 18 weeks. Isotretinoin reduced the volume of rhinophyma (assessed objectively using molds of the noses) by 9–23%, but did not restore normal skin contours in advanced cases.

The authors report good results in five cases and consider this their treatment of choice.

New surgical adjuncts in the treatment of rhinophyma: the microdebrider and FloSeal®. Kaushik V, Tahery J, Malik TH, Jones PH. J Laryngol Otol 2003; 117: 551–2.

This is a report of a single case treated using this approach. The microdebrider is a powered rotary shaving device. FloSeal is a haemostatic mixture of thrombin and gelatin applied topically after the surgery. The use of these adjuncts allowed precise sculpting and immediate hemostasis.

Surgical treatment of rhinophyma with the Shaw scalpel. Eisen RF, Katz AE, Bohigian RK, Grande DJ. Arch Dermatol 1986; 122: 307–9.

The Shaw scalpel is a device in which a scalpel blade can be heated. A rhinophyma was treated using a temperature of 150°C to achieve hemostasis while paring. Contours were then refined using a CO_2 laser and light dermabrasion.

Rhinophyma, associated with carcinoma, treated successfully with radiation. Plenk HP. Plast Reconstruct Surg 1995; 95: 559–62.

Two patients with basal cell carcinoma complicating rhinophyma had complete control of both conditions by radiotherapy using orthovoltage X-radiation. The authors suggest that this modality might be useful for rhinophyma alone.

Rhinophyma treated with kilovoltage photons. Skala M, Delaney G, Towell V, Vladica N. Australas J Dermatol 2005; 46: 88–9.

A rhinophyma was successfully treated with 90-kV photons to a total dose of 40 Gy in 20 daily fractions.

Treatment of rhinophyma with the Versajet Hydrosurgery System. Taghizadeh R, Mackay SP, Gilbert PM. J Plast Reconstruct Aesthet Surg 2008; 61: 330–3.

Six patients were treated successfully.

The Versajet Hydrosurgery System is a novel surgical device which uses a high-velocity jet of water for excision and vacuum aspiration of water and debris.

Rocky Mountain spotted fever and other rickettsial infections

George G Kihiczak, Robert A Schwartz

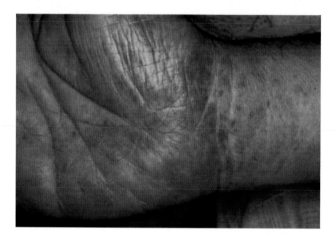

The Rickettsiae are a family of obligate intracellular bacteria that cause infections with a diverse array of clinical presentations. They may be divided into the spotted fevers, including Rocky Mountain spotted fever, the typhus group, rickettsialpox, Q fever, and erhlichiosis.

RICKETTSIAL SPOTTED FEVERS

These include African tick bite fever (*R. africae*), Astrakhan fever, (*R. conorii*), Flinders Island spotted fever (*R. honei*), Indian tick typhus (*R. conorii*), Israeli spotted fever (*R. conorii*), Japanese spotted fever (*R. japonica*), Mediterranean spotted fever (*R. conorii*), Queensland tick typhus (*R. australis*), Rocky Mountain spotted fever (*R. rickettsii*), and Siberian tick typhus (*R. sibirica*).

ROCKY MOUNTAIN SPOTTED FEVER

Rocky Mountain spotted fever is caused by *R. rickettsii* and is endemic to almost all areas of the USA. A classic triad seen early on in the course of the disease consists of tick bite, rash, and fever. The characteristic rash is pink macules that appear on the wrists and ankles, become petechial and purpuric, and then progress to the palms, soles, extremities, and trunk, sparing the face. The rash does not appear until the third day and is absent in nearly 10% of patients. Atypical rashes, confined to one region of the body, may be seen. Fever, myalgias, and severe headaches are present in most cases; bilateral calf pain is the most common presenting complaint. Gastrointestinal symptoms such as abdominal pains, diarrhea, nausea, and vomiting occur in nearly half of patients, usually early in the course of the illness. This often leads to misdiagnosis or delay in therapy. Vascular injury to the appendix, gallbladder, and small intestine has been reported, in some cases mimicking acute cholecystitis.

Prognosis is related to the timely diagnosis and initiation of effective treatment.

Prevention is achieved by avoiding areas with ticks. Covering skin with long protective clothing reduces the risk of exposure. Clothing may be impregnated with acaricidal compounds for added protection. Any uncovered skin should be treated with topical insect repellants prior to activities in high-risk areas. Unfortunately, most insect repellants are effective for only short periods and need to be reapplied frequently. Thorough skin examinations should be conducted on a regular basis, at least twice daily in endemic areas, and any ticks removed. The scalp, axillary, and pubic hair requires particularly careful examination. There is currently no effective vaccine, although immunogenic surface protein antigens have been cloned and sequenced.

MANAGEMENT STRATEGY

Doxycycline is the best first-line agent for treating RMSF and other spotted fevers, as shown by extensive research data and clinical experience. In pregnant patients *chloramphenicol* is the therapy of choice as an alternative to tetracyclines (although serious side effects such as agranulocytosis may occur). Supportive care is also an important component in successful treatment. A high-protein diet, adequate hydration, and continuous monitoring of blood volume are critical. In cases in which renal, pulmonary, or cardiac complications occur, other specialized therapies may be required.

Clinical suspicion of a spotted fever is sufficient to warrant treatment. Serologic confirmation should not delay the initiation of appropriate therapy. Diagnosis is difficult, as the characteristic rash is not a reliable sign of disease and the classic triad is often not evident. The spotted fevers progress rapidly and therefore immediate treatment is required initially (ideally in the first 3–4 days). Doxycycline is the medication of choice, administered at a dose of 100 mg twice daily in adults. Children 8 years and older should receive 4 mg/kg daily. These oral antibiotics are taken for a minimum of 7 days and are continued until the patient is afebrile for a minimum of 48 hours. Within 24 hours of the initiation of treatment a response may be observed. Within the first 36–48 hours considerable clinical improvement is seen, and apyrexia is often achieved by 72 hours. Death occurs at a higher rate in those untreated beyond 5 days of illness onset. Of note, early discontinuation of therapy may result in relapse. RMSF has a case-fatality rate as high as 30% in certain untreated patients. Even with treatment, hospitalization rates of 72% and case-fatality rates of 4% are seen.

Tetracycline (500 mg every 6 hours, maximum dose 2 g) is efficacious but is contraindicated in patients with renal failure, during pregnancy, and in children under 8 years of age. Chloramphenicol (50–75 mg/kg daily, divided into four doses) is the recommended treatment for pregnant women and children under 8. However, there are limited data on this treatment and relapses have occurred.

In severe cases intravenous antibiotics and hospitalization are required. Supportive measures including fluid maintenance, intravenous hydration, nutritional support, and oxygen supplementation are essential in severe cases. In some cases anuria, oliguria, or renal failure may necessitate hemodialysis.

Fatal cases of Rocky Mountain spotted fever in family clusters – three states, 2003. MMWR Morb Mortal Wkly Rep 2004; 53: 407–10.

During the summer of 2003, three families had more than one member with RMSF and a child died from RMSF. These cases highlight the need for rapid diagnosis and antimicrobial therapy in patients with RMSF. Moreover, the diagnosis of RMSF should be considered in family members and contacts of patients with RMSF who present with fevers.

SPECIFIC INVESTIGATIONS

> ▶ Skin biopsy, direct immunofluorescence/ immunoperoxidase
> ▶ Serologic testing for anti-rickettsial antibodies
> ▶ Polymerase chain reaction (PCR)
> ▶ Liver function tests
> ▶ Complete blood count

Diagnosis is most often based on clinical presentation, as patients may have a history of a tick bite after spending time in an endemic area. Clinical suspicion requires the rapid initiation of therapy even when confirmatory tests are pending, as mortality increases when treatment is delayed. Direct immunofluorescence or immunoperoxidase staining of skin biopsy specimens is a relatively quick way of diagnosing RMSF. Serologic tests, including indirect immunofluorescence, latex agglutination, and enzyme immunoassay, that detect anti-rickettsial antibodies are available. However, these tests usually yield negative readings in the critical first days of the disease as antibodies are not detectable until 7–10 days after the onset of the illness. Confirmation of the diagnosis using acute and convalescent-phase serum samples is possible with these tests. The indirect hemagglutination antibody and immunofluorescent antibody tests are most useful because of their high sensitivity and specificity. The immunofluorescent test is especially useful because of its capacity to assess IgG and IgM levels.

A highly specific and sensitive polymerase chain reaction (PCR) assay for the detection of spotted fever and typhus group of *Rickettsiae* was recently developed to provide rapid confirmation of the diagnosis when rickettsial loads are low.

A complete blood count and liver function tests should obtained. Most patients will have some degree of anemia or leukopenia, though in some cases the white blood count may be elevated. Thrombocytopenia may occur in severe cases. Hepatic enzymes, bilirubin, and lactate dehydrogenase are often elevated.

Blood cultures or skin biopsy specimen may be used to confirm the diagnosis, but are not helpful in the initial diagnosis of spotted fevers owing to the length of time they require for results.

Rickettsiae do not stain well with Gram stain, and instead should be stained with Giemsa, Machiavello's or Castaneda's stains.

Laboratory diagnosis of Rocky Mountain spotted fever. Walker DH, Burday MS, Folds JD. South Med J 1980; 73: 1143–6.

Immunofluorescence staining of 16 skin biopsies proved this test to be the best for early diagnosis of RMSF. A specificity of 100% and sensitivity of 70% were reported.

Immunofluorescence must be conducted within 48 hour after initiating antirickettsial therapy.

Immunoperoxidase and immunofluorescent staining of *Rickettsia rickettsii* **in skin biopsies: a comparative study.** Procop GW, Burchette JL, Howell DN, Sexton DJ. Arch Pathol Lab Med 1997; 121: 894–9.

Immunofluorescent staining for *R. rickettsii* and immunoperoxidase staining for *R. rickettsii* on formalin-fixed, paraffin-embedded skin biopsies were compared in 26 patients. Sensitivity and specificity were equivalent for both techniques. Immunofluorescent staining provided faster results, but immunoperoxidase staining had the benefit of easier antigen localization and allowed simultaneous examination of histopathology.

Polymerase chain reaction-based diagnosis of Mediterranean spotted fever in serum and tissue samples. Leitner M, Yitzhaki S, Rzotkiewicz S, Keysary A. Am J Trop Med Hyg 2002; 67: 166–9.

The diagnosis of Mediterranean spotted fever via nested PCR was developed through the use of specific primers derived from a *Rickettsia conorii* 17-kDa protein gene. Both serum and tissue samples may be used for this test.

Spotless rickettsiosis caused by *Rickettsia slovaca* **and associated** *Dermacentor* **ticks.** Raoult D, Lakos A, Fenollar F, Beytout J, Brouqui P, Fournier PE. Clin Infect Dis 2002; 34: 1331–6.

PCR confirmed *Rickettsia slovaca* infections in 17 of 67 patients with scalp lesions and enlarged cervical lymph nodes following a *Dermacentor* tick bite.

A highly sensitive and specific real-time PCR assay for the detection of spotted fever and typhus group *Rickettsiae.* Stenos J, Graves SR, Unsworth NB. Am J Trop Hyg 2005; 73: 1083–5.

PCR was developed to target the citrate synthase gene of *Rickettsiae.* This is a quantitative assay that can confirm the diagnosis of a spotted disease when rickettsial numbers are low, and makes possible the enumeration of rickettsiae in clinical specimens as well. *R. akari, R. australis, R. conorii, R. honei, 'R. marmionii', R. sibirica, R. rickettsii, R. typhus,* and *R. prowazekii* all were detectable by this PCR.

FIRST-LINE THERAPIES

> ▶ Doxycycline or tetracycline   C
> ▶ Chloramphenicol (in pregnant patients)   D

Rickettsia rickettsii is sensitive to tetracyclines, chloramphenicol, and rifampin. Doxycycline is the therapy of choice and should be administered early in the illness. Adults and children weighing 45 kg or more should take 100 doses of doxycycline at 12-hour intervals either orally or intravenously. Children weighing less than 45.4 kg should receive 2.2 mg/kg body weight per dose administered twice daily.

Erythromycin versus tetracycline for treatment of Mediterranean spotted fever. Munoz-Espin T, Lopez-Pares P, Espejo-Arenas E, Font-Creus B, Martinez-Vila I, Travería-Casanova J, et al. Arch Dis Child 1986; 6: 1027–9.

A randomized trial assessed erythromycin stearate versus tetracycline hydrochloride in 81 children with Mediterranean spotted fever. Treatment with tetracycline led to a significantly more rapid disappearance of clinical symptoms and fever than did erythromycin.

Relapse of rickettsial Mediterranean spotted fever and murine typhus after treatment with chloramphenicol. Shaked Y, Samra Y, Maier MK, Rubinstein E. J Infect 1989; 18: 35–7.

Ten of 24 patients treated with chloramphenicol had a relapse, which did not occur in any of the 108 patients treated with tetracycline.

Analysis of risk factors for fatal Rocky Mountain spotted fever: evidence for superiority of tetracyclines for therapy. Holman RC, Paddock CD, Curns AT, Krebs JW, McQuiston JH, Childs JE. J Infect Dis 2001; 184: 1437–44.

The US national surveillance of 1981–1998 recorded 6388 patients with Rocky Mountain spotted fever. A higher risk of death was found in patients treated exclusively with chloramphenicol, in patients who received treatment 5 or more days after onset of symptoms, and in older patients.

Should tetracycline be contraindicated for therapy of presumed RMSF in children less than 9 years of age? Abramson JS, Givner LB. Pediatrics 1990; 86: 123–4.

Tetracycline-related teeth staining is dose related. Minimal tooth discoloration was observed in children below the age of 5 treated with fewer than six courses (6 days per course) of tetracycline. Chloraphenicol is not recommended because of the risk of aplastic anemia and other serious complications. The authors hold that the benefits outweigh the risks when it comes to the use of tetracycline in children less than 9 years old with RMSF.

Rocky Mountain spotted fever: a clinician's dilemma. Masters EJ, Olson GS, Weiner SJ, Paddock CD. Arch Intern Med 2003; 163: 769–74.

The outcome of RMSF is directly related to the speed of treatment initiation. Failure to diagnose and treat stems from the follow characteristics at presentation: (1) absence of a skin rash, (2) absence of a tick bite by history, (3) inappropriate geographic and seasonal exclusion, (4) misdiagnosis due to non-specific symptoms, and (5) failure to treat with appropriate doses of doxycycline. The mortality rate reported was 6.5% for patients treated within 5 days of disease onset and 22.9% for those treated 5 days or more after onset (Therapeutic delay and mortality in cases of Rocky Mountain spotted fever. Kirkland KB, Wilkinson WE, Sexton DJ. Clin Infect Dis 1995; 20: 1118–21).

SECOND-LINE THERAPIES

▶ Chloramphenicol (in non-pregnant patients)	C
▶ Azithromycin	B
▶ Clarithromycin	B
▶ Ciprofloxacin	B

Analysis of risk factors for fatal Rocky Mountain spotted fever: evidence for superiority of tetracyclines for therapy. Holman RC, Paddock CD, Curns AT, Krebs JW, McQuiston JH, Childs JE. J Infect Dis 2001; 184: 1437–44.

A study of RMSF derived from reports received by the Centers for Disease Control and Prevention by state health departments and private physicians consisting of 5600 confirmed and probable cases occurring from 1981 to 1998. Age, race, and time of treatment with respect to onset of illness were used to stratify the patient population. Four treatments groups were studied: tetracycline without chloramphenicol; chloramphenicol without tetracycline; chloramphenicol with tetracycline; and neither chloramphenicol nor tetracycline.

Patients with RMSF, regardless of the stratified group, who did not receive tetracycline-only treatment, those treated with chloramphenicol only, and those who did not receive treatment with either a tetracycline or chloramphenicol had a significantly increased risk of death.

Coexistent medical conditions and an array of risk factors that may predispose patients to a more severe course were not considered. However, this report maintains that the use of tetracycline antibiotics early in the course of illness significantly reduces the risk of death in patients with RMSF.

Clarithromycin versus azithromycin in the treatment of Mediterranean spotted fever in children: a randomized controlled trial. Cascio A, Colomba C, Antinori S, Paterson DL, Titone L. Clin Infect Dis 2002; 34: 154–8.

This open-label randomized controlled trial compared azithromycin (10 mg/kg daily in one dose for 3 days) and clarithromycin (15 mg/kg daily in two divided doses for 7 days) in the treatment of Mediterranean spotted fever in children. Both these agents may be suitable for children 8 years old and under.

THIRD-LINE THERAPIES

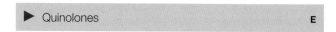

▶ Quinolones	E

Evaluation of the antirickettsial activities of fluoroquinolones. Keren G, Hzhaki A, Oron C, Keysarg A. Drugs 1995; 49: 208–10.

Rickettsia conorii and other *Rickettsia* spp. were inhibited by fluoroquinolones at concentrations <1 mg/mL in in-vitro tissue cultures. This study is suggestive of the usefulness of fluoroquinolones in the treatment of rickettsial diseases; in-vivo human studies are not available and further studies are required.

TYPHUS GROUP

MANAGEMENT STRATEGY

Epidemic typhus

Epidemic typhus is caused by *R. prowazekii*, transmitted via the body louse. Recommended treatment is oral doxycycline (200 mg daily for 5 days) or intravenously in more severe cases. Chloramphenicol is effective also. Prevention is crucial and can be achieved through bathing, washing clothes, and the use of insecticides.

Murine typhus

Murine typhus (or endemic typhus) is due to *R. typhi*, transmitted via the rat flea and the rat louse. Doxycycline taken orally at 200 mg daily for 7–15 days or until 3 days of defervescence is recommended. Chloramphenicol may also be effective, though relapses have been reported. Prevention is achieved through the use of insecticides and controlling the rat population.

Scrub typhus

Scrub typhus is caused by *R. tsutsugamushi*, transmitted via larval mites. Tetracyclines are recommended in adults: doxycycline (200 mg daily) or tetracycline (2 g daily) for 2–14 days. Chloramphenicol, albeit also effective, does not act as quickly as the tetracyclines.

SPECIFIC INVESTIGATIONS

> **Epidemic typhus**
> ▶ Serology: microimmunofluorescent and plate microagglutination tests
>
> **Murine typhus**
> ▶ Serology: indirect fluorescent antibody, latex agglutination, solid-phase immunoassay
>
> **Scrub typhus**
> ▶ Serology: indirect fluorescent antibody test

FIRST-LINE THERAPIES

> **Epidemic typhus**
> ▶ Doxycycline   A
>
> **Murine typhus**
> ▶ Doxycycline   A
>
> **Scrub typhus**
> ▶ Doxycycline   A
> ▶ Azithromycin   A
> ▶ Rifampicin (Rifampin)   A

Comparison of the effectiveness of five different antibiotic regimens on infection with *Rickettsia typhi*: therapeutic data from 87 cases. Gikas A, Doukakis S, Pediaditis J, Kastanakis S, Manios A, Tselentis Y. Am J Trop Med Hyg 2004; 70: 576–9.

A retrospective study of five different antibiotic regimens used in 87 patients with endemic typhus. Mean time to defervescence was 2.9 days for doxycycline, 4 days for chloramphenicol, and 4.2 days for ciprofloxacin.

Pediatric scrub typhus in Thailand: a study of 73 confirmed cases. Silpapojakul K, Varachit B, Silpapojakul K. Trans Roy Soc Trop Med Hyg 2004; 98: 354–9.

A study of 73 children with a mean age of 9 years afflicted with scrub typhus demonstrated that defervescence began 1 day (median) following doxycycline and 3 days after chloramphenicol. Those receiving other antibiotics or no treatment had a median of 5 days until defervescence.

Doxycycline and rifampicin for mild scrub-typhus infections in northern Thailand: a randomized trial. Watt G, Kantipong P, Jongaskul K, Watcharapichat P, Phulsuksombati D, Strickman D. Lancet 2000; 356: 1057–61.

A randomized study of adults with mild scrub typhus in which patients received oral doxycycline 200 mg daily (n=28), oral rifampicin 600 mg daily (n=26), or oral rifampicin 900 mg daily (n=24). Patients treated with rifampicin at either dosage demonstrated a significantly shorter median duration of pyrexia than the doxycycline patients.

Doxycycline versus azithromycin for treatment of leptospirosis and scrub typhus. Phimda K, Hoontrakul S, Suttinont C, Chareonwat S, Losuwanaluk K, Chueasuwanchai S, et al. Antimicrob Agents Chemother 2007; 51: 3259–63.

A randomized controlled trial in which 296 patients were randomly allocated to receive either a 7-day course of doxycycline or a 3-day course of azithromycin. The group studied included 57 patients (19.3%) with scrub typhus, 14 (4.7%) with murine typhus, 69 (23.3%) with leptospirosis, and 11 (3.7%) with both leptospirosis and a rickettsial infection. Both regimens demonstrated similar effectiveness and fever clearance times. Doxycycline is an effective choice for scrub typhus and leptospirosis, whereas azithromycin is effective, has fewer adverse effects, but is more expensive.

SECOND-LINE THERAPIES

> **Epidemic typhus**
> ▶ Chloramphenicol   D
>
> **Murine typhus**
> ▶ Chloramphenicol   D
>
> **Scrub typhus**
> ▶ Chloramphenicol   D

RICKETTSIALPOX

MANAGEMENT STRATEGY

Rickettsialpox is due to *R. akari*. The house mouse is the reservoir, and mites transmit the bacteria to humans. This is a self-limited disease. Treatment in adults is doxycycline (200 mg daily) for 2–5 days.

SPECIFIC INVESTIGATIONS

> ▶ Serology: complement fixation

FIRST-LINE THERAPIES

> ▶ Doxycycline   A

Rickettsialpox: report of an outbreak and a contemporary review. Brettman LR, Lewin S, Holzman RS, Goldman WD, Marr JS, Kechijian P, et al. Medicine 1981; 60: 363–72.

Antibiotics shorten the duration of symptoms to 24–48 hours.

Q FEVER

Q fever is caused by *Coxiella burnetti*. Transmission to humans occurs via aerosolized urine, feces, or birth products of ungulates (hoofed mammals).

MANAGEMENT STRATEGY

Acute Q fever

The treatment of choice in adults is doxycycline (200 mg daily for 2–3 weeks). In vitro the disease has been susceptible to quinolones, chloramphenicol, rifampin, and trimethoprim-sulfamethoxazole.

Chronic Q fever

May be associated with endocarditis which is resistant to treatment, owing to the bacteriostatic rather than the bactericidal effects of antibiotics on *C. burnetti*. A 3-year course of quinolone and doxycycline has been proposed. Hydroxychloroquine, when combined with doxycycline, may increase bactericidal activity.

SPECIFIC INVESTIGATIONS

Acute Q fever
▶ Serology: complement fixation, immunofluorescent antibody
▶ PCR

Chronic Q fever
▶ Echocardiography
▶ Serology

High throughput detection of *Coxiella burnetii* by real-time PCR with internal control system and automated DNA preparation. Panning M, Kilwinski J, Greiner-Fischer S, Peters M, Kramme S, Frangoulidis D, et al. BMC Microbiol 2008; 8: 77.

A sensitive real-time PCR was established for the rapid screening of *C. burnetii* in local outbreaks. Although serology is the gold standard for diagnosis it is inadequate for early case detection.

FIRST-LINE THERAPIES

Acute Q fever
▶ β-Lactams   B
▶ Doxycycline   B
▶ Macrolides   B
▶ Quinolones   B

Chronic Q fever
▶ Quinolone and doxycycline   B
▶ Doxycycline and hydroxychloroquine   B

Q fever: epidemiology, clinical features and prognosis. A study from 1983 to 1999 in the South of Spain. Alarcon A, Villanueva JL, Viciana P, López-Cortés L, Torronteras R, Bernabeu M, et al. J Infect 2003; 47: 110–16.

The authors retrospectively studied 231 cases of acute Q fever. All antimicrobial treatments (β-lactams, doxycycline, macrolides, and quinolones) failed to reduce the duration of fever. Antibiotics administered within the first 2 weeks of illness were more effective.

Q fever in the Greek island of Crete: epidemiology, clinical and therapeutic data from 98 cases. Tselentis Y, Gikas A, Kofteridis D, Psaroulaki A, Tselentis Y, et al. Clin Infect Dis 1995; 20: 1311–16.

Ninety-eight cases of Q fever were studied retrospectively. No difference in the duration of fever was observed with either tetracycline or erythromycin. However, this may have been due to delay in initiating tetracycline therapy.

Comparison of different antibiotic regimens for therapy of 32 cases of Q fever endocarditis. Levy PY, Drancourt M, Etienne J, Auvergnat JC, Beytout J, Sainty JM, et al. Antimicrob Agents Chemother 1991; 35: 533–7.

A study of 32 cases of Q fever endocarditis in France between 1985 and 1989. Doxycycline and a quinolone had a better effect on mortality than doxycycline used alone. The authors advise a minimum treatment duration of 3 years.

Treatment of Q fever endocarditis: comparison of 2 regimens containing doxycycline and ofloxacin or hydroxychloroquine. Raoult D, Houpikian P, Tissot Dupont H, Riss JM, Arditi-Djiane J, Brouqui P. Arch Intern Med 1999; 159: 167–73.

Treatment with doxycycline and quinolone was compared with doxycycline and hydroxychloroquine in 35 patients with Q fever endocarditis. Doxycycline in combination with hydroxychloroquine for at minimum of 18 months leads to a reduction in the duration of therapy and the number of relapses.

EHRLICHIOSIS

The ehrlichioses consists of two tickborne diseases: human monocytic ehrlichiosis due to *E. chaffeensis*, and human granulocytic erhlichiosis due to *E. equi*. Both are found in mammalian reservoirs (deer, dogs, horses) and are transmitted via ticks.

MANAGEMENT STRATEGY

Doxycycline (100 mg orally twice daily for adults, or 4 mg/kg daily in children 8 years of age and older) is the treatment of choice. The treatment ought to be continued for a minimum of 7 days and for 3 days following defervescence.

SPECIFIC INVESTIGATIONS

▶ Serology: immunofluorescent antibody

FIRST-LINE THERAPIES

▶ Doxycycline   A

Human granulocytic ehrlichiosis: a case series from a medical center in New York State. Aguero-Rosenfeld ME, Horowitz HW, Wormser GP, McKenna DF, Nowakowski J, Muñoz J, et al. Ann Intern Med 1996; 125: 904–8.

A study of 18 patients with human granulocytic erhlichiosis all successfully treated with doxycycline.

The importance of early treatment with doxycycline in human ehrlichiosis. Hamburg BJ, Storch GA, Micek ST, Kollef MH. Medicine (Baltimore) 2008; 87: 53–60.

Patients who were started on doxycycline within the first 24 hours of hospital admission did much better than those who did not have empiric doxycycline therapy. A low therapeutic threshold was encouraged, especially in endemic regions.

SECOND-LINE THERAPIES

▶ Rifampin (rifampicin)   D

Successful treatment of human granulocytic ehrlichiosis in children using rifampin. Krause PJ, Corrow CL, Bakken JS. Pediatrics 2003; 112: 252–3.

Rifampin was successfully used in the treatment of two cases of human granulocytic ehrlichiosis in children.

Evidence Levels: **A** Double-blind study **B** Clinical trial ≥ 20 subjects **C** Clinical trial < 20 subjects **D** Series ≥ 5 subjects **E** Anecdotal case reports

Rosacea

John Berth-Jones

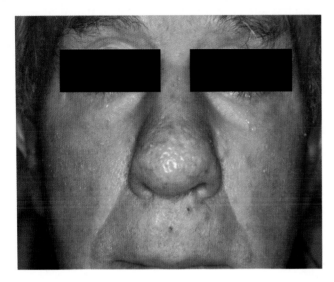

Rosacea is a common inflammatory skin disease. The eruption is generally confined to the face, principally the cheeks, forehead, nose, and chin. In some cases lesions may extend on to the scalp, and occasionally also onto the neck and the upper part of the body. A common early feature is flushing, often accompanied by a burning sensation. Inflammatory lesions (papulation and pustulation) are characteristic and may become florid. Vascular changes (telangiectasia and erythema) are also frequently observed. These are initially mild, but may later become very conspicuous. Other later features are the development of lymphedema, thickening, and induration. On the nose and, less often the ears, forehead or chin, hypertrophy and lymphedema of subcutaneous tissue may develop into distinct swellings known as phymas, of which rhinophyma is most familiar. Ocular involvement is frequent and manifests as a sensation of grittiness, which may be accompanied by conjunctivitis, blepharitis, episcleritis, chalazion, hordeolum, iritis, and occasionally severe keratitis. The etiology and pathogenesis of rosacea remain poorly understood. Hopefully, improvements in our understanding of the etiology will one day facilitate a more rational approach to treatment, which has so far developed rather empirically.

MANAGEMENT STRATEGY

Patients may find it beneficial to *avoid alcohol, spicy food, hot drinks*, etc. which may induce flushing and promote the development of telangiectasia. Exposure to irritants should be avoided, and emollients can be helpful. *Cosmetic camouflage* of the erythema and telangiectasia can be helpful. *Facial massage* may promote lymphatic drainage and reduce the development of lymphedema. Papulation, pustulation, and erythema can be effectively suppressed using a variety of topical and systemic *antibiotics, retinoids,* and other agents described below. Unfortunately, these modalities are usually not very effective for suppressing flushing and have little effect on established

telangiectasia. Telangiectasia and erythema can be effectively treated by physical measures to ablate the vessels, such as *intense pulsed light or vascular lasers*. Flushing is usually the most difficult feature to treat, but sometimes improves during treatment of telangiectasia. Ocular rosacea is often treated symptomatically with a range of 'artificial tears' – the ophthalmic equivalent of emollients. *Systemic tetracyclines*, used as for cutaneous rosacea, and topical ophthalmic formulations of fusidic acid are also helpful. The use of *retinoids f*or rosacea requires special care in patients with eye involvement and may be poorly tolerated. Treatments are discussed below in sections focused on inflammatory rosacea, erythematotelangiectatic rosacea, flushing, lymphedema, ocular rosacea, and rosacea fulminans. Treatments for rhinophyma and perioral dermatitis are described in separate chapters.

SPECIFIC INVESTIGATIONS

In selected cases
▶ Urinary 5-HIAA to exclude carcinoid syndrome
▶ Serology to exclude lupus

INFLAMMATORY ROSACEA

FIRST-LINE TREATMENTS

▶ Topical metronidazole	A
▶ Topical azelaic acid	A
▶ Oral tetracyclines	A
▶ Oral erythromycin	C
▶ Emollients	C

Treatment of rosacea with 1% metronidazole cream. A double-blind study. Nielson PG. Br J Dermatol 1983; 108: 327–32.

Eighty-one patients were treated with 1% metronidazole cream or vehicle for 2 months. Metronidazole cream was significantly more effective than placebo in suppression of inflammatory lesions and erythema.

The efficacy of metronidazole 1% cream once daily compared with metronidazole cream twice daily and their vehicles in rosacea: a double-blind clinical trial. Jorizzo JL, Lebwohl M, Tobey RE. J Am Acad Dermatol 1998; 39: 502–4.

This study also demonstrated improvements in numbers of inflammatory lesions and in erythema relative to placebo. However, there was no apparent difference between once-daily and twice-daily application.

Topical metronidazole maintains remissions of rosacea. Dahl MV, Katz HI, Krueger GG, Millikan LE, Odom RB, Parker F, et al. Arch Dermatol 1998; 134: 679–83.

Eighty-eight subjects who had responded to treatment with systemic tetracycline and topical metronidazole were randomized to receive 0.75% metronidazole gel or placebo gel for 6 months. In those applying the metronidazole, 23% developed a relapse of papulopustular lesions, and 55% a worsening of erythema, compared to 42% and 74% of subjects, respectively, in the placebo gel group.

A randomized, double-blind, placebo-controlled trial of the combined effect of doxycycline hyclate 20 mg tablets and metronidazole 0.75% topical lotion in the treatment of rosacea. Sanchez J, Somolinos AL, Almodovar PI, Webster G, Bradshaw M, Powala C. J Am Acad Dermatol 2005; 53: 791–7.

Combinations of topical and systemic treatment are often used and seem likely to be more effective than either used alone. In this study the addition of low-dose (20 mg) doxycycline improved the response to topical metronidazole.

Topical azelaic acid in the treatment of rosacea. Carmichael AJ, Marks R, Graupe KA, Zaumseil RP. J Dermatol Treat 1993; 4: 19–22.

Topical azelaic acid 20% cream was shown to be more effective than the base alone in a double-blind, controlled, split-face study with 33 patients. Treatment was given for 9 weeks and improvement was seen in papules, pustules, and erythema, but not telangiectasia.

Double-blind comparison of azelaic acid 20% cream and its vehicle in treatment of papulo-pustular rosacea. Bjerke R, Fyrand O, Graupe K. Acta Dermatol Venereol 1999; 79: 456–9.

A 3-month randomized, double-blind study compared the efficacy and safety of azelaic acid 20% cream, applied twice daily, with its vehicle in 116 patients. Azelaic acid cream produced significantly greater mean reductions in total inflammatory lesions than did vehicle: 73.4% vs 50.6%, respectively. Erythema also responded.

A comparison of topical azelaic acid 20% cream and topical metronidazole 0.75% cream in the treatment of patients with papulopustular rosacea. Maddin S. J Am Acad Dermatol 1999; 40: 961–5.

A double-blind, randomized, split-face study with 40 patients comparing topical azelaic acid 20% cream with metronidazole 0.75% cream, each applied twice daily for 15 weeks. The treatments were similarly effective.

A comparison of 15% azelaic acid gel and 0.75% metronidazole gel in the topical treatment of papulopustular rosacea. Elewski BE, Fleischer AB, Pariser DM. Arch Dermatol 2003; 139: 1444–50.

A double-blind study on 251 patients with papulopustular rosacea. In these formulations, azelaic acid proved superior to metronidazole for reducing inflammatory lesions and erythema. Metronidazole was somewhat better tolerated.

A clinical trial of tetracycline in rosacea. Sneddon IB. Br J Dermatol 1966; 78: 649–52.

A double-blind trial with 78 evaluable subjects comparing tetracycline 250 mg twice daily with placebo after 4 weeks' treatment. There was a significantly superior response to active treatment, even though a pronounced placebo effect was observed. During subsequent follow-up it was found that some patients could be completely controlled using only 100 mg daily.

Safety of long-term tetracycline therapy for acne. Sauer GC. Arch Dermatol 1976; 112: 1603–5.

A study of 325 patients treated with oral tetracycline for 3 years or more showed the drug was generally well tolerated. However, elevated bilirubin and alkaline phosphatase levels were found in approximately 5% of cases (the majority being minimally so, or returning to normal on repeat testing), suggesting that liver function should be monitored in patients on long-term therapy. One patient developed mild jaundice while taking 500 mg of tetracycline daily.

Two randomized phase III clinical trials evaluating anti-inflammatory dose doxycycline (40-mg doxycycline, USP capsules) administered once daily for treatment of rosacea. Del Rosso JQ, Webster GF, Jackson M, Rendon M, Rich P, Torok H, et al. J Am Acad Dermatol 2007; 56: 791–802.

Doxycycline appears to be effective even at low dose.

A double-blind study of 1% metronidazole cream versus systemic oxytetracycline therapy for rosacea. Nielsen PG. Br J Dermatol 1983; 109: 63–5.

A randomized, double-blind trial in which 51 patients were treated for 2 months with 1% metronidazole cream and placebo tablets, or with oxytetracycline 250 mg twice daily and placebo cream. Improvement occurred in 90% of the patients. There was no significant difference between the treatments.

Steroid rosacea in prepubertal children. Weston WL, Morelli JG. Arch Pediatr Adolesc Med 2000; 154: 62–4.

A retrospective evaluation of 106 children younger than 13 years with steroid rosacea. Abrupt cessation of topical corticosteroid use and initiation of treatment with oral erythromycin stearate for 4 weeks produced complete clearing in 86% of children within 4 weeks and in 100% by 8 weeks.

The efficacy of oral tetracyclines seems to be well established, although most of the trials on the use of these antibiotics have been against active comparators rather than placebo. Both tetracycline and oxytetracycline are generally used at the dose of 250–500 mg twice daily in rosacea. Other systemic tetracyclines, such as minocycline 100 mg daily, doxycycline 100 mg daily, and lymecycline 408 mg daily, are also often prescribed. These offer the advantage of once-daily administration and their absorption is less influenced by dietary calcium, so they can be taken with food. Erythromycin 250–500 mg twice daily is also often prescribed and widely held to be effective, and can be useful when rosacea occurs in children, for whom tetracyclines are contraindicated.

Beneficial use of Cetaphil moisturizing cream as part of a daily skin care regimen for individuals with rosacea. Laquieze S, Czernielewski J, Baltas E. J Dermatol Treat 2007; 18: 158–62.

Twice-daily application of a moisturizer appeared beneficial in this open study on 20 patients.

SECOND-LINE TREATMENTS

▶ Topical erythromycin	C
▶ Topical clindamycin	C
▶ Oral metronidazole	A
▶ Topical benzoyl peroxide	A
▶ Ampicillin	A
▶ Azithromycin	B

Topically applied erythromycin in rosacea. Mills OH, Kligman AM. Arch Dermatol 1976; 112: 553–4.

A 2% solution applied twice daily to 15 patients produced a 50–100% improvement in 87% of cases, and treatment was effective by 4 weeks. Once-daily application was sufficient once the disease was controlled.

670

Evidence Levels: **A** Double-blind study **B** Clinical trial ≥ 20 subjects **C** Clinical trial < 20 subjects **D** Series ≥ 5 subjects **E** Anecdotal case reports

Treatment of rosacea: topical clindamycin versus oral tetracycline. Wilkin JK, DeWitt S. Int J Dermatol 1993; 32: 65–7.

A randomized, blinded trial comparing topical clindamycin lotion twice daily with oral tetracycline in 43 patients evaluated over 12 weeks. Similar improvements were found in both groups, although clindamycin was superior in eradication of pustules.

Double-blind, randomized, vehicle-controlled clinical trial of once-daily benzoyl peroxide/clindamycin topical gel in the treatment of patients with moderate to severe rosacea. Breneman D, Savin R, VandePol C, Vamvakias G, Levy S, Leyden J. Int J Dermatol 2004; 43: 381–7.

This combination of 5% benzoyl peroxide and 1% clindamycin was effective and well tolerated.

Treatment of rosacea by metronidazole. Pye RJ, Burton JL. Lancet 1976; 1: 1211–12.

A double-blind, placebo-controlled, parallel-group trial demonstrating the efficacy of oral metronidazole 200 mg twice daily after 6 weeks of treatment. Ten out of 14 patients treated with metronidazole showed a good response.

A double-blinded trial of metronidazole versus oxytetracycline therapy for rosacea. Saihan EM, Burton JL. Br J Dermatol 1980; 102: 443–5.

Forty patients were treated for 12 weeks with oxytetracycline 250 mg twice daily or metronidazole 200 mg twice daily. On both drugs the degree of improvement was greater after 12 weeks than after 6 weeks. There was no significant difference between them.

Although metronidazole is generally well tolerated and it has been used long term, there is a risk of peripheral neuropathy if it is used for longer than 3 months.

Topical treatment of acne rosacea with benzoyl peroxide acetone gel. Montes LF, Cordero AA, Kriner J. Cutis 1983; 32: 185–90.

Benzoyl peroxide gel (5% increasing to 10%) was significantly superior to vehicle, although it was poorly tolerated and there was a high drop-out rate.

Comparative effectiveness of tetracycline and ampicillin in rosacea. A controlled trial. Marks R, Ellis J. Lancet 1971; 2: 1049–52.

A double-blind, placebo-controlled trial lasting 6 weeks and completed by 56 patients. Both antibiotics were significantly more effective than placebo. Tetracycline was apparently (but not significantly) more effective than ampicillin.

A novel treatment for acne vulgaris and rosacea. Elewski BE. J Eur Acad Dermatol Venereol 2000; 14: 423–4.

Ten patients were treated in an open study of azithromycin, 500 mg on day 1, followed by 250 mg/day for 4 consecutive days beginning on the first and 15th days of each month for 3 months. All patients improved, and nine were clear by 3 months.

Therapeutic potential of azithromycin in rosacea. Bakar O, Demircay Z, Gurbuz O. Int J Dermatol 2004; 43: 151–4.

In a 12-week open study on 18 patients, azithromycin was used at a dose of 500 mg/day for 3 consecutive days each week for the first 4 weeks, 250 mg/day on 3 days for the next 4 weeks, and 500 mg once weekly for the last 4 weeks. Both inflammatory lesions and erythema improved markedly in the 14 evaluable subjects.

Oral use of azithromycin for the treatment of acne rosacea. Fernandez-Obregon A. Arch Dermatol 2004; 140: 489–90.

Ten patients responded well to azithromycin 250 mg/day for 3 days each week (Monday, Wednesday and Friday), within 4 weeks. Ocular symptoms also improved.

Azithromycin has a relatively long half-life and is therefore suited to this sort of regimen.

THIRD-LINE TREATMENTS

▶ Systemic isotretinoin	B
▶ Topical tretinoin	C
▶ Topical adapalene	B
▶ Topical sulfur	B
▶ Topical corticosteroids	D
▶ Topical ketoconazole	D
▶ Systemic ketoconazole	D
▶ Topical bifonazole	D
▶ Photodynamic therapy	D
▶ Spironolactone	D
▶ Demodex eradication	B
▶ *Helicobacter pylori* eradication	D
▶ Sunscreens	E
▶ Topical tacrolimus	C
▶ Topical pimecrolimus	D
▶ Octreotide	C
▶ Inhibition of ovulation	C
▶ Topical NADH	C
▶ Topical 1-methylnicotinamide	C
▶ Oral nicotinamide with zinc	C
▶ Zinc sulphate	B
▶ Trichloroacetic acid peels	E

Treatment of rosacea with isotretinoin. Hoting E, Paul E, Plewig G. Int J Dermatol 1986; 25: 660–3.

This open study on 92 patients is the largest on the use of isotretinoin in rosacea. Results were beneficial, although seven patients were intolerant of the drug.

Continuous microdose isotretinoin in adult recalcitrant rosacea. Hofer T. Clin Exp Dermatol 2004; 29: 204–5.

In this report on 12 patients, isotretinoin was commenced at 10 or 20 mg daily for a period of 4–6 months, then reduced individually to lower doses. The treatment was well tolerated and quality of life, assessed using the Dermatology Life Quality Index, was improved relative to a control group.

There have been several reports of the use of isotretinoin at doses of 10–60 mg/day or 0.5–1 mg/kg/day for 6–28 weeks. Variable relapse rates have been reported after discontinuing the drug, and there being a trend towards more frequent relapse in those given lower total doses. However, doses often need to be kept low to avoid aggravating ocular symptoms. Partly for this reason, other investigators have advocated the use of continuous low-dose therapy with isotretinoin.

Topical tretinoin for rosacea; a preliminary report. Kligman AM. J Dermatol Treat 1993; 4: 71–3.

Topical tretinoin 0.025% for 6–12 months improved rosacea in about 70% of cases in this open study with 19 patients. Improvement was seen in telangiectasia as well as the erythematous and papulosquamous lesions.

A comparison of the efficacy of topical tretinoin and low-dose oral isotretinoin in rosacea. Ertl GA, Levine N, Kligman AM. Arch Dermatol 1994; 130: 319–24.

In this study on 22 patients, topical tretinoin (0.025% cream), low-dose isotretinoin (10 mg/day) and a combination of both these treatments appeared equally effective after 16 weeks.

Adapalene vs. metronidazole gel for the treatment of rosacea. Altinyazar HC, Koca R, Tekin NS, Estürk E. Int J Dermatol 2005; 44: 252–5.

In an investigator-blinded, parallel-group trial with 55 patients using adapalene 0.1% gel produced significant reductions in inflammatory lesions, with results similar to those of metronidazole 0.75% gel.

Topical treatment with sulfur 10% for rosacea. Blom I, Hornmark A-M. Acta Dermatol Venereol 1984; 64: 358–9.

A randomized study with 40 patients. Treatment duration was 4 weeks. Topical sulfur 10% in a cream base (Diprobase) was as effective as oral lymecycline 150 mg/day. A greater reduction in inflammatory lesions was observed in the group treated with sulfur, although there were a greater number of lesions at baseline in this group.

The treatment of rosacea: the safety and efficacy of sodium sulfacetamide 10% and sulfur 5% lotion (Novacet) is demonstrated in a double-blind study. Saunder DN, Miller R, Gratton D, Danby W, Griffiths C, Phillips S. J Dermatol Treat 1997; 8: 79–85.

The efficacy of a lotion of 10% sodium sulfacetamide and 5% sulfur was demonstrated in an 8-week double-blind, randomized, vehicle-controlled, parallel-group, multicenter study of 103 patients.

Comparative study of triamcinolone acetonide and hydrocortisone 17-butyrate in rosacea with special regard to the rebound phenomenon. Go MJ, Wuite J. Dermatologica 1976; 152: 239–46.

The place of steroids in rosacea is ill defined and probably very limited, although their use has been reported in conjunction with standard treatments. In this study with 19 subjects, topical steroids given in conjunction with tetracycline did not cause a rebound phenomenon when the steroids were discontinued.

Treatment of rosacea with ketoconazole. Utas S, Unver U. J Eur Acad Dermatol Venereol 1997; 8: 69–70.

A double-blind, placebo-controlled study of oral ketoconazole 400 mg/day, ketoconazole 2% cream, and both treatments combined in 53 patients. Improvement was reported in all three actively treated groups after 2 weeks.

Treatment of rosacea with bifonazole cream: a preliminary report. Veraldi S, Schianchi-Veraldi R. Ann Ital Derm Clin Sper 1990; 44: 169–71.

Topical bifonazole 1% cream was used successfully in eight cases of rosacea, with no recurrence at 3 months.

Photodynamic therapy in a series of rosacea patients. Bryld LE, Jemec GB. J Eur Acad Dermatol Venereol 2007; 21: 1199–202.

A series of 17 patients with rosacea refractory to previous therapy were treated with PDT using 16% methyl aminolevulinic acid (Metvix) cream applied for 3 hours, followed by 37 J/cm² of red light. Initially patients received one or two treatments at an interval of 1 week, and up to four treatments were used on each treated area if required. A good response was observed in 10 cases.

Oral spironolactone therapy in male patients with rosacea. Aizawa H, Niimura M. J Dermatol 1992; 19: 293–7.

Spironolactone at a dose of 50 mg/day for 4 weeks was reported to benefit seven of 13 male patients with rosacea. Two of the patients did not tolerate the drug.

Demodex folliculorum and topical treatment: action evaluated by standardized skin surface biopsy. Forton F, Seys B, Marchal JL, Song AM. Br J Dermatol 1998; 138: 461–6.

There have been several reports of increased numbers of *Demodex* mites in rosacea – circumstantial evidence to suggest they might be implicated in the pathogenesis in some cases. This has provided a rationale for the use of a range of therapies aimed at eradication of the mites. This study of 34 patients with high *Demodex* carriage compared the miticidal effect of topical metronidazole, permethrin, sulfur, lindane, crotamiton, and benzyl benzoate. Benzyl benzoate and crotamiton had particular effects on the mite population, suggesting that they may be appropriate treatment for some cases of rosacea and 'rosacea-like demodecosis'.

A pilot study of 5% permethrin cream versus 0.75% metronidazole gel in acne rosacea. Signore RJ. Cutis 1995; 56: 177–9.

Six patients who applied 5% permethrin cream to one side of the face and 0.75% metronidazole gel to the other showed similar responses to the two topical agents.

Permethrin 5% cream versus metronidazole 0.75% gel for the treatment of papulopustular rosacea. A randomized double-blind placebo-controlled study. Koçak M, Yagli S, Vahapoglu G, Eksioglu M. Dermatology 2002; 205: 265–70.

Permethrin 5% cream was compared with metronidazole 0.75% gel and placebo, applied twice daily for 2 months in a randomized parallel-group study on 63 subjects. Permethrin was more effective in improving erythema and papules than placebo, and as effective as metronidazole 0.75% gel, but had no effect on telangiectasia, rhinophyma, or pustules. The reduction in demodex counts was significantly greater with permethrin than with the other treatments.

Treatment of rosacea-like demodicidosis with oral ivermectin and topical permethrin cream. Forstinger C, Kittler H, Binder M. J Am Acad Dermatol 1999; 41: 775–7.

A patient suffering from a follicular, papulopustular, facial eruption with a long history of unsuccessful treatment responded to ivermectin 200 µg/kg. This was followed by once-weekly application of 5% permethrin cream to prevent reinfestation.

A study on *Demodex folliculorum* in rosacea. Abd-El-Al AM, Bayoumy AM, Abou Salem EA. J Egypt Soc Parasitol 1997; 27: 183–95.

An open-label study showing benefit from 10% crotamiton cream.

***Helicobacter pylori* eradication treatment reduces the severity of rosacea.** Utas S, Ozbakir O, Turasan A, Utas C. J Am Acad Dermatol 1999; 40: 433–5.

Thirteen patients with rosacea having evidence of *H. pylori* infection received a course of amoxicillin 500 mg three times daily for 2 weeks, metronidazole 500 mg three times daily for

2 weeks, and bismuth subcitrate 300 mg four times daily for 4 weeks. There was a significant reduction in the severity of the rosacea at the end of treatment.

Several investigators have proposed an association between H. pylori *and rosacea, although this remains highly controversial.*

The response of rosacea to eradication of Helicobacter pylori. Son SW, Kim IH, Oh CH, Kim JG. Br J Dermatol 1999; 140: 984–5.

Twenty cases of rosacea were treated with amoxicillin 2.25 g/day for 2 weeks, clarithromycin 1.5 g/day for 2 weeks, and nizatidine 300 mg/day for 6 weeks. The 13 who had evidence of *H. pylori* infection demonstrated significantly greater improvement in erythema than the seven who did not.

The effect of the treatment of *Helicobacter pylori* infection on rosacea. Bamford JL, Tilden RL, Blankush JL, Gangeness DE. Arch Dermatol 1999; 135: 659–63.

A randomized, double-blind placebo-controlled trial of *H. pylori* eradication with clarithromycin and omeprazole or placebo. There was no difference in the rosacea between the two groups at 60 days.

Effective sunscreen ingredients and cutaneous irritation in patients with rosacea. Nichols K, Desai N, Lebwohl MG. Cutis 1998; 61: 344–6.

Patients with rosacea are particularly susceptible to the irritation caused by sunscreen ingredients. Formulations with protective constituents, such as dimethicone and cyclomethicone, may be preferable.

Epidemiological studies of the influence of sunlight on the skin. Berg M. Photodermatology 1989; 6: 80–4.

Individuals with rosacea experienced improvement more often than impairment from exposure to sunlight.

Tacrolimus ointment for the treatment of steroid-induced rosacea: a preliminary report. Goldman D. J Am Acad Dermatol 2001; 44: 995–8.

Corticoid-induced rosacea resolved in three patients after 7–10 days of treatment with topical tacrolimus 0.075% ointment in conjunction with avoidance of topical corticoids and other possible exacerbating factors.

The use of 1% pimecrolimus cream for the treatment of steroid-induced rosacea. Chu CY. Br J Dermatol 2005; 152: 396–9.

Two patients with steroid-induced rosacea responded to topical pimecrolimus.

Pimecrolimus for treatment of acne rosacea. Crawford KM, Russ B, Bostrom P. Skinmed 2005; 4: 147–50.

An open-label study on 12 patients. Improvements were seen in erythema and papulopustular lesions.

Pimecrolimus cream 1% for papulopustular rosacea: a randomized vehicle-controlled double-blind trial. Weissenbacher S, Merkl J, Hildebrandt B, Wollenberg A, Braeutigem M, Ring J, et al. Br J Dermatol 2007: 156: 728–732.

Pimecrolimus was no more effective than placebo.

Tacrolimus effect on rosacea. Bamford JTM, Elliott BA, Haller IV. J Am Acad Dermatol 2004; 50: 107–8.

Topical tacrolimus 0.1% reduced erythema but not papulopustular lesions in this open study with 24 subjects.

Induction of rosaceiform dermatitis during treatment of facial inflammatory dermatoses with tacrolimus ointment. Antille C, Saurat JH, Lübbe J. Arch Dermatol 2004; 140: 457–60.

Rosacea-like eruptions developed or worsened in six patients treating facial dermatoses with tacrolimus.

Topical tacrolimus and pimecrolimus have both been reported to induce rosacea-like eruptions. If there is a role for these topical agents in the management of rosacea, this remains to be clarified.

Incidental control of rosacea by somatostatin. Piérard-Franchimont C, Quatresooz P, Piérard GE. Dermatology 2003; 206: 249–51.

A report of four cases of rosacea which improved during incidental treatment of diabetic retinopathy with a long-acting octreotide injection (Sandostatine) 20 mg monthly.

Octreotide is a somatostatin analog known to be highly active in suppressing the secretion of vasoactive hormones by carcinoid tumors, and reduces the flushing associated with the carcinoid syndrome. It is also worth observing that carcinoid syndrome has occasionally been misdiagnosed as rosacea in the past.

Effect of oral inhibitors of ovulation in treatment of rosacea and dermatitis perioralis in women. Spirov G, Berova N, Vassilev D. Aust J Dermatol 1971; 12: 149–54.

Inhibition of ovulation with an oral contraceptive was associated with improvement of rosacea in 90% of 30 women. An open, uncontrolled study.

Topical application of NADH for the treatment of rosacea and contact dermatitis. Wozniacka A, Sysa-Jedrzejowska A, Adamus J, Gebicki J. Clin Exp Dermatol 2003; 28: 61–3.

Ten cases of rosacea were treated in an open study with 1% NADH in an ointment base. Nine showed some degree of improvement. The response was proposed to be due to the antioxidant properties of NADH.

Topical application of 1-methylnicotinamide in the treatment of rosacea: a pilot study. Wozniacka A, Sysa-Jedrzejowska A, Adamus J, Gebicki J. Clin Exp Dermatol 2005; 30: 632–5.

This compound is a metabolite of nicotinamide with anti-inflammatory properties. Thirty-four patients were treated twice daily with a gel containing 0.25% methylnicotinamide in this open-label pilot study. Improvement was good in nine cases and moderate in 17.

The Nicomide Improvement in Clinical Outcomes Study (NICOS): results of an 8-week trial. Niren NM, Torok HM. Cutis 2006; 77: 17–28.

This compound formulation (Nicomide), comprising nicotinamide 750 mg, zinc 25 mg, copper 1.5 mg, and folic acid 500 μg, was reported as effective in an open-label study on 198 patients with acne vulgaris and/or rosacea.

Oral zinc sulfate in the treatment of rosacea: a double-blind, placebo-controlled study. Sharquie KE, Najim RA, Al-Salman HN. Int J Dermatol 2006; 45: 857–61.

Zinc sulfate 100 mg/day proved more effective than placebo in this crossover trial with 25 patients.

This was a small study with limited power and an apparently pronounced carry-over effect in the group treated with zinc in the first treatment period.

Low-strength trichloroacetic acid in the treatment of rosacea. Auada-Souto MP, Velho PE. J Eur Acad Dermatol Venereol 2007; 21: 1443–5.

In a series of three cases both papulopustular and erythematotelangiectatic features improved after a peel using 10–20% TCA, followed by self-treatment at home using 10% TCA once, twice, and three times a week during the second, third, and fourth months, respectively.

ERYTHEMATOTELANGIECTATIC ROSACEA

▶ Cosmetic camouflage	C
▶ Intense pulsed light	B
▶ Vascular lasers	C
▶ Ondansetron	E

Decorative cosmetics improve the quality of life in patients with disfiguring skin diseases. Boehncke WH, Ochsendorf F, Paeslack I, Kaufmann R, Zollner TM. Eur J Dermatol 2002; 12: 577–80.

Twenty women with a range of dermatoses, including nine with rosacea, completed the DLQI quality of life questionnaire before and after instruction by a cosmetician. The mean score improved from 9.2 to 5.5.

Objective and quantitative improvement of rosacea-associated erythema after intense pulsed light treatment. Mark KA, Sparacio RM, Voigt A, Marenus K, Sarnoff DS. Dermatol Surg 2003; 29: 600–4.

Objective assessments were performed on four subjects before and after IPL therapy for rosacea. Five treatments at 3-week intervals were undertaken using the Photoderm VL machine, with a 515 nm filter, a single pulse of 3 ms duration, and various fluences. Facial blood flow was reduced by 30%, the area of the cheek occupied by telangiectasia was reduced by 29%, and erythema intensity was reduced by 21%.

Treatment of rosacea with intense pulsed light. Taub AF. J Drugs Dermatol 2003; 2: 254–9.

Thirty-two patients underwent one to seven treatments. Eighty-three percent had reduced redness, 75% noted reduced flushing, and 64% noted fewer acneiform breakouts. The treatment was well tolerated.

Treatment of facial vascular lesions with intense pulsed light. Angermeier MC. J Cutan Laser Ther 1999; 1: 95–100.

Two hundred patients with facial pathologies were treated with an intense pulsed light source (PhotoDerm VL) using various treatment parameters. Indications included telangiectasia, hemangiomas, rosacea, and port wine stains. After one to four treatment sessions 75–100% clearance was achieved. Side effects were minimal with no instances of scarring, and were considered less frequent than with laser treatment.

Intense pulsed light (IPL) seems to have emerged as the treatment of choice for rosacea telangiectasia. It can improve not only telangiectasia, but also erythema and flushing. IPL is also generally better tolerated than lasers. Some expertise is required for optimal results.

Selective destruction of facial telangiectasia using a copper vapor laser. Key JM, Waner M. Arch Otololaryngol Head Neck Surg 1992; 118: 509–13.

Twenty patients with facial telangiectasia were treated with the 578-nm option of a copper vapor laser in an office setting. Eighteen experienced satisfactory clearance.

Argon laser treatment of the red nose. Dicken CH. J Dermatol Surg Oncol 1990; 16: 33–6.

A good result was reported in seven patients with telangiectasia due to rosacea.

Flash lamp pumped dye laser for rosacea-associated telangiectasia and erythema. Lowe NJ, Behr KL, Fitzpatrick R, Goldman M, Ruiz-Esparza J. J Dermatol Surg Oncol 1991; 17: 522–5.

This laser gave good or excellent reduction of telangiectasia and erythema and better overall appearance in 24 out of 27 patients after one to three treatments. Papulation and pustulation were also improved.

Pulsed dye laser therapy for rosacea. Tan ST, Bialostocki A, Armstrong JR. Br J Plast Surg 2004; 57: 303–10.

Forty patients were treated and all considered that the treatment was worthwhile. When improvement in erythema and telangiectasis was assessed on a five-point scale by an independent panel of 10, there was a mean score of 3.7, i.e., between slight (3) and moderate (4) improvement.

How laser surgery can help your rosacea patients. West T. Skin Aging 1998; March: 43–6.

A review of the use of lasers and intense pulsed light for rosacea telangiectasia. Intense pulsed light is considered to require more operator skill than the KTP or pulsed dye lasers. This article includes recommended parameters for the use of lasers and intense pulsed light.

The response of erythematous rosacea to ondansetron. Wollina U. Br J Dermatol 1999; 140: 561–2.

Two cases of resistant rosacea responded to the serotonin receptor antagonist ondansetron. This drug, which is a 5-HT antagonist, is used mainly as an antiemetic during chemotherapy. It was initially given intravenously at a dose of 12 mg daily, and later orally at doses of 4–8 mg twice daily. Erythema and also ocular symptoms improved.

Improvement of erythema and flushing has also been reported with granisetron (see below).

ROSACEA FLUSHING

The flushing associated with rosacea is often the most difficult symptom to treat. This symptom often persists even when the inflammatory component is effectively treated. However, some improvement of flushing is not uncommon when erythematotelangiectatic disease is treated with intense pulsed light or lasers. A range of pharmacological approaches have proved beneficial in some cases.

▶ Clonidine	D
▶ β-Blockers	D
▶ Naloxone	D
▶ Rilmenidine	D
▶ Cosmesis	C
▶ Pulsed dye laser	D
▶ Intense pulsed light	D
▶ Hypnosis	E
▶ Oxymetazoline	E
▶ Granisetron	D

Clonidine and facial flushing in rosacea. Cunliffe WJ, Dodman B, Binner JG. Br Med J 1977; 1: 105.

Clonidine 0.05 mg bd was compared with placebo in a crossover trial with 17 subjects. Five of them reported an improvement in the severity and frequency of flushing while on clonidine.

Flushing in rosacea: a possible mechanism. Guarrera M, Parodi A, Cipriani C, Divano C, Rebora A. Arch Dermatol Res 1982; 272: 311–16.

A study of possible pharmacological inhibitors of rosacea flushing. A single 0.15 mg dose of clonidine inhibited the flushing induced by ingestion of 100 mL beer in all five patients tested. The testing was undertaken 1 hour after the oral dose, so that the blood level of clonidine was at its peak during the investigation.

Effect of subdepressor clonidine on flushing reactions in rosacea. Change in malar thermal circulation index during provoked flushing reactions. Wilkin JK. Arch Dermatol 1983; 119: 211–14.

Clonidine can reduce menopausal flushing. In this study clonidine 0.05 mg given orally twice daily did not suppress the flushing reactions provoked by water at 60°C, red wine, and chocolate. Clonidine did reduce the temperature of malar skin, suggesting a vasoconstrictor effect.

Rilmenidine in rosacea: a double-blind study versus placebo. Grosshans E, Michel C, Arcade B, Cribier B. Ann Dermatol Venereol 1997; 124: 687–91.

This is a centrally acting hypotensive drug similar in action to clonidine but with less tendency to cause sedation. In this trial with 34 evaluable subjects the reduction in flushing was higher on rilmenidine 1 mg daily than with placebo, but the difference was not quite significant (p=0.076).

Effect of nadolol on flushing reactions in rosacea. Wilkin JK. J Am Acad Dermatol 1989; 20: 202–5.

A placebo-controlled trial of nadolol 40 mg daily. Spontaneous flushing and flushing provoked in the laboratory by challenges with hot drinks, alcohol, and nicotinic acid were evaluated in 15 subjects. Nadolol had no effect on objective measurements of provoked flushing. There was a trend towards improvement in patient-reported spontaneous flushing.

Alcohol-induced rosacea flushing blocked by naloxone. Bernstein JE, Soltani K. Br J Dermatol 1982; 107: 59–61.

In an experimental setting five subjects with rosacea were investigated to determine whether alcohol-induced rosacea flushing could be inhibited by naloxone 0.8 mg subcutaneously, placebo injection, or chlorpheniramine 12 mg orally. Naloxone effectively prevented alcohol-induced rosacea flushing. Chlorpheniramine or placebo had no consistent effect. This suggests that there may be a role for opioid antagonists in inhibition of this reaction.

Treatment of rosacea with intense pulsed light. Taub AF. J Drugs Dermatol 2003; 2: 254–9.

Thirty-two consecutive patients with Fitzpatrick skin types I–III underwent one to seven treatments with intense pulsed light: 83% had reduced redness, 75% noted reduced flushing and improved skin texture, and 64% noted fewer acneiform breakouts.

Pulsed dye laser treatment of rosacea improves erythema, symptomatology, and quality of life. Tan SR, Tope WD. J Am Acad Dermatol 2004; 51: 592–9.

Sixteen patients with erythematotelangiectatic rosacea were treated with the pulsed dye laser, 15 of them on two occasions. Not only telangiectasia and erythema, but also symptoms including flushing, burning, and stinging, were improved.

The use of intense pulsed light is discussed above under treatment of telangiectasia. It would seem plausible that the pulsed dye laser and IPL may reduce flushing as a secondary effect by reducing the number of dilated capillaries.

Hypnosis in dermatology. Shenefelt PD. Arch Dermatol 2000; 136: 393–9.

Hypnosis has been reported to improve the blushing associated with rosacea.

This is a comprehensive review of the many potential applications for hypnosis in dermatology.

Successful treatment of the erythema and flushing of rosacea using a topically applied selective alpha1-adrenergic receptor agonist, oxymetazoline. Shanler SD, Ondo AL. Arch Dermatol 2007; 143: 1369–71.

Two cases of erythematotelangiectatic rosacea were treated with a commercially available 0.05% solution of oxymetazoline hydrochloride applied once daily to the face. Redness and flushing were markedly improved.

Influence of the 5-HT3 receptor antagonist granisetron on erythema and flushing tendency in rosacea patients. Jansen T. Kosmetische Medizin 2005; 26: 22–4.

Both symptoms improved in a series of 10 patients treated with this antiemetic agent.

ROSACEA LYMPHEDEMA (MORBIHAN'S DISEASE)

This is a particularly refractory, chronic form of rosacea which has received little attention in the literature. Indurated edema develops mainly over the upper half of the face. Treatment is difficult and the evidence base is very limited. Measures that are generally employed include control of underlying inflammatory rosacea using broad-spectrum antibiotics, and facial massage to improve lymphatic drainage.

▶ Broad-spectrum antibiotics	E
▶ Facial massage	E
▶ Isotretinoin with ketotifen and H_1 antagonist	E
▶ Prednisolone with metronidazole	E
▶ CO_2 laser blepharoplasty	E
▶ Surgical debulking of the eyelids	E

The treatment of rosaceous lymphoedema. Jansen T, Plewig G. Clin Exp Dermatol 1997; 22: 57.

Jansen and Plewig have suggested the use of low-dose isotretinoin 0.1–0.2 mg/kg/day over a period of 2–4 months, which may be combined with ketotifen 1–2 mg daily and a potent H_1 antihistamine.

Persistent facial swelling in a patient with rosacea. Scerri L, Saihan EM. Arch Dermatol 1995; 131: 1069–74.

A marked reduction in facial swelling was reported in one case from a reducing course of prednisolone, starting at 30 mg daily and metronidazole 400 mg/day over a 4-month period, followed by metronidazole 200 mg/day.

Morbihan's disease: treatment with CO_2 laser blepharoplasty. Bechara FG, Jansen T, Losch R, Altmeyer P, Hoffmann K. J Dermatol 2004; 31: 113–15.

CO_2 laser blepharoplasty led to good cosmetic results and reduced visual impairment.

Chronic eyelid lymphedema and acne rosacea. Report of two cases. Bernardini FP, Kersten RC, Khouri LM, Moin M, Kulwin DR, Mutasin DF. Ophthalmology 2000; 107: 2220–3.

Surgical debulking of the affected soft tissue resulted in very satisfactory cosmetic and functional improvement in both patients.

OCULAR ROSACEA

Ocular involvement in rosacea is very common and may even be seen in isolation or before the onset of cutaneous features. Symptoms are most frequently related to the occurrence of blepharitis, episcleritis, chalazion, or hordeolum. Rosacea keratitis can be a serious complication and may occur in adults and children. Severe or refractory cases of ocular disease require specialist ophthalmologic supervision. Particular care is required if systemic retinoids are to be used for inflammatory rosacea when ocular features are present. Retinoids impair meibomian gland secretion, impairing tear film formation and aggravating the dryness and 'grittiness' of the eyes.

▶ Tear substitutes, e.g., carbomers, liquid paraffin, hypromellose	C
▶ Oral tetracyclines	A
▶ Fucidic acid (topical)	C
▶ *H. pylori* eradication	D
▶ Odansetron	E

Oxytetracycline in the treatment of ocular rosacea: a double-blind trial. Bartholomew RS, Reid BJ, Cheesbrough MJ, Macdonald M, Galloway NR. Br J Ophthalmol 1982; 66: 386–8.

Thirty-five patients were investigated in a trial of systemic oxytetracycline, 250 mg twice daily for 6 weeks. Oxytetracycline produced a significantly higher number of remissions than placebo.

Efficacy of doxycycline and tetracycline in ocular rosacea. Frucht-Pery J, Sagi E, Hemo I, Ever-Hadani P. Am J Ophthalmol 1993; 116: 88–92.

Twenty-four patients were randomized to receive doxycycline 100 mg/day or tetracycline 1 g/day. Both groups improved. At 6 weeks all patients except one had symptomatic improvement.

Effects of minocycline on the ocular flora of patients with acne rosacea or seborrheic blepharitis. Ta CN, Shine WE, McCulley JP, Pandya A, Trattler W, Norbury JW. Cornea 2003; 22: 545–8.

Six patients with rosacea and meibomianitis had marked improvement.

Placebo controlled trial of fusidic acid gel and oxytetracycline for recurrent blepharitis and rosacea. Seal DV, Wright P, Ficker L, Hagan K, Troski M, Menday P. Br J Ophthalmol 1995; 79: 42–5.

Seventy-five percent of patients with blepharitis and associated rosacea were symptomatically improved by fusidic acid gel and 50% by oxytetracycline, but fewer (35%) appeared to benefit from combined treatment.

Ocular rosacea and treatment of symptomatic *Helicobacter pylori* infection: a case series. Dakovic Z, Vesic S, Vukovic J, Milenkovic S, Jankovic-Terzic K, Dukic S, et al. Acta Dermatovenerol Alp Panonica Adriat 2007; 16: 83–6.

Ocular disease responded better than cutaneous rosacea to eradication of *H. pylori* in this series of seven patients.

The response of erythematous rosacea to ondansetron. Wollina U. Br J Dermatol 1999; 140: 561–2.

Two cases of resistant rosacea responded to the serotonin receptor antagonist ondansetron. This drug, which is a 5-HT antagonist, is used mainly as an antiemetic during chemotherapy. It was initially given intravenously at a dose of 12 mg daily, and later orally at doses of 4–8 mg twice daily. Erythema and also ocular symptoms improved.

ROSACEA FULMINANS

Rosacea fulminans (pyoderma faciale) is a very severe facial eruption of sudden onset with prominent pustulation and abscess formation. In addition to conventional treatment modalities for rosacea, a short course of systemic steroids is often indicated to reduce the acute inflammation. Isotretinoin seems to be useful in this condition.

▶ Systemic corticosteroids	C
▶ Topical corticosteroids	D
▶ Isotretinoin	C
▶ Systemic antibiotics	C

Pyoderma faciale: a review and report of 20 additional cases: is it rosacea? Plewig G, Jansen T, Kligman AM. Arch Dermatol 1992; 128: 1611–17.

Ten of these 20 patients were hospitalized to commence treatment. Prednisolone was commenced at 1 mg/kg/day for 1–2 weeks before adding isotretinoin 0.2–0.5 mg/kg/day. The corticosteroid was then tapered off over 2–3 weeks and the isotretinoin continued for 3–4 months.

Treatment of rosacea fulminans with isotretinoin and topical alclometasone dipropionate. Veraldi S, Scarabelli G, Rizzitelli G, Caputo R. Eur J Dermatol 1996; 6: 94–6.

Five cases were treated successfully with this combination. Alclometasone dipropionate cream (a moderate-potency corticosteroid) was applied twice daily for 10 days then daily for 10 days. The initial dose of isotretinoin was 0.5 mg/kg/day for 1 month followed by 0.7 mg/kg/day for 3 months. Combined cyproterone acetate/ethinylestradiol was used as a contraceptive.

Marked improvement was observed after a month and complete resolution after 4 months.

Pyoderma faciale – a clinical study of 29 patients. Massa MC, Su WP. J Am Acad Dermatol 1982; 6: 84–91.

Thirteen of these patients were hospitalized. All were treated with antibiotics, most frequently tetracycline, minocycline, or erythromycin. Vleminckx packs (containing sulfur, calcium polysulfide, and calcium thiosulfate) were used for 21 cases and were considered the most effective topical treatment. Other modalities employed included benzoyl peroxide and UVB.

Evidence Levels: **A** Double-blind study **B** Clinical trial ≥ 20 subjects **C** Clinical trial < 20 subjects **D** Series ≥ 5 subjects **E** Anecdotal case reports

Sarcoidosis

Pascal G Ferzli, Warren R Heymann

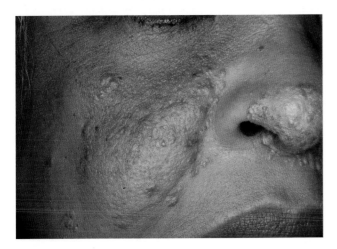

Sarcoidosis is a multisystem disease of unknown etiology characterized histologically by non-caseating granulomas. It is considered to be immune mediated, with a Th1-predominant cytokine profile. Skin manifestations are observed in approximately 25% of cases. Recently, sarcoidosis has been reported to develop following exposure to inorganic particles in the environment. The use of polymerase chain reaction (PCR) techniques has also led to the identification of mycobacterial and propionibacterial DNA and RNA in sarcoidal tissue. Sarcoidosis may be the end result of immune responses to those or other specific triggers. The age of genetic analysis will allow us to identify individuals with a greater risk for developing sarcoidosis based on their genotypic variation. Therapy for erythema nodosum associated with sarcoidosis is addressed in the chapter on erythema nodosum.

MANAGEMENT STRATEGY

The treatment of cutaneous sarcoidosis depends on the type and extent of lesions present and is directed at suppressing the formation of granulomas. Guidelines for treating extracutaneous involvement can be found elsewhere, but it should be recognized that therapy for internal involvement may take precedence over skin disease and that response to treatment may be variable, depending on the type of tissue involved.

In small papular or extremely localized sarcoidosis, treatment with *potent topical corticosteroids* or *intralesional triamcinolone acetonide* (3.3–10 mg/mL) is reasonable. If this is ineffective or involvement is more diffuse, *oral chloroquine* (initial dose 250 mg twice daily) or *hydroxychloroquine* (initial dose 200 mg twice daily) may be effective. If no response is seen with antimalarials, or disfiguring lesions are present, *oral prednisone* can be used at a dose of 1 mg/kg daily (maximum 60 mg) for up to 3 months, and then tapered if improvement or a stable level is reached, to a maintenance dose of 5–10 mg on alternate days for several months. Periodic escalations in dose are necessary with flares.

Methotrexate may be used as a corticosteroid-sparing agent or as monotherapy in those patients with lupus pernio, ulcer-

ative sarcoidosis, or severe disease that has not responded to prednisone. Initial doses of 15–20 mg weekly are favored. *Thalidomide, azathioprine, chlorambucil, isotretinoin,* or *allopurinol* could be considered if methotrexate fails in this subset of patients. Azathioprine and chlorambucil are better studied in patients with pulmonary sarcoidosis. Thalidomide seems to be more effective than isotretinoin and allopurinol in cutaneous disease. Reported failures are described with etretinate and allopurinol.

Biologic agents that inhibit tumor necrosis factor (TNF)-α are new therapeutic modalities that should be reserved for recalcitrant cutaneous sarcoidosis. Infliximab may be more effective than adalimumab, but may be associated with a higher rate of infection and autoimmune disease. Etanercept does not appear to be useful for the treatment of sarcoidosis, but some studies have reported on its potential role in patients developing sarcoidosis, or in relapse of pre-existing sarcoidosis.

Leflunomide has shown promise in the treatment of cutaneous sarcoidosis unresponsive to other therapies, but further studies are needed to establish its long-term usefulness.

Localized disease that does not respond to topical or intralesional corticosteroids, or in those cases in which the use of systemic antimalarials or corticosteroids is undesirable, may represent a niche for other modalities, such as *excision, laser, or intralesional chloroquine.*

SPECIFIC INVESTIGATIONS

- ▶ Special stains, cultures, and polarization of biopsy specimens
- ▶ Electrolytes, blood urea nitrogen, creatinine, serum calcium, liver function tests, complete blood count, 24-hour urine calcium, and serum angiotensin-converting enzyme (ACE)
- ▶ Ophthalmologic evaluation, including slit-lamp examination
- ▶ Chest radiograph, pulmonary function tests
- ▶ Electrocardiogram
- ▶ FDG PET* is useful in identifying sites for diagnostic biopsy (for patients without apparent lung involvement)
- ▶ MRI with gadolinium (neurological sarcoidosis may occur without any other internal organ involvement)
- ▶ Bone density scans in patients on long-term oral corticosteroids

* Denotes F-fluorodeoxyglucose positron-emission tomography

Sarcoidosis. Iannuzzi MC, Rybicki BA, Teirstein AS. N Engl J Med 2007; 357: 2153–65.

A thorough review of the literature that discusses advances in the diagnosis and treatment of sarcoidosis and the challenges that clinicians may encounter.

Cutaneous sarcoidosis therapy updated. Badgwell C, Rosen T. J Am Acad Dermatol 2007; 56: 69–83.

The initiation of sarcoidal granuloma formation involves the deposition of poorly soluble antigenic material into tissue, which is processed by antigen-presenting cells. Although no specific antigen has been identified, the primary immune response causing sarcoidosis is Th1: elevated IFN-γ, IL-2, and IL-12.

Genotype-corrected reference values for serum angiotensin-converting enzyme. Biller H, Zissel G, Ruprecht B, Nauck M, Busse Grawitz A, Müller-Quernheim J. Eur Respir J 2006; 28: 1085–90.

In this study, 159 Caucasian patients donated blood for ACE genotype analysis and ACE levels. The authors report that the deletion (D)/insertion (I) genotype is the factor that has the greatest impact on ACE level. They found that ACE genotypes and phenotypes correlated significantly: the highest ACE levels were found in patients with the D/D genotype, whereas patients with the I/I genotype had the lowest. They emphasize the need to use the new genotype-corrected reference values in order to study and follow sarcoidosis patients undergoing therapy.

FIRST-LINE THERAPIES

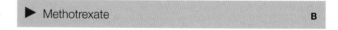

▶ Topical corticosteroids	C
▶ Intralesional corticosteroids	C
▶ Oral corticosteroids	C
▶ Chloroquine	B
▶ Hydroxychloroquine	C

Sarcoidosis in a preschooler with only skin and joint involvement. Fetil E, Ozkan S, Ilknur T, Kavukçu S, Kusku E, Lebe B. Pediatr Dermatol 2003; 20: 416–18.

A 3-year-old boy presented with cutaneous sarcoidosis in the form of lichenoid papules on the trunk and extremities, associated with tender swelling of the ankle and wrist joints. Topical steroid therapy led to remission of the cutaneous lesions, but there was no change in the joints involved.

Potent topical corticosteroid use is reported to be of some value in anecdotal reports. Most authors believe that intralesional corticosteroids are more effective, yet this too is anecdotal. Small lesions would be optimal candidates, but lupus pernio has also been reported to respond.

A case of scar sarcoidosis of the eyelid. Kim YJ, Kim YD. Korean J Ophthalmol 2006; 20: 238–40.

A 29-year-old man presented with a mass on his right eyelid that was biopsied and found to be sarcoidosis. The patient had no other findings of systemic sarcoidosis. A total of 0.6 mL of intralesional triamcinolone 40 mg/mL was injected at 1 cm intervals along the eyelid. Dramatic improvement of the lesion had occurred when he returned for his 1-month follow-up: he received an additional 1 mL of triamcinolone at the same site, which resolved the lesion completely.

Anecdotal reports suggest small, papular sarcoid responds best. The strength of triamcinolone acetonide varies from 2 to 40 mg/mL, and frequency varies from weekly to monthly.

Evidence-based therapy for cutaneous sarcoidosis. Baughman RP, Lower EE. Clin Dermatol 2007; 25: 334–40.

Whereas the recommended starting dose of prednisone for pulmonary sarcoidosis is suggested to be 20–40 mg daily, the dose and duration of treatment for cutaneous sarcoidosis has not been established. The authors suggest using this as a benchmark and tapering the steroid dose after 1 or 2 months to one that controls the disease while avoiding toxicity. They report that the need for long-term systemic corticosteroids for treatment of chronic sarcoidosis occurs in about a quarter of patients.

Another suggested regimen of prednisone in cutaneous sarcoidosis is 30 mg on alternate days until the granulomas fade. The dose is then tapered over several months to 15 mg on alternate days. Recurrences are managed by increasing back to the initial dose. Other protocols report a good response with prednisone 30–40 mg daily, with a gradual taper to 10–20 mg on alternate days for 1 year, or prednisone 1 mg/kg daily (maximum 60 mg) for 8–12 weeks, with a taper to 0.25 mg/kg daily continued for 6 months.

Patients on long-term oral corticosteroids should be started on bisphosphonates and undergo yearly bone density scans in order to prevent osteoporosis. If there is no contraindication, they should also be started on Pneumocystis carinii pneumonia (PCP) prophylaxis with appropriate antibiotics.

Treatment of cutaneous sarcoidosis with chloroquine: review of the literature. Zic JA, Horowitz DH, Arzubiaga C, King LE. Arch Dermatol 1991; 127: 1034–40.

A review of the efficacy and safety of chloroquine in the treatment of cutaneous sarcoidosis. The article cites four studies – three open clinical trials and one case series – that support the use of chloroquine. The authors recommend an initial dose of 250 mg twice daily for 14 days, then 250 mg daily for long-term suppression, though most studies have used 500 mg daily for several months. Relapses after discontinuation of treatment are frequent.

Hydroxychloroquine is effective therapy for control of cutaneous sarcoidal granulomas. Jones EJ, Callen JP. J Am Acad Dermatol 1990; 23: 487–9.

Seventeen patients were treated with 200 mg daily or 400 mg daily of hydroxychloroquine. Cutaneous lesions regressed in 12 patients within 4–12 weeks, and three patients had a partial response. Of the 12 patients with the best response, six had a recurrence after a dosage reduction or discontinuation.

Hydroxychloroquine may have a better safety profile than chloroquine; however, chloroquine has been better studied in sarcoidosis. Furthermore, a case series of 15 patients has documented a poor response to hydroxychloroquine at 500–1000 mg daily.

SECOND LINE THERAPIES

▶ Methotrexate	B

Methotrexate is steroid sparing in acute sarcoidosis: results of a double blind, randomized trial. Baughman RP, Winget DB, Lower EE. Sarcoidosis Vasc Diffuse Lung Dis 2000; 17: 60–6.

Twenty-four patients with new-onset symptomatic pulmonary disease were randomized to receive either methotrexate or placebo, in addition to their prednisone. Although only 15 patients received at least 6 months of therapy, the methotrexate group required less prednisone than the placebo group. There was no difference in toxicity between the methotrexate and the placebo groups.

To date, this is the only randomized placebo-controlled trial for the treatment of sarcoidosis with methotrexate. A favorable response is usually expected after several months of therapy, and the dose can be tapered weekly after 4–6 months.

Some studies indicate that methotrexate may be particularly useful for those with ulcerative sarcoidosis.

Evidence Levels: **A** Double-blind study **B** Clinical trial ≥ 20 subjects **C** Clinical trial < 20 subjects **D** Series ≥ 5 subjects **E** Anecdotal case reports

Prolonged use of methotrexate for sarcoidosis. Lower EE, Baughman RP. Arch Intern Med 1995; 155: 846–51.

Fifty patients were treated with methotrexate, 10 mg weekly, for a minimum of 2 years. Most patients did not have cutaneous involvement, but in those who did a good response was seen. In many patients methotrexate was used in conjunction with prednisone, with favorable results.

THIRD-LINE THERAPIES

▶ Thalidomide	D
▶ Allopurinol	D
▶ Isotretinoin	E
▶ Azathioprine	E
▶ Chlorambucil	E
▶ Quinacrine	D
▶ Minocycline, doxycycline	D
▶ Clofazimine	E
▶ Fumaric acid esters	E
▶ Topical tacrolimus	E
▶ Intralesional chloroquine	E
▶ Excision	D
▶ Laser	E
▶ Melatonin	D
▶ Pentoxifylline	E
▶ Leflunomide	D
▶ Infliximab	D
▶ Adalimumab	E
▶ Etanercept	E
▶ Medium-dose UVA1	E

Treatment of cutaneous sarcoidosis with thalidomide. Nguyen YT, Dupuy A, Cordoliani F, Vignon-Pennamen MD, Lebbé C, Morel P, et al. J Am Acad Dermatol 2004; 50: 235–41.

A retrospective evaluation of 12 patients with cutaneous sarcoidosis, two with systemic involvement, 10 of whom were treated successfully with a treatment duration of 2 to more than 16 months with a daily dose of thalidomide ranging from 50–200 mg daily. Two patients received combined therapy with oral corticosteroids (dose ranging from 7.5 to 30 mg daily), one patient used potent topical corticosteroids, and one received combined therapy with methotrexate (dose 25 mg weekly). The average response time was 2–3 months. The main adverse effect noted in this series was deep venous thrombosis in one patient.

A case of cutaneous acral sarcoidosis with response to allopurinol. Antony F, Layton AM. Br J Dermatol 2000; 142: 1052–3.

A 38-year-old Afro-Caribbean man with painful sarcoidal nodules around the ends of his fingers (but no evidence of sarcoidal arthritis) had a partial response to oral and intralesional steroids with subsequent recurrence of his lesions. He had no improvement with hydroxychloroquine, methotrexate, or azathioprine. He was started on allopurinol 100 mg twice daily, which was increased to 300 mg daily after 3 weeks. This resulted in sustained objective clinical improvement.

A few case reports demonstrate resolution of truncal and extremity plaques of sarcoidosis after 12 weeks of allopurinol.

Cutaneous sarcoidosis: complete remission after oral isotretinoin therapy. Georgiou S, Monastirli A, Pasmatzi E, Tsambaos D. Acta Dermatol Venereol 1998; 78: 457–9.

A 31-year-old woman with nodules and plaques on the trunk and extremities showed a complete remission with 8 months of isotretinoin at 1 mg/kg daily; 15-month follow-up revealed continuing remission.

Two other cases report improvement with a 30-week course (0.67–1.34 mg/kg daily) and a 6-month course (0.4–1 mg/kg daily), respectively, of isotretinoin.

Long-term use of azathioprine as a steroid-sparing treatment. Hof DG, Hof PC, Godfrey WA. Am J Respir Crit Care Med 1996; 153: 870A.

Of the 21 patients in this study, eight had 'multisystem' involvement and one had skin-only involvement. All patients with extrapulmonary disease achieved a complete remission with azathioprine and a tapering dose of prednisone.

Chlorambucil treatment of sarcoidosis. Israel HL, McComb BL. Sarcoidosis. 1991; 8: 35–41.

In this study, 31 patients received chlorambucil because complicating diseases prevented them from received corticosteroids, or they did not respond to them. Marked improvement was noted in 15 patients, moderate improvement in 13 patients, but relapses were very common upon discontinuation. No immune suppression-related side effects were noted.

Scar sarcoidosis following tattooing of the lips treated with mepacrine. Yesudian PD, Azurdia RM. Clin Exp Dermatol 2004; 29: 552–4.

A 50-year-old woman with disfiguring scar sarcoidosis of the lips responded poorly to steroids and was unable to tolerate hydroxychloroquine; she was started on mepacrine 100 mg daily with significant remission to practically normal lip margins. She has had no flares in 10 months of follow-up visits.

The yellow discoloration of the skin and sclera observed with quinacrine (one-third of patients) makes chloroquine and hydroxychloroquine better alternatives.

The use of tetracyclines for the treatment of sarcoidosis. Bachelez H, Senet P, Cadranel J, Kaoukhov A, Dubertret L. Arch Dermatol 2001; 137: 69–73.

Twelve patients with cutaneous sarcoidosis, three of whom had systemic involvement, were treated with minocycline at a daily dose of 200 mg for a median duration of 12 months. Ten patients showed a response, eight complete and two partial; one patient's symptoms remained stable and one patient's disease progressed. For patients experiencing relapse after discontinuation of minocycline, doxycycline was used, resulting in remission.

Disseminated small-node cutaneous sarcoidosis. Schwarzenbach R, Djawari D. Dtsch Med Wochenschr 2000; 125: 560–2.

An 83-year-old woman with cutaneous sarcoidosis without systemic involvement was treated with clofazimine 300 mg daily tapered over 4 months, with resolution of cutaneous findings.

Successful treatment of recalcitrant cutaneous sarcoidosis with fumaric acid esters. Nowack U, Gambichler T, Hanefeld C, Kastner U, Altmeyer P. BMC Dermatol 2002; 24: 215.

Report of three patients with cutaneous sarcoidosis treated with fumaric acid esters for 4–12 months, resulting in complete clearance of cutaneous lesions.

Successful topical treatment of cutaneous sarcoidosis with tacrolimus. Gutzmer R, Volker B, Kapp A, Werfel T. Hautarzt 2003; 54: 1193–7.

Topical tacrolimus was used for cutaneous sarcoidosis of the face for 3 months, with nearly complete remission lasting for at least 4 months.

Intralesional chloroquine for the treatment of cutaneous sarcoidosis. Liedtka JE. Int J Dermatol 1996; 35: 682–3.

Multiple injections of intralesional chloroquine hydrochloride (50 mg/mL) were effective in treating five lesions in a single patient, with minimal side effects.

Cutaneous nasal sarcoidosis – treatment by excision and split-skin grafting. Goldin JH, Jawad SMA, Reis AP. J Laryngol Otol 1983; 97: 1053–6.

Split-thickness and full-thickness skin grafts, dermabrasion, and primary closure have been attempted, with mixed results. Surgery has been used in ulcerative and non-ulcerative sarcoidosis.

CO_2 laser vaporization for disfiguring lupus pernio. Young HS, Chalmers RJ, Griffiths CE, August PJ. J Cosmet Laser Ther 2002; 4: 87–90.

CO_2 laser resurfacing was used in two patients with lupus pernio, with a favorable cosmetic result.

Flashlamp pulsed dye laser and Q-switched ruby laser were beneficial in one case report of lupus pernio. However, exacerbations of lupus pernio, namely generalized ulceration in treated and untreated lesions, have been reported following this therapy.

Scar sarcoidosis in a child: case report of successful treatment with the pulsed dye laser. Holzmann RD, Astner S, Forschner T, Sterry G. Dermatol Surg 2008; 34: 393–6.

A 10-year-old boy with a 1.0 cm lesion of varicella zoster-induced scar sarcoidosis on the left cheek had not responded to systemic antibiotics or systemic steroids. Clinical remission occurred after three pulsed dye laser treatments at 6-week intervals which consisted of two to four pulses using a 595-nm wavelength and a 0.5 ms pulse duration. At 12 months' follow-up there was no evidence of recurrence, although the varicella scar became more visible once the sarcoidosis disappeared.

Melatonin is a safe and effective treatment for chronic pulmonary and extrapulmonary sarcoidosis. Pignone AM, Rosso AD, Fiori G, Matucci-Cerinic M, Becucci A, Tempestini A, et al. J Pineal Res 2006; 41: 95–100.

Melatonin was given for 2 years to 18 chronic sarcoid patients at a dose of 20 mg/day during the first year and 10 mg/day during the second year. Normalization of ACE levels was found in patients receiving melatonin. Hilar adenopathy resolved completely in eight patients, and parenchymal lesions were improved in all. Skin lesions, present in three patients, completely disappeared after 24 months of treatment. No side effects were reported.

Melatonin may increase drowsiness, and has been associated with hypothermia, hypotension, and bradycardia.

Pentoxifylline in treatment of sarcoidosis. Zabel P, Entzian P, Dalhoff K, Schlaak M. Am J Respir Crit Care Med 1997; 155: 1665–9.

Twenty-three previously untreated patients with pulmonary sarcoidosis were given pentoxifylline at 25 mg/kg/day. Of 18 patients that remained, 11 demonstrated improvement in their pulmonary function. Major side effects included mild bleeding diathesis, gastrointestinal symptoms, and restlessness.

Leflunomide for chronic sarcoidosis. Baughman RP, Lower EE. Sarcoidosis Vasc Diffuse Lung Dis 2004; 21: 43–8.

In a case series study, 32 patients with sarcoidosis involving the eye, lung and/or skin were treated with leflunomide. Remission (complete and partial) was seen in 12 of 17 patients treated with leflunomide, and 13 of 15 patients treated with leflunomide and methotrexate. An initial dose of leflunomide 100 mg/day for 3 days was followed by 20 mg daily after that.

Adverse events included gastrointestinal problems (diarrhea, abdominal pain, nausea, vomiting, elevated liver function tests). Hypersensitivity reactions, including erythema multiforme and Stevens–Johnson syndrome, have also been reported.

Treatment of sarcoidosis with infliximab. Doty JD, Mazur JE, Judson MA. Chest 2005; 127: 1064–71.

Ten patients with sarcoidosis recalcitrant to previous therapies were treated with infliximab. Infliximab is administered via intravenous infusion in doses ranging from 3 to 10 mg/kg/dose at 0, 2, 6, and every 8–10 weeks after that. Nine of 10 patients reported subjective improvement of their lesions, and all 10 were found to have objective measures of improvement. All five patients with lupus pernio experienced significant improvement or clearance of the lesions.

Infliximab has been shown to increase the risk of tuberculosis reactivation, of granulomatous infections, lymphomas, and autoimmune disease. Therapy is expensive, costing up to thousands of dollars per infusion.

Adalimumab for treatment of cutaneous sarcoidosis. Heffernan MP, Smith DI. Arch Dermatol 2006; 142: 17–19.

A 46-year-old black woman with cutaneous sarcoidosis in the form of papules on the nose and ulcerating nodules on the legs had failed local therapy with topical clobetasol and intralesional kenalog, plaquenil, and pentoxifylline. She did not tolerate minocycline. Adalimumab was administered at a dose of 40 mg subcutaneously once weekly. After 10 weeks the nodules on her legs were completely healed, and the lesions on her nose were significantly improved.

Another case report highlights the successful use of adalimumab in a 55-year-old woman with ulcerative cutaneous sarcoidosis.

Etanercept does not appear to be useful for the treatment of sarcoidosis. In a double-blind randomized trial it showed no improvement in the treatment of ocular sarcoidosis. There are also a few reports of the new development or relapse of sarcoidosis in patients treated with etanercept.

Etanercept ameliorates sarcoidosis, arthritis and skin disease. Khanna D, Liebling MR, Louie JS. J Rheumatol 2003; 30: 1864–7.

Case report of a patient with therapy-resistant sarcoidosis responding to etanercept.

More recently, a double-blind randomized trial for treatment of ocular sarcoidosis with etanercept showed no comparative improvement in the sarcoidal lesions. Also, sarcoidosis was reported to develop in a patient with ankylosing spondylitis after being treated with etanercept.

Cutaneous sarcoidosis treated with medium-dose UVA1. Mahnke N, Medve-Koenigs K, Berneburg M, Ruzicka T, Neumann NJ. J Am Acad Dermatol 2004; 50: 978–9.

An 82-year-old woman with cutaneous sarcoidosis affecting 80% of her body surface was treated with medium-dose UVA1 radiation four times weekly. She received 20 J/cm^2 for the first three treatment sessions, 40 J/cm^2 for the following 12 sessions, and then 60 J/cm^2 for the next 35 sessions. After 50 sessions, nearly all lesions had resolved. This was proved with skin biopsies 5 months after the end of the phototherapy.

This is a singular case report: no other studies have tried to reproduce the results reported here.

Scabies

William FG Tucker

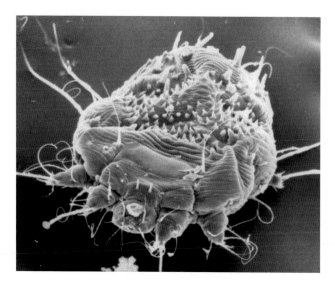

Scabies is a characteristically pruritic skin condition due to infestation by the itch mite *Sarcoptes scabiei*. Patients can be of any age or social strata, and personal hygiene is no guarantor of freedom from infection. Heavy parasitization results in crusted or 'Norwegian scabies,' and tends to occur in the elderly, people who are mentally disadvantaged, the immunocompromised, and those unable to scratch.

MANAGEMENT STRATEGY

Infection with the scabies mite results from close personal contact with an infected individual, and generally requires prolonged skin-to-skin contact, such as handholding, sexual intercourse, and/or sharing a bed. Where an infected person is heavily colonized, as in crusted scabies, their clothing and surroundings can become sufficiently contaminated with live mites as to cause a significant hazard to their attendants and companions.

Because newly infected patients do not begin to itch until 4–8 weeks after being infested, and may have little or no visible rash, the infection is passed on easily and unintentionally. Once sensitized to the mite, reinfestation results in immediate symptoms. Equally, itching can continue for a week or two after mite cure. Secondary impetiginization is common in children.

Itching at night and when warm is a hallmark feature.

Suspicion is the prerequisite for disease control because many patients are assumed by family physicians and other medical attendants to have eczema or other skin disorders.

Total isolation from other people is clearly unnecessary with a causative organism that cannot jump or fly, and can survive for only approximately 72 hours away from the skin.

Topical application of antiscabetic agents is standard practice. *Sulfur* was the first effective agent and is still used in many countries, and when nothing else is suitable, as in very young infants. *Benzoyl benzoate* has been the mainstay of therapy, and is cheap and effective if used properly. It has an unfortunate tendency to cause eczematous rashes after repeat applications, and has fallen from favor in most western countries. *Lindane (γ-benzene hexachloride)* was in very widespread use until recently, and is very effective. Unfortunately, it accumulates in body fat stores and has been implicated in causing neurologic damage in infants; it has been withdrawn in the UK. Where lindane is used, the risk of toxicity is reduced by not bathing before treatment, showering 12 hours later, and not having more than two treatments per month. *Malathion* is well tolerated and has the theoretic advantage of prolonged retention in the epidermis, so that reinfection may be reduced. *Permethrin* has been the latest agent to be used and seems to be well tolerated and effective. Readers who are gardeners will recognize these agents, and realize their limitations.

Crotamiton is favored in primary care because it is also antipruritic. *Monosulfiram soap* was reported effective, but has been withdrawn from the UK market.

With all topical agents the key to success is to ensure that adequate concentrations of the scabicide are in contact with the skin for long periods. It is generally accepted that the face and scalp do not need treatment except in infants and the immunocompromised, although some may argue this is a source of treatment failure. Other reservoirs of infection include the subungual areas. What is essential is that *all intimates of the patient, whether apparently infected or not, are treated* at about the same time. Many clinicians find a simple explanatory leaflet, which can also emphasize the need to *launder clothes and bedding*, helpful.

What should be done if this does not work, there is severe eczematization, and/or compliance is doubtful? Oral therapy would seem to be the answer, and *ivermectin* in single doses of 200 µg/kg has been shown to be very effective in a number of studies, although it is no more effective than *properly applied permethrin*. It is unlicensed for this use in humans, but is used in animal 'mange' and is widely and safely used in onchocerciasis.

SPECIFIC INVESTIGATIONS

► Visualization of mites and burrows

The one specific investigation for scabies is to isolate the mite; nothing is more guaranteed to ensure compliance than to show a patient their co-dweller under the bench microscope. Dermatologists take a great delight in capturing their quarry, and each will be an advocate of one particular method. With standard scabies, burrows are generally easiest to find around the hands, and the mite can often be seen as a dark dot at one end. With the aid of a blunt needle or sewing pin, the mite is then winkled out and placed on a glass slide. It should be noted that hypodermic needles are useless for this purpose because they slice and shred the mite! Alternatively, the burrow is carefully scraped or shaved with a 15 Bard–Parker blade and the slice of stratum corneum placed on a glass slide with some immersion oil. As the slide warms up the mite can be seen moving, and her eggs may also be seen. Both methods require practice and skill. Scraping/shaving is the test of choice in crusted scabies. If you have neither the time, the equipment, nor the expertise for this, mite presence can be proved in a number of other ways. Skin biopsy is often illuminating, particularly because the mite may be a surprise finding. A dermatoscope can actually enable you to visualize the mite in situ, and is a useful aid in visiting elderly persons in residential homes; there is a characteristic 'delta' appearance at one end.

682

The single most useful piece of portable diagnostic equipment is a fountain pen. A blob of ink is carefully applied to a suspected burrow, left for a minute or so, and wiped off with an isopropyl alcohol swab. If a burrow is present, then capillary action will have led to tracking of the ink into the burrow, leaving a wiggly line. Less traditional doctors substitute felt-tip pens with apparent success. Tetracycline solution has been used for the same purpose, along with a UV lamp, but why complicate matters?

Laboratory testing will frequently show a mild eosinophilia in peripheral blood.

FIRST-LINE THERAPIES

▶ Permethrin 5% cream	A
▶ Malathion 0.5% lotion	C
▶ Benzyl benzoate	B
▶ Lindane	A

Permethrin 5% dermal cream: a new treatment for scabies. Taplin D, Meinking TL, Porcelain SL, Castillero PM, Chen JA. J Am Acad Dermatol 1986; 15: 995–1001.

Fifty-two patients in a rural community in Panama with a high endemic scabies infection rate were randomly selected, with microscopic confirmation of mite presence in all but five. They were given a single head-to-toe application of either lindane 1% lotion or permethrin 5% cream. Microscopic confirmation of cure was sought at 2 and 4 weeks, with permethrin coming out ahead and curing 21 of 23 patients, compared to a cure rate of 15 of the 24 patients treated with lindane.

Sarcoptes scabiei **infestation treated with malathion liquid.** Hanna NF, Clay JC, Harris JRW. Br J Vener Dis 1978; 54: 354.

An uncontrolled study using 0.5% malathion liquid in 30 patients, yielding an 83% cure rate at 4 weeks. Surprisingly, as this has become the recommended first-line treatment for scabies in the *British National Formulary*, there has been a dearth of randomized controlled trials showing its efficacy.

A family based study on the treatment of scabies with benzyl benzoate and sulphur ointment. Gulati PV, Singh KP. Ind J Dermatol Venereol Leprol 1978; 44: 269–73.

One hundred and fifty-eight clinically diagnosed patients were randomly allocated to use either 25% benzyl benzoate emulsion or 5% sulfur ointment. Treatment was applied at least three times over 24 hours. The sulfur seems to have been marginally more effective.

Interventions for treating scabies. Strong M, Johnstone PW. Cochrane Databases of Systematic Review 2007, Issue 3, Art No: CD000 320. DOI: 10.1002?14651858.CD.000320.PS2.

A very comprehensive review of all published work, but with strict exclusion criteria: 50 of 70 studies were excluded! Recently updated. Overall, permethrin comes out best.

SECOND-LINE THERAPIES

▶ Sulfur	B
▶ Crotamiton	B
▶ Ivermectin	A

Therapeutic efficacy, secondary effects, and patient acceptability of 10% sulfur in either pork fat or cold cream for the treatment of scabies. Avila-Romay A, Alvarez-Franco M, Ruiz-Maldonada R. Pediatr Dermatol 1991; 8: 64–6.

Readers will be pleased to learn that cold cream came out best, with no clinical failures at day 10 in the 26 patients (of 51) assigned to this arm of the trial. Interestingly, there were more side effects, such as pruritus and burning sensations, in the pork-fat group. However, sulfur was effective and cheap.

Permethrin versus crotamiton and lindane in the treatment of scabies. Amer M, El-Gharib I. Int J Dermatol 1992; 31: 357–8.

Comparison of crotamiton 10% cream (Eurax) and permethrin 5% cream (Elimite) for the treatment of scabies in children. Taplin D, Meinking TL, Chen JA, Sanchez R. Pediatr Dermatol 1990; 7: 67–73.

Both these studies show superior efficacy for permethrin, with clinical cures of 91 of 97 vs 72 of 97 patients. The Taplin et al. study also measured parasitic cure, and by this outcome permethrin was much more effective, curing 42 of 47 vs 28 of 47.

Tratamiento de la escabiasis con ivermectina por via oral. Macotela-Ruiz E, Pena-Gonzalez G. Gac Med Mex 1993; 129: 201–5.

This randomized trial compared the treatment of 55 patients with a clinical diagnosis of scabies with either a single dose of ivermectin 200 µg/kg or placebo. After 7 days the code was broken because there was such a significant improvement in the treated group: 23 of 29 vs four of 26.

Comparison of ivermectin and benzyl benzoate for treatment of scabies. Glaziou P, Cartel JL, Alzieu P, Briot C, Moulia-Pelat JP, Martin PM. Trop Med Parasitol 1993; 44: 331–2.

A randomized study in French Polynesia comparing a single dose of 100 µg/kg ivermectin with 10% benzyl benzoate lotion applied below the neck and repeated 12 hours later. Both were equally effective.

Treatment of scabies with ivermectin. Offidani A, Cellini A, Simonetti O, Fumelli C. Eur J Dermatol 1999; 9: 100–1.

Six patients with heavy mite infestation received a single dose of 200 µg/kg ivermectin. All were clinically cured.

A comparative trial of oral ivermectin and topical permethrin in the treatment of scabies. Usha V, Gopalakrishnan Nair TV. J Am Acad Dermatol 2000; 42: 236–40.

In this trial in 88 patients, permethrin came out better for cure at 2 weeks.

Safety of and compliance with community-based ivermectin therapy. Pacque M, Munoz B, Greene BM, White AT, Dukuly Z, Taylor HR. Lancet 1990; 335: 1377–80.

Adverse reactions after large-scale treatment of onchocerciasis with ivermectin: combined results from eight community trials. De Sole G, Remme J, Awadzi K, Accorsi S, Alley ES, Ba O, et al. J WHO 1989; 67: 707–19.

In both studies ivermectin was remarkably well tolerated, even in repeated courses.

Deaths associated with ivermectin treatment of scabies. Barkwell R, Shields S. Lancet 1997; 349: 1144–5.

This is the only 'fly in the ointment' with ivermectin: the authors report on the treatment of 47 elderly, mentally disadvantaged residents of an institution with a single dose of ivermectin at 150–200 µg/kg body weight. All had failed to respond to multiple earlier courses of lindane and crotamiton. All were cured, but over the next 6 months 15 died from a number of causes, whereas only five died in an equivalent, matched population within the same unit. Many patients were taking other drugs, raising the possibility of interactions.

THIRD-LINE THERAPIES

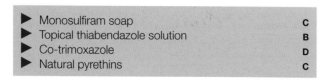

▶ Monosulfiram soap		**C**
▶ Topical thiabendazole solution		**B**
▶ Co-trimoxazole		**D**
▶ Natural pyrethins		**C**

Control of scabies by use of soap impregnated with tetraethylthiuram monosulphide ('tetmosol'). Gordon RM, Davey TH, Unsworth K, Hellier FF, Parry SC, Alexander JB. Br Med J 1944; 2: 803–6.

A bath a day for 6 days using 20% tetmosol soap cured all six patients; three baths on alternate days cured 88 of 110 patients.

Presumably the limiting factor in wartime Britain was the lack of hot bathwater!

Scabies prophylaxis using 'tetmosol' soap. Mellanby K. Br Med J 1945; 1: 38–9.

A non-randomized open study carried out in a large mental hospital showed significant reductions in infection rates.

Where has this soap gone?

Topically applied thiabendazole in the treatment of scabies. Hernandez-Perez E. Arch Dermatol 1976; 112: 1400–1.

Forty patients with scabies were treated with a single external application of a 10% suspension of thiabendazole. Thirty-two (80%) seemed to be cleared, but six needed a second course.

Perhaps worth trying when patients have had adverse reactions to other topical agents.

A trial of cotrimoxazole in scabies. Shashindran CH, Gandhi IS, Lal S. Br J Dermatol 1979; 100: 483.

Unlike pediculosis, where there is some evidence of benefit, this did not seem to work. The potential toxicity of co-trimoxazole is also of concern.

Efficacy and tolerability of natural synergised pyrethrins in a new thermo labile foam formulation in topical treatment of scabies: a prospective randomized, investigator-blinded, comparative trial vs permethrin cream. Amerio P, Capizzi R, Milan M. Eur J Dermatol 2003; 13: 69–71.

Forty patients received either 5% permethrin cream or a foam formulation of 0.16% pyrethrins synergized with piperonil butoxide, designed for head and pubic lice. It was equally effective, and significantly easy to apply.

As compliance is the essential component of successful scabies treatment, expect to see more of this product.

Evidence Levels: **A** Double-blind study   **B** Clinical trial ≥ 20 subjects   **C** Clinical trial < 20 subjects   **D** Series ≥ 5 subjects   **E** Anecdotal case reports

Scleredema

Amy E Helms, Stephen E Helms, Robert T Brodell

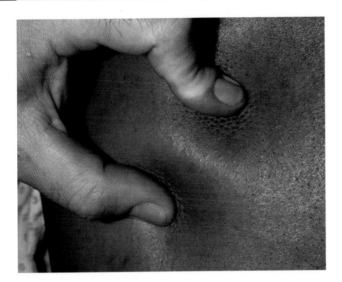

Scleredema (scleredema adultorum or scleredema of Buschke) is a connective tissue disorder characterized by progressive, symmetric induration and thickening of the skin secondary to increased amounts of collagen and glycosaminoglycans. Clinically, scleredema most commonly involves the posterior neck, shoulders, trunk, face, and arms. The three clinical forms are: scleredema following acute viral or bacterial infection, which usually resolves spontaneously in 6 months to 2 years; scleredema associated with diabetes mellitus, which persists indefinitely; and scleredema associated with malignancy (monoclonal gammopathy, insulinoma, and carcinoma of the gallbladder).

MANAGEMENT STRATEGY

Treatment of scleredema is difficult. There are case-based data to support the effectiveness of several therapies. In many cases a frank discussion with the patient regarding the limitations of treatment, cost, and side effects will lead to a decision to withhold treatment. This is particularly appropriate in patients with the post-infectious form, which can resolve spontaneously without specific treatment. Of course, the identification of a specific etiology, such as streptococcal pharyngitis, should lead to appropriate antibiotic treatment, even without evidence that this would alter the rate of clearing in this self-limited form of scleredema. In the forms associated with diabetes mellitus and monoclonal gammopathy, however, progressive involvement can lead to discomfort, unsightly thickening, and even systemic complications such as restrictive pulmonary function, dysphagia secondary to tongue swelling, and cardiac arrhythmias. In these cases, patients will demand treatment.

Bath or cream psoralen PUVA is recommended as initial therapy in moderately severe disease, and more recently, narrowband UVB as well as UVA1 has shown to be moderately effective. *Electron beam therapy* would be the primary recom-mendation for patients with severe disease, especially cases with restrictive pulmonary function. Alternative therapies include *ciclosporin* and *high-dose penicillin*. Antidiabetic therapy has no effect on the evolution of scleredema in diabetics, as the progression of scleredema has been found to be unrelated to control of serum glucose levels.

Scleredema: a review of thirty cases. Venencie PY, Powell FC, Su D, Perry HO. J Am Acad Dermatol 1984; 11: 128–34.

Mucinoses. Rongioletti F, Rebora A. In: Bolognia J, Jorizzo J, Rapini R, eds. Dermatology, 2nd edn. Edinburgh: Elsevier, 2008.

SPECIFIC INVESTIGATIONS

> ▶ Fasting blood sugar, glucose tolerance test, hemoglobin A1c (glycosylated hemoglobin)
> ▶ Serum protein electrophoresis, immuno-electrophoresis
> ▶ Antistreptolysin O, bacterial culture, other efforts to identify an acute infectious agent, erythrocyte sedimentation rate

Scleredema adultorum due to streptococcal infection. Alp H, Orbak Z, Aktas A. Pediatr Int 2003; 45: 101–3.

In 65–95% of cases scleredema occurs within a few days to 6 weeks after an acute febrile illness. Of these infections, 58% are streptococcal. They may present as tonsillitis, pharyngitis, scarlet fever, erysipelas, cervical adenitis, pneumonia, otitis media, pyoderma, impetigo, or rheumatic fever. Appropriate studies will rapidly help determine whether one of these is the cause of scleredema.

As 50% of cases of scleredema occur in childhood, the term adultorum is a misnomer.

Monoclonal gammopathy in scleredema: observations in three cases. Kovary PM, Vakilzadeh F, Macher E, Zaun H, Merk H, Goerz G. Arch Dermatol 1981; 117: 536–9.

Immunoelectrophoresis studies in six patients with severe persistent scleredema revealed that three of them also had a monoclonal gammopathy, and many subsequent reports have also confirmed this association. The skin manifestations often precede the development of the gammopathy, and thus it is recommended that immunoelectrophoresis be performed at regular intervals in all cases of widespread scleredema.

Scleredema associated with carcinoma of the gall bladder. Manchanda Y, Das S, Sharma VK, Srivastava DN. Br J Dermatol 2005; 152: 1373–4.

Scleredema has been reported to be associated with internal malignancies and was seen in a female with carcinoma of the gallbladder.

When clinically indicated, an evaluation for internal malignancies may be appropriate.

Scleredema and diabetes mellitus. Fleischmajer R. Arch Dermatol 1970; 101: 21–6.

Scleredema in patients with diabetes mellitus generally follows a progressive course that is unrelated to control of serum glucose levels.

> ▶ Identify and treat any underlying disease (diabetes mellitus, monoclonal gammopathy, acute infection) **D**
> ▶ Conservative management using the principle 'Do no harm' **D**

Scleredema: a review of thirty-three cases. Venencie PY, Powell FC, Su D, Perry HO. J Am Acad Dermatol 1984; 11: 128–34.

A review of 33 cases of scleredema in which systemic corticosteroids, methotrexate, and D-penicillamine had no effect on the disease course. Both diabetic and non-diabetic patients were studied, and although some patients in both groups had mild complications such as dysphagia and ECG changes, the authors emphasize that, for the most part, scleredema is a mild disease that does not pose a threat to overall health.

Scleredema adultorum. Not always a benign self-limited disease. Curtis AC, Shulak BM. Arch Dermatol 1965; 92: 526–41.

A review of 223 scleredema patients revealed that 25% had had symptoms for more than 2 years. The following were found to have no therapeutic benefit: calcium gluconate, estradiol, fever, hot baths, hyaluronidase, nicotinic acid, ovarian extract, para-amino benzoate, penicillin, pituitary extract, corticosteroids, thyroid hormone, and vitamin D.

Because of the expense and potential side effects of the second-line therapies discussed below, as well as the recognition that many patients with mild scleredema either improve without treatment or do not respond to the therapy, a policy of 'do no harm' and withholding of treatment is recommended in patients with mild disease.

SECOND-LINE THERAPIES

> ▶ Narrowband UVB phototherapy **E**
> ▶ UVA1 phototherapy **D**
> ▶ Electron beam therapy **E**
> ▶ Bath PUVA and cream PUVA **E**
> ▶ High-dose penicillin **E**
> ▶ Ciclosporin **E**
> ▶ Extracorporeal photophoresis **E**

Scleredema adultorum treated with narrow-band ultraviolet B phototherapy. Xiao T, Yang Z, He C, Chen H. J Dermatol 2007; 34: 270–2.

A 56-year-old Chinese man with scleredema was treated with NB-UVB at an initial dose of $0.2 J/cm^2$. This was increased by 25% per treatment and was administered three times weekly. Significant improvement was seen after 10 treatments and the patient received a total of 54 exposures ($33.8 J/cm^2$ dose). Beneficial effects were still evident at 14 months' follow-up. NB-UVB phototherapy has several advantages over PUVA. It has shorter irradiation times, no need for protective glasses following treatment, and a reduced risk of photocarcinogenesis. Further large-scale studies are needed to define the role of NB-UVB in scleredema.

UVA1 phototherapy for cutaneous diseases: an experience of 92 cases in the United States. Tuchinda C, Kerr H, Taylor C, Jacobe H, Bergamo B, Elmets C, et al. Photodermatol Photoimmunol Photomed 2006; 22: 247–53.

In this retrospective study, six patients with scleredema adultorum were treated with UVA1 phototherapy (five received low-dose regimens and one a medium-dose regimen). One patient developed polymorphous light eruption and therapy was discontinued. Moderate to good responses were seen in four out of five patients treated. In recalcitrant cases UVA1 phototherapy should be considered as a therapeutic option.

Scleredema of Buschke successfully treated with electron beam therapy. Tamburin LM, Pena JR, Meredith R. Arch Dermatol 1998; 134: 419–22.

A patient with scleredema and insulin-dependent diabetes mellitus experienced complete resolution of skin induration after receiving electron beam therapy twice weekly for 36 days. Prior treatment with topical, intralesional, and systemic corticosteroids had failed. This patient also suffered significant restrictive pulmonary disease thought to be secondary to scleredema, and pulmonary function tests following electron beam therapy revealed a marked improvement in lung function. This treatment should be considered in patients with severe persistent disease and systemic complications.

Electron-beam therapy in scleredema adultorum with associated monoclonal hypergammaglobulinaemia. Angeli-Besson C, Koeppel M, Jacquet P, Andrac L, Sayag J. Br J Dermatol 1994; 130: 394–7.

Ten sessions of electron beam therapy produced significant clinical improvement in the skin lesions of a patient with scleredema associated with IgA κ monoclonal gammopathy. A trial of factor XIII and cyclofenil had proved unsuccessful in this patient. Although the patient had initially responded to systemic corticosteroids, she subsequently became resistant and the condition progressed. At that point, electron beam therapy was begun.

Bath-PUVA therapy in three patients with scleredema adultorum. Hager CM, Sobhi HA, Hunzelmann N, Wickenhauser C, Scharenberg R, Krieg T, et al. J Am Acad Dermatol 1998; 38: 240–2.

Bath PUVA therapy (median of 59 treatments) produced substantial clinical improvement in three patients with scleredema. Although one patient did not have a history of diabetes mellitus or preceding infection, the remaining two had diabetes. The successful use of bath PUVA in these cases may be significant, as diabetic patients with scleredema tend to have a long unremitting course without treatment.

Cream PUVA therapy for scleredema adultorum. Grundmann-Kollmann M, Ochsendorf F, Zollner TM, Spieth K, Kaufmann R, Podda M. Br J Dermatol 2000; 142: 1058–9.

Cream PUVA therapy (35 irradiations) produced marked clinical improvement and softening of the skin in a patient with a 10-year history of scleredema who also suffered non-insulin-dependent diabetes mellitus. Bath PUVA was contraindicated in this patient because of coronary artery disease, and prior treatment with intravenous penicillin was unsuccessful. Cream PUVA therapy is easier to administer than bath PUVA and may become an important treatment option for scleredema.

Persistent scleredema of Buschke in a diabetic: improvement with high-dose penicillin. Krasagakis K, Hettmannsperger U,

Trautmann C, Tebbe B, Garbe C. Br J Dermatol 1996; 134: 597–8.

High-dose (3×10^6 IU daily) intravenous penicillin for 7 days led to a reduction in the degree of scleredema in a patient with comorbid severe diabetes mellitus. The antifibrotic action of penicillin, leading to reduced dermal thickness, is postulated to be the mechanism of action in this case. The observation that treatment with erythromycin was not effective in this patient and that antibiotics in general have not been successful in treating scleredema supports the role of an antifibrotic rather than an antibiotic action of penicillin at work in this case.

Cyclosporine in scleredema. Mattheou-Vakali G, Ioannides D, Thomas T, Lazaridou E, Tsogas P, Minas A. J Am Acad Dermatol 1996; 35: 990–1.

Ciclosporin at a dose of 5 mg/kg daily for 5 weeks was effective in completely clearing scleredema in two patients, neither of whom had coexistent monoclonal gammopathy or diabetes mellitus. Both patients presented with the post-infectious form of scleredema and thus would probably have experienced resolution of their symptoms even without treatment.

Scleredema associated with paraproteinemia treated by extracorporeal photophoresis. Stables GI, Taylor PC, Highet AS. Br J Dermatol 2000; 142: 781–3.

A patient with scleredema associated with paraproteinemia demonstrated a significant improvement in skin lesions following treatment with extracorporeal photophoresis. When the treatment sessions were reduced from two per month to one, the patient's condition deteriorated, suggesting that the improvement was due to therapy rather than spontaneous resolution. Because scleredema associated with paraproteinemia usually has a progressive course, this treatment should be considered in patients with a similar presentation.

Beneficial effect of aggressive low-density lipoprotein apheresis in a familial hypercholesterolemic patient with severe diabetic scleredema. Koga N. Ther Apher 2001; 5: 506–12.

A 59-year-old woman with diabetic scleredema and familial hypercholesterolemia, treated with weekly LDL apheresis over a period of 3 years, had significant improvement in her scleredema when her lipid levels were reduced to normal. Histopathologic as well as clinical improvement was noted. The author concluded that LDL apheresis therapy is an effective second-line treatment for resistant diabetic scleredema.

Treatment with chemotherapy of scleredema associated with IgA myeloma. Santos-Juanes J, Osuna CG, Iglesias JR, De Quiros JF, del Río JS. Int J Dermatol 2001; 40: 720–1.

A 70-year-old woman with IgA myeloma and scleredema was treated with oral melphalan and prednisone over a 6-month period. During the 18 months she was followed, clinical evidence of softening of the indurated and taut skin was observed. Similar cases were cited in which chemotherapy for myeloma resulted in significant improvement of associated scleredema.

Scleroderma

Sameh S Zaghloul, Najat Marraiki, Mark JD Goodfield

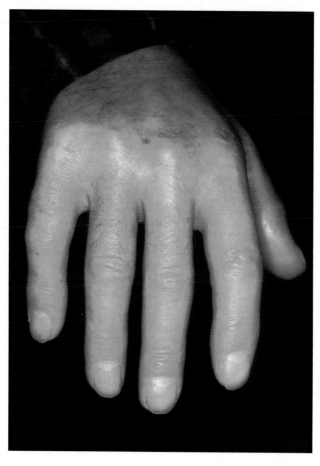

Systemic sclerosis (SSc) is a rare multisystem disease characterized by skin fibrosis, autoantibody production, and vascular abnormalities often leading to visceral disease. It can affect any organ system, particularly the gastrointestinal tract, kidney, heart, and lungs. Patients typically present with cutaneous sclerosis or Raynaud's phenomenon (RP). The degree of skin involvement defines the clinical subset of the disease. Diffuse cutaneous SSc (dcSSc) involves the skin proximal to the neck, elbows, or knees, whereas involvement distal to these sites is known as limited cutaneous SSc (lcSSc); some authors include an intermediate group.

MANAGEMENT STRATEGY

Limited cutaneous and diffuse cutaneous SSc, with different severities and survivals, have been recognized as distinct subsets. Some authors have suggested an intermediate cutaneous form with intermediate survival.

In most cases cutaneous lesions and RP precede systemic involvement. The face and hands are typically involved, with patients displaying a characteristic shiny appearance of the skin and complaining of increased skin stiffness or rigidity. To date, no treatment has proved effective in modifying the course of the disease and there is no specific therapy for the skin, although dry skin should be cared for daily using *emollient creams. Topical 0.025–0.05% tretinoin* may improve the perioral radial furrows and facial tightening.

UVA phototherapy (PUVA and UVA1) has been reported to be effective in reducing skin thickness. *Vasodilators* such as *nifedipine* reduce vasospasm and improve peripheral blood flow. Also, *losartan*, an antagonist of angiotensin II receptor type I, has been found to be effective in reducing the severity and frequency of attacks of RP. *Parenteral prostacyclin* analogs such as *iloprost* also improve both the severity and frequency of RP. Both *low-dose prednisolone* 20 mg/day and *methotrexate* 15–25 mg/week have been shown to reduce skin thickness scores. *Ciclosporin* 3–4 mg/kg/day may improve skin induration but has no effect on internal organ involvement. It should be used with caution as renal involvement with SSc is not uncommon. *Cyclophosphamide* 1–2 mg/kg/day is of proven value in reducing skin scores and preventing the development of lung fibrosis and other complications. Respiratory complications of SSc develop in roughly 30% of patients. Pulmonary hypertension (PAH) may occur and should be confirmed by appropriate investigation. Iloprost infusions have also been shown to reduce PAH. *Angiotensin-converting enzyme (ACE) inhibitors* are particularly effective in reducing the renal complications of the disease, and early treatment may prevent the onset of renal failure. *Proton pump inhibitors* treat esophageal disease effectively. Recent randomized controlled trials have suggested that oral minocycline and D-penicillamine are not effective in SSc. Although SSc carries a high case-specific mortality, there have been significant advances in the management of skin, renal, and pulmonary complications. The identification of novel signaling pathways and mediators that are altered in systemic sclerosis and contribute to tissue damage allows their selective targeting. This in turn opens the door for novel therapeutic strategies using novel compounds, or innovative ways of using already approved drugs.

SPECIFIC INVESTIGATIONS

- ▶ Skin biopsy
- ▶ Renal function tests
- ▶ Anticentromere and anti-Scl-70 antibodies
- ▶ Chest X-ray
- ▶ Pulmonary function tests
- ▶ Echocardiography

Evidence-based guidelines for the use of immunologic tests: Anticentromere, Scl-70, and nucleolar antibodies. Basu D, Reveille JD. Autoimmunity 2005; 38: 65–72.

Anti-Scl-70 antibodies are very useful in distinguishing systemic sclerosis (SSc) patients from healthy controls, from patients with other connective tissue diseases, and from unaffected family members. Among patients with SSc, anti-Scl-70 positivity is useful in predicting those at higher risk for diffuse cutaneous involvement and interstitial fibrosis/ restrictive lung disease, though the latter has not been universally observed.

Once a patient is determined as being anti-Scl-70 positive or negative, there is little justification for serial determinations.

Scleroderma – clinical and pathological advances. Denton CP, Black C. Best Pract Res Clin Rheumatol 2004; 18: 271–90.

Evidence Levels: **A** Double-blind study **B** Clinical trial ≥ 20 subjects **C** Clinical trial < 20 subjects **D** Series ≥ 5 subjects **E** Anecdotal case reports

This review focuses on the current assessment and treatment of SSc patients. It recommends that all patients with SSc should be regularly screened for pulmonary disease. Regular monitoring of blood pressure improves outcome.

FIRST-LINE THERAPIES

▶ Nifedipine	**A**
▶ Iloprost	**A**
▶ ACE inhibitors	**B**

Iloprost for the treatment of systemic sclerosis. Hachulla E, Launay D, Hatron P-Y. Presse Med 2008; 37: 831–9.

An imbalance between prostacyclin (PGI_2) and thromboxane A_2 is observed in patients with scleroderma. Iloprost is a stable analog of PGI_2 with a plasma half-life of 20–30 minutes. Intravenous iloprost is effective in the treatment of Raynaud's phenomenon related to scleroderma, reducing the frequency and severity of attacks. It also appears useful for the treatment of digital ulcers. Intravenous iloprost improves kidney vasospasm in patients with scleroderma. The possible benefits of sequential intravenous iloprost on the natural course of scleroderma require further investigation.

Calcium channel blockers for Raynaud's phenomenon. Thompson AE, Pope JE. Rheumatology 2005; 44: 145–50.

Calcium channel blockers yield moderate clinical improvement in the severity and frequency of Raynaud's attacks, with an average decrease of 2.8–5.0 attacks per week and a 33% improvement in the severity of attacks compared with placebo.

Outcome of renal crisis in systemic sclerosis: relation to availability of angiotensin converting enzyme (ACE) inhibitors. Steen VD, Costantino JP, Shapiro AP, Medsger TA Jr. Ann Intern Med 1990; 113: 352–7.

Patients with systemic sclerosis who develop hypertension should be treated with an ACE inhibitor. Improved survival and successful discontinuation of dialysis are possible when ACE inhibitors are used to treat scleroderma renal crisis.

SECOND-LINE THERAPIES

▶ Methotrexate	**A**
▶ Cyclophosphamide	**B**
▶ Prednisolone	**B**
▶ Losartan	**B**
▶ Acitretin	**C**
▶ Colchicine	**C**
▶ UVA	**C**

Evaluation of oral methotrexate in the treatment of systemic sclerosis. Sumanth K, Sharma M, Vinod K, Khaitan BK, Kapoor A, Tejasvi T. Int J Dermatol 2007; 46: 218–23.

Thirty-three patients with systemic sclerosis were included in a clinical trial to evaluate the efficacy of oral methotrexate. It was concluded that MTX for 6 months only provides subjective improvement, and further studies after 1 year of treatment with MTX are recommended.

Randomized placebo controlled trial of methotrexate in systemic sclerosis. Das SN, Alam MR, Islam N, Rahman MH, Sutradhar SR, Rahman S, et al. Mymensingh Med J 2005; 14: 71–4.

Clinical improvement following treatment was observed in 33.33% of patients in the MTX group but none in the placebo group, but this difference was not statistically significant. Anorexia, nausea, and occasional vomiting were common side effects in MTX group and subsided in most cases with the passage of time, despite the continuation of therapy.

A randomized, controlled trial of methotrexate versus placebo in early diffuse scleroderma. Pope JE, Bellamy N, Seibold JR, Baron M, Ellman M, Carette S, et al. Arthritis Rheum 2001; 44: 1351–8.

In this trial 35 patients received between 7.5 mg and 50 mg weekly doses of MTX versus 36 patients who received placebo, and no significant differences were found between the groups. However, there was a significant improvement in the severity of skin involvement in the first few months in those treated with MTX.

The efficacy of oral cyclophosphamide plus prednisolone in early diffuse systemic sclerosis. Calguneri M, Apras S, Ozbalkan Z, Ertenli I, Kiraz S, Ozturk MA, et al. Clin Rheumatol 2003; 22: 289–94.

In this study 27 patients with early diffuse SSc were treated with oral cyclophosphamide (1–2 mg/kg/day) plus oral prednisolone (40 mg every other day) between the years 1995 and 1998. The results regarding the efficacy and toxicity of cyclophosphamide were compared with those of 22 early SSc patients who had been treated with oral D-penicillamine between 1992 and 1995. There was a significant improvement in the skin score, maximal oral opening, flexion index, predicted forced vital capacity (FVC), and carbon monoxide diffusing capacity (DLCO) in the cyclophosphamide group. The decrease in skin score in the cyclophosphamide group started earlier than in the D-penicillamine group.

Randomized unblinded trial of cyclophosphamide versus azathioprine in the treatment of systemic sclerosis. Nadashkevich O, Davis P, Fritzler M, Kovalenko W. Clin Rheumatol 2006; 25: 205–12.

Thirty patients were assigned to receive oral CYC (2 mg/kg daily for 12 months and then maintained on 1 mg/kg daily) and 30 patients were assigned to receive oral AZA (2.5 mg/kg daily for 12 months and then maintained on 2 mg/kg daily). During the first 6 months of the trial the patients also received prednisolone, which was started at a dosage of 15 mg daily and tapered to zero by the end of the sixth month. This study showed that CYC is a promising disease-modifying medication for SSc, as it exhibited a positive influence on the evolution of disease.

Treatment of early diffuse cutaneous systemic sclerosis patients in Japan by low-dose corticosteroids for skin involvement. Takehara K. Clin Exp Rheumatol 2004; 22: S87–9.

Twenty-three patients with early dcSSc were treated with 20 mg/kg of prednisolone, with a significant reduction in skin scores.

The vitamin A derivative etretinate improves skin sclerosis in patients with systemic sclerosis. Ikeda T, Uede K, Hashizume H, Furukawa F. J Dermatol Sci 2004; 34: 62–6.

This small study of 31 patients showed that patients taking oral etretinate had significant improvements in skin thickness compared to patients not taking etretinate.

Losartan therapy for Raynaud's phenomenon and scleroderma: clinical and biochemical findings in a fifteen-week, randomized, parallel-group, controlled trial. Dziadzio M, Denton CP, Smith R, Blann HK, Bowers E, Black CM. Arthritis Rheum 1999; 42: 2646–55.

Losartan is an antagonist of angiotensin II receptor type I. In this randomized controlled trial 25 patients with primary RP and 27 with RP secondary to SSc were treated with either losartan (50 mg/day) or nifedipine (40 mg/day). Losartan reduced the frequency and severity of RP.

Therapeutic management of acral manifestations of systemic sclerosis. Meyer MF, Daigeler A, Lehnhardt M, Steinau H-U, Klein HH. Med Klin 2007; 102: 209–18.

Patients with acral manifestations of systemic sclerosis are ideally treated by a team that includes a rheumatologist, dermatologist, hand surgeon, physiotherapist, and, eventually, a psychologist. Calcium channel antagonists, α_1-adrenergic blockade with prazosin, and prostacyclin analogs were proved to be effective in the treatment of scleroderma-related Raynaud's phenomenon. Losartan, an angiotensin II receptor inhibitor, and fluoxetine, a selective serotonin reuptake inhibitor, have been beneficial for systemic sclerosis-associated Raynaud's phenomenon in pilot studies.

Long-term evaluation of colchicine in the treatment of scleroderma. Alarcon-Segovia D, Ramos-Niembro F, Ibanez de Kasep G, Alcocer J, Perez-Tamayo R. J Rheumatol 1979; 6: 705–12.

In this early uncontrolled study, 19 patients with dSSc were treated with colchicine, 10.1 mg/week, with a follow-up of 19–57 months. They reported improvement in skin elasticity, mouth opening and finger mobility, and a reduction in dysphagia.

Different low doses of broad-band UVA in the treatment of morphea and systemic sclerosis. El-Mofty M, Mostafa W, El-Darouty M, Bosseila M, Nada H, Yousef R, et al. Photodermatol Photoimmunol Photomed 2004; 20: 148–56.

Fifteen patients complaining of SS received 20 sessions of UVA (320–400 nm); all improved clinically.

UVA is well tolerated and there is experimental evidence that UVA1 may be beneficial. Further trials are required to confirm efficacy.

THIRD-LINE THERAPIES

▶ Extracorporeal photochemotherapy	B
▶ Ciclosporin	C
▶ Thalidomide	D
▶ Etanercept	D
▶ Minocycline	F

Systemic Sclerosis Study Group. A randomized, double-blind, placebo-controlled trial of photopheresis in systemic sclerosis. Knobler RM, French LE, Kim Y, Bisaccia E, Graninger W, Nahavandi H, et al. J Am Acad Dermatol 2006; 54: 793–9.

This randomized, double-blind, placebo-controlled clinical trial was conducted at 16 investigational sites in the United States, Canada, and Europe. Sixty-four patients with typical clinical and histologic findings of scleroderma, of less than 2 years' duration, were studied to evaluate the efficacy of photopheresis in the treatment of patients with systemic sclerosis.

Photopheresis induced significant improvement of skin and joint involvement in patients with scleroderma of recent onset.

Ciclosporin in systemic sclerosis. Clements PJ, Lachenbruch PA, Sterz M, Danovitch G, Hawkins R, Ippoliti A, et al. Arthritis Rheum 1993; 36: 75–83.

Ciclosporin is an immunosuppressive drug that selectively inhibits the release of IL-2, which has been shown to be increased in SSc serum. This study showed that ciclosporin may improve skin induration, but had no effect on internal organ involvement.

The high incidence of nephrotoxicity with ciclosporin therapy reduces its use in SSc where renal crisis may occur.

Immune stimulation in scleroderma patients treated with thalidomide. Oliver SJ, Moreira A, Kaplan G. Clin Immunol 2000; 97: 109–20.

Eleven patients with SSc were treated with thalidomide in a 12-week open-label, dose-escalating study. Thalidomide appears to induce immune stimulation in SSc patients in association with clinical changes. However, it remains to be shown whether long-term enhancement of immune responses in SSc patients is clinically beneficial.

Reduced fibrosis and normalisation of skin structure in scleroderma patients treated with thalidomide. [Abstract.] Oliver SJ, Moreira A, Kaplan G. Arthritis Rheum 1999; 42: s187.

An open trial on 10 patients. Improvement was noted in skin repigmentation and healing of digital ulcers.

Etanercept as treatment for diffuse scleroderma: a pilot study. [Abstract.] Ellman MH, McDonald PA, Hayes FA. Arthritis Rheum 2000; 43: s392.

This targeted fusion protein blocks TNF-α. Four out of 10 patients treated with etanercept 25 mg subcutaneously twice weekly had improvements of skin scores and healing of digital ulcers.

Minocycline in early diffuse scleroderma. Le CH, Morales A, Trentham DE. Lancet 1998; 352: 1755–6.

Eleven patients with early SSc were treated with minocycline (100 mg daily for 4 weeks; 200 mg daily for 11 months). Four patients showed complete resolution of skin involvement after 9 and 12 months of therapy.

A more recent study reported that minocycline is not an effective therapy for SSc (see below).

Minocycline is not effective in systemic sclerosis: results of an open-label multicenter trial. Mayes MD, O'Donnell D, Rothfield NF, Csuka ME. Arthritis Rheum 2004; 50: 553–7.

In this open-label trial involving 36 patients no significant change in skin score was found.

OTHER: INTERNAL ORGAN INVOLVEMENT

Prostacyclin for pulmonary hypertension in adults. Paramothayan NS, Lasserson TJ, Wells AU, Walters EH. Cochrane Database Syst Rev (2): CD002994, 2005.

There is evidence that intravenous prostacyclin in addition to conventional therapy at tolerable doses optimized by titration, can confer some short-term benefits (up to 12 weeks of treatment) in exercise capacity, NYHA functional class, and cardiopulmonary hemodynamics. There is also some evidence that patients with more severe disease based on NYHA functional class showed a greater response to treatment.

Review of bosentan in the management of pulmonary arterial hypertension. Gabbay E, Fraser J, McNeil K. Vasc Health Risk Manage 2007; 3: 887–900.

Bosentan was the first endothelin receptor antagonist approved for use in PAH. Clinical studies have shown that in PAH the use of bosentan is associated with improved exercise capacity, WHO functional class, cardiopulmonary hemodynamics, and quality of life, and delayed time to clinical worsening compared to placebo. Further, long-term studies have demonstrated improved survival with the use of bosentan compared to historical controls, although there are no placebo-controlled data confirming a survival benefit.

Bosentan therapy for pulmonary arterial hypertension. Rubin LJ, Badesch DB, Barst RJ, Galie N, Black CM, Keogh A, et al. N Engl J Med 2002; 346: 896–903.

In this randomised control trial of patients with PAH, the dual endothelin receptor antagonist bosentan improved exercise capacity. SSc patients with PAH were shown to have improved exercise capacity on subgroup analysis.

Interstitial lung disease associated with systemic sclerosis: what is the evidence for efficacy of cyclophosphamide? Berezne A, Valeyre D, Ranque B, Guillevin L, Mouthon L. Ann NY Acad Sci 2007; 1110: 271–84.

Since 1993, the beneficial effect of oral or intravenous cyclophosphamide (CYC) in the treatment of SSc-related ILD has been reported in retrospective studies, one showing improvement of pulmonary function test scores and/or chest CT at 1 year, and improvement of survival at 16 months. The results of two controlled trials were recently reported. The Scleroderma Lung Study, a prospective randomized placebo-controlled trial, included 158 patients, of whom 145 completed at least 6 months of treatment. The course of forced vital capacity (primary outcome) adjusted at 1 year was significantly better in the group treated with oral CYC (p<0.03), although the effect of CYC was minor.

Cyclophosphamide is associated with pulmonary function and survival benefit in patients with scleroderma and alveolitis. White B, Moore WC, Wigley FM, Xiai HQ, Wise RA. Ann Intern Med 2000; 132: 947–54.

This retrospective cohort study involving 103 patients with SSc showed that lung inflammation (alveolitis) treated with cyclophosphamide improves lung function outcome and survival.

Renal transplantation in scleroderma. Chang YJ, Spiera H. Medicine 1999; 78: 382–5.

A retrospective study from data collected by the United Network for Organ Sharing (UNOS) Scientific Renal Transplant Registry. Between 1987 and 1997, 86 patients with SSc had renal transplantation. At 5-year follow-up, 47% of the patients were still alive. Patients whose renal function does not improve with ACE inhibitors should be considered for transplantation.

Autologous stem cell transplantation in the treatment of systemic sclerosis: report from the EBMT/EULAR Registry. Farge D, Passweg J, van Laar JM, Marjanovic Z, Besenthal C, Finke J, et al. Ann Rheum Dis 2004; 63: 974–81.

The use of stem cell transplantation to treat severe SSc is currently being studied. Prospective randomized controlled trials are awaited.

Omeprazole in the long-term treatment of severe gastro-oesophageal reflux disease in patients with systemic sclerosis. Hendel L. Aliment Pharmacol Ther 1992; 6: 565–77.

Twenty-five patients treated with omeprazole showed significant improvement of GI symptoms.

Sebaceous hyperplasia

Agustin Martin-Clavijo, John Berth-Jones

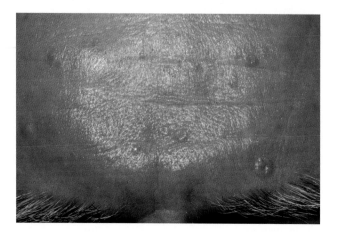

Sebaceous hyperplasia is a common benign condition. It affects adults of middle age and older and its incidence increases with age. It presents as single or multiple soft yellow papules, often with central umbilication, mainly on the face (commonly the nose, cheeks, and forehead), but it can present in other areas such as the chest, areola, mouth, and genitalia. Its frequency is increased in immunocompromised patients, especially after transplantation in patients on ciclosporin and corticosteroids.

Alta prevalencia de hiperplasias sebaceas en transplantados renales. Perez-Espana L, Prats I, Sanz A, Mayor M. Nefrologia 2003; 23: 179–80.

The authors looked at 163 renal transplant patients, of whom 25.9% had sebaceous hyperplasia. This was greatest in patients on ciclosporin. However, other immunosuppressants (azathioprine, mycophenolate mofetil, and tacrolimus) showed no significant increase in the incidence of sebaceous hyperplasia.

MANAGEMENT STRATEGY

This is a benign condition with no potential for malignant transformation. Lesions are asymptomatic and therefore need treatment only for cosmetic reasons. We normally use *cautery (electrodesiccation) or cryotherapy* as a first-line therapy, and it is often valuable to treat some test lesions to assess patient satisfaction prior to widespread treatment. Other treatments include *surgical excision, photodynamic therapy, laser, isotretinoin,* and *chemical peels.* It is important to stress to the patient the risk of scarring with many of these techniques.

SPECIFIC INVESTIGATIONS

No specific investigations are usually needed, as this is a clinical diagnosis. The differential diagnosis includes rhinophyma, nevus sebaceous, basal cell carcinoma, dermal nevus, plane warts, lupus miliaris disseminatus faciei, and syringoma. If the diagnosis is uncertain, a biopsy will show enlargement of individual glands with increased numbers of fully mature lobules with no atypia or dysplasia.

FIRST-LINE THERAPIES

▶ Conservative management/cosmetic camouflage	E
▶ Electrodesiccation/cautery	C
▶ Cryotherapy	E

Guidelines of care for cryosurgery. American Academy of Dermatology Committee on Guidelines of Care. J Am Acad Dermatol 1994; 31: 648–53.

The authors include sebaceous hyperplasia as a condition treatable with cryotherapy.

Surgical pearl: Intralesional electrodesiccation of sebaceous hyperplasia. Bader RS, Scarborough DA. J Am Acad Dermatol 2000; 42: 127–8.

The authors describe the technique for intralesional electrodesiccation. They have used it on more than 30 patients with no recurrences after 7 months.

SECOND-LINE THERAPIES

▶ Isotretinoin	C
▶ Photodynamic therapy	C

Premature familial sebaceous hyperplasia: Successful response to oral isotretinoin in three patients. Grimalt R, Ferrando J, Mascaro JM. J Am Acad Dermatol 1997; 37: 996–8.

Three closely related patients with premature familial sebaceous hyperplasia were treated with isotretinoin 1 mg/kg/day for 6 weeks. Response was maintained with isotretinoin 20 mg on alternate days in one case and isotretinoin gel 0.05% in the others. Follow-up was for 5 months.

Isotretinoin for the treatment of sebaceous hyperplasia. Grekin RC, Ellis CN. Cutis 1987; 34: 90–2.

Two patients were treated with isotretinoin. Both had a good response but relapsed after the treatment was withdrawn, needing maintenance treatment. The first patient received 20 mg daily with a maintenance dose of 10 mg on alternate days; the second received 40 mg on alternate days with a maintenance dose of 40 mg twice a week.

Photodynamic therapy of sebaceous hyperplasia with topical 5-aminolaevulenic acid and slide projector. Horio T, Horio O, Miyaichi-Hashimoto H, Ohnuki M, Isei T. Br J Dermatol 2003; 148: 1270–90.

The authors treated one patient with photodynamic therapy. The response was good, with no scarring or hyperpigmentation at 12 months' follow-up.

Treatment of sebaceous gland hyperplasia by photodynamic therapy with 5-aminolevulinic acid and a blue light source or intense pulsed light source. Gold MH, Bradshaw VL, Boring MM, Bridges TM, Biron JA, Lewis TL. J Drugs Dermatol 2004; 3: S6–9.

Twelve patients were randomized to topical aminolevulinic acid and either blue light or intense pulsed light. They had four treatments at 1 month intervals. Both treatment arms had more than 50% reduction in the number of the lesions without recurrence at 12 weeks' follow-up.

Evidence Levels: **A** Double-blind study **B** Clinical trial ≥ 20 subjects **C** Clinical trial < 20 subjects **D** Series ≥ 5 subjects **E** Anecdotal case reports

THIRD-LINE THERAPIES

▶ Topical aminolevulinic acid and pulsed dye laser	D
▶ Diode laser	D
▶ Pulsed dye laser	D
▶ Argon laser	E
▶ Carbon dioxide laser	E
▶ Erbium:YAG laser	E
▶ Bichloroacetic acid	C
▶ Surgery/curettage	E

Photodynamic therapy with topical aminolevulenic acid and pulsed dye laser irradiation for sebaceous hyperplasia. Alster TS, Tanzi EL. J Drugs Dermatol 2003; 2: 501–4.

Ten patients were treated with topical 5-ALA followed 1 hour later by the 595 nm pulsed dye laser. They were compared with untreated lesions and laser-only treated lesions. Laser PDT treatment yielded the best results; 70% of lesions had total clearing after one treatment, the remaining 30% after two treatments.

Sebaceous hyperplasia treated with a 1450-nm diode laser. No D, McLaren M, Chotzen V, Kilmer SL. Dermatol Surg 2004; 30: 382–4.

The authors treated 10 patients. Both objective and subjective improvement was noted in the majority of patients, with very few side effects.

Elucidating the pulsed-dye laser treatment of sebaceous hyperplasia in vivo with real-time confocal scanning laser microscopy. Aghassi D, Gonzalez E, Anderson RR, Rajadhyaksha M, Gonzalez S. J Am Acad Dermatol 2000; 43: 49–53.

The authors treated 29 lesions on seven different patients with pulsed-dye laser. There was improvement in 93% of lesions and complete clearance in 28%. No scarring or hyperpigmentation was noted. However, 28% of the lesions reappeared and 7% returned to their original size.

A three year experience with the argon laser in dermatotherapy. Landthaler M, Haina D, Waidelich W, Braun-Falco O. J Dermatol Surg Oncol 1984; 10: 456–61.

The authors report on 477 patients with different cutaneous lesions treated with an argon laser, including sebaceous hyperplasia.

Sebaceous gland hyperplasia as a side effect of cyclosporin A. Treatment with the CO_2 laser. Walther T, Hohenleutner U, Landthaler M. Dtsch Med Wochenschr 1998; 123: 798–800.

This article reports the treatment of a patient with CO_2 laser. The lesions cleared without scarring.

Controlled cosmetic dermal ablation in the facial region with the erbium:YAG laser. Riedel F, Bergler W, Baker-Schreyer A, Stein E, Hormann K. HNO 1999; 47: 101–6.

This article looks at 216 patients with different facial lesions. The authors report good-to-excellent results with sebaceous hyperplasia.

The treatment of benign sebaceous hyperplasia with the topical application of bichloracetic acid. Rosian R, Goslen JB, Brodell RT. J Dermatol Surg Oncol 1991; 17: 876–9.

The authors treated 67 lesions in 20 patients: 66 cleared after one application of 100% bichloracetic acid, with minimal scarring.

Surgical removal

Occasionally, sebaceous hyperplasia is treated surgically. This has the advantage of providing tissue for histology when there is any doubt about the diagnosis.

Seborrheic eczema

Jason Williams, Ian Coulson

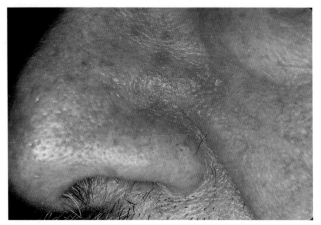

From Lebwohl MG. The Skin and Systemic Disease: A Color Atlas, 2nd edn. Churchill Livingstone 2003, with permission of Elsevier.

Seborrheic eczema is a chronic dermatitis affecting between 3% and 10% of adults. The signs and symptoms comprise erythema, greasy scaling, pruritus, burning, and dryness in a typical distribution pattern affecting the scalp, the face – particularly the nasolabial folds, eyebrows and ears – the upper trunk, and the flexures. Seborrheic eczema can also affect infants up to the age of 3–4 months in the diaper area. It is reported to account for up to 3.5% of dermatology specialist outpatient consultations and is more common in patients with Parkinson's disease, particularly those with neuroleptic-induced disease, and chronic alcoholics. It is particularly severe and recalcitrant in patients with HIV infection. Although the etiology is yet to be fully elucidated, three important factors are *Malassezia* yeasts, sebaceous triglycerides, and individual susceptibility.

MANAGEMENT STRATEGY

Seborrheic eczema is a chronic relapsing dermatitis. It responds to a variety of immunosuppressive therapies, but there are no cures.

Seborrheic eczema of the face is dry and flaky, so that soap avoidance and substitution with a *light emollient cleanser* (soap substitute) will help. Facial and flexural disease responds to *mild topical corticosteroids* alone or in combination with a variety of *topical antipityrosporal agents such as miconazole, clotrimazole, ketoconazole, itraconazole, ciclopiroxolamine, or sulfur*. An ointment containing *lithium gluconate/lithium succinate* may also be helpful. Studies have demonstrated short-term efficacy with the topical calcineurin inhibitors *tacrolimus* and *pimecrolimus*. Recent studies have suggested that *terbinafine cream* and *metronidazole gel* may also be beneficial. Resistant cases may respond to a short course of *oral itraconazole*. Scalp seborrheic dermatitis can be helped with *topical azoles, zinc pyrithione, selenium sulfide, corticosteroid and tar* shampoos, or a *propylene glycol* preparation formulated for scalp use. Severe cases with marked hyperkeratosis or pityriasis amiantacea may require topical keratolytics such as *salicylic acid ointment* or *coconut compound ointment*.

SPECIFIC INVESTIGATIONS

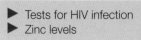

▶ Tests for HIV infection
▶ Zinc levels

In neonates and children consider acrodermatitis enteropathica or transient neonatal zinc deficiency, which can mimic recalcitrant seborrheic dermatitis. A similar eruption in parenterally fed adults can occur due to zinc deficiency.

Cutaneous findings in HIV-1 positive patients: a 42-month prospective study. Smith KJ, Skelton HG, Yeager J, Ledsky R, McCarthy W, Baxter D, et al. J Am Acad Dermatol 1994; 31: 746–54.

In this study of 912 HIV-positive patients, seborrheic dermatitis was the third most common skin disorder diagnosed (53% of cases).

Seborrheic dermatitis in neuroleptic-induced parkinsonism. Binder RL, Jonelis FJ. Arch Dermatol 1983; 119: 473–5.

Comparison of 42 hospitalized patients with drug-induced parkinsonism using psychiatric patients as controls showed an incidence of seborrheic dermatitis of 59.5% in those with parkinsonism, compared to 15% in the control group.

Cutaneous changes in chronic alcoholics. Rao GS. Indian J Dermatol Venereol Leprol 2004; 70: 317

In this study of 200 alcoholic patients attending for alcohol detoxification, seborrheic dermatitis was the second most common skin disorder (11.5% of cases).

NON-SCALP DISEASE

FIRST-LINE THERAPIES

▶ Topical ketoconazole	A
▶ Topical hydrocortisone	A

Double-blind treatment of seborrhoeic dermatitis with 2% ketoconazole cream. Skinner RB, Noah PW, Taylor RM, Zanolli MD, West S, Guin JD, et al. J Am Acad Dermatol 1985; 12: 852–6.

This paper reports a controlled double-blind trial in 37 patients; there was a 75–95% improvement in 18 of 20 patients treated with the ketoconazole cream compared to a vehicle control for a 4-week treatment period.

Ketoconazole 2% cream versus hydrocortisone 1% cream in the treatment of seborrhoeic dermatitis. A double-blind comparative study. Stratigos JD, Antoniou C, Katsambas A, Böhler K, Fritsch P, Schmölz A, et al. J Am Acad Dermatol 1988; 19: 850–3.

In a double-blind study, 72 patients were treated daily for 4 weeks with either 2% ketoconazole cream or 1% hydrocortisone cream; 80.5% of the ketoconazole group showed a significant improvement in all symptoms compared to 94.4% of the hydrocortisone group. There was no significant difference between the two groups in relapse rates at 2 and 4 weeks following treatment.

SECOND-LINE THERAPIES

▶ Lithium succinate/lithium gluconate	A
▶ Topical ciclopiroxolamine cream	A
▶ Tacrolimus 0.1% ointment	C
▶ Pimecrolimus cream	B

A double-blind, placebo-controlled, multicenter trial of lithium succinate ointment in the treatment of seborrhoeic dermatitis. Multicenter trial group. The Efalith Multicenter Trial Group. J Am Acad Dermatol 1992; 26: 452–7.

A multicenter, placebo-controlled, double-blind study in 227 patients showed that lithium succinate ointment was significantly more effective than placebo in treating all symptoms of non-scalp seborrheic dermatitis.

Lithium gluconate 8% vs ketoconazole 2% in the treatment of seborrhoeic dermatitis: a multicentre, randomized study. Dreno B, Chosidow O, Revuz J, Moyse D. Br J Dermatol 2003; 148: 1230–6.

A randomized, non-inferiority study comparing 8% lithium gluconate and ketoconazole 2% in moderate to severe seborrheic dermatitis for 2 months; 269 patients were treated. Lithium was 22% more effective than ketoconazole in giving complete remission of seborrheic dermatitis.

Randomized, placebo-controlled, double-blind study on clinical efficacy of ciclopiroxolamine 1% cream in facial seborrhoeic dermatitis. Dupuy P, Maurette C, Amoric JC, Chosidow O. Br J Dermatol 2001; 144: 1033–7.

One hundred and twenty-seven patients were randomized to receive either 1% ciclopiroxolamine cream twice daily for 28 days, followed by once-daily application for a further 28 days, or placebo. At the end of the treatment, 43 patients (63%) in the ciclopiroxolamine group responded.

An open pilot study using tacrolimus ointment in the treatment of seborrheic dermatitis. Meshkinpour A, Sun J, Weinstein G. J Am Acad Dermatol 2003; 49: 145–7.

In this study 18 patients used 0.1% tacrolimus twice a day for 28 days or until complete clearance of their seborrheic dermatitis was achieved: 61% showed 100% clearance and 39% showed 70–90% clearance.

Pimecrolimus cream 1% vs. betamethasone 17-valerate 0.1% cream in the treatment of seborrhoeic dermatitis. A randomized open-label clinical trial. Rigopoulos D, Ioannides D, Kalogeromitros D, Gregoriou S, Katsambas A. Br J Dermatol 2004; 151: 1071–5.

Twenty patients with seborrheic dermatitis were included in this study, 11 in the pimecrolimus 1% cream group and nine in the betamethasone 17-valerate 0.1% cream group. Similar efficacy was seen in both groups, but pruritus returned more slowly on discontinuation of treatment in the pimecrolimus group.

The authors point out that betamethasone is a potent corticosteroid and not to be recommended for long-term facial use.

THIRD-LINE THERAPIES

▶ Oral itraconazole	B
▶ Phototherapy	E

▶ Benzoyl peroxide	C
▶ Oral terbinafine	A
▶ Topical terbinafine	D
▶ Metronidazole gel	B

Itraconazole in the treatment of seborrhoeic dermatitis: a new treatment modality. Baysal V, Yildirim M, Ozcanli C, Ceyhan M. Int J Dermatol 2004; 43: 63–6.

Twenty-eight patients took 200 mg itraconazole daily for 1 month followed by 200 mg daily for 2 days each of the following 11 months. Nineteen patients showed complete improvement (>71% clear), six showed moderate and three a slight improvement.

Narrow-band ultraviolet B (TL-01) phototherapy is an effective and safe treatment option for patients with severe seborrhoeic dermatitis. Pirkhammer D, Seeber A, Honigsmann H, Tanew A. Br J Dermatol 2000; 143: 964–8.

In this study 18 patients were treated three times weekly until complete clearing or to a maximum of 8 weeks. Six showed complete clearance and 12 marked improvement.

Benzoyl peroxide in seborrheic dermatitis. Bonnetblanc JM, Bernard P. Arch Dermatol 1986; 122: 752.

Twenty-eight of 30 patients showed improvement with 1 week's use of 2.5% benzoyl peroxide preparation. All relapsed within 2–12 weeks of stopping treatment.

Evaluation of the efficacy and tolerability of oral terbinafine in patients with seborrhoeic dermatitis. A multicentre, randomized, investigator-blinded, placebo-controlled trial. Scaparro E, Quadri G, Virno G, Orifici C, Milani M. Br J Dermatol 2001; 144: 854–7.

Sixty patients with moderate to severe seborrheic dermatitis were treated with terbinafine 250 mg daily for 4 weeks, or a moisturizing cream twice daily. Terbinafine statistically reduced severity scores compared to baseline and placebo.

Oral terbinafine in the treatment of multi-site seborrheic dermatitis: a multicentre, double-blind placebo-controlled study. Vena GA, Micala G, Santoianni P, Cassano N, Peruzzi E. Int J Immunopathol Pharmacol 2005; 18: 745–53.

One hundred and seventy-four patients with seborrheic dermatitis in three or more areas were randomized to receive either terbinafine 250 mg once daily or placebo for 6 weeks. Terbinafine was statistically more effective (achieving 50% improvement) than placebo in patients with non-exposed sites affected (70% vs 45%). There was no statistical difference in patients with lesions on exposed sites.

Efficacy of terbinafine 1% cream on seborrheic dermatitis. Gündüz K, Inanir I, Sacar H. J Dermatol 2005; 32: 22–5.

Thirty-five patients with seborrheic dermatitis were treated with terbinafine 1% cream twice daily for 4 weeks. Complete remission was seen in 32% of cases.

The efficacy of 1% metronidazole gel in facial seborrheic dermatitis: a double blind study. Siadat AH, Iraji F, Shahmoradi Z, Enshaieh S, Taheri A. Indian J Dermatol Venereol Leprol 2006; 72: 266–9

Fifty-six patients applied either 1% metronidazole gel or vehicle twice daily for 8 weeks. Metronidazole gel was significantly more effective than vehicle at reducing severity scores.

Is metronidazole 0.75% gel effective in the treatment of seborrheic dermatitis? A double-blind, placebo controlled study. Ozcan H, Seyhan M, Yologlu S. Eur J Dermatol 2007; 17: 313–16.

In this study of 67 patients with mild to moderate seborrheic dermatitis there was no difference between treatment with metronidazole 0.75% gel and that with placebo over a 4-week period. Disease returned within 4 weeks of stopping treatment.

Metronidazole 0.75% gel vs. ketoconazole 2% cream in the treatment of facial seborrheic dermatitis: a randomized, double blind study. Seckin D, Gurbuz O, Akin O. J Eur Acad Dermatol Venereol 2007; 21: 345–50.

Sixty patients with facial seborrheic dermatitis used either 0.75% metronidazole gel (with ketoconazole cream as vehicle) or 2% ketoconazole cream (with metronidazole gel as vehicle) for 4 weeks. Around 80% improvement was noted in both groups, with no statistical difference.

SCALP DISEASE

FIRST-LINE THERAPIES

▶ Ketoconazole shampoo	A
▶ Ciclopirox shampoo	A
▶ Zinc pyrithione shampoo	B

Successful treatment and prophylaxis of scalp seborrhoeic dermatitis and dandruff with 2% ketoconazole shampoo: results of a multicentre, double-blind, placebo-controlled trial. Peter RU, Richarz-Barthauer U. Br J Dermatol 1995; 132: 441–5.

Five hundred and seventy-five patients with moderate to severe scalp seborrheic dermatitis and dandruff were treated with 2% ketoconazole shampoo twice weekly for 2 months, producing clearance in 88%. Responders were then randomized to active treatment or placebo once weekly. There were fewer relapses in the ketoconazole prophylactic treatment group after 6 months.

Safety and efficacy of ciclopirox 1% shampoo for the treatment of seborrheic dermatitis of the scalp in the US population: results of a double-blind, vehicle-controlled trial. Lebwohl M, Plott T. Int J Dermatol 2004; 43: 17–20.

When 499 patients with seborrheic dermatitis of the scalp were randomized to apply either ciclopirox shampoo 1% or vehicle twice weekly for 4 weeks, ciclopirox was found to be significantly more effective than vehicle.

Clinical efficacies of shampoos containing ciclopirox olamine (1.5%) and ketoconazole (2%) in the treatment of seborrheic dermatitis. Ratnavel RC, Squire RA, Boorman GC. J Dermatol Treat 2007; 18: 88–96.

This randomized, double-blind study enrolled 350 patients to compare 1.5% ciclopirox shampoo with 2% ketoconazole shampoo and placebo over a period of 4 weeks. Ciclopirox shampoo and ketoconazole shampoo were both significantly more effective than placebo, with ciclopirox *probably* the most effective.

The effects of a shampoo containing zinc pyrithione on the control of dandruff. Marks R, Pearse AD, Walker AP. Br J Dermatol 1985; 112: 415–22.

Thirty-two patients with dandruff were treated with a shampoo containing 1% zinc pyrithione to half the scalp, the other half being washed in a shampoo with base alone. Each scalp was washed one, three, six, or nine times. The actively treated group showed a progressive reduction in dandruff on the actively treated side. The difference was statistically significant after three, six, and nine washes.

SECOND-LINE THERAPIES

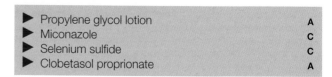

▶ Propylene glycol lotion	A
▶ Miconazole	C
▶ Selenium sulfide	C
▶ Clobetasol proprionate	A

Propylene glycol in the treatment of seborrhoeic dermatitis of the scalp: a double-blind study. Faergemann J. Cutis 1988; 42: 69–71.

Thirty-nine patients with scalp seborrheic dermatitis were treated in a double-blind controlled study with 15% propylene glycol in a base of 50% ethanol and 35% water or vehicle alone: 89% in the group treated with propylene glycol showed healing, compared to 32% in the control group.

A randomized, double-blind, placebo-controlled trial of ketoconazole 2% shampoo versus selenium sulfide 2.5% shampoo in the treatment of moderate to severe dandruff. Danby FW, Maddin WS, Margeson LJ, Rosenthal D. J Am Acad Dermatol 1993; 29: 1008–12.

A total of 236 patients were included in the study. Both medicated shampoos were statistically better than placebo in treating scaling and itching. However, ketoconazole was superior to selenium shampoo.

Seborrhoeic dermatitis and *Pityrosporum orbiculare*: treatment of seborrhoeic dermatitis of the scalp with miconazole-hydrocortisone (Daktacort), miconazole and hydrocortisone. Faergemann J. Br J Dermatol 1986; 114: 695–700.

Sixty-seven patients were treated twice daily for 6 weeks and those cured received prophylactic treatment twice monthly for 3 months. Nineteen of 21 patients were cured in the Daktacort group, 15 of 22 in the miconazole group, and 17 of 24 in the hydrocortisone group. Daktacort and miconazole were significantly better than hydrocortisone for prophylaxis.

Clobetasol propionate shampoo 0.05% in the treatment of seborrheic dermatitis of the scalp: results of a pilot study. Reygagne P, Poncet M, Sidou F, Soto P. Cutis 2007; 79: 397–403.

Fifty-five patients were enrolled in this study comparing clobetasol propionate shampoo applied for 2.5, 5, or 10 minutes; clobetasol propionate vehicle applied for 10 minutes; and ketoconazole foaming gel applied for 5 minutes before rinsing off. Treatments were applied twice weekly for 4 weeks. All active treatments were more effective than vehicle. There was no difference between 5- and 10-minute application times for the clobetasol propionate shampoo.

The authors would like to stress that clobetasol propionate shampoo is a superpotent steroid and may not be considered suitable for long-term use.

Seborrheic keratosis

Richard J Motley

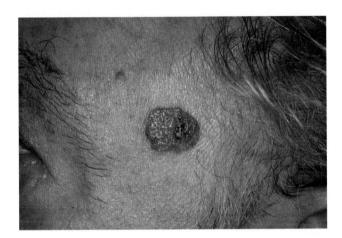

Seborrheic keratosis is a benign, exophytic, warty, lightly pigmented growth of the skin surface that becomes increasingly common with age. Found mainly on the trunk, often at sites of pressure, it is a cosmetic nuisance and rarely a cause for diagnostic confusion. Several variants exist and are described below.

MANAGEMENT STRATEGY

Many patients present with seborrheic keratoses because of concern about possible melanoma, and reassurance may be all that is required. Occasionally the lesion can become 'irritated' and show erythema, crusting, and itching. In this case the appearance may resemble a pyogenic granuloma or squamous cell carcinoma.

Where treatment is requested there are several options and the choice will depend on patient and physician preference. *Surgical excision*, although effective, is never the treatment of choice and usually indicates that the physician failed to make the correct clinical diagnosis or is unfamiliar with alternative treatments. When the diagnosis is in doubt then material should be taken for histologic examination, preferably by a '*shave*' or *tangential biopsy* technique or by *sharp curettage*. Blunt curettage provides poor material for histologic assessment. *Cautery* is very effective at softening the lesion and often allows it to be removed with minimal effort, the heat separating the lesion at the dermoepidermal junction. The 'melting' of the lesion observed after the application of heat is almost diagnostic. Smaller lesions can be 'flicked off' the skin using a traditional curette, often without local anesthesia. Heat can be applied to the surface of the lesion followed by curettage, and for superficial lesions 'curettage' can be achieved using a cotton gauze swab to wipe away the softened lesion. Cautery can also be used after shave excision to treat any tissue remnants. With all these treatments the aim is to remove the lesion, but little of the underlying skin surface.

Cryotherapy using a liquid nitrogen spray is an alternative method of treatment. Liquid nitrogen is sprayed onto the lesion until it is frozen, and then continued for 5–10 seconds. It can be undertaken without local anesthesia because freezing reduces sensation of pain, and this can be an advantage when treating multiple lesions. After a day or two the treated lesion blisters and crumbles away. The underlying wound heals over after several days and is often quite exudative, requiring daily cleansing by the patient. Overall the recovery period is longer and the wound slower to heal than following curettage and cautery. Whereas following cautery hyperpigmentation is common, following cryotherapy, hypopigmentation occurs. For this reason it is not recommended in black people.

Seborrheic keratosis variants

Senile or 'solar' lentigines can be considered to be flat versions of the seborrheic keratosis. Sometimes referred to as 'age' or 'liver' spots, these small pigmented papules and plaques are more commonly seen on areas of frequent sun exposure, such as the face and dorsa of the hands. Their true nature can be recognized by the slight velvety texture to the lesional surface, which is best seen with tangential lighting. This indicates that the lesion is not a true lentigo but a superficial keratosis. These lesions are amenable to very minor treatments. Topical *tretinoin* cream can be effective. Other treatments include light abrasion with an *exfoliating cream*, *light dermabrasion* or *laser resurfacing, cryotherapy,* or *chemical peels* using trichloroacetic acid or phenol. A favorite treatment is minimal cautery followed by 'curettage' with a cotton gauze swab. This leaves an erythematous superficial wound that heals rapidly.

Dermatosis papulosa nigra is commonly seen on the cheeks of black adults. These small seborrheic warts are easily treated by light cautery or diathermy followed by cotton gauze curettage, but patients should be warned about the possibility of hyperpigmentation.

Stucco keratoses are small grayish-white seborrheic keratoses which are typically found on the forearms and lower legs and are easily removed with curettage without bleeding. The edge of these lesions is often curled up away from the skin surface.

Giant seborrheic keratoses are large lesions, usually found on the scalp, and are often several centimeters in diameter.

Multiple seborrheic keratoses

Seborrheic keratoses may have a familial tendency, especially when multiple. It is these patients who are often the most challenging to treat – and also the most affected by their condition. Many middle-aged to elderly patients will not undress for sporting activities such as swimming because they are embarrassed by the appearance of their skin. Patients not infrequently present with multiple lesions and request their complete removal. In these circumstances it is reasonable to offer several different types of treatment so that the patient can determine their preference.

The sudden onset of multiple seborrheic keratoses may be associated with underlying malignancy – the sign of Leser–Trelat – and should prompt a full clinical examination for underlying malignancy.

SPECIFIC INVESTIGATIONS

▶ Consider the sign of Leser–Trelat and investigate for underlying malignancy

Sign of Leser–Trelat. Schwartz RA. J Am Acad Dermatol 1996; 35: 88–95.

The sign of Leser–Trelat is rare. The sudden eruption of multiple seborrheic keratoses or their rapid increase in size is caused by a malignancy. Its association with malignant acanthosis nigricans, seen in 35% of patients, is one of several of its features that support its legitimacy as a true paraneoplastic disorder.

FIRST-LINE THERAPIES

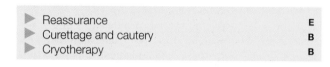

▶ Reassurance	E
▶ Curettage and cautery	B
▶ Cryotherapy	B

Curettage of small basal cell papillomas with the disposable ring curette is superior to conventional treatment. Long CC, Motley RJ, Holt PJ. Br J Dermatol 1994; 131: 732–3.

Ring curettage followed by aluminum chloride 25% in 70% isopropyl alcohol gave a superior cosmetic result compared to using a traditional curette and light cautery.

Skin tumours: seborrhoeic warts. Motley R. Dermatol Pract 1997; 5: 6–7.

A practical review of treatment options.

Cutaneous cryotherapy: principles and practice. Dawber R, Colver G, Jackson A, eds. London: Martin Dunitz, 1997.

A well-illustrated practical guide to all that is cutaneous cryosurgery, including seborrheic warts!

Treatment of superficial surgical wounds after removal of seborrhoeic keratoses: a single-blinded randomized-controlled study. Goetze S, Ziemer M, Lipman RD, Elsner P. Dermatol Surg 2006; 32; 661–8.

Hydrocolloid dressings produced superior healing of superficial wounds following curettage of seborrhoeic keratoses.

SECOND-LINE THERAPIES

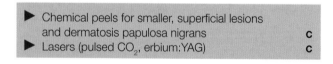

▶ Chemical peels for smaller, superficial lesions and dermatosis papulosa nigrans	C
▶ Lasers (pulsed CO_2, erbium:YAG)	C

Focal trichloroacetic acid peel method for benign pigmented lesions in dark-skinned patients. Chun EY, Lee JB, Lee KH. Dermatol Surg 2004; 30; 512–16.

After cleansing the skin with alcohol, 65% trichloroacetic acid was applied focally to seborrheic keratoses using a sharpened wooden applicator, to create evenly frosted spots on each lesion. Crusts separated from the skin with gentle washing after 4–7 days, and healing was complete 10–14 days later. Twenty-three patients required a mean of 1.5 treatments, and in 57% of these the results were rated as excellent.

Use of the Alexandrite laser for treatment of seborrhoeic keratoses. Mehrabi D, Brodell RT. Dermatol Surg 2002; 28: 437–9.

A patient with multiple seborrheic keratoses was treated in four sessions with a normal-mode Alexandrite laser (755 nm wavelength) spot size 8 mm, fluence 100 J/cm². The entire surface of each lesion was treated in a checkerboard fashion.

Twelve-day follow-up revealed excellent cosmetic resolution of the lesions with minimal scarring and hypopigmentation, especially compared to areas previously treated with liquid nitrogen cryotherapy.

Use of a long-pulse Alexandrite laser in the treatment of superficial pigmented lesions. Trafeli JP, Kwan JM, Meehan KJ, Domankevitz Y, Gilbert S, Malomo K, et al. Dermatol Surg 2007; 33: 1477–82.

Patients with solar lentigines were treated with a long-pulse Alexandrite laser (755 nm wavelength). Optimal settings were spot size 10 mm, pulse duration 3 ms, fluence 22 J/cm² (without skin cooling). The authors advocate undertaking some initial test spots and observing the result after 10 minutes before proceeding to treat an entire area. The desired endpoint is a slight darkening of each lesion and/or perilesional erythema. Treated lesions darken and crust and fall off within about 10 days.

Treatment of verruca vulgaris, seborrheic keratoses, lentigines, and actinic cheilitis. Clinical advantage of the CO_2 laser superpulsed mode. Fitzpatrick RE, Goldman MP, Ruiz-Esparza J. J Dermatol Surg Oncol 1994; 20; 449–56.

Continuous and superpulsed CO_2 lasers were compared in their effect on a variety of lesions, including seborrheic keratoses. Ideal parameters prevent unwanted thermal damage.

Ablation of cutaneous lesions using an erbium: YAG laser. Khatri KA. J Cosmet Laser Ther 2003; 5; 150–3.

Erbium:YAG laser was used to remove multiple benign skin lesions and found to be safe and effective for this purpose.

532-nm diode laser treatment of seborrhoeic keratoses with color enhancement. Gulbertson GR. Dermatol Surg 2008; 34: 525–8.

A red color marker was applied to seborrheic keratoses to enhance the laser absorption prior to treatment with a 532-nm diode laser; 93% of lesions responded completely.

THIRD-LINE THERAPIES

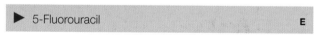

▶ 5-Fluorouracil	E

Giant seborrhoeic keratosis on the frontal scalp treated with topical fluorouracil. Tsuji T, Morita A. J Dermatol 1995; 22: 74–5.

An unusual giant scalp seborrheic keratosis was successfully treated with topical fluorouracil.

Seborrhoeic keratoses: a study comparing the standard cryosurgery with topical calcipotriene, topical tazorotene and topical imiquimod. Herron MD, Bowen AR, Krueger GG. Int J Dermatol 2006; 43: 300–2.

One treatment with cryotherapy was effective and acceptable to all patients. In seven out of 15 patients tazarotene 0.1% applied twice daily produced clinical improvement.

Use of a keratolytic agent with occlusion for topical treatment of hyperkeratotic seborrhoeic keratoses. Burkhart CG, Burkhart CN. Skinmed 2008; 1; 15–18.

A topical 50% urea-containing product applied under occlusion was combined with superficial scraping to remove hyperkeratotic seborrheic keratoses on the trunk and extremities.

Sporotrichosis

Mahreen Ameen, Wanda Sonia Robles

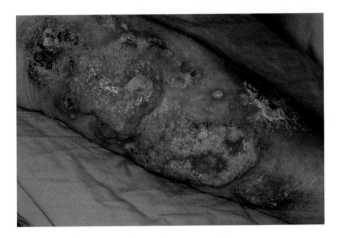

Sporotrichosis is a deep cutaneous fungal infection caused by *Sporothrix schenckii*, a rapidly growing dimorphic saprophytic fungus found in soil and plant matter. It can affect both humans and animals and is prevalent worldwide, but is more common in the tropics. Disseminated infection, particularly to osteoarticular structures and viscera, is a risk in the immunocompromised and an emerging problem in those with advanced HIV infection. Infection is usually sporadic, but outbreaks may occur from contaminated soil and wood. Cutaneous lesions develop following traumatic inoculation of *S. schenckii*. Infection is therefore more common in certain occupations, such as horticulturists, carpenters and miners. Fifteen percent of cases occur in children under 10 years of age. The initial lesion appears at the site of injury as an erythematous, ulcerated, or verrucous nodule. Lesions can be localized and are known as fixed-type sporotrichosis. The more common presentation is the lymphocutaneous form, where there is nodular lymphangitic spread.

MANAGEMENT STRATEGY

Although there have been cases describing the spontaneous remission of sporotrichosis, it is usual practice to treat. Treatment includes *local measures (hyperthermia), saturated solution of potassium iodide (SSKI), azoles, terbinafine*, and *amphotericin B*. Historically, uncomplicated lymphangitic and fixed forms of sporotrichosis have been treated with high-dose SSKI, beginning with five drops three times daily and increased as tolerated to 10–50 drops three times daily (equivalent to 250 mg–1 g three times daily). Treatment is continued for 3–4 weeks after clinical cure. The mechanism of action of potassium iodide is not known, but it is highly effective, with reported cure rates ranging from 80% to 100%. It is also inexpensive, and is first-line treatment for sporotrichosis in most developing countries. However, it is inconvenient to administer and side effects are common, including metallic taste, nausea, abdominal pain, and salivary gland enlargement.

Itraconazole is first-line therapy in countries where it is affordable. It should be started at a loading dose of 200 mg three times daily for 3 days, followed by 200–400 mg daily. Cure rates for cutaneous and lymphocutaneous infection are

high, generally 90–100%. High-dose *terbinafine* (500 mg twice daily) produces similar efficacy, although there is less clinical experience with its use. *Fluconazole* therapy (400–800 mg daily) gives response rates of 63–71% and is therefore recommended for second-line therapy only. Ketoconazole is ineffective for the treatment of sporotrichosis.

There are no clinical trials to guide therapy for disseminated or meningeal sporotrichosis. On the basis of case reports parenteral amphotericin B (AmB) is the preferred treatment (AmB deoxycholate 0.7 mg/kg daily, or as a lipid formulation 3.0–5.0 mg/kg daily). A lipid formulation of AmB is recommended for meningeal infection. Following AmB induction therapy, itraconazole (200 mg twice daily) is given as maintenance therapy.

Local hyperthermia (using infrared and far infrared wavelengths to heat tissues to 42–43°C) is known to be effective, although there are few reports of its use. It has a useful role in those for whom systemic therapies are contraindicated.

SPECIFIC INVESTIGATIONS

▶ Culture
▶ Histology
▶ Serology for HIV infection (where relevant)

Direct microscopy of infected material is futile because the infective organisms are scarce in tissue. Culture is the most sensitive means of diagnosis and is characteristically rapid, with growth usually seen within 3–5 days. Infected material, consisting of pus or biopsy tissue from a lesion, is inoculated onto Sabouraud's dextrose agar at 25°C. The colonies are initially white or creamy with a wrinkled surface, which becomes progressively darker to a brown or black color. The diagnosis is confirmed by demonstrating dimorphism, or conversion to the yeast phase. This is best achieved by incubation at 37°C on brain–heart infusion agar, which produces oval or cigar-shaped yeasts. Histopathology reveals a mixed granulomatous and pyogenic inflammatory response with pseudoepitheliomatous hyperplasia. The fungus is sometimes visualized with periodic acid–Schiff staining and is associated with extracellular *Sporothrix* asteroid bodies, consisting of yeast surrounded by radiating eosinophilic spicules. Polymerase chain reaction is able to detect the fungus even in lesions with few parasites.

FIRST-LINE THERAPIES

▶ Itraconazole	B
▶ Potassium iodide	B
▶ Terbinafine	B
▶ Amphotericin B (for disseminated sporotrichosis)	E

The following reviews summarize the clinical features and management of sporotrichosis.

Clinical practice guidelines for the management of sporotrichosis: 2007 update by the Infectious Diseases Society of America. Kauffman CA, Bustamante B, Chapman SW, Pappas PG. Clin Infect Dis 2007; 45: 1255–65.

For cutaneous and lymphocutaneous infection in developed countries the first-line recommended therapy is itraconazole 200 mg daily, continued for 2–4 weeks after all lesions have resolved. Usually a 3–6-month course of treatment is recommended. Patients who fail to respond can be given either high-dose itraconazole 200 mg twice daily, terbinafine 500 mg twice daily, or saturated solution of potassium iodide (SSKI initiated at a dose of five drops three times daily and increased as tolerated to 40–50 drops three times daily). Children can be treated with the same drugs at a dose of 6–10 mg/kg for itraconazole (maximum 400 mg daily) and a maximum of 1 drop/kg of SSKI. Fluconazole should only be used in patients who cannot tolerate any of these treatments. Local hyperthermia can be used for fixed lesions in those in whom oral therapy is contraindicated, such as pregnant women. Amphotericin B is recommended first-line therapy for severe pulmonary or osteoarticular infection, disseminated, and meningeal sporotrichosis. After the initial response itraconazole is recommended as step-down therapy and should be given to complete a total of at least 12 months of treatment. Amphotericin B is also the drug of choice for severe infection in pregnancy.

Disseminated sporotrichosis and *Sporothrix schenckii* fungemia as the initial presentation of human immunodeficiency virus infection. Al-Tawfiq JA, Wools KK. Clin Infect Dis 1998; 26: 1403–6.

There are a growing number of reports of *S. schenckii* infection in the HIV-infected population. Disease usually starts as a localized cutaneous lesion which subsequently disseminates. This article presents a case report of disseminated sporotrichosis in an HIV-infected patient followed by a review of the literature and discussion of treatment options for such patients.

Al-Tawfiq et al. revised the treatment of sporotrichosis in AIDS patients, suggesting amphotericin B as the drug of choice, and itraconazole for use as maintenance therapy.

Potassium iodide in dermatology: a 19th century drug for the 21st century: uses, pharmacology, adverse effects, and contraindications. Sterling JB, Heymann WR. J Am Acad Dermatol 2000; 43: 691–7.

This article reviews the pharmacology and adverse effects of potassium iodide as a therapeutic agent. It discusses contraindications to its use, which include a history of thyroid or kidney disease, and pregnancy.

Disseminated sporotrichosis associated with treatment with immunosuppressants and tumor necrosis factor-alpha antagonists. Gottlieb GS, Lesser CF, Holmes KK, Wald A. Clin Infect Dis 2003; 37: 838–40.

An adult male developed disseminated infection following treatment with multiple immunosuppressants, including etanercept and infliximab, for inflammatory arthritis. He was subsequently treated with a lipid formulation of amphotericin B.

With the increasing availability and use of anti-TNF-α agents there is an increased risk of sporotrichosis presented with disseminated infection rather than indolent cutaneous lesions only.

Sporotrichosis: a forgotten disease in the drug research agenda. Bustamante B, Campos PE. Exp Rev Anti Infect Ther 2004; 2: 85–94.

This article appraises the current therapeutic options for the management of sporotrichosis. The authors emphasize the need for more effective drug therapies, and of evaluating new drugs in large, randomized clinical trials, given the emergence of more serious disease forms such as disseminated sporotrichosis in AIDS patients.

Epidemiology of sporotrichosis: a study of 304 cases in Brazil. Da Rosa AC, Scroferneker ML, Vettorato R, Gervini RL, Vettorato G, Weber A. J Am Acad Dermatol 2005; 52: 451–9.

A retrospective analysis over a 35-year period (1967–2002) describing 304 mycologically confirmed cases. The majority were successfully treated with potassium iodide. Multifocal and extracutaneous involvement is also described, as well as unusual sites of infection.

This article describes the characteristic clinical features of a large number of cases from an endemic region.

Sporotrichosis. Ramos-e-Silva M, Vasconcelos C, Carneiro S, Cestari T. Clin Dermatol 2007; 25: 181–7.

A recent and comprehensive review article. The authors conclude that itraconazole is the most effective therapy for cutaneous and lymphocutaneous sporotrichosis.

Treatment of sporotrichosis with itraconazole. Sharkey-Mathis PK, Kauffman CA, Graybill JR, Stevens DA, Hostetler JS, Cloud G, et al.; NIAID Mycoses Study Group. Am J Med 1993; 95: 279–85.

Twenty-seven cases (lymphocutaneous, n=9; osteoarticular, n=15; pulmonary, n=3) were treated with itraconazole 100–600 mg daily for 3–18 months; 83% responded to treatment, but 28% of those who responded subsequently relapsed 1–7 months after treatment cessation. The rest remained disease free over follow-up periods of 6–42 months (mean 17.6 months). Itraconazole was well tolerated

Cutaneous sporotrichosis. Intermittent treatment (pulses) with itraconazole. Bonifaz A, Fierro L, Saúl A, Ponce RM. Eur J Dermatol 2008; 8: 61–4.

Five patients received pulse itraconazole 400 mg daily for 1 week at 3-week intervals. Clinical and mycological cure was obtained in four patients after a mean of 3.5 pulses. Treatment was well tolerated, with no adverse effects or biochemical abnormalities. The authors emphasize that pulse therapy produces high efficacy with a reduction in total drug dosage required.

Potassium iodide remains the most effective therapy for cutaneous sporotrichosis. Sandhu K, Gupta S. J Dermatol Treat 2003; 14: 200–2.

Case report of a patient with cutaneous sporotrichosis that failed to respond to an adequate course of itraconazole but responded dramatically to treatment with a saturated solution of potassium iodide.

This report illustrates that potassium iodide is often more efficacious than itraconazole, although there have been no comparative studies.

Cutaneous sporotrichosis in Himachal Pradesh, India. Mahajan VK, Sharma NL, Sharma RC, Gupta ML, Garg G, Kanga AK. Mycoses 2005; 48: 25–31.

One hundred and three cases of the lymphocutaneous and fixed cutaneous varieties of sporotrichosis are described during the period 1990–2002. Potassium iodide was used as first-line treatment, and in 93% of patients healing of lesions occurred in 4–32 weeks (average 8.7 weeks) without significant side effects. Itraconazole was used in 12 patients, and was also highly effective.

Sporotrichosis in Uttarakhand (India): a report of nine cases. Agarwal S, Gopal K, Umesh, Kumar B. Int J Dermatol 2008; 47: 367–71.

Of nine cases (lymphocutaneous form, n=5; fixed cutaneous form, n=4), eight were successfully treated with SSKI for 12–16 weeks. A single patient who was pregnant was treated with thermotherapy.

Potassium iodide is the preferred treatment option because of its low cost. However, it is contraindicated in pregnancy because of potential toxicity to the fetal thyroid. Azoles are teratogenic.

Comparative evaluation of the efficacy and safety of two doses of terbinafine (500 and 1000 mg/day) in the treatment of cutaneous or lymphocutaneous sporotrichosis. Chapman SW, Pappas P, Kauffmann C, Smith EB, Dietze R, Tiraboschi-Foss N, et al. Mycoses 2004; 47: 62–8.

This was a multicenter, randomized, double-blind trial evaluating the safety and efficacy of oral terbinafine for the treatment of cutaneous and lymphocutaneous sporotrichosis. Patients were treated with either 500 mg daily (n=28) or 1000 mg daily (n=35) for a maximum of 24 weeks. Cure was significantly higher in the higher-dose treatment group (87% vs 52%, p=0.004), with no relapses 24 weeks after treatment cessation. By contrast, there were six relapses in the lower-dose group.

Terbinafine has fungicidal activity and therefore continuing treatment beyond mycological cure may not be required, although studies have yet to demonstrate this.

Therapeutic potential of terbinafine in subcutaneous and systemic mycoses. Hay RJ. Br J Dermatol 1999; 141: 36–40.

Terbinafine 500 mg once or twice daily was highly effective, and the average time to negative culture was 12 weeks (range 4–32 weeks).

Cutaneous and meningeal sporotrichosis in a HIV patient. Vilela R, Souza GF, Fernandes Cota G, Mendoza L. Rev Iberoam Micol 2007; 24: 161–3.

A case report from Brazil of a patient with advanced HIV infection who presented with multiple ulcerated nodules. *S. schenckii* was isolated from the skin as well as the spinal fluid. Treatment consisted of amphotericin B (1.0 mg/kg/day) and a total dose of 650 mg was given. The skin lesions and neurological condition improved within 1 week of treatment.

Sporotrichosis in childhood: clinical and therapeutic experience in 25 patients. Bonifaz A, Saúl A, Paredes-Solis V, Fierro L, Rosales A, Palacios C, et al. Pediatr Dermatol 2007; 24: 369–72.

The mean age of this cohort of affected children was 9.3 years. Two-thirds were affected with the lymphocutaneous form, and the upper limbs and face were most commonly involved. Nineteen children were cured clinically and mycologically with potassium iodide, three with itraconazole, and one with heat therapy.

SECOND-LINE THERAPIES

| ▶ Fluconazole | B |
| ▶ Local hyperthermia | D |

A Pan-American 5-year study of fluconazole therapy for deep mycoses in the immunocompetent host. Diaz M, Negroni R, Montero-Gei F, Castro LG, Sampaio SA, Borelli D, et al.; Pan-American Study Group. Clin Infect Dis 1992; 14: S68–76.

An open-label multicenter trial of fluconazole administered at a dose of 200–400 mg daily to 19 patients with sporotrichosis produced a 63% cure rate. The vast majority of patients required a 400 mg daily dose. Treatment was well tolerated.

Treatment of lymphocutaneous and visceral sporotrichosis with fluconazole. Kauffman CA, Pappas PG, McKinsey DS, Greenfield RA, Perfect JR, Cloud GA, et al. Clin Infect Dis 1996; 22: 46–50.

This clinical trial involved 14 patients with lymphocutaneous infection and 16 with osteoarticular or visceral sporotrichosis. Eleven of the 30 patients had previously been treated with other forms of antifungal therapy without success. Most patients were treated with fluconazole 400 mg/day. Four patients received 200 mg/day and another four received 800 mg/day; 71% of patients (10/14) with lymphocutaneous sporotrichosis were cured. However, only 31% (5/16) with osteoarticular or visceral sporotrichosis responded to treatment.

This paper concluded that fluconazole is only modestly effective for the treatment of sporotrichosis, and perhaps should be considered second-line therapy in patients who are unable to take itraconazole.

Hyperthermic treatment of sporotrichosis: experimental use of infrared and far infrared rays. Hiruma M, Kawada A, Noguchi H, Ishibashi A, Conti Díaz IA. Mycoses 1992; 35: 293–9.

Pocket warmers and infrared and far infrared rays were used to treat 14 cases of sporotrichosis, seven in children and seven in adults. Daily applications of heat were applied to the lesions and the devices warmed tissues to 42–43°C. All lesions treated with pocket warmers were facial lesions in children. Infrared and far infrared rays generated more heat than pocket warmers, allowing the duration of a single treatment to be reduced by three-quarters to only a single 15-minute treatment daily. The overall cure rate was 71%.

The efficacy for this form of treatment has not been satisfactorily evaluated. However, it has an important role in the treatment of infection in those who are unable to take systemic therapy.

Squamous cell carcinoma

Heidi A Waldorf

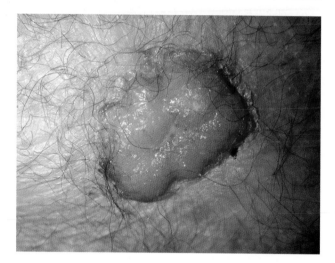

Squamous cell carcinoma (SCC) is a malignant neoplasm arising from epithelial keratinocytes of the skin and mucous membranes that generally appears as an erythematous, keratotic papule or nodule which may become ulcerated. Although it is most commonly associated with chronic sun exposure in light-skinned individuals, squamous cell carcinoma can arise secondary to scarring processes (burns, chronic ulcers, hidradenitis suppurativa), chemical carcinogens (arsenic, tobacco tar, hydrocarbons), human papillomavirus (types 16, 18, 30, 33, 35), and ionizing radiation exposure (X-rays, γ-rays, radium). Immunosuppression due to disease or drug therapy is an instigating factor.

MANAGEMENT STRATEGY

The management of squamous cell carcinoma depends on the histopathologic classification and clinical setting. The risk of local recurrence and of metastasis is correlated with poor histologic differentiation, perineural invasion, tumor size (>2 cm), tumor depth (>4 mm), tumor location (lip, ear, temple, genitalia), treatment modality, history of recurrence, host immunosuppression, and precipitating factors other than UV light. Regional lymphadenopathy is a poor prognostic sign.

Accurate histopathologic diagnosis is the most critical investigation. The differential diagnosis may include verruca vulgaris, actinic keratosis, squamous cell carcinoma in situ (Bowen's disease), and keratoacanthoma (these conditions are described in separate chapters). Specimens for histopathologic diagnosis should include epidermis and dermis. A deep curette or scoop shave biopsy is generally sufficient, but an incisional or excisional biopsy is useful if there is concern regarding obtaining adequate tissue.

Regional lymph node palpation is performed when an aggressive tumor is suspected, based on the criteria specified above. In the absence of palpable lymphadenopathy, additional radiologic and surgical studies are performed if deep invasion (bone, cartilage, parotid) or perineural spread is suspected.

Small superficial squamous cell carcinoma may be effectively treated using a destructive modality. *Cryosurgery* destroys tumor if it is frozen to −40 to −70°C – generally two cycles of at least 60-seconds' thaw time. *Curettage and electrodesiccation* involves a sequence of three curette scrapings and electrodesiccations. A margin of 3 or 4 mm around the tumor should be treated with cryosurgery and with curettage and desiccation. Adequately treated lesions often require several weeks to heal and may leave hypopigmented, atrophic, or hypertrophic scars. Cosmetically sensitive areas, concave surfaces, and skin prone to keloid formation should be avoided. Cure rates are highly technique dependent.

Standard surgical excision, utilizing 3–4 mm margins beyond the clinically apparent tumor, is a reasonable option for well-demarcated squamous cell carcinomas, particularly of the trunk and extremities. Recent studies have suggested that light curettage of the lesion prior to excision, traditionally used to better define tumor margins, may not be efficacious. Extensive tumors of the limbs involving bone may require amputation.

The gold standard for treatment of squamous cell carcinoma is *Mohs' micrographic surgery*, a technique in which the surgeon also acts as pathologist. The tumor is extirpated in a series of thin layers which are precisely oriented, horizontally sectioned, and immediately processed for evaluation. The process is continued until all margins are clear to maximize tumor eradication and tissue conservation. Indications for Mohs' micrographic surgery include tumor size, location (cosmetically or functionally sensitive, high recurrence rate), indistinct margins, history of recurrence, aggressive histopathology, and young patient age. *Adjuvant radiation therapy* following Mohs' micrographic surgery should be considered for facial squamous cell carcinoma >2 cm in diameter and those with perineural spread.

Although the use of radiation therapy as a primary modality has decreased, it remains a good treatment option for selected patients, particularly those of advanced age or at poor surgical risk, with uncomplicated tumors of the head and neck. A total of 4000–7000 cGy is given sequentially over several weeks. One standard schedule is administration of 500 cGy three to five times per week over 2–6 weeks. Complications include hypopigmentation, telangiectasia, loss of adnexa, radiation dermatitis, and late (10–20 years) tumor recurrence.

For patients with squamous cell carcinoma not amenable to surgical extirpation or radiation due to advanced disease stage or large number of lesions, *topical therapy with imiquimod or 5-fluorouracil, intralesional therapy with bleomycin, 5-fluorouracil or interferon, or systemic therapy with retinoids or interferon* may be effective. *Photodynamic therapy*, most commonly using topical porphyrins followed by selective irradiation with visible light, is another alternative. Systemic regimens including *monoclonal antibodies* and *protein kinase inhibitors* are also being studied for inoperable tumors.

SPECIFIC INVESTIGATIONS

- ▶ Histopathology
- ▶ Physical examination for lymphadenopathy
- ▶ Radiologic examination (MRI, CT scan)
- ▶ Sentinel lymph node biopsy

Evidence Levels: **A** Double-blind study **B** Clinical trial ≥ 20 subjects **C** Clinical trial < 20 subjects **D** Series ≥ 5 subjects **E** Anecdotal case reports

Surgical Pearl: Obtaining a clean histopathologic specimen using a ring curette. Madan V, Dawn G. J Am Acad Dermatol 2007; 56: S103–4.

Standard curette biopsy may produce fragmented tissue and hence be suboptimal for diagnosis of squamous cell carcinoma. The authors suggest a more reliable method using the sharp edge of a disposable ring curette held in a 'fountain pen technique' to delineate the margins of the lesion and achieve sufficient depth.

Reliability of the histopathologic diagnosis of keratinocyte carcinomas. Jagdeo J, Weinstock MA, Piepkorn M, Bingham S. J Am Acad Dermatol 2007; 57: 279–84.

A prospective blinded study of 3926 specimens assigned a diagnosis by local pathologists and one or both (355 slides) central dermatopathologists. Intraobserver agreement was highest for basal cell carcinoma and lowest in the categories of invasive squamous cell carcinoma, squamous cell carcinoma in situ, and actinic keratosis, suggesting that the diagnostic boundaries of these diagnoses are imprecisely defined.

Epidermal growth factor receptor: a novel biomarker for aggressive head and neck cutaneous squamous cell carcinoma. Ch'ng S, Low I, Ng D, Brasch H, Sullivan M, Davis P, et al. Hum Pathol 2008; 39: 344–9.

Using immunohistochemistry and fluorescence in situ hybridization, epidermal growth factor (EGF) receptor protein over-expression was detected in 36% of primary squamous cell carcinomas without metastases, 79% of primary squamous cell carcinomas with subsequent metastases, and 47% of squamous cell carcinomas with metastatic nodal disease. Multivariate analysis showed EGF receptor over-expression to be an independent prognostic factor for subsequent metastases. Future study is needed, but this finding could have important prognostic and therapeutic implications for high-risk tumors.

Parotid and cervical nodal status predict prognosis for patients with head and neck metastatic cutaneous squamous cell carcinoma. Ch'ng S, Maitra A, Allison RS, Chaplin JM, Gregor RT, Lea R, et al. J Surg Oncol 2008; 98: 101–5.

Survival rates were measured and multivariate analysis performed retrospectively on 170 patients with head and neck metastatic cutaneous squamous cell carcinoma to test a comprehensive clinical staging system. Overall, the 5-year survival rate was 69% and the locoregional recurrence rate was 36%. The presence of parotid or neck disease, immunosuppression, and the uptake of radiotherapy statistically reduced survival. Higher parotid or neck disease category worsened the prognosis further.

High-risk cutaneous squamous cell carcinoma without palpable lymphadenopathy: is there a therapeutic role for elective neck dissection? Marinez JC, Cook JL. Dermatol Surg 2007; 33: 410–20.

A literature review suggested that patients with cutaneous squamous cell carcinoma who underwent elective node dissection had no proven survival benefit over those who are initially staged as node negative and undergo therapeutic neck dissection after the development of apparent regional disease.

Nonmelanoma cutaneous malignancy with regional metastasis. Chu A, Osguthorpe JD. Otolaryngol Head Neck Surg 2003; 128: 663–73.

This is a retrospective study of 28 patients who underwent a variable combination of parotidectomy, neck dissection, and postoperative radiation for management of regional metastasis from non-melanoma cutaneous malignancies of the head and neck. Only 39% of these patients were disease free at a mean follow-up of 34 months, indicating that patients with regional metastasis have a poor prognosis even with aggressive treatment.

Sentinel node biopsy for high-risk nonmelanoma cutaneous malignancy. Wagner JD, Evdokimow DZ, Weisberger E, Moore D, Chuang TY, Wenck S, et al. Arch Dermatol 2004; 140: 75–9.

A study population of 24 patients with high-risk non-melanoma cutaneous malignancies, the majority squamous cell carcinoma (n=17), underwent preoperative dermatolymphoscintigraphy and sentinel lymphadenectomy. Although these patients had non-palpable lymph nodes at presentation, 29.2% had tumor-positive sentinel nodes. The sensitivity of the sentinel node procedure was 88%, and the specificity 100%.

Sentinel lymph node biopsy for high risk cutaneous squamous cell carcinoma: case series and review of the literature. Renzi C, Caggiati A, Manooranperampil TJ, Passarelli F, Tartaglione G, Pennasilico GM et al. Eur J Surg Oncol 2007; 33: 364–9.

In a consecutive series of 22 clinically node-negative high-risk cutaneous squamous cell carcinoma patients who underwent sentinel lymph node biopsy (SLNB), 4.5% (one patient) had histologically positive nodes and developed a recurrence during follow-up. SLNB-negative patients had no metastases at a median follow-up of 17 months. Literature review revealed an incidence of positive sentinel nodes ranging from 12.5% to 44.4%. Analysis combining the results of this series and 61 patients from previous reports found in the literature supported the concept of SLNB for high-risk cutaneous squamous cell carcinoma.

FIRST-LINE THERAPIES

▶ Curettage and electrodesiccation	C
▶ Cryosurgery	C
▶ Standard excision	B
▶ Mohs' micrographic surgery	B
▶ Radiation therapy	C

Cryosurgery for cutaneous malignancy. An update. Kuflik EG. Dermatol Surg 1997; 23: 1081–7.

A review article outlining the techniques and advantages of cryotherapy, including low cost and speed.

Surgical margins for excision of primary squamous cell carcinoma. Brodland DG, Zitelli JA. J Am Acad Dermatol 1992; 27: 241–8.

Based on a prospective study of subclinical microscopic tumor extension, it was recommended that minimal margins of 4 mm be taken around clinical borders of squamous cell carcinoma. Margins of at least 6 mm were proposed for tumors 2 cm or larger, histologic grade 2 or higher, with invasion of subcutaneous tissue, and/or location in high-risk areas.

Efficacy of curettage before excision in clearing surgical margins of nonmelanoma skin cancer. Chiller K, Passaro D, McCalmont T, Vin-Christian MD. Arch Dermatol 2000; 136: 1327–32.

A retrospective, non-randomized case–control series of 1983 basal cell carcinomas and 849 squamous cell carcinomas treated with pre-excisional curettage followed by simple excision. Pre-excisional curettage reduced the frequency of tumor margin involvement compared to non-curetted lesions for basal cell carcinomas, but not squamous cell carcinomas.

Cutaneous squamous cell carcinoma treated with Mohs micrographic surgery in Australia I. Experience over 10 years. Leibovitch I, Huilgol S, Selva D, Hill D, Richards S, Paver R. J Am Acad Dermatol 2005; 53: 253–60.

In a prospective multicenter case series of 1263 patients with cutaneous squamous cell carcinoma treated with Mohs' micrographic surgery, recurrent tumors were larger than the primary tumors, had larger post-excision defects, required more Mohs' stages, and had more cases of subclinical extension. Recurrence rate was 2.6% for primary SCC and 5.9% for previously recurrent SCC.

Cutaneous squamous cell carcinoma treated with Mohs micrographic surgery in Australia II. Perineural invasion. Leibovitch I, Huilgol SC, Selva D, Hill D, Richards S, Paver R. J Am Acad Dermatol 2005; 53: 2612–16.

Of 1177 squamous cell carcinoma patients treated with Mohs' micrographic surgery in a prospective multicenter case series, 70 were found to have perineural invasion. Perineural invasion was more common in men, in previously recurrent tumors, and in moderately and poorly differentiated histologic subtypes. Perineural invasion was associated with larger tumor size, postoperative defect size, subclinical extension, and mean number of Mohs' stages.

Prognostic factors for local recurrence, metastasis, and survival rates in squamous cell carcinoma of the skin, ear, and lip, implications for treatment modality selection. Rowe DE, Carroll RJ, Day CL. J Am Acad Dermatol 1992; 26: 976–90.

A review of all studies since 1940 revealed lower recurrence rates for Mohs' micrographic surgery than for other modalities, including standard excision for primary squamous cell carcinoma of the skin and lip (3.1% vs 10.9%), of the ear (5.3% vs 18.7%), with diameter >2 cm (25.2% vs 41.7%), with perineural involvement (0% vs 47%), poorly differentiated (32.6% vs 53.6%), and squamous cell carcinoma locally recurrent after previous treatment (10% vs 23.3%).

What is the role of adjuvant radiotherapy in the treatment of cutaneous squamous cell carcinoma with perineural invasion? Han A, Ratner D. Cancer 2007; 109: 1053–9.

This literature review concluded that the extent of perineural tumor involvement may be helpful in determining the role of adjuvant radiation therapy after surgery. Squamous cell carcinoma with microscopic perineural invasion had local control rates of 78–87% versus 50–55% for those with extensive perineural invasion.

Office-based radiation therapy for cutaneous carcinoma: evaluation of 710 treatments. Hernandez-Machin B, Borrego L, Gil-Garcia M, Hernandez BH. Int J Dermatol 2007; 46: 453–9.

A retrospective study of 604 basal cell carcinomas and 106 squamous cell carcinomas irradiated between 1971 and 1996 revealed cure rates for squamous cell carcinoma of 92.7% at 5 years and 78.6% at 15 years, suggesting that radiation therapy is an effective first option in many cases.

SECOND-LINE THERAPIES

▶ Topical imiquimod	**B**
▶ Topical 5-fluorouracil	**D**
▶ Intralesional 5-fluorouracil	**B**
▶ Electrochemotherapy with bleomycin	**B**
▶ Intralesional interferon-α	**C**

Successful treatment with topical 0.5% fluorouracil and imiquimod 5% cream in the treatment of a patient with actinic keratoses and a squamous cell carcinoma. Torok HM. J Am Acad Dermatol 2004; 50: 129.

A case report of clinical clearance of multiple actinic keratoses and a 1.2 × 1.2 cm squamous cell carcinoma of the scalp using concomitant application of 0.5% 5-fluorouracil cream at night and 5% imiquimod cream in the morning for 2 weeks in a patient who had previously failed treatment with imiquimod alone. There was no recurrence at 1 year.

Topical imiquimod therapy for basal and squamous cell carcinomas: a clinical experience. Tillman DK, Carroll MT. Cutis 2007; 79: 241–8.

Twenty squamous cell carcinoma lesions on 19 patients were treated with biopsy alone or biopsy plus curettage, followed by imiquimod 5% cream five times weekly for 6 weeks. At 26 months two SCCs had residual tumor or recurrence on repeat biopsy.

Imiquimod 5% cream in the treatment of Bowen's disease and invasive squamous cell carcinoma. Peris K, Micantonio T, Fargnoli MC, Lozzi GP, Chimenti S. J Am Acad Dermatol 2006; 55: 324–7.

This open-label clinical trial used imiquimod 5% cream five times a week for up to 16 weeks to treat seven invasive squamous cell carcinoma lesions on 10 patients. Five sites (71.4%) showed complete clinicopathologic regression and two (28.6%) partial regression at 16 weeks. There were no recurrences at a mean of 31 months' follow-up.

Intratumoral chemotherapy with fluorouracil/epinephrine injectable gel: a nonsurgical treatment of cutaneous squamous cell carcinoma. Kraus S, Miller BH, Swinehart JM, Shavin JS, Georgouras KE, Jenner DA, et al. J Am Acad Dermatol 1998; 38: 438–42.

One biopsy-proven squamous cell carcinoma on each of 25 patients was treated weekly over 6 weeks with up to 1 mL of a 5-fluorouracil/epinephrine/bovine collagen gel. Histology of the tumor site and margins at 4 months revealed clearance in 96% of the 23 patients available for follow-up, with good to excellent cosmetic results.

A previous study by this group resulted in 91% cure.

Treatment of cutaneous and subcutaneous tumors with electrochemotherapy using intralesional bleomycin. Heller R, Jaroszeski MJ, Reintgen DS, Puleo CA, DeConti RC, Gilbert RA, et al. Cancer 1998; 83: 148–57.

In 34 patients 130 of 143 (91%) tumor nodules had a complete response, defined clinically and by random biopsies, to intralesional injection of bleomycin followed by the direct application of electric pulses.

Effective treatment of cutaneous and subcutaneous malignant tumours by electrochemotherapy. Mir LM, Glass LF, Sersa G, Teissié J, Domenge C, Miklavcic D, et al. Br J Cancer 1998; 77: 2336–42.

Evidence Levels: A Double-blind study **B** Clinical trial ≥ 20 subjects **C** Clinical trial < 20 subjects **D** Series ≥ 5 subjects **E** Anecdotal case reports

A prospective clinical trial of 291 tumors, including 87 squamous cell carcinomas of the head and neck, in 50 patients revealed clinical complete responses in 154 (56.4%) and partial responses in 79 (28.9%) of all tumors using electrochemotherapy with intralesional bleomycin. Follow-up was limited to 1 month after treatment.

Treatment of cutaneous squamous cell carcinomas by intralesional interferon alpha-2b therapy. Edwards L, Berman B, Rapini RP, Whiting DA, Tyring S, Greenway HT Jr, et al. Arch Dermatol 1992; 128: 1486–9.

In an open-label study a complete histologic response rate of 88.2% was achieved for 36 actinically induced primary squamous cell carcinomas <2.0 cm in diameter (28 invasive, eight in situ), 18 weeks after completing a 3-week course of intralesional injection of 1.5 million units of interferon-α_{2b} three times a week.

THIRD-LINE THERAPIES

▶ Amputation	D
▶ Photodynamic therapy	C
▶ Systemic retinoids	B
▶ Systemic interferon-α	C
▶ Protein kinase inhibitors	E
▶ Chemoradiation	E

Squamous cell carcinoma arising in osteomyelitis and chronic wounds. Treatment with Mohs' micrographic surgery vs. amputation. Kirsner RS, Spencer J, Falanga V, Garland LE, Kerdel FA. Dermatol Surg 1996; 22: 1015–18.

Patients with extensive local or metastatic squamous cell carcinoma of the leg involving bone may require amputation if Mohs' micrographic surgery would render the remaining limb unstable.

A review of laser and photodynamic therapy for the treatment of nonmelanoma skin cancer. Marmur ES, Schmults CD, Goldberg DJ. Dermatol Surg 2004; 30: 264–71.

Photodynamic therapy involves the administration of a photosensitizer preferentially absorbed in tumor tissue followed by selective irradiation with visible light. The most common treatment protocol involves application of topical 20% aminolevulinic acid followed by exposure to an incoherent light source. When used to treat squamous cell carcinoma, photodynamic therapy achieves only an 8% clearance rate and has a recurrence rate of 82%. Although useful in certain populations, this modality remains inferior to standard surgical excision.

A good review article.

Long-term treatment of photoaged human skin with topical tretinoic acid improves epidermal cell atypia and thickens the collagen band in papillary dermis. Cho S, Lowe L, Hamilton TA, Fisher GJ, Vorhees JJ, Kang S. J Am Acad Dermatol 2005; 53: 769–74.

Thirty-four caucasian women with photoaged skin treated daily with 0.05% retinoic acid for at least 6 months (mean duration 2.3 years) had improved epidermal cellular atypia on histopathology in 73% of cases by one evaluator and 85% of cases by the other evaluator, consistent with the ability of retinoic acid to act as a chemopreventive agent in epithelial

carcinogenesis. The authors also discussed the ability of topical tretinoin in vivo to prevent ultraviolet-induction of c-Jun, a proto-oncoprotein that is elevated in human squamous cell carcinoma.

13-cis-retinoic acid and interferon alpha-2a: effective combination therapy for advanced squamous cell carcinoma of the skin. Lippman SM, Parkinson DR, Itri LM, Weber RS, Schantz SP, Ota DM, et al. J Natl Cancer Inst 1992; 84: 235–41.

Of 28 patients with inoperable cutaneous squamous cell carcinoma, 19 (68%) had a partial response and seven (25%) had a complete response to a regimen of oral isotretinoin, 1 mg/kg daily, and subcutaneous interferon-α_{2a}, 3 million units daily. The major dose-limiting side effect was fatigue.

Beneficial effect of low-dose systemic retinoid in combination with topical tretinoin for the treatment and prophylaxis of premalignant and malignant skin lesions in renal transplant recipients. Rook AH, Jaworsky C, Nguyen T. Transplantation 1995; 59: 714–19.

In a study of 11 renal allograft patients a combination of topical tretinoin cream and oral etretinate, 10 mg daily, significantly reduced the number of existing lesions and reduced the recurrence rate of new squamous cell carcinomas.

Acitretin suppression of squamous cell carcinoma: case report and literature review. Lebwohl M, Tannis C, Carrasco D. J Dermatol Treat 2003; 14; 3–6.

A 40-year-old man with a history of severe psoriasis began developing numerous cutaneous squamous cell carcinomas after treatment with psoralen and ultraviolet A (PUVA) for 4.5 years. Because of a flare in his psoriasis he was started on 25 mg daily of acitretin, which resulted in a dramatic reduction in the number of squamous cell carcinomas. This report reviews the mechanism by which retinoids are thought to act and describes how oral retinoids may be an important therapy in patients at risk for developing multiple cutaneous malignancies.

Oral retinoid use reduces cutaneous squamous cell carcinoma risk in patients with psoriasis treated with psoralen-UVA: a nested cohort study. Nijsten TEC, Stern RS. J Am Acad Dermatol 2003; 49: 644–50.

To assess whether oral retinoids reduce the risk of developing cutaneous squamous cell carcinoma, a nested cohort of 135 patients participating in the PUVA follow-up study with at least 1 year of substantial retinoid use was identified. Each patient's tumor incidence during retinoid therapy was compared to the incidence of squamous cell carcinoma development in periods of no use. Overall, a 30% reduction in squamous cell carcinoma incidence was noted when patients were on oral retinoid therapy.

Retinoids (isotretinoin, acitretin) may play a role in the treatment of patients with squamous cell carcinoma not amenable to surgical extirpation owing to advanced stage of disease or large number of lesions. Several studies have shown an overall response rate of about 70%. Systemic retinoids may play a greater role in chemoprevention of new and recurrent malignancies in susceptible individuals, such as organ transplant recipients and those with xeroderma pigmentosum, than in treatment.

Cutaneous squamous cell carcinoma responding serially to single-agent cetuximab. Suen JK, Bressler L, Shord SS, Warso M, Villano JL. Anticancer Drugs 2007; 18: 827–9.

A case report of repeated responses to cetuximab, a monoclonal antibody that binds to human epidermal growth factor receptor, in a patient with non-resectable squamous cell carcinoma with strong human epidermal growth factor receptor expression. This therapy may have a palliative role in recurrent or metastatic cancers.

The promise of molecular targeted therapies: Protein kinase inhibitors in the treatment of cutaneous malignancies. Kondapalli L, Soltani K, Lacouture ME. J Am Acad Dermatol 2005; 53: 291–302.

Protein kinases mediate most signal transduction pathways in malignant cells to increase proliferation, invasion, and metastasis. This review outlines the rationale for the use of protein kinase inhibitors on cutaneous malignancies, including squamous cell carcinoma.

Chemoradiation using low-dose cisplatin and 5-fluorouracil in locally advanced squamous cell carcinoma of the skin: A report of two cases. Fujisawa T, Umchayashi Y, Ichikawa E, Kawachi Y, Otsuka F. J Am Acad Dermatol 2006; 55: S81–5.

Two case studies of locally invasive squamous cell carcinomas metastatic to regional lymph nodes were treated with IV cisplatin and 5-fluorouracil concurrent with either conventional fractionated radiation therapy or external beam radiation. Although the primary tumors of both patients initially underwent complete regression, one patient required resection of a local recurrence at 5 years. The other developed lung metastases and died of disseminated disease at 18 months.

Staphylococcal scalded skin syndrome

Dimitra Koch, Saleem M Taibjee

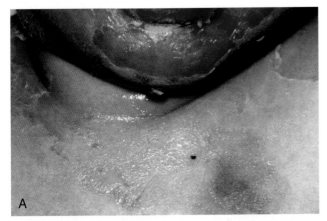

A

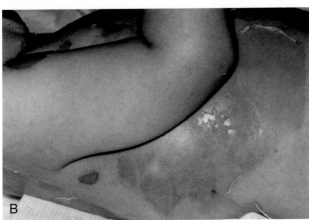

B

Staphylococcal scalded skin syndrome (SSSS) is a blistering condition triggered by exfoliative toxin-producing *Staphylococcus aureus*, and most commonly affects neonates and children under the age of 6 years. It presents only rarely in adults, usually in association with renal failure or immunocompromise, and possibly NSAID use. In healthy infants mortality is uncommon, with reported rates up to 3%, contrasting with up to 50–60% in adults with comorbidity.

SSSS is caused by hematogenous spread of exfoliative toxin (ET) produced by *S. aureus*, most commonly phage group II (types 3A, 3B, 3C, 55, 71), including both methicillin-sensitive and methicillin-resistant (MRSA) strains. ET, a serine protease, specifically cleaves the desmosomal protein desmoglein-1, leading to disruption of keratinocyte adhesion. Increased susceptibility to SSSS in neonates and adults with renal failure, and in immunocompromised individuals, is thought to be due to impaired renal clearance of ET or low titers of ET-specific antibodies, respectively.

Clinical features include a prodrome of malaise, irritability, and fever. Skin manifestations develop within 24–48 hours. Tender erythema is followed by superficial, flaccid blistering, most pronounced in flexural and periorificial areas. The Nikolsky sign is positive. Mucosal surfaces are not involved. With successful treatment SSSS resolves over 10–14 days.

Bullae rupture to leave an exudative surface, followed by desquamation and re-epithelialization without scarring.

Typically the causative organism cannot be cultured from affected skin, as this is a toxin-mediated disease. However, in some cases it may be possible to culture ET-producing *S. aureus* from extracutaneous sites, most commonly the nasopharynx, but also the conjunctivae, umbilicus, rectum, and blood. Histology of affected skin typically shows a superficial, subcorneal blister, absence of epidermal necrosis, and minimal inflammation. Frozen section of the blister roof is an alternative method of confirming the superficial level of cleavage and may facilitate more rapid diagnosis.

The main differential diagnosis is the Stevens–Johnson syndrome–toxic epidermal necrolysis spectrum, in which targetoid skin lesions, mucosal involvement, and a deeper level of blistering with full-thickness epidermal necrosis are distinguishing features.

SPECIFIC INVESTIGATIONS

> ▶ Nose, throat and skin swabs for bacterial culture and sensitivities
> ▶ Culture from suspected site of primary infection
> ▶ Blood cultures
> ▶ Full blood count
> ▶ Serum urea, creatinine and electrolytes
> ▶ Skin biopsy or frozen section of blister roof
> ▶ Screening contacts for *S. aureus* carriage

Isolating *Staphylococcus aureus* from children with suspected staphylococcal scalded skin syndrome is not clinically useful. Ladhani S, Robbie S, Chapple DS, Joannou CL, Evans RW. Pediatr Infect Dis J 2003; 22: 284–6.

S. aureus was isolated from skin lesions in patients with suspected generalized SSSS over a 4-year period. Polymerase chain reaction for *eta* and *etb* genes and Western blotting confirmed ET-producing strains in only 17 of 54 (31%) of isolates.

Failure to isolate ET-producing S. aureus *from affected skin does not exclude the diagnosis of SSSS.*

MANAGEMENT STRATEGY

Treatment includes *antibiotic therapy* in combination with *supportive measures* addressing electrolyte and fluid balance, temperature regulation, nutrition, analgesia, and skin care. *Bland emollients* such as 50:50 white soft paraffin/liquid paraffin should be applied regularly to reduce friction and insensible fluid losses. *Non-adherent dressings* are used to cover denuded areas, with avoidance of adhesive tapes directly to skin. Systemic β-lactamase-resistant antibiotics are necessary to eradicate the causative *S. aureus* strain. Patients with extensive SSSS require hospital admission and intravenous antibiotics, converting to oral once clinical improvement is established. In view of the growing emergence of resistant *S. aureus* strains, in particular MRSA, antibiotic choice should be guided by the local microbiology team.

SSSS outbreaks on maternity and neonatal units are reported. Strict infection control measures are advisable, including patient isolation, barrier nursing, and hand-washing. Screening programs may identify *S. aureus* carriers among patient contacts, including healthcare workers. Colonized individuals require treatment with *topical antiseptics* such as *chlorhexidine*, with nasal carriage eradicated by topical antibiotics.

Early hospital discharge and cross-infection. Bell FG, Fenton PA. Lancet 1993; 342: 120.

An outbreak of SSSS due to ET-producing *S. aureus* carriage by a paediatrician.

This was not initially recognized, since many cases presented following hospital discharge.

Nosocomial outbreak of staphylococcal scalded skin syndrome in neonates: epidemiological investigation and control. El Helali N, Carbonne A, Naas T, Kerneis S, Fresco O, Giovangrandi Y, et al. J Hosp Infect 2005; 61: 130–8.

An SSSS outbreak affecting 13 neonates in a maternity unit. Temporary removal from duty of a nurse with chronic hand dermatitis confirmed as a carrier of the causative ET-producing *S. aureus* with infection control measures (patient isolation, barrier-nursing, chlorhexidine hand-washing, treatment of carriers with nasal mupirocin and chlorhexidine showers), controlled the outbreak. All affected neonates were successfully treated with oxacillin.

Healthcare workers are an important potential source of outbreaks.

SPECIFIC THERAPY

The choice of antibiotic therapy should be guided by local incidence of multidrug-resistant *S. aureus* strains and microbiology advice.

FIRST-LINE THERAPIES

▶ β-Lactamase-resistant penicillins, e.g., flucloxacillin **D**

Outbreak of staphylococcal scalded skin syndrome among neonates. Dancer SJ, Simmons NA, Poston SM, Noble WC. J Infect 1988; 16: 87–103.

Twelve neonates were successfully treated with intravenous flucloxacillin (50 mg/kg total daily dose at age <7 days, 75 mg/kg at age >7 days).

Staphylococcal scalded skin syndrome in healthy adults. Patel GK, Varma S, Finlay AY. Br J Dermatol 2000; 142: 1253–5.

Two healthy adults with generalized SSSS were successfully treated with oral flucloxacillin 500 mg four times daily for 10 days and topical 2% mupirocin for nasal carriage.

Staphylococcal scalded skin syndrome as a complication of septic arthritis. Sladden MJ, Mortimer NJ, Elston G, Newey M, Harman KE. Clin Exp Dermatol 2007; 32: 754–5.

An adult developed septic arthritis and SSSS following knee arthroscopy, successfully treated with high-dose intravenous flucloxacillin and benzylpenicillin.

The patient was on an NSAID prior to surgery.

SECOND-LINE THERAPIES

▶ Glycopeptide antibiotic, e.g., vancomycin **E**

A clinical and microbiological comparison of *Staphylococcus aureus* toxic shock and scalded skin syndromes in children. Chi CY, Wang SM, Lin HC, Liu CC. Clin Infect Dis 2006; 42: 181–5.

All *S. aureus* strains isolated from 16 Taiwanese children with either SSSS or staphylococcal toxic shock syndrome expressed macrolide resistance genes, and community-acquired MRSA genes in 11 (69%). In vitro susceptibility testing demonstrated all *S. aureus* isolates were sensitive to vancomycin, gentamicin, doxycycline, and trimethoprim-sulfamethoxazole.

Most isolates were resistant to clindamycin. The clinical efficacy of trimethoprim-sulfamethoxazole in SSSS needs to be established.

Staphylococcal scalded skin syndrome in the course of lupus nephritis. Rydzewska-Rosolowska A, Brzosko S, Borawski J, Mysliwiec M. Nephrology 2008; 13: 265–6.

An adult with SLE, antiphospholipid syndrome, and chronic renal failure, receiving pulsed cyclophosphamide and prednisolone, developed SSSS due to MRSA. She recovered with intravenous vancomycin therapy (750 mg every 48 hours).

A reduced vancomycin dosage is required in renal failure.

Staphylococcal scalded skin syndrome in an adult due to methicillin-resistant *Staphylococcus aureus.* Ito Y, Yoh MF, Toda K, Shimazaki M, Nakamura T, Morita E. J Infect Chemother 2002; 8: 256–61.

An adult with diabetes mellitus and metastatic renal cell carcinoma developed cholecystitis and SSSS due to ET-producing MRSA, successfully treated with a combination of intravenous vancomycin and teicoplanin, and percutaneous transhepatic gallbladder drainage.

THIRD-LINE THERAPIES

▶ Quinolones	**E**
▶ Tetracyclines	**E**
▶ Cephalosporins	**E**
▶ Aminoglycosides	**E**
▶ Pooled human immunoglobulin	**E**
▶ Fresh-frozen plasma	**E**

Antimicrobial agent of susceptibilities and antiseptic resistance gene distribution among methicillin-resistant staphylococcal aureus isolates from patients with impetigo and staphylococcal scalded skin syndrome. Noguchi N, Nakaminami H, Nishijima S, Kurokawa I, So H, Sasatsu M. J Clin Microbiol 2006; 44: 2119–25.

A Japanese study of MRSA, including 76 strains isolated from patients with impetigo and SSSS, of which 75 (99%) were community acquired (C-MRSA). C-MRSA strains frequently demonstrated evolution of multidrug resistance (95% gentamicin- and 80% clarithromycin-resistant), although all remained susceptible to levofloxacin and minocycline; 71 of 76 (93.5%) C-MRSA strains were susceptible to cationic antiseptic agents, contrasting with 112 of 207 (54%) hospital-acquired MRSA.

Staphylococcal scalded skin syndrome in two very low birth weight infants. Haveman LM, Fleer A, Gerards LJ. J Perinat Med 2003; 31: 515–19.

Two preterm neonates were successfully treated with intravenous cefazolin and gentamicin, switching to flucloxacillin in one patient following culture results.

Adult staphylococcus scalded skin syndrome in a peritoneal dialysis patient. Suzuki R, Iwasaki S, Ito Y, Hasegawa T, Yamamoto T, Ideura T, et al. Clin Exp Nephrol 2003; 7: 77–80.

An adult undergoing peritoneal dialysis developed acute peritonitis, initially treated with intraperitoneal and intravenous vancomycin (0.5 g/day each, 1 g/day total). He subsequently developed SSSS with septic shock, successfully treated with intravenous amikacin (100 mg/day) for 1 day, followed by cefoperazone with sulbactam.

Staphylococcal scalded skin syndrome caused by exfoliative toxin B-producing methicillin-resistant *Staphylococcus aureus*. Yokota S, Imagawa T, Katakura S, Mitsuda T, Arai K. Eur J Pediatr 1996; 155: 722.

A 6-month-old infant with SSSS due to ET-B-producing MRSA was successfully treated, according to sensitivity, with oral minocycline 5 mg/kg daily.

Note that tetracyclines are usually contraindicated in children <12 years.

Staphylococcal scalded skin syndrome in an extremely premature neonate: a case report with a brief review of the literature. Kapoor V, Travadi J, Braye S. J Pediatr Child Health 2008; 44: 374–6.

A premature neonate with SSSS was successfully treated with intravenous flucloxacillin and a single dose of intravenous immunoglobulin 1 g/kg in view of transient low IgG levels.

Severe staphylococcal scalded skin syndrome in children. Blyth M, Estela C, Young ER. Burns 2008; 34: 98–103.

Four children with severe SSSS were successfully treated with a regimen including intravenous penicillinase-resistant penicillin and fresh frozen plasma, postulated to possess anti-toxin properties.

Steatocystoma multiplex

Roy A Palmer, Martin Keefe

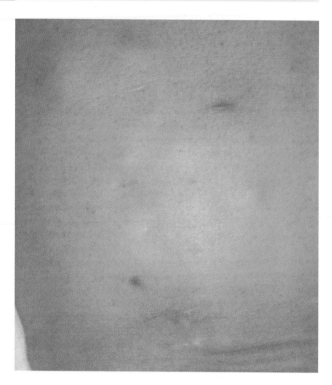

Although probably genetically heterogeneous, steatocystoma multiplex often demonstrates an autosomal dominant pattern of inheritance. It is characterized by the development in adolescence or early adulthood of cysts on the trunk and proximal limbs, or in some patients on the face and scalp. These are true 'sebaceous cysts': they contain sebum, and sebaceous gland lobules are present in the walls. Overlap with eruptive vellus hair cysts and association with pachyonychia congenita type II have been reported.

MANAGEMENT STRATEGY

The cysts persist indefinitely. Although usually a minor cosmetic problem, they can be highly disfiguring. Paradoxically, those patients who would benefit the most from treatment are sometimes regarded as being unsuitable for surgery because they have too many cysts to excise. The *surgical* technique described below is quick, and so can be used on large numbers of lesions in one session. It produces good cosmetic results.

Lesions can become inflamed, due to rupture of the cyst wall with leakage of the contents into the dermis, or because of bacterial infection. Suppuration and scarring may follow. The clinical picture then resembles cystic acne and is called steatocystoma multiplex suppurativum. Oral *isotretinoin* is an effective treatment for inflammatory lesions but not for non-inflamed cysts. This suggests it operates by a direct anti-inflammatory effect rather than by reducing the sebum excretion rate. Alternatively, inflamed cysts can be treated with *incision and drainage, intralesional triamcinolone, tetracycline* 1 g/day, or *minocycline* 100–200 mg/day.

Topical treatment is largely ineffective because it does not penetrate to reach the cyst wall.

SPECIFIC INVESTIGATIONS

> ▶ Skin biopsy if diagnosis is in doubt

FIRST-LINE THERAPIES

Inflamed lesions
▶ Isotretinoin	D
▶ Antibiotics	E
▶ Incision and drainage	E

Lesions not inflamed
▶ Surgical incision and extraction of cyst wall	D

Steatocystoma multiplex suppurativum: treatment with isotretinoin. Schwartz JL, Goldsmith LA. Cutis 1984; 34: 149–53.

The treatment of steatocystoma multiplex suppurativum with isotretinoin. Statham BN, Cunliffe WJ. Br J Dermatol 1984; 111: 246.

Isotretinoin in the treatment of steatocystoma multiplex: a possible adverse reaction. Rosen BL, Broadkin RH. Cutis 1986; 115: 115–20.

Steatocystoma multiplex treated with isotretinoin: a delayed response. Mortiz DL, Silverman RA. Cutis 1988; 42: 437–9.

Treatment of steatocystoma multiplex and pseudofolliculitis barbae with isotretinoin. Friedman SJ. Cutis 1987; 39: 506–7.

These five papers report a total of seven patients treated with oral isotretinoin, at a dose of approximately 1 mg/kg/day for about 20 weeks. Inflammation of cysts was greatly reduced. Non-inflammatory lesions were unaffected, and in one patient appeared to increase in size and number. One successfully treated patient relapsed 10 weeks after ceasing therapy, but other patients did not relapse during a follow-up period of up to 8 months.

Successful treatment of steatocystoma multiplex by simple surgery. Keefe M, Leppard BJ, Royle G. Br J Dermatol 1992; 127: 41–4.

Five generations with steatocystoma multiplex congenita: a treatment regimen. Pamoukian VN, Westreich M. Plast Reconstruct Surg 1997; 99: 1142–6.

Surgical pearl: mini-incisions for the extraction of steatocystoma multiplex. Schmook T, Burg G, Hafner J. J Am Acad Dermatol 2001; 44: 1041–2.

A simple surgical technique for the treatment of steatocystoma multiplex. Kaya TI, Ikizoglu G, Kokturk A, Tursen U. Int J Dermatol 2001; 40: 785–8.

Suggestion for the treatment of steatocystoma multiplex located exclusively on the face. Duzova AN, Senturk GB. Int J Dermatol 2004; 43: 60–2.

Evidence Levels: **A** Double-blind study   **B** Clinical trial ≥ 20 subjects   **C** Clinical trial < 20 subjects   **D** Series ≥ 5 subjects   **E** Anecdotal case reports

The vein hook successfully used for eradication of steatocystoma multiplex. Lee SJ, Choe YS, Park BC, Lee WJ, Kim do W. Dermatol Surg 2007; 33: 82–4.

These six reports describe variants of a simple surgical technique for non-inflamed cysts. Local, regional, general or no anesthesia is used, depending on the exact technique and the number of cysts being treated. In most cases a 1–10 mm incision is made with a surgical blade, the contents of the cyst are expressed, then fine artery forceps are passed through the opening to grasp the base of the cyst, which is pulled out. The incisions heal by secondary intention. Good cosmetic results and a very low recurrence rate are reported.

Excision of cysts and aspiration have also been described.

SECOND-LINE THERAPIES

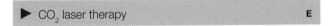

▶ CO_2 laser therapy   E

CO_2 laser therapy for steatocystoma multiplex. Krahenbuhl A, Eichmann A, Pfaltz M. Dermatologica 1991; 183: 294–6.

'Fairly good' results were reported.

THIRD-LINE THERAPIES

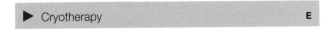

▶ Cryotherapy   E

Treatment of lesions of steatocystoma multiplex and other epidermal cysts by cryosurgery. Notowicz A. J Dermatol Surg Oncol 1980; 6: 98–9.

Three or four days after cryotherapy, the necrotic skin overlying the cyst was removed and the intact cyst expressed through the opening.

Stoma care

Calum Lyon

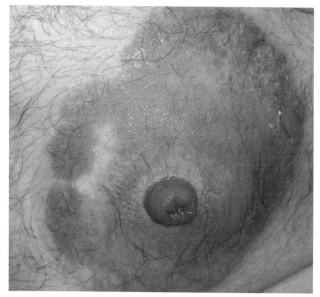

From Griffiths CE, Tranfaqlia MG and Kang S. Prolonged occlusion in the treatment of psoriasis: a clinical and immunohistologic study. J Am Acad Dermatol 1995; 32: 618–22, with permission of Elsevier.

Stomas are artificial openings created to maintain proper drainage from internal structures. The most common are colostomies, ileostomies, and urostomies (ileal conduits), formed as either a temporary or a permanent measure. They are ideally produced electively, having been correctly sited by a stoma nurse specialist, but may be created under emergency conditions. Even with the best of preventative measures dermatologic problems will occur in over 50% of patients at some time. These are mostly irritant reactions to body fluids, particularly in the higher-output stomas (ileostomy and urostomy), but a range of common skin disorders, infections, or any dermatosis exacerbated by trauma or irritation may also be seen.

MANAGEMENT STRATEGY

Although all irritant reactions share similar histological features, the clinical appearance depends on the type of stoma and the source of irritation. Ileostomies have a high output containing degradative enzymes and irritant bile acids, so that severe dermatitis and erosions may be seen. Irritated colostomies generally have a milder dermatitis, often due to occlusion, but sizeable hypergranulating polyps and acanthomas can occur where there are leaks. Urostomy dermatitis may also be erosive because of the high output and ileal mucus production, predisposing to leaks. Chronic papillomatous dermatitis is a distinct eruption comprising aggregating hyperplastic papulonodules that usually affects leaking urostomies. It responds to appliance modifications and acidification of the urine. Input from an expert stoma nurse is essential when managing irritant reactions. They can advise on the most appropriate appliance, so that mechanical trauma to the skin or stoma and exposure of normal skin to effluent can be avoided.

Patients anxious to avoid leaks, smells, etc., sometimes wear bags too tightly or change them excessively, frequently resulting in skin damage and irritation. The stoma nurse specialist is trained to identify and resolve such issues. It is appropriate to treat symptomatic irritant inflammation with anti-inflammatory preparations such as *topical corticosteroids, tacrolimus,* or *pimecrolimus.* The choice of vehicle is very important, as oily creams etc., will prevent proper adhesion and cause leaks. Products useful on peristomal skin include a range of aqueous lotions and gels formulated for scalp, ear or eye disorders, as well as corticosteroid in carmellose-sodium paste (Orabase), normally admininstered for intraoral use. *Flurandrenolide tape,* an occlusive corticosteroid therapy, is particularly useful because the stoma device can be applied over the tape. Leaks and inflammation are sometimes inevitable despite appliance changes. It may be necessary to use topical anti-inflammatories intermittently, with care taken to avoid steroid atrophy. Hypergranulation can be treated with *silver nitrate, cryotherapy,* or *excision (shave or curettage) and electrodesiccation.*

Allergic contact dermatitis is rare, as ostomy manufacturers strive to minimize allergens in their products. When it occurs it is mostly due to perfumed deodorizers and excipients in topical products (e.g., biocides in wet wipes). Usage tests are particularly helpful in identifying the offending product, even if patch testing fails to identify the precise allergen. Treatment is as for irritant reactions.

Skin infection is not uncommon in the moist and warm environment under a stoma bag, especially folliculitis in those who shave their abdomens. All rashes should be swabbed, because bacterial infection can present as a nonspecific dermatitis under occlusion, and pre-existing rashes can become secondarily infected. Treatment involves careful hygiene and the use of specific antimicrobials.

Pre-existing skin disorders may occur in the skin surrounding the stoma. Dermatologic disorders that particularly affect stomas are psoriasis, seborrheic dermatitis, cutaneous Crohn's disease, pyoderma gangrenosum, lichen sclerosus, and eczema.

SPECIFIC INVESTIGATIONS

- ▶ Skin biopsy
- ▶ Wound culture
- ▶ Patch testing & usage test

The spectrum of skin disorders in abdominal stoma patients. Lyon CC, Smith AJ, Griffiths CEM, Beck MH. Br J Dermatol 2000; 143: 1248–60.

This large cohort study documented the many different types of skin disorder that can occur around a stoma. Initial evaluations for patients presenting with inflammation include a bacterial swab, because infections are relatively common and easy to treat. Allergic contact hypersensitivity should be suspected in any patient with persistent disease that is unresponsive to treatment. And finally, in any peristomal skin disorder with ulceration or a papular component, a biopsy should be performed.

A comprehensive review discussing the various different pathologies that can occur with a stoma, and how to evaluate them.

Results of a nationwide prospective audit of stoma complications within 3 weeks of surgery. Cottam J, Richards K, Hasted A, Blackman A. Colorectal Dis 2007; 9: 834–8.

Evidence Levels: **A** Double-blind study **B** Clinical trial ≥ 20 subjects **C** Clinical trial < 20 subjects **D** Series ≥ 5 subjects **E** Anecdotal case reports

A prospective audit of stomas – analysis of risk factors and complications and their management. Arumugam PJ, Bevan L, Macdonald L, Watkins AJ, Morgan AR, Beynon J, et al. Colorectal Dis 2003; 5: 49–52.

Healthy peristomal skin is dependent on good surgical technique, with more problems being associated with short stomas (<10 mm) and after emergency procedures. Body mass index and diabetes are significantly associated with skin problems.

Peristomal allergic contact dermatitis – case report and review of the literature. Martin JA, Hughes TM, Stone NM. Contact Dermatitis 2005; 52: 273–5.

Case report detailing sensitivity to Gantrez resin in a stoma barrier paste, and a review of previously reported allergens.

FIRST-LINE THERAPIES

▶ Change appliance	D
▶ Absorbent powders	D
▶ Antibiotics	D
▶ Topical corticosteroids	B

Dermatologic considerations of stoma care. Rothstein MS. J Am Acad Dermatol 1986; 15: 411–32.

Ill-fitting devices can cause stoma and skin irritation. The chemical irritation caused from the stomal effluent, mechanical irritation, and contact dermatitis can all be alleviated by replacing the stoma device at the earliest sign of irritation. Additionally, careful drying of the skin after washing and the use of absorbent powders will alleviate irritation caused by intertrigo and ill-fitting devices. Infection is another cause of complications, and treatment depends on the causative organism.

Peristomal dermatoses; a novel indication for topical steroid lotions. Lyon CC, Smith AJ, Griffiths CEM, Beck MH. J Am Acad Dermatol 2000; 43: 679–82.

This large clinical study demonstrated the benefits of treating inflammatory peristomal skin diseases with topical corticosteroids formulated in an aqueous alcohol lotion. This formulation was found advantageous because it did not interfere with adhesion of the ostomy bag to the skin, allowing treatment of the skin disease as well as correct bag application.

SECOND-LINE THERAPIES

▶ Intralesional corticosteroids	E
▶ Tacrolimus ointment or pimecrolimus cream	E
▶ Amikacin gel	C
▶ Sucralfate	C

Topical sucralfate in the management of peristomal skin disease: an open study. Lyon CC, Stapelton M, Smith AJ, Griffiths CE, Beck MH. Clin Exp Dermatol 2000: 25; 584–8.

The authors demonstrated the ability of sucralfate to help treat peristomal erosions. Sucralfate is a basic aluminum salt of sucrose octasulfate that polymerizes in acidic environments and provides a viscous barrier on mucosal surfaces. Sucralfate was effective for erosions and irritation caused by either feces or urine. However, it was ineffective for peristomal pyoderma gangrenosum.

Peristomal pyoderma gangrenosum. Keltz M, Lebwohl M, Bishop S. J Am Acad Dermatol 1992; 27: 360–4.

A patient with peristomal pyoderma gangrenosum is described who responded well to intralesional corticosteroids.

This article also discusses the difficulties in diagnosing peristomal pyoderma gangrenosum.

Topical tacrolimus in the management of peristomal pyoderma gangrenosum. Lyon CC, Stapelton M, Smith AJ, Mendelsohn S, Beck MH, Griffiths CE. J Dermatol Treat 2001; 12: 13–17.

Topical tacrolimus (0.3% in carmellose sodium paste) in conjunction with other treatments was found to rapidly heal pyoderma gangrenosum.

Amikacin gel administration in the treatment of peristomal dermatitis. La Torre F, Nicolai AP. Drugs Exp Clin Res 1998; 24: 153–7.

Local daily application of amikacin sulfate 5% gel was successful in patients with moderate to severe peristomal dermatitis.

THIRD-LINE THERAPIES

▶ Topical cromolyn sodium	E
▶ Oral dapsone	E
▶ Ciclosporin	D
▶ Tumor necrosis factor (TNF)-blocking drugs	E
▶ Collagen injections	E
▶ Lipectomy	E
▶ Cholestyramine	E

Clinical features and treatment of peristomal pyoderma gangrenosum. Hughes AP, Jackson JM, Callen JP. JAMA 2000; 284: 1546–8.

Peristomal pyoderma gangrenosum is a difficult and frequently misdiagnosed condition. It was observed in this study that six of seven patients required either dapsone, topical cromolyn sodium, ciclosporin, mycophenolate mofetil, or infliximab, and that these treatments are beneficial in treating peristomal pyoderma gangrenosum rather than other peristomal ulcers.

Paraileostomy recontouring by collagen sealant injection: a novel approach to one aspect of ileostomy morbidity. Report of a case. Smith GH, Skipworth RJ, Terrace JD, Helal B, Stewart KJ, Anderson DN. Dis Colon Rectum 2007; 50: 1719–23.

Peristomal dermal deformity such as skin creasing and scarring makes appliance placement troublesome. The authors report a case of a dermal contour defect that was successfully treated with intradermal injections of collagen.

Troublesome colostomies and urinary stomas treated with suction assisted lipectomy. Samdal F, Amlamd PF, Bakka A, Aasen AO. Eur J Surg 1995; 161: 361–4.

This study demonstrated the usefulness of syringe-assisted lipectomy for stomas with significant leakage. The ability to reduce the amount of leakage and irritation led to significant patient satisfaction.

Treatment of skin irritation around enterostomies with cholestyramine ointment. Rodriguez JT, Huang TL, Ferry GD, Klish WJ, Harberg FJ, Nichols BL. J Pediatr 1976; 88: 659–61.

This study found that the irritation caused by stomas can be treated with cholestyramine ointment.

Striae

Jonathan E Blume

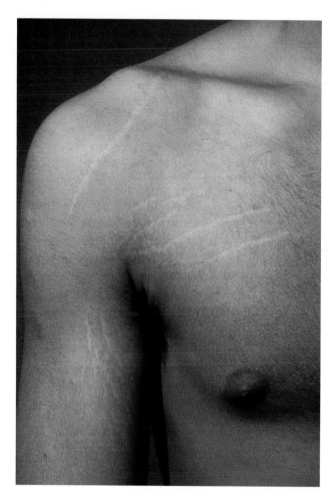

Striae distensae are common lesions that are of significant cosmetic concern to many patients. Striae are initially slightly elevated and have a pink to violaceous color. Over time, these striae rubra evolve into striae alba, which are white, atrophic, linear bands of skin. They are considered by most to be atrophic dermal scars and are probably the result of a combination of factors, including genetics, mechanical stress, and hormones (e.g., cortisol and estrogen).

MANAGEMENT STRATEGIES

The goal of treatment is gradual, incremental improvement. In general, 'older' striae alba respond more slowly and less dramatically to therapy than 'newer' striae rubra. The best results are achieved by combining multiple treatment modalities.

Several studies have shown that *topical tretinoin* improves the appearance of striae. Based on these reports, striae rubra respond better to this therapy. Although not formally investigated, it is expected that *other topical retinoids (e.g., tazarotene, adapalene)* may also provide some improvement.

Non-ablative lasers probably produce improvement by stimulating an increase in dermal collagen and elastin. The *pulsed dye laser* is the one that has been most studied. Early reports suggest that this laser is helpful for both striae rubra and striae alba. However, more recent studies suggest that improvement is more common in early striae that are pink to red in color.

The *excimer laser, intense pulsed light,* and *glycolic acid products* appear to be the most promising treatments for mature striae.

SPECIFIC INVESTIGATIONS

> ▶ Thorough history and physical examination
> ▶ Skin biopsy (not generally necessary)
> ▶ Serum adrenocorticotropin (ACTH) levels, 24-hour urine free cortisol level, plasma cortisol levels

The diagnosis and cause of striae are usually straightforward to elucidate. When the lesions are particularly severe and the cause is unknown, laboratory testing to exclude Cushing's syndrome is advised. Occasionally, striae may be confused with linear focal elastosis, which is stria-like, slightly palpable, yellow bands commonly found on the lower back of older adults. Histological evaluation, with specific attention given to the elastic fiber content, will clearly differentiate these two entities.

FIRST-LINE THERAPIES

> ▶ Observation   **D**

Adolescent striae. Ammar NM, Roa B, Schwartz RA, Janniger CK. Cutis 2000; 65: 69–70.

Striae cutis distensae. Nigam PK. Int J Dermatol 1989; 28: 426–7.

It is well known that striae tend to become less conspicuous with time. Thus, reassurance may be all that is required for the patient who is not overly concerned about his or her striae.

SECOND-LINE THERAPIES

> ▶ Topical tretinoin   **B**
> ▶ Pulsed dye laser (585 nm)   **C**

Topical tretinoin 0.1% for pregnancy-related abdominal striae: an open-label, multicenter, prospective study. Rangel O, Aries I, García E, Lopez-Padilla S. Adv Ther 2001; 18: 181–6.

Twenty patients who were 1 week post delivery applied tretinoin cream 0.1% once a day for 3 months to half of the abdomen: 80% noted a marked or moderate improvement. Measured striae decreased by 20% in length and by 23% in width.

Topical tretinoin for management of early striae. Kang S. J Am Acad Dermatol 1998; 38: S90–2.

Twenty-six patients with early erythematous striae were randomized to either tretinoin cream 0.1% or placebo for 24 weeks: 80% of the patients in the treatment arm experienced improvement or marked improvement, with reduced length and width of striae.

Topical tretinoin (retinoic acid) improves early stretch marks. Kang S, Kim KJ, Griffiths CEM, Wong TA, Talwar HS, Fisher GJ, et al. Arch Dermatol 1996; 132: 519–26.

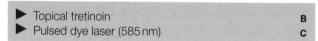

Evidence Levels: **A** Double-blind study   **B** Clinical trial ≥ 20 subjects   **C** Clinical trial < 20 subjects   **D** Series ≥ 5 subjects   **E** Anecdotal case reports

In this double-blind study, 22 patients with early striae applied either tretinoin cream 0.1% or placebo cream daily for 6 months: 80% of the patients who used tretinoin showed improvement or marked improvement.

Low-dose tretinoin does not improve striae distensae: a double-blind, placebo-controlled study. Pribanich S, Simpson FG, Held B, Yarbrough CL, White SN. Cutis 1994; 54: 121–4.

No difference was noted in the treatment group compared with the control group.

It should be noted that this study was very small (only 11 subjects) and that low-dose tretinoin (0.025% cream) was used.

Treatment of striae distensae with topical tretinoin. Elson ML. J Dermatol Surg Oncol 1990; 16: 267–70.

All patients applied Retin-A cream 0.1% once a day for 12 weeks: 15 of 16 patients experienced significant improvement, and some had total resolution. Although not specifically quantified, some of the patients who showed improvement had striae alba.

Treatment of striae rubra and striae alba with the 585-nm pulsed-dye laser. Jiménez G, Flores F, Berman B, Gunja-Smith Z. Dermatol Surg 2003; 29: 362–5.

Nine patients with striae rubra and 11 patients with striae alba were treated at baseline and again at 6 weeks. The treatment was moderately effective in reducing the erythema of striae rubra, but no improvement was noted in late-stage striae. The authors warn against using the pulsed dye laser in patients with skin types V and VI.

Comparison of the 585 nm pulsed dye laser and the short pulsed CO_2 laser in the treatment of striae distensae in skin types IV and VI. Nouri K, Romagosa R, Chartier T, Bowes L, Spencer JM. Dermatol Surg 1999; 25: 368–70.

This study confirmed that laser treatment for patients with skin types IV, V, or VI should be avoided, or used only with extreme caution.

Treatment of mature striae with the pulsed dye laser. Nehal KS, Lichtenstein DA, Kamino H, Levine VJ, Ashinoff R. J Cutan Laser Ther 1999; 1: 41–4.

Five patients with late-stage striae were treated with multiple sessions of the pulsed dye laser. All five felt that their striae had improved. However, physician, photographic, textural, and histologic assessments could not confirm this improvement.

Treatment of stretch marks with the 585-nm flashlamp-pumped pulsed dye laser. McDaniel DH, Ash K, Zukowski M. Dermatol Surg 1996; 22: 332–7.

Thirty-nine striae were treated once with the pulsed dye laser. Except for one stria, all were of the alba type. All of the striae showed at least minimal improvement that continued for 6 or more months after the treatment.

THIRD-LINE THERAPIES

▶ Excimer laser (308 nm)	C
▶ Intense pulsed light	C
▶ Copper bromide laser (577–511 nm)	C
▶ 1064-nm Nd:YAG laser	C
▶ Radiofrequency and 585-nm pulsed dye laser	B
▶ 20% glycolic acid/0.05% tretinoin	C

▶ 20% glycolic acid/10% L-ascorbic acid	C
▶ 70% glycolic acid gel/40% trichloroacetic acid (TCA) chemical peel	D
▶ *Centella asiatica* extract	A
▶ Microdermabrasion	E

The safety and efficacy of the 308-nm excimer laser for pigment correction of hypopigmented scars and striae alba. Alexiades-Armenakas MR, Bernstein LJ, Friedman PM, Geronemus RG. Arch Dermatol 2004; 104: 955–60.

In this randomized controlled trial, nine patients with striae alba experienced re-pigmentation after treatment with the excimer laser. The pigment normalization is temporary and requires maintenance treatment every 1–4 months.

Intense pulsed light in the treatment of striae distensae. Hernández-Pérez E, Colombo-Charrier E, Valencia-Ibiett E. Dermatol Surg 2002; 28: 1124–30.

In this prospective study, 15 women with late-stage striae of the abdomen were treated with five sessions of intense pulsed light. All patients showed clinical and microscopic improvement in their striae.

Two-year follow-up results of copper bromide laser treatment of striae. Longo L, Postiglione MG, Marangoni O, Melato M. J Clin Laser Med Surg 2003; 21: 157–60.

Thirteen of 15 patients experienced improvement in their striae that remained after 1–2 years. One-third of the patients had total disappearance of selected striae.

Stretch marks: treatment using the 1,064-nm Nd:YAG laser. Goldman A, Rossato F, Prati C. Dermatol Surg 2008; 34: 686–91.

Twenty patients with striae rubra were treated with the 1064-nm Nd:YAG laser; all considered the results satisfactory, and a majority (55%) found the results to be excellent.

Radiofrequency and 585-nm pulsed dye laser treatment of striae distensae: a report of 37 Asian patients. Suh DH, Chang KY, Son HC, Ryu JH, Lee SJ, Song KY. Dermatol Surg 2007: 33: 29–34.

Thirty-seven patients were treated with one session of radiofrequency (Thermage) and three monthly sessions of the 585-nm pulsed dye laser. A majority of patients (89.2%) showed 'good or very good' improvement.

Comparison of topical therapy for striae alba (20% glycolic acid/0.05% tretinoin versus 20% glycolic acid/10% L-ascorbic acid). Ash K, Lord J, Zukowski M, McDaniel DH. Dermatol Surg 1998; 24: 849–56.

Ten patients with skin types I–V and abdominal and thigh striae associated with childbirth applied glycolic acid in the morning and either tretinoin or L-ascorbic acid in the evening for a total of 12 weeks. All patients felt that they had improvement of their striae.

Chemical peel of nonfacial skin using glycolic acid gel augmented with TCA and neutralized based on visual staging. Cook KK, Cook WR. Dermatol Surg 2000; 26: 994–9.

The authors comment on their experience treating over 3100 patients with non-facial peels using a combination of 70% glycolic acid gel combined with 40% TCA. It is reported that striae, including atrophic hypopigmented striae, can be improved with this treatment.

Prophylaxis of striae gravidarum with a topical formulation: a double blind trial. Mallol J, Belda MA, Costa D, Noval A, Sola M. Int J Cosmet Sci 1991; 3: 51–7.

One hundred pregnant women applied either trofolastin cream (contains *C. asiatica*, α-tocopherol, and collagen–elastin hydrolysates) or placebo daily from 12 weeks' gestation until labor. The product, which is only available in Europe, helped women who already had striae from developing additional striae in pregnancy.

Extracts of C. asiatica, *a medicinal plant, are widely used outside the USA for many dermatologic conditions, including striae, kelo-ids, hypertrophic scars, chronic venous insufficiency, leprosy sores, slow-healing wounds, and cellulitis.*

Laser therapy of stretch marks. McDaniel DH. Dermatol Clin 2002; 20: 67–76.

The author states that microdermabrasion has become part of the adjunctive armamentarium for striae, often combined with laser, topical agents, and chemical peels.

Evidence Levels: **A** Double-blind study **B** Clinical trial ≥ 20 subjects **C** Clinical trial < 20 subjects **D** Series ≥ 5 subjects **E** Anecdotal case reports

Subacute cutaneous lupus erythematosus

Jeffrey P Callen

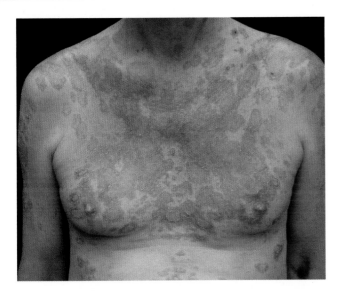

Subacute cutaneous lupus erythematosus (SCLE) is a non-scarring, non-atrophic variant of lupus erythematosus that was first distinguished from other cutaneous variants in 1979. In the original article Sontheimer et al. (1979) described two subsets: patients with annular disease, and patients with papulosquamous disease. It might be debated whether tumid LE belongs to the SCLE subset of LE, because these patients have non-scarring lesions; however, they have chronic disease and rarely manifest a positive serology, in contrast to the patient with SCLE in whom ANA positivity is frequent and the anti-Ro (SS-A) antibody is common. At least half of the patients with SCLE have or develop four or more of the features that allow classification as systemic LE. In general, however, their prognosis is better than that of unselected patients with systemic LE

MANAGEMENT STRATEGY

Therapy of cutaneous lesions in patients with LE involves both an empiric and a scientific approach. Unfortunately, there are few double-blind, placebo-controlled trials of drugs used in the treatment of cutaneous LE.

The goals of management of discoid lupus erythematosus (DLE) or SCLE are to improve the patient's appearance and prevent the development of deforming scars, atrophy, or dyspigmentation. In addition, the majority of patients with SCLE have disease that primarily affects their skin, and may be reassured that their prognosis is relatively benign. Cosmetic problems are often of major importance to the patient with cutaneous LE. Dyspigmentation may follow both DLE and SCLE, and may be effectively hidden by agents such as Covermark or Dermablend.

Once a diagnosis of subcutaneous LE has been made, management must involve *sun avoidance* and *sun protection*, and *elimination of medications that might be responsible for the skin*

lesions. Treatment with the most benign drugs possible should be stressed. *Topical corticosteroids* and *oral antimalarials* are the most commonly prescribed medications. Although *systemic corticosteroids* may be highly effective, attempts should be made to reduce their dosage and use other medications in their place to avoid corticosteroid side effects.

SPECIFIC INVESTIGATIONS

▶ Thorough evaluation to exclude systemic disease
▶ History of drug ingestion that might be responsible for the disease
▶ History of smoking

The cornerstone of the management of DLE and SCLE is correct diagnosis and thorough evaluation. The patient should have a careful history, physical examination, and laboratory studies directed at uncovering systemic manifestations that might occur in LE. The risk of serious systemic involvement (renal, central nervous system, or cardiopulmonary involvement) in patients with SCLE is probably around 10%, though many patients with SCLE – more than 50% – have sufficient criteria to classify them as having systemic lupus erythematosus (SLE).

Subacute cutaneous lupus erythematosus associated with hydrochlorothiazide therapy. Reed BR, Huff JC, Jones SK, Orton PW, Lee LA, Norris DA. Ann Intern Med 1985; 103: 49–51.

This was the first report that linked a drug (hydrochlorthiazide) to SCLE. Discontinuation of the drug led to a clearing of the disease.

Subacute cutaneous lupus erythematosus induced or exacerbated by terbinafine: a report of five cases. Callen JP, Hughes AP, Kulp-Shorten CL. Arch Dermatol 2001; 137: 1196–8.

This report links terbinafine to SCLE. Four of the five patients did not have documented onychomycosis. Also, this report suggests that patients with a prior history of LE or photosensitivity may be predisposed to the development of this eruption.

Drug-induced, Ro/SSA-positive cutaneous lupus erythematosus. Srivastava M, Rencic A, Diglio G, Santana H, Bonitz P, Watson R, et al. Arch Dermatol 2003; 139: 45–9.

This study detailed only patients with cutaneous disease who were anti-Ro/SS-A positive. However, they found that among 70 such patients, 15 had a link to a new drug within 6 months of the diagnosis of SCLE. Most of these instances were linked to antihypertensive agents, but two patients with statin-induced disease were reported.

A complete list of the patient's medications will assist in the exclusion of drug-induced cutaneous LE. Drugs that have been linked as causes of SCLE primarily include antihypertensive agents such as hydrochlorothiazide, calcium channel blockers, and angiotensin-converting enzyme inhibitors. In addition, there are multiple reports of terbinafine and tumor necrosis factor-α (TNF-α) inhibitors that have been linked to the development of SCLE. Because of the growing list of agents linked to SCLE development or exacerbation, any newly introduced drug should be considered as a possible trigger.

Drug-induced subacute cutaneous lupus erythematosus: a paradigm for bedside-to-bench patient-oriented translational clinical investigation. Sontheimer RD, Henderson CL, Grau RH. Arch Dermatol Res. 2009; 301: 65–70.

This report details a literature review of 71 cases of drug-induced SCLE. Antihypertensive medications and antifungals are the most commonly reported medicines. The reaction often occurs after months of therapy and most of the implicated agents are photosensitizers.

Although reports of antifungal medications as causes of SCLE are numerically greater, the most frequently implicated drug remains hydrochlorothiazide.

Report of an association between discoid lupus erythematosus and smoking. Gallego H, Crutchfield CE III, Lewis EJ, Gallego HJ. Cutis 1999; 63: 231–4.

These authors suggest that cutaneous LE is more severe in patients who smoke.

Patients with cutaneous lupus erythematosus who smoke are less responsive to antimalarial treatment. Jewell ML, McCauliffe DP. J Am Acad Dermatol 2000; 42: 983–7.

These authors compared antimalarial-responsive patients to those who did not respond. Their results indicate that patients with cutaneous LE who smoke are significantly less likely to respond to antimalarial therapy.

Patients who smoke should be encouraged to stop for the benefit of their skin disease. In personal observations, the author has noted a marked improvement in some patients who take this advice.

FIRST-LINE THERAPIES

▶ Cosmetics	E
▶ Sunscreens and protective clothing	C
▶ Topical corticosteroids	E
▶ Antimalarials	B
▶ Topical retinoids	E
▶ Topical tacrolimus or pimecrolimus	D

Experimental reproduction of skin lesions in lupus erythematosus by UVA and UVB radiation. Lehmann P, Holze E, Kind P, Goerz G, Plewig G. J Am Acad Dermatol 1990; 22: 181–7.

The action spectrum was defined by photoprovocation testing and includes UVA, UVB, and occasionally visible light.

Broad-spectrum sunscreens, protective clothing, and sun avoidance are important parts of any therapeutic regimen.

Evaluation of the capacity of sunscreens to photoprotect lupus erythematosus patients by employing the photoprovocation test. Stege H, Budde MA, Grether S, Krutmann J. Photodermatol Photoimmunol Photomed 2000; 16: 256–9.

These authors examined the capacity of three sunscreens to prevent the development of skin lesions by provocative phototesting. Although each of the three sunscreens tested prevented lesions, the extent to which they did so varied greatly. The sunscreen that was most effective contained Octocrylene as the UVB protectant, Mexoryl SX, Mexoryl XL, and Parsol 1789 as UVA protectants, and titanium oxide. This sunscreen's SPF was 60. Their study was of only 11 patients (nine men and two women), of whom eight had SCLE and three had DLE.

Intralesional triamcinolone is effective for discoid lupus erythematosus of the palms and soles. Callen JP. J Rheumatol 1985; 12: 630–3.

Intralesional injections of corticosteroids are often effective in patients with lesions that are refractory to topical corticosteroids. Small amounts of triamcinolone acetonide may be injected with a 30-gauge needle into multiple areas. These injections are often very effective in control of the lesions, but do not prevent the development of new lesions.

The potential for cutaneous atrophy and/or dyspigmentation similar to that seen with the disease should be discussed with the patient; however, in most cases an experienced dermatologist is able to inject without a great risk. Alternative agents for intralesional injection have not been well tested.

The association of the two antimalarials chloroquine and quinacrine for treatment-resistent chronic and subacute cutaneous lupus erythematosus. Feldmann R, Salomon D, Saurat JH. Dermatology 1994; 189: 425–7.

The first-line therapy is the use of an antimalarial drug. The antimalarial preferred by the author is hydroxychloroquine sulfate (Plaquenil). This drug is used in doses of 200 mg orally once or twice daily, or in a dose of less than 6.5 mg/kg daily. The onset of action of the antimalarial agents is roughly 4–8 weeks, and for this reason some physicians have advocated higher initial loading doses. Hydroxychloroquine is also of benefit for the joint symptoms and malaise that may accompany SCLE. Hydroxychloroquine is less toxic, but also less effective than chloroquine phosphate (Aralen), which is used in doses of 250–500 mg daily. Thus patients who fail to respond fully to hydroxychloroquine may be switched to chloroquine, but the two should not be used together because of the concern that ophthalmologic toxicity may be enhanced. Another antimalarial, quinacrine hydrochloride (Atabrine), may add benefit to either hydroxychloroquine or chloroquine, and is not associated with ophthalmologic toxicity. This agent is not readily available, but several compounding pharmacies in the USA have it.

Hydroxychloroquine sulfate treatment is associated with later onset of systemic lupus erythematosus. James JA, Kim-Howard XR, Bruner BF, Jonsson MK, McClain MT, Arbuckle MR, et al. Lupus 2007; 16: 401–9.

This is a retrospective analysis of a prior cohort of 130 US military personnel who later met ACR criteria for classification of SLE. Patients treated with hydroxychloroquine prior to a diagnosis of SLE had a significantly longer time between the onset of the first clinical symptom (often cutaneous disease) and the development of SLE criteria (median: 1.08 versus 0.29 years). Patients treated with prednisone before diagnosis also more slowly satisfied the classification criteria. The difference in median times between patients who received NSAIDs before diagnosis, as opposed to those who did not, was not statistically different. Patients treated with hydroxychloroquine also had a lower rate of autoantibody accumulation and fewer autoantibody specificities both at and after diagnosis. These findings suggest that early hydroxychloroquine use is associated with delayed onset of SLE.

This is an important observation by which dermatologists might justify the use of antimalarials early in the course of disease, even for localized lesions.

Cutaneous lupus treated with topical tretinoin: a case report. Seiger E, Roland S, Goldman S. Cutis 1991; 47: 351–5.

This is a case report of hypertrophic lupus erythematosus treated with topical tretinoin.

Treatment of localized discoid lupus erythematosus with tazarotene. Edwards KR, Burke WA. J Am Acad Dermatol 1999; 41: 1049–50.

Several other topical agents might be of use in individual patients with SCLE. None of these agents has been tested in any systematic manner. It appears that they are more likely to be effective in chronic cutaneous LE. Other topical non-steroidal agents that might be considered in the future would be tacrolimus and imiquimod.

Evidence Levels: **A** Double-blind study **B** Clinical trial ≥ 20 subjects **C** Clinical trial < 20 subjects **D** Series ≥ 5 subjects **E** Anecdotal case reports

Topical tacrolimus therapy of resistant cutaneous lesions in lupus erythematosus: a possible alternative. Lampropoulos CE, Sangle S, Harrison P, Hughes GR, D'Cruz DP. Rheumatology 2004; 43: 1383–5.

This is an open-label study of 12 patients with various types of cutaneous lesion who had disease that was recalcitrant to previous therapies, including systemic therapies. The patients with a malar photosensitive eruption responded best, and those with discoid LE lesions responded less well. Two of the four patients with SCLE included in this study responded to therapy with topical tacrolimus.

Pimecrolimus 1% cream for cutaneous lupus erythematosus. Kreuter A, Gambichler T, Breuckmann F, Pawlak FM, Stücker M, Bader A, et al. J Am Acad Dermatol 2004; 51: 407–10.

This is an open-label study of 11 patients with various forms of cutaneous LE. The two patients with SCLE in this study had excellent responses. These patients differ from those in the tacrolimus study in that they were not selected for recalcitrant disease, and therefore this method of selection may have been associated with an improved response rate.

SECOND-LINE THERAPIES

▶ Dapsone	E
▶ Gold	B
▶ Antibiotics	E
▶ Thalidomide	B
▶ Retinoids	C
▶ Immunosuppressive agents – methotrexate, azathioprine, mycophenolate mofetil	C

Dapsone is an effective therapy for the skin lesions of subacute cutaneous lupus erythematosus and urticarial vasculitis in a patient with C2 deficiency. Holtman J, Neustadt D, Callen JP. J Rheumatol 1990; 17: 122–5.

A case of SLE with acute, subacute and chronic cutaneous lesions successfully treated with dapsone. Neri R, Mosca M, Bernacchi E, Bombardieri S. Lupus 1999; 8: 240–3.

Dapsone, given in doses of 25–200 mg daily, has been useful for SCLE lesions and for the vasculitic lesions that may accompany SCLE, as well as for patients with bullous LE.

Treatment of chronic discoid lupus erythematosus with an oral gold compound (auranofin). Dalziel K, Going G, Cartwright PH, Marks R, Beveridge GW, Rowell NR. Br J Dermatol 1986; 115: 211–16.

Nineteen of 23 patients in this open study responded to oral gold, with complete resolution of lesions in four of them.

The author's personal experience with a small number of patients has been encouraging. Auranofin is begun at a dose of 3 mg daily, and after 1 week this may be increased to twice daily if the patient experiences no problems with nausea, diarrhea, or headache. Monitoring with regular complete blood counts and urinalysis is suggested. The author has seen one patient with a lichenoid drug eruption presumed to be due to the auranofin.

Long-term cefuroxime axetil in subacute cutaneous lupus erythematosus. A report of three cases. Rudnicka L, Szymanska E, Walecka I, Stowinska M. Dermatology 2000; 200: 129–31.

A variety of antibiotics have been used for the treatment of SCLE. Rudnicka et al. reported that the antibiotic cefuroxime axetil at a dose of 500 mg daily resulted in the clearing of skin lesions in three patients with SCLE. Cefuroxime axetil is a second-generation β-lactamase oral cephalosporin. Others must replicate this observation before it can be recommended for widespread use, but it is a relatively benign form of treatment.

Sulfasalazine in the treatment of cutaneous lupus erythematosus: open trial in six cases. [Abstract.] LaGrange S, Piette J-C, Becherel P-A, Cacoub P, Frances C. Lupus 1998; 7: 21.

LaGrange et al. noted a drug eruption in five of six patients treated with sulfasalazine, and in only two patients did they feel that there was a beneficial effect.

Thalidomide in the treatment of cutaneous lupus erythematosus refractory to conventional therapy. Ordi-Ros J, Cortes F, Cucurull E, Mauri M, Buján S, Vilardell M. J Rheumatol 2000; 27: 1429–33.

Six of seven patients treated with long-term low-dose thalidomide experienced marked resolution or complete clearing of cutaneous lesions in an average of 2.2 months. Sedation, constipation, weight gain, intermittent shaking, and paresthesias occurred.

Low-dose thalidomide therapy for refractory cutaneous lesions of lupus erythematosus. Housman TS, Jorizzo JL, McCarty MA, Grummer SE, Fleischer AB Jr, Sutej PG. Arch Dermatol 2003; 139: 50–4.

This is a retrospective analysis of 23 patients treated with thalidomide for at least 1 month for various skin lesions of LE, including three patients with SCLE; 74% had complete resolution of their disease, but with discontinuation of thalidomide relapse was frequent. Neurological toxicity was common, occurring in five patients as documented by nerve conduction studies.

Long-term thalidomide use in refractory cutaneous lesions of lupus erythematosus: a series of 65 Brazilian patients. Coelho A, Souto MI, Cardoso CR, Salgado DR, Schmal TR, Waddington Cruz M, et al. Lupus 2005; 14: 434–9.

Sixty-three patients (98.9%) presented complete or partial improvement with thalidomide therapy. Drowsiness occurred in 50 patients (77%). Twenty-eight (43.2%) presented with neuropathy symptoms. Nerve conduction studies were done in 21 (75%) of them and were abnormal in 12 (57%). With the interruption of thalidomide, 24 (82.5%) had complete or partial improvement of neuropathy symptoms and 23 (82%) had cutaneous relapse. There were no significant differences in treatment duration, age, total dose and systemic versus cutaneous LE between those who did or did not develop neuropathy.

Thalidomide in cutaneous lupus erythematosus. Pelle MT, Werth VP. Am J Clin Dermatol 2003; 4: 379–87.

This is an excellent compilation of reports of the use of thalidomide for cutaneous lupus erythematosus.

Thalidomide has recently become more available and is being used with some regularity for patients with cutaneous LE. Its mechanism of action is believed to involve a reduction in inflammatory mediators, particularly TNF-α and Fas ligand. Open-label trials suggest that it is highly effective, and may result in an increase in the lymphocyte count and a reduction in C-reactive protein level. Induction with 100–300 mg daily at bedtime results in improve-

ment in 90% of patients who are able to tolerate the drug. Toxicity commonly associated with thalidomide use includes drowsiness, headache, weight gain, amenorrhea, and dizziness. Drowsiness and dizziness may persist during the following day. Neuropathy, usually sensory, may limit the ability of patients to continue thalidomide on a long-term basis. Neuropathy may be reversible, but there are patients whose neuropathy has progressed despite stopping the drug. Whether nerve conduction studies should be performed at the onset of therapy and periodically is not known, but in their recent summary paper, Pelle and Werth suggest this study at baseline and every 6 months while on therapy. The author chooses not to perform nerve conduction studies unless symptoms develop. Thalidomide is a potent teratogen, and accordingly the company has developed a program to prevent the chance of pregnancy in patients exposed to the drug. This requires that the prescribing physician and the pharmacy be registered with the company, and that the patient use extra precautions in taking the drug. No more than a 1-month supply may be prescribed at any one time. Unfortunately, the response to thalidomide is not durable in most patients; therefore long-term, low-dose maintenance therapy may be necessary.

Mechanism-oriented assessment of isotretinoin in chronic or subacute cutaneous lupus erythematosus. Newton RC, Jorizzo JL, Solomon AR, Sanchez RL, Daniels JC, Bell JD, et al. Arch Dermatol 1986; 122: 180–6.

Eight of 10 patients with cutaneous LE had an excellent response to oral isotretinoin 80 mg daily for 16 weeks.

Treatment of cutaneous lupus erythematosus with etretinate. Ruzicka T, Meurer M, Brown-Falco O. Acta Dermatol Venereol 1985; 65: 324–9.

Eleven of 19 patients with cutaneous lupus erythematosus had excellent results after 2–6 weeks of treatment with etretinate.

Oral retinoids are effective in many patients who have failed to respond to previous less toxic therapies. Isotretinoin and acitretin (formerly etretinate was used) have both been used in doses similar to those used for acne vulgaris or psoriasis, respectively. The response is not durable, and after short courses the patient will still need further suppressive therapy. These agents are particularly helpful in patients with hypertrophic lesions of chronic cutaneous LE. Experience in SCLE is limited.

Azathioprine: an effective, corticosteroid-sparing therapy for patients with recalcitrant cutaneous lupus erythematosus or with recalcitrant cutaneous leukocytoclastic vasculitis. Callen JP, Spencer LV, Burruss JB, Holtman J. Arch Dermatol 1991; 127: 515–22.

Three of six patients with chronic cutaneous LE had an excellent response to azathioprine, permitting prednisone doses to be reduced.

Mycophenolate sodium for subacute cutaneous lupus erythematosus resistant to standard therapy. Kreuter A, Tomi NS, Weiner SM, Huger M, Altmeyer P, Gambichler T. Br J Dermatol 2007; 156: 1321–7.

This was a prospective, non-randomized, open-label pilot study to evaluate the efficacy of mycophenolate sodium monotherapy in patients with recalcitrant subacute SCLE. Monotherapy with oral enteric-coated mycophenolate sodium 1440 mg daily was given for a total of 3 months. Treatment outcome was evaluated by means of the Cutaneous Lupus Erythematosus Disease Area and Severity Index (CLASI). Assessment included the monitoring of adverse effects and clinical laboratory parameters. Ten patients with active SCLE resistant to at least one standard therapy were included in the

trial. Mycophenolate sodium led to a remarkable improvement of skin lesions, resulting in a significant reduction in the mean CLASI from the beginning to the end of therapy. Clinical improvement was confirmed by ultrasonographic assessments and colorimetry. No serious side effects were noted.

This report used measures of response that are validated. In addition, photodocumentation was provided for two patients and is convincing. A double-blind, placebo-controlled trial needs to be performed.

Mycophenolate mofetil for non-renal manifestations of systemic lupus erythematosus: a systematic review. Mok CC. Scand J Rheumatol 2007; 36: 329–37.

This systematic review dealt with other aspects of systemic lupus erythematosus, but noted that the reports dealing with MMF use for cutaneous disease were conflicting.

The author has patients who have seemed to have some response to MMF, but ability to manage patients with this agent as a sole therapy is mixed, just as the reports in the literature suggest.

Efficacy and safety of methotrexate in recalcitrant cutaneous lupus erythematosus: results of a retrospective study in 43 patients. Wenzel J, Brähler S, Bauer R, Bieber T, Tüting T. Br J Dermatol 2005; 153: 157–62.

Among 139 patients with cutaneous LE seen between 2001 and 2003, 43 were treated with low-dose methotrexate. This led to a highly significant (p<0.01) decline in disease activity. An improvement of the cutaneous lesions was recorded in nearly all patients treated with MTX (42 of 43; 98%). Severe side effects necessitating discontinuation of treatment were recorded in seven patients (16%), which quickly resolved when MTX was discontinued. Life-threatening complications were not observed. Intravenous application was tolerated better than oral administration. Interestingly, we observed a significant increase in circulating lymphocyte numbers in patients with lymphopenia prior to MTX treatment.

This is a large number of patients with excellent improvement. This agent has not been as successful in the patients the author has treated.

Treatment of discoid and subacute cutaneous lupus erythematosus with cyclophosphamide. Schulz EJ, Menter MA. Br J Dermatol 1971; 85: 60–5.

Several cytotoxic agents have been reported to be beneficial for the control of cutaneous LE lesions. Azathioprine has perhaps had the greatest number of reports, but methotrexate and mycophenolate mofetil have also been reported to benefit patients with 'recalcitrant' disease. Individual reports have suggested that cyclophosphamide may be effective.

THIRD-LINE THERAPIES

▶ Clofazimine	A
▶ Phenytoin	B
▶ High-dose intravenous immunoglobulin	C
▶ Cytokine therapy	D
▶ Rituximab	E

Clofazimine (Lamprene) in the treatment of discoid lupus erythematosus. Krivanek JFC, Paver WKA, Kossard S, Cains G. Australas J Dermatol 1976; 17: 108–10.

Clofazimine failed to demonstrate efficacy in all but one report.

Evidence Levels: **A** Double-blind study **B** Clinical trial ≥ 20 subjects **C** Clinical trial < 20 subjects **D** Series ≥ 5 subjects **E** Anecdotal case reports

Double-blind, randomized, controlled clinical trial of clofazimine compared with chloroquine in patients with systemic lupus erythematosus. Bezerra EL, Vilar MJ, da Trindade Neto PB, Sato EI. Arthritis Rheum 2005; 52: 3073–8.

This is a randomized controlled trial comparing clofazimine to chloroquine. Twenty-seven of 33 patients who were randomized completed 6 months of treatment. The groups were homogeneous and comparable in terms of demographic and clinical characteristics. Five CFZ-treated patients and one CDP-treated patient (p=0.15) dropped out because of the development of severe lupus flare. At the end of the study, 12 CFZ-treated patients (75%) and 14 CDP-treated patients (82.4%) had complete or near-complete remission of skin lesions; intention-to-treat analysis showed no significant difference in the response rates between groups. Side effects, mainly skin and gastrointestinal events, were frequent in both groups, but no patients had to discontinue their treatment.

In the author's opinion, careful analysis of this report does not justify the conclusion rendered above. More patients treated with clofazimine had LE flares, and the responses were not comparable. In addition, the numbers of patients is quite small. The results of this study do not warrant the use of clofazimine

Phenytoin in the treatment of discoid lupus erythematosus. Rodriquez-Castellanos MA, Rubio JB, Gomez JFB, Mendoza AG. Arch Dermatol 1995; 131: 620–1.

This group studied 93 patients with cutaneous LE and observed excellent results in 90%. They administered oral phenytoin 300 mg daily to their patients for up to 6 months. Relapse occurred in at least one-third of patients for whom follow-up data were available, but prolonged remission of 6–12 months was noted in 33 patients. Toxicity was minimal in prevalence and severity.

The author has not tried this agent in patients with cutaneous LE.

Intravenous immunoglobulin (IVIg) for therapy-resistant cutaneous lupus erythematosus. Goodfield M, Davison K, Bowden K. J Dermatol Treat 2004; 15: 46–50.

This is an open-label study of 12 patients with various forms of cutaneous LE, all of whom had SLE. Three of the patients had SCLE. Of the 10 evaluable patients, five had excellent responses, two had partial responses, and three had limited or no responses. One patient developed an acute cutaneous vasculitis; otherwise, there were no significant adverse reactions.

High-dose intravenous immunoglobulin has been used successfully – 1 g/kg daily for 2 consecutive days monthly was administered to these patients who had failed to respond to multiple previous therapies. Although there might be an excellent response in some patients, the response is often short-lived. Toxicity is minimal, but this therapy is extremely expensive.

Response of discoid and subacute cutaneous lupus erythematosus to recombinant interferon alpha-2a. Nicolas J-F, Thivolet J, Kanitkis J, Lyonnet S. J Invest Dermatol 1990; 95: 142S–5S.

Interferon-α has been used successfully; however, all patients on this regimen developed toxicity and long-term remission was rarely achieved.

Treatment of severe cutaneous lupus erythematosus with a chimeric CD4 monoclonal antibody, cM-T412. Prinz JC, Meurer M, Reiter C, Rieber EP, Plewig G, Riethmüller G. J Am Acad Dermatol 1996; 34: 244–52.

Prinz and colleagues used chimeric CD4 monoclonal antibody infusions in five patients with severe, refractory cutaneous LE. Long-lasting improvement was noted, with a restoration of responsiveness to conventional treatments.

If other cytokines can be administered and result in the restoration of response to less toxic therapy, then perhaps we will be able to induce remission with one agent and maintain it with another.

Regression of subacute cutaneous lupus erythematosus in a patient with rheumatoid arthritis treated with a biologic tumor necrosis factor alpha-blocking agent: comment on the article by Pisetsky and the letter from Aringer et al. Fautrel B, Foltz V, Frances C, Bourgeois P, Rozenberg S. Arthritis Rheum 2002; 46: 1408–9.

This is a single case report. There have been multiple reports linking TNF-α antagonists to the development of cutaneous as well as systemic LE.

There are many new biologic agents that might prove to be useful for cutaneous LE. Caution should be used with the TNF antagonists, however, because although an individual case of benefit has been reported, there are many patients in whom these drugs have resulted in development of the disease. Properly conducted observational studies followed by placebo-controlled trials will be helpful.

Case reports of etanercept in inflammatory dermatoses. Norman R, Greenberg RG, Jackson JM. J Am Acad Dermatol 2006; 54: S139–42.

Among the four patients reported, one had SCLE and was said to have a good response.

Successful treatment of refractory skin manifestations of systemic lupus erythematosus with rituximab: report of a case. Uthman I, Taher A, Abbas O, Menassa J, Ghosn S. Dermatology 2008; 216: 257–9.

This is a single case report using an anti-CD20 antibody to treat SLE.

Leflunomide in subacute cutaneous lupus erythematosus – two sides of a coin. Suess A, Sticherling M. Int J Dermatol 2008; 47: 83–6.

This report describes two patients, one in whom leflunomide was effective and one in whom it resulted in a flare of the disease.

Although it is intriguing to use a new chemotherapeutic agent that has a similar mechanism to methotrexate, there are more cases linked to exacerbation or flare of disease.

Subcorneal pustular dermatosis

Rebecca CC Brooke, Robert JG Chalmers

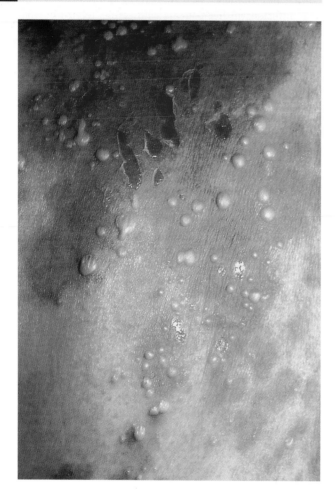

Subcorneal pustular dermatosis is a rare, chronic neutrophilic dermatosis of unknown etiology in which flaccid pustules and vesicopustules, classically forming a hypopyon, arise in crops on truncal and flexural skin. The condition occurs at any age, more commonly in females, and usually follows a relapsing and remitting course, but generally the patient remains systemically well. Long-term follow-up is required because monoclonal IgA paraproteinemia or myeloma may occur many years after presentation. The condition may be difficult to differentiate from other vesicopustular dermatoses, and some cases may develop into pustular psoriasis.

MANAGEMENT STRATEGY

Dapsone is the treatment of choice (25–200 mg daily) and normally results in resolution of the rash within 4 weeks; the drug usually needs to be continued long term because relapse is common on withdrawal of therapy. After control is gained, the dose should be tapered to the lowest required to maintain remission. Other sulfones (*sulfapyridine, salazosulfapyridine*) have also been reported to be beneficial in isolated reports.

In a proportion of cases the response to dapsone is poor; *retinoids* (formerly etretinate, now replaced by acitretin) have been substituted with success, using an initial dose of 0.5–1.0 mg/kg daily and then reducing to the lowest dose that will maintain control. Alternatively, for those unable to tolerate dapsone in the dose required, retinoids have been added to dapsone; this has enabled lower doses of each to be used. There are a few case reports detailing good response to *phototherapy – psoralen and UVA (PUVA), narrowband UVB, or broadband UVB –* in combination with dapsone or retinoids.

Both *topical* and *systemic corticosteroids* have been reported to provide some degree of control in isolated cases. Unacceptably high doses of systemic corticosteroids may be required, but combination with *dapsone, ciclosporin, vitamin E, or antibiotics (minocycline, tetracycline)* may allow control with lower doses.

Subcorneal pustular dermatosis tends to run a chronic course. Maintenance of a continuing beneficial response may be difficult, as may be inferred from the extensive range of treatment options described. Although dapsone appears to offer the best chance of a good therapeutic response, treatment regimens for this condition have not been formally evaluated.

Immunofluorescence studies have shown that a subset of patients have intraepidermal deposits of IgA. These have been given various alternative designations, including IgA pemphigus, intraepidermal IgA pustulosis, or intercellular IgA dermatosis, and in a number of them desmocollin 1 has been identified as the target antigen.

SPECIFIC INVESTIGATIONS

- ▶ Full blood count
- ▶ Immunoglobulin levels
- ▶ Immunoelectrophoresis
- ▶ Bence–Jones protein
- ▶ Autoantibodies
- ▶ Biopsy with immunofluorescence

Subcorneal pustular dermatosis: 50 years on. Cheng S, Edmonds E, Ben-Gashir M, Yu RC. Clin Exp Dermatol 2008; 33: 229–33.

Subcorneal pustular dermatosis: a clinical study of ten patients. Lutz ME, Daoud MS, McEvoy MT, Gibson LE. Cutis 1998; 61: 203–8.

Four of seven patients tested had paraproteinemia, three of IgA and one of IgG type. A further three had subcorneal deposits of IgA on direct immunofluorescence.

Subcorneal pustular dermatosis (Sneddon–Wilkinson disease) in association with a monoclonal IgA gammopathy: a report and review of the literature. Kasha EE, Epinette WW. J Am Acad Dermatol 1988; 19: 854–8.

Subcorneal pustular dermatosis and IgA λ myeloma: an uncommon association but probably not coincidental. Vaccaro M, Cannavò SP, Guarneri F. Eur J Dermatol 1999; 9: 644–6.

A case report of IgA λ myeloma. Treatment of the underlying myeloma had no effect on the skin disease.

Sneddon–Wilkinson disease in association with rheumatoid arthritis. Butt A, Burge SM. Br J Dermatol 1995; 132: 313–15.

A useful overview of all reported cases associated with either seronegative or seropositive arthritis.

Evidence Levels: **A** Double-blind study **B** Clinical trial ≥ 20 subjects **C** Clinical trial < 20 subjects **D** Series ≥ 5 subjects **E** Anecdotal case reports

Subcorneal pustular dermatosis. Reed J, Wilkinson J. Clin Dermatol 2000; 18: 301–13.

Review, with detailed tables of associations and differential diagnoses.

Intraepidermal IgA pustulosis. Wallach D. J Am Acad Dermatol 1992; 27: 993–1000.

Overview of all reported cases.

Subcorneal pustular dermatosis has also been reported in association with pyoderma gangrenosum, Crohn's disease, ulcerative colitis, systemic lupus erythematosus, morphea, myeloproliferative disorders, hyperthyroidism, multiple sclerosis, solid tumors, and infections, particularly mycoplasma. Isolated reports detail resolution with treatment of the associated disorder. Two drugs have been implicated: diltiazem and thiols (bucillamine or gold sodium thiomalate). In one case the condition arose at the site of injection of recombinant human granulocyte–macrophage colony-stimulating factor.

FIRST-LINE THERAPIES

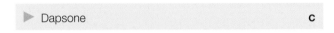

| ▷ Dapsone | C |

Subcorneal pustular dermatosis. Sneddon IB, Wilkinson DS. Br J Dermatol 1956; 68: 385–93.

Three of six patients responded to dapsone 50–100 mg daily.

Sneddon–Wilkinson disease in association with rheumatoid arthritis. Butt A, Burge SM. Br J Dermatol 1995; 132: 313–15.

A further five patients who responded to dapsone.

Dapsone is the treatment of choice, with over 20 reports of successful control. Combination with other drugs has been reported to be helpful.

Subcorneal pustular dermatosis and IgA gammopathy. Burrows D, Bingham EA. Br J Dermatol 1984; 111: 91–3.

The addition of etretinate enabled control in a patient intolerant of higher-dose dapsone.

Subcorneal pustular dermatosis treated with PUVA therapy. Bauwens M, De Coninck A, Roseeuw D. Dermatology 1999; 198: 203–5.

A patient resistant to dapsone alone responded well to combination with PUVA.

Sneddon–Wilkinson disease. Four case reports. Launay F, Albes B, Bayle P, Carriere M, Lamant L, Bazex J. Rev Med Interne 2004; 25: 154–9.

Three patients responded to dapsone, one to etretinate.

Subcorneal pustular dermatosis in a young boy. Garg BR, Sait MA, Baruah MC. Indian J Dermatol 1985; 30: 21–3.

Report of dapsone use in a child.

SECOND-LINE THERAPIES

▶ Sulfones	D
▶ Corticosteroids	D
▶ Etretinate (no longer marketed)	D
▶ Acitretin	E
▶ PUVA	D
▶ Narrowband UVB	E
▶ Broadband UVB	E

Subcorneal pustular dermatosis. Sneddon IB, Wilkinson DS. Br J Dermatol 1956; 68: 385–93.

Two patients were controlled on sulfapyridine 1 g twice daily.

Pyoderma gangrenosum followed by subcorneal pustular dermatosis in a patient with IgA paraproteinemia. Kohl PK, Hartschuh W, Tilgen W, Frosch PJ. J Am Acad Dermatol 1991; 24: 325–8.

Sulfasalazine (salazosulfapyridine) 3 g daily provided control in this patient.

Subcorneal pustular dermatosis in children. Johnson SAM, Cripps DJ. Arch Dermatol 1974; 109: 73–7.

Two children were controlled but not cleared with topical and systemic corticosteroids.

Role of tumour necrosis factor-α in Sneddon–Wilkinson subcorneal pustular dermatosis. Grob JJ, Mege JL, Capo C, Jancovicci E, Fournerie JR, Bongrand P, et al. J Am Acad Dermatol 1991; 25: 944–7.

Methylprednisolone induced remission in this patient who failed to respond to dapsone, etretinate, or plasma exchange. A maintenance dose of 12 mg daily was required.

An unusual severe case of subcorneal pustular dermatosis treated with cyclosporine and prednisolone. Zachariae CO, Rossen K, Weismann K. Acta Dermatol Venereol 2000; 80: 386–7.

After failure with dapsone and prednisolone (because of abnormal liver enzymes), ciclosporin (400 mg daily) was substituted for dapsone; onset of resolution was swift, and ciclosporin was stopped after 3 weeks; prednisolone was slowly tapered off over 2 months, with no recurrence.

Treatment of subcorneal pustulosis by etretinate. Iandoli R, Monfrecola G. Dermatologica 1987; 175: 235–8.

A patient who failed to respond to dapsone 300 mg daily and topical corticosteroids responded well to etretinate 1 mg/kg daily. A maintenance dose of 0.75 mg/kg daily was required.

Successful treatment of subcorneal pustular dermatosis (Sneddon–Wilkinson disease) by acitretin: report of a case. Marlière V, Beylot-Barry M, Beylot C, Doutre M-S. Dermatology 1999; 199: 153–5.

This paper reviews the use of retinoids for subcorneal pustular dermatosis.

Subcorneal pustular dermatosis treated with PUVA therapy. Bauwens M, De Coninck A, Roseeuw D. Dermatology 1999; 198: 203–5.

This paper contains a useful overview of PUVA therapy.

Subcorneal pustular dermatosis (Sneddon–Wilkinson disease) treated with narrowband (TL-01) UVB phototherapy. Cameron H, Dawe RS. Br J Dermatol 1997; 137: 150–1.

This patient was initially controlled with minocycline 200 mg daily and topical corticosteroids, but suffered a flare that was poorly responsive. Narrowband UVB phototherapy enabled corticosteroids to be withdrawn and control maintained with minocycline alone.

Subcorneal pustular dermatosis responsive to narrowband (TL-01) UVB phototherapy. Orton DI, George SA. Br J Dermatol 1997; 137: 149–50.

After long-term PUVA treatment this patient achieved a satisfactory response with narrowband UVB phototherapy.

Subcorneal pustular dermatosis treated with phototherapy. Park YK, Park HY, Bang DS, Cho CK. Int J Dermatol 1986; 25: 124–6.

After failure of dapsone, prednisolone, and topical fluocinolone acetonide, lasting remission was achieved with broadband UVB.

THIRD-LINE THERAPIES

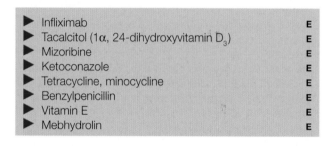

▶ Infliximab	E
▶ Tacalcitol (1α, 24-dihydroxyvitamin D₃)	E
▶ Mizoribine	E
▶ Ketoconazole	E
▶ Tetracycline, minocycline	E
▶ Benzylpenicillin	E
▶ Vitamin E	E
▶ Mebhydrolin	E

Infliximab (anti-tumor necrosis factor alpha antibody): a novel, highly effective treatment of recalcitrant subcorneal pustular dermatosis (Sneddon–Wilkinson disease). Voigtlander C, Luftl M, Schuler G, Hertl M. Arch Dermatol 2001; 137: 1571–4.

After suitable work-up, IV infliximab at a dose of 5 mg/kg over 2 hours was given after therapeutic trials of multiple agents failed, enabling oral methylprednisolone to be withdrawn and the dose of acitretin to be stabilized at 0.4 mg/kg daily. After 14 days the patient developed new pustules and a second dose of infliximab was given, again with excellent results. Over a 3-month period complete remission was achieved with oral methylprednisolone and acitretin.

Recalcitrant subcorneal pustular dermatosis and bullous pemphigoid treated with mizoribine, an immunosuppressive, purine biosynthesis inhibitor. Kono T, Terashima T, Oura H, Ishii M, Taniguchi S, Muramatsu T. Br J Dermatol 2000; 143: 1328–30.

Two patients responded to mizoribine (Bredinin) 150 mg daily, one to mizoribine alone, the other with combined prednisolone 50 mg and mizoribine 150 mg daily.

A case of subcorneal pustular dermatosis treated with tacalcitol (1alpha,24-dihydroxyvitamin D₃). Kawaguchi M, Mitsuhashi Y, Kondo S. J Dermatol. 2000; 27: 669–72.

Topical vitamin D₃ led to sustained resolution of lesions.

Ketoconazole as a therapeutic modality in subcorneal pustular dermatosis. Verma KK, Pasricha JS. Acta Dermatol Venereol 1977; 77: 407–8.

After failing to respond to dapsone a patient achieved remission using ketoconazole 200 mg daily. Although initially started in conjunction with dapsone, on withdrawal she flared and was controlled subsequently on ketoconazole alone.

Subcorneal pustular dermatosis (Sneddon–Wilkinson). Mandel EH, Gonzales V. Arch Dermatol 1969; 99: 246–7.

Tetracycline 250 mg four times daily controlled new pustule formation.

Cutaneous manifestations of neutrophilic disease. Vignon-Pennamen MD, Wallach D. Dermatologica 1991; 183: 255–64.

An overview of seven cases with various neutrophilic dermatoses.

Subcorneal pustular dermatosis with polyarthritis. Lin RY, Schwartz RA, Lambert WC. Cutis 1986; 37: 123–6.

Intravenous benzylpenicillin (20 million units daily) plus topical triamcinolone resolved both the arthritis and the rash over a period of 8 days. No follow-up information given.

Subcorneal pustular dermatosis controlled by vitamin E. Ayres S, Mihan R. Arch Dermatol 1974; 109: 74.

Vitamin E (400 IU D-α-tocopheryl acetate), when added to prednisolone 40 mg daily, enabled the dosage of prednisolone to be reduced to 5 mg daily.

Subcorneale pustulose Sneddon Wilkinson, therapie mit Mebhydrolin. Dorittke P, Wassilew SW. Z Hautkrankheiten 1988; 63: 1025–7.

Mebhydrolin 50 mg three times daily was successful.

Subcutaneous fat necrosis of the newborn

Bernice R Krafchik

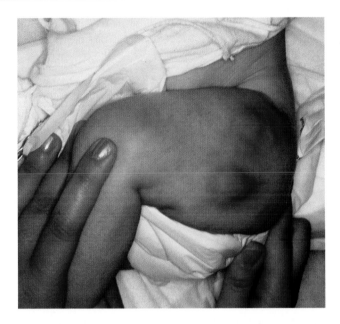

Subcutaneous fat necrosis (SFN) is a rare, self-limiting skin disease that occurs mainly in neonates. It affects areas where fat tissue is found and is thought to arise from perinatal stress. It usually resolves spontaneously within 3–6 months with no scarring; occasionally small pits remain. Treatment is seldom necessary, except in rare instances when liquefaction of the fat tissue occurs, or when hypercalcemia develops.

MANAGEMENT STRATEGY

Biopsy is usually not warranted as the clinical picture is typical. MRI scans often demonstrate characteristic features. The lesions of SFN heal within a few months, leaving normal skin or small pitted scars, and very occasionally an absence of fat tissue in the affected areas. The rare occurrence of liquefaction in the lesions is treated by removal of the liquid with a large-bore needle.

Hypercalcemia and hypercalciuria may develop (in about one-third of patients in one series who were admitted to the hospital). Rarely thrombocytopenia, hypoglycemia, and hypervitaminosis D may also be seen. Hypercalcemia is diagnosed by blood sampling, which is routinely performed in patients with SFN or if symptoms supervene. The symptoms are nonspecific and consist of fever, vomiting, lethargy, constipation, feeding difficulties, failure to thrive, and seizures. In normal infants or those with perinatal stress, the calcium levels may be low in the first 2 weeks. It is important to monitor those with SFN weekly with repeated serum calcium levels, or if there is any increase in value biweekly for up to 6 months to ensure that hypercalcemia does not occur.

Treatment regimens are determined by the levels of hypercalcemia, and hypercalciuria. If serum levels are marginally raised, monitoring the serum and urine calcium may be all that is necessary and a spontaneous return to normal levels usually occurs. If the increased levels persist or rise further, treatment should be instigated. Mild hypercalcemia is treated by the *withdrawal of vitamin D* and by using a *low-calcium diet*. This is best accomplished by *breastfeeding*, as breast milk is low in both vitamin D and calcium. If this is not possible or helpful, a formula low in calcium with no vitamin D should be tried. If a reduction in calcium does not occur or the levels continue to rise, *intravenous saline* at 1.5 times the maintenance requirement is given, to promote the renal excretion of calcium. This is augmented with *furosemide* (a diuretic), which further promotes excretion. Other options for non-responders include *calcitonin* (4–8 IU/kg every 6–12 hours), *bisphosphonates (pamidronate)*, and *oral corticosteroids* (hydrocortisone or prednisone). The latter treatments should be instituted with the help of a pediatric endocrinologist.

SPECIFIC INVESTIGATIONS

> ▶ Follow serum and urine calcium for 6 months
> ▶ If hypercalcemia occurs, calcium should be monitored biweekly
> ▶ Monitor calcium/creatinine ratio in the urine
> ▶ Ultrasound of kidneys for nephrocalcinosis and nephrolithiasis; other organs may be involved and should be checked radiologically

MRI and ultrasound findings of subcutaneous fat necrosis of the newborn. Vasireddy S, Long SD, Sacheti B, Mayforth RD. Pediatric Radiol 2008; 89: Epub.

This article discusses the US and MRI findings of SFN.

Radiological case of the month. Subcutaneous fat necrosis of the newborn. Bellini C, Oddone M, Biscaldi E, Serra G. Arch Pediatr Adolesc Med 2001; 155: 1381–2.

A report of the diagnosis of SFN made from an MRI examination. The characteristics on MRI are typical. This procedure precludes the need for biopsy.

Subcutaneous fat necrosis of the newborn: be aware of hypercalcaemia. Borgia F, De Pasquale L, Cacace C, Meo P, Guarneri C, Cannavo SP. J Paediatr Child Health 2006; 42: 316–18.

A report on the extracutaneous and cutaneous features of SFN. The associated metabolic complications include hypoglycemia, thrombocytopenia, hypertriglyceridemia, anemia, and hypercalcemia. The delayed onset of hypercalcemia, 1–6 months after the development of the skin manifestations, and its frequent lack of symptoms necessitates prolonged follow-up to prevent toxic effects on the cardiovascular and renal systems and metastatic calcification.

Complications of subcutaneous fat necrosis of the newborn: a case report and review of the literature. Tran JT, Sheth AP. Pediatr Dermatol 2003; 20: 257–61.

This article discusses the rare extracutaneous complications of SFN, including hypercalcemia, thrombocytopenia, hypertriglyceridemia, and hypoglycemia. The authors describe the first case where all of these were encountered in the same infant. Physicians should be aware of all these complications.

FIRST-LINE THERAPIES

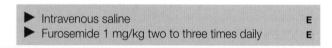

▶ No treatment for the majority of patients	C
▶ If mild hypercalcemia develops with or without symptoms, treatment should be instigated	
▶ Low calcium diet and low vitamin D (either breast milk or formula)	C

Subcutaneous fat necrosis of the newborn: a review of 11 cases. Burden AD, Krafchik BR. Pediatr Dermatol 1999; 16: 384–7.

A review of SFN in patients requiring hospitalization. Ten of 11 patients had been delivered by cesarean section for fetal distress, and four of 11 developed hypercalcemia. Patients should be monitored for 5 months, even if the lesions of SFN have disappeared.

SECOND-LINE THERAPIES

▶ Intravenous saline	E
▶ Furosemide 1 mg/kg two to three times daily	E

Subcutaneous fat necrosis of the newborn following hypothermia and complicated by pain and hypercalcaemia. Wiadrowski TP, Marshman G. Australas J Dermatol 2001; 42: 207–10.

A female infant was delivered with complications of severe meconium aspiration and birth asphyxia. She was diagnosed with SFN, which was complicated by pain resistant to treatment with opiates. Asymptomatic hypercalcemia was noted at 7 weeks on periodic testing, and treated by rehydration, diuretics, prednisolone, etidronate, and a low-calcium and vitamin D diet. Treatment of hypercalcemia in SFN is reviewed.

Subcutaneous fat necrosis of the newborn: hypercalcaemia with hepatic and atrial myocardial calcification. Dudink J, Walther FJ, Beekman RP. Arch Dis Child 2003; 88: 343–5.

This case report discusses the various treatments of SFN and the calcification of organs that may result from severe involvement. The need to monitor serum levels of calcium is stressed.

THIRD-LINE THERAPIES

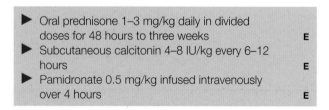

▶ Oral prednisone 1–3 mg/kg daily in divided doses for 48 hours to three weeks	E
▶ Subcutaneous calcitonin 4–8 IU/kg every 6–12 hours	E
▶ Pamidronate 0.5 mg/kg infused intravenously over 4 hours	E

Subcutaneous fat necrosis of the newborn. Singalavanija S, Limponsanurak W, Wannaprasert T. J Med Assoc Thai 2007; 90: 1214–22.

This article discusses seven cases of SFN, all term babies: there were four males and three females. Five (70%) had perinatal asphyxia. The mean age of onset was 14 days (range 3–42 days). The locations of SFN were the back (three cases), shoulder (two), arm (two), buttock (one), and neck (one). Skin biopsy was performed in three cases and was compatible with subcutaneous fat necrosis. Treatment was supportive, with close monitoring of serum calcium. Hypercalcemia was seen in five cases (70%) and three were treated with oral prednisolone. Cutaneous lesions of all cases resolved without sequelae.

Intravenous bisphosphonate for hypercalcemia accompanying subcutaneous fat necrosis: a novel treatment approach. Khan N, Licata A, Rogers D. Clin Pediatr (Phila) 2001; 40: 217–19.

Oral bisphosphonates are poorly absorbed. This is the first report of intravenous administration of a bisphosphonate that resulted in fast normalization of the hypercalcemia from SFN. The drug acts by slowing the calcium turnover from bone.

Subcutaneous fat necrosis with hypercalcemia. Vijayakumar M, Prahlad N, Nammalwar BR, Shanmughasundharam R. Indian Pediatr 2006; 43: 360–3.

A report of a 28-day-old infant with SFN, hypercalcemia, and nephrocalcinosis who was managed with intravenous saline followed by furosemide, oral prednisolone, potassium citrate, and etidronate.

Pamidronate: Treatment for severe hypercalcemia in neonatal subcutaneous fat necrosis. Alos N, Eugène D, Fillion M, Powell J, Kokta V, Chabot G. Horm Res 2006; 65: 289–94.

This report reviews the various treatments of hypercalcemia in SFN, including hydration, furosemide, and corticosteroids, citing one report only on the use of intravenous bisphosphonates. They describe four newborns with SFN complicated by severe hypercalcemia. All had ionized calcium levels higher than 1.4 mmol/L, associated with high urinary calcium/creatinine ratios and high 1,25-dihydroxyvitamin D levels. Despite treatment with IV fluids, a low-calcium diet, and furosemide, calcium levels remained high. Four doses (0.25–0.50 mg/kg/dose) of pamidronate were given. Urinary calcium/creatinine ratios and calcium levels decreased within 48–96 hours. 1,25-Dihydroxyvitamin D levels normalized with resolution of the skin lesions. No persistent nephrocalcinosis was observed. To prevent nephrocalcinosis, pamidronate might be considered as first-line treatment for severe hypercalcemia in SFN.

Expanding role of bisphosphonate therapy in children. Shoemaker LR. J Pediatr 1999; 134: 264–7.

The initial report of improvement with bisphosphonates appeared over 30 years ago, but pediatric experience has been limited. Although the first adverse effects on the growing skeleton have been exaggerated, physicians should warn parents that careful monitoring is important.

Sweet's syndrome

Samuel L Chachkin, Joel M Gelfand, William D James

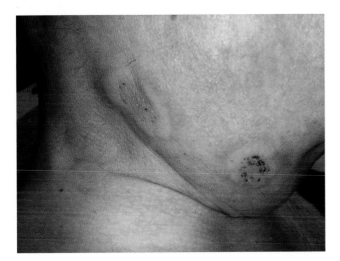

Sweet's syndrome is a neutrophilic dermatosis, characterized clinically by multiple painful, well-demarcated, non-scarring erythematous plaques or pustules on the face, neck, upper trunk, and extremities. There can be a pseudovesicular appearance. Fever, leukocytosis, arthralgias, myalgias, headaches, and general malaise may occur. Oral, ocular, and internal organ involvement is rare. Histologically, there is a diffuse neutrophilic infiltrate in the upper dermis without evidence of primary leukocytoclastic vasculitis. Neutrophilic dermatosis of the dorsal hands (NDDH) is a recently identified entity and is classified as an anatomically limited subset of Sweet's syndrome.

MANAGEMENT STRATEGY

Sweet's syndrome is often idiopathic, but may be associated with malignancy (most commonly acute myelogenous leukemia, but also lymphomas, dysproteinemias, and carcinomas), inflammatory bowel disease, infection (commonly *Streptococcus* or *Yersinia*), medication, and pregnancy. A work-up including skin biopsy, complete physical examination, and laboratory studies is indicated. Treatment of the underlying associated condition or discontinuation of the causative medication may lead to resolution of skin lesions. The standard treatment for Sweet's syndrome is *corticosteroids*. For patients with contraindications to corticosteroids, or for therapeutic failures, second-line therapies may be used.

SPECIFIC INVESTIGATIONS

▶ History and physical examination
▶ Complete blood count with differential and erythrocyte sedimentation rate
▶ Medical work-up including cultures as indicated by history and physical examination
▶ Pregnancy test (in women of childbearing potential)
▶ Thorough medication history

Sweet's syndrome revisited: a review of disease concepts. Cohen PR, Kurzrock R. Int J Dermatol 2003; 42: 761–78.
An excellent review of the literature.

The relationship between neutrophilic dermatosis of the dorsal hands and Sweet syndrome: Report of 9 cases and comparison to atypical pyoderma gangrenosum. Walling HW, Snipes CJ, Gerami P, Piette WW. Arch Dermatol 2006; 142: 57–63.
A report of nine cases of NDDH. All 43 cases of NDDH reported previously in the literature are also assessed.

Histiocytoid Sweet Syndrome. Heymann WR. J Am Acad Dermatol 2009; (in press).
The term 'histiocytoid' Sweet Syndrome refers to the histologic presence of immature neutrophils; the clinical implications are identical to those of the classical Sweet Syndrome.

FIRST-LINE THERAPIES

▶ Oral corticosteroids	C
▶ Topical and intralesional corticosteroids	C

Sweet's syndrome: a review of current treatment options. Cohen PR, Kurzrock R. Am J Clin Dermatol 2002; 3: 117–31.
A review of the literature regarding treatment for Sweet's syndrome.
Corticosteroid therapy (oral prednisone 0.5–1.5 mg/kg daily tapered over 4–6 weeks) results in rapid relief of systemic symptoms (e.g. within 1–2 days) and skin lesions within 3–9 days. Up to one-third of patients will relapse.
High-potency topical corticosteroids and intralesional corticosteroids may be useful as monotherapy for patients with limited or mild disease, or as adjuvant treatment.

SECOND-LINE THERAPIES

▶ Potassium iodide	C
▶ Colchicine	C
▶ Indometacin	C
▶ Pulse intravenous corticosteroids	D
▶ Dapsone	D
▶ Clofazimine	D
▶ Doxycycline	E
▶ Metronidazole	E

Potassium iodide in dermatology: a 19th century drug for the 21st century – uses, pharmacology, adverse effects, and contraindications. Sterling JB, Heymann WR. J Am Acad Dermatol 2000; 43: 691–7.
The usual dosage is 40–60 mg orally three times a day up to 300 mg three times a day. A supersaturated solution of potassium iodide (SSKI) may also be used. Start at three drops orally three times daily and increase by one drop per dose up to 10 drops (500 mg) three times daily until clear, then taper. SSKI is contraindicated in pregnancy, hyperkalemia, and in patients with renal disease. Baseline thyroid function tests and periodic monitoring are required for patients on SSKI.

Long-term suppression of chronic Sweet's syndrome with colchicine. Ritter S, George R, Serwatka LM, Elston DM. J Am Acad Dermatol 2002; 47: 323–4.

A case report of successful long-term treatment using colchicine.

Indomethacin treatment of eighteen patients with Sweet's syndrome. Jeanfils S, Joly P, Young P, Le Corvaisier-Pieto C, Thomine E, Lauret P. J Am Acad Dermatol 1997; 36: 436–9.

A prospective open-label uncontrolled study of 18 patients treated with indometacin 150 mg daily for 7 days, followed by 100 mg daily from days 7 to 21. Seventeen of 18 patients responded within 48 hours, and no relapses occurred.

Association of acute neutrophilic dermatosis and myelodysplastic syndrome with (6;9) chromosome translocation: a case report and review of the literature. Megarbane B, Bodemer C, Valensi F, Radford-Weiss I, Fraitag S, MacIntyre E, et al. Br J Dermatol 2000; 143: 1322–4.

Pulse corticosteroid therapy has been successful for refractory and/or recurrent Sweet's syndrome. Intravenous doses of methylprednisolone up to 1000 mg daily for 3–5 days have been used, followed by a low-dose tapering schedule of an oral corticosteroid with or without another immunosuppressant.

Sweet's syndrome and malignancy in the UK. Bourke JF, Keohane S, Long CC, Kemmett D, Davies M, Zaki I, et al. Br J Dermatol 1997; 137: 609–13.

A review of 87 cases with Sweet's syndrome. Dapsone was used successfully as first-line therapy in five of six cases.

Dapsone is used as monotherapy or combination therapy. Initial oral doses range from 100 to 200 mg daily.

Sweet's syndrome in association with generalized granuloma annulare in a patient with previous breast cancer. Anthony F, Holden CA. Clin Exp Dermatol 2001; 26: 668–70.

A case report of Sweet's syndrome successfully treated with clofazimine.

Clofazimine 200 mg daily for 4 weeks followed by 100 mg daily for 4 weeks has been reported to be an effective dosage regimen in six patients.

Sweet's syndrome. Amichai B, Lazarov A, Halevy S. J Am Acad Dermatol 1995; 33: 144–5.

Case report of a patient with Sweet's syndrome associated with a chlamydial infection who responded to tetracycline.

Tetracycline, doxycycline, and minocycline have been effective in cases of Sweet's syndrome with and without associated Chlamydia *or* Yersinia *spp. infections. Interestingly, there are several reports of minocycline as a cause of Sweet's syndrome.*

Sweet's syndrome in association with Crohn's disease: report of a case and review of the literature. Rappaport A, Shaked M, Landau M, Dolev E. Dis Colon Rectum 2001; 44: 1526–9.

Case report of a patient successfully treated with metronidazole and prednisone.

THIRD-LINE THERAPIES

▶ Ciclosporin	E
▶ Interferon	E
▶ Cyclophosphamide	E
▶ Chlorambucil	E
▶ Etretinate	E
▶ Etanercept	E
▶ Thalidomide	E
▶ Anakinra	E
▶ IVIG	E

Peripheral ulcerative keratitis – an extracutaneous neutrophilic disorder: report of a patient with rheumatoid arthritis, pustular vasculitis, pyoderma gangrenosum, and Sweet's syndrome with an excellent response to cyclosporine therapy. Wilson DM, John GR, Callen JP. J Am Acad Dermatol 1999; 40: 331–4.

Case report of a patient with Sweet's syndrome who responded to ciclosporin.

Initial doses of 2–10 mg/kg daily have been used successfully. Ciclosporin should generally be limited to short-term use given its potential renal toxicity when used chronically.

Systemic interferon-alpha treatment for idiopathic Sweet's syndrome. Bianchi L, Masi M, Hagman JH, Piemonte P, Orlandi A. Clin Exp Dermatol 1999; 24: 443–5.

Case report of one patient who responded to interferon-α 3 million units intramuscularly three times weekly plus hydroxycarbamide (hydroxyurea) 500 mg twice daily for 30 days, tapered to 500 mg daily for 30 days. The patient then maintained remission for 2 years with intramuscular interferon-α as monotherapy.

Lymphocytic infiltrates as a presenting feature of Sweet's syndrome with myelodysplasia and response to cyclophosphamide. Evans AV, Sabroe RA, Liddell K, Russell-Jones R. Br J Dermatol 2002; 146: 1087–90.

Case report of one patient who responded to oral cyclophosphamide 50 mg daily, with an occasional need for oral prednisolone to alleviate exacerbations.

Treatment of recurrent Sweet's syndrome with coexisting rheumatoid arthritis with the tumor necrosis factor antagonist etanercept. Yamauchi P, Turner L, Lowe N, Gindi V, Jackson JM. J Am Acad Dermatol 2006; 54: S122–5

Case report of two patients with rheumatoid arthritis associated Sweet's syndrome who had significant clearing with etanercept.

Thalidomide in the treatment of recalcitrant Sweet's syndrome associated with myelodysplasia. Browning C, Dixon J, Malone J, Callen J. J Am Acad Dermatol 2005; 53: S135–8

Case report of a patient with refractory Sweet's syndrome which cleared completely with thalidomide 100 mg daily.

The use of pulse methylprednisolone and chlorambucil in the treatment of Sweet's syndrome. Case JD, Smith SZ, Callen JP. Cutis 1989; 44: 125–9.

Case report of chronic and relapsing Sweet's syndrome successfully treated with pulse intravenous methylprednisolone. Remission was maintained with oral chlorambucil 4 mg daily.

Efficacy of anakinra, an IL1 receptor antagonist, in refractory Sweet syndrome. Delluc A, Limal N, Puèchal X, Francès C, Piette JC, Cacoub P. Ann Rheum Dis 2008; 67: 278.

Case report of chronic Sweet's syndrome, refractory to multiple medications, which demonstrated a rapid and sustained response to anakinra 100 mg/day, combined with prednisone 10 mg daily.

Evidence Levels: **A** Double-blind study **B** Clinical trial ≥ 20 subjects **C** Clinical trial < 20 subjects **D** Series ≥ 5 subjects **E** Anecdotal case reports

Pediatric Sweet syndrome and immunodeficiency successfully treated with intravenous immunoglobulin. Haliasos E, Soder B, Rubenstein D, Henderson W, Morell D. Pediatric Dermatology 2005: 22: 530–5.

Case report of an immunodeficient child successfully treated with IVIG and dapsone. The initial IVIG dose was 1 mg/kg. This was lowered to 0.5 mg/kg, and given at 3-week intervals, with dapsone added for small residual papulopustules.

Sweet's syndrome in a patient with idiopathic myelofibrosis and thymoma–myasthenia gravis–immunodeficiency complex: efficacy of treatment with etretinate. Altomare G, Capella GL, Frigerio E. Haematologica 1996; 81: 54–8.

Case report of one patient who responded to etretinate 50 mg daily.

Etretinate has been withdrawn in some countries and replaced by acitretin, but there are no indexed reports using acitretin in Sweet's syndrome.

Syphilis

Miguel Sanchez

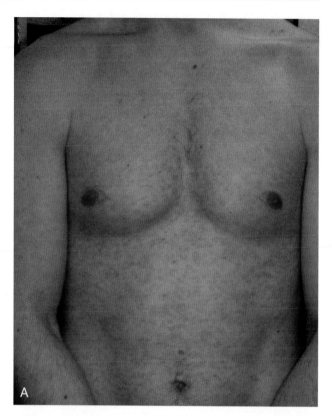

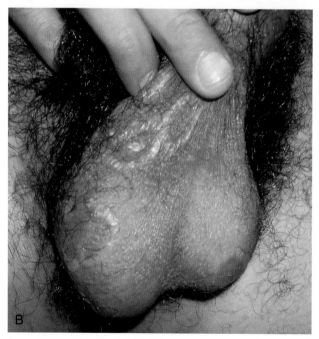

Syphilis (Lues) is a chronic systemic infection with a variable clinical course caused by the motile, corkscrew-shaped human spirochete *Treponema pallidum* (ssp. *pallidum*). The World Health Organization estimates that at least 12 million people worldwide are infected with syphilis. In adults, the infection is transmitted almost exclusively through sexual contact with infectious mucocutaneous lesions, and only rarely through transfusion or accidental inoculation. About one-third of persons become infected after a single episode of unprotected sexual intercourse with a partner who has infectious syphilis.

MANAGEMENT STRATEGY

Accurate staging of syphilis is required before choosing the treatment regimen. The course of the infection is divided into three clinically distinct stages and two asymptomatic epidemiologic stages. The *primary stage* begins with the appearance of a chancre at the site of treponemal penetration, usually after an incubation period of approximately 3 weeks (range 10–90 days). The *secondary stage* usually presents with an eruption that appears 2–10 weeks after the onset of the chancre. The clinical manifestations of secondary syphilis heal in 4–12 weeks, at which point the patient is asymptomatic and the infection is only diagnosable through a positive serologic test (*latent syphilis*). *Latent syphilis* is classified as early (<1 year in duration) or late (>1–2 years in duration). Latent cases in which the onset of infection cannot be determined are diagnosed as syphilis of *indeterminate duration*. Although patients during the latent stage are not infectious, approximately 25% will develop one or more relapses of highly infectious secondary syphilis lesions, usually during the first year. Nearly 60% of these patients cannot recall the presence of an eruption, and about 25% fail to remember having had a chancre. Without treatment about one-third of untreated patients with latent syphilis progress to *tertiary syphilis* (cardiovascular disease, neurosyphilis, or gummata).

Parenteral penicillin G is the treatment of choice for all stages, but the selected preparation, dose, and duration of treatment depend on the clinical stage and disease manifestations. The recommended treatment for patients with primary, secondary, or early latent syphilis is a single dose of benzathine penicillin G, 2.4 million IU, intramuscularly. For patients with syphilis of indeterminate duration, late latent syphilis, or tertiary syphilis, this regimen should be repeated weekly for three doses. Patients who are pregnant or HIV seropositive should be treated only with penicillin, and should be desensitized to penicillin if there is a history of previous allergy. Other patients who are allergic to penicillin may be treated orally with tetracycline (500 mg four times daily), doxycycline (100 mg twice daily), or erythromycin (500 mg four times daily) for 14 days for early syphilis, or 28 days for late latent syphilis. Treatment efficacy should be evaluated by serologic and clinical examinations at 6 and 12 months and, if needed, 24 months in healthy patients, and at 3-month intervals for the first year and annually thereafter in HIV-seropositive patients. Serologic serum titers should decline fourfold within 6 months after treatment for primary or secondary syphilis; they may decrease more slowly in late syphilis, and in patients with new early syphilis who had previously been treated for syphilitic infection. Patients whose non-treponemal test titers increase fourfold from baseline or a preceding test, or do not decrease fourfold within 12 months of treatment, are considered to have failed treatment. Such patients should be evaluated with a CNS examination and retreated accordingly with regimens for late latent syphilis or for neurosyphilis.

Penicillin is the only drug to be proved effective for neurosyphilis, and these patients should be treated with intravenous aqueous crystalline penicillin G 18–24 million IU daily, administered as 3–4 million IU every 4 hours. An alternative regimen is a 10-day course of procaine benzylpenicillin (procaine penicillin), 2–4 million IU, administered as a single daily intramuscular injection in addition to oral probenecid 500 mg four times daily.

SPECIFIC INVESTIGATIONS

▶ Darkfield microscopy
▶ Direct fluorescence antibody test
▶ Serologic tests
▶ CSF examination

Comparison of methods for the detection of *Treponema pallidum* in lesions of early syphilis. Cummings MC, Lukehart SA, Marra C, Smith BL, Shaffer J, Demeo LR, et al. Sex Transm Dis 1996; 23: 366–9.

Definitive diagnosis of syphilis rests on the demonstration of spirochetes in the exudate of a chancre by darkfield examination or direct fluorescence antibody staining, or in biopsied skin treated with silver stains.

Laboratory methods of diagnosis of syphilis for the beginning of the third millennium. Wicher K, Horowitz HW, Wicher V. Microbes Infect 1999; 1: 1035–49.

The diagnosis of syphilis is confirmed with serologic tests. The less costly, easier to perform, highly sensitive but less specific non-treponemal tests, such as the Venereal Disease Research Laboratory (VDRL) and the rapid plasma reagin (RPR) tests, are widely used for screening. These assays use cardiolipin antigens to detect antibodies to *T. pallidum*, and may be falsely reactive (2% of tests) in patients with narcotic abuse, connective tissue disease, viral and spirochetal infections, malignancy, and other acute infections and systemic illnesses. Therefore, a reactive VDRL or RPR result should be confirmed with a treponemal test, such as the fluorescent treponemal antibody absorbed (FTA-ABS) assay and the microhemagglutination assay for antibody to *T. pallidum* (MHA-TP). Treponemal tests are highly specific as well as sensitive, but are rarely reactive in some connective tissue diseases and other treponemal infections. However, the presence of reactive non-treponemal and treponemal serologic tests in a patient provides compelling evidence for a presumptive diagnosis of syphilis. Because enzyme immunoassays (EIA) are as easy to perform as non-treponemal tests and are as sensitive and more specific than non-treponemal tests, they are becoming the standard test for syphilis screening. Non-treponemal tests, however, should continue to be used to monitor treatment response.

In most cases non-treponemal tests become non-reactive with time after treatment, but in some patients low titers persist indefinitely (a serofast reaction). On the other hand, treponemal tests remain reactive in the majority of patients for life, regardless of treatment or disease activity, with the exception of 15–25% of patients treated for primary syphilis, in whom these tests become non-reactive within 2–3 years.

Current controversies in the management of adult syphilis. Stoner BP. Clin Infect Dis 2007; 44: 130–46.

Treponemal EIAs are screening tests. Causes of a positive EIA-IgG with non-reactive non-treponemal tests include untreated, late-latent syphilis, previously treated syphilis, partially treated syphilis resulting from antibiotic treatment of other infections, or a biological false-positive result.

Reactive EIA-IgG tests should be confirmed with both non-treponemal and a second treponemal test. If either of these two other tests is reactive, and previous treatment of syphilis cannot be verified, the patients should be treated for syphilis.

Treatment failure occurs when there is a fourfold increase in the RPR titer; or a titer persistently 1:64; or if there is clinical progression of the disease in the absence of re-infection. *Relapse* occurs when there is a fourfold reduction in the RPR titer, followed by a return to the original titer or a higher titer. *Serofast status* or *treatment non-response* occurs when there is a twofold change in the RPR titer over at least 6 months in early syphilis. Neurosyphilis should be excluded in any patient with treatment failure or relapse and considered for serofast status.

Sexually transmitted diseases treatment guidelines 2006. Centers for Disease Control and Prevention. Morb Mort Week Rep 2006; 55: 22–29.

Some HIV-infected patients can have atypical serologic test results (i.e., unusually high, unusually low, or fluctuating titers) A treponemal screening test should have a standard non-treponemal test with titer to guide patient management decisions. If the non-treponemal test is negative, then a different treponemal test should be performed to confirm the results of the initial test. If a second treponemal test is positive, treatment decisions should be discussed in consultation with a specialist.

CSF examination is indicated to exclude neurosyphilis in patients with neurologic signs, cardiovascular syphilis, gummata, iritis, auditory symptoms, HIV infection (late latent syphilis and syphilis of unknown duration), treatment failure, or slow decline in serologic titers after treatment with a medication other than penicillin.

A diagnosis of symptomatic neurosyphilis depends on the presence of neurologic manifestations or symptoms and a combinations of reactive serologic test results, elevated CSF cell count (>5 white blood cell count/mm^3) or protein, or a reactive VDRL-CSF. When contamination with blood can be excluded a reactive CSF is considered diagnostic, but negative results may also occur in the presence of neurosyphilis. The CSF FTA-ABS is highly sensitive but less specific in neurosyphilis than the VDRL-CSF, so that a negative CSF FTA-ABS test virtually excludes neurosyphilis.

Syphilis and HIV: a dangerous combination. Lynn WA, Lightman S. Lancet Infect Dis 2004; 4: 456–66.

All patients with syphilis should be tested for HIV antibodies and then retested in 3 months, as therapeutic management of syphilis in HIV-infected persons differs because of their higher rates of treatment failure and relapse. Additionally, HIV-infected patients should be regularly screened for syphilis. Contact with the primary chancre of a person co-infected with HIV and *T. pallidum* enhances the transmission of HIV infection. There is an increased rate of early neurological and ophthalmic involvement. HIV infection can exacerbate the progression of syphilis and increase the risk of developing neurosyphilis.

In most HIV-infected patients, serologic tests are accurate and reliable to follow the response to treatment. Unusually high or low serologic titers may be seen in some co-infected patients. Delayed seroconversion is rare and requires diagnostic confirmation of the clinical presentation by biopsy and direct microscopy.

Cerebrospinal fluid abnormalities in patients with syphilis: association with clinical and laboratory features. Marra CM, Maxwell CL, Smith SL. J Infect Dis 2004; 189: 369–76.

Regardless of the stage of syphilis, HIV-infection status, or previous antibiotic treatment, in this multicenter prospective study of 326 patients with syphilis evaluated by lumbar puncture, the risk of neurosyphilis (defined as either a positive CSF-VDRL or a CSF WBC count >20 cells/μL) was significantly higher with a serum RPR titer 1:32. Among HIV-infected patients, neurosyphilis was six times more likely to occur in patients with a serum RPR titer 1:32 and 3.1 times more likely to occur in patients with a CD4 cell count 350 cells/μL.

CSF examination should be strongly considered in all patients at any stage of syphilis with a serum RPR titer 1:32, especially those who are also infected with HIV.

Neurosyphilis in a clinical cohort of HIV-1-infected patients. Ghanem KG, Moore RD, Erbelding EJ, Zenilman J, Gebo KA. AIDS 2008; 22: 1145–51.

Forty-one cases of neurosyphilis were diagnosed among 231 new syphilis cases with CD4 cell counts <350 cells/mL at the time of diagnosis. Highly active antiretroviral therapy before the diagnosis of syphilis reduced the odds of neurosyphilis by 65%. The median time to neurosyphilis was 9 months. Despite treatment of neurosyphilis with recommended regimens, only 38% had resolution of all CSF abnormalities on follow-up lumbar puncture within 12 months, and at 1 year 38% had persistence of their major symptom requiring re-treatment.

FIRST-LINE THERAPIES

▶ Benzathine penicillin	A
▶ Procaine penicillin plus probenecid	A

Penicillin in the treatment of syphilis. The experience of three decades. Idsøe O, Guthe T, Willcox RR. Bull WHO 1972; 47: 1–68.

In studies totaling 1381 patients with seronegative primary syphilis, 97% of treated patients were clinically well and serologically negative. Treatment failures were attributed to re-infection.

Relapse of secondary syphilis after benzathine penicillin G: molecular analysis. Myint M, Bashiri H, Harrington RD, Marra CM. Sex Transm Dis 2004; 31: 196–9.

Relapses of infectious syphilis after treatment with the recommended doses of penicillin is rare but does occur. For this reason, it is important to follow treated patients both clinically and serologically. These patients respond to higher and more prolonged doses of penicillin.

Efficacy of treatment for syphilis in pregnancy. Alexander JM, Sheffield JS, Sanchez PJ, Mayfield J, Wendel GD Jr. Obstet Gynecol 1999; 93: 5–8.

The Centers for Disease Control recommended regimens for the treatment of maternal syphilis infection were found to prevent congenital syphilis in 98.2% of cases (27/27 with primary syphilis, 71/75 with secondary syphilis, 100/102 with early latent syphilis, and 136/136 with late latent syphilis).

A randomized trial of enhanced therapy for early syphilis in patients with and without human immunodeficiency virus infection. Rolfs RT, Joesoef MR, Hendershot EF, Rompalo AM, Augenbraun MH, Chiu M, et al. N Engl J Med 1997; 337: 307–14.

In a multicenter randomized, double-blind trial of 501 syphilis patients, which included 101 HIV-infected patients, treatment with 2 g of amoxicillin and 500 mg of probenecid three times a day for 10 days in addition to benzathine penicillin was not superior to treatment with benzathine penicillin alone.

The non-treponemal titer does not decline by a twofold dilution in 15% of patients with early syphilis tested 1 year after treatment with the recommended penicillin regimens.

Review of current evidence and comparison of guidelines for effective syphilis treatment in Europe. Parkes R, Renton A, Meheus A, Laukamm-Josten U. Int J STD AIDS 2004; 15: 73–88.

In some European countries, such as England, the recommended treatment is daily procaine benzylpenicillin (procaine penicillin) injections with or without oral probenecid for 8–21 days, depending on the stage of the disease.

SECOND-LINE THERAPIES

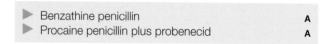

▶ Tetracycline	B
▶ Doxycycline	B
▶ Amoxicillin plus probenecid	B
▶ Ceftriaxone	B

National guideline for the management of early syphilis. Clinical Effectiveness Group (Association of Genitourinary Medicine and the Medical Society for the Study of Venereal Diseases). Sex Trans Infect 1999; 75: S29–33.

The recommended treatment for primary, secondary, or early latent syphilis in immunocompetent persons who are allergic to penicillin is orally administered doxycycline, 100 mg twice daily, or tetracycline 500 mg four times daily for 14 days. Amoxicillin 500 mg four times daily plus probenecid 500 mg four times daily for 14 days is not as effective as parenteral penicillin owing to poorer compliance with this regimen.

Doxycycline 100 mg by mouth twice daily for 28 days is recommended for immunocompetent patients with uncomplicated late latent syphilis or syphilis of unknown duration. Some experts prefer a dose of 200 mg twice daily.

Sexually transmitted diseases treatment guidelines 2006. Centers for Disease Control and Prevention l. Morb Mort Week Rep 2006; 55: 22–29.

Patients receiving alternatives to parenteral penicillin should have close follow-up. In HIV-infected persons, treatment with doxycycline, ceftriaxone, or azithromycin must be carefully considered because data are limited.

Ceftriaxone therapy for syphilis: report from the emerging infections network. Augenbraun M, Workowski K. Clin Infect Dis 1999; 29: 1337–8.

A single injection of 1 g ceftriaxone is not effective for treating infectious syphilis. Daily or alternate-day injections for 8–10 days appear to be efficacious, but more data are needed to evaluate late failures.

Response of HIV-infected patients with asymptomatic syphilis to intensive intramuscular therapy with ceftriaxone or procaine penicillin. Smith NH, Musher DM, Huang DB, Rodriguez PS, Dowell ME, Ace W, et al. Int J STD AIDS 2004; 15: 328–32.

In this prospective pilot study of 31 HIV-infected patients with latent syphilis or syphilis of unknown duration, a four-fold or greater decline in serologic titers occurred in 71% (10 of 14) of patients treated with a daily 1 g intramuscular injection of ceftriaxone for 15 days and 70% (seven of 10) of those treated with a daily 2.4 million units intramuscular injection of procaine penicillin (plus probenecid 500 mg orally four times daily) for 15 days. Two penicillin-treated and one ceftriaxone-treated patient relapsed, and two patients failed ceftriaxone therapy. Three penicillin-treated, and two ceftriaxone-treated patients remained serofast.

A pilot study evaluating ceftriaxone and penicillin G as treatment agents for neurosyphilis in human immunodeficiency virus-infected individuals. Marra CM, Boutin P, McArthur JC, Hurwitz S, Simpson PA, Haslett JA, et al. Clin Infect Dis 2000; 30: 540–4.

There was no difference in CSF abnormalities after treatment with intravenous ceftriaxone or intravenous penicillin in HIV-seropositive patients with neurosyphilis.

Syphilis and human immunodeficiency virus (HIV)-1 coinfection: influence on CD4 T-cell count, HIV-1 viral load, and treatment response. Kofoed K, Gerstoft J, Mathiesen LR, Benfield T. Sex Transm Dis 2006; 33: 143–8.

There was no difference in serologic response rates between 15 patients treated with penicillin and 25 treated with doxycycline for infectious syphilis.

CD4 cell count decreased significantly during infection in patients with primary and secondary stages of syphilis, but both the CD4 cell count and HIV-RNA increased in the overall group following treatment.

THIRD-LINE THERAPIES

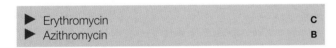

▶ Erythromycin	C
▶ Azithromycin	B

Single-dose azithromycin versus penicillin G benzathine for the treatment of early syphilis. Riedner G, Rusizoka M, Todd J, Maboko L, Hoelscher M, Mmbando D, et al. N Engl J Med 2005; 353: 1236–44.

Three hundred and twenty-eight subjects (25 with primary and 303 with either secondary or latent syphilis with high RPR titer of at least 1:8) were randomly treated with either 2 g of azithromycin orally (163 subjects) or 2.4 million units of benzathine penicillin G intramuscularly (165 subjects); 97.7% of the azithromycin group and 95.0% percent of the penicillin group were clinically cured. At 3 months cure rates were 59.4% in the azithromycin group and 59.5% in the penicillin group, and at 6 months were 85.5% and 81.5%, respectively. In this study a 2 g dose of azithromycin was as effective as a standard dose of benzathine penicillin G.

Azithromycin-resistant syphilis infection: San Francisco, California, 2000–2004. Mitchell SJ, Engelman J, Kent CK, Lukehart SA, Godornes C, Klausner JD. Clin Infect Dis 2006; 42: 337–45.

Molecular screening of 124 samples from San Francisco identified 46 azithromycin-resistant *T. pallidum* isolates and 72 wild-type *T. pallidum* isolates. In total, 52 case patients and 72 control patients were identified. All case patients were male and either gay or bisexual, and 31% (16 of 52) were HIV infected. There was no evidence for a sexual network or demographic differences between cases and controls. However, seven patients had recently used azithromycin, compared to one control patient. Surveillance data demonstrated that the prevalence of azithromycin-resistant *T. pallidum* increased from 0% in 2000 to 56% in 2004.

Macrolide resistance in *Treponema pallidum* in the United States and Ireland. Lukehart SA, Godornes C, Molini BJ, Sonnett P, Hopkins S, Mulcahy F, et al. N Engl J Med 2004; 351: 154–8.

A mutation that makes *T. pallidum* resistant to azithromycin was identified with the use of a restriction-digestion assay in 15 of 17 samples (88%) from Dublin, 12 of 55 samples (22%) from San Francisco, three of 23 samples (13%) from Seattle, and two of 19 samples (11%) from Baltimore. The study suggests that a mutated strain was either introduced into a sexual network or has been selected for among persons who engage in high-risk behavior.

Azithromycin resistance in *Treponema pallidum*. Katz KA, Klausner JD. Curr Opin Infect Dis 2008; 21: 83–91.

Azithromycin resistance in *T. pallidum* is increasing in the United States, Canada, and Ireland. Closer observation for treatment failures is needed in patients treated with azithromycin.

Successful prevention of syphilis infection with azithromycin in both HIV-negative and HIV-positive individuals, San Francisco 1999–2003. Klausner JD, Steiner K, Kohn R. In: Program and abstracts of the 2004 National STD Prevention Conference (Philadelphia). Atlanta: Centers for Disease Control and Prevention, 2004. [Abstract A02B.]

Azithromycin is effective as a single 2 g oral dose in the prevention of disease in sexual partners of patients with infectious syphilis.

Azithromycin treatment failures in syphilis infections – San Francisco, California, 2002–2003. Centers for Disease Control and Prevention. Morb Mort Week Rep 2004; 53: 197–198.

Treatment of eight patients with either primary syphilis or seronegative contacts of partners with syphilis with a single 2 g dose of azithromycin failed to prevent progression to symptomatic or serologic infection, or to heal the chancres. Five of the patients were HIV-infected. A 2 g dose of azithromycin is an alternative to doxycycline for penicillin-allergic patients with early syphilis, but only when close follow-up can be ensured, because treatment efficacy is not well documented and has not been studied in HIV-infected persons.

Syringomata

James AA Langtry

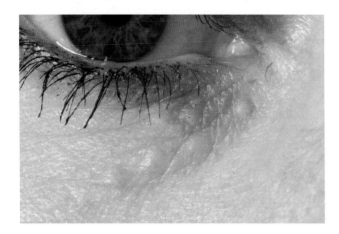

Syringomata are benign appendageal tumors of the intraepidermal eccrine sweat duct which have a characteristic histologic appearance. The typical clinical presentation is of individual skin- or tan-colored papules, with a rounded or flat surface, 1–5 mm in diameter. Single tumors can occur, but more commonly they are multiple and symmetric, more common in females and from adolescence onwards. Syringomata most often involve the lower eyelids, although they may occur at other sites, including the cheeks, axillae, abdomen, and vulva. A linear distribution, familial occurrence, a variant associated with Down's syndrome, as well as generalized forms have all been described. Frequent onset around puberty and reports of symptoms during pregnancy or menstruation have led to immunohistochemical studies of estrogen and progesterone receptors, with varying results and uncertain relevance.

MANAGEMENT STRATEGY

Syringomata of the eyelids and cheeks are in a prominent site, may appear conspicuous, and treatment may be sought to improve appearance. The syringomata are situated in the upper to mid dermis. Available treatments aim to remove or flatten the papule produced by each syringoma. All are ablative modalities and include surgical excision with primary suturing. As some patients are troubled by a few individual lesions, *excision* of these may be an option. The modalities are: scissor excision with secondary intention healing; surgical excision of the entire cosmetic unit of the lower eyelids in patients who would also benefit from lower eyelid blepharoplasty; *electrocautery*; *electrodesiccation*; *intralesional electrodesiccation*; *dermabrasion*; *cryotherapy*; and ablation with CO_2 *or erbium:YAG laser*.

Local anesthesia is needed prior to treatment, and this may be topical, or by local injections with or without nerve blocks. Local anesthetic injections producing a field block are most commonly employed, as good anesthesia is helpful when using ablative treatments near the eye. Patients should be warned about the possibility of postoperative bruising. Eye protection is of paramount importance, and specific precautions relevant to the use of lasers must be taken if laser treatment is used.

Ablative treatments will produce some degree of scarring and the aim is to make this imperceptible and produce an excellent cosmetic result. Possible sequelae, including scarring and hypo- or hyperpigmentation (especially with increasing skin pigmentation), should always be discussed prior to treatment.

There are no studies comparing different treatment modalities for syringomata, and very few long-term follow-up data on which to base recommendations for treatment. On the basis of experience and the limited evidence available, it is not necessary to have the latest and most expensive technology to achieve good results. Expertise and good outcomes with simple, 'low-tech' methods are as important as with 'high-tech' modalities. Each has benefits as well as pitfalls for the novice or unwary. It is more important to be expert in the use and application of one or more modalities than to 'have a go' at them all.

SPECIFIC INVESTIGATIONS

The clinical features of periorbital syringomata are usually typical and a skin biopsy may be useful to confirm the diagnosis, as well as in situations of diagnostic uncertainty.

FIRST-LINE THERAPIES

▶ Surgical excision	E
▶ Snip excision and secondary intention healing	E
▶ Electrocautery	E
▶ Intralesional electrodesiccation	D
▶ CO_2 laser	D

Cosmetic dermatologic surgery, 2nd edn. Stegman SS, Tromovitch TA, Glogau RG, eds. Chicago: Year Book Medical, 1992; 32.

A commonsense approach to treatment of syringomata, advocating the use of surgical excision, electrosurgery, or laser.

An easy method for removal of syringoma. Maloney ME. J Dermatol Surg Oncol 1982; 8: 973–5.

A single case is reported with a good outcome following removal of four to six lesions per session, in 12 sessions over 5 months.

A good photographic demonstration of the removal of periorbital syringomata with fine ophthalmic spring-action scissors.

True electrocautery in the treatment of syringomas and other benign cutaneous lesions. Langtry JAA, Carruthers JA. J Cutan Med Surg 1997; 2: 60–3.

The technique of electrocautery is described and good results reported in a number of benign skin lesions, including syringomata.

Intralesional electrodesiccation of syringomas. Karma P, Benedetto AV. Dermatol Surg 1997; 23: 921–4.

Twelve patients were treated with electrodesiccation via a fine electrode into the center of the syringoma, with the aim of localizing the effect and minimizing scarring. All reported excellent results and no recurrence after a follow-up of 18–48 months. Two patients with Fitzpatrick skin type IV had focal hyperpigmentation, which cleared in 2–3 months.

Treatment of multiple facial syringomas with the carbon dioxide (CO_2) laser. Wang JI, Roenigk HH Jr. Dermatol Surg 1999; 25: 136–9.

A description of 10 patients treated with CO_2 laser reporting excellent results. Patients with more lesions needed more treatment sessions. The median follow-up was 16 months, and one patient had new syringomata at other periorbital sites 18 months after treatment. Erythema lasted 6–12 weeks in all patients. One patient with Fitzpatrick type IV skin had minimal focal areas of hyperpigmentation, which cleared after 2–3 months.

SECOND-LINE THERAPIES

▶ Electrodesiccation and curettage	E
▶ Cryotherapy	E
▶ Combination of CO_2 laser and trichloroacetic acid	D

Syringoma: removal by electrodesiccation and curettage. Stevenson TR, Swanson SA. Am Plast Surg 1985; 15: 151–4.

The technique is described and well illustrated. Good results are reported, but there is no description of numbers of patients treated, clinical details, or follow-up data using this technique.

Cryosurgery. Dawber RPR. In: Lask GP, Moy RL, eds. Principles and techniques of cutaneous surgery. New York: McGraw-Hill, 1996; 154.

Syringoma is listed as a condition treatable by cryotherapy. *Details are not given and periorbital syringomata are not specifically mentioned.*

A new treatment for syringoma. Combination of carbon dioxide laser and trichloroacetic acid. Kang H, Kim NS, Kim YB, Shim WC. Dermatol Surg 1998; 24: 1370–4.

This study evaluates the histopathology and efficacy of combined CO_2 laser and 50% trichloroacetic acid treatment in 20 Korean patients with periorbital syringomata. Results were reported as excellent (11 patients), good (six), and fair (three), without complications such as scarring, infection, or textural change, using the technique detailed.

THIRD-LINE THERAPIES

▶ Dermabrasion	E
▶ Trichloroacetic acid	E
▶ Topical atropine	E
▶ Topical tretinoin	E

Dermabrasion by diamond fraises revolving at 85000 revolutions per minute. Fulton JE. J Dermatol Surg Oncol 1978; 4: 777–9.

High-speed dermabrasion is described and good results are reported in 65 patients with acne scarring, actinic damage, adenoma sebaceum, and syringomata.

The treatment of eruptive syringomas in an African American patient with a combination of trichlororacetic acid and CO_2 laser destruction. Frazier CC, Camacho AP, Cockerell CJ. Dermatol Surg 2001; 27: 489–92.

A single case report of eruptive facial syringomata in an African-American woman treated by 35% trichloroacetic acid peel, followed 2 weeks later by CO_2 laser, with acceptable cosmetic results and without significant side effects.

Eruptive pruritic syringomas: treatment with topical atropine. Sanchez TS, Dauden E, Casas AP, Garcia-Diez A. J Am Acad Dermatol 2001; 44: 148–9.

A single case report of pruritic syringomata of the chest and neck improving with topical 1% atropine.

Eruptive syringoma: treatment with topical tretinoin. Gomez MI, Perez B, Azana JM, Nunez M, Ledo A. Dermatology 1994; 189: 105–6.

Tinea capitis

Elisabeth M Higgins

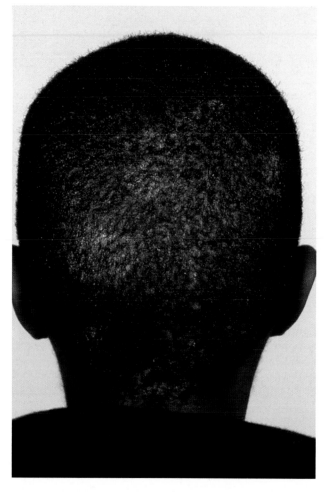

Tinea capitis (scalp ringworm) is the term used to describe a fungal infection of the scalp caused by dermatophyte species. Infections may be passed from person to person (so-called anthropophilic, in which man is the primary host) or acquired from animals (zoophilic). Several different species of fungi may be responsible, predominantly *Microsporum* and *Trichophyton* species, and can be identified by their varied characteristics on microscopy and culture. Species that invade only the inside of the hair shaft are termed endothrix infections, whereas those that invade both the inside and the outside of the hair shaft are responsible for ectothrix infections. The disease is most prevalent in children and usually presents with areas of scaling and alopecia, with a varying degree of inflammation. There may be associated cervical lymphadenopathy. Some species of dermatophyte induce a very inflammatory, pustular reaction, which may lead to scarring and permanent alopecia. However, this is fortunately relatively rare with modern treatment regimens, in which full regrowth of hair is the norm.

MANAGEMENT STRATEGY

Treatment of tinea capitis is aimed at eradicating the organism to prevent the spread of infection and minimize scarring. Established infections cannot be treated topically and oral therapy is required. In many countries, including the UK, *griseofulvin* remains the only licensed oral antifungal agent for use in tinea capitis in children. Although only weakly fungistatic, griseofulvin is effective in the treatment of most varieties of tinea capitis, but may need to be given in high doses over a prolonged period. Each case should be monitored to ensure adequate treatment and eradication of the organism. Traditionally this has been done using Wood's light examination, but this is only viable in cases due to species that fluoresce (e.g., *Microsporum* infections). An increasing number of cases in the UK and North America today are due to the emergence of *Trichophyton tonsurans*, a non-fluorescent endothrix species. Treatment response therefore has to be followed mycologically, by sending specimens to the laboratory. Mycological cure should be the gold standard of treatment.

In recent years the azoles *itraconazole, ketoconazole,* and *fluconazole,* and the allylamine *terbinafine* have become available for systemic use. Many studies have demonstrated that these agents have at least equal efficacy to *griseofulvin* in a variety of types of tinea capitis, and treatment times are often shorter. Although these agents are more expensive, shorter treatment regimens may help compliance and reduce the spread of infection.

Over the past decade, the use of intermittent or pulsed treatment regimens using *fluconazole* or *itraconazole* have been explored. This treatment strategy is based on the long half-life of the drugs in keratin. Such regimens do not appear to confer any benefit in terms of cure rates, but may reduce the total cost of treatment.

There are variations in the response of different dermatophyte species to the different antifungal agents, and treatment should be tailored accordingly. Overall, *griseofulvin* appears superior in the clearance of *Microsporum* infections, but newer agents appear more effective against *Trichophyton*. However, so far no agent has been shown to achieve a 100% cure rate, which remains the ultimate objective of any treatment strategy.

Ectothrix infections are generally caused by *Microsporum* species, most notably the zoophilic *M. canis* or the anthropophilic *M. audouinii*, and almost always occur in children. Griseofulvin remains the treatment of choice at a dose of 10–20 mg/kg/day, but clearance may be slow and treatment should be continued for as long as necessary, which is at least 6 weeks, but may be 12–16 weeks, and monitored as outlined above. Itraconazole may be considered an alternative, although there are licensing restrictions in some countries.

Endothrix infections, most commonly with *T. tonsurans* or *T. violaceum,* are more prevalent in children, but may occasionally occur in adults (usually the contacts/carers of children). Higher-dose regimens of *griseofulvin* tend to be required to achieve cure. The newer *azoles* and *terbinafine* appear to achieve cure more rapidly (usually in 4 weeks). In adults with tinea capitis due to *Trichophyton* species, *terbinafine* 250 mg/day for 4 weeks is the treatment of choice. Although unlicensed in children, the current *British National Formulary* gives the dosing schedule for *terbinafine* in tinea capitis, in recognition of its widespread use (<20 kg, 62.5 mg/day; 20–40 kg, 125 mg/day; >40 kg, 250 mg/day). Current evidence suggests that either this or itraconazole should become the treatment of choice in children with *Trichophyton* infections.

Topical antifungal creams and shampoos are sometimes used in conjunction with oral therapy, with the aim of reducing the time that the patient is infectious.

In the current urban epidemics of *T. tonsurans*, asymptomatic infection in household contacts is posing a significant problem in re-infection/relapse, and there is merit in screening all family members (including adults) where practical.

Ketoconazole or selenium sulphide shampoos may reduce infectivity.

SPECIFIC INVESTIGATIONS

> ▶ Examination of hair and scalp scale by direct microscopy and culture
> ▶ Direct observation under Wood's light for fluorescence
> ▶ Screen contacts, especially siblings, where possible

Diagnosis in colour: Medical mycology. Midgley G, Clayton Y, Hay RJ. London: Mosby-Wolfe, 1997; 9–15, 38–50.

Fungal infection: diagnosis and management. Richardson MD, Warnock DW. Oxford: Blackwell, 2003; 21, 87.

Scalp hairs infected by *M. audouinii*, *M. canis* and *T. schoenleinii* fluoresce bright green under Wood's light. Direct microscopic examination of hairs reveals arthrospores of the fungus either inside (endothrix) or on the outside of the hair shaft. Individual dermatophyte species can be identified by specific appearances in culture.

Screening for asymptomatic carriage of *Trichophyton tonsurans* in household contacts of patients with tinea capitis: results of 209 patients from south London. White JM, Higgins EM, Fuller LC. J Eur Acad Dermatol Venereol 2007; 21: 1061–4.

More than 50% of household contacts in this study had positive fungal cultures (7.1% overt infection and 44.5% silent fungal carriage). Children under 16 were most likely to be affected (p<0.001), especially girls (p<0.01).

Treatment of tinea capitis often needs to be started before laboratory confirmation is obtained. Treatment should be started on the basis of clinical evidence, but appropriate mycology samples should always be sent prior to initiation of therapy.

FIRST-LINE THERAPIES

> ▶ Griseofulvin   A
> ▶ Terbinafine   A
> ▶ Itraconazole   A

Terbinafine hydrochloride oral granules versus oral griseofulvin suspension in children with tinea capitis: Results of two randomised investigator-blinded, multicenter, international, controlled trials. Elewski BE, Cáceres HW, Deleon L, El Shimy S, Hunter JA, Korotkiy N, et al. J Am Acad Dermatol 2008; Mar 29 [epub ahead of print].

A multicenter investigator-blinded, randomized controlled study with two arms compared 6 weeks' griseofulvin 10–20 mg/kg/day (n = 509) with terbinafine 5–8 mg/kg/day (n = 1040). All children had microscopy-proven tinea capitis. Rates of complete cure (45.1% vs 33.01%) and mycological cure (61.55 vs 55.5%) were significantly higher for terbinafine than for griseofulvin (p<0.05). Higher doses of griseofulvin (>20 mg/kg/day) did not appear to produce a greater cure rate than more conventional doses. Subgroup analysis revealed that terbinafine was significantly better than griseofulvin for all cure rates (clinical, mycological, and complete) among patients with *T. tonsurans* infection but not for *M. canis* (p<0.001). In contrast, for *M. canis*, mycological and clinical cure rates were significantly better with griseofulvin (p<0.05).

Fifty percent of patients in each group reported mild side effects with treatment, but there was no significant effect on liver transaminases.

This largest pediatric study to date highlights the safety and efficacy of a new formulation of terbinafine in the treatment of tinea capitis in children. However, limitations of the study were not using a standard dose of griseofulvin in each center, inconsistency in the use of adjuvant topical therapy, and the inclusion of more than one causal species. Subanalysis shows a clear differentiation in response rates between organisms, and therapy should probably be tailored, with terbinafine being the treatment of choice in T. tonsurans *infection, while griseofulvin is superior in* Microsporum *infections.*

Systemic anti-fungal therapy for tinea capitis in children. González U, Seaton T, Bergus G, Jacobson J, Martínez-Mónzon C. Cochrane Database Syst Rev. 2007; 4: CD004685.

An analysis of 21 randomized control trials involving 1812 subjects under the age of 18 years, in which systemic antifungal therapy was used in mycologically proven tinea capitis. In view of varying susceptibilities, studies were evaluated according to the causal organism.

For *Trichophyton* species: *terbinafine* given on a weight-related dosage schedule for 4 weeks showed similar efficacy to *griseofulvin* given for 8 weeks in three studies involving 382 subjects (RR 1.09; 95% CI 0.95–1.26). Itraconazole and griseofulvin given for 6 weeks showed similar cure rates in a study of 35 children (RR 1.06; 95% CI 0.81–1.39). However, *itraconazole* given for short periods may also be as effective as griseofulvin given for 6 weeks (RR 0.89; 95% CI 0.76–1.04), and both itraconazole and terbinafine given for 2–3 weeks were equally effective in two studies involving 160 participants (RR 0.93; 95% CI 0.72–1.19).

For *Microsporum* species: overall, no difference was found between the efficacy of griseofulvin and that of terbinafine in clearance of *Microsporum* infections, but there was little evidence on the use of systemic agents in this species that met the study inclusion criteria.

The authors conclude that terbinafine and itraconazole are probably preferable to griseofulvin in the treatment of Trichophyton *tinea capitis because of the shorter treatment duration, even though these agents are more expensive and may not always be available in a pediatric formulation.*

Meta-analysis: griseofulvin efficacy in the treatment of tinea capitis. Gupta AK, Cooper EA, Bowen JE. J Drugs Dermatol 2008; 7: 369–72.

An analysis of seven studies involving 438 patients revealed that the overall mean efficacy (based on mycological cure) of griseofulvin given for 6–8 weeks was 73.4% (± 7%). Higher doses (>18 mg/kg) were reported to have greater efficacy. However, subanalysis on the basis of species involved showed that the mean efficacy in the treatment of *Trichophyton* species was 67.6% (± 9%) (five studies, n = 396), compared to 88.1% (± 5%) (two studies, n = 42) for *Microsporum* infection.

Although this review confirms that griseofulvin remains an effective therapy in tinea capitis, there is clear superiority in treating Microsporum *infections. However, qualitative data for its use against this organism are comparatively sparse.*

Itraconazole in the treatment of tinea capitis caused by *Microsporum canis*: experience in a large cohort. Ginter-Hanselmayer G, Smolie J, Gupta A. Paediatr Dermatol 2004; 21: 499–502.

An open study of 163 children with mycologically proven *M. canis* tinea capitis, 55 of whom had previously received terbinafine without successful clearance. All children received itraconazole 5 mg/kg/day either as a capsule or as a suspension. All children achieved complete cure after a mean period of 39 ± 12 days (range 10–77 days). Treatment was well tolerated, with only minor side effects.

This study shows that itraconazole is a well-tolerated alternative to griseofulvin in children with M. canis *tinea capitis.*

SECOND-LINE THERAPIES

▶ Fluconazole	**B**
▶ Short-duration terbinafine	**B**
▶ Short-duration itraconazole	**B**

Therapeutic options for the treatment of tinea capitis caused by *Trichophyton* species: griseofulvin versus the new oral antifungal agents, terbinafine, itraconazole and fluconazole. Gupta AK, Adam P, Dlova N, Lynde CW, Hofstader S, Morar N, et al. Paediatr Dermatol 2001: 18: 433–8.

A multicenter prospective, randomized single-blinded study of 200 children comparing the efficacy of griseofulvin 20 mg/kg/day for 6 weeks, terbinafine (62.5–250 mg/day according to weight) for 2 weeks, *itraconazole* 5 mg/kg/day for 2 weeks, or fluconazole 6 mg/kg/day for 2 weeks. Patients on the shorter regimens were evaluated 2 weeks after the end of treatment and given an extra week of treatment if clinically indicated. All children had either *T. tonsurans* or *T. violaceum* infection. Evaluation at 12 weeks revealed no significant difference in the mycological cure rates between the groups (92% for griseofulvin, 94% for terbinafine, 86% for *itraconazole*, and 84% for fluconazole (p < 0.33)). However, side effects (mostly nausea and GI upset) were only noted in the griseofulvin group.

This study shows that short-duration therapy with itraconazole, fluconazole, and terbinafine is as effective as high-dose standard-duration griseofulvin in the treatment of Trichophyton *tinea capitis, and newer agents appear better tolerated.*

Therapeutic options for the treatment of tinea capitis: griseofulvin versus fluconazole. Dastghaib L, Azizzadeh M, Jafari P. J Dermatol Treat 2005; 16: 43–6.

A randomized prospective, single-blind study of 40 patients aged 1–16 years with mycologically proven tinea capitis (40% *T. violaceum*, 40% *T. verrucosum*, 20% *M. canis*) showed no significant difference in overall cure rates (clinical and mycological) between fluconazole 5 mg/kg/day for 4 weeks and griseofulvin 15 mg/kg/day for 6 weeks (78% and 76%, respectively). Subgroup analysis of response by species showed significant variability in cure rates, griseofulvin being superior in *Microsporum* infections (75% vs 25%), but fluconazole being superior in *Trichophyton* species (93% vs 79%).

In this study both drugs show similar efficacy but Trichophyton *infections responded best. Of the small number of cases (8) of* Microsporum *infection, one of four on griseofulvin and two of four on fluconazole failed to clear. However, the greater availability and lower cost still favor the use of griseofulvin in many countries.*

Once weekly fluconazole is effective in children in the treatment of tinea capitis: a prospective multi-centre study. Gupta AK, Dlova N, Taborda P, Morar N, Taborda V, Lynde CW, et al. Br J Dermatol 2000; 142: 965–8.

An open, multicenter assessment of 61 children treated with oral fluconazole 8 mg/kg once weekly for 8 weeks (extended for a further 4 weeks if clinically indicated). Causal organisms were *T. violaceum* (33), *T. tonsurans* (11), and *M. canis* (17). All 44 children with *Trichophyton* infections had mycological and clinical cure at 16 weeks after the start of treatment; the majority (35/44) only required 8 weeks of therapy, but nine out of 33 of the *T. violaceum* group required treatment for 12 weeks. Twelve out of 17 of the *M. canis* group were clinically clear after 8 weeks. Treatment was extended for a total of 12 weeks in one and 16 weeks in three patients, but overall 16 of 17 children in this group had complete cure 2 months after the end of therapy. One child had asymptomatic and reversible elevation of liver function tests.

Short duration treatment with terbinafine for tinea capitis caused by *Trichophyton* or *Microsporum* species. Hamm H, Schwinn A, Brautigan M, Weidinger G. Br J Dermatol 1999; 140: 480–2.

A double-blind study of 35 children comparing the efficacy of 1 or 2 weeks of oral terbinafine, 62.5–250 mg/day according to weight. Patients were followed up for 12 weeks and non-responders were given an additional 4 weeks of therapy. Twenty-three children had *Trichophyton* infections (12 *T. tonsurans*) and 12 had *M. canis* infection; cure rates after 1 and 2 weeks of therapy were 86% and 56%, respectively. However, only one of the 12 children with *Microsporum* infection responded initially, although a further four cleared with 4 more weeks of treatment.

Short-duration (2 weeks) and intermittent treatment regimens show remarkable clearance rates, particularly in infections with Trichophyton *species, and may offer a significant cost saving.*

THIRD-LINE THERAPIES

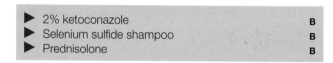

▶ 2% ketoconazole	**B**
▶ Selenium sulfide shampoo	**B**
▶ Prednisolone	**B**

Treatment of kerions. Honig PJ, Caputo GL, Leyden JJ, McGinley K, Selbst SM, McGravey AR. Paediatr Dermatol 1994; 11: 69–71.

Thirty patients with kerions were randomly assigned to receive treatment with either griseofulvin alone, griseofulvin plus prednisolone, griseovulvin plus erythromycin, or griseofulvin plus prednisolone and erythromycin. Although the degree of scale and pruritus was lessened by prednisolone and erythromycin, the total time taken for the kerion to flatten was unchanged.

A randomised comparative trial of treatment of kerion celsi with griseofulvin plus oral prednisolone vs. griseofulvin alone. Hussain I, Muzzafar F, Rashid T, Jahangir M, Haroon TS. Med Mycol 1999; 37: 97–9.

A randomized study of 30 patients with scalp kerion comparing treatment with griseofulvin and prednisolone to griseofulvin alone. Evaluation at 12 weeks revealed similar cure rates in both groups.

Although traditionally many clinicians have used prednisolone to reduce the inflammation of kerions, in an effort to minimize scarring and hence the possibility of permanent alopecia, the little evidence that exists does not support its use. Kerion formation is not uncommon in the current spate of T. tonsurans *infections in the UK. However, scarring is exceptionally rare. It is the author's practice not to use prednisolone in tinea capitis, full regrowth of hair being the norm.*

Successful treatment of tinea capitis with 2% ketoconazole shampoo. Greer DL. Int J Dermatol 2000; 39: 302–4.

Sixteen children aged 3–6 years with *T. tonsurans* tinea capitis were treated with 2% ketoconazole shampoo daily for 8 weeks. All showed clinical improvement, some as early as 2 weeks. Six of 15 (40%) had negative cultures at 8 weeks and five (33%) remained clear 1 year later.

Comparison of 1% and 2.5% selenium sulphide in the treatment of tinea capitis. Gibbens TG, Murray MM, Baker RC. Arch Pediatr Adolesc Med 1995; 149: 808–11.

A randomized controlled trial of 54 patients showing that selenium sulfide, as either a lotion or a shampoo, reduces surface counts of dermatophytes in children being treated with griseofulvin 15 mg/kg/day.

Selenium sulphide: adjunctive treatment for tinea capitis. Allen HB, Honig PJ, Leyden JJ, McGinley KJ. Pediatrics 1992; 69: 81–3.

Selenium sulfide has been shown to be sporicidal in vitro. In children with tinea capitis being treated with griseofulvin the additional use of twice-weekly selenium sulfide shampoo resulted in negative cultures at 2 weeks in 15 of 16 children, in contrast to those treated with griseofulvin alone or in combination with a bland shampoo or topical clotrimazole, who all had positive cultures at 2 weeks (and up to 8 weeks later).

These small studies support the use of an antifungal shampoo to reduce surface counts of the organism, and therefore aid clearance and possibly reduce the risk of transmission. If systemic therapy is contraindicated or unavailable, there may be a limited benefit in using 2% ketoconazole shampoo alone.

Tinea pedis and skin dermatophytosis

L Claire Fuller

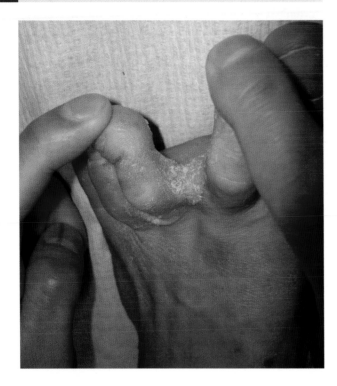

Tinea pedis (athlete's foot) describes a dermatophyte infection of the soles of the feet and interdigital spaces; tinea cruris, an infection of the groin; tinea facei, the face; and tinea corporis the rest of the skin.

MANAGEMENT STRATEGY

Tinea pedis rarely causes significant morbidity and certainly not mortality, but there is some evidence that it acts as a portal of entry for bacteria that produce bacterial cellulitis. *Topical antifungal treatment (with topical azoles or allylamines) of tinea pedis* is generally adequate, as it is for small areas of tinea corporis and cruris, but for extensive infections, and especially those in immunosuppressed patients, oral therapy may be required. Several antifungal topical therapies are available without prescription, and the vast majority of the disease burden is likely to be managed without intervention from medical personnel. However, relapse from inadequate therapy is a common event in tinea pedis, albeit less so in other body sites. Reinfection can also occur in about 10% of cases. Certain clinical forms of tinea pedis are more resistant to treatment and may require oral therapy with systemic antifungals such as *terbinafine, fluconazole, or itraconazole*. Severe macerated forms of tinea pedis may well be superinfected with bacteria justifying concomitant antibiotic therapy, although some topical antifungal agents have in vitro antibacterial activity, such as *ciclopiroxolamine*.

Chronic dermatomycoses of the foot as risk factors for acute bacterial cellulitis of the leg: a case–control study. Roujeau JC, Sigurgeirsson B, Korting HC, Kerl H, Paul C. Dermatology 2004; 209: 301–7.

Two hundred and forty-three patients with acute bacterial cellulitis and 467 age- and gender-matched controls were investigated and mycology-proven tinea pedis was shown to be a significant risk factor for cellulitis (odds ratio OR 2.4; p<0.001). Interdigital tinea pedis conferred the highest risk (OR 3.2, p<0.001) followed by onychomycosis (OR 2.2, p<0.001) and then plantar-type tinea pedis (OR 1.2, p=0.005). A previous history of cellulitis, venous insufficiency, and leg edema was also reported to increase the risk.

SPECIFIC INVESTIGATIONS

> ► Skin scrapings for mycological microscopy and culture
> ► Skin swabs for bacteriology

The lesions should be scraped carefully, harvesting surface scale with a no. 15 blade or banana-shaped knife. The active edges of large lesions are likely to yield more scale. Avoiding the application of emollients prior to sampling aids sample collection. Blister and pustule tops may be ruptured and the contents swabbed and placed directly onto agar plates.

Clinical signs and procedures in dermatology. Marks R, Dykes P, Motley R. London: Taylor & Francis, 1993.

The principal organisms responsible for tinea pedis are *Trichophyton rubrum*, *Trichophyton mentagrophytes* and *Epidermophyton floccosum*. Not all scaly eruptions are due to tinea, so confirming the presence of a dermatophyte enables the instigation of relevant, targeted therapy and avoids causing unwanted side effects in non-fungal cases.

Frequency of culture-proven dermatophyte infection in patients with suspected tinea pedis. Fuchs A, Fiedler J, Lebwohl M, Sapadin A, Rudikoff D, Lefkovits A, et al. Am J Med Sci 2004; 327: 77–8.

Culture-positive rates in 874 patients suspected of having tinea pedis were only 32%.

Many clinicians will scrape a scaly rash or an acral eruption to rule out a tinea contribution, so this is probably an appropriately low positive result.

Macerated tinea pedis may well be superinfected with bacteria.

Interdigital athlete's foot. The interaction of dermatophytes and resident bacteria. Leyden JJ, Kligman AM. Arch Dermatol 1978; 114: 1466–72.

Quantitative cultures of 140 cases of interdigital 'athlete's foot' showed that as the clinical disease became more macerated, increasing numbers of resident aerobic organisms, such as large colony diphtheroids, were present.

FIRST-LINE THERAPIES

Topical

► Clotrimazole (azole)	A
► Miconazole (azole)	A

Evidence Levels: **A** Double-blind study **B** Clinical trial ≥ 20 subjects **C** Clinical trial < 20 subjects **D** Series ≥ 5 subjects **E** Anecdotal case reports

Systematic review of topical treatments for fungal infections of the skin and nails of the feet. Hart R, Bell-Syer SE, Crawford F, Torgerson DJ, Young P, Russell I. Br Med J 1999; 319: 79–82.

This rigorous review found 17 placebo-controlled trials for azoles with an estimated pooled risk of failure to cure of 0.54, versus 12 trials of allylamines against placebo with a rate of 0.3 of failure to cure. There are 12 randomized controlled trials of azoles against allylamines, and although allylamines are slightly more effective than azoles and undecanoic acid, they are more expensive, so the authors recommended first to treat with azoles topically and to use allylamines only in treatment failures. This saves £1.94 (sterling) for each cured patient.

SECOND-LINE THERAPIES

Topical

▶ Terbinafine 1% (allylamine) as either cream, solution, gel or film forming solution (FFS)   A
▶ Cicolpirox   A

Comparable efficacy and safety of various topical formulations of terbinafine in tinea pedis irrespective of the treatment regimen: results of a meta-analysis. Korting HC, Kiencke P, Nelles S, Rychlik R. Am J Clin Dermatol 2007; 8: 357–64.

An efficacy analysis from 19 eligible studies involving nearly 3000 patients demonstrated that mycological cure rates with terbinafine were significantly superior to those of placebo, but no significant differences were shown between the different formulations, durations of therapy, or frequencies of application. Regimens varied from a single application of the FFS to 4 weeks once or twice daily of the other formulations. Ten randomized controlled studies compared terbinafine with an active control, and although clinical and mycological cure rates were slightly higher with terbinafine, this did not reach statistical significance.

Ciclopirox gel in the treatment of patients with interdigital tinea pedis. Aly R, Fisher G, Katz I, Levine N, Lookingbill DP, Lowe N, et al. Int J Dermatol 2003; 42: 29–35.

Three hundred and seventy-four subjects with mild to moderate tinea pedis were enrolled and randomized to one of two treatment groups: ciclopirox gel 0.77%, or ciclopirox gel vehicle, applied twice daily for 28 days. Eighty-five percent of ciclopirox subjects were mycologically cured, compared to only 16% of vehicle subjects 2 weeks post treatment.

THIRD-LINE THERAPIES

Topical

▶ 40% urea cream   C

The use of 40% urea cream in the treatment of moccasin tinea pedis. Elewski BE, Haley HR, Robbins CM. Cutis 2004; 73: 355–7.

Twelve patients with moccasin-type tinea pedis were treated with 40% urea cream once daily as an adjunct to the topical antifungal ciclopirox cream twice daily. At 3 weeks a 100% cure rate was shown.

Systemic

▶ Terbinafine   A
▶ Itraconazole   A
▶ Fluconazole   A
▶ Griseofulvin   A

Short-term itraconazole versus terbinafine in the treatment of tinea pedis or manus. Tausch I, Decroix J, Gwiezdzinski Z, Urbanowski S, Baran E, Ziarkiewicz M, et al. Int J Dermatol 1998; 37: 140–2.

A double-blind randomized multicenter phase 3 study involving 300 patients with palmar-type tinea pedis (moccasin) or manum using 200 mg itraconazole twice daily for 7 days versus 250 mg terbinafine once daily for 14 days, showed no difference in the mycological cure rates of 79% verses 80%. Side effects were reported in 14% of the itraconazole group and 19% of the terbinafine group, with no clinically relevant changes in laboratory variables evaluated.

Although this is a high dose of itraconazole this is shown both to be efficacious and safe in the treatment of tinea pedis.

A multicentre (double-blind) comparative study to assess the safety and efficacy of fluconazole and griseofulvin in the treatment of tinea corporis and tinea cruris. Faergemann J, Mork NJ, Haglund A, Odegard T. Br J Dermatol 1997; 13: 575–7.

Two hundred and thirty patients were entered into a double-blind, parallel-group study comparing fluconazole 150 mg once weekly with griseofulvin 500 mg once daily for 4–6 weeks in the treatment tinea corporis or tinea cruris. Mycological cure was achieved in 78% of the fluconazole group compared to 80% in the griseofulvin group.

Efficacy and safety of short-term itraconazole in tinea pedis: a double-blind, randomized, placebo-controlled trial. Svejgaard E, Avnstorp C, Wanscher B, Nilsson J, Heremans A. Dermatology 1998; 197: 368–72.

Seventy-two patients with moccasin-type tinea pedis were randomized to receive either itraconazole 200 mg twice daily for 1 week or placebo. After 8 weeks of follow-up mycological cure rates were 56% versus 8% (p<0.001) in favor of itraconazole, and clinical cure rates 75% verses 11% (p<0.001).

Short-term treatment showed that itraconazole is significantly more effective than placebo in treating tinea pedis.

Therapy with fluconazole for tinea corporis, tinea cruris, and tinea pedis. Montero-Gei F, Perera A. Clin Infect Dis 1992; 14: S77–81.

Twenty patients each with tinea corporis and/or tinea cruris and 20 patients with tinea pedis were treated with a single dose of 150 mg fluconazole and followed weekly. A further dose was administered each week in the persisting presence of clinical evidence of infection, to a maximum of four doses. In tinea corporis/cruris 70% required two doses, 20% three doses, and 10% four doses. At 30 days mycological clearance was observed in 95%. In tinea pedis 20% needed two doses, 20% three, and 60% four doses, with mycological clearance at 30 days observed in 75%.

Safety and efficacy of short-duration oral terbinafine for the treatment of tinea corporis or tinea cruris in subjects with HIV infection or diabetes. Rich P, Houpt KR, LaMarca A,

Loven KH, Marbury TC, Matheson R, et al.; Tinea Corporis/ Tinea Cruris Research Group. Cutis 2001; 68: 15–22.

A small prospective open-label study randomly treated six HIV-positive and eight diabetic adult patients with tinea corporis or tinea cruris using oral terbinafine 250 mg once daily for either 1 or 2 weeks. At 6 weeks, of the 11 patients that had full mycological results available for analysis, all the HIV-positive patients and 83% of diabetic patients achieved mycological clearance. There was no difference observed between 1 or 2 weeks' treatment, and the drug was well tolerated.

Tinea unguium

Antonella Tosti, Bianca Maria Piraccini

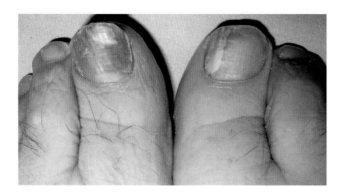

Onychomycosis accounts for about half of all nail abnormalities and a third of all fungal infections of the skin. It affects about the 10% of the general population, with figures that vary in different areas of the world. About 85% of cases of onychomycosis result from dermatophyte invasion of the nail (tinea unguium), the most common responsible agent being *Trichophyton rubrum*, followed by *Trichophyton interdigitale*. The prevalence of onychomycosis increases with age, and the toenails are most frequently affected. Tinea pedis plantaris or interdigitale are associated with onychomycosis in most patients and, if not concomitantly treated, may be the source of recurrence.

Predisposing factors for onychomycosis include old age, diabetes, HIV infection, peripheral vascular impairment and peripheral neuropathies, podiatric abnormalities, sports activities, and traumatic nail disorders.

Factors influencing coexistence of toenail onychomycosis with tinea pedis and other dermatomycoses: a survey of 2761 patients. Szepietowski JC, Reich A, Garlowska E, Kulig M, Baran E; Onychomycosis Epidemiology Study Group. Arch Dermatol 2006; 142: 1279–84.

This study evaluated the presence of skin dermatophyte infections in 2761 patients with dermatophyte onychomycosis. Coexistence of tinea pedis and toenail onychomycosis was found in 933 patients (33.8%). Other concomitant fungal skin infections were tinea cruris, tinea corporis, and tinea manuum.

SPECIFIC INVESTIGATIONS

▶ Direct microscopy of 40% KOH preparations of subungual scales
▶ Cultures of nail scrapings in sabouraud-agar-cloramphenicol and sabouraud-agar-cloramphenicol + acitidione media
▶ Histopathology of PAS-stained nail clippings

The diagnosis of onychomycosis always requires laboratory confirmation, as differential diagnosis from psoriasis or traumatic onychodystrophy is often impossible on a clinical basis.

Fungal elements in the affected nails can be detected using KOH preparations of the nail samples or histopathology of PAS-stained nail clippings.

Cost-effectiveness of diagnostic tests for toenail onychomycosis: a repeated-measure, single-blinded, cross-sectional evaluation of 7 diagnostic tests. Lilly KK, Koshnick RL, Grill JP, Khalil ZM, Nelson DB, Warshaw EM. J Am Acad Dermatol 2006; 55: 620–6.

This study compared the cost-effectiveness (sensitivity related to cost) of the most commonly used diagnostic tests for onychomycosis. KOH and PAS were equally sensitive, with KOH being less expensive but requiring practitioners proficient in direct microscopy techniques.

KOH preparations or histopathology of PAS-stained nail clippings do not permit identification of the responsible fungus. This can only be done using cultures in Sabouraud's dextrose agar plus chloramphenicol, with and without cycloheximide. A negative mycological result does not rule out onychomycosis, as direct microscopy is negative in up to 10% of cases and culture in up to 30%. KOH and cultures should be repeated in negative cases when the clinical features are highly suggestive for tinea unguium.

Correct sampling of nail debris is mandatory for obtaining reliable mycological results. In the most common variety of onychomycosis, the distal subungual type, culture sensitivity improves the more proximal the location of the sample.

Fast and sensitive detection of *Trichophyton rubrum* DNA from the nail samples of patients with onychomycosis by a double-round polymerase chain reaction-based assay. Gupta AK, Zaman M, Singh J. Br J Dermatol 2007; 157: 698–703.

Trichophyton rubrum was identified in 62 nails with onychomycosis both by cultures in Sabouraud's agar and by genotyping methods using DNA extracted directly from nails. *T. rubrum* culture was positive in 22.6% of samples, compared with 59.7% *T. rubrum* DNA detection using PCR assays.

Although several recent reports underline the high sensitivity and rapidity of polymerase chain reaction (PCR) assays, cultures remain the best and most cost-effective technique for laboratory identification of fungi.

MANAGEMENT STRATEGY

Different clinical patterns of nail infection result from the way in which fungi colonize the nail and the extent. In distal subungual onychomycosis (DSO), the most common type, fungi reach the nail from the hyponychium and colonize the nail bed, producing onycholysis and subungual hyperkeratosis. In proximal subungual onychomycosis (PSO), fungi penetrate the nail matrix via the proximal nail fold and colonize the deep portion of proximal nail plate, resulting in a subungual white patch located in the lunula area. In white superficial onychomycosis (WSO), fungi are localized on the nail plate surface and produce whitish opaque, friable areas on the nail plate. The type of nail invasion depends on both the causative fungus and host susceptibility.

The goals for antifungal therapy are mycological cure and a normal-looking nail. Clinical cure, which requires several months owing to slow nail growth, can be impossible to achieve because of the frequent association of onychomycosis with traumatic nail dystrophies, which are not influenced by treatment. Immediately after treatment with systemic agents, which usually lasts 3 months, it is common to observe a still abnormal nail: signs of a good response to treatment are the arrest of proximal progression of the onychomycosis and a proximal area of normal-appearing nail.

Treatment of onychomycosis depends on the clinical type of the onychomycosis, the number of affected nails, and the severity of involvement. A systemic treatment with either *terbinafine, itraconazole or fluconazole* is always required in PSO and in DSO involving the lunula region. WSO and DSO limited to the distal nail can be treated with a topical agent such as *amorolfine or ciclopirox. Combined systemic and topical treatment* increases the cure rate.

Terbinafine is an allylamine with fungicidal properties. Interactions of terbinafine with other drugs are extremely rare. Adverse effects may involve gastrointestinal function and the skin. Patients with known lupus erythematosus or photosensitivity are predisposed to drug-induced or drug-exacerbated disease. Terbinafine is administered at a dose of 250 mg daily; treatment duration is 6 weeks for fingernails and 12 weeks for toenails. Clinical trials have repeatedly demonstrated a higher efficacy of terbinafine compared to other antifungal treatments. A meta-analysis of 18 studies on terbinafine for onychomycosis showed a mycological cure rate of 76%.

Terbinafine persists in the nail for at least 30 weeks after the completion of treatment, and is effective also when administered as pulse regimen at a dose of 250 mg for 1 week per month every 2 or 3 months.

Itraconazole is a synthetic triazole with fungistatic activity and a broad spectrum of action. It is administered as pulse therapy at a dose of 400 mg daily for 1 week a month. Treatment duration is 6 weeks for fingernails and 12 weeks for toenails. The drug should be administered with a high-fat meal and/or an acidic beverage to improve its absorption. Agents that increase gastric alkalinity reduce absorption. With itraconazole the basis of some drug interactions is the inhibition/induction of the cytochrome P450-linked enzyme 3A4 (CYP 3A4). Adverse effects may involve gastrointestinal symptoms. The use of itraconazole may be associated with congestive heart failure. A meta-analysis of six studies on pulse itraconazole for onychomycosis showed a mycological cure rate of 63%.

Fluconazole is a bis-triazole broad-spectrum fungistatic drug with high oral bioavailability. It is administered as pulse treatment, with regimens ranging from 150 to 450 mg once a week for 6 (fingernails) to 9 (toenails) months. Fluconazole inhibits cytochrome P450-linked enzymes (CYP 3A4 and CYP 2C9), intensifying the action of many other drugs. Adverse effects may involve gastrointestinal symptoms. A meta-analysis of three studies on fluconazole for onychomycosis showed a mycological cure rate of 48%.

Two transungual delivery systems are currently marketed: *amorolfine* 5% nail lacquer (not approved in the USA) and *ciclopiroxolamine* 8% nail lacquer. Amorolfine is applied once a week, whereas ciclopiroxolamine is applied daily. Long-term (6–12 months) monotherapy has been used in the treatment of white superficial onychomycosis and distal subungual onychomycosis limited to the distal nail of a few digits. The clinical efficacy of monotherapy with nail lacquers ranges from 40 to 55%. Nail lacquers are also used in association with oral treatment to increase cure rates.

Systemic therapies can also be combined with *surgical or chemical debulking of the thickened* nail plate. *Photodynamic therapy* after application on the nails of a solution of ALA methyl ester in aqueous cream has been recently reported effective on *T. rubrum* onychomycosis, suggesting a future alternative to systemic antifungals.

Poor prognostic factors of onychomycosis include areas of nail involvement >50%, involvement of the lateral portion of the nail, subungual hyperkeratosis thicker than 2 mm, white/yellow or orange/brown streaks in the nail (including dermatophytoma), diffuse nail involvement that includes the matrix, and immunosuppression.

Recurrence (relapse or reinfection) of onychomycosis is not uncommon, with reported rates ranging from 10% to 53%.

FIRST-LINE THERAPIES

▶ Systemic terbinafine 250 mg/die (for 6 weeks for fingernails and 12 weeks for toenails)

Onychomycosis: diagnosis and definition of cure. Scher RK, Tavakkol A, Sigurgeirsson B, Hay RJ, Joseph WS, Tosti A, et al. J Am Acad Dermatol 2007; 56: 939–44.

This article points out the multiple problems clinicians have when dealing with papers about the treatment of onychomycosis and promotes guidelines for the correct management of this condition, including criteria for the diagnosis of dermatophyte onychomycosis, a list of poor prognostic factors, criteria for assessing cure, and risk of relapses.

Cumulative meta-analysis of systemic antifungal agents for the treatment of onychomycosis. Gupta AK, Ryder JE, Johnson AM. Br J Dermatol 2004; 150: 537–44.

A cumulative meta-analysis of the randomized controlled trials on antimycotic agents for onychomycosis was performed to determine cure rates of the different antifungals. Mycological cure rates were terbinafine 78 ± 6% to 76 ± 3%; itraconazole pulse 75 ± 10% to 63 ± 7%; fluconazole 53 ± 6% to 48 ± 5%. Terbinafine seems therefore the most effective antifungal for onychomycosis and has the most enduring efficacy over the years.

The successful treatment of *Trichophyton rubrum* nail bed (distal subungual) onychomycosis with intermittent pulse-dosed terbinafine. Zaias N, Rebell G. Arch Dermatol 2004; 140: 691–5.

This study evaluated the efficacy of intermittent administration of oral terbinafine (250 mg/day for 7 consecutive days every 2–4 months) in distal subungual onychomycosis and showed that terbinafine is effective also when administered as pulse regimen at a dose of 250 mg for 1 week a month every 2 or 3 months.

SECOND-LINE THERAPIES

▶ Systemic itraconazole 400 mg/week (for 6 weeks for fingernails and 12 weeks for toenails)
▶ Systemic fluconazole 300–450 mg/week (for 6 months for fingernails and 9 months for toenails)

Evidence Levels: **A** Double-blind study **B** Clinical trial ≥ 20 subjects **C** Clinical trial < 20 subjects **D** Series ≥ 5 subjects **E** Anecdotal case reports

Itraconazole for the treatment of onychomycosis. Gupta AK, De Doncker P, Scher RK, Haneke E, Daniel CR 3rd, André J, et al. Int J Dermatol 1998; 37: 303–8.

Both continuous and pulsed therapy regimens are safe, with few adverse effects. Compared to continuous therapy, the pulse regimen has an improved adverse-effects profile, is more cost-effective, and is preferred by many patients.

A double-blind, randomized study to compare the efficacy and safety of terbinafine (Lamisil) with fluconazole (Diflucan) in the treatment of onychomycosis. Havu V, Heikkilä H, Kuokkanen K, Nuutinen M, Rantanen T, Saari S, et al. Br J Dermatol 2000; 142: 97–102.

Terbinafine 250 mg daily for 12 weeks is significantly more effective in the treatment of onychomycosis than fluconazole 150 mg once weekly for either 12 or 24 weeks.

The safety of oral antifungal treatments for superficial dermatophytosis and onychomycosis: a meta-analysis. Chang CH, Young-Xu Y, Kurth T, Orav JE, Chan AK. Am J Med 2007; 120: 791–8.

All studies published before 31 December 2005 were reviewed to assess the risks of treatment withdrawal and the incidence of liver adverse effects with antifungals in onychomycosis. Treatment discontinuation due to adverse events was 3.44% for continuous terbinafine, 2.58% for pulse itraconazole, and 5.76% for intermittent fluconazole 300–450 mg/week. The risk of asymptomatic elevation of serum transaminase not requiring treatment discontinuation was less than 2.0% for all treatment regimens evaluated.

THIRD-LINE THERAPIES

▶ Systemic terbinafine 250 mg/die (for 6 weeks for fingernails and 12 weeks for toenails) and topical amorolfine nail lacquer once a week for 6–12 months
▶ Systemic terbinafine 250 mg/die (for 6 weeks for fingernails and 12 weeks for toenails) associated with periodic nail debridement
▶ Photodynamic therapy

A multicentre, randomized, controlled study of the efficacy, safety and cost-effectiveness of a combination therapy with amorolfine nail lacquer and oral terbinafine compared with oral terbinafine alone for the treatment of onychomycosis with matrix involvement. Baran R, Sigurgeirsson B, de Berker D, Kaufmann R, Lecha M, Faergemann J, et al. Br J Dermatol 2007; 157: 149–57.

This randomized study evaluated clinical cure and negative mycology at 18 months in patients with dermatophytic toenail onychomycosis and matrix involvement undergoing treatment with either a combination of amorolfine 5% nail lacquer once weekly for 12 months plus terbinafine 250 mg once daily for 3 months, or terbinafine alone once daily for 3 months. The results showed a significantly higher success rate in patients treated with the combination (59.2% vs 45.0%).

Treatment of toenail onychomycosis with oral terbinafine plus aggressive debridement: IRON-CLAD, a large, randomized, open-label, multicenter trial. Jennings MB, Pollak R, Harkless LB, Kianifard F, Tavakkol A. J Am Podiatr Med Assoc 2006; 96: 465–73.

This study evaluated the efficacy of oral terbinafine (250 mg/day for 12 weeks) with and without debridement of the affected nail. Mycological and clinical cure rates at week 48 were higher in the terbinafine plus debridement group than in the terbinafine-only group, although significance was reached only for clinical cure (59.8% vs 51.4%).

Successful treatment of toenail onychomycosis with photodynamic therapy. Watanabe D, Kawamura C, Masuda Y, Akita Y, Tamada Y, Matsumoto Y, et al. Arch Dermatol 2008; 144: 19–21.

Available information indicates that *Trichophyton rubrum* is a possible target of photodynamic therapy as almost 50% of the fungal growth could be inhibited in vitro. This article reports complete cure of dermatophyte onychomycosis of the great toenails in two patients, which were irradiated seven and six times, respectively, with pulsed laser light at a wavelength of 630 nm at 100 J/cm^2 using an excimer-dye laser, after the application of a 20% solution of ALA methyl ester in aqueous cream.

Tinea versicolor
(pityriasis versicolor)

Aditya K Gupta, Elizabeth A Cooper

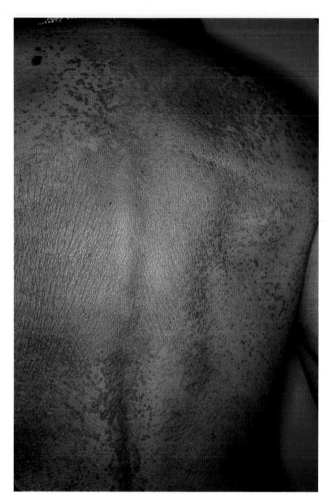

Pityriasis (tinea) versicolor (PV) has a worldwide distribution, though the prevalence is higher in tropical climates than in temperate ones (30–40% versus 1–4%, respectively). PV is caused by the lipophilic yeast species *Malassezia*. *Malassezia* organisms are a normal part of human commensal skin flora, and PV results when they are converted from the yeast phase to a mycelial phase which is able to infect the stratum corneum, producing the characteristic hypo- or hyperpigmented lesions.

Infection is associated with sebaceous gland activity, hence infection is most often seen in adults and post-pubescent adolescents, rarely in prepubescent children. An equal prevalence between the sexes has been noted. Predisposing factors include high temperature and humidity, malnutrition, the use of oral contraceptives, hyperhidrosis, genetic susceptibility, increased plasma cortisol levels, and immunodeficiency.

Initially only two species under the genus name *Pityrosporum* were described. Genetic research in the 1990s confirmed at least seven species of *Malassezia*, and more have been discovered since. The most common species contributing to PV lesions are *M. globosa* (50–60%), *M. sympodialis* (3–59%), *M. furfur*, and *M. slooffiae* (1–10% each). It is not currently known whether the clinical pattern of infection or antifungal susceptibility vary between the different infecting species.

MANAGEMENT STRATEGY

Topical treatment is the first-line therapy in most cases. *Topical azoles* formulated as gels, creams, solutions, or shampoos (ketoconazole, fluconazole, bifonazole, clotrimazole, miconazole, etc.) have demonstrated efficacy for PV. The allylamine *terbinafine* has several topical formulations (solution, cream, gel, or spray) that have been used effectively, as have formulations of the benzylamine *butenafine*. *Topical ciclopirox* provides both antifungal and anti-inflammatory activity against *Malassezia*.

Systemic antifungal therapies may be warranted in severe cases, or cases with widespread body involvement, patients with recurrent disease, or those who are immunocompromised. Patients may also prefer a short-duration oral therapy to frequent application of a topical agent.

Second-line therapy for cases refractive to topical therapy may be treated with oral antifungals. *Ketoconazole, itraconazole,* and *fluconazole* show high efficacy in the literature. However, in contrast to topical terbinafine, oral terbinafine is not effective, and nor is griseofulvin.

Treatment does not vary with hyperpigmented versus hypopigmented disease. Although fungal organisms may be eradicated after 2–4 weeks of therapy, it may take significantly longer before the skin's normal pigmentation is restored, particularly with hypopigmented lesions.[5]

Relapse of PV is common owing to endogenous host factors: recurrence rates have been reported as high as 60–90% 2 years after treatment. Both ketoconazole (a single 400 mg dose or 200 mg daily for 3 days once monthly) and itraconazole (a single 400 mg dose once monthly for 6 months) have been used in prophylactic regimens for PV, though ketoconazole is not used because of its potential for hepatotoxicity.

SPECIFIC INVESTIGATIONS

> ► Direct microscopy on KOH specimens
> ► Wood's light

Malassezia organisms should be identified by skin scrapings for definitive diagnosis, and are easily identified where microscopic examination of skin scrapings reveals fungal hyphae in a typical 'spaghetti and meatball' pattern. PV lesions fluoresce yellow/green or gold under Wood's light; however, the examination is positive in only one-third of all PV cases, most likely when the causative organism is *M. furfur*.

FIRST-LINE THERAPY

Topical antifungals	
► Ketoconazole	A
► Bifonazole	A
► Terbinafine	A
► Clotrimazole	A
► Econazole	A
► Oxiconazole	A
► Ciclopirox	A
► Tioconazole	B

Evidence Levels: **A** Double-blind study   **B** Clinical trial ≥ 20 subjects   **C** Clinical trial < 20 subjects   **D** Series ≥ 5 subjects   **E** Anecdotal case reports

▶ Butenafine	A
▶ Selenium sulfide 2.5%	A
▶ Fluconazole shampoo	A
▶ Zinc pyrithione shampoo	B

Pityriasis versicolor: a review of pharmacological treatment options. Gupta AK, Kogan N, Batra R. Exp Opin Pharmacother 2005; 6: 165–78.

A thorough summary of published information regarding the use of topical therapies. Azole topical agents have shown good mycological cure, clinical cure, and complete cure in many double-blind randomized clinical trials, as have the nonspecific topical agents (zinc pyrithione shampoo, selenium sulfide, etc.) and terbinafine.

Flutrimazole shampoo 1% versus ketoconazole shampoo 2% in the treatment of pityriasis versicolor. A randomized double-blind comparative trial. Rigopoulos D, Gregoriou S, Kontochristopoulos G, Ifantides A, Katsambas A. Mycoses 2007; 50: 193–5.

Randomized double-blind assignment to either flutrimazole or ketoconazole shampoo, applied to head and body, left on for 5 minutes before rinsing; application repeated daily for 14 days. No significant difference was found in clinical response between treatments at day 28 (flutrimazole: 86.25; ketoconazole: 88.5%) or clinical/mycological cure (flutrimazole: 75.9%; ketoconazole: 80.8%).

Clinical efficacy and tolerability of terbinafine in patients with pityriasis versicolor. Aste N, Pau M, Pinna AL, Colombo MD, Biggio P. Mycoses 1991; 34: 353–7.

A randomized, single-blind trial of 1% terbinafine cream versus 1% bifonazole cream, applied twice daily for 2–4 weeks, with follow-up 2 weeks after the end of treatment. At the end of the study, 100% of terbinafine patients and 95% of bifonazole patients had mycological and clinical cure.

Double-blind comparison of 2% ketoconazole cream and placebo in the treatment of tinea versicolor. Savin RC, Horwitz SN. J Am Acad Dermatol 1986; 15: 500–3.

A randomized, double-blind trial of 2% ketoconazole cream versus vehicle cream, once daily for approximately 2 weeks, with follow-up at 8 weeks post treatment: 98% of ketoconazole patients responded clinically to therapy versus 28% of placebo patients; 37/43 ketoconazole responders continued to the end of follow-up, and all patients remained cured.

Butenafine: an update of its use in superficial mycoses. Gupta AK. Skin Ther Lett 2002; 7: 1–2, 5.

Butenafine is a safe and effective synthetic benzylamine antifungal agent, applied once daily for 2 weeks. The effectiveness lasted 4 weeks after the termination of therapy, which suggests retention of the drug in the skin.

SECOND-LINE THERAPY

Oral antifungals	
▶ Itraconazole	A
▶ Ketoconazole	A
▶ Fluconazole	A
Oral prophylaxis	
▶ Itraconazole	A

Comparison of a single 400 mg dose versus a 7-day 200 mg daily dose of itraconazole in the treatment of tinea versicolor. Kose O, Bulent Tastan H, Riza Gur A, Kurumlu Z. J Dermatol Treat 2002; 13: 77–9.

A randomized open-label trial of a single dose of itraconazole 400 mg versus itraconazole 200 mg daily for 7 days. Mycological cure rates at week 6 for both regimens were greater than 80%, and clinical cure was 70–80% for the two regimens. There was no significant difference between regimens in outcomes.

Fluconazole vs. itraconazole in the treatment of tinea versicolor. Montero-Gei F, Robles ME, Suchil P. Int J Dermatol 1999; 38: 601–3.

A randomized open-label trial of a single dose of fluconazole 450 mg, two 300 mg doses of fluconazole given 1 week apart, and itraconazole 200 mg daily for 7 days. Mycological cure rates seen at day 30 were 70%, 97%, and 80%, respectively (a significant difference between the two fluconazole doses), dropping to 55%, 77%, and 78% at day 60. Clinical cure rates at day 60 were 52%, 70%, and 74%, respectively.

Single-dose fluconazole versus itraconazole in pityriasis versicolor. Partap R, Kaur I, Chakrabarti A, Kumar B. Dermatology 2004; 208: 55–9.

A randomized trial of patients with 15% or more skin surface area involvement, comparing single doses of fluconazole (400 mg) and itraconazole (400 mg). At week 8, fluconazole showed a greater proportion of patients with reduced scaling and no residual pigmentation compared to itraconazole (65% and 20% vs 35% and 5%, respectively), though the difference did not reach statistical significance. Mycological cure for fluconazole was also higher than for itraconazole (65% vs 20%). Relapse was seen in both groups (fluconazole 35%, itraconazole 60%).

Fluconazole versus ketoconazole in the treatment of tinea versicolor. Farschian M, Yaghoobi R, Samadi K. J Dermatol Treat 2002; 13: 73–6.

A randomized, double-blind clinical trial of fluconazole 300 mg once weekly for 2 weeks vs 400 mg ketoconazole once weekly for 2 weeks (at least 25% of trunk affected). Mycological cure rates for fluconazole and ketoconazole at week 8 were 90% and 88%, respectively, reducing to 82% and 78%, respectively, at week 12.

Comparison between fluconazole and ketoconazole effectivity in the treatment of pityriasis versicolor. Yazdanpanah MJ, Azizi H, Suizi B. Mycoses 2007; 50: 311–13.

A randomized trial of single-dose ketoconazole 400 mg versus a fluconazole 300 mg dose once weekly for 2 weeks in patients with >25% body area affected. Clinical improvement rates 30 days after the start of treatment in the two groups were 87.9% and 81.5%, respectively (p=0.37).

Efficacy of itraconazole in the prophylactic treatment of pityriasis (tinea) versicolor. Faergemann J, Gupta AK, Al Mofadi A, Abanami A, Shareaah AA, Marynissen G. Arch Dermatol 2002; 138: 69–73.

Patients achieving mycological cure after open treatment with itraconazole 200 mg once daily for 7 days entered a double-blind, placebo-controlled trial of itraconazole prophylaxis (itraconazole or placebo: 200 mg twice daily

1 day per month for 6 consecutive months). At the end of prophylaxis, 88% of itraconazole patients remained mycologically negative, compared to only 57% of placebo-treated patients (p<0.001).

THIRD-LINE THERAPY

▶ Naftifine (topical allylamine)	B
▶ Pramiconazole (oral triazole)	C
▶ Isotretinoin (oral retinoid)	E

Naftifine solution (1%) in the treatment of pityriasis versicolor in Zambia. Hira SK, Abraham MS, Mwinga A, Kamanga J, Schmidt C. Mycosen 1986; 29: 378–81.

An open clinical trial using 1% naftifine solution for either 3 days or 6 days, applying nightly after a bath, with a follow-up period of 6 weeks. In the 3-day treatment 43.3% had clinical cure and 30% had mycological cure. In the 6-day group, clinical cure was 90.3% and mycological cure was 82.3%. A small number of patients experienced dryness or mild irritation during treatment, but did not require interruption of treatment.

The efficacy of oral treatment with pramiconazole in pityriasis versicolor: a phase IIa trial. Faergemann J, Ausma J, Vandeplassche L, Borgers M. Br J Dermatol 2007; 156: 1362–402.

A new oral triazole showing promise in *Malassezia* infection. A preliminary phase II trial in 19 subjects showed that a single dose of 200 mg pramiconazole given over 3 consecutive days provided 100% mycological cure at day 30. No serious adverse events occurred, but nine patients reported adverse events (3/9 being headache), with a majority being mild and not related to pramiconazole.

Not currently approved or marketed. As more data accumulates, the level of evidence may alter.

Tinea versicolor clearance with oral isotretinoin therapy. Bartell H, Ransdell BL, Ali A. J Drugs Dermatol 2006; 5: 74–5.

A single case report of a 14-year-old boy presenting with acne vulgaris recalcitrant to oral antibiotic therapy, who also presented with PV infection on the upper back and shoulders. One month after starting oral isotretinoin 40 mg twice daily, the PV lesions had completely resolved. Resolution attributed to the sebum-altering properties of isotretinoin.

The use of isotretinoin cannot be advocated because of the potential for serious side effects, particularly in females. However, where concomitant PV and acne requiring isotretinoin are presented, no additional medication may be required for the PV infection.

Toxic epidermal necrolysis and Stevens–Johnson syndrome

Nicholas M Craven, Daniel Creamer

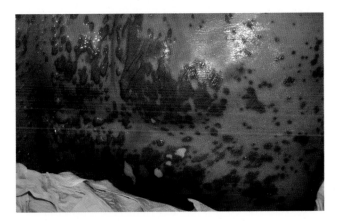

Toxic epidermal necrolysis (TEN) and Stevens–Johnson syndrome (SJS) form a spectrum of rare, potentially life-threatening conditions manifesting widespread erythematous macules or atypical target lesions and severe erosions of mucous membranes. Confluence of cutaneous lesions leads to epidermal loss, which by definition involves less than 10% of total body surface area (BSA) in SJS, 10–30% in overlap cases, and more than 30% in TEN. Complications develop similar to those seen after burns. In most cases TEN and SJS can be attributed to a drug reaction.

MANAGEMENT STRATEGY

The causative drug should be identified and discontinued. In general, drugs introduced in the 4 weeks before the onset of symptoms are usually responsible. If in doubt, all drugs should be stopped if possible.

The patient should be managed in a burns unit or appropriate high-dependency unit. Supportive therapy is directed at fluid replacement, maintaining a warm environment to reduce heat loss, topical antiseptic preparations, hydrocolloid dressings or skin substitutes to reduce colonization of the skin, and regular monitoring for sepsis. *Fluid replacement* requirements depend on the extent of involvement of the skin and mucous membranes, and may be 5–7 L in the first 24 hours. Peripheral lines are preferable to central lines, which increase the risk of sepsis. *Nutritional support* may require fine-bore nasogastric tube feeding until the oral mucosa has healed. All lines should be checked daily for signs of infection, changed at least every 3 days, and the tips of all discarded lines and catheters sent for culture. *Antibiotics* should not be given routinely as this may promote resistance. If signs of sepsis develop (rising or falling temperature, rigors, hypotension, fall in urine output, deterioration of respiratory status, diabetic control, or level of consciousness),

initial antibiotic therapy can be guided by the results of swabs taken from the skin and mucous membranes. Necrolytic epidermis should be removed gently once it starts to fold over to reduce the risk of infection.

Ophthalmologic review should be obtained as soon as possible after diagnosis to minimize the risk of conjunctival scarring and blindness. Regular instillation of antiseptic eye drops and separation of newly forming synechiae are required. Oral and nasal debris should be cleaned regularly and an antiseptic mouthwash used several times a day.

Analgesia with opiates is often required, and care should be taken to monitor for respiratory depression. Respiratory failure may develop, requiring ventilation in an intensive care facility.

The use of *systemic corticosteroids* in the management of TEN and SJS remains controversial (see below). Several reports suggest that the use of corticosteroids increases morbidity and mortality, usually by increasing the risk of sepsis. Conversely, a number of case reports and short studies advocate the use of high-dose corticosteroids in the early stages of the evolution of these conditions. It is therefore possible that high-dose corticosteroids may prove beneficial in aborting further epithelial loss in patients with evolving SJS/TEN, but this has not yet been tested in a randomized controlled trial. Nevertheless, it is generally accepted that continuing administration of corticosteroids is counterproductive once extensive skin loss has occurred.

Several other potential disease-modifying treatments (*intravenous immunoglobulin* – IVIG, *ciclosporin, pentoxifylline,* plasmapheresis, cyclophosphamide) have been reported in small numbers of patients, but there is currently no strong evidence base for recommending any specific intervention other than supportive care.

Survivors of TEN and SJS and their close relatives should *avoid exposure to the culprit drug and related* compounds.

SPECIFIC INVESTIGATIONS

► Histology
► Biochemical and hematological monitoring

Established TEN can usually be diagnosed clinically. Biopsy and immunofluorescence of an affected area of skin can exclude conditions such as staphylococcal scalded skin syndrome and paraneoplastic pemphigus. Histologic examination of the roof of a fresh blister (even on frozen section specimens) may be adequate to distinguish TEN from staphylococcal scalded skin syndrome.

Supportive care involves regular monitoring of full blood count, urea, creatinine, electrolytes (including calcium and phosphate), transaminases, glucose, blood gases, swabs from infected areas and flexures, blood and urine cultures, and urine output.

Pulmonary complications in toxic epidermal necrolysis: a prospective clinical study. Lebargy F, Wolkenstein P, Gisselbrecht M, Lange F, Fleury-Feith J, Delclaux C, et al. Intens Care Med 1997; 23: 1237–44.

Dyspnea, bronchial hypersecretion, and marked hypoxemia in the presence of a normal chest radiograph suggests bronchial injury from TEN, indicating a likely need for ventilation and a poor prognosis.

Incidence of Stevens–Johnson syndrome and toxic epidermal necrolysis in patients with the acquired immunodeficiency syndrome in Germany. Rzany B, Mockenhaupt M, Stocker U, Hamouda O, Schöpf E. Arch Dermatol 1993; 129: 1059.

Patients with AIDS have an incidence of SJS/TEN of around 1:1000 per year, compared to an incidence in the total population of 1.2–1.4 per 10^6 per annum.

HIV testing should be considered for high-risk patients presenting with TEN/SJS.

Medication use and the risk of Stevens–Johnson syndrome or toxic epidermal necrolysis. Roujeau J-C, Kelly JP, Naldi L, Rzany B, Stern RS, Anderson T, et al. N Engl J Med 1995; 333: 1600–7.

The main culprit drugs are sulfonamides, anticonvulsants, oxicam non-steroidal anti-inflammatory drugs (NSAIDs), allopurinol, chlormezanone, and corticosteroids, but the excess risk associated with the use of these drugs is less than five cases per million users per week.

SCORTEN: a severity-of-illness score for toxic epidermal necrolysis. Bastuji-Garin S, Fouchard N, Bertocchi M, Roujeau JC, Revuz J, Wolkenstein P. J Invest Dermatol 2000; 115: 149–53.

Assessment of seven clinical parameters within the first 24 hours of admission (age over 40; history of malignancy; tachycardia >120 bpm; skin loss >10%; urea >10 mmol/L; glucose >14 mmol/L; bicarbonate <20 mmol/L) can be used to predict risk of mortality (score 0 or 1: 3% risk of death; 2: 12%; 3: 35%; 4: 58%; 5+: 90%).

FIRST-LINE THERAPIES

▶ Supportive measures	E
▶ Withdrawal of culprit drug	E
▶ Analgesia	E
▶ Bioengineered skin substitute	C

Toxic epidermal necrolysis: current evidence, practical management and future directions. Chave TA, Mortimer NJ, Sladden MJ, Hall AP, Hutchinson PE. Br J Dermatol 2005; 153: 241–53.

An extensive review article covering all aspects of TEN. Advice on management issues is based on available evidence and covers all aspects of supportive care, in addition to specific interventions such as IVIG, ciclosporin and corticosteroids.

Toxic epidermal necrolysis and Stevens–Johnson syndrome: does early withdrawal of causative drugs decrease the risk of death? Garcia-Doval I, LeCleach L, Bocquet H, Otero XL, Roujeau JC. Arch Dermatol 2000; 136: 323–7.

Early discontinuation of the causative drug improved prognosis in this study of 113 patients.

A multicenter review of toxic epidermal necrolysis treated in U.S. burn centers at the end of the twentieth century. Palmieri TL, Greenhalgh DG, Saffle JR, Spence RJ, Peck MD, Jeng JC, et al. J Burn Care Rehab 2002; 23: 87–96.

A retrospective multicentre study of 199 patients admitted with TEN to 15 burn centers from 1995 to 2000. Overall mortality was 32%, increasing to 51% for patients transferred to a burn center more than 1 week after the onset of TEN.

There are several studies (but no controlled trials) showing benefit from early transfer of TEN patients to specialist units.

Toxic epidermal necrolysis: use of Biobrane for skin coverage reduces pain, improves mobilization and decreases infection in elderly patients. Boorboor P, Vogt PM, Bechara FG, Alkandari Q, Aust M, Gohritz A, et al. Burns 2008; 34: 487–92.

A comparative study of two dressing regimens in 14 TEN patients managed in a burns unit. In eight patients denuded skin was covered with paraffin gauze, which was changed daily; in six patients the exposed dermis was covered with Biobrane, a biosynthetic wound dressing, which was left undisturbed following application. Assessment of a range of clinical parameters demonstrated a significant reduction in pain and significantly enhanced mobility in the Biobrane group compared to the control group. Speed of re-epithelialization, duration of hospital stay, and mortality were not significantly different in the two groups.

SECOND-LINE THERAPIES

▶ Ciclosporin	C
▶ Systemic corticosteroids	C
▶ Intravenous immunoglobulin	C

Treatment of toxic epidermal necrolysis with ciclosporin A. Arévalo JM, Lorente JA, González-Herrada C, Jiménez-Reyes J. J Trauma 2000; 48: 473–8.

An improved outcome is reported in 11 consecutive patients with TEN treated with ciclosporin 3 mg/kg daily, compared to six historical controls treated with cyclophosphamide and corticosteroids. Both groups were of comparable age, with similar extent of skin loss and delay between onset of TEN and admission. Patients treated with ciclosporin had more rapid re-epithelialization, were less likely to suffer multiorgan failure, and had a lower mortality (0 of 11 vs three of six).

Toxic epidermal necrolysis treated with cyclosporin. Hewitt J, Ormerod AD. Clin Exp Dermatol 1992; 17: 264–5.

Two cases of TEN improving on ciclosporin. One followed an upper respiratory tract infection treated with Dequacaine lozenges and pholcodeine linctus, and was treated with 3.6 mg/kg daily (route not stated). The other followed amoxicillin treatment for an upper respiratory tract infection (treated with 3 mg/kg daily orally), and recurred following ciprofloxacin treatment for a urinary infection, again resolving on ciclosporin 5 mg/kg.

There are now several reports of the successful use of ciclosporin in TEN. Because most of the hazards of this drug are associated with long-term use it seems logical to use high doses in TEN, as treatment will only be needed for a few days.

Improved burn center survival of patients with toxic epidermal necrolysis managed without corticosteroids. Halebian PH, Corder VJ, Madden MR, Finklestein JL, Shires GT. Ann Surg 1986; 204: 503–12.

Fifteen consecutive TEN patients treated in a burns unit with supportive measures had an overall mortality rate of only 33%, compared to 66% in the historical control group treated with corticosteroids. Eleven of the 'non-corticosteroid' group had nevertheless been started on corticosteroids by the referring institutions prior to arrival at the burns unit.

Evidence Levels: A Double-blind study   B Clinical trial ≥ 20 subjects   C Clinical trial < 20 subjects   D Series ≥ 5 subjects   E Anecdotal case reports

Erythema multiforme in children. Response to treatment with systemic corticosteroids. Rasmussen JE. Br J Dermatol 1976; 95: 181–6.

A retrospective study comparing the progress of 17 children with SJS treated with prednisolone 40–80 mg/m² with 15 given supportive care only. Both groups were similar in terms of age, sex, and extent of cutaneous and mucosal involvement. The corticosteroid group had more complications (mostly infections) and a longer mean duration of hospitalization (21 vs 13 days) than the non-corticosteroid group. No patients died.

It is likely that a number of these cases recorded as having iris lesions would now be classified as bullous erythema multiforme rather than SJS.

Characteristics of toxic epidermal necrolysis in patients undergoing long-term glucocorticoid therapy. Guibal F, Bastuji-Garin S, Chosidow O, Saiag P, Revuz J, Roujeau JC. Arch Dermatol 1995; 131: 669–72.

TEN can occur in patients already taking high-dose corticosteroids. The onset of TEN is delayed following exposure to the culprit drug, but its progression is not halted.

High-dose systemic corticosteroids can arrest recurrences of severe mucocutaneous erythema multiforme. Martinez AE, Atherton DJ. Pediatr Dermatol 2000; 17: 87–90.

Two children, one with SJS and one with bullous erythema multiforme (typical target lesions), were subject to recurrent attacks, which appeared to be abated by intravenous methylprednisolone (20 mg/kg daily for 3 days), commenced within 24–48 hours of the onset of skin signs.

Corticosteroid therapy in an additional 13 cases of Stevens-Johnson syndrome: a total series of 67 cases. Tripathi A, Ditto AM, Grammer LC, Greenberger PA, McGrath KG, Zeiss CR, et al. Allergy Asthma Proc 2000; 21: 101–5.

Latest in a series of reports from this group. Thirteen patients with SJS were treated with intravenous methylprednisolone 160–240 mg daily on admission to the unit (1–14 days after onset of symptoms). One patient died from unrelated causes; all others survived. This extends to 67 the authors' series of patients with SJS treated with corticosteroids.

Clinical descriptions are incomplete, but surprisingly few of the patients had bullous lesions. It is possible that a significant number of these 67 patients would be classified by dermatologists as having hypersensitivity syndrome rather than SJS.

Effects of treatments on the mortality of Stevens–Johnson syndrome and toxic epidermal necrolysis: A retrospective study on patients included in the prospective EuroSCAR study. Schneck J, Fagot JP, Sekula P, Sassolas B, Roujeau JC, Mockenhaupt M. J Am Acad Dermatol 2008; 58: 33–40.

A large multicenter retrospective study of treatment of 281 patients with TEN enrolled in EuroSCAR (a case–control study of risk factors for severe cutaneous adverse reactions) showed no significant effect on mortality with the administration of IVIG, but a trend for beneficial effect of corticosteroids considered to be worthy of further exploration.

Inhibition of toxic epidermal necrolysis by blockade of CD95 with human intravenous immunoglobulin. Viard I, Wehrli P, Bullani R, Schneider P, Holler N, Salomon D, et al. Science 1998; 282: 490–3.

A series of 10 consecutive patients with TEN treated with IVIG at 0.2–0.75 g/kg daily for 4 days. Progression of skin disease stopped within 24–48 hours, and all patients survived.

Intravenous immunoglobulin treatment for Stevens–Johnson syndrome and toxic epidermal necrolysis: a prospective noncomparative study showing no benefit on mortality or progression. Bachot N, Revuz J, Roujeau JC. Arch Dermatol 2003; 139: 33–6.

A prospective open trial of 34 patients with SJS, TEN, or overlap treated with IVIG 2 g/kg over 2 days; 11 deaths occurred (32%; mostly elderly patients with impaired renal function), compared to a predicted mortality of 8.2 deaths based on SCORTEN data. No measurable effect was observed on the progression of epidermal detachment or on the speed of re-epithelialization.

Treatment of toxic epidermal necrolysis with high-dose intravenous immunoglobulins: multicenter retrospective analysis of 48 consecutive cases. Prins C, Kerdel FA, Padilla RS, Hunziker T, Chimenti S, Viard I, et al. Arch Dermatol 2003; 139: 26–32.

A multicenter retrospective analysis of 48 consecutive TEN patients treated with IVIG, mean dose 2.7 g/kg. Treatment was associated with a rapid cessation of skin and mucosal detachment in 43 patients (90%) and survival in 42 (88%). It was noted that patients who responded to IVIG had received treatment earlier in the course of disease and had higher doses of IVIG. The authors therefore recommend early treatment with IVIG at a total dose of 3 g/kg over 3 consecutive days (1 g/kg daily for 3 days).

Intravenous immunoglobulin does not improve outcome in toxic epidermal necrolysis. Shortt R, Gomez M, Mittman N, Cartotto R. J Burn Care Rehab 2004; 25: 246–55.

Outcome data for 16 patients with TEN treated with IVIG were compared with those of 16 historical controls treated without IVIG. The mortality rate of the IVIG group was 25%, compared to 38% in the control group (not statistically significant). There were no significant differences between the groups with respect to the duration of hospital stay, duration of ventilation, the incidence of sepsis, or time to healing. There was a trend towards less severe wound progression in patients who received IVIG.

As with all data on treatment of TEN, interpretation of the available literature is limited by lack of uniformity in the treatment regimens used, by the lack of adequate control data, and/or by the relatively small size of the studies.

THIRD-LINE THERAPIES

| ▶ Plasmapheresis | C |
| ▶ Pentoxifylline | E |

Plasmapheresis as an adjunct treatment in toxic epidermal necrolysis. Egan CA, Grant WJ, Morris SE, Saffle JR, Zone JJ. J Am Acad Dermatol 1999; 40: 458–61.

A retrospective study of 16 patients, six of whom were selected for plasmapheresis (one to four treatments) based on rapid progression of disease in the 24 hours after admission. None of the patients treated with plasmapheresis died, whereas four of the other 10 patients did.

Lack of significant treatment effect of plasma exchange in the treatment of drug-induced toxic epidermal necrolysis? Furubacke A, Berlin G, Anderson C, Sjoberg F. Intens Care Med 1999; 25: 1307–10.

A comparison of outcome in eight patients with TEN affecting 12–100% body surface area who received one to eight plasma exchange treatments with the results from two other centers that used almost identical treatment protocols but without plasma exchange showed no benefit in terms of mortality (12.5%), time to re-epithelialization, or duration of stay in the burns intensive care unit. The authors concluded that the results did not support the use of plasma exchange in the treatment of TEN.

Plasma exchange in patients with toxic epidermal necrolysis. Bamichas G, Natse T, Christidou F, Stangou M, Karagianni A, Koukourikos S, et al. Ther Apher 2002; 6: 225–8.

A retrospective study of 13 patients with TEN involving 17–100% body surface area treated with two to five sessions of plasmapheresis either daily or on alternate days. Three patients died (mortality rate 23%).

Pentoxifylline in toxic epidermal necrolysis and Stevens–Johnson syndrome. Sanclemente G, De La Roche CA, Escobar CE, Falabella R. Int J Dermatol 1999; 38: 878–9.

Two children with SJS and SJS/TEN overlap were treated with intravenous pentoxifylline 12 mg/kg daily. In both cases skin loss stopped on commencement of treatment, and in one of the children the skin deteriorated when pentoxifylline was temporarily discontinued.

Randomised comparison of thalidomide versus placebo in toxic epidermal necrolysis. Wolkenstein P, Latarjet J, Roujeau J-C, Duguet C, Boudeau S, Vaillant L, et al. Lancet 1998; 352: 1586–9.

Patients with TEN were randomized to either a 5-day course of thalidomide 400 mg daily (12 patients) or placebo (10 patients). The study was stopped early because of excess mortality in the treatment arm.

Transient acantholytic dermatosis

(Grover's disease)

Stuart C Murray, Susan M Burge

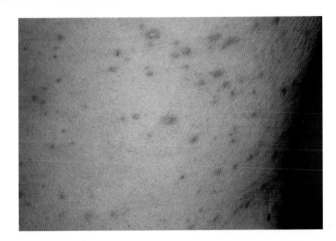

Grover's disease is an acquired pruritic, papulovesicular eruption characterized histologically by focal acantholytic dyskeratosis. It is predominantly self-limiting. It is more common in middle-aged and elderly people, especially men, and involves mainly the trunk. The evolution is acute or chronic. The etiology is unknown, but excessive UV exposure, heat, sweating, and ionizing radiation are linked to the disease.

MANAGEMENT STRATEGY

Grover's disease is an uncommon disorder characterized by discrete erythematous, edematous papulovesicles or keratotic papules. The duration of the eruption may be weeks to months and it may be persistent or recurrent. Pruritus of variable intensity is experienced by most patients and may be out of proportion to the clinical signs. Constitutional symptoms are usually absent.

Treatment is difficult. There have been no large clinical trials and reports are based on small numbers.

Patients should be advised to *avoid excessive sun exposure, strenuous exercise, heat, and occlusive fabrics*. In mild cases, simple antipruritic measures such as *avoidance of soap, simple emollients, and soothing baths with bath oils or colloidal oatmeal* may be of benefit. *Wet compresses with zinc oxide, calamine, or topical corticosteroids* may help to relieve the itching. *Antihistamines* may aid in the control of pruritus, but do not prevent the development of new lesions.

Topical calcipotriol (ointment) twice daily 50 μg/g may be helpful after 3–4 weeks of treatment. *Topical vitamin A acid (retinoic acid)* is of limited use owing to skin irritation.

Systemic therapy may be indicated in more extensive and persistent disease. *Oral vitamin A* has been recommended in the past. The aromatic retinoid *acitretin* been used successfully in doses of 0.5 mg/kg daily. *Isotretinoin* 40 mg daily has been used for periods ranging from 2 to 12 weeks. It may be administered on a reducing regimen if the initial response is rapid,

with a maintenance dose of 10 mg daily. Side effects include dry skin, cheilitis, teratogenicity, and elevation of cholesterol and triglycerides.

Systemic corticosteroids have been used to suppress inflammation and pruritus, but relapses frequently occur on drug withdrawal.

Psoralen with UVA (PUVA) may be useful, but an initial exacerbation may occur. There are anecdotal reports of the success of narrowband UVB and of medium-dose ultraviolet A1 phototherapy.

Tropical 5-fluorouricil, dapsone, antibiotics, and cryotherapy are ineffective.

SPECIFIC INVESTIGATIONS

> ▶ Skin biopsy

Acantholysis is the characteristic epidermal change. The histologic changes may mimic Darier's disease, pemphigus, and Hailey–Hailey disease. Hyperkeratosis, parakeratosis, and spongiosis are other common epidermal changes.

FIRST-LINE THERAPIES

▶ Emollients	E
▶ Avoid heat/sweating	D
▶ Tropical corticosteroids	D
▶ Antihistamines	D

Transient acantholytic dermatosis. Heenan PJ, Quirk CJ. Br J Dermatol 1980; 102: 515–20.

This study looked at a series of 24 cases of transient acantholytic dermatosis. Most of them required tropical fluorinated corticosteroids to control the pruritus, and two required intermittent courses of oral corticosteroids. Antihistamines were of limited value in controlling the pruritus.

Incidence of transient acantholytic dermatosis (Grover's disease) in a hospital setting. French LE, Piletta PA, Etienne A, Salomon D, Saurat JH. Dermatology 1999; 198: 410–1.

A prospective study of 28 hospital inpatients diagnosed with Grover's disease. In over 80% of cases the duration of hospitalization exceeded 2 weeks and was associated with strict bed rest. The authors suggested a sweat-related pathogenesis.

Transient acantholytic dermatosis (Grover's disease). Hu H, Michel B, Farber EM. Arch Dermatol 1985; 121: 1439–41.

Seven cases of Grover's disease are presented in this article, which demonstrated a causal association with heat and sweating. Five of the cases are reported to have responded to topical corticosteroids.

SECOND-LINE THERAPIES

▶ Isotretinoin/acitretin	D
▶ Systemic corticosteroids	D
▶ PUVA	E
▶ Vitamin A	D

Persistent acantholytic dermatosis. Dodd HJ, Sarkany I. Clin Exp Dermatol 1984; 9: 431–4.

A case report of a 41-year-old man with a 5-year history of an itchy truncal and lower limb rash consistent with persistent acantholytic dermatosis. Bath emollients and aqueous cream BP afforded minor relief. Etretinate (50 mg daily) cleared the skin lesions and reduced the itching.

Etretinate has been replaced by its active metabolite acitretin. Lower doses of the latter may be effective.

Grover's disease treated with isotretinoin. Helfman RJ, Gables C. J Am Acad Dermatol 1985; 12: 981–4.

Four patients with biopsy-proven Grover's disease responded to 40 mg daily of isotretinoin for 2–4 months. In two patients most lesions had cleared after 3–4 weeks of treatment. Their dose was reduced by 10 mg daily for a further 8 weeks. One patient required 40 mg daily for 8 weeks. These patients remained in remission for up to 10 months after treatment. The final patient obtained partial relief and then discontinued treatment because of elevated triglycerides.

Transient acantholytic dermatosis treated with isotretinoin. Mancuso A, Cohen EH. Int J Dermatol 1989; 28: 58–9.

A 48-year-old man with severe pruritus had a 2-month history of Grover's disease. Systemic corticosteroids initially relieved his symptoms. On discontinuation of prednisone he relapsed. Isotretinoin was commenced at an initial dose of 1 mg/kg daily (40 mg twice daily) and then reduced to 40 mg daily due to adverse effects. He had improved by 6 weeks. Lesions and pruritus resolved after 3 months of therapy.

Response of transient acantholytic dermatosis to photochemotherapy. Paul BS, Arndt KA. Arch Dermatol 1984; 120: 121–2.

A 59-year-old man with persistent Grover's disease was unresponsive to oral prednisone and vitamin A (300 000 units daily). PUVA was initiated with 50 mg (0.6 mg/kg) methoxsalen and 2 J/cm^2 of UVA. Treatment was twice weekly and the UVA dosage was increased by 0.5 J/cm^2 with each treatment. The patient experienced a flare after four treatments, but improved by week 6, with maximal improvement by week 8. Therapy was then tapered off over the following 4 weeks, with complete clearing. No recurrence had occurred 25 months after therapy.

Photochemotherapy beyond psoriasis. Honig B, Morison WL, Karp D. J Am Acad Dermatol 1994; 31: 775–90.

The authors comment that Grover's disease may occur in patients receiving PUVA for other skin conditions. Continuation of PUVA clears the rash, with the pruritus resolving within 10 treatments and the eruption clearing within 20–30 treatments. No numbers are supplied.

Reports show that approximately 10 treatments are required for resolution of pruritus and 20–30 treatments may be needed to clear the eruption. Paradoxically, Grover's disease may complicate PUVA prescribed for other conditions.

Treatment of transient acantholytic dermatosis. Rohr JR, Quirk CJ. Arch Dermatol 1979; 115: 1033–4.

Eight patients were treated with vitamin A 50 000 units three times a day for up to 2 weeks; all patients responded. Once initial improvement was noted the dose was reduced to 50 000 units daily as maintenance or for several weeks. No signs of toxicity were noted. One patient required reinstitution of the drug owing to recurrence on cessation of treatment.

THIRD-LINE THERAPIES

▶ Calcipotriol	E
▶ Tacalcitol	E
▶ Trichloroacetic acid	E
▶ Antibiotic ointment	E
▶ UVA1	E

Treatment of Grover's disease with calcipotriol (Dovonex). Keohane SG, Cork MJ. Br J Dermatol 1995; 132: 832–3.

A 50-year-old man had a 13-month history of Grover's disease. He responded poorly to oxytetracycline, topical corticosteroids, dapsone, and etretinate. Lesions cleared following hospitalization and prednisone 100 mg daily, but he relapsed with any reduction in dose. Oral corticosteroids were stopped and he was commenced on an alternating regimen of calcipotriol ointment and 0.025% betamethasone valerate ointment. There was complete clearance of lesions after 1 month of treatment, but the disease relapsed when treatment was stopped.

Successful treatment of Grover's disease with calcipotriol. Mota AV, Correia TM, Lopes JM, Guimaraes JM. Eur J Dermatol 1998; 8: 33–5.

Case report of an 84-year-old man with a 2-year history of Grover's disease. He improved significantly despite initial moderate irritation following a 3-week course of calcipotriol 50 µg/g twice daily. Lesions did not recur during a 6-month follow-up.

Treatment of Grover's disease with tacalcitol. Hayashi H. Clin Exp Dermatol 2002; 27: 160.

A 31-year-old man with a 2-month history of Grover's disease that failed to respond to topical corticosteroid was commenced on tacalcitol ointment twice daily. He improved dramatically within 1 week and was in remission after 1 month.

Effective treatment of persistent Grover's disease with trichloroacetic acid peeling. Kouba DJ, Dasgeb B, Deng AC, Gaspari AA. Dermatol Surg 2006; 32: 1083–8.

A 46-year-old woman had a 6-month history of progressive Grover's disease with intractable pruritus. She failed to respond to topical calcipotriene (Dovonex). She was treated with an even, light application of 40% (w/v) TCA – single-pass strokes with TCA-dampened gauze. Individual lesions of Grover's disease were identified and were re-treated with 40% TCA using a cotton-tipped applicator. Three weeks post procedure she had re-epithelialized and was disease free, and was still in remission 8 months later.

The authors stress that practitioners not accustomed to using TCA in office applications should use low-strength formulations such as 20–30% to avoid scarring.

Antibiotic ointment in the treatment of Grover disease. Julliard KN, Milburn PB. Cutis 2007; 80: 72–4.

Six of nine patients with Grover's disease (four biopsy proven) had major or total resolution of the lesions following the daily application of a triple antibiotic ointment (active compound not supplied) to affected areas for 1 month. Follow-up varied between 3 and 72 months.

Medium-dose ultraviolet A1 phototherapy in transient acantholytic dermatosis (Grover's disease). Breuckmann F, Appelhans C, Altmeyer P, Kreuter A. J Am Acad Dermatol 2005; 52: 169–70.

Evidence Levels: **A** Double-blind study **B** Clinical trial ≥ 20 subjects **C** Clinical trial < 20 subjects **D** Series ≥ 5 subjects **E** Anecdotal case reports

A 78-year-old man with persistent Grover's disease had failed to respond to topical and oral corticosteroids. He was treated with a medium-dose UVA1 cold light monophototherapy containing a special filtering and cooling system (21°C). Irradiation (50 J/cm, 1.9 J/cm/min; 26 min), six times weekly for 3 weeks, then three times weekly for 3 weeks. Total 24 treatments, cumulative dose 1200 J/cm²). Complete remission was achieved after 4 weeks, with no subsequent relapse.

Trichotillomania

Leslie G Millard

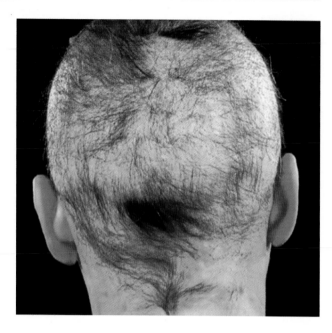

The term trichotillomania was first used by Hallopeau in 1889 and is derived from the Greek *thrix* (hair), *tillein* (to pull out) and *mania* (madness). Literally, it means a morbid craving to pull out hair. Psychiatric classification lists trichotillomania under impulse-control disorders in company with compulsive gambling. Now the definition must encompass a broader spectrum of additional psychopathologies, such as obsessive–compulsive disorder, body dysmorphic disorder, and mood disorders. The revised diagnostic criteria for trichotillomania include the following:

- Recurrent pulling out of ones own hair resulting in hair loss
- An increasing sense of tension immediately before pulling out the hair or when attempting to resist this behaviour
- Pleasure, gratification or relief when pulling out the hair
- The disturbance is not better accounted for by another mental disorder
- The disturbance provokes clinically marked distress and/or impairment in occupational, social, or other areas of functioning.

MANAGEMENT STRATEGY

The management of this complaint is complex because it is a product of various psychopathologies. Management centers on three issues. First, the diagnosis of the hair defect; second, the diagnostic grouping and the presence of other psychopathologies, such as depression; and third, the presence of complications such as trichobezoar.

Trichotillomania is seen in both children and adults. The latter may also have additional classifiable psychiatric illnesses, which distorts any attempt to make this a homogeneous entity. There appear to be two distinct populations: those who present in childhood, mainly between the ages of 5 and 12 years, and chronic cases presenting as adults who have continued hair-pulling activity from adolescence or developed the disorder in early adult life. The early-onset group, usually between the ages of 2 and 10 years, show benign, self-limiting behavior and most are probably suffering a habit disorder, perhaps as an extension of hair-twirling activity and childhood stress. There is an association with nail biting, thumb sucking, skin picking, nose picking, lip biting, and cheek chewing. In children, there is an association with anxiety and dysthymia, learning disability, and iron deficiency.

The adolescent group are much more likely to be female (ratios of up to 3.5:1). The psychopathology may be related to parent relationships, school difficulties, especially bullying, body image changes, and increasingly parental and sexual abuse. The adult age groups are associated with greater psychopathology and show a distinct female preponderance (up to 15:1). This remains true for different racial groups. There is a significant association of trichotillomania with obsessive–compulsive disorder and/or depressive illness.

The hair-pulling activity is either a conscious, deliberate act or subconscious, in some children being part of a hypnagogic (dreamlike) state. Most adult patients describe a deliberate act following an increased sense of tension before hair pulling and a sense of relief immediately afterwards. Hair pulling and plucking is commonest from the scalp, but not as a response to scalp symptoms. Most pull hair from the vertex, but temporal, occipital, and frontal hair loss in children may be more obvious on the side of manual dominance. The hair loss may be minimal – commonly a solitary patch, but visible hair thinning may progress to extensive depilation in adult women.

The hairs are short, irregular, broken, and distorted and feel like stubble. In alopecia areata the hair is much smoother. The clinical differentiation is made easier using a dermatoscope. This technique will also identify the compulsive hair shavers and cutters. The patterns of plucking start from a single point or are linear, in wave-like activity. Children will pluck the eyebrows and eyelashes, but adults will pluck hair on the torso and pubic areas. Children pluck hair as a distracted activity, whereas adults are more conscious and secretive. This may become more like a compulsion, with elaboration of the rituals using instruments such as tweezers.

Patients disguise the defects using wigs, false eyelashes, and semi-permanent wearing of hats and scarves. The psychosocial effects of hair loss are a reluctance to date or play sports, and causes significant social isolation. Chronic folliculitis of the chin, chest, pubic areas, or thighs may be the presenting complaint as a result of secretive plucking.

The hair root alone may be eaten (trichorhizophagia) as a secretive activity, and in a few patients the whole hair is eaten (trichophagia). Occasionally hair may be seen stuck between the teeth. Patients who eat more hair tend to swallow the longer strands, and a small percentage develop gastrointestinal trichobezoars. These are seen almost exclusively girls and young women; they have a high morbidity, with chronicity and complications which can be fatal. Children with trichotillomania who present with abdominal pain, weight loss, nausea, vomiting, anorexia, and foul breath should be investigated. Gastric trichobezoars may cause intestinal bleeding, pancreatitis, or obstructive symptoms.

Children with trichotillomania can be managed with *supportive psychotherapy*, and eventual spontaneous resolution can be expected. *Habit retraining* may be beneficial in adults. Combining *SSRI antidepressants* and *clomipramine* with psychological modalities may benefit older patients. Combining modern atypical neuroleptics such as *olanzapine* and *risperidone* with SSRIs has been beneficial.

Evidence Levels: A Double-blind study B Clinical trial ≥ 20 subjects C Clinical trial < 20 subjects D Series ≥ 5 subjects E Anecdotal case reports

SPECIFIC INVESTIGATIONS

> ► Dermatoscopy
> ► Hair microscopy
> ► Scalp biopsy
> ► Full blood count and ferritin
> ► If appropriate, investigate trichobezoar

Trichotillomania: a histopathological study in 66 patients. Muller SA. J Am Acad Dermatol 1990; 23: 56–62.

A description of definitive signs on scalp biopsy: empty follicles, follicular keratin debris, and trichomalacia. These features differentiate trichotillomania from alopecia areata and obsessive hair cutting.

Hair dermatoscopy and microscopy differentiates plucked, broken hair seen in trichotillomania from cut hair in compulsive hair cutters, and from exclamation mark hairs in alopecia areata.

Diagnosis and management of trichotillomania in children and adolescents. Bruce T. Paediatr Drugs 2005; 7: 365–76.

Gastrointestinal bezoars: sonographic and CT characteristics. Ripolles T. Am J Roentgenol 2001; 177: 65–9.

Characteristics of non-invasive investigations.

Laparoscopic removal of huge gastric trichobezoar. Shami S. Surg Laparosc Tech 2007; 17: 197–200.

Direct vision of a suspect lesion and endoscopic removal are described.

FIRST-LINE THERAPIES

> ► Supportive psychotherapy   A
> ► Cognitive therapy and directive training   B
> ► SSRI medication   C

For most children supportive empathic therapy accompanied by elucidation of stress factors is sufficient.

Trichotillomania and related disorders in children and adolescents. Hanna GL. Child Psychiatry 1997; 27: 255–68.

Psychological factors and therapy in children.

Trichotillomania treatment. Van Hasselt VB. Sourcebook of psychological treatment for adult disorders. New York: Plenum Press, 1996; 657–87.

Use of psychological therapies and SSRI drugs can improve 60% of adult cases of trichotillomania.

Use of psychotropic drugs in dermatology. Gupta MA. Dermatol Clin 2000; 18: 711–25.

Clomipramine was more effective than SSRIs, although more side effects were present. Citalopram over 12 weeks was effective in one-third of patients over 3 months.

SECOND-LINE THERAPIES

> ► Behaviour therapy/habit retraining   B
> ► Combined psychological and drug therapy   B
> ► Atypical neuroleptics   C

Treatment of trichotillomania with behavioural therapy or fluoxetine: a randomized waiting list study. Van Minnen A, Hoogduin KA, Keijsers GP, Hellenbrand I, Hendriks GJ. Arch Gen Psychiatry 2003; 60: 517–22.

Behavioral therapy was significantly better than fluoxetine (60 mg/day), which did provide some symptom relief.

Behavioural treatment of trichotillomania: two-year follow-up results. Keijsers GP, van Minnen A, Hoogduin CA, Klaassen BN, Hendriks MJ, Tanis-Jacobs J. Behav Res Ther 2006; 44: 359–70.

The manual-based behavioral therapy consisted of self-control procedures offered in six sessions. The area of the patch of trichotillomania was assessed and was reduced by 49% and 70% at 3 months and 2 years. Better 2-year follow-up results were associated with lower pretreatment levels of depressive symptoms and with complete abstinence from hair pulling immediately after treatment.

Single modality versus dual modality treatment for trichotillomania. Dougherty D. J Clin Psychiatry 2006; 67: 1086–92.

Habit reversal and SSRI drug therapy together were better than either alone.

Systematic review: Pharmacological and behavioural treatment for trichotillomania. Block M, Landeros-Weisenberger A, Dombrowski P, Kelmendi B, Wegner R, Nudel J, et al. Biol Psychiatry 2007; 62: 839–46.

Olanzapine in doses up to 10 mg/day improved hair pulling by 66%, and risperidone augmented the response to SSRIs in some patients. Close control of the drugs is necessary.

THIRD-LINE THERAPIES

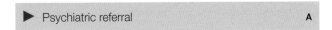
> ► Psychiatric referral   A

Systematic review: Pharmacological and behavioural treatment for trichotillomania. Block M, Landeros-Weisenberger A, Dombrowski P, Kelmendi B, Wegner R, Nudel J, et al. Biol Psychiatry 2007; 62: 839–46.

In adults, major depressive illness is present in 14% and 15% show an anxiety disorder. Substance abuse and eating disorders may also be associated.

Tuberculosis and tuberculids

Anita Takwale, John Berth-Jones

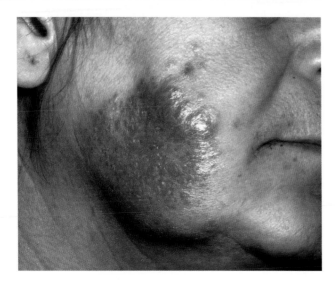

Cutaneous tuberculosis (TB) has a variety of presentations. Primary infection of the skin with *Mycobacterium tuberculosis* may occur by inoculation from an exogenous source, giving rise to tuberculous chancre, warty tuberculosis, or lupus vulgaris. Secondary cutaneous tuberculosis, from an endogenous source, may give rise to acute miliary tuberculosis, lupus vulgaris, or tuberculous gumma by hematogenous spread, to scrofuloderma via contiguous spread, or to periorificial tuberculosis via auto-inoculation. Tuberculids, e.g., lichen scrofulosorum, papulonecrotic tuberculid, erythema induratum (of Bazin), and erythema nodosum, are immunologically mediated phenomena regarded as manifestations of tuberculosis at a site remote from the active infection. On occasions mycobacterial antigens can be detected by PCR in biopsy material from these eruptions.

MANAGEMENT STRATEGY

An accurate and early diagnosis of tuberculosis is important for its effective management. Characteristic clinical and histopathologic findings along with a positive culture have always remained the gold standard. Until recently the tuberculin skin tests (TST) have been in widespread use for detection of TB, but false-positive responses due to reactivity caused by infection with non-tuberculous mycobacteria or bacillus Calmette–Guérin (BCG) limit their use.

Polymerase chain reaction (PCR) has become a valuable tool in the rapid identification of these slow-growing organisms. There has also been a growing interest in interferon-γ assays for mycobacterial detection in cutaneous tuberculosis. These tests, which include the enzyme-linked immunosorbent assay, e.g., QuantiFERON-TB (QFT) (gold test) and the enzyme-linked immunospot assay (e.g., T-spot-TB test) are being used commonly in pulmonary TB.

All patients with documented cutaneous tuberculosis should be evaluated further for pulmonary and other extrapulmonary disease. HIV testing should be considered in widespread lesions, and in cases of multidrug-resistant mycobacteria.

The improvement in general health and nutrition and the public health aspects of tracing sources are important in management. The aim of treatment is to cure the disease as rapidly as possible. The standard treatment regimens recommended are based on controlled trials carried out for pulmonary tuberculosis. The standard 6-month regimen for adults comprises *rifampicin* (10 mg/kg), *isoniazid* (INH) (5 mg/kg), *pyrazinamide* (35 mg/kg), and *ethambutol* (15 mg/kg) for the initial 2 months, followed by rifampicin and INH for a further 4 months in the 'continuation phase'. Ethambutol can be omitted in patients with a low risk of resistance to INH. In countries where the resources to provide rifampicin are not available, ethambutol and isoniazid are recommended by the World Health Organization for the continuation phase. Occasionally longer treatment regimens may be necessary to achieve a complete cure.

In HIV-infected patients the continuation phase may need to be extended for 7 or more months. Cases of multidrug-resistant tuberculosis should be managed at specialist centers.

Other measures may also be used. The *excision* of small lesions of lupus vulgaris or warty tuberculosis, if diagnosed early, may be effective. Local destruction of small residual nodules of lupus vulgaris may have a place in the management. Surgery may be useful in scrofuloderma. Plastic surgery may help the disfigurement left by treated lupus vulgaris.

SPECIFIC INVESTIGATIONS

- ▶ Skin biopsy for histopathology and tissue or pus for culture for *M. tuberculosis*
- ▶ Tuberculin skin test
- ▶ Polymerase chain reaction for *M. tuberculosis* DNA in skin
- ▶ Interferon-γ-based assays
- ▶ Screening for tuberculosis at other sites: chest X-ray; cultures of sputum, early morning urine, etc.

Detection of *Mycobacterium tuberculosis* complex DNA by the polymerase chain reaction for rapid diagnosis of cutaneous tuberculosis. Margall N, Baselga E, Coll P, Barnadas MA, de Moragas JM, Prats G. Br J Dermatol 1996; 135: 231–6.

Of 48 paraffin-embedded specimens from 32 patients with different variants of cutaneous tuberculosis 37 (77%) were positive for the *M. tuberculosis* complex DNA.

Clinical utility of an interferon-γ-based assay for mycobacterial detection in papulonecrotic tuberculid. Tanaka R, Matsuura H, Kobashi Y, Fujimoto W. Br J Dermatol 2007; 156: 169–71.

A case report of a 37-year-old patient with papulonecrotic tuberculid in whom mycobacterial DNA was not detected by PCR but supported by Quantiferon-TB-2G.

Usefulness of the Quantiferon test in the confirmation of latent tuberculosis in association with erythema induratum. Angus J, Roberts C, Kulkarni K, Leach I, Murphy R. Br J Dermatol 2007; 157: 1267–304.

A 14-year old boy with a clinical and histopathologic diagnosis of erythema induratum, a negative tuberculin test, and a positive interferon-based test had successful resolution of lesions after antituberculous treatment.

FIRST-LINE THERAPIES

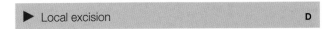

▶ Antituberculous drugs   **A**

Treatment of tuberculosis: guidelines for national programmes. Geneva: World Health Organisation, 2003.

The essential anti-TB drugs recommended are INH (H) (5 mg/kg), rifampin (R) (10 mg/kg), pyrazinamide (Z) (25 mg/kg), streptomycin (S) (15 mg/kg), ethambutol (E) (15 mg/kg), and thiacetazone (T) (2.5 mg/kg). A common regimen employed is 2 months of HRZE then 6 months of HE.

Chemotherapy and management of tuberculosis in the United Kingdom: recommendations 1998. Joint Tuberculosis Committee of the British Thoracic Society. Thorax 1998; 53: 536–48.

The committee recommend an initial phase of 2 months treatment with four drugs: INH (5 mg/kg), rifampin (10 mg/kg), pyrazinamide (35 mg/kg), and ethambutol (15 mg/kg). This is followed by a continuation phase of 4 months using INH and rifampin for pulmonary and extrapulmonary tuberculosis. The fourth drug (ethambutol) can be omitted in patients with a low risk of resistance to INH.

Comparative efficacy of drug regimens in skin tuberculosis. Ramesh V, Misra RS, Saxena U, Mukherjee A. Clin Exp Dermatol 1991; 16: 106–9.

Three antituberculous drug regimens were employed to study the response in 90 patients with cutaneous tuberculosis. The first two regimens contained rifampin (adults 450 mg, children 15 mg/kg), INH (adults 300 mg, children 5 mg/kg) and either pyrazinamide (adults 1500 mg, children 30 mg/kg) or thiacetazone (adults 150 mg, children 4 mg/kg); the third regimen had rifampin and INH only. The patients with lupus vulgaris and warty tuberculosis cleared with all three regimens in 4 and 5 months for localized and generalized disease, respectively. Patients with scrofuloderma responded well to both triple-drug regimens, with the skin lesions subsiding completely within 5 months in the localized and 6 months in the widespread forms of the disease. However, 9–10 months treatment was necessary in the group receiving isoniazid and rifampin.

SECOND-LINE THERAPIES

▶ Local excision   **D**

Scrofuloderma of the lower extremity treated with wide resection: a case report and review of the literature. Connolly B, Pitcher JD Jr, Roth B, Youngberg RA, Devine J. Am J Orthop 1999; 28: 417–20.

A report on an immunocompromised patient who presented with scrofuloderma of the lower extremity. This failed to resolve with the standard antituberculous regimen consisting of four drugs: INH, rifampin, pyrazinamide, and ethambutol for 2 months, followed by INH and rifampin for 3 months, but was then successfully treated with wide resection under spinal anesthesia.

Lupus vulgaris of the ear lobe. Okazaki M, Sakurai A. Ann Plast Surg 1997; 39: 643–6.

A 59-year-old woman with an initial diagnosis of hemangioma had surgical treatment followed by antituberculous therapy (INH, rifampin, and pyridoxine for 9 months) for lupus vulgaris of the earlobe.

Primary inoculation tuberculosis. Hooker RP, Eberts TJ, Strickland JA. J Hand Surg [Am] 1979; 4: 270–3.

A case of primary inoculation tuberculosis of the finger is reported, in which Mantoux test conversion reverted after prompt surgical and medical treatment with INH (300 mg/day) for 1 year and ethambutol (200 mg/day) for the initial 3 months.

Urticaria and angioedema

Frances Humphreys

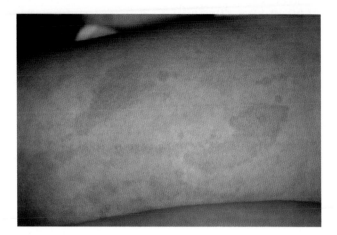

Urticaria is the result of transient leakage of plasma from the dermal vasculature and is characterized by short-lived, itchy, raised wheals due to dermal edema. In angioedema the swelling is deeper, resulting in more diffuse and prolonged edema, particularly affecting the face. These conditions are defined as chronic if symptoms have lasted longer than 6 weeks.

Hereditary angioedema (HAO) and the physical urticarias are dealt with separately in Chapters 92 and 175, respectively.

MANAGEMENT STRATEGY

Explanation of the nature and prognosis of the disorder is important. Most patients with chronic urticaria become asymptomatic within 2 years. Patients with a longer history and those with coexisting physical urticarias are less likely to remit. It is important to exclude causative and exacerbating factors, particularly drugs (i.e., aspirin, non-steroidal anti-inflammatories (NSAIDs), angiotensin-converting enzyme (ACE) inhibitors). IgE-mediated allergy is rarely a cause of chronic symptoms and does not need to be tested for routinely. Blood tests and chest radiography should only be performed if history or examination dictate. There is an increased incidence of positive thyroid autoantibodies in chronic urticaria (CU) patients and some evidence of an increased incidence of celiac disease in children. Of patients with CU 30–40% have a positive autologous serum skin test providing evidence of autoimmunity. This test is not performed in routine practice. HAO should be excluded in those with angioedema without urticaria by measuring the C4 and C1 esterase inhibitor levels. Individual urticarial lesions lasting over 24 hours may indicate urticarial vasculitis, necessitating skin biopsy and appropriate investigation if confirmed.

Potent non-sedating antihistamines are the mainstay of treatment and are usually given regularly, but occasionally as required for intermittent symptoms. Many patients show a diurnal variation in symptoms, and timing of once-daily treatment should be adjusted accordingly. In practice *acrivastine,*

cetirizine/levocetirizine, fexofenadine, loratadine/desloratadine, and *mizolastine* are all effective. Individual responses to different antihistamines reportedly vary and tachyphylaxis is reported, so changing H_1 antagonists is warranted. Increasing the dose of an individual antihistamine, combining two different long-acting ones 12 hours apart, or adding a short-acting antihistamine for breakthrough symptoms, can all be useful maneuvers. Sedative antihistamines can be useful at night, particularly for nocturnal pruritus.

There is increasing evidence of some benefit of adding *leukotriene antagonists* to H_1 antihistamines in some patients, although some trials have failed to confirm this. There is some evidence that pseudoallergen-free *diets* may help in urticaria. It seems logical to try a low-salicylate diet for a 4-week assessment period in patients who report exacerbation of symptoms with aspirin or NSAIDs. *Systemic corticosteroids* do not help all patients with urticaria and, if introduced and effective in CU, can be very difficult to withdraw. A short course of prednisolone 20–30 mg daily for 3 days can reduce the severity and time course of attacks of angioedema and acute urticaria. *Intramuscular epinephrine (adrenaline)* is not routinely used, but may be necessary for severe angioedema affecting the upper respiratory tract.

H_2 *antagonists* have been used in combination with H_1 antagonists, but their benefit in practice is disappointing. Patients with confirmed *Helicobacter pylori* infection have a greater chance of remission of urticaria after successful eradication therapy.

Limited evidence exists for other drugs such as *doxepin* (a tricyclic with H_1 antagonist properties), *nifedipine, psoralen and UVA (PUVA), sulfasalazine,* and *warfarin.* Non-hereditary angioedema has been treated with *stanozolol* and *tranexamic acid. Dipyridamole* has been used in combination with an H_1 antagonist. Some authors have used *thyroxine,* with variable results. The potential benefits of therapies for which evidence is poor must be weighed against possible side effects.

There is now good evidence for an autoimmune etiology in chronic urticaria. Because most patients have a self-limiting and non-life-threatening condition, *immunosuppressive therapy* is not indicated for the majority. In those with severe and unremitting problems who are experiencing considerable morbidity associated with the condition, *ciclosporin, plasmapheresis,* and *intravenous immunoglobulin* have all now been shown to be effective. The benefit of such treatment may be short-lived. A recent open study has shown that 4 weeks of ciclosporin gives the same degree of benefit as 12 weeks of treatment.

Mycophenalate mofetil and *tacrolimus* have been used for patients with very severe symptoms in open studies. Three patients with very severe angioedema have been treated with *omalizumab.*

SPECIFIC INVESTIGATIONS

> ▶ None; or
> ▶ Screening tests based on history and physical examination
> ▶ C4 and C1 esterase inhibitor in angioedema without urticaria
> ▶ Thyroid function and thyroid antibodies
> ▶ Screening for celiac disease in children

Guidelines for evaluation and management of urticaria in adults and children. Grattan CE, Humphreys F. Br J Dermatol 2007; 157: 1116–23.

Evidence Levels: **A** Double-blind study **B** Clinical trial ≥ 20 subjects **C** Clinical trial < 20 subjects **D** Series ≥ 5 subjects **E** Anecdotal case reports

The effectiveness of a history-based diagnostic approach in chronic urticaria and angioedema. Kozel MMA, Mekkes JR, Bossuyt PMM, Bos JD. Arch Dermatol 1998; 134: 1575–80.

This prospective study of 238 new patients with chronic urticaria and/or angioedema found that extensive laboratory investigation did not contribute to finding an underlying cause for urticaria compared to limited laboratory investigation based on the history.

Syndrome of idiopathic chronic urticaria and angioedema with thyroid autoimmunity: a study of 90 patients. Leznoff A, Sussman GL. J Allergy Clin Immunol 1989; 84: 66–71.

This study found that 90 of 624 patients with chronic idiopathic urticaria and angioedema had evidence of thyroid autoimmunity, compared to an expected number of 37; p<0.01.

Chronic urticaria and associated coeliac disease in children: a case control study. Caminiti L, Passalacqua G, Magazzu G, Comisi F, Vita D, Barberio G, et al. Paediatr Allergy Immunol 2005; 16: 428–32.

This study of 79 children with chronic urticaria that responded poorly to treatment and 2545 controls found that 5% of patients and 0.67% of controls, respectively, had celiac disease. In the four children with celiac disease a gluten-free diet led to improvement of the urticaria.

FIRST-LINE THERAPIES

▶ Non-sedating H₁ antagonists	A

There are many double-blind studies of non-sedating antihistamines showing efficacy, but few high-quality comparative studies.

Chronic urticaria: assessment of current treatment. Wedi B, Kapp A. Exp Rev Clin Immunol 2005; 1: 459–73.

This review lists 31 randomized controlled trials of non-sedating antihistamines the majority of which show a significant effect compared with placebo. The authors point out that most studies are of patients with only mild/moderate disease, as those with severe disease are unable to have a treatment-free washout period.

SECOND-LINE THERAPIES

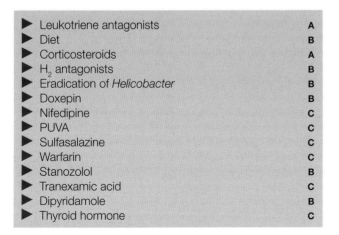

▶ Leukotriene antagonists	A
▶ Diet	B
▶ Corticosteroids	A
▶ H₂ antagonists	B
▶ Eradication of *Helicobacter*	B
▶ Doxepin	B
▶ Nifedipine	C
▶ PUVA	C
▶ Sulfasalazine	C
▶ Warfarin	C
▶ Stanozolol	B
▶ Tranexamic acid	C
▶ Dipyridamole	B
▶ Thyroid hormone	C

Desloratidine in combination with montelukast in the treatment of chronic urticaria: a randomized, double-blind, placebo-controlled study. Nettis E, Colanardi MC, Paradiso MT, Ferrannini A. Clin Exp Allergy 2004; 34: 1401–7.

This double-blind study of 81 patients with chronic urticaria compared desloratadine 5 mg daily plus placebo with desloratadine 5 mg daily plus montelukast 10 mg daily, and with placebo alone over a 6-week treatment period. Both active treatment groups were more effective than placebo; desloratadine plus montelukast improved symptoms and quality of life more than desloratadine alone, but did not affect the number of urticarial episodes.

Urticaria is also reported as a side effect of leukotriene antagonists.

Pseudoallergen-free diet in the treatment of chronic urticaria. Zuberbier T, Chantraine-Hess S, Hartmann K, Czarnetski BM. Acta Dermatol Venereol 1995; 75: 484–7.

In an open study of 64 patients with CU, 73% improved on a 2-week pseudoallergen-avoidance diet. Only 19% reacted to pseudoallergens on provocation testing. An additive-free, stringently controlled diet may provide a means of treating some patients with chronic urticaria.

Outpatient management of acute urticaria: the role of prednisone. Pollack CV, Romano TJ. Ann Emerg Med 1995; 26: 547–51.

Forty-three patients with acute urticaria of <24 hours duration were treated with intramuscular diphenhydramine and discharged on either regular hydroxyzine plus placebo or hydroxyzine plus prednisolone 20 mg 12-hourly for 4 days. Symptoms of itch and extent of rash were statistically more improved in the group treated with prednisone at 2 and 5 days.

Cimetidine and chlorpheniramine in the treatment of chronic idiopathic urticaria: a multi-centre randomized double-blind study. Bleehan SS, Thomas SE, Greaves MW, Newton J, Kennedy CT, Hindley F, et al. Br J Dermatol 1987; 117: 81–8.

Forty patients whose symptoms were not abolished by treatment with chlorpheniramine (chlorphenamine) alone were treated with either chlorpheniramine and placebo or chlorpheniramine and cimetidine 400 mg four times daily. A significant improvement in wheals and pruritus was shown for the active treatment.

The effect of antibiotic therapy for patients infected with *Helicobacter pylori* who have chronic urticaria. Federman DG, Kirsner RS, Moriarty JP, Concato J. J Am Acad Dermatol 2003; 49: 861–4.

This review looks at 10 studies of patients with chronic urticaria and evidence of *H. pylori* infection. Successful eradication of *H. pylori* was statistically associated with remission of urticaria.

Double-blind crossover study comparing doxepin with diphenhydramine for the treatment of chronic urticaria. Green SL, Reed CE, Schroeter AL. J Am Acad Dermatol 1985; 12: 669–75.

Fifty patients with CU were treated with doxepin 10 mg three times daily compared to diphenhydramine 25 mg three times daily, with control of symptoms in 74% and 10%, respectively.

In practice, sedation can limit the usefulness of this drug.

Therapy of chronic idiopathic urticaria with nifedipine: demonstration of beneficial effect in a double-blinded, placebo-controlled, crossover trial. Bressler RB, Sowell K, Huston DP. J Allergy Clin Immunol 1989; 83: 756–63.

Ten patients with refractory urticaria had nifedipine (up to 20 mg three times daily) or placebo added to their treatment for 4 weeks. A beneficial effect was shown in seven patients who completed the study.

Treatment of chronic urticaria with PUVA or UVA plus placebo: a double-blind study. Olafsson JH, Larkö O, Roupe G, Granerus G, Bengtsson U. Arch Dermatol Res 1986; 278: 228–31.

This study showed improvement with PUVA and UVA plus placebo, suggesting either a therapeutic effect of UVA or a placebo effect.

Successful treatment of recalcitrant urticaria with sulfasalazine. McGirt LY, Vasagar K, Gober LM, Saini SS, Beck LA. Arch Dermatol 2006; 142: 1337–42.

In this open study 19 patients with CU unresponsive to H$_1$ antagonists were treated with sulfasalazine; 14 improved.

This drug can exacerbate urticaria, particularly in aspirin-sensitive subjects.

Warfarin treatment of chronic idiopathic urticaria and angio-oedema. Parslew R, Pryce D, Ashworth J, Friedmann PS. Clin Exp Allergy 2000; 30: 1161–5.

Six of eight treatment-resistant patients showed a therapeutic effect of warfarin in an open study. Three responders then took part in a double-blind study, which confirmed an improvement in pruritus and angioedema scores.

Stanozolol in chronic urticaria: a double blind, placebo controlled trial. Parsad D, Pandhi R, Juneja A. J Dermatol 2001; 28: 299–302.

Fifty-eight patients with refractory urticaria were treated with either cetirizine and placebo or cetirizine plus stanozolol 2 mg twice daily. Severity scores were used and a significant difference was found for the active group, 17 of whom became asymptomatic, compared to seven in the placebo group.

Non-hereditary angioedema treated with tranexamic acid. Munch EP, Weeke B. Allergy 1985; 40: 92–7.

In this small double-blind study nine of 10 patients with frequent attacks of angioedema showed improvement with tranexamic acid.

Efficacy and safety of desloratidine combined with dipyridamole in the treatment of chronic urticaria. Khalif AT, Liu X, Sheng W, Tan J, Abdalla AN. J Eur Acad Dermatol Venereol 2008; 22: 487–92.

In a randomized double-blind study 64 patients with urticaria were treated either with desloratadine alone or desloratadine and dipyridamole 25 mg three times daily. The active group showed higher rates of clinical effectiveness.

Improvement of chronic idiopathic urticaria with L-thyroxine: a new TSH role in immune response? Aversano M, Caizzo P, Iorio G, Ponticiello L, Lagana B, Leccese F. Allergy 2005; 60: 489–93.

In an open study 20 patients with chronic idiopathic urticaria and autoimmune thyroiditis were treated with L-thyroxine, whether euthyroid or hypothyroid. In 16 patients the urticaria improved.

THIRD-LINE THERAPIES

▶ Ciclosporin	A
▶ Plasmapheresis	C
▶ Intravenous immunoglobulin	C
▶ Mycophenylate mofetil	C
▶ Tacrolimus	C
▶ Omalizumab	E

Ciclosporin in chronic idiopathic urticaria: a double blind, randomized, placebo-controlled trial. Vena GA, Cassano N, Colombo D, Peruzzi E, Pigatto P; NEO-I-30 Study Group. J Am Acad Dermatol 2006; 55: 705–9.

Ninety-nine patients with severe CIU were treated with ciclosporin for 16 weeks or for 8 weeks followed by 8 weeks' placebo, or placebo for 16 weeks. All groups took cetirizine. Ciclosporin was started at a dose of 5 mg/kg and reduced in two steps to 3 mg/kg by day 28. Symptom scores improved significantly in both ciclosporin groups.

Plasmapheresis for severe, unremitting, chronic urticaria. Grattan CE, Francis DM, Slater NG, Barlow RJ, Greaves MW. Lancet 1992; 339: 1078–80.

Eight patients with severe disease and serum histamine-releasing activity underwent plasmapheresis, with beneficial effect in six.

Intravenous immunoglobulin in autoimmune chronic urticaria. O'Donnell BF, Barr RM, Black AK, Francis DM, Kermani F, Niimi N, et al. Br J Dermatol 1998; 138: 101–6.

An open, uncontrolled study showed benefit in nine of 10 patients with severe CIU and evidence of autoimmunity: 0.4 g/kg was used daily for 5 days.

Treatment of severe chronic idiopathic urticaria with oral mycophenylate mofetil in patients not responding to antihistamines and/or corticosteroids. Shahar E, Bergman R, Guttman-Yassky E, Pollack S. Int J Dermatol 2006; 45: 1224–7.

In this open study of nine severe cases, mycophenylate mofetil 1000 mg twice daily was given for 12 weeks; patients continued with antihistamines and steroids as necessary. There was a significant reduction in the urticaria activity score, and all patients were able to stop prednisolone.

Tacrolimus in the treatment of severe chronic idiopathic urticaria: an open-label prospective study. Kessel A, Bamberger E, Toubi E. J Am Acad Dermatol 2005; 52: 145–8.

In this open study 12 of 17 patients improved with 12 weeks' treatment with oral tacrolimus.

Successful treatment of 3 patients with recurrent idiopathic angioedema with omalizamab. Sands MF, Blume JW, Schwartz SA. J Allergy Clin Immunol 2007; 120: 979–81.

Three patients with very severe angioedema, two of whom were asthmatic and two of whom had received lisinopril in the past, were treated with the recombinant humanized monoclonal anti-IgE antibody omalizamab, a treatment for moderate to severe asthma. All three patients showed a rapid improvement.

Varicella

Christine Soon, John Berth-Jones

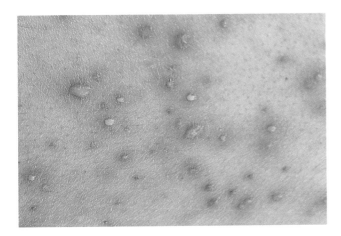

Varicella, or chickenpox, is the exanthematic illness caused by infection with the herpes virus varicella zoster (VZV). It is common and highly contagious. Varicella has a typical incubation period of 10–14 days. The disease spreads by direct person-to-person contact or by airborne droplets. Fever and malaise can precede the development of erythema, papules, and vesicles. The vesicles tend to appear in crops over 2–4 days in a centripetal distribution, and crust over before healing. The mucosae are often involved, and pruritus is often a prominent feature. The disease is infectious from 48 hours before the rash appears until the vesicles crust.

Varicella occurs most commonly in young children. Systemic symptoms are usually mild, although complications may occur. In patients with atopic dermatitis, varicella may closely resemble eczema herpeticum. In adolescents, adults, and immunocompromised individuals of any age it is a more severe disease with a higher complication rate. Treatment is most commonly recommended in this group of individuals. Potential complications include secondary bacterial infection of the skin, bacterial pneumonia, and varicella pneumonitis. Rare complications of varicella include aseptic meningitis, encephalitis, cerebellar ataxia, myocarditis, corneal lesions, nephritis, arthritis, acute glomerulonephritis, Reye's syndrome, bleeding diathesis, and hepatitis. Herpes zoster (shingles), a delayed complication of varicella, is the subject of a separate chapter.

MANAGEMENT STRATEGY

In the USA, *routine vaccination* of all healthy persons 12 months of age or older who have not had varicella is now recommended. This is a live, attenuated vaccine and is implemented as a routine two-dose program. The first dose is administered at age 12–15 months and the second dose at age 4–6 years. A second dose catch-up vaccination is recommended for those who had previously received one dose, including children, adolescents, and adults. Post-exposure immunization may also be effective for household contacts if given within 3 days of the appearance of the rash in the index case. In the UK, vaccination is recommended for non-immune healthcare workers and other carers who are in frequent contact with individuals (mainly immunocompromised patients) who would be especially vulnerable to the infection, the purpose being to protect these vulnerable individuals.

In *healthy children* below the age of 12 years, symptomatic treatment is all that is generally required. Acetaminophen (paracetamol) is suitable. Aspirin should be avoided because of the risk of Reye's syndrome. If a child is the second affected case in a family the illness can run a more severe course and antiviral therapy should be considered. Oral *aciclovir* is the antiviral of choice and should be started within 24 hours of the rash developing.

In *healthy adolescents and adults*, oral aciclovir commenced within 24 hours of development of the rash has been shown to be beneficial. Heavy smokers and people with chronic lung disease are at greater risk of developing complications, particularly varicella pneumonitis. Treatment with aciclovir should be given if they are seen within 24 hours of the rash developing. There is no evidence to suggest significant benefit if treatment is started after 24 hours in cases where infection is following the normal course and there are no complications. These patients should be treated symptomatically and advised to return promptly if they deteriorate. Patients with complications require hospital assessment.

Pregnant women are more likely to develop severe or complicated disease. Those who are not immune to varicella should avoid contact with varicella and zoster, and if this occurs they should report the contact immediately. Non-immune pregnant women who have had contact with a person with varicella should receive specific *varicella zoster immunoglobulin (VZIG)*. VZIG is effective up to 10 days after contact. This has been shown to prevent varicella or modify disease severity. It also reduces the risk of fetal transmission if disease develops. Fetal infection between 3 and 28 weeks' gestation may cause the fetal varicella syndrome (including developmental abnormalities of the eyes and central nervous system). This occurs in an estimated 0.91% of pregnancies complicated by chickenpox during the first 20 weeks of gestation. The risk is probably greatest when infection occurs between 13 and 20 weeks. During the first trimester the use of aciclovir carries a theoretical risk of possible teratogenesis, although it is not a recognized teratogen. Beyond 20 weeks' gestation oral aciclovir can be unequivocally recommended if the patient is seen within 24 hours of the onset of the rash. Pregnant women who are smokers, have chronic lung disease, are taking steroids, or are in the latter half of pregnancy are at greater risk of developing systemic symptoms. Hospitalization should be considered in late pregnancy and in women with chest or neurological symptoms, a hemorrhagic rash, bleeding, or very severe disease with a dense rash and mucosal lesions.

Neonates whose mothers had varicella 7 days before to 7 days after delivery should be given prophylaxis with VZIG. Neonates with varicella whose mothers developed varicella within 7 days prior to delivery may develop severe disease and should be treated with intravenous aciclovir. Treatment should also be considered within 48 hours of development of the rash in other infants with congenital varicella (rash within 16 days of delivery) and severe clinical disease.

Immunocompromised individuals exposed to varicella should be given prophylactic VZIG. It is most effective when given within 72 hours, but may still modify disease if given up to 10 days after exposure. All immunocompromised and immunodeficient patients who develop varicella, including those on oral corticosteroids or with a history of oral corticosteroid intake for more than 3 weeks in the preceding 3 months, should be admitted to hospital and treated with intravenous aciclovir, as they are at risk of severe disease and complications. Resistance to aciclovir can occur in immunocompromised individuals following long-term aciclovir therapy. In patients with proven aciclovir-resistant VZV strains, intravenous *foscarnet* is currently the antiviral agent of choice.

Newer anti-VZV drugs have been developed. These include *valaciclovir, famciclovir, and brivudin,* although they are currently only licensed for use in herpes zoster.

SPECIFIC INVESTIGATIONS

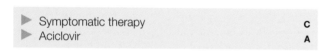

> ▶ Virology on vesicle fluid
> ▶ Serology on acute and convalescent sera

The diagnosis of viral infections. Kangro HO. In: Parker MT, Collier LH, eds. Topley and Wilson's principles of bacteriology, virology, and immunity. London: Edward Arnold, 1999; 227–42.

This is a general review of diagnostic virology, including VZV. The virus can be identified by electron microscopy, immune electron microscopy, tissue culture or shell viral culture, immunofluorescence, immunostaining, or detection of viral DNA by PCR.

FIRST-LINE THERAPIES

▶ Symptomatic therapy	C
▶ Aciclovir	A

Acyclovir for treating varicella in otherwise healthy children and adolescents. Klassen TP, Belseck EM, Wiebe N, Hartling L. Cochrane Database Syst Rev 2004; CD002980.

This systematic review concluded that aciclovir initiated within 24 hours after rash onset shows a therapeutic benefit in reducing the length of time with fever and the maximum number of lesions in immunocompetent children. There were no clinically important differences in the number of complications and adverse effects between aciclovir and placebo groups.

The use of oral acyclovir in otherwise healthy children with varicella. Hall CB, Granoff DM, Gromisch DS, Halsey NA, Kohl S, Marcuse EK, et al. Pediatrics 1993; 91: 674–6.

A helpful review article with treatment recommendations. Oral aciclovir is safe, but the cost–benefit ratio of treatment in otherwise healthy children remains to be established. Treatment initiated within 24 hours of onset will typically reduce fever duration by 1 day, and also reduce the severity of the eruption.

Symptomatic treatment with analgesics and topical agents such as calamine lotion or crotamiton cream and daily baths are all that is required in most children.

When required, aciclovir is the antiviral of choice for varicella infection. It is usually given orally. In children up to 12 years of age it is given at a dose of 20 mg/kg 6-hourly (to a maximum of 800 mg/ dose) for 5 days. In adolescents and adults the dose is 800 mg five times daily for 7 days. Aciclovir is given intravenously in severe disease and in immunocompromised individuals.

Acyclovir treatment of varicella in otherwise healthy adolescents. Balfour HH Jr, Rotbart HA, Feldman S, Dunkle LM, Feder HM Jr, Prober CG, et al. J Pediatr 1992; 120: 627–33.

A double-blind, placebo-controlled trial with 62 evaluable subjects. Aciclovir, 800 mg orally four times per day for 5 days, significantly reduced the severity and duration of the illness.

Treatment of adult varicella with oral aciclovir: A randomized, placebo-controlled trial. Wallace MR, Bowler WA, Murray NB, Brodine SK, Oldfield EC III. Ann Intern Med 1992; 117: 358–63.

A study of 148 evaluable military personnel hospitalized for varicella and treated with aciclovir, 800 mg orally five times per day for 7 days, or placebo. Patients treated within 24 hours of onset of the rash had fewer lesions and shorter time to crusting. Treatment after 24 hours had no effect on the disease.

SECOND-LINE THERAPIES

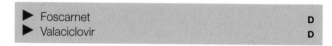

▶ Foscarnet	D
▶ Valaciclovir	D

Foscarnet therapy in five patients with AIDS and aciclovir resistant varicella zoster virus infection. Safrin S, Berger TG, Wolfe PR, Wosby CB, Mills J, Biron KK. Ann Intern Med 1991; 115: 19–21.

Five patients with AIDS and aciclovir-resistant VZV were treated with foscarnet. Four had healing of the lesions and negative cultures during therapy. Fluorescent antigen testing remained positive in two patients: one healed completely, but the other had concomitant clinical failure of therapy.

Foscarnet is used in patients who have developed resistance to aciclovir. The dose is 40 mg/kg 8-hourly in 1-hour transfusions for 10 days.

Varicella in a pediatric heart transplant population on nonsteriod maintenance immunosuppression. Dodd DA, Burger J, Edwards KM, Dummer JS. Pediatrics 2001; 108: E80.

Six of 14 pediatric heart transplant patients with varicella were treated with oral valaciclovir, dose range from 61 to 88 mg/kg/day, for 7 days, one with oral aciclovir for 10 days and seven with intravenous aciclovir for 3 days followed by oral aciclovir for 7 days. All treatment regimens were well tolerated, without complications.

PROPHYLAXIS

▶ Vaccines	A
▶ Varicella zoster immunoglobulin	B
▶ Intravenous immunoglobulin	C
▶ Aciclovir	A

Prevention of varicella. Recommendations of the Advisory Committee on Immunization Practices (ACIP). Marin M, Güris D, Chaves SS, Schmid S, Seward JF. MMWR Recommendations and Reports June 22, 2007 / 56 (RR04); 1–40. http://www.cdc.gov/mmwr/pdf/rr/rr5604.pdf

A comprehensive overview of the available strategies for prophylaxis.

Oka/Merck varicella vaccine in healthy children: Final report of a 2-year efficacy study and 7-year follow-up studies. Kuter BJ, Weibel RE, Guess HA, Matthews H, Morton DH, Neff BJ, et al. Vaccine 1991; 9: 643–7.

A large placebo-controlled trial in children aged 1–14 years demonstrating the varicella vaccine to be 70–90% effective for preventing varicella and more than 95% effective for preventing severe varicella.

Safety and immunogenicity of a combination measles, mumps, rubella and varicella vaccine (ProQuad). Kuter BJ, Hoffman Brown ML, Hartzel J, Williams WR, Eves KA, et al.; Study Group for ProQuad. Hum Vaccin 2006; 2: 205–14.

A single dose of combination measles, mumps, rubella and varicella vaccine (ProQuad) was evaluated in five clinical trials. A single dose in 12–23-month-old children was shown to be as immunogenic as a single dose of MMR II (measles, mumps, and rubella combination vaccine) and Varivax (varicella vaccine) and is well tolerated in a 1- or 2-dose schedule.

Evaluation of varicella zoster immune globulin: Protection of immunosuppressed children after household exposure to varicella. Zaia JA, Levin MJ, Preblud SR, Leszcynski J, Wright CG, Ellis RJ, et al. J Infect Dis 1983; 147: 737–43.

VZIG is effective for prophylaxis.

Intravenous immunoglobulin prophylaxis in children with acute leukaemia following exposure to varicella. Chen SH, Liang DC. Pediatr Hematol Oncol 1992; 9: 347–51.

Five children with leukemia received a single dose (200 mg/kg) of intravenous immunoglobulin within 3 days of exposure to varicella. None developed the infection. IVIG appears to be an effective and safe alternative when hyperimmune zoster immunoglobulin or varicella zoster immunoglobulin is unavailable.

Postexposure prophylaxis of varicella in family contact by oral acyclovir. Asano Y, Yoshikawa T, Suga S, Kobayashi I, Nakashima T, Yazaki T, et al. J. Pediatrics 1993; 92: 219–22.

Twenty-five children were treated with oral aciclovir 40 or 80 mg/kg daily in four divided doses, 7–9 days after household exposure to varicella. Twenty-five age-matched control subjects who had been exposed but did not receive treatment were also followed. Twenty of the 25 treated subjects were protected from disease, but four of them failed to seroconvert. All 25 controls developed varicella.

Although its efficacy is not as well established as that of VZIG, oral aciclovir also seems likely to be effective in post-exposure prophylaxis. It is given approximately 9 days after exposure for 1 week, and may abort the disease or reduce its severity. However, seroconversion and subsequent immunity may also be suppressed.

Antiviral prophylaxis and treatment in chickenpox. A review prepared for the UK Advisory Group on Chickenpox on behalf of the British Society for the Study of Infection. Ogilvie MM. J Infect 1998; 36: 31–8.

A review of the use of varicella zoster immunoglobulin, live attenuated varicella vaccine, and aciclovir. Oral aciclovir is only considered effective if begun within 24 hours of rash onset. It is recommended for treatment of varicella in otherwise healthy adults and adolescents, but not for routine use in children under 13 years of age unless they are sibling contacts or have other medical conditions. Aciclovir has a high therapeutic index and good safety profile, but caution is advised with use in pregnancy.

Chickenpox in pregnancy. Green-top Guideline No. 13. Royal College of Obstetricians and Gynaecologists. September 2007. http://www.rcog.org.uk/resources/Public/pdf/greentop13_chickenpox0907.pdf

Current UK guideline on the treatment of pregnant women with varicella and advice on post-exposure prophylaxis. VZIG is recommended for post-exposure prophylaxis. Oral aciclovir is recommended if patients present within 24 hours of the rash and are at more than 20 weeks' gestation. If delivery occurs within 7 days of maternal infection, or if the mother develops chickenpox within 7 days of giving birth, the neonate should be given VZIG. The infant should be monitored for signs of infection for 28 days after the onset of maternal infection. If neonatal infection occurs, it should be treated with aciclovir.

Viral exanthems: rubella, roseola, rubeola, enterovirus

Leah Belazarian, Lauren Alberta-Wszolek, Karen Wiss

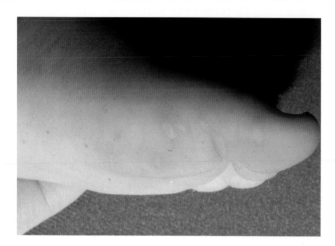

RUBELLA

Rubella (German measles, 3-day measles) is usually a mild disease of low-grade fever, generalized erythematous macules and papules, and generalized lymphadenopathy. It is caused by an enveloped RNA virus of the Togaviridae family.

MANAGEMENT STRATEGY

In children there is typically no prodrome. In adolescents and adults, a prodrome of fever, malaise, sore throat, nausea, anorexia, and generalized lymphadenopathy is often seen. The pink erythematous macules and papules start on the face and neck and spread from the neck down and out in a centrifugal fashion within 1–2 days. The lesions disappear from the face and neck and down in 2–3 days. An enanthem, called Forchheimer spots, consisting of petechiae on the hard palate, may accompany the rash.

Rubella is a self-limited illness that resolves spontaneously. The treatment is *supportive* in most cases. Some individuals, especially teenagers and adults, may have transient polyarthralgia and polyarthritis. Thrombocytopenia and encephalitis are extremely rare. Maternal rubella during the first trimester of pregnancy can result in fetal death or the congenital rubella syndrome. The main fetal anomalies include eye findings (cataracts, glaucoma, microphthalmia, and chorioretinitis), sensorineural deafness, cardiac abnormalities (patent ductus arteriosus, atrial septal defects, ventricular septal defects), pulmonic stenosis, and blueberry muffin lesions (extramedullary hematopoiesis).

It can be difficult to distinguish rubella from other viral exanthems, in particular enteroviruses. Rubella may also mimic measles and infection by parvovirus B19, human herpesvirus-6 (HHV-6), and arboviruses. It is essential that the correct diagnosis is confirmed during pregnancy with suspected congenital infection.

Rubella virus can be isolated from the nose and throat in postnatal infection, and from blood, urine, cerebrospinal fluid, and throat in congenitally infected infants. Antibody testing for rubella-specific IgM will suggest recent infection. A fourfold or greater increase in antibody titer between acute and convalescent IgG titers over several months also suggests infection. Identification of viral RNA by reverse transcription-polymerase chain reaction (RT-PCR) from nasopharyngeal swabs or urine samples has also been established as a method of detection. Children with rubella should be *excluded from school for 7 days after onset of the rash*. *Rubella vaccine* is recommended in combination with the measles and mumps vaccine, with or without varicella vaccine (MMR or MMRV) at 12–15 months of age, with a second dose at school entry between 4 and 6 years of age. Postpubertal females can be tested for rubella IgG antibody and vaccinated. Because the vaccine contains live virus, it should not be given to pregnant women.

SPECIFIC INVESTIGATIONS

- ▶ Viral culture
- ▶ Acute IgM antibody titers
- ▶ Acute and convalescent IgG antibody titers
- ▶ Polymerase chain reaction (PCR)

Rubella virus replication and links to teratogenicity. Lee JY, Bowden DS. Clin Microbiol Rev 2000; 13: 571–87.

The virus has been readily grown in tissue culture and has some unusual features of replication that probably play a role in the teratogenesis.

Comparison of four methods using throat swabs to confirm rubella virus infection. Zhu Z, Xu WB, Abernathy ES, Chen MH, Zheng Q, Wang T, et al. J Clin Microbiol 2007; 45: 2847–52.

Direct reverse transcription PCR followed by southern hybridization was the most sensitive method for detecting rubella virus, compared to viral culture/RT-PCR, immunofluorescence, and replicon-based methods.

FIRST-LINE THERAPIES

▶ Antipyretics – acetaminophen (paracetamol), ibuprofen	E
▶ Analgesics – non-steroidal anti-inflammatory drugs (NSAIDs)	E
▶ School avoidance for 7 days	A
▶ Immunization	A

The epidemiological profile of rubella and congenital rubella syndrome in the United States, 1998–2004: the evidence for absence of endemic transmission. Reef SE, Redd SB, Abernathy E, Zimmerman L, Icenogle JP. Clin Infect Dis 2006; 43: S126–32.

Since the advent of the national rubella vaccination program, epidemiologic evidence strongly supports that rubella virus is no longer endemic in the United States.

The safety and immunogenicity of a quadrivalent measles, mumps, rubella and varicella vaccine in healthy children: a study of manufacturing consistency and persistence of antibody. Lieberman JM, Williams WR, Miller JM, Black S, Shinefield H, Henderson F, et al. Pediatr Infect Dis J 2006; 25: 615–22.

MMRV and MMR + V administered concomitantly have comparable immunogenicity and safety profiles. Both combination vaccines are well tolerated and have long-term persistence of antibodies in the pediatric population.

ROSEOLA

Roseola infantum (exanthem subitum, sixth disease) is an exanthem of young childhood caused by primary infection with HHV-6 or -7. The clinical findings include high fever in a well-appearing child, and a rash with defervescence. The exanthem consists of pink macules and papules that spread from neck down to the trunk and proximal extremities.

MANAGEMENT STRATEGY

Roseola is an illness of children aged between 6 and 36 months. The first sign of illness is a high fever (>39.5°C) that persists for 3–7 days. This is followed by pink macules and papules on the trunk that last hours to days. *Typically, no treatment is necessary* and the illness resolves spontaneously in a few days. Febrile seizures are commonly seen in infants during the febrile phase of the illness. These infants usually require emergency room care.

Identification of virus, either HHV-6 or HHV-7, by culture from the peripheral blood, is currently available only in specialized research laboratories. Amplification of the viruses by polymerase chain reaction (PCR) is available. However, it can be difficult to distinguish active from latent infection, or from chronic persistence. PCR of plasma has been shown to be sensitive and specific for diagnosing primary HHV-6 infection in immunocompetent children. HHV-6 IgM serology is available, but is not very reliable by itself. Seroconversion of IgG antibody in sera collected 2–3 weeks apart with a fourfold increase in titer can be more reliable. There is considerable cross-reactivity between HHV-6, HHV-7, and cytomegaloviruses.

Most individuals harbor HHV-6 and HHV-7 in their saliva throughout their lives. Reactivation of the virus may cause more severe disease, especially in immunocompromised hosts. Reactivation may manifest as fever, bone marrow suppression, hepatitis, pneumonia, lymphoproliferative disorders, and encephalitis. In these patients, *ganciclovir* and *foscarnet* have been recommended by some authors. Ganciclovir and foscarnet are inhibitors of HHV-6 replication in vitro. Individual case reports have suggested benefit from these agents in ill patients.

SPECIFIC INVESTIGATIONS

- ▶ None
- ▶ HHV-6 IgM
- ▶ HHV-6 IgG – acute and convalescent titers
- ▶ PCR for HHV-6

Early diagnosis of primary human herpesvirus 6 infection in childhood: serology, polymerase chain reaction, and virus load. Chiu SS, Cheung CY, Tse CY, Peiris M. J Infect Dis 1998; 178: 1250–6.

Using a combination of these methods improves the sensitivity of diagnosing primary HHV-6 infection.

▶ Antipyretics – acetaminophen, ibuprofen	**E**

SECOND-LINE THERAPIES

▶ Ganciclovir	**D**
▶ Foscarnet	**D**

Determination of antiviral efficacy against lymphotropic herpesviruses utilizing flow cytometry. Long MC, Bidanset DJ, Williams SL, Kushner NL, Kern ER. Antiviral Res 2003; 58: 149–57.

Flow cytometry was used successfully to evaluate HHV-6 and showed inhibition by foscarnet and ganciclovir.

Human herpesvirus type 6 and human herpesvirus type 7 infections of the central nervous system. Dewhurst S. Herpes 2004; 11: 105A–11A.

Ganciclovir and foscarnet may be used for managing HHV-6-related disease. Ganciclovir, but not foscarnet, may be useful for HHV-7-related illness.

Antiviral prophylaxis may prevent human herpesvirus-6 reactivation in bone marrow transplant recipients. Rapaport D, Engelhard D, Tagger G, Or R, Frenkel N. Transpl Infect Dis 2002; 4: 10–16.

In six bone marrow transplant recipients, ganciclovir prevented HHV-6 reactivation.

RUBEOLA

Rubeola (measles) is a systemic illness caused by a paramyxovirus. The clinical signs and symptoms consist of fever, cough, coryza, conjunctivitis, morbilliform rash, and Koplik spots. Complications include pneumonia, croup, diarrhea, acute encephalitis, brain damage, and death from respiratory and neurologic complications. Subacute sclerosing panencephalitis (SSPE) due to persistent measles infection is a rare degenerative neurologic disease that can occur years after the original infection.

MANAGEMENT STRATEGY

The measles rash consists of erythematous macules and papules that begin along the hairline and behind the ears and spread down the body. A pathognomonic enanthem called Koplik spots occurs before the onset of the rash. It is important to distinguish the measles rash from other viral infections, in particular enterovirus infections. Drug eruptions and Kawasaki disease are frequently considered in the differential diagnosis.

Perhaps most clinically useful is a rapid diagnostic technique with immunofluorescence obtained by collecting desquamated nasal mucosa cells. Measles-specific IgM antibody tests from sera collected at the onset of the eruption can be quite useful. Although diagnosis will be delayed, acute and convalescent IgG antibody can be obtained. Measles virus can also be isolated from nasopharyngeal secretions during the febrile phase of the illness.

Children with measles need to be *isolated for 4 days after the onset of the rash*. In the United States and the UK, suspected cases of measles should be *notified* to the appropriate monitoring authorities.

Measles *vaccine* contains live attenuated virus and is recommended as part of the MMR (or MMRV) vaccine at 12–15 months of age, and again at 4–6 years. It can also be given as a measles-only formulation. The vaccine is very effective. Two doses are usually recommended for maximum immunity.

Individuals with poor nutritional states are at greatest risk for complications from measles. *Dietary supplementation with vitamin A* may reduce the morbidity and mortality of the disease. Vitamin A should be given to children aged 6 months to 2 years who are hospitalized for complications of measles. Any children with measles who are immunocompromised, have vitamin A deficiency or malnutrition, or have recently emigrated from areas with high mortality rates for measles are candidates for treatment. Vitamin A supplementation is recommended by the World Health Organization in all communities in which vitamin A deficiency is a problem. The dose suggested is 100 000–200 000 IU as a single oral dose. The dose is given the next day and at 4 weeks if there is clinical evidence or great risk for vitamin A deficiency.

Immunoglobulin prophylaxis can prevent or modify measles in a susceptible person within 6 days of exposure. It is recommended for susceptible household contacts, especially if those contacts are younger than 1 year of age or are pregnant or immunocompromised.

Measles virus is susceptible to *ribavirin* in vitro. It has been given intravenously and nasally to treat immunocompromised children with severe illness.

SPECIFIC INVESTIGATIONS

> ▶ Immunofluorescence
> ▶ IgM antibody
> ▶ IgG antibody – acute and convalescent
> ▶ Viral culture
> ▶ Polymerase chain reaction (PCR)

Development and evaluation of a real-time PCR assay for rapid identification and semi-quantitation of measles virus. Thomas B, Beard S, Jin L, Brown KE, Brown DW. J Med Virol 2007; 79: 1587–92.

Real-time PCR of a variety of clinical samples, including oral fluids, sera, urine, throat swabs, blood samples, and nasopharyngeal aspirates, is a sensitive and specific method of detection for measles virus.

Recommendations from an ad hoc meeting of the WHO Measles and Rubella Laboratory Network (LabNet) on use of alternative diagnostic samples for measles and rubella surveillance. Centers for Disease Control and Prevention (CDC). MMWR Morb Mortal Wkly Rep 2008; 57: 657–60.

Serum-based assays remain the gold standard for detection of measles and rubella virus antibodies. However, alternative sampling techniques, including dried blood spots or oral fluid samples, are viable options for measles and rubella surveillance in parts of the world if serum cannot be obtained. The United States will continue to use serum-based assays or reverse transcription-polymerase chain reaction (RT-PCR) of nasopharyngeal swabs or urine samples for virus detection.

FIRST-LINE THERAPIES

> ▶ Antipyretics – acetaminophen, ibuprofen   **E**
> ▶ Report to local or state health department   **A**
> ▶ Measles vaccine   **A**

Measles surveillance in the United States: an overview. Guris D, Harpaz R, Redd SB, Smith NJ, Papania MJ. J Infect Dis 2004; 189: S177–84.

The elimination of measles is facilitated by reporting and investigation of all suspected measles cases.

Feasibility of global measles eradication after interruption of transmission in the Americas. de Quadros CA, Andrus JK, Danovaro-Holliday MC, Castillo-Solórzano C. Exp Rev Vaccines 2008; 7: 355–62.

Vaccination programs have dramatically reduced measles rates in the world, but some 345 000 deaths still occur each year. Global eradication is possible if appropriate strategies are implemented. Two-dose schedules are needed to eliminate the disease.

Measles – United States, January 1–April 25, 2008. Redd SB, Kutty PK, Parker AA, LeBaron CW, Barskey AE, Seward JF, et al. MMWR Morb Mortal Wkly Rep 2008; 57: 494–8.

Measles was declared eradicated from the United States in 2000 as the result of a successful immunization program, yet 20 million cases of measles occur each year worldwide: 64 confirmed cases were reported to the CDC in the first 4 months of 2008. This upsurge was due to importation of measles from other countries into the United States, in patients who were unvaccinated or had unknown or undocumented vaccination status. Maintaining high levels of vaccination is essential in preventing measles transmission, as the risk for imported disease and outbreaks remains.

SECOND-LINE THERAPIES

> ▶ Oral vitamin A   **A**
> ▶ Immunoglobulin prophylaxis   **A**
> ▶ Ribavirin   **D**

Vitamin A for the treatment of children with measles – a systematic review. D'Souza RM, D'Souza R. J Trop Pediatr 2002; 48: 323–7.

A meta-analysis of randomized controlled trials comparing vitamin A with placebo concluded that 200 000 IU repeated on 2 days should be used for measles treatment in areas where case fatalities are high.

Inhibitors of measles virus. Barnard DL. Antivir Chem Chemother 2004; 15: 111–19.

Oral or intravenous ribavirin given alone or in combination with immunoglobulin has shown variable efficacy in treating severe cases of measles. Effective antiviral therapies are desperately needed.

ENTEROVIRUSES

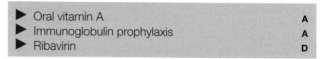

Enteroviruses are a group of non-enveloped single-stranded RNA viruses that includes coxsackieviruses A and B, enteroviruses 68–71, echoviruses, and polioviruses. As polio has been eliminated, non-polioviruses are the main concern. Peaks occur during the summer and fall, transmission is via the orofecal route, and distribution is worldwide. Young children are the most frequently affected. There is a wide spectrum of clinical disease, including mild fever, upper respiratory tract infections, aseptic meningitis, myocarditis, and encephalitis, as well as more specific syndromes such as hand, foot, and mouth disease, herpangina, hemorrhagic conjunctivitis, and pleurodynia.

MANAGEMENT STRATEGY

The majority of enterovirus infections are mild and self-limited. Commonly, fever, malaise, diarrhea, vomiting, and upper respiratory symptoms are noted. The exanthem is typically a non-pruritic morbilliform eruption and often has a petechial component.

Hand, foot, and mouth disease is most commonly caused by coxsackievirus A16. There is a prodrome of fever, malaise, and sore throat. Painful red macules, which become vesicles, develop on the tongue, soft palate, uvula, and tonsillar pillars. Ovoid-shaped vesicles with a surrounding rim of erythema may be noted on the hands, feet, and buttocks. The disease is usually self-limited. Epidemics in Taiwan, caused by enterovirus 71, led to deaths as a result of pulmonary hemorrhage and edema, meningitis, encephalitis, myocarditis, and flaccid paralysis.

Herpangina may present with a similar prodrome. White-gray vesicles with a rim of erythema are later observed on the soft palate, uvula, and tonsillar pillars. Typically fewer than 20 lesions are noted.

Enteroviral infections may be diagnosed by viral culture of the oropharynx or stool, and sometimes the blood, CSF, urine, or tissue. The specific serotype can usually be identified. Disadvantages to viral culture include low sensitivity and the fact that it may take up to 8 days to grow (although they grow faster than most other viruses). Serology is not routinely used to diagnose enteroviral infections, but is commercially available for many enteroviruses. Because all enteroviruses share common genomic sequences, polymerase chain reaction (PCR) can be used to detect almost all enterovirus serotypes.

Treatment of most enteroviral infections, hand, foot, and mouth disease, and herpangina consists of hydration and pain control. Enteroviral infections can be of particular concern in the newborn period and in immunosuppressed patients. Because antibodies do play a role in immunity to enterovirus infections, immunoglobulin has been used by some for severe life-threatening illness in these populations. It is not used for self-limited non-life-threatening infections. Pleconaril is an antiviral drug that prevents viral attaching and uncoating, and has the potential to improve morbidity and mortality associated with enterovirus infection. At present its use is limited to severe life-threatening enteroviral infections and enteroviral meningitis.

SPECIFIC INVESTIGATIONS

> ▶ Viral culture
> ▶ Enteroviral PCR

Enterovirus infections: A review of clinical presentation, diagnosis, and treatment. Stalkup JR, Chilukuri S. Dermatol Clin 2002; 20: 217–23.

Viral culture is the traditional method of confirming enteroviral infection; however, studies have shown that PCR is an even more sensitive diagnostic tool.

FIRST-LINE THERAPIES

> ▶ Antipyretics such as acetaminophen or ibuprofen   E
> ▶ Analgesics   E
> ▶ Hydration   E

SECOND-LINE THERAPIES

> ▶ Immunoglobulin   C
> ▶ Pleconaril   B

Enteroviral infections in children with malignant disease: A 5-year study in a single institution. Moschovi MA, Katsibardi K, Theodoridou M, Michos MG, Tsakris A, Spanakis N, et al. J Infect 2007; 54: 387–92.

Intravenous immunoglobulin improved the viremia associated with severe enteroviral infections.

Enteroviral meningitis: natural history and outcome of pleconaril therapy. Desmond RA, Accortt NA, Talley L, Villano SA, Soong SJ, Whitley RJ. Antimicrob Agents Chemother 2006; 50: 2409–14.

Pleconaril shortened the course of illness in a subgroup of patients with enteroviral meningitis.

Viral warts

Imtiaz Ahmed

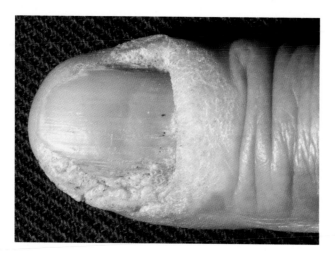

This common disease is caused by infection with various strains of the human papillomavirus. Children present most commonly with warts on the hands and feet. Presentation is often as verruca vulgaris (common warts). Plane warts are frequently seen on the dorsum of the hands or on the face. Genital warts are considered in another chapter.

MANAGEMENT STRATEGY

Most warts will resolve spontaneously with time. However, treatment is demanded by patients, and in the case of children by their parents, for various reasons. Warts may be painful, an object of ridicule, lead to loss of confidence and distorted self-image, worry about loss of employment, a cosmetic concern, or a public health and safety issue. Immunosuppressed patients may have extensive and resistant warts. Before presenting to the physician, patients have usually treated themselves with over-the-counter preparations containing keratolytics or caustics. *Salicylic acid* in various concentration and different bases is the most commonly used and can be applied with or without occlusion. It may cause irritation of the surrounding skin. *Formaldehyde soaks, glutaraldehyde solution,* or *silver nitrate pencils* are also available.

When seen by a physician, the diagnosis and the possibility of spontaneous resolution should be explained. The patient should be educated on how to apply the topical preparations accurately. Keeping the warts well pared down using a file or pumice stone after soaking is important. When patients are referred to a dermatologist, *liquid nitrogen cryotherapy* is one of the most common treatments used. Cryotherapy can be applied with a cotton bud or a cryospray. The wart is frozen from the centre to include a 2-mm rim and the freeze maintained for 5 seconds. Cryotherapy is usually repeated at 1–3-weekly intervals. Hyperkeratotic warts should be pared before cryotherapy, and plantar warts treated by two freeze–thaw cycles. This treatment is painful and not well tolerated by very young children. The warts can be sore or occasionally blister afterwards. In pigmented skin, post-treatment hypo- and hyperpigmentation

can be a problem. Liquid nitrogen cryotherapy can be combined with topical preparations. Cryotherapy with *carbon dioxide snow* or *dimethylether* applicators does not produce temperatures as low as liquid nitrogen and is considered less effective.

If cryotherapy is not successful then various other options are available. *Immunotherapy* with topical application of *diphencyprone* or *squaric acid* and *intralesional mumps/candida* antigen can be effective. Treatment may need to be repeated several times before a response is obtained. *Intralesional bleomycin* using a solution containing 1 IU/mL of bleomycin can be injected into the wart or the solution applied to the wart and then repeatedly pricked through with a lancet. This treatment is quite painful and should only be done by someone with experience. *Surgical excision, CO₂ laser ablation or curettage, and cautery* of troublesome and resistant single warts can be attempted, but the risk of scarring and recurrence in the scar can be a problem. *Pulse dye laser* treatment, by theoretically targeting the rich capillary network in the wart, is sometimes effective.

Other treatments, such as oral *high-dose cimetidine, oral retinoids, topical retinoids* for plane warts, *topical 5-fluorouracil,* and oral levamisole can be tried. In some published series cimetidine has been shown to be effective, particularly in children; however, controlled trials have not shown an advantage over placebo. *Localized heat therapy* using various devices has been effective in some cases. *Photodynamic therapy* using 5-aminolevulinic acid or other photosensitizers may find a place in treatment of resistant warts. *Topical imiquimod* has not lived up to the initial enthusiasm, perhaps due to poor penetration. *Hypnotherapy* and *suggestion* have been described to work and may be tried as a first or last resort, depending, perhaps, on the suggestibility of the physician. *Duct tape occlusion* may work on the same principle or by some other unknown mechanism.

FIRST-LINE THERAPIES

▶ Salicylic acid preparations	B
▶ Glutaraldehyde	B
▶ Silver nitrate	B

An assessment of methods of treating viral warts by comparative treatment trials based on a standard design. Bunney MH, Nolan MW, Williams DA. Br J Dermatol 1976; 94: 667–79.

This is the seminal work on the treatment of warts, describing a series of 11 trials on 1802 patients. In a randomized blind trial involving 389 patients with hand warts, salicylic acid with lactic acid (SAL) paint was as effective as liquid nitrogen cryotherapy performed by the physician. Patients having both treatments concurrently had a better cure rate (78%). The SAL paint comprised one part (17%) salicylic acid, one part (17%) lactic acid, and four parts (66%) of flexible collodion. In another study of 382 plantar warts, 84% of patients with simple plantar warts (n=296) were cured after 12 weeks of regular SAL paint application. In a separate study (n=94), mosaic plantar warts showed a 44% clearance with SAL paint compared to 47% of patients applying 10% glutaraldehyde.

Monochloroacetic acid and 60% salicylic acid as a treatment for simple plantar warts: effectiveness and mode

of action. Steele K, Shirodaria P, O'Hare M, Merrett JD, Irwin WG, Simpson DIH, et al. Br J Dermatol 1988; 118: 537–44.

In this double-blind study of 57 patients with plantar warts, a preparation of monochloroacetic acid and 60% salicylic acid ointment was applied to the wart and left on for 1 week. After this single application, 19 (66%) were cured at week 6 assessment, compared to five (18%) in the placebo group. In view of the severe irritant effect of this preparation, it had to be applied very carefully. In the active group a significant number of patients complained of pain, and one patient developed cellulitis.

Local treatment for cutaneous warts. Gibbs S, Harvey I, Sterling JC, Stark R. Cochrane Database Syst Rev. 2003; (3): CD001781.

Fifty-two trials fulfilled the criteria for inclusion in this review. The best evidence was for the use of preparations containing salicylic acid. Data pooled from six placebo-controlled trials showed a cure rate of 75% in the salicylic acid group compared to 48% in the placebo group.

Efficacy of silver nitrate pencils in the treatment of common warts. Yazar S, Basaran E. J Dermatol 1994; 21: 329–33.

A randomized, placebo-controlled study with 35 patients in each group showed that 1 month after treatment 15 (43%) patients were cleared of warts by three applications of a silver nitrate pencil at 3-day intervals. Only four (11%) of the placebo group responded.

Efficacy of 10% silver nitrate solution in the treatment of common warts: a placebo-controlled, randomized, clinical trial. Sedgheh E, Nader D, Esmaeel J, Bahdor S. Int J Dermatol 2007; 46: 215–17.

In this trial a 10% solution of silver nitrate was applied for 3 weeks on alternate days and carried on for 6 weeks if required by the patient. Of 30 patients, 19 (63%) achieved complete clearance after 6 weeks in the active group.

SECOND-LINE THERAPY

▶ Liquid nitrogen cryotherapy	B

An assessment of methods of treating viral warts by comparative treatment trials based on a standard design. Bunney MH, Nolan MW, Williams DA. Br J Dermatol 1976; 94: 667–79.

This series of trials described a standardized method of cryotherapy using liquid nitrogen applied to the wart with a cotton wool bud just smaller than the wart, using slight vertical pressure, until a frozen halo appeared around its base (5–30 s, according to the thickness of the wart). After 3 months of cryotherapy at 3-week intervals the cure rate in hand warts was 68.6% with liquid nitrogen alone, and 78% when combined with nightly applications of SAL (number of patients in each group around 100). In a separate trial comparing cure rates for hand warts treated when cryotherapy was performed at 2-, 3-, or 4-week intervals for 3 months, the authors conclude that the cure rate for 4-weekly treatments (40%) was significantly less than that for the 2- or 3-weekly treatment groups (78%, 75%).

Value of a second freeze-thaw cycle in cryotherapy of common warts. Berth-Jones J, Bourke J, Eglitis H, Harper C, Kirk P, Pavord S, et al. Br J Dermatol 1994; 131: 883–6.

This randomized parallel-group study of 300 patients suggests that a double freeze–thaw cycle in the cryotherapy of plantar warts (n=121) may be considerably more effective than a single freeze.

Cryotherapy of common viral warts at intervals of 1, 2 and 3 weeks. Bourke JF, Berth-Jones J, Hutchinson PE. Br J Dermatol 1995; 132: 433–6.

This study carried out on 225 patients showed that the cure rate (45%) with liquid nitrogen cryotherapy of hand and foot warts is related to the number of treatments received and independent of the interval between treatments.

Liquid nitrogen cryotherapy of common warts: cryo-spray versus cotton wool bud. Ahmed I, Agarwal S, Ilchyshyn A, Charles-Holmes S, Berth-Jones J. Br J Dermatol 2001; 144: 1006–9.

This prospective study of 363 patients compared cotton wool bud application with cryospray. The authors conclude that cryotherapy with liquid nitrogen for hand and foot warts is equally effective when applied with a cotton wool bud or by means of a cryospray (47% and 44%, respectively) after 3 months of treatment.

THIRD-LINE THERAPIES

Local

▶ Immunotherapy with diphencyprone		C
▶ Immunotherapy with squaric acid dibutylester		C
▶ Immunotherapy with mumps or candida antigen		D
▶ Intralesional bleomycin		A
▶ Intralesional zinc sulphate		B
▶ Surgery, curettage and cautery and laser treatment		C
▶ Topical imiquimod		C
▶ Topical 5-fluorouracil		A
▶ Photodynamic therapy		A
▶ Topical tretinoin		B
▶ Intralesional interferon		C
▶ Formaldehyde soaks		C
▶ Localized heat therapy		C
▶ Intralesional formic acid		B
▶ Topical α-lactalbumin-oleic acid		A
▶ Duct tape application		B
▶ Sodium salicylate iontophoresis		D
▶ Fig tree latex therapy		B
▶ Topical 20% zinc oxide ointment		A

Systemic and others

▶ Oral cimetidine		C
▶ Oral levamisole		A
▶ Oral zinc sulphate		B
▶ Oral retinoids		C
▶ Hypnotherapy		C
▶ Smoke from leaves of *Populus euphratica* olivier		B

Anecdotal reports

▶ Cidofovir		E
▶ Vitamin D3 derivatives		E
▶ Imiquimod and salicylic acid		E

Local

Recalcitrant viral warts treated by diphencyprone immunotherapy. Buckley DA, Keane FM, Munn SE, Fuller LC, Higgins EM, Du Vivier AW. Br J Dermatol 1999; 141: 292–6.

This is a retrospective case series of 60 patients with resistant hand and foot warts. Forty-two of 48 (88%) patients who attended regularly cleared after a mean of five treatments (range 1–22). A concentration of 0.01–6% diphencyprone was used after initial sensitization, and treatments performed at an interval of 1–4 weeks. Painful local blistering (n=11), blistering at site of sensitization (n=9), and a pompholyx-like or more generalized eczematous eruption (n=11) were significant adverse events. Six patients withdrew because of side effects.

In another retrospective series 211 patients were sensitized for treatment of recalcitrant palmoplantar and periungual warts. Out of 154 evaluable patients, 135 (87.7%) cleared completely with an average of five treatments over a 6-month period. (Upitis JA, Krol A. J Cutan Med Surg 2002; 6: 214–17.)

A further case series of 111 patients with resistant warts having up to eight weekly treatments revealed a 60% response rate, with 49 complete and 18 partial remissions. (Rampen FH, Steijlen PM. Dermatology 1996; 193: 236–8.)

Squaric acid immunotherapy for warts in children. Silverberg NB, Lim JK, Paller AS, Mancini AJ. J Am Acad Dermatol 2000; 42: 803–8.

This is a retrospective series of 61 children with warts, treated by home application with squaric acid dibutylester (SADBE) after initial sensitization. The treatment was carried out for between 3 and 7 nights a week for at least 3 months, at a starting concentration of 0.2%. Eleven patients had concomitant therapies. Thirty-four (59%) patients cleared completely and 11 (19%) improved with the treatment. Only two patients had to discontinue treatment because of side effects.

Another retrospective case series of 29 patients showed a 69% clearance with SADBE contact immunotherapy when treated at 2-weekly intervals by a physician. (Lee AN, Mallory SB. J Am Acad Dermatol 1999; 41: 595–9.)

Immunotherapy for recalcitrant warts in children using intralesional mumps or candida antigens. Clifton MM, Johnson SM, Robertson PK, Kincannon J, Horn TD. Pediatr Dermatol 2003; 20: 268–71.

In this study 47 patients with recalcitrant warts were treated intralesionally with mumps or candida antiserum at 3-week intervals, with an average of 3.8 treatments to the largest wart. A complete response in the treated wart was seen in 22 patients (47%); 14 of these experienced resolution of all distant warts as well.

Another study comparing standard treatment with intralesional Candida albicans allergenic extract showed complete clearing in 44 of 87 patients (51%) after an average of 2.3 treatments. In the standard treatment group 46 of 95 patients (48%) cleared after an average of 1.6 treatments. (Signore RJ. Cutis 2002; 7: 185–92.)

A further study showed that 146 of 206 (70.9%) patients treated with a combined candida, mumps, and trichophyton antigen cleared after an average of 4.7 treatments. (Johnson SM, Horn TD. J Drugs Dermatol 2004; 3: 263–5.)

Bleomycin in the treatment of recalcitrant warts. Shumer SM, O'Keefe EJ. J Am Acad Dermatol 1983; 9: 91–6.

In this double-blind, placebo-controlled crossover trial, intralesional injections of bleomycin (1 IU/mL) or saline placebo were performed on two occasions, 2 weeks apart. The warts persisting after two treatments were then treated with the other agent. Twenty-nine of the 40 patients treated with bleomycin cleared, compared to none in the placebo group. Large plantar warts and periungual warts were significantly painful and tender after bleomycin injection.

In two more recent case series intralesional bleomycin sulfate was injected for the treatment of verruca plantaris. (Salk R, Douglas TS. J Am Podiatr Med Assoc 2006; 9: 220–5; and Bleomycin treatment for verrucae. Price NM. SKINmed: Dermatology for the Clinician 2007; 6: 166–71); the overall success of was 87% and 96%, respectively, after a maximum of five treatments.

Dermojet delivery of bleomycin has also shown a similar efficacy of 90% complete or partial clearance after five treatments. (Dermojet delivery of bleomycin for the treatment of recalcitrant plantar warts. Agius E, Mooney JM, Bezzina AC, Yu RC. J Dermatol Treat 2006; 17: 112–16.)

Treatment of viral warts by intralesional injection of zinc sulphate. Sharquie KA, Al-Nuaimy AA. Ann Saudi Med 2002; 22: 26–8.

In this study 2% zinc sulfate solution was injected up to three times at 2-weekly intervals in 173 warts. In 53 patients 98% of the warts responded, whereas in the 176 control warts no spontaneous clearance developed. In the other arm of the study 143 warts in 47 patients were treated with intralesional hypertonic (7%) saline at 2-weekly intervals, with a cure rate of 8% after five treatments. Injection of zinc sulfate solution was more painful than the hypertonic saline, and both injections produced inflammation and pigmentation.

Long-term follow-up evaluation of patients with electrosurgically treated warts. Gibbs RC, Scheiner AM. Cutis 1978; 21: 383–4.

Curettage can be an effective treatment for single or small numbers of warts, particularly filiform warts. Destruction with electrocautery can be tried but is painful and can result in scarring. A questionnaire study looked at the response of warts on extremities following electrocautery and curettage under local anesthesia: 100 questionnaires were sent and 23 were returned, in which 22 warts had responded to treatment and the warts had not recurred.

Pulsed-dye laser versus conventional therapy in the treatment of warts: A prospective randomized trial. Robson KJ, Cunningham NM, Kruzan KL, Patel DS, Kreiter CD, O'Donnell MJ, et al. J Am Acad Dermatol 2000; 43: 275–80.

In this trial of 40 patients pulse dye laser or cryotherapy treatment was performed at 1-month intervals. The response rates after four treatments were similar (66% vs 70%, respectively) in the two groups.

Pulsed-dye laser therapy for viral warts. Kenton-Smith J, Tan ST. Br J Plast Surg 1999; 52: 554–8.

In this series of 28 patients, 95 of 103 recalcitrant warts (>2 years' duration, and failed to respond to at least one conventional treatment) cleared after a mean of 2.1 treatments. A power setting of 6–9 J/cm^2 was used, spot size 5–7 mm, spots overlapped by 1 mm, treatment extending 5 mm beyond the clinical margin of the wart, and there were three passes over each area.

Evidence Levels: **A** Double-blind study **B** Clinical trial ≥ 20 subjects **C** Clinical trial < 20 subjects **D** Series ≥ 5 subjects **E** Anecdotal case reports

Successful treatment of recalcitrant warts in pediatric patients with carbon dioxide laser. Serour F, Somekh E. Eur J Pediatr Surg 2003; 13: 219–23.

In this case series of 40 children (mean age 12.7 years) 54 warts were treated with CO_2 laser ablation under local anesthesia or ring block. Healing time was 4–5 weeks. There was no recurrence at 12 months. No significant or disabling scarring was noticed, but hypopigmentation was noticed in 11 (27.5%) cases.

Er:YAG laser followed by topical podophyllotoxin for hard-to-treat palmoplantar warts. Wollina U. J Cosmet Laser Ther 2003; 5: 35–7.

Recalcitrant warts in 35 patients were ablated once with Er:YAG laser and then treated with topical podophyllotoxin for up to six cycles (one cycle=3 days on, 4 days off topical application). Complete resolution was observed in 31 patients (88.6%). Mild burning and prickling was noted during podophyllotoxin treatment.

A controlled trial on the use of topical 5-fluorouracil on viral warts. Hursthouse MW. Br J Dermatol 1975; 92: 93–5.

This was a placebo-controlled, double-blind, right–left comparison of 5-FU applied daily under occlusion for 4 weeks in 60 patients, including 40 children. In 48 assessable patients, 29 (60%) in the active group cleared, compared to eight (17%) in the placebo group. Onycholysis occurred in 11 patients with fingertip or periungual warts treated with 5-FU.

Topical 5% 5-fluorouracil cream in the treatment of plantar warts: A prospective randomised and controlled clinical study. Salk RS, Grogan KA, Chang TJ. J Drugs Dermatol 2006; 5: 418–24.

In this trial 40 patients were randomized to either 5% 5-FU with tape occlusion or tape occlusion alone with regular debridement for 12 weeks. Of 20 patients in the active group, 19 achieved complete cure, whereas only two of 20 in the tape occlusion-only group were cured.

Topical treatment of warts and mollusca with imiquimod. Hengge UR, Goos M. Ann Intern Med 2000; 132: 95.

In this open trial, 28 of 50 (56%) patients were cleared of their recalcitrant warts after a mean treatment of 9.5 weeks. Some of these patients were immunosuppressed.

In another uncontrolled study of resistant warts, 10 of 37 patients cleared after a mean treatment of 19 weeks with imiquimod applied twice daily. (Topical 5% imiquimod long-term treatment of cutaneous warts resistant to standard therapy modalities. Grussendorf-Conen EI, Jacobs S, Rübben A, Dethlefsen U. Dermatolog. 2002; 205: 139–45.)

Photodynamic therapy with 5-aminolaevulinic acid or placebo for recalcitrant foot and hand warts: randomised double-blind trial. Stender I-M, Na R, Fogh H, Gluud C, Wulf HC. Lancet 2000; 355: 963–6.

In this study 5-ALA photodynamic therapy (PDT) was compared with placebo in a blinded, randomized fashion in the treatment of resistant warts. Three treatments were done at weekly intervals and repeated if the warts persisted 4 weeks after the last treatment. Sixty-four of 104 (56%) warts cleared in the active group, whereas 47 of 102 (42%) warts cleared in the group exposed to placebo and light. The pain associated with the treatment was significant and classed as unbearable in some cases. The authors conclude that ALA PDT is superior to placebo PDT.

Evaluation of the efficacy and safety of 0.05% tretinoin cream in the treatment of plane warts in Arab children. Kubeyinje EP. J Dermatol Treat 1996; 7: 21–2.

In a randomized controlled study of 25 children 85% of warts cleared, compared to 32% in controls.

Treatment of verrucae with alpha-2 interferon. Berman B, Davis-Reed L, Silverstein L, Jaliman D, France D, Lebwohl M. J Infect Dis 1986; 154: 328–30.

In this study of recalcitrant warts, patients were given 0.1 mL of either 10^5 units of IFN or placebo injection into the wart. Single warts were treated in eight patients. Three of the four patients treated with IFN were cured after a course of nine injections given over a period of 3 weeks, compared to one of four patients in the placebo group.

Treatment of plantar warts in children. Vickers CFH. Br Med J 1961; 2: 743–5.

A survey of 646 children with plantar warts showed that 3% formalin foot-soaks for 15–20 minutes each night for 6–8 weeks cured 80% of all plantar warts up to 1 cm in diameter.

Controlled localized heat therapy in cutaneous warts. Stern P, Levine N. Arch Dermatol 1992; 128: 945–8.

In this controlled, randomized trial, 13 patients with 29 warts were treated by a hand-held radiofrequency heat generator device. They were treated on between one and four occasions for 30 seconds so that a temperature of 50°C was achieved in the warts. Twenty-five of the 29 (86%) treated warts cleared, compared to seven of 17 (41%) control warts.

Nd:YAG laser hyperthermia in the treatment of recalcitrant verrucae vulgares (Regensburg's technique). Pfau A, Abd el Raheem TA, Baumler W, Hohenleutner U, Landthaler M. Acta Dermatol Venereol 1994; 74: 212–14.

Hyperthermia of the warts achieved by this method was effective in a 54-year-old woman with recalcitrant verrucae vulgares on the little finger of her right hand and on her left sole. Laser energy was applied twice, with an interval of 6 weeks. Laser output power was 10 W, spot size 8 mm, and irradiation time up to 20 seconds.

Topical formic acid puncture technique for the treatment of common warts. Bhat RM, Vidya K, Kamath G. Int J Dermatol 2001; 40: 415–19.

This was an non-randomized, placebo-controlled trial of 100 patients with common warts comparing 85% formic acid puncture technique with saline placebo. A maximum number of 12 treatments were done on alternate days, and 46 (92%) of the patients in the active group showed clearance after a mean of 4.6 treatments. In the placebo group only three (6%) cleared after a mean of 11.6 treatments. A mild sensation of burning was felt by all patients with formic acid, and six patients in this group developed secondary infection requiring systemic antibiotics.

Treatment of skin papillomas with topical α-lactalbumin-oleic acid. Gustafsson L, Leijonhufvud I, Aronsson A, Mossberg A-K, Svanborg C. N Engl J Med 2004; 350: 2663–72.

In this randomized, placebo-controlled, double-blind study of 40 patients with warts, 20 patients were randomized to topical application of α-lactalbumin-oleic acid under occlusion for 3 weeks. The active agent is a complex produced by binding of α-lactalbumin (from human milk) and oleic acid, which can induce apoptosis in transformed cell lines. Wart volume was reduced by >75% in all 20 patients in the active group, compared to only three of 20 in the placebo group.

The efficacy of duct tape vs cryotherapy in the treatment of verruca vulgaris (the common wart). Focht DR III, Spicer C, Fairchok MP. Arch Pediatr Adolesc Med 2002; 156: 971–4.

Fifty-one patients were randomized to either cryotherapy or duct tape occlusion of one target wart. Cryotherapy was done with a 10-second freeze for a maximum of six treatments every 2–3 weeks. Duct tape was applied every 6 days, the wart being debrided upon removal of the tape, for a maximum of 2 months. Twenty-two (85%) of 26 patients in the duct tape arm had complete resolution of their warts, compared to 15 (60%) of 25 in the cryotherapy group.

A more recent placebo-controlled study has not shown a significant effect of duct tape occlusion in school children. (de Haen M, Spigt MG, van Uden CJT, van Neer P, Feron FJM, Knottnerus A. Arch Paediatr Adolesc Med 2006; 160: 1121–25.)

A similar double-blind randomized controlled trial in adults showed no difference between duct tape and mole skin occlusion. (Wenner R, Askari SK, Cham PMH, Kedrowski DA, Liu A, Warshaw EM. Arch Dermatol 2007; 143: 309–13.)

Treatment of plantar verrucae using 2% sodium salicylate iontophoresis. Soroko YT, Repking MC, Clemment JA, Mitchell PL, Berg RL. Phys Ther 2002; 82: 1184–91.

Twenty patients with plantar warts were treated using 2% sodium salicylate solution with iontophoresis on three occasions 1 week apart, and assessed 3 months after treatment. One patient had complete clearance of their warts, three demonstrated a large reduction in wart area, and 12 exhibited a measurable reduction in wart area.

Comparative study of fig tree efficacy in the treatment of common warts (verruca vulgaris) vs. cryotherapy. Bohlooli S, Mohebipoor A, Mohammadi S, Kouhnavard M, Pashapoor S. Int J Dermatol 2007; 46: 524–6.

In this open prospective left/right comparative study, fig tree latex was applied to warts on one side and cryotherapy on the other side. Self-application of fig tree latex three times daily for at least 4 days resulted in 44% clearance rate, compared to 56% clearance in the cryotherapy group.

Topical zinc oxide vs. salicylic acid-lactic acid combination in the treatment of warts. Khattar JA, Musharrafieh UM, Tamim H, Hamadeh GN. Int J Dermatol 2007; 46: 427–30.

Forty-four patients were randomized to apply either 20% zinc oxide ointment or a 15% salicylic acid combination twice daily for up to 3 months. In the zinc oxide group 50% patients were cured, compared to 42% in the salicylic acid arm.

Systemic and other

Cimetidine therapy for recalcitrant warts in adults. Glass AT, Solomon BA. Arch Dermatol 1996; 132: 680–2.

An open, uncontrolled prospective study of cimetidine, 30–40mg/kg/day, in 20 adult patients with recalcitrant warts. Of the 18 patients who completed 3 months of treatment, 16 (84%) had either dramatic improvement or complete resolution. The treatment was well tolerated.

Cimetidine therapy for warts: A placebo-controlled, double-blind study. Yilmaz E, Alpsoy E, Basaran E. J Am Acad Dermatol 1996; 34: 1005–7.

In this randomized placebo-controlled, double-blind study, 70 patients with multiple warts received either cimetidine 25–40 mg/kg/day or placebo for 3 months. Most patients had previously received conventional treatment for their warts and not responded. Of the 54 evaluable patients, the cure rates in the active and placebo groups were similar (32% and 30.7%, respectively).

Another double-blind placebo-controlled study showed a similar result. The authors, however, suggested a trend towards efficacy in younger patients. (Rogers CJ, et al. J Am Acad Dermatol 1999; 41: 123–7.)

Comparison of combination of cimetidine and levamisole with cimetidine alone in the treatment of recalcitrant warts. Parsad D, Saini R, Negi KS. Australas J Dermatol 1999; 40: 93–5.

In this double-blind study 48 patients were randomized to either high-dose cimetidine alone or in combination with levamisole for 12 weeks. The dose of levamisole was 150 mg on 2 consecutive days per week. In the levamisole plus cimetidine group, 15 (71%) patients were cured compared to eight (38%) in the cimetidine-only group. In the levamisole group, mild side effects were recorded in four patients; however, severe nausea led to withdrawal from the study in two patients.

Verrucae treated by levamisole. Amer M, Tosson Z, Soliman A, Selim AG, Salem A, Al-Gendy AA. Int J Dermatol 1991; 30: 738–40.

A double-blind placebo-controlled study of oral levamisole given at a dose of 5 mg/kg on 3 consecutive days every 2 weeks for up to 5 months in 40 patients with viral warts. In the active treatment group 12 (60%) patients showed complete resolution, compared to one (5%) in the control group.

Another placebo-controlled study of 49 patients with common warts (Schou M, Helin P. Acta Dermatovener (Stockholm) 1977; 57: 449–54) treated with a similar regimen of levamisole failed to show any significant effect.

Oral zinc sulphate in the treatment of recalcitrant viral warts: randomized placebo-controlled clinical trial. Al-Gurairi FT, Al-Waiz M, Sharquie KE. Br J Dermatol 2002; 146: 423–31.

Forty patients with recalcitrant warts were treated with oral zinc sulfate at a dose of 10 mg/kg/day up to a maximum of 600 mg/day for up to 2 months. Almost all patients who completed the study (20 of 23) responded with complete clearance. None in the placebo group responded. All patients suffered with nausea, but not severe enough to discontinue treatment. It was perhaps relevant that all patients with warts had a significantly lower serum zinc level (mean 62.5 ± 10.72) than that of a matched healthy population (mean 87.8 ± 10.06).

Treatment of extensive warts with etretinate: A clinical trial of 20 children. Gelmetti C, Cerri D, Schiuma AA, Menni S. Pediatr Dermatol 1987; 4: 254–8.

This was an open study of 20 children (mean age 8.5 years) with resistant common warts (11), plane warts (2), plantar warts (1), genital warts (3), and mixed (3). A dose of 1 mg/kg/day was given for a maximum of 3 months. Sixteen children cleared and were free of warts at review after 12 months. The other four children had significant improvement. None of the children stopped treatment because of side effects, but one child had transient alopecia which recovered after discontinuation of treatment.

Effects of hypnotic, placebo, and salicylic acid treatments on wart regression. Spanos NP, Williams V, Gwynn MI. Psychosom Med 1990; 52: 109–14.

Patients were randomized to undergo hypnotic suggestion, topical salicylic acid, placebo, or no treatment for their warts for 6 weeks. Six of 10 subjects in the hypnotic group lost one or more wart, compared to four of the remaining 30 patients.

Smoke from leaves of *Populus euphratica* Olivier vs. conventional cryotherapy for the treatment of cutaneous warts: a pilot, randomized, single-blind, prospective study. Rahimi AR, Emad M, Rezaian GR. Int J Dermatol 2008; 47: 393–7.

Consecutive wart patients were randomized to treatment with leaves of the euphratica tree or conventional cryotherapy once weekly for a maximum of 10 treatments. At 22 weeks 16 of 24 (68%) patients treated with smoke from euphratica leaves were cured, compared to 13 of 28 (46%) treated with cryotherapy.

Anecdotal reports

Refractory HPV associated oral warts treated topically with 1–3% cidofovir solutions in HIV-1 infected patients. Husk R, Zouboulis CC, Sander-Bahr C. Br J Dermatol 2005; 152: 590–1.

Intravenous cidofovir for recalcitrant verruca vulgaris in the setting of HIV. Hivnor C, Shepard JW, Shapiro MS, Vittorio CC. Arch Dermatol. 2004; 140: 13–14.

Large plantar wart caused by HPV-66 and resolution by topical cidofovir therapy. Davis MD, Gostout BS, McGovern RM, Persing DH, Schut RL, Pittelkow MR. J Am Acad Dermatol. 2000; 43: 340–3.

Anecdotal reports of wart resolution in HIV with cidofovir.

Topical vitamin D3 derivatives for recalcitrant warts in three immunocompromised patients. Egawa K, Ono T. Br J Dermatol 2004; 150: 374–6.

Anecdotal reports of topical maxacalcitol under occlusion being effective in patients with HTLV-1 infection, SLE and Crohns disease.

There are a few reports of imiquimod combined with salicylic acid being effective in resistant warts, presumably by allowing the imiquimod to penetrate the wart more effectively.

Vitiligo

Suhail M Hadi, James M Spencer

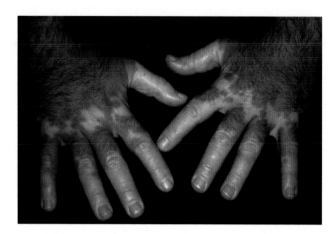

Vitiligo is an acquired idiopathic hypomelanotic disorder in which localized areas are devoid of melanocytes, resulting in depigmented macules which are often symmetrically distributed. The disease has 1–3% worldwide prevalence, with no predilection for age, sex, or race. About 50% of cases start before 20 years of age. Vitiligo can be quite psychologically and socially distressing, and in some cultures results in affected individuals being ostracized. This can lead to severe impairment of a patient's life, particularly if the visible areas of the body (face, hands) are involved. Because of lack of melanin pigment there is an increased risk of sunburn and a theoretic increased risk of skin cancer in the amelanotic areas, and there is an association with ocular abnormalities, especially iritis.

There are many hypotheses to explain the etiology of vitiligo: autoimmune, autocytotoxic (toxic metabolites), neural, hereditary, and environmental factors. The autoimmune theory is supported by the association with a number of autoimmune diseases – thyroid disease, diabetes mellitus, Addison's disease, and pernicious anemia – the finding of organ-specific autoantibodies and circulating antimelanocyte autoantibodies, and, in addition, evidence of cellular immunity by immunohistologic study of perilesional skin and T-cell analysis of peripheral blood. Vitiligo might be induced or exacerbated by drugs, with topical imiquimod being a recent example.

Recent studies have shown that genes play an important role in the pathogenesis of vitiligo. Vitiligo susceptibility genes have been discovered and need further study in the hope that this might help in disease management and prevention. Guidance and support groups can play an important role in alleviating patients' suffering and improving their self-esteem. Lastly, reassurance and psychological therapy may have a positive impact on the progression of the disease.

MANAGEMENT STRATEGY

Even though vitiligo does not cause physical impairment, the associated substantial disfigurement can cause serious emotional stress for the patient, which necessitates treatment. Protection of the vitiliginous areas with sun block is important because of the increased vulnerability of the lesional skin to the effects of ultraviolet light, which makes it more sensitive to sunburn. Cosmetic improvement can be achieved by acceptable camouflage products and self-tanning lotions, and might have psychosocial benefits.

Although vitiligo is a notoriously challenging disease to treat, there are several options. More than one treatment modality should be tried for many months before a patient is deemed resistant to therapy.

Associated autoimmune disease should be looked for. Recommended blood tests include thyroid studies, antinuclear antibodies (ANA), and screening for other organ-specific autoantibodies, fasting blood glucose levels, and complete blood count with indices for pernicious anemia. In generalized vitiligo reversal of helper T cells and suppressor T-cell ratio has been identified.

Treatment options include *topical corticosteroids* and *topical low-dose 8-methoxypsoralen (8-MOP) (0.1%) with UVA* for small, localized patches. For widespread disease, *systemic therapy with 8-MOP, 5-MOP, 4,5,8-trimethylpsoralen or a combination of these, along with sunlight or artificial UVA,* may be beneficial. If the patients do not achieve visible repigmentation after 25–30 sessions with a given psoralen, an alternative therapy should be sought. Topical and systemic PUVA therapy may require 100–300 treatment sessions to achieve complete repigmentation. *Narrowband UVB radiation* and *5-MOP with UVA* have been shown to be effective alternatives to conventional PUVA, with fewer phototoxic effects. Studies have shown that narrowband UVB light stimulates the migration and proliferation of melanocytes, which might explain the beneficial effect of this treatment modality in vitiligo.

L-*Phenylalanine, khellin with UVA, and pseudocatalase with UVA* are other alternative treatments that may be beneficial for some patients. *Topical calcipotriene* has been used in combination with topical corticosteroids, with narrowband UVB, and with PUVA, with some success. The most recent effective and approved therapy for vitiligo is the *308-nm excimer laser* with or without *topical calcineurin antagonists* (tacrolimus and pimecrolimus). The pattern of repigmentation differs with different treatment modalities: it can be perifollicular, marginal, or diffuse.

For patients with refractory segmental or localized disease, thin split-thickness and suction blister *epidermal grafting* have been reported to be the most effective transplantation methods. Single hair grafting is effective for eyelid and eyebrow disease. Other surgical methods are autologous non-cultured melanocyte–keratinocyte cell transplantation and cultured pure melanocyte suspension.

Cosmetic tattooing is used for localized stable vitiligo, especially of the mucosal type.

Patients with extensive disease (>50% body area) who desire permanent matching of skin color but for whom repigmentation is not possible can be depigmented with *20% monobenzyl ether of hydroquinone*, twice daily for 9–12 months. The results are excellent but irreversible. For vitiligo universalis, treatment with topical 4-methoxyphenol and the Q-switched ruby laser has been effective. The psychological impact of the disease being a stigmatizing condition, the effect on the patient's quality of life should be addressed.

Evidence Levels: **A** Double-blind study **B** Clinical trial ≥ 20 subjects **C** Clinical trial < 20 subjects **D** Series ≥ 5 subjects **E** Anecdotal case reports

SPECIFIC INVESTIGATIONS

▶ Antinuclear antibodies (ANA)
▶ Complete blood count with indices
▶ Fasting blood glucose
▶ Thyroid-stimulating hormone (TSH) and thyroid autoantibodies
▶ Immunohistopathology of skin

Occurrence of organ-specific and systemic autoimmune diseases among the first- and second-degree relatives of Caucasian patients with connective tissue diseases: report of data obtained through direct patient interviews. Mosca M, Carli L, d'Ascanio A, Tani C, Talarico R, Baldini C, et al. Clin Rheumatol 2008; 27: 1045–8.

To study familial aggregation of systemic and/or organ-specific autoimmune diseases, 626 patients were involved; 50% of patients vs 25% of controls were found to have at least one relative with an autoimmune disease.

Clinical and immunological studies in vitiligo in the United Arab Emirates. Galadari I, Bener A, Hadi S, Lestringant GG. Allerg Immunol (Paris) 1997; 29: 297–9.

Sixty-five patients with vitiligo were evaluated. A positive family history of vitiligo was found in 19% of patients. An association with other autoimmune diseases was found in 6%.

Autoimmune diseases in vitiligo: do anti-nuclear antibodies (ANA) decrease thyroid volume? Zettinig G, Tanew A, Fischer G, Mayr W, Dudczak R, Weissel M. Clin Exp Immunol 2003; 131: 347–54.

In this study, 106 patients with vitiligo and 38 controls were evaluated. Autoimmune thyroiditis (AT) was significantly more frequent in vitiligo (21% vs 3%). Vitiligo may precede AT by 4–35 years. Vitiligo patients with elevated ANA had significantly smaller thyroid volume than those with normal ANA. No statistically significant association with HLA was found in vitiligo patients.

Histopathologic features in vitiligo. Kim YC, Kim YJ, Kang HY, Sohn S, Lee ES. Am J Dermatopathol 2008; 30: 112–16.

One hundred patients with vitiligo and 30 patients with nevus depigmentosus were studied. There were fewer melanocytes and melanin in vitiligo. There was more basal hypopigmentation and dermal inflammation in vitiligo than in the perilesional normal skin.

Inflammatory changes in vitiligo: stage I and II depigmentation. Sharquie KE, Mehenna SH, Naji AA, Al-Azzawi H. Am J Dermatopathol 2004; 26: 108–12.

Epon-embedded sections from 25 patients with vitiligo and 11 normal volunteers were studied. Focal spongiosis was found in 48% of vitiligo patients (marginal areas and stage I vitiligo). An epidermal mononuclear cell infiltrate was found in 80% of both marginal skin and stage I vitiligo. The number of inflammatory cells was more than in stage II vitiligo and uninvolved skin. Thus, the authors concluded that vitiligo is an inflammatory disease and the epidermal lymphocytic infiltrate is most likely the primary immunologic event.

New insights into the pathogenesis of vitiligo: imbalance of epidermal cytokines at sites of lesions. Moretti S, Spallanzani A, Amato L, Hautmann G, Gallerani I, Fabiani M, et al. Pigment Cell Res 2002; 15: 87–92.

In vitiligo the expression of epidermal cytokines may be modified compared to normal skin. Fifteen patients with active non-segmental vitiligo were evaluated. Compared to perilesional, non-lesional, and healthy skin, in vitiligo skin there was significantly lower expression of keratinocyte-derived cytokines with stimulatory activity on melanocytes, e.g., granulocyte–monocyte colony-stimulating factor, and significantly higher expression of keratinocyte-derived cytokines with inhibitory activity on melanocytes, e.g., interleukin-6 and tumor necrosis factor-α.

The majority of patients with vitiligo do not have an accompanying systemic disease, but directed medical history and blood tests are helpful to identify high-risk individuals who require further evaluation.

FIRST-LINE THERAPIES

▶ Topical corticosteroids	A
▶ Topical photochemotherapy	B
▶ Systemic photochemotherapy	A
▶ Narrowband UVB (NBUVB)	A
▶ 308-nm excimer laser	B
▶ Topical tacrolimus or pimecrolimus	B
▶ Topical tacrolimus plus 308-nm excimer laser	A
▶ Topical calcineurin antagonists plus NBUVB	A
▶ Topical calcipotriene and narrowband UVB	C
▶ Monochromatic excimer light	B
▶ Topical tacalcitol plus sunlight	E
▶ Narrowband UVB microphototherapy	B

A double-blind randomized trial of 0.1% tacrolimus vs 0.05% clobetasol for the treatment of childhood vitiligo. Lepe V, Moncada B, Castanedo-Cazares JP, Torres-Alvarez MB, Ortiz CA, Torres-Rubalcava AB. Arch Dermatol 2003; 139: 581–5.

Twenty patients with vitiligo were treated for 2 months: 90% experienced some repigmentation. The mean percentage of repigmentation was 49.3% for clobetasol and 41.3% for tacrolimus. The authors concluded that tacrolimus is almost as effective as clobetasol and is better for sensitive areas (eyelids) because, unlike clobetasol, it does not cause skin atrophy.

Ophthalmologic examination should be performed after starting topical corticosteroids on the eyelids.

Treatment of vitiligo with UV-B radiation vs topical psoralen plus UV-A. Westerhof W, Nieuweboer-Krobotova L. Arch Dermatol 1997; 133: 1525–8.

Patients with extensive vitiligo were treated with topical PUVA for 4 months (n=28) or 311-nm UVB radiation for 4 months (n=78). Forty-six percent of patients treated with topical PUVA and 67% of patients treated with the 311-nm UVB showed repigmentation. The authors concluded that narrowband UVB is as efficient as topical PUVA but with fewer adverse effects.

Randomized double-blind trial of treatment of vitiligo: efficacy of psoralen-UV-A therapy vs narrowband-UV-B therapy. Yones SS, Palmer RA, Garibaldinos TM, Hawk JL. Arch Dermatol 2007; 143: 643–6.

This study involved 56 patients with vitiligo. Narrowband UVB was superior to PUVA in producing >50% pigmentation (64% vs 36%).

Narrow-band UVB for the treatment of generalized vitiligo in children. Kanwar AJ, Dogra S. Clin Exp Dermatol 2005; 30: 332–6.

Twenty-six children 5–14 years old with generalized vitiligo were treated with narrowband UVB three times per week for a maximum of 1 year; 75% developed marked to complete repigmentation.

Efficacy, predictors of response, and long-term follow-up in patients with vitiligo treated with narrowband UVB phototherapy. Nicolaidou E, Antoniou C, Stratigos AJ, Stefanaki C, Katsambas AD. J Am Acad Dermatol 2007; 56: 274–8.

Seventy patients with vitiligo were treated with narrowband UVB twice weekly: >75% pigmentation was achieved in 34.4% of those with lesions on the face. Pigmentation was stable in 14.3% of patients 4 years after cessation of treatment.

Treatment of vitiligo using the 308-nm excimer laser. Hadi S, Tinio P, Al-Ghaithi K, Al-Qari H, Al-Helalat M, Lebwohl M, et al. Photomed Laser Surg 2006; 24: 354–7.

Two hundred and twenty-one patches of vitiligo in 97 patients were treated with this laser; 50.6% of patients achieved 75% pigmentation or more, 64.3% achieved 50% pigmentation or more. Lesions on the face respond best. UV-sensitive areas of the body (face, neck, and trunk) tended to respond much better than UV-resistant areas (bony prominences, extremities).

The excimer laser, emitting light at 308 nm, has recently become available as a new form of phototherapy. The laser light emitted from this laser is in the UVB range. It is possible that the light–tissue interaction is different when the light is given in the form of laser light rather than conventional incoherent light, and may produce a superior result.

Tacrolimus ointment promotes repigmentation of vitiligo in children: a review of 57 cases. Silverberg NB, Lin P, Travis L, Farley-Li J, Mancini AJ, Wagner AM, et al. J Am Acad Dermatol 2004; 51: 760–6.

Fifty-seven children with vitiligo were treated with topical tacrolimus for at least 3 months. Tacrolimus was effective for childhood vitiligo, especially on the head and neck (89% response rate). Sixty-three percent of patients with lesions on the extremities responded.

Combined excimer laser and topical tacrolimus for the treatment of vitiligo: a pilot study. Kawalek AZ, Spencer JM, Phelps RG. Dermatol Surg 2004; 30: 130–5.

Twenty-four patches in eight patients with vitiligo (elbows, knees) were treated with the excimer laser three times a week for 24 sessions or 10 weeks. In addition, topical tacrolimus 0.1% ointment and placebo were applied to randomized patches twice daily throughout the trial. Fifty percent of patches treated with combination excimer laser and tacrolimus achieved a successful response (75% pigmentation), compared to 20% for the placebo group.

The efficacy of pimecrolimus 1% cream plus narrow-band ultraviolet B in the treatment of vitiligo: A double-blind, placebo-controlled clinical trial. Esfandiarpour I, Ekhlasi A, Farajzadeh S, Shamsadini S. J Dermatol Treat 2008; 16: 1–5.

This study involved 68 patients. A combination of NB-UVB with pimecrolimus induced better pigmentation of facial lesions than did NB-UVB alone (64.3% vs 25.1%).

Topical calcipotriene and narrowband ultraviolet B in the treatment of vitiligo. Kullavanijaya P, Lim HW. Photodermatol Photoimmunol Photomed 2004; 20: 248–51.

Twenty patients with symmetrical vitiligo were treated with narrowband UVB three times per week; in addition, calcipotriene ointment was applied to lesions on one side of the body. Nine of 17 patients who completed the study achieved appreciably better pigmentation on the UVB plus calcipotriene side.

Comparison between 308-nm monochromatic excimer light and narrowband UVB phototherapy (311–313 nm) in the treatment of vitiligo – a multicentre controlled study. Casacci M, Thomas P, Pacifico A, Bonnevalle A, Paro Vidolin A, Leone G. J Eur Acad Dermatol Venereol 2007; 21: 956–63.

Twenty-one patients were involved in this comparative study. Treatment was given twice weekly for 6 months. The 308-nm monochromatic excimer light was found to be more effective than NB-UVB.

The light from the 308 nm monochromatic excimer light can treat large areas within a short time.

First case report of topical tacalcitol for vitiligo repigmentation. Amano H, Abe M, Ishikawa O. Pediatr Dermatol 2008; 25: 262–4.

A combination of tacalcitol (vitamin D$_3$ ointment) and sunlight induced complete pigmentation of vitiliginous patches in a child.

Narrow-band UV-B micro-phototherapy: a new treatment for vitiligo. Menchini G, Tsoureli-Nikita E, Hercogova J. J Eur Acad Dermatol Venereol 2003; 17: 171–7.

A total of 734 patients with vitiligo (segmental and nonsegmental) underwent a mean of 24 sessions of focused beam narrowband UVB (microphototherapy – Bioskin) over 12 months. Approximately 70% achieved normal pigmentation on more than 75% of the treated areas.

SECOND-LINE THERAPIES

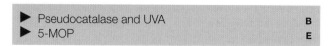

| ▶ Pseudocatalase and UVA | B |
| ▶ 5-MOP | E |

From basic research to the bedside: efficacy of topical treatment with pseudocatalase PC-KUS in 71 children with vitiligo. Schallreuter KU, Krüger C, Würfel BA, Panske A, Wood JM. Int J Dermatol 2008; 47: 743–53.

Seventy-one children with vitiligo were studied using low-dose, narrowband UVB-activated pseudocatalase. Topical pseudocatalase was applied to the entire body twice daily and 100% cessation was observed in 70 of the 71 children. More than 75% repigmentation was seen in 66 of 71 patients on the face and/or neck. This shows that narrowband UVB-activated pseudocatalase is an effective treatment for childhood vitiligo.

5-Methoxypsoralen. A review of its effects in psoriasis and vitiligo. McNeely W, Goak KL. Drugs 1998; 56: 667–90.

Treatment with oral 5-MOP (not available in the USA) and oral 8-MOP resulted in similar lesion clearance rates. Patients treated with 5-MOP often required a greater total UV exposure than 8-MOP recipients. Short-term cutaneous and gastrointestinal side effects were markedly less with 5-MOP, although the long-term tolerability of this treatment has not yet been established.

THIRD-LINE THERAPIES

▶ Monobenzyl ether of hydroquinone (MBEHQ)	C
▶ l-Phenylalanine and UVA	B
▶ Khellin and UVA (KUVA)	B
▶ Topical fluorouracil	B
▶ Surgical grafting	B
▶ Ruby laser	C
▶ Cosmetic tattooing	B

Monobenzyl ether of hydroquinone. Moser D, Parrish J, Fitzpatrick T. Br J Dermatol 1977; 97: 669–79.

Of 18 patients treated with MBEHQ therapy twice daily over a 1-year period, eight achieved complete depigmentation, three had marked but not complete depigmentation, and the remaining seven had either poor or no depigmentation. The depigmentation is permanent. Major side effects are erythema, pruritus, contact dermatitis, and complete and irreversible depigmentation at the application sites and also at remote sites.

A case study to evaluate the treatment of vitiligo with khellin encapsulated in l-phenylalanine stabilized phosphatidylcholine liposomes in combination with ultraviolet light therapy. de Leeuw J, van der Beek N, Maierhofer G, Neugebauer WD. Eur J Dermatol 2003 13: 474–7.

The efficacy of treatment with khellin encapsulated in l-phenylalanine-stabilized phosphatidylcholine liposomes in combination with UVA/UVB light was assessed in 74 patients with vitiligo; 72% of treated lesions showed 50–100% repigmentation. The control group who received light therapy alone showed hardly any result.

Comparative evaluation of the therapeutic efficacy of dermabrasion, dermabrasion combined with topical 5% 5-fluorouracil cream, and dermabrasion combined with topical placentrex gel in localized stable vitiligo. Sethi S, Mahajan BB, Gupta RR, Ohri A. Int J Dermatol 2007; 46: 875–9.

Thirty patients with localized stable vitiligo were studied. Dermabrasion combined with 5-fluorouracil gave the best results (73.33%).

A systematic review of autologous transplantation methods in vitiligo. Njoo MD, Westerhof W, Bos JD, Bossuyt PM. Arch Dermatol 1998; 134: 1543–9.

Sixty-three studies were analyzed: 16 on minigrafting, 13 on split-thickness grafting, 15 on grafting of epidermal blisters, 17 on grafting of cultured melanocytes, and two on grafting of non-cultured epidermal suspension. The highest mean success rates were achieved with split-skin grafting and epidermal blister grafting. No controlled trials were included. No conclusion could be drawn about the effectiveness of culturing techniques because of the small sample sizes studied. *A good review article.*

Autologous melanocyte transfer via epidermal grafts for lip vitiligo. Gupta S, Goel A, Kanwar AJ, Kumar B. Int J Dermatol 2006; 45: 747–50.

Twenty-six patients with lip vitiligo were treated. Suction blisters were used followed by photochemotherapy. Complete pigmentation was achieved in 92% of the patients.

Treatment of vitiligo by transplantation of cultured pure melanocyte suspension: analysis of 120 cases. Chen YF, Yang PY, Hu DN, Kuo FS, Hung CS, Hung CM. J Am Acad Dermatol 2004; 51: 68–74.

A total of 120 patients were treated with transplantation of autologous cultured pure melanocyte suspension after CO_2 laser abrasion. Overall, 90–100% coverage was achieved in 84% of patients with stable localized vitiligo and in 54% of patients with stable generalized vitiligo, but only 14% of patients with active generalized vitiligo achieved good repigmentation.

Repigmentation of vitiligo with punch grafting and narrow-band UV-B (311 nm) – a prospective study. Lahiri K, Malakar S, Sarma N, Banerjee U. Int J Dermatol 2006; 45: 649–55.

Punch grafts were used to treat 66 patients with stable refractory vitiligo in different regions, followed by narrow-band UVB. Successful pigmentation was achieved in 86.36% of cases.

Comparison of minipunch grafting versus split-skin grafting in chronic stable vitiligo. Khandpur S, Sharma VK, Manchanda Y. Dermatol Surg 2005; 31: 436–41.

Sixty-four patients with stable vitiligo were involved in the study. Grafting was followed by PUVAsol. Split-skin grafting gave much better repigmentation and cosmetic matching than minipunch grafting (83.3% of patients vs 44.1%).

Subjective and objective evaluation of noncultured epidermal cellular grafting for repigmenting vitiligo. van Geel N, Vander Haeghen Y, Vervaet C, Naeyaert JM. Ongenae K. Dermatology 2006; 213: 23–9.

Non-cultured autologous melanocytes and keratinocytes were used to treat 40 patients with stable refractory vitiligo: 70% or more repigmentation was noted in 62% of patients.

Single hair grafting for the treatment for vitiligo. Na GY, Seo SK, Choi SK. J Am Acad Dermatol 1998; 38: 580–4.

Fourteen of 17 patients with localized/segmental vitiligo and one of four patients with generalized vitiligo achieved perifollicular pigmentation. Single hair grafting is especially effective for small vitiliginous areas, and on hairy parts of the skin such as the eyelids and eyebrows.

Depigmentation therapy in vitiligo universalis with topical 4-methoxyphenol and the Q-switched ruby laser. Njoo MD, Vodegel RM, Westerhof W. J Am Acad Dermatol 2000; 42: 760–9.

Eleven of 16 patients treated with 4-methoxyphenol (4-MP) cream twice daily achieved total depigmentation within 6–24 months. Four of the patients had recurrences after a treatment-free period of between 2 and 36 months. Four of the five patients who did not respond to 4-MP were subsequently successfully treated with the Q-switched ruby (QSR) laser. Nine of 13 patients treated between twice and 10 times with the QSR laser achieved total depigmentation. Three of the four unresponsive patients had successful depigmentation with the 4-MP cream.

Evaluation of cosmetic tattooing in localized stable vitiligo. Mahajan BB, Garg G, Gupta RR. J Dermatol 2002; 29: 726–30.

Thirty patients with localized, stable vitiligo – 19 with skin lesions, nine with mucosal lesions, and two with both skin and mucosal lesions – were treated and followed up for 6 months. Color matching was considered excellent in 23 cases (76.7%). Excellent results were achieved in all mucosal patches.

Vulvodynia

Bethanee J Schlosser, Ginat W Mirowski

Vulvodynia is defined by the International Society for the Study of Vulvovaginal Disease (ISSVD) as 'vulvar discomfort, most often described as burning pain, occurring in the absence of relevant visible findings or a specific, clinically identifiable neurologic disorder.' It describes a group of symptoms, including burning, stinging, irritation, and rawness, but does not indicate a specific etiology. Vulvodynia is a complex disorder of unknown etiology attributed to altered sensory perception and is a diagnosis of exclusion. Terms previously used include burning vulva syndrome, vestibular adenitis, vulvar vestibulitis syndrome, dysesthetic vulvodynia, essential vulvodynia, and general or localized vulvar dysesthesia. Current classification divides vulvodynia into generalized and localized types which are subcategorized into provoked (requiring physical stimulus to elicit pain), unprovoked (pain in the absence of stimulus), and mixed (provoked and unprovoked).

A thorough examination and appropriate laboratory testing should be performed to exclude infections and dermatoses. Neurologic conditions and referred pain from the genitourinary or gastrointestinal tracts should also be excluded. This chapter will focus on strategies for the management of vulvodynia.

MANAGEMENT STRATEGY

Management should focus on excluding other etiologies of vulvar pain. Symptomatic relief is a priority. In addition to the physical discomfort, patients also find vulvodynia psychologically distressing and socially embarrassing. A multidisciplinary approach to the treatment of vulvodynia includes dermatology, gynecology, rehabilitation medicine, physical therapy, neurology, gastroenterology, urology, and others as indicated.

Once vulvodynia is diagnosed, appropriate treatment may be instituted. The mainstay of treatment is the use of low-dose antidepressant regimens with *amitriptyline, imipramine,* and *desipramine,* and anticonvulsants such as *gabapentin.* Relief may not be immediate, and the patient should be advised to undergo an adequate course of therapy before determining treatment failure. Surgical interventions should be reserved for the treatment of refractory cases of localized vulvodynia using vestibulectomy.

SPECIFIC INVESTIGATIONS

- ▶ Clinical visual and manual examination of the vulva, vagina, oral cavity, conjunctivae, total body skin, scalp, and nails
- ▶ Clinical palpation of inguinal lymph nodes
- ▶ Sensory testing for light touch and Q-Tip evaluation of the vulva and vaginal vestibule
- ▶ Normal saline wet mount of vaginal secretions (*Trichomonas vaginalis*, bacterial vaginosis, atrophic vaginitis)
- ▶ pH assessment of vaginal secretions (bacterial vaginosis, atrophic vaginitis)

- ▶ Whiff test (bacterial vaginosis)
- ▶ KOH microscopic examination (fungi, scabies infestation)
- ▶ Microbiologic cultures (bacterial, fungal, viral)
- ▶ Tape test, if perirectal pruritus present (*Enterobius vermicularis*, pinworms)
- ▶ Papanicolaou smear
- ▶ Colposcopy of vulva (*Candida* species, dysplasia)
- ▶ Biopsy, if primary skin lesion present
- ▶ Blood glucose
- ▶ Trial of hormone replacement therapy
- ▶ Patch testing (allergic contact dermatitis)
- ▶ Evaluation for the presence of primary or concomitant psychiatric disorders

2003 ISSVD terminology and classification of vulvodynia: a historical perspective. Moyal-Barracco M, Lynch PJ. J Reprod Med 2004; 49: 772–7.

A summary of the definition and clinical classification of vulvar pain.

The vulvodynia guideline. Haefner HK, Collins ME, Davis GD, Edwards L, Foster DC, Hartmann ED, et al. J Low Genit Tract Dis 2005; 9: 40–51.

This review of the literature provides information on the diagnosis and treatment of vulvodynia.

Vulvodynia: strategies for treatment. Goldstein AT, Marinoff SC, Haefner HK. Clin Obstet Gynecol 2005; 48: 769–85.

A review of the epidemiology, etiology, and clinical approach to the treatment of vulvodynia.

FIRST-LINE THERAPIES

▶ Low-dose antidepressants (amitriptyline, desipramine, etc.)	B
▶ Topical lidocaine	B
▶ Anticonvulsants (gabapentin, pregabalin)	C

Response to treatment in dysaesthetic vulvodynia. Munday PE, McKay M. J Obstet Gynaecol 2001; 21: 610–13.

Thirty-two women were treated with a tricyclic antidepressant and behavioral interventions: a complete response was recorded in 47% after 6 months.

Treatment of vulvodynia with tricyclic antidepressants: efficacy and associated factors. Reed BD, Caron AM, Gorenflo DW, Haefner HK. J Low Genit Tract Dis 2006; 10: 245–51.

A prospective cohort study of 209 women diagnosed with vulvodynia and treated initially with a tricyclic antidepressant (amitriptyline in 183 patients, desipramine in 23, and others in three). Of 83 women taking a tricyclic antidepressant at first follow-up (median 3.2 months), 59.3% improved by >50% versus 38% of women not taking a tricyclic antidepressant.

Overnight 5% lidocaine ointment for treatment of vulvar vestibulitis. Zolnoun DA, Hartmann KE, Steege JF. Obstet Gynecol 2003; 102: 84–7.

Sixty-one women with vulvar vestibulitis were instructed to place a cotton ball coated with 5% lidocaine ointment in the vestibule and apply the ointment to the affected areas nightly for an average of 7 weeks: 57% reported a 50% or greater reduction in pain with intercourse. Nearly two-thirds of the women who were unable to have intercourse prior to treatment reported the ability to have intercourse after treatment.

Evaluation of gabapentin in the treatment of generalized vulvodynia, unprovoked. Harris G, Horowitz B, Borgida A. J Reprod Med 2007; 52: 103–6.

A retrospective chart review of 152 women diagnosed with generalized vulvodynia, treated with gabapentin as monotherapy and followed for at least 30 months; 64% experienced at least 80% resolution of symptoms; 32% did not have adequate resolution. Sleep disturbance was the only comorbidity found to negatively affect gabapentin efficacy. There was a trend towards a less favorable response to gabapentin in patients with longer periods of untreated vulvodynia.

Pregabalin-induced remission in a 62-year-old woman with a 20-year history of vulvodynia. Jerome L. Pain Res Manage 2007; 12: 212–14.

Case report of a 62-year-old woman with a 20-year history of vulvodynia recalcitrant to other medications who responded positively to pregabalin.

SECOND-LINE THERAPIES

▶ Electromyographic biofeedback	B
▶ Nitroglycerin cream	B
▶ Acupuncture	C

Treating vulvar vestibulitis with electromyographic biofeedback of pelvic floor musculature. McKay E, Kaufman RH, Doctor U, Berkova Z, Glazer H, Redko V. J Reprod Med 2001; 46: 337–42.

Twenty-nine patients performed biofeedback-assisted pelvic floor muscle rehabilitation exercises. Of the 29 women, 20 (69%) became sexually active and 24 (83%) reported negligible or mild pain. Five of the 29 did not show any significant improvement.

EMG biofeedback versus topical lidocaine gel: a randomized study for the treatment of women with vulvar vestibulitis. Danielsson I, Torstensson T, Brodda-Jansen G, Bohm-Starke N. Acta Obstet Gynecol Scand 2006; 85: 1360–7.

A prospective, randomized study of 46 women with vulvar vestibulitis treated with either electromyographic biofeedback or topical lidocaine for 4 months. Both groups showed statistically significant improvements on vestibular pain measurements, sexual functioning, and psychosocial adjustment at 12 months' follow-up. No differences were detected between the treatment groups. Compliance with electromyographic biofeedback training was low.

Safety and efficacy of topical nitroglycerin for treatment of vulvar pain in women with vulvodynia: a pilot study. Walsh KE, Berman JR, Berman LA, Vierregger K. J Gend Specif Med 2002; 5: 21–7.

Thirty-four women were treated with 0.2% nitroglycerin cream applied directly to the skin of the affected area at least three times per week, 5–10 minutes prior to sexual relations. Nearly all reported a significant improvement in pain.

Acupuncture for the treatment of vulvar vestibulitis: a pilot study. Danielsson I, Sjoberg I, Ostman C. Acta Obstet Gynecol Scand 2001; 80: 437–41.

Fourteen young women with vulvar vestibulitis were enrolled in the study, and 13 completed the acupuncture treatment a total of 10 times. For evaluation, quality of life (QOL) assessments were made before starting the treatment and then at 1 week and 3 months post treatment. The treatment was well tolerated, and QOL measurements were all significantly higher both after the last acupuncture and at 3 months, compared to pretreatment measures.

THIRD-LINE THERAPIES

▶ Urinary oxalate reduction therapy	B
▶ Surgery	D
▶ Botulinum toxin A	E
▶ Hypnosis	E
▶ Psychotherapy	E
▶ Spinal cord stimulator	E

Influence of dietary oxalates on the risk of adult-onset vulvodynia. Harlow BL, Abenhaim HA, Vitonis AF, Harnack L. J Reprod Med 2008; 53: 171–8.

A population-based, case–control study of women with and without vulvodynia: 242 vulvodynia cases and 242 controls were assessed for dietary oxalate consumption in order to calculate the odds ratio for developing vulvodynia as a result of self-reported consumption of dietary oxalate. No differences were observed in oxalate consumption patterns between patients and controls. There was no increase in the risk of developing vulvodynia with increasing tertiles of estimated oxalate intake.

Pudendal canal syndrome as a cause of vulvodynia and its treatment by pudendal nerve decompression. Shafik A. Eur J Obstet Gynecol Reprod Biol 1998; 80: 215–20.

Eleven women with vulvodynia ranging in age from 28 to 53 years had a significant increase in pudendal nerve terminal motor latency, and motor and sensory changes suggested a pudendal canal syndrome. Pudendal nerve block, as a diagnostic and therapeutic test, effected temporary pain relief. Pudendal nerve decompression was performed via a fasciotomy to release the pudendal nerve in the ischiorectal fossa. Vulvar pain disappeared in nine of the 11 patients. Stress urinary incontinence was relieved in four of six patients, anal reflex normalized in five of seven, and vulvar and perineal hypoesthesia in four of six.

A randomized comparison of group cognitive-behavioral therapy, surface electromyographic biofeedback, and vestibulectomy in the treatment of dyspareunia resulting from vulvar vestibulitis. Bergeron S, Binik YM, Khalife S, Pagidas K, Glazer HI, Meana M, et al. Pain 2001; 91: 297–306.

Seventy-eight women were randomly assigned to a 12-week trial of group cognitive behavioral therapy, EMG biofeedback, or vestibulectomy. After 6 months, completers of the study had statistically significant reductions on pain measures regardless of treatment assignment; the vestibulectomy group was slightly more successful than the two other groups.

Vestibulectomy for vulvar vestibulitis. Gaunt G, Good A, Stanhope CR. J Reprod Med 2003; 48: 591–5.

A retrospective chart review of 42 patients post vestibulectomy at the Mayo Clinic from 1992 to 2001. Thirty-eight (90%) had a significant improvement in their symptoms.

Evidence Levels: **A** Double-blind study **B** Clinical trial ≥ 20 subjects **C** Clinical trial < 20 subjects **D** Series ≥ 5 subjects **E** Anecdotal case reports

Botulinum toxin A for the management of vulvodynia. Yoon H, Chung WS, Shim BS. Int J Impot Res 2007; 19: 84–7.

A case series of seven patients with vulvodynia who underwent injection of botulinum toxin A to the vestibule, levator ani muscle, or perineal body (20–40 U per site) every 2 weeks as needed for symptoms. Pain resolved completely in all patients. Two required only one injection, and five patients required two. Subjective pain scores improved from 8.3 to 1.4. No recurrence was documented on follow-up (mean 11.6 months, range 4 to 24 months).

Effectiveness of hypnosis for the treatment of vulvar vestibulitis syndrome: a preliminary investigation. Pukall C, Kandyba K, Amsel R, Khalife S, Binik Y. J Sex Med 2007; 4: 417–25.

A case series of eight women with vulvar vestibulitis syndrome who underwent six hypnotherapy sessions. Pain and psychosexual questionnaires were administered at baseline and 1 and 6 months after treatment. Significant reductions in gynecologic examination pain and intercourse pain were noted. Overall sexual function and satisfaction increased after treatment. Patients reported satisfaction with treatment and rated the achieved pain reduction as average.

Spinal cord stimulation for intractable vulvar pain. A case report. Whiteside JL, Walters MD, Mekhail N. J Reprod Med 2003; 48: 821–3.

A 21-year-old woman failed to respond to a partial vulvar vestibulectomy with Bartholin gland excision but had temporary relief following bilateral hypogastric plexus blocks. A permanent spinal cord stimulator was implanted and gave sustained symptom relief.

Wells' syndrome
(Syn. Eosinophilic cellulitis)

Emma C Benton, Ian Coulson

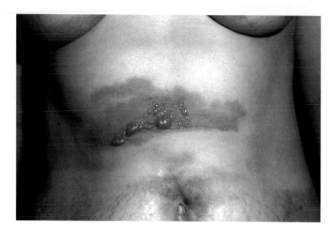

Wells' syndrome or eosinophilic cellulitis is a rare condition, first described by the London dermatologist George Wells in 1971; it is a 'recurrent granulomatous dermatitis with eosinophilia' and is of unknown etiology, but there are several disease associations as well as drug-induced disease. The condition can be recurrent, and although thought to be sporadic, familial patterns have been reported. The typical presentation of eosinophilic cellulitis is of lesions resembling an acute bacterial cellulitis. Patients are usually afebrile, however. Erythematous patches and plaques are the commonest clinical type, but papulonodular and bullous types are described. Histologic features are characterized by edema, flame figures, and a marked eosinophilic dermal infiltrate. The usual course is of a pruritic sensation, followed rapidly by indurated, erythematous plaques of edema with violaceous edges and even blistering. The lesions progress over a few days, resolving without scarring within 8 weeks, often showing a green hue during resolution. The plaques can occur anywhere on the skin and may be solitary or multiple.

MANAGEMENT STRATEGY

Although there is no known cause, several precipitating factors have been suggested (Table 1). Some of the associations are well reported, others anecdotal and possibly fortuitous. The TNF antagonists etanercept and adalimumab may induce Wells' syndrome localized to injection sites; a Wells' syndrome-like disorder has been associated with minocycline administration.

If an underlying systemic disease is identified this will require treatment in its own right. Suspect culprit drugs should be withdrawn.

The most frequently reported mode of therapy is with *systemic corticosteroids*, used at moderate dose to gain control of symptoms, followed by tapering, although cases may resolve spontaneously. As with bullous pemphigoid, localized disease may respond to *superpotent topical steroids*. The H_1 antihistamine with anti-eosinophil action *cetirizine* has been used with success. *Minocycline, dapsone, antimalarials, and ciclosporin* have shown benefit in anecdotal reports. *Sulfasalazine* with oral corticosteroids proved effective in a case with ulcerative colitis. A case associated with HIV infection responded to *interferon-α*.

SPECIFIC INVESTIGATIONS

> ▶ Peripheral blood eosinophil count
> ▶ Skin biopsy
> ▶ Look for known associations of the disease

Wells' syndrome: a clinical and histopathologic review of seven cases. Moossavi M, Mehregan DR. Int J Dermatol 2003; 42: 62–7.

The authors stress the dynamic features of Wells' syndrome histopathology, starting with dermal edema and infiltration of eosinophils, the development of 'flame figures,' and finishing with the appearance of phagocytic histiocytes.

Two cases of bullous eosinophilic cellulitis. Ling TC, Antony F, Holden CA, Al-Dawoud A, Coulson IH. Br J Dermatol 2002; 146: 160–1.

The authors present two cases in which blistering was a striking feature – negative direct immunofluorescence distinguishes bullous Wells' syndrome from pemphigoid.

Exaggerated insect bite reaction exacerbated by a pyogenic infection in a patient with chronic lymphocytic leukaemia. Walker P, Long D, James C, Marshman G. Australas J Dermatol 2007; 48: 165–9.

Eosinophilic cellulitis associated with molluscum contagiosum. Hamamoto Y, Ichimiya M, Yoshikawa Y, Muto M. Br J Dermatol 2004; 151: 1279–81.

Wells' syndrome associated with ulcerative colitis: a case report and literature review. Sakaria SS, Ravi A, Swerlick R, Sitaraman S. J Gastroenterol 2007; 42: 250–2.

Bullous eosinophilic cellulitis associated with ulcerative colitis: effective treatment with sulfasalazine and glucocorticoids. Utikal J, Peitsch WK, Kemmler N, Booken N, Hildenbrand R, Gladisch R, et al. Br J Dermatol 2007 156: 764–6.

Table 1 Reported associations

Infections – bacterial, viral (HIV, herpes simplex, molluscum contagiosum) parasitic (ascaris, toxocariasis)
Insect bite reactions
Ulcerative colitis
Leukemia
Lymphoma
Solid cancers (lung and colon)
Angioimmunoblastic lymphadenopathy
Hypereosinophilic syndrome
Drugs

Eosinophilic cellulitis as a presenting feature of chronic eosinophilic leukaemia, secondary to a deletion on chromosome 4q12 creating the FIP1L1-PDGFRA fusion gene.

Davis RF, Dusanjh P, Majid A, Fletcher A, Wardlaw A, Siebert R, et al. Br J Dermatol 2006; 155: 1087–9.

Eosinophilic cellulitis (Wells' syndrome) in association with angioimmunoblastic lymphadenopathy. Renner R, Kauer F, Treudler R, Niederwieser D, Simon JC. Acta Dermatol Venereol 2007; 87: 525–8

Eosinophilic cellulitis (Wells' syndrome) as a cutaneous reaction to the administration of adalimumab. Boura P, Sarantopoulos A, Lefaki I, Skendros P, Papadopoulos P. Ann Rheum Dis 2006; 65: 839–40.

Eosinophilic cellulitis like reaction to subcutaneous etanercept injection. Winfield H, Lain E, Horn T, Hoskyn J. Arch Dermatol 2006; 142: 218–20.

Eosinophilic cellulitis (Wells' syndrome) associated with colon carcinoma. Hirsch K, Ludwig RJ, Wolter M, Zollner TM, Hardt K, Kaufmann R, et al. J Dtsch Dermatol Ges 2005; 3: 530–1.

Some of the associations are based on single case reports and may be coincidental.

FIRST-LINE TREATMENT

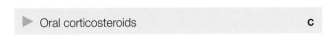

▷ Oral corticosteroids	C

Recurrent granulomatous dermatitis with eosinophilia. Wells GC. Trans St Johns Hosp Dermatol Soc 1971; 57: 46–56.

Eosinophilic cellulitis. Wells GC, Smith NP. Br J Dermatol 1979; 100: 101–9.

Wells' first publications on the disease. Oral prednisolone, ranging in doses of 20–40 mg/day, is a reasonable starting point, tapering the dose until control and hopefully eventual spontaneous resolution.

SECOND-LINE TREATMENT

▶ Cetirizine	E
▶ Ciclosporin	E
▶ Dapsone	E
▶ Interferon-α_{2a}	E
▶ Minocycline	E
▶ Sulfasalazine	E

Eosinophilic cellulitis in a child successfully treated with cetirizine. Aroni K, Aivaliotis M, Liossi A, Davaris P. Acta Dermatol Venereol 1999; 79: 332.

There are several reports of Wells' syndrome in children. Concerns regarding growth retardation have prompted other treatment strategies: cetirizine 10 mg daily has been used successfully in a child.

Cetirizine 10–30 mg/day would be a reasonable consideration in adults.

Eosinophilic cellulitis (Wells' syndrome) successfully treated with low-dose cyclosporine. Herr H, Koh JK. J Korean Med Sci 2001; 16: 664–8.

A report of ciclosporin use in an adult with Wells' syndrome: 2.5–5 mg/kg/day was used.

Eosinophilic cellulitis case report: treatment options. Lee MW, Nixon RL. Australas J Dermatol 1994; 35: 95–7.

Dapsone was added to oral steroids and antihistamines as a steroid sparing agent, as monotherapy with steroids alone gained inadequate control.

50–150 mg/day would be an appropriate trial.

Eosinophilic cellulitis (Wells' syndrome): treatment with minocycline. Stam-Westerveld EB, Daenen S, Van der Meer JB, Jonkman MF. Acta Dermatol Venereol 1998; 78: 157.

Minocycline, 200 mg daily, was used to control disease and 100 mg daily was used as maintenance.

Niacinamide was used in combination at 500 mg four times a day as in some of the bullous pemphigoid treatment regimens.

Interferon alfa treatment of a patient with eosinophilic cellulitis and HIV infection. Husak R, Goerdt S, Orfanos CE. N Engl J Med 1997 28; 337: 641–2.

Failure to control HIV-associated Wells' syndrome with steroids prompted a trial of interferon-α_{2a} treatment, starting with 3 million units on alternate days and increasing to 18 million units to gain control. Eventually 3 million units twice a week retained disease control.

Bullous eosinophilic cellulitis associated with ulcerative colitis: effective treatment with sulfasalazine and glucocorticoids. Utikal J, Peitsch WK, Kemmler N, Booken N, Hildenbrand R, Gladisch R, et al. Br J Dermatol 2007; 156: 764–6.

Wells' syndrome activity waxed and waned in parallel with the activity of the colitis. Salazopyrine was added to oral steroids, with benefit to both bowel and skin.

Xanthomas

Lucile E White, Marcelo G Horenstein, Christopher R Shea

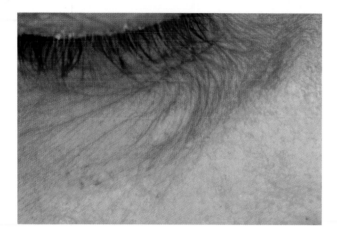

Xanthomas are flat, yellow plaques or nodules consisting of abnormal lipid deposition. Clinically, xanthomas can be classified as eruptive, tuberoeruptive, tuberous, tendinous, or plane. Plane xanthomas are the most common and include xanthelasma palpebrarum, xanthoma striatum palmaris, and intertriginous xanthomas. Necrobiotic xanthogranulomas are scarring, commonly ulcerated nodules with a predilection for the periorbital areas, and associated with paraproteinemia.

MANAGEMENT STRATEGY

Xanthomas may be idiopathic or a sign of underlying hyperlipidemia. It is necessary to *diagnose and treat the underlying disease*, not only to reduce the size of the xanthomas but also to reduce the risk of atherosclerosis associated with lipoprotein disorders. Treatment of the hyperlipidemia initially consists of *diet and lipid-lowering agents* such as statins, fibrates, bile-acid binding resins, probucol, or nicotinic acid. The lipid-lowering effects of these agents are well documented, but few studies document the efficacy of these drugs at resolving xanthomas, thus limiting an evidence-based evaluation of what would appear to be a rational management approach. Anecdotally, eruptive xanthomas typically appear to resolve within weeks of initiating systemic treatment, tuberous xanthomas after some months, but tendinous xanthomas may take years to resolve or even persist indefinitely. *Surgery or locally destructive modalities* can be used for idiopathic or unresponsive xanthomas.

SPECIFIC INVESTIGATIONS

► Serum lipid panel of cholesterol, triglycerides, VLDL, LDL, and HDL
► Gas–liquid and high-performance liquid chromatography to diagnose sitosterolemia
► Capillary gas chromatography of urine to diagnose cerebrotendinous xanthomatosis
► Serum protein electrophoresis, immunoelectrophoresis, or immunofixation to detect M proteins

Excluding an underlying condition is essential in the management of most clinical forms of xanthoma. Eruptive xanthomas typically occur in the setting of hypertriglyceridemia. Hypertriglyceridemia can be the result of lipoprotein lipase deficiency, familial hyperlipoproteinemia, or secondary causes such as diabetes mellitus, alcohol ingestion, or exogenous estrogens. Tuberoeruptive and tuberous xanthomas represent parts of a spectrum and are seen most commonly in the setting of familial dysbetalipoproteinemia. Tuberous xanthomas may also be a presentation of homozygous familial hypercholesterolemia, cerebrotendinous xanthomatosis (associated with ataxia), or sitosterolemia. Patients with sitosterolemia and cerebrotendinous xanthomatosis may have normal serum lipid panels; therefore, diagnosis may require liquid chromatography for plant sterols or urinary gas chromatography. Tendinous xanthomas may also occur with cerebrotendinous xanthomatosis, sitosterolemia or, more commonly, heterozygous familial hypercholesterolemia. Certain xanthomas are diagnostic for an inherited hyperlipidemia: xanthoma striatum palmaris for familial dysbetalipoproteinemia, and intertriginous xanthomas for homozygous familial hypercholesterolemia. With these clinical presentations, a serum lipid panel should be ordered to confirm these diagnoses. Xanthelasma palpebrarum, a type of plane xanthoma, has a less definite association with hyperlipidemia, levels of total cholesterol being elevated in only about half of those affected. Less commonly, plane xanthomas can signal a monoclonal gammopathy. In this situation, the differential diagnosis of necrobiotic xanthogranuloma with paraproteinemia, a condition usually associated with lymphoproliferative disorders, should be considered.

Dermal, subcutaneous, and tendon xanthomas: diagnostic markers for specific lipoprotein disorders. Cruz PD, East C, Bergstresser PR. J Am Acad Dermatol 1988; 19: 95–111.

Normocholesterolemic xanthomatosis. Parker F. Arch Dermatol 1986; 122: 1253–6.

Sitosterolaemia and xanthomatosis in a child. Cheng WF, Yuen YP, Chow CB, Au KM, Chan YW, Tam SC. Hong Kong Med J 2003; 9: 206–9.

Capillary gas chromatography of urine samples in diagnosing cerebrotendinous xanthomatosis. Bouwes Bavinck JN, Vermeer BJ, Gevers Leuen JA, Koopman BJ, Wolthers BG. Arch Dermatol 1986; 122: 1269–72.

The pathogenesis and clinical significance of xanthelasma palpebrarum. Bergman R. J Am Acad Dermatol 1994; 30: 236–42.

Monoclonal gammopathies and skin disorders. Daoud MS, Lust JA, Kyle RA, Pittelkow MR. J Am Acad Dermatol 1999; 40: 507–38.

Evidence Levels: **A** Double-blind study **B** Clinical trial ≥ 20 subjects **C** Clinical trial < 20 subjects **D** Series ≥ 5 subjects **E** Anecdotal case reports

FIRST-LINE THERAPIES

> ► Low-fat diet and systemic lipid-lowering therapy –
> statins, bile-acid binding resins, fibrates, and/or
> nicotinic acid   **B**

Opposite effects on serum cholesteryl ester transfer protein levels between long-term treatments with pravastatin and probucol in patients with primary hypercholesterolemia. Inazu A, Koizumi J, Kajinami K, Kiyohar T, Chichibu K, Mabuchi H. Atherosclerosis 1999; 145: 405–13.

This prospective study examined whether pravastatin or probucol was better at regressing tendon xanthomas and xanthelasma in patients with primary hypercholesterolemia. In both the pravastatin and the probucol groups, xanthelasma regressed in two of four patients. Achilles tendon xanthoma regressed in four of five patients treated with pravastatin and two of five patients on probucol.

A comparative study of the therapeutic effect of probucol and pravastatin on xanthelasma. Fujita M, Shirai K. J Dermatol 1996; 23: 598–602.

Fifty-four patients were treated with probucol or pravastatin. Xanthelasmas regressed in 13 of 36 patients treated with probucol and one of 18 patients treated with pravastatin. Total cholesterol levels decreased in both treatment groups, but HDL cholesterol decreased only in those treated with probucol.

Effects of probucol on xanthomata regression in familial hypercholesterolemia. Yamamoto A, Matsuzawa Y, Yokoyama S, Funahashi T, Yamamura T, Kishino B. Am J Cardiol 1986; 57: H29–35.

This study examined 51 patients with familial hypercholesterolemia, including eight homozygotes. Patients were treated with combinations of probucol, cholestyramine, clofibrate, and compactin. The sizes of Achilles tendon xanthomas were reduced in all patients who received probucol. Probucol possibly reduces the size of HDL particles, increasing reverse cholesterol transport.

Use of combined diet and colestipol in long-term (7–7½ years) treatment of patients with type II hyperlipoproteinemia. Kuo PT, Kiyoshi H, Kostis JB, Moreyra AE. Circulation 1979; 59: 199–212.

Twenty-one patients with atherosclerosis and cutaneous, tendinous, or corneal xanthomas were followed for up to 7.5 years. Patients were placed on a low-fat, low-cholesterol diet and colestipol, a bile-acid binding resin. This regimen caused tendinous xanthomas to disappear in two of 11 patients and improve in nine. Xanthelasmas disappeared in two of four patients and improved in two of four.

SECOND-LINE THERAPIES

> ► Surgery   **B**
> ► CO_2 laser   **B**
> ► Erbium:YAG laser   **C**
> ► Pulsed dye laser   **B**
> ► Argon laser   **B**
> ► Q-switched Nd:YAG laser   **D**
> ► KTP laser   **D**

Treatment of xanthelasma by excision with secondary intention healing. Eedy DJ. Clin Exp Dermatol 1996; 21: 273–5.

Xanthelasmas were removed in 28 patients by scissor excision. After 18 months, two patients, one with hypercholesterolemia and one with primary biliary cirrhosis, had recurrence. One patient developed scarring. No ectropion developed.

Xanthelasma: follow-up on results after surgical excision. Mendelson BC, Masson JK. Plast Reconstruct Surg 1976; 58: 535–8.

Surgical excision of xanthelasma was performed in 100 patients. Twenty-six of 68 patients (38%) who were having their lesions treated for the first time had a recurrence. Factors that predicted recurrence were systemic hyperlipidemia, involvement of all four eyelids, and a previous history of recurrent xanthelasma.

Xanthelasma palpebrarum. Parkes ML, Waller TS. Laryngoscope 1984; 94: 1238–40.

Parkes and Waller review several different methods of excision, suggesting that routine blepharoplasty with staged excisions achieves the best results.

Upper and lower eyelid reconstruction for severe disfiguring necrobiotic xanthogranuloma. Schaudig U, Al-Samir K. Orbit 2004; 23: 65–76.

Severe cicatricial eyelid deformation caused by necrobiotic xanthogranuloma can be treated successfully by excision and free skin grafting.

Xanthelasma palpebrarum: treatment with the ultrapulsed CO_2 laser. Raulin C, Schoenermark MP, Werner S, Greve B. Lasers Surg Med 1999; 24: 122–7.

Ultrapulsed CO_2 laser delivers high energy in short pulses and reduces the risk of scarring and hyperpigmentation seen with continuous-mode CO_2 lasers. Twenty-three patients with 52 xanthelasmas were treated. All lesions were removed completely. One patient experienced mild erythema for 4 months, but no permanent hyperpigmentation or ectropion developed. Three patients had recurrent lesions at an average follow-up time of 10 months.

Xanthelasma palpebrarum: treatment with the erbium: YAG laser. Borelli C, Kaudewitz P. Lasers Surg Med 2001; 29: 260–4.

Fifteen patients with 33 xanthelasmas were treated with an Er:YAG laser at settings between of 300 mJ, 2 Hz for a 2 mm spot size and 1200 mJ, 6 Hz for a 10 mm spot size. All xanthelasmas were removed completely. Postoperative erythema resolved within 2 weeks. No scarring or ectropion developed. No lesions recurred over a 7–12-month follow-up period.

Treatment of diffuse plane xanthoma of the face with erbium:YAG laser. Lorenz S, Hohenleutner S, Hohenleutner U, Landthaler M. Arch Dermatol 2001; 137: 1413–15.

A patient presented with diffuse plane xanthomas of the entire face and neck which were partially cleared by the Er:YAG laser. Two months later, a second treatment was performed for persistent lesions. The treated lesions did not recur over a 12-month follow-up. Because of the risk of scarring, her neck and earlobe region were not treated.

New operative technique for treatment of xanthelasma palpebrarum: laser-inverted resurfacing: preliminary report. Levy JL, Trelles MA. Ann Plast Surg. 2003; 50: 339–43.

The authors propose the use of pulsed Er:YAG vaporization of the lipomatous tissue off the inner surface of the eyelid after incision and eversion of the incised tissue to expose the xanthelasma. In two patients treated by this technique no recurrence was seen in up to 1 year of follow-up.

Treatment of xanthelasma palpebrarum by 1064-nm Q-switched Nd:YAG laser: a study of 11 cases. Fusade T. Br J Dermatol 2008; 158: 84–7.

The results after even a single treatment were good or excellent in eight of 11 patients (in 26 of 38 lesions), and healing was rapid.

Treatment of xanthelasma palpebrarum with argon laser photocoagulation. Basar E, Oguz H, Ozdemir H, Ozkan S, Uslu H. Int Ophthalmol 2004; 25: 9–11.

Twenty-four patients with 40 xanthelasmas were treated with an argon laser at settings of 500 μm, 0.1–0.2 s, and 900 mW. Complete removal of all lesions occurred with one to four sessions at intervals of 2–3 weeks. Six lesions recurred over 8–12 months and required re-treatment. Erythema persisted for 1 month in 8 lesions. Hyperpigmentation occurred in one patient and persisted for 3 months, and hypopigmentation occurred in two lesions. No bleeding, infections, or ectropion occurred.

Histopathological study of xanthelasma palpebrarum after pulsed dye laser. Soliman M. J Eur Acad Dermatol Venereol 2004; 18: 19–33.

Twenty-six patients were treated with fluences ranging from 6.5 to 8 J/cm², a spot size of 5 mm, and a pulse width of 450 ms. All patients experienced very good to excellent clinical improvement with one to three treatments at 3–4-week intervals.

KTP laser coagulation for xanthelasma palpebrarum. Berger C, Kopera D. J Dtsch Dermatol Ges 2005; 3: 775–9.

The authors employed the potassium titanyl phosphate (KTP) laser (532 nm) to treat 14 patients with xanthelasma palpebrarum on 33 eyelids. Over 70% of patients tolerated laser irradiation without analgesia, and 85.7% showed reduction of lesions after one to three treatment sessions, without reported side effects.

THIRD-LINE THERAPIES

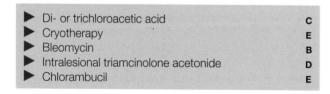

▶ Di- or trichloroacetic acid	C
▶ Cryotherapy	E
▶ Bleomycin	B
▶ Intralesional triamcinolone acetonide	D
▶ Chlorambucil	E

Treatment of xanthelasma palpebrarum with bichloracetic acid. Haygood LJ, Bennett JD, Brodell RT. Dermatol Surg 1998; 24: 1027–31.

Ten of 13 patients with 25 lesions had complete clearing with the application of bichloroacetic acid. Five lesions

recurred and required a second treatment to achieve complete resolution. No complications were reported.

Evaluation of three different strengths of trichloroacetic acid in xanthelasma palpebrarum. Haque MU, Ramesh V. J Dermatol Treat 2006; 17: 48–50.

Three strengths of TCA were tested on 51 patients. For papulonodular lesions, on average, about two applications were required with 100% or 70% TCA, versus about four applications with 50% TCA. For flat plaques an average of approximately 1.50 applications of 100% or 70% TCA sufficed, versus about three applications with 50% TCA. Macular lesions responded to a single application of all strengths of TCA studied.

Koebner phenomenon in xanthelasma after treatment with trichloroacetic acid. Akhyani M, Daneshpazhooh M, Jafari AK, Naraghi ZS, Farahani F, Toosi S. Dermatol Online J 2006; 12: 12.

Despite initial improvement, a 47-year-old woman noticed extension of biopsy-proven xanthelasma lesions at the site of TCA treatment. Physicians should be aware of the possibility of an isomorphic (Koebner) response when treating xanthelasma palpebrarum with TCA.

Cryotherapy may be effective for eyelid xanthoma. Hawk JL. Clin Exp Dermatol 2000; 25: 351.

One patient was treated with liquid nitrogen applied for 0.5–1 seconds. Treatment was carefully limited to only the yellow areas. Previous treatment with trichloroacetic acid had been unsuccessful.

Therapeutic effect and pathology changing of eyelid xanthelasma by bleomycin A5. Meng RH, Meng Y, Yang L, Sun L, Sun WR, Liu HM. Zhonghua Yan Ke Za Zhi 2005; 41: 231–3.

Twenty-five randomly selected outpatients received intralesional injections of 0.2 mL of 0.4% bleomycin solution every 10 days. In five other cases one eye received bleomycin injection once and the contralateral eye was left untreated as a negative control. The 25 bleomycin-treated xanthelasmas were reported to disappear completely, without adverse sequelae.

Local corticosteroid treatment of eyelid and orbital xanthogranuloma. Elner VM, Mintz R, Demirci H, Hassan AS. Trans Am Ophthalmol Soc 2005; 103: 69–73.

Six patients received two intralesional injections of triamcinolone acetonide (40 mg/mL) for eyelid and orbital necrobiotic xanthogranuloma (four patients) or adult-onset xanthogranuloma (two patients). Local control was obtained in all six cases, with a reduction of symptoms and signs of the disease in five; no complications were noted.

Necrobiotic xanthogranuloma treated with chlorambucil. Torabian SZ, Fazel N, Knuttle R. Dermatol Online J 2006; 12: 11.

A 56-year-old man with a 5-year history of multiple necrobiotic xanthogranulomas involving the periorbital area, extremities, and trunk was treated with chlorambucil at 2 mg/day, later increased to 4 mg/day, which resulted in complete resolution of the lesions.

Xeroderma pigmentosum

Deborah Tamura, John J DiGiovanna, Kenneth H Kraemer

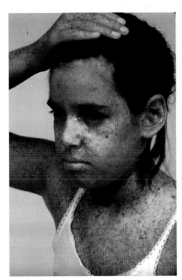

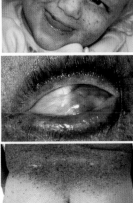

Xeroderma pigmentosum (XP) is a rare autosomal recessive disorder characterized by cellular hypersensitivity to the damaging effects of ultraviolet (UV) radiation, resulting in a 1000-fold increased risk of skin cancers. The cancers often develop in the first decade of life. About half of patients present with acute photosensitivity manifested as exaggerated reactions to minimal sun exposure with acute erythema and blistering. These burns can be so severe that child abuse or neglect is suspected. Patients who do not have these acute reactions often develop early freckle-like pigmentation before the age of 2. This may be accompanied by a dry 'aged appearance' to the skin, cheilitis, and photophobia. The eyes are particularly vulnerable in XP patients. Sun damage to the eyes includes dry eye, ectropion, pterygia, pinguecula, corneal scarring leading to blindness, and cancer of the lids, sclera, or cornea. Cancers can also occur on the lips and tip of the tongue.

The progressive skin and eye damage seen in patients with this disorder is due to their inability to repair UV-induced DNA damage in sun-exposed tissues. XP patients have mutations in one of the eight genes (*XPA, XPB, XPC, XPD, XPE, XPF,* and *XPG*) of the nucleotide excision repair pathway (NER) or in DNA polymerase eta (XP variant). The NER pathway is critical for the identification, removal, and repair of UV-induced DNA damage, while polymerase eta bypasses unrepaired DNA damage.

Approximately 20% of patients with XP have progressive neurodegeneration, characterized by loss of deep tendon reflexes, progressive sensorineural deafness, motor abnormalities, and impaired cognition. This primary neurodegeneration may begin in infancy or may not start to develop until the second decade of life. MRI shows progressive dilation of the ventricles and loss of gray matter of the brain.

MANAGEMENT STRATEGY

Diagnosis

It is important to establish the clinical diagnosis as early in life as possible. Xeroderma pigmentosum should be suspected in a child presenting with a history of freckling on sun-exposed skin before age 2, severe sunburn after minimal sun exposure, photophobia, or skin or eye cancer. Some children may present with developmental delays, in addition to the skin findings.

Laboratory testing can be performed on cultured fibroblasts obtained from a small skin biopsy. The cells of XP patients in culture are extremely sensitive to the killing effects of UV. At present there are no CLIA-certified laboratories in the United States performing UV sensitivity testing for XP; however, a laboratory is under development at the University of Medicine and Dentistry of New Jersey. DNA testing for mutations in several of the XP genes is available on a limited basis (www.genetests.org).

Environmental management

The most critical management goal for XP is UV protection. Although XP patients do not repair damage from UV in exposed tissues, they react normally to visible light. Patients and their families can be taught to recognize and avoid sources of UV radiation and how to institute protective measures in their home, school, and other areas where the patient will spend long periods of time. The use of *high SPF sunblock* that blocks both UVB and UVA wavelengths, protective clothing (long-sleeved shirts, long pants, hats that cover the ears) and UV-blocking sunglasses with side shields is extremely important and should be regularly reinforced with the families and patients, when the diagnosis of XP is suspected or confirmed.

Environmental levels of UV can be measured with relatively inexpensive handheld UV meters; they measure levels of both UVB (short-wavelength UV 290–320 nm) and UVA (long-wavelength UV 320–400 nm). Although the UVB radiation is more damaging, UVA radiation can also produce DNA damage, so protection from all UV wavelengths is desirable. Having the ability to directly measure UV in the environment provides patients and families with a greater ability to ensure safer surroundings for the patient.

UV protection in the home, school, and work environment begins with educating the family about sources of UV. The major source is the sun. Although window glass blocks most UVB wavelengths, UVA can pass through glass (along with visible light wavelengths). Extremely sensitive XP patients have burned through window glass. *UV-blocking window films* can be installed on home and vehicle windows. The Americans with Disability Act (ADA) and other laws and regulations mandate that children with XP should be provided with a safe educational environment. Windows in rooms where XP patients will be spending substantial amounts of time, such as in day care or school, should be shielded. In addition, schools should make accommodations for XP children during fire drills and physical education activities. As leaving the building during these activities is not safe for children with XP, schools should develop an individualized plan for them (individualized educational plan, IEP) to keep them protected from UV sources but involved in these activities.

Like other patients with 'invisible disorders,' patients with XP should wear medical alert bracelets and carry an information card about the condition in their purse or wallet. Information about MedicAlert ID jewelry is available at www.medicalert.org/home/Homegradient.aspx.

Unshielded fluorescent lighting and halogen lights pose potential UV hazards to XP patients. In the home, replacement of unshielded fluorescent bulbs with incandescent lights or placing *plastic shielding over fluorescent bulbs* can substantially reduce the ambient levels of UV. Replacing all halogen lights with incandescent lights is recommended, as halogen lights emit substantial levels of UVB.

Applying protective agents such as sunscreen, sun block, sun-protective lip balms and makeup, should be a daily routine for XP patients. Many effective sun-protective agents are on the market and contain sun blocks such as zinc oxide or titanium dioxide, or various sunscreen agents. XP patients should use a preparation with an SPF (sun protection factor) of at least 15 or higher that offers broad UVA and UVB protection. The first application of the day should cover all body skin surface areas that could be exposed, and the preparation should be reapplied to uncovered skin (usually face, ears, neck and hands) several times during the day. As there is a wide variety of sun-protective agents with different formulations, consistencies, and fragrances, finding one that is most acceptable to the XP patient may take some trial and error.

Clothing for XP patients should cover as much skin surface as possible and should include long pants, long-sleeved shirts, socks, and closed-toe shoes. If they are going outside during the day, gloves or mittens should be worn, as well as large-brimmed hats that cover the ears. Clothing material should be tightly woven: denim is effective. A simple test of the effectiveness of UV protection by clothing is to hold the material up to a bright light. If visible light can pass through the material then UV can also pass through. Clothing that blocks all visible light is recommended. Clothing made from sun-blocking material is commercially available, but may be expensive. One alternative is a commonly available laundry additive, manufactured in the United States by the Rit Corporation, which is advertised to increase the ability of clothing to block UV radiation. Regular washing of outer clothing (pants, shirts, jackets, socks, gloves, and hats) with this additive is recommended to increase UV protection. There are similar agents available in Japan, Australia, and Europe.

As the cornea and sclera of XP patients are also subject to UV damage, patients should wear *UV-blocking sunglasses* when they are in areas of potential exposure. The glasses should 'wrap around' the eyes, providing protection to the sides of the eyes, and should be large enough to fully protect both lids.

Vitamin D is produced in the skin by UV exposure and can also be obtained by eating vitamin D-rich foods such as milk and fish. Whereas young active XP patients may maintain normal vitamin D levels with diet alone, for very well-protected XP patients vitamin D levels may be periodically monitored. *Vitamin D-containing vitamin supplements* can be used if serum levels of 25-OH vitamin D are low.

XP patients should not use any type of tobacco product and should be protected from secondhand smoke. The benzo[a]pyrene derivatives and other carcinogens found in tobacco products and smoke induce DNA damage repaired by the NER pathway, putting the XP patient at risk for respiratory tract cancers.

The most challenging aspect of managing UV exposure is the substantial lifestyle adjustment necessary to provide a UV-safe environment. Patients should avoid outdoor activities during daylight hours, and should strictly avoid being outside between 10 am and 2 pm. Identifying appropriate indoor play and sports activities for the affected XP child while continuing to meet the needs of unaffected family members can be a considerable challenge.

Obtaining affordable health insurance and workplace accommodations are a few of the challenges adults with XP face. As with any chronic illness, the family and patient will need to go through a period of adjustment to the lifestyle limitations of the condition. The patient may be eligible for Social Security Disability Insurance or other medical assistance. Referring the patient and family to the several XP support groups helps them connect with other affected families and not feel as isolated; these groups also sponsor UV-safe family activities. Websites for these organizations are: The XP Family Support Group: *www.xpfamilysupport.org/joomla/*; The Xeroderma Pigmentosum Support Group UK: *www.xpsupport-group.org.uk/*; The Xeroderma Pigmentosum Society: *www.xps.org/*. In situations where psychosocial pathologies exist (substance abuse or domestic violence), or if the family is having extreme difficulty coping with the diagnosis, a referral to social services or a therapist may be advisable.

Medical and surgical management

The dermatologist, the patient and their family will need to cooperate in skin surveillance. Teaching the signs and symptoms of premalignant and malignant lesions will enable earlier identification by patients and families and prompt removal of smaller more easily resectable tumors. Depending on the rate of new tumor development, a full skin examination should be scheduled every 3–6 months. If the patient or family becomes concerned about rapidly evolving lesions, it may be necessary to schedule more frequent visits. Baseline whole-body photographs of the patient and close-up photographs of lesions with a ruler in the image for size comparison can help track skin changes. These images can be stored on CDs and copies can be given to the family for use at home and kept in the patient's chart.

Premalignant lesions, including actinic keratoses, can be treated with *cryotherapy, topical 5-fluorouracil (5-FU)*, or topical *imiquimod.* Care needs to be taken when using topical 5-FU or imiquimod as field treatments to ensure that any existing skin cancers are adequately treated. When using field treatments over large areas there is a risk of treating the superficial areas of cancers but leaving deeper areas untreated. Well-controlled studies of topical field treatments in XP patients have not been published.

Dermabrasion or *dermatome shaving* has been used to remove the superficial photodamaged layers. Theoretically, these procedures allow epidermal replacement of severely damaged cells by cells arising from the deeper, less damaged adnexal structures. Additional preventative measures have been used in XP patients, including *chemoprevention with retinoids* (isotretinoin, etretinate, or acitretin). A longitudinal study of a small number of XP patients performed at the National Institutes of Health found that oral retinoid therapy was effective in reducing the number of new skin cancers. However, there were many side effects in these patients, especially at the higher drug dosages.

Early and adequate treatment of skin cancers before they enlarge or spread is extremely important. All suspected tumors should be biopsied and quickly removed. Standard techniques, including *curettage and desiccation, surgical excision*, and *cryosurgical ablation*, can be used for small superficial lesions. Owing to the extensive poikilodermatous changes and scarring in XP patients, it can be difficult to differentiate recurrent from new lesions; in addition, recurrent lesions can eventually result in large invasive tumors with extensive tissue destruction. *Mohs' micrographic surgery* is an excellent method for combining effective tumor removal with tissue sparing. If the surgical defect is large, it can be closed using plastic surgical techniques. XP patients are at high risk for the development of future skin cancers, so skin-sparing approaches should be a high priority in the surgical plan. As the surrounding skin is likely to be severely sun damaged, moving tissue with flaps can be complicated because of the presence of pre-cancers or small skin cancers in the surrounding skin. Despite their hypersensitivity to UV, many XP patients have demonstrated a normal response to *X-ray therapy* when it is used to treat recurrent skin and eye cancers.

Ophthalmologic management is extremely important to preserve eyesight. Most ophthalmologic problems in XP patients occur in the surface structures of the eye. One of the earliest symptoms of XP in young children can be photophobia and conjunctivitis. Because all the exposed parts of the eye (and the supporting tissues) are susceptible to UV damage, precancerous and cancerous lesions can arise on the cornea, sclera, lids, and conjunctiva. Secondary to UV damage on the cornea, XP patients will develop 'dry eye,' leading to keratitis and conjunctival inflammation. Ectropion of the lids, resulting in defects of eye closure, can occur secondary to atrophy of the eyelids and surgical removal of malignancies from the periocular skin. Ectropion can exacerbate dryness, and, if left untreated, this chronic process leads to corneal ulceration, scarring, and opacification of the cornea, with resultant blindness. *Corneal transplants* have been performed in some XP patients, but they frequently experienced rejection because of vascularization of the area. XP patients should have a thorough ophthalmologic examination at least yearly, which can include Schirmer's testing for dry eye and assessment of lid closure. Eye lubricants, including *artificial tears*, are usually recommended, along with lubricating ointments at night in cases with poor lid closure.

Approximately 20% of XP patients develop progressive neurologic disease. The development of symptoms and rate of progression vary greatly among patients, with the most severe cases developing symptoms in early childhood (De Santis–Cacchione syndrome). The first symptom of XP neurologic disease is loss of deep tendon reflexes, most notably in the lower extremities. This may be noted in early childhood and be the only symptom for many years. Routine checking of deep tendon reflexes during skin examinations can help identify patients at risk for neurologic disease. Symptoms of progressive neurologic disease include cognitive decline, mobility difficulties, and ataxia and falls; eventually a wheelchair and other assistive devices may be needed. Death from aspiration pneumonia or other complications of severe debilitation can occur in patients with significant neurologic disease.

Progressive sensorineural hearing loss in XP patients may be diagnosed as early as the first decade of life and may first be suspected secondary to falling grades in school. The hearing loss is helped with *hearing aids*, and assisted-hearing systems may be used in the classroom. XP patients should have regular audiology examinations.

XP patients have a significantly increased risk of developing cancers on the lips and squamous cell carcinoma on the tip of the tongue. Telangiectasia on the tip of the tongue is an early UV-induced change seen in XP patients. The tongue and lips should be evaluated during the regular skin examination, and patients should be promptly referred to oral surgery if a suspicious lesion is noted.

XP patients have an approximately 50-fold increased risk of developing primary central nervous system tumors. These have responded to full-dose *X-ray therapy* with normal skin reaction in many patients. However, as some XP cell lines have shown increased sensitivity to X-irradiation, a small test dose might be advised prior to full exposure.

With improved healthcare, XP patients are marrying and having children. XP is an autosomal recessive condition that requires two abnormal alleles for an individual to be affected. XP heterozygotes are clinically unaffected and would be rare in the general population. Therefore, the chance of an XP patient having an affected child would be very low when conception is between non-blood-related individuals. However, when an XP patient is contemplating pregnancy, referral for *genetic counseling* should be considered to give the patient and spouse an opportunity to discuss testing and monitoring during the pregnancy.

In conclusion, the optimal management of XP patients is a *multidisciplinary process* involving a number of medical specialties, along with active cooperation and input from the patient and their family. In the past XP patients had significantly shortened life expectancy; however, with early diagnosis, good UV protection, and adequate management of skin cancers, people with XP are living well into adulthood, working in the community, and raising families.

SPECIFIC INVESTIGATIONS

> ▶ Clinical skin examination to monitor for skin cancers
> ▶ High index of suspicion with early biopsy for diagnosis of possible skin cancers
> ▶ Ophthalmologic examinations
> ▶ Neurologic examinations
> ▶ Audiologic examinations
> ▶ UV sensitivity testing on cultured fibroblasts

Xeroderma pigmentosum: Cutaneous, ocular and neurologic abnormalities in 830 published cases. Kraemer KH, Lee MM, Scotto J. Arch Dermatol 1987; 123: 241–50.

Xeroderma pigmentosum in: GeneReviews at GeneTests: Medical Genetics Information Resource [database online]. Wattendorf D, Kraemer KH. (updated May 2008) Seattle: University of Washington, 1997–2005. Available at http://www.genetests.org

Neurologic disease in xeroderma pigmentosum – documentation of the late onset of the juvenile onset form. Robbins JH, Brumback RA, Mendiones M, Barrett SF, Carl JR, Cho S, et al. Brain 1991; 114: 1335–61.

Ocular manifestations in the inherited DNA repair disorders. Dolfus H, Porto F, Caussade C, Speeg-Schatz C, Sahel J, Grosshans E, et al. Surv Opthalmol 2003; 48: 107–22.

Xeroderma pigmentosum – bridging a gap between clinic and laboratory. Moriwaki SI, Kraemer K. Photodermatol Photoimmunol Photomed 2001; 17: 47–54.

Hereditary diseases of genome instability and DNA repair. Ruenger TM, DiGiovanna JJ, Kraemer KH. In: Wolff K, Goldsmith LA, Katz SI, Gilchrest BA, Paller AS, Leffel DJ., eds. Fitzpatrick's dermatology in general medicine, 7th edn. New York: McGraw-Hill, 2008; 1311–25.

Rare diseases provide rare insights into DNA repair pathways TFIIH, aging and cancer. Bohr VA, Sander M, Kraemer K. DNA Repair 2005; 4: 293–302.

Understanding xeroderma pigmentosum. Clinical Center, National Cancer Institute: http://clinicalcenter.nih.gov/ccc/patient_education/pepubs/xp7_17.pdf

This patient information booklet is written in lay terms for patients, family members, and healthcare providers.

FIRST-LINE THERAPIES

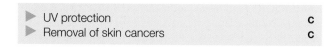

▶ UV protection	C
▶ Removal of skin cancers	C

Normal vitamin D levels can be maintained despite rigourous photoprotection: 6 years experience with xeroderma pigmentosum. Sollito RB, Kraemer KH, DiGiovanna JJ. J Am Acad Dermatol 1997; 37: 942–7

Eight XP patients who wore protective clothing and sunscreens when outdoors had levels of vitamin D (25-OH and 1,25-OH) measured over a 6-year period: all maintained adequate levels of vitamin D.

Xeroderma pigmentosum, trichothiodystrophy and Cockayne syndrome: a complex genotype–phenotype relationship. Kraemer KH, Patronas NJ, Schiffmann R, Brooks BP, Tamura D, DiGiovanna JJ. Neuroscience 2007; 145: 1388–96.

Review article discussing three diseases associated with deficient DNA repair. The article compares and contrasts the features of the diseases and discusses the known etiology of the conditions.

Prevention of skin cancer in xeroderma pigmentosum: The physician as advocate. Cox S, Roberts L, Bergstresser P. J Am Acad Dermatol 1993; 29: 1045–6.

Discusses facial resurfacing and the role of the physician in assessing a UV-safe environment.

SECOND-LINE THERAPIES

▶ Topical imiquimod	E
▶ Topical 5-fluorouracil	E
▶ Oral retinoid therapy	C

Cancer protection in xeroderma pigmentosum variant. Somos S, Farkas B, Schneider I. Anticancer Res 1999; 19: 2195–200.

A brother and sister were diagnosed with XP as adults. The brother died secondary to SCC metastases. His sister was treated with isotretinoin and a 25% reduction in new tumor development was observed.

Therapeutic response of a brother and sister with xeroderma pigmentosum to imiquimod 5% cream. Weisberg NK, Varghese M. Dermatol Surg 2002; 28: 518–23.

Siblings diagnosed with XP failed chemoprophylaxis for dozens of tumors with oral retinoids. Treatment with imiquimod 5% cream was initiated three times per week for several months. Both patients experienced a reduction in new tumor development and resolution of multiple existing basal cell carcinomas. Interestingly, one sibling demonstrated a robust inflammatory response and the other had little visible reaction.

5% 5-Fluorouracil cream for the treatment of small superficial basal cell carcinoma: efficacy, tolerability, cosmetic outcome and patient satisfaction. Gross K, Kircik L, Kricorian G. Dermatol Surg 2007; 33: 433–40.

This study evaluated the efficacy, tolerability, cosmetic outcome, and patient satisfaction of 5% 5-FU treatment for superficial basal cell carcinomas in 29 patients. Histologic cure rate was 90% and patients were generally very satisfied with the treatment. These were not XP patients.

Prevention of skin cancer with oral 13-cis retinoic acid in xeroderma pigmentosum. Kraemer KH, DiGiovanna JJ, Moshell AN, Tarone RE, Peck GL. N Engl J Med 1988; 318: 1633–7.

Five XP patients were treated for a total of 2 years with high-dose (2 mg/kg/day) isotretinoin. The patients had a total of 121 tumors before treatment and only 25 occurred during treatment. The tumor frequency increased 8.5-fold after the drug was discontinued. However, there were significant side effects, including cutaneous, triglyceride, liver function, or skeletal problems.

Spinal cord astrocytoma in a patient with xeroderma pigmentosum: 9-year survival with radiation and isotretinoin therapy. DiGiovanna JJ, Patronas N, Katz D, Abangan D, Kraemer KH. J Cutan Med Surg 1998; 2: 153–8.

Case report of an XP patient who received radiation therapy for a spinal cord astrocytoma, with normal cutaneous response to standard dosages.

THIRD-LINE THERAPIES

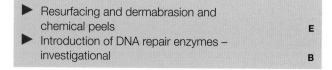

▶ Resurfacing and dermabrasion and chemical peels	E
▶ Introduction of DNA repair enzymes – investigational	B

Is facial resurfacing with monoblock full-thickness skin graft a remedy in xeroderma pigmentosum? Ergun S, Cek DI, Demirkesen C. Am Soc Plast Surg 2002; 110: 1290–93.

Case report of an XP patient who had multiple skin grafts and experienced tumor recurrence which originated under the graft.

The role of dermabrasion and chemical peels in the treatment of patients with xeroderma pigmentosum. Nelson BR, Fader DJ, Gillard M, Baker S, Johnson TM. J Am Acad Dermatol 1995; 32: 623–6.

Case report of two XP patients treated periodically with trichloroacetic acid chemical peels; one also underwent dermabrasion. Both procedures provided some prophylactic effects, with the dermabrasion having better results. Before and after pictures are presented.

Effect of topically applied T4 endonuclease V in liposomes on skin cancer in xeroderma pigmentosum: a randomized study. Yarosh D, Klein J, O'Connor A, Hawk J, Rafal E, Wolf P; Xeroderma Pigmentosum Study Group. Lancet 2001; 357: 926–9.

This was a double-blind multicenter study randomly assigning 20 XP patients for treatment or placebo. The patients in the treatment arm noted a reduction in the development of actinic keratoses and basal cell carcinomas. There were no significant side effects. This medication is still awaiting approval by the US FDA.

Evidence Levels: **A** Double-blind study **B** Clinical trial ≥ 20 subjects **C** Clinical trial < 20 subjects **D** Series ≥ 5 subjects **E** Anecdotal case reports

Xerosis

Jason Williams, Ian Coulson

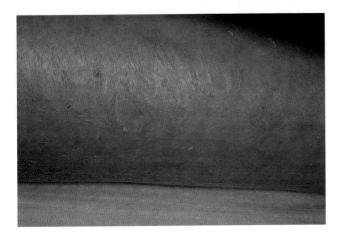

Xerosis is the term used to describe a condition where there is a rough, dry textural feel to the skin, accompanied by fine scaling and sometimes fine fissuring. Increasing xerosis is usually accompanied by increasing itch. It is a descriptive term, not a diagnosis – it may result from a combination of environmental conditions (low humidity, degreasing of the skin by excessive bathing, soap or detergent use), genetic disorders of keratinization (ichthyoses), Down syndrome (12% of patients), atopic eczema, endocrine disease states (hypothyroidism), diabetes mellitus (39% of patients), celiac disease, and a host of underlying disease states such as chronic renal failure, liver disease (including 69% of patients with primary biliary cirrhosis), malnutrition, anorexia nervosa (58% of patients), essential fatty acid deficiency, Sjögren's syndrome (56% of patients), HIV infection, lymphoma, and carcinomatosis (especially hematologic). It is more common in the elderly. Drugs are occasionally implicated. It is reported to be more frequent in winter months.

MANAGEMENT STRATEGY

Initial evaluation should seek to distinguish simple xerosis from a genetic ichthyosis, although management is similar for both conditions. Family history, distribution, and morphology will help to differentiate the two. A history of weight loss, dietary history, and body mass index may give clues towards an underlying metabolic or malabsorptive disorder. Dry eyes and mouth may indicate underlying Sjögren's syndrome. History and clinical examination should seek symptoms and signs of hypothyroidism, diabetes mellitus, and chronic renal disease. Drug use and sexual contact history may reveal HIV infection. Xerosis is an almost universal accompaniment of atopic eczema.

The mainstay of therapy for xerosis after any underlying disorders (if possible) are corrected are *improvement of the humidity* in the patient's environment, *avoidance of exacerbating factors* such as soap and detergents, and the use of *emollients or humectants*.

Low environmental humidity both at home and work will exacerbate xerosis of any cause. Arid air is a problem in air-conditioned homes, offices, and vehicles. Hot dry air directed to the lower legs during the winter in the front of automobiles is a common cause of lower leg xerosis. In the home or workplace humidifiers can be fitted over radiators; alternatively, placing wet towels or containers of water over them will increase air humidity.

Soaps and detergents degrease the skin, reduce epidermal thickness, and increase scale and itch, and so are best avoided, and light emollient cleansers (soap substitutes) are suggested in their place. Bathing in tepid water is often preferred by patients, and patting the skin dry will produce less scale and dryness than vigorous toweling.

Emollients (which simply produce an impervious film over the epidermis and prevent 'transpiration') and humectants (such as lactic acid, urea, or glycerine that hold water in the epidermis osmotically) are the mainstays of therapy. Few good comparative studies exist for the most common type of xerosis, which is surprising because they are the most frequently used dermatological products! They should be used liberally and as frequently as possible and applied in the direction of hair growth; emollients are particularly valuable after bathing or showering to hold water in the epidermis. Light emollients for use in the shower or bath may be preferred to *bath oils* by some. Choice of emollient is entirely personal to the patient – a pack with small amounts of a variety of products for home trial or a self-selection 'tub tray' for the clinic is likely to enhance compliance.

Agents containing α-*hydroxy acids (AHAs)* may offer some advantages over conventional paraffin-based emollients, but this may be at the expense of irritation in some people. Low-concentration *salicylic acid* may help reduce scale in more severe xerosis, but it is essential to remember that systemic absorption and salicylism can occur.

Topical retinoids have only been used in the more severe ichthyoses and are too irritating for use in xerosis. Systemic therapies have little part to play in most patients.

SPECIFIC INVESTIGATIONS

▶ Thyroid function tests
▶ Renal function tests
▶ Random glucose
▶ Consider tests for Sjögren's syndrome, HIV infection, malignancies, and malabsorption, if clinically indicated
▶ Drug history

Sjögren's syndrome: a retrospective review of the cutaneous features of 93 patients by the Italian Group of Immunodermatology. Bernacchi E, Amato L, Parodi A, Cottoni F, Rubegni P, De Pità O, et al. Clin Exp Rheumatol 2004; 22: 55–62.

Over half of 93 patients with Sjögren's syndrome had xerosis and its presence correlated with the presence of SSA and SSB antibodies.

HIV-associated pruritus: etiology and management. Singh F, Rudikoff D. Am J Clin Dermatol 2003; 4: 177–88.

Xerosis is one of the more common causes of itch in HIV infection and AIDS.

Non infectious skin conditions associated with diabetes mellitus: a prospective study of 308 cases. Diris N, Colomb M, Leymarie F, Durlach V, Caron J, Bernard P. Ann Dermatol Venereol 2003; 130: 1009–14.

Xerosis was noted in 39% of 309 patients.

The mucocutaneous manifestations associated with celiac disease in childhood and adolescence. Seyhan M, Erdem T, Ertekin V, Selimoglu MA. Paediatr Dermatol 2007; 24: 28–33.

Xerosis from lithium carbonate. Hoxtell E, Dahl MV. Arch Dermatol 1975; 111: 1073–4.

Litt's Drug Eruption Reference Manual, 10th edn. (Litt JZ, ed. London: Taylor & Francis, 2004) lists in excess of 150 drugs (from acebutolol to zonisamide!) that have been implicated in causing xerosis. Cimetidine, protease inhibitors, statins, and nicotinamide are perhaps the best known.

FIRST-LINE THERAPIES

▶ Soap avoidance	A
▶ Humidification	C
▶ Emollients	B
▶ Bath oils	B

Emollients improve treatment results with topical corticosteroids in childhood atopic dermatitis: a randomized comparative study. Szczepanowska J, Reich A, Szepietowski JC. Pediatr Allergy Immunol 2008; 19: 614–8.

In a study of 52 children with atopic dermatitis, those applying emollients concurrently with topical corticosteroids had significantly improved xerosis.

How useful are soap substitutes? Berth-Jones J, Graham-Brown RAC. J Dermatol Treat 1992; 3: 9–11.

Thirty-eight subjects with atopic dermatitis, psoriasis, or senile xerosis were treated with emulsifying ointment BP or Wash E45 as soap substitutes. Dryness and itching improved in both groups. Wash E45 was considered more effective as a cleanser.

The effect of washing on the thickness of the stratum corneum in normal and atopic individuals. White MI, McEwan Jenkinson D, Lloyd DH. Br J Dermatol 1987; 116: 525–30.

A histological study confirming that stratum corneum thickness was reduced by washing with soap in both normal and atopic individuals. The stratum corneum was thinner in the atopic individuals than in controls at baseline, and was almost completely removed in the atopics by the use of soap.

The value of oil baths for adjuvant basic therapy of inflammatory dermatoses with dry, barrier-disrupted skin. Melnik B, Braun-Falco O. Hautarzt 1996; 47: 665–72.

The use of oil baths with emollients is an integral and indispensable constituent of maintenance therapy in dry skin conditions, atopic eczema, and inflammatory dermatoses.

A new technique for evaluating bath oil in the treatment of dry skin. Stanfield JW, Levy J, Kyriakopoulos AA, Waldman PM. Cutis 1981; 28: 458–60.

A comparative study confirming that bath oils are superior to soap for lower leg xerosis in the elderly.

SECOND-LINE THERAPIES

▶ Urea-containing creams	A
▶ Lactic acid-containing creams	A
▶ Ammonium lactate creams	A
▶ AHA creams	B
▶ Thyroxine cream	D

A double-blind comparison of two creams containing urea as the active ingredient. Assessment of efficacy and side effects by non-invasive techniques and a clinical scoring scheme. Serup J. Acta Dermatol Venereol (Stockh) 1992; 177: 34–43.

A comparison of 3% and 10% urea cream showed that both were effective at reducing scale, dryness, and laboratory parameters (transepidermal water loss and colorimetric changes). The 10% cream was better at restoring the skin's water barrier function.

Clinical evaluation of 40% urea and 12% ammonium lactate in the treatment of xerosis. Ademola J, Frazier C, Kim SJ, Theaux C, Saudez X. Am J Clin Dermatol 2002; 3: 217–22.

A double-blind study comparing 40% urea cream with 12% ammonium lactate cream showing superiority of the urea cream. Flexural irritation was a problem.

Many urea-containing products contain lower concentrations than used in this study.

A controlled two-center study of lactate 12 percent lotion and a petrolatum-based creme in patients with xerosis. Wehr R, Krochmal L, Bagatell F, Ragsdale W. Cutis 1986; 37: 205–7.

Lactate lotion 12% was significantly more effective than a petrolatum-based cream in reducing the severity of xerosis during treatment and post-treatment phases.

Comparative efficacy of 12% ammonium lactate lotion and 5% lactic acid lotion in the treatment of moderate to severe xerosis. Rogers RS III, Callen J, Wehr R, Krochmal L. J Am Acad Dermatol 1989; 21: 714–16.

This comparative study of twice-daily application of 5% lactic acid vs 12% ammonium lactate lotion showed superiority of 12% ammonium lactate in reducing the severity of xerosis.

A double-blind clinical trial comparing the efficacy and safety of pure lanolin versus ammonium lactate 12% cream for the treatment of moderate to severe foot xerosis. Jennings MB, Alfieri DM, Parker ER, Jackman L, Goodwin S, Lesczczynski C. Cutis 2003; 71: 78–82.

A study showing equivalence of a petrolatum compound and 12% ammonium lactate cream for foot xerosis.

A prospective, randomized, controlled double-blind study of a moisturizer for xerosis of the feet in patients with diabetes. Pham HT, Exelbert L, Segal-Owens AC, Veves A. Ostomy Wound Manage 2002; 48: 30–6.

A cream containing 10% urea and 4% lactic acid was statistically more effective than base control in treating foot xerosis in 40 diabetic patients after twice-daily treatment for 4 weeks.

Evidence Levels: **A** Double-blind study **B** Clinical trial ≥ 20 subjects **C** Clinical trial < 20 subjects **D** Series ≥ 5 subjects **E** Anecdotal case reports

An evaluation of the effect of an alpha hydroxy acid-blend skin cream in the cosmetic improvement of symptoms of moderate to severe xerosis, epidermolytic hyperkeratosis, and ichthyosis. Kempers S, Katz HI, Wildnauer R, Green B. Cutis 1998; 61: 347–50.

Twenty subjects completed a course of treatment with either regular or extra-strength AHA-blend cream on a test site compared with a currently marketed, non-AHA moisturizing lotion on a control site. Improvements were significant compared to baseline and compared to sites treated with the control lotion, but the AHA cream did cause some local mild to moderate adverse effects; all subjects were able to continue using the test product for the duration of the study.

Xerosis in hypothyroidism: a potential role for the use of topical thyroid hormone in euthyroid patients. Heymann WR, Gans EH, Manders SM, Green JJ, Haimowitz JE. Med Hypotheses 2001; 57: 736–9.

Euthyroid patients with xerosis were treated with an emollient to one leg and the same base with 7.5 μg/g thyroxine and the same concentration of tri-iodothyronine. In 20 of 24 patients the control- and the thyroid hormone-treated sides showed similar improvement. The authors hypothesize on a mechanism whereby topical thyroxine should help xerosis and propose further studies to optimize delivery and concentration.

Yellow nail syndrome

Robert Baran

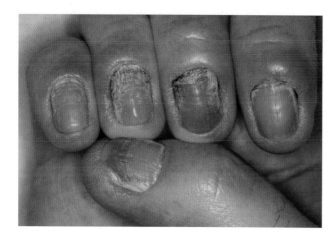

The yellow nail syndrome (YNS) is an uncommon disorder of unknown etiology characterized by the triad of yellow nails, lymphedema, and respiratory tract involvement. The term was originally used to describe the association of slow-growing yellow nails with primary lymphedema. Pleural effusion was later recognized to be an additional sign of the syndrome. Since then, other respiratory conditions, such as bronchiectasis, sinusitis, bronchitis, and chronic respiratory infections, have been associated with the disorder. Although all the three signs that classically characterize the triad of YNS do not occur in every patient, the presence of typical nail alterations should be considered an absolute requirement for the diagnosis. The complete triad is seen in 25% of patients, lymphedema in 40%, and pleural effusions in only 2% of patients with yellow nails. A variant of yellow nails can also be seen in HIV infection.

MANAGEMENT STRATEGY

Although YNS may resolve spontaneously, treatment is often sought by sufferers. Yellow nails are unsightly, discolored, hard, show transverse overcurvature, and are slow growing. Paronychia and onycholysis can be observed.

Underlying diseases such as respiratory disorders, malignancy, infections, immunologic and hematologic abnormalities, endocrine, connective tissue and renal abnormalities, and miscellaneous disorders, including penicillamine therapy, should be sought. Improvement of any underlying disorder (for example, lymphedema) may also result in improvement of the nail plate.

There are no large series or randomized trials in the treatment of yellow nail syndrome. *Oral vitamin E* has been used as monotherapy. The oral azole antifungals *itraconazole and fluconazole* have also been reported to be effective, both alone or in combination with vitamin E. *Matrix steroid injections* have been successfully employed. *Octreotide, zinc, and medium chain fatty acid triglyceride supplements* have been used in anecdotal reports.

SPECIFIC INVESTIGATIONS

▶ Rule out nail fungal infection or *Pseudomonas* infection
▶ Complete blood count
▶ Urinalysis, proteinuria
▶ Immunoelectrophoresis
▶ TSH
▶ Serum rheumatoid factor
▶ Chemistry profile with blood creatinine
▶ Sinus and chest radiography
▶ ENT and pulmonary investigations
▶ Liver enzymes, alkaline phosphatase

There are anecdotal reports of YNS with tuberculosis, solid carcinoma, and lymphomas.

FIRST-LINE THERAPIES

▷ α-Tocopherol	**D**
▷ Itraconazole or fluconazole	**C**
▷ Treatment of the concomitant disorder	**E**

Yellow nail syndrome. Response to vitamin E. Ayres S, Mihan R. Arch Dermatol 1973; 108: 267–8.

Vitamin E at dosages ranging from 600 to 1200 IU daily can induce complete clearing of the nail changes.

The new oral antifungal drugs in the treatment of the yellow nail syndrome. Baran R. Br J Dermatol 2002; 147: 189–91.

Itraconazole pulse therapy or, better, fluconazole combined with vitamin E, produces a positive effect of this treatment on nail growth.

Combination of fluconazole and α-tocopherol in the treatment of yellow-nail-syndrome. Baran R, Thomas L. J Drugs Dermatol 2009; 8: 276–8.

Complete cure has been obtained in 18–24 months. However, there is still a wide discrepancy between the response of the nail to treatment and the remaining signs, which are usually unimproved.

SECOND-LINE THERAPIES

▶ Intradermal triamcinolone injections in the proximal nail matrix	**C**
▶ Physiotherapy	**E**

The yellow nail syndrome (report on 55 cases). Samman PD. Trans St John's Hosp Dermatol Soc 1973; 59: 37–8.

Repeated intradermal trimacinolone injections in the proximal nail matrix may be very effective.

Syndrome des ongles jaunes d'évolution favorable: rôle de la kinésithérapie respiratoire? Fournier C, Just N, Leroy S, Wallaert B. Rev Mal Resp 2003; 20: 969–72.

Besides the nail manifestations, the patient had bilateral bronchiectasis. Daily physiotherapy with bronchial drainage led to a progressive improvement in the respiratory signs. The nail abnormalities disappeared after 2 years of treatment.

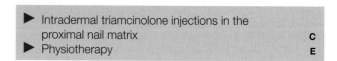

Evidence Levels: **A** Double-blind study **B** Clinical trial ≥ 20 subjects **C** Clinical trial < 20 subjects **D** Series ≥ 5 subjects **E** Anecdotal case reports

Improvement in lymphatic function and partial resolution of nails after complete decongestive physiotherapy in yellow nail syndrome. Szolnoky G, Lakatos B, Husz S, Dobozy A. Int J Dermatol 2005; 44: 501–3.

Manual lymphatic drainage was performed on each leg for 45 min and multilayered compression bandaging was subsequently applied. This was repeated daily for 2 weeks, except at weekends, when the compression was not accompanied by massage. The edema reduction and the increase in lymph flow were associated with an improvement in the appearance of the toenail plates. Fingernails failed to show any change.

THIRD-LINE THERAPIES

▶ Oral zinc supplementation	E
▶ Dietary treatment	E
▶ Octreotide treatment	E

Yellow nail syndrome cured by zinc supplementation. Arroyo JF, Cohen ML. Clin Exp Dermatol 1992; 18: 62–4.

Total resolution of yellow nails and lymphedema was observed following oral zinc supplementation for 2 years.

Yellow nail syndrome in a 10-year-old girl. Gocmen A, Kucukosmanoglu O, Kiper N, Karaduman A, Ozcelik U. Turk J Pediatr 1997; 39: 105–9.

A low-fat diet supplemented with medium chain triglycerides brought moderate improvement in the lymphedema of the lower extremities.

Successful octreotide treatment of chylous pleural effusion and lymphedema in the yellow nail syndrome. Makrilakis K, Pavlatos S, Giannikopoulos G, Toubanakis C, Katsilambros N. Ann Intern Med 2004; 141: 246–7.

Octreotide, a somatostatin analog, was effective in a classic case of YNS with yellow nails, lymphedema of the lower extremities, and recurrent chylous pleural effusion.

Index

Index

Note: Readers are recommended when considering drug therapies, to look up specific drug types (e.g. antidepressants), any subtypes/subgroups (e.g. selective serotonin reuptake inhibitors), and specific generic names (e.g. fluoxetine).

D

DAB-IL-2 (denileukin diftitox; diphtheria toxin targeted to IL-2 receptor)
  cutaneous T-cell lymphoma, 472
  psoriasis, 634
dacarbazine (DTIC)
  melanoma, 425, 427–8
  necrolytic migratory erythema, 483
daclizumab (mAb to IL-2 receptor alpha)
  bullous pemphigoid, 110
  epidermolysis bullosa acquisita, 211
  erythrodermic T-cell leukemia/lymphoma, 232
  graft-versus-host disease, 272
  mucous membrane pemphigoid, 458
dactylitis, blistering distal, 104
dalbavancin, MRSA, 452–3
dalfopristin–quinipristin MRSA, 449
danazol
  actinic dermatitis (chronic), 147, 148
  autoimmune progesterone dermatitis, 69, 70–1
  cholinergic urticaria and pruritus, 554, 558
  granulomatous cheilitis, 286
  hereditary angioedema, 292, 294, 295
dapsone
  acne vulgaris, 9
  aphthous stomatitis, 50, 53
  Behçet's disease, 85, 86
  bullous pemphigoid, 108
  delayed pressure urticaria, 555
  dermatitis herpetiformis, 172, 173
  eosinophilic fasciitis, 198
  epidermolysis bullosa acquisita, 209
  erythema dyschromicum perstans, 216
  erythema nodosum, 224–5
  follicular mucinosis, 253
  folliculitis (spinulosa) decalvans, 258, 259, 354
  granuloma annulare, 277
  granuloma faciale, 280
  Hailey–Hailey disease, 288
  herpes gestationis, 597
  hidradenitis suppurativa, 310
  leukocytoclastic vasculitis, 375, 376
  linear IgA bullous dermatosis, 393, 394
  lupus erythematosus (cutaneous)
    discoid, 188, 190
    subacute, 719
  mucous membrane pemphigoid, 456–7
  panniculitis
    $α_1$-antitrypsin deficiency, 518
    lupus panniculitis, 514
  pityriasis lichenoides et varioliformis acuta, 570
  pityriasis rosea, 572
  pyoderma gangrenosum, 640
  relapsing polychondritis, 658, 659, 660
  subcorneal pustular dermatosis, 722
  Sweet's syndrome, 728
  Well's syndrome, 785
daptomycin, MRSA, 453
Darier disease, 159–61
Dead Sea products, radiation dermatitis, 649
deafness (hearing loss), xeroderma pigmentosum, 791
debridement
  Darier's disease, 160
  decubitus ulcers, 162, 163, 164

with maggots see maggot therapy
  reactive perforating collagenosis, 546
  rhinophyma, 663
  tinea unguium, 745
decolonization, MRSA, 449, 450, 451–2
decongestive therapy
  lymphedema, 410, 411
  pretibial myxedema, 601
  yellow nail syndrome, 796–7
decubitus ulcers, 162–6
DEET (diethyl-m-toluamide)
  bedbugs, 532
  malaria vector, 97
Degos disease, 422–3
delayed pressure urticaria, 553, 555, 556
delivery in pruritic urticarial papules and plaques of pregnancy, early, 594–5
delusional parasitosis, 167–9
Demodex folliculorum and rosacea, 672
dengue viruses, 96
denileukin diftitox see DAB-IL-2
dental interventions, hereditary angioedema relapse following, 292, 295
2′-deoxycoformicin
  Langerhans' cell histiocytosis, 359
  mycosis fungoides, 468, 472
1-deoxygalactonojirimycin, 247, 249
depigmented areas in vitiligo, 776, 777
depilation/epilation
  hypertrichosis and hirsutism, 321, 322–3
  pseudofolliculitis barbae, 620, 621, 622–3
dermabrasion
  actinic dermatitis (chronic), 147, 148
  actinic keratosis, 14, 17
  amyloidosis, 156
  Darier's disease, 160
  Hailey–Hailey disease, 288
  melasma, 435
  nevoid basal cell carcinoma syndrome, 495
  palmoplantar keratoderma, 507, 509
  porokeratosis, 586
  seborrheic, 694–6
  striae, 716
  syringomata, 735
  vitiligo, 779
  xeroderma pigmentosum, 782
dermal fat graft, morphea, 448
dermatitis (eczema) see acrodermatitis; chondrodermatitis nodularis helicis; neurodermatitis circumscripta; photodermatoses
dermatitis (eczema)
  allergic contact, 27–30
  atopic see atopic dermatitis
  autoimmune progesterone, 69–71
  chronic actinic (CAD), 27, 28, 29, 146–8
  decubitus, 163
  diaper, 120, 121, 183–4
  discoid, 185–7
  dyshidrotic, 581–3
  estrogen, 70
  exfoliative, 228–32
  granulomatous, recurrent, 784, 785
  perioral, 547–8
  radiation, 648–9
  stoma-related, 712, 713
  subcorneal pustular, 722–4
  tropical rat mite, 531
  see also eczema herpeticum; eczema tyloticum

dermatitis artefacta, 170–1
dermatitis–eosinophilia syndrome, 230
dermatitis herpetiformis, 172–3
Dermatobia hominis, 474, 475
dermatofibroma protuberans and keloids, differentiation, 346
dermatography, alopecia areata, 31, 35
dermatologic non-disease, 175–7
dermatomyositis, 178–82
  paraneoplastic, 229
dermatonecrosis see necrosis
dermatophytosis see tinea
derm(at)oscopy
  atypical nevus, 65, 66
  Becker's nevus, 83
  Bowen's disease, 105
  malignant melanoma, 424, 426
  pigmented purpuric dermatoses, 125
  porokeratosis, 585
  pseudofolliculitis barbae, 621
  trichotillomania, 757
dermatosis papulosa nigra, 697
dermographism, symptomatic, 553–4, 555–6
dermoplasty, nasal septal, 297
dermoscopy see dermatoscopy
desensitization, cold urticaria, 554
desferrioxamine, porphyria cutanea tarda, 588
desipramine
  body dysmorphic disorder, 176
  vitiligo, 781
desloratadine, urticaria, 761, 762
  delayed pressure, 555
dexamethasone
  aphthous stomatitis, 50
  bullous pemphigoid, 109
  cholestasis of pregnancy, 611
  5-fluorouracil/glycolic peel, 586
  granuloma faciale, 279
  leprosy reactions, 372
  melasma, 434
  papular urticaria, 532
dexpanthenol, radiation dermatitis, 649
diabetes mellitus
  bullous pemphigoid and, 108
  cholesterol emboli syndrome, 400
  granuloma annulare, 275, 277
  keratosis pilaris and, 353
  necrobiosis lipoidica, 478, 479, 480, 481
  neuropathy, and leg/foot ulcers, 360, 361
  palmoplantar pustulosis and, 510
  prurigo pigmentosa, 606
  pruritus vulvae, 618
  reactive perforating collagenosis, 544
  scleredema and, 685, 686–7, 687
  tinea pedis, 741–2
  xerosis, 793
dialysis
  cholestatic pruritus, 610
  Fabry disease, 248
  see also hemodialysis
diamond fraise dermabrasion
  porokeratosis, 586
  syringomata, 735
diaper dermatitis, 120, 121, 183–4
diathermy, neurofibromatosis type 1, 488, 489
dichloroacetic acid (bichloroacetic acid)
  sebaceous hyperplasia, 693
  xanthelasma palpebrum, 788